Carol McKinney

EDITED BY

FRANK H. KRUSEN, M.D.,
F.A.C.P., Dr. Med. (h.c.),
L.L.D. (hon.), F.R.S.M. (hon.)

Emeritus Chairman, Department of Physical Medicine
and Rehabilitation, Mayo Clinic; Emeritus Professor of
Physical Medicine and Rehabilitation, Mayo Graduate School
of Medicine, University of Minnesota; Emeritus Professor
of Physical Medicine and Rehabilitation, Temple University
School of Medicine; Formerly Professor of Physical Medicine
and Rehabilitation, Tufts University School of Medicine

ASSOCIATE EDITORS

FREDERIC J. KOTTKE, M.D., Ph.D.

Professor and Head, Department of Physical Medicine and
Rehabilitation, University of Minnesota Medical School

PAUL M. ELLWOOD, JR., M.D.

Executive Director, American Rehabilitation Foundation

PUBLISHED UNDER THE AUSPICES OF
THE AMERICAN REHABILITATION FOUNDATION

HANDBOOK OF

PHYSICAL MEDICINE
and
REHABILITATION

Second Edition

W. B. SAUNDERS COMPANY
PHILADELPHIA   LONDON   TORONTO

W. B. Saunders Company: West Washington Square
Philadelphia, Pa. 19105

12 Dyott Street
London, WC1A 1DB

833 Oxford Street
Toronto 18, Ontario

Handbook of Physical Medicine and Rehabilitation   ISBN 0-7216-5571-8

Print No.:   9   8   7   6   5   4

CONTRIBUTORS

THEODORE M. COLE, M.D.
Associate Professor, Department of Physical Medicine and Rehabilitation, University of Minnesota Medical School. Consultant, University of Minnesota Hospitals.

EARL C. ELKINS, B.S., M.D.
Emeritus Professor of Physical Medicine and Rehabilitation, Mayo Graduate School of Medicine, University of Minnesota. Emeritus Consultant, Department of Physical Medicine and Rehabilitation, Mayo Clinic. Consultant, Rochester State Hospital. Secretary-Treasurer, American Board of Physical Medicine and Rehabilitation.

PAUL M. ELLWOOD, JR., M.D.
Clinical Associate Professor of Neurology and Pediatrics and Clinical Professor of Physical Medicine and Rehabilitation, University of Minnesota.

WILBERT E. FORDYCE, PH.D.
Professor (Psychology) of Rehabilitation Medicine, University of Washington School of Medicine.

HUBERT L. GERSTMAN, D.ED.
Assistant Professor, Physical and Rehabilitation Medicine, Tufts University School of Medicine. Clinical Director, Speech, Hearing and Language Center, New England Medical Center Hospitals, Boston.

HENRY GOEHL, PH.D.
Professor of Speech, Temple University. Consultant, The Woods Schools. Consultant, Veterans Administration Outpatient Clinic, Philadelphia.

ROBERT C. GOODPASTURE, B.E., M.ENG.
Formerly Executive Vice-President, National Industries for the Blind.

H. FREDERIC HELMHOLZ, JR., M.D.
Associate Professor, Physiology, Mayo Graduate School, University of Minnesota. Staff Member, Mayo Clinic, Rochester, Minnesota.

CARL D. HERMAN, A.B., M.D.
Clinical Assistant Professor in Physical Medicine and Rehabilitation (in Psychiatry), Temple University School of Medicine. Staff Psychiatrist, Moss Rehabilitation Hospital, Philadelphia. Clinical Assistant in Psychiatry, Albert Einstein Medical Center, Northern Division, Philadelphia.

MASAYOSHI ITOH, M.D., M.P.H.
Associate Professor of Rehabilitation Medicine, School of Medicine, New York University. Assistant Director, Department of Rehabilitation Medicine, Goldwater Memorial Hospital, New York University Medical Center.

v

ERNEST W. JOHNSON, M.D.
Professor and Chairman, Department of Physical Medicine, Ohio State University.

MILAND E. KNAPP, M.D., M.A. (B.S., M.B.)
Clinical Professor of Physical Medicine and Rehabilitation, University of Minnesota School of Medicine. Consultant, Metropolitan Medical Center and Hennepin County General Hospital, Minneapolis, Minnesota.

MICHAEL KOSIAK, M.D.
Clinical Assistant Professor, Department of Physical Medicine and Rehabilitation, University of Minnesota Medical School. Director, Department of Physical Medicine and Rehabilitation, St. Paul-Ramsey Hospital. Director, Department of Physical Medicine and Rehabilitation, St. John's Hospital, St. Paul, Minnesota.

FREDERIC J. KOTTKE, M.D., PH.D.
Professor and Head, Department of Physical Medicine and Rehabilitation, University of Minnesota Medical School. Head, Department of Physical Medicine and Rehabilitation, University of Minnesota Hospitals.

FRANK H. KRUSEN, M.D., DR. MED. (H.C.), L.L.D. (HON.), F.A.C.P., F.R.S.M. (HON.)
Emeritus Chairman, Department of Physical Medicine and Rehabilitation, Mayo Clinic. Emeritus Professor of Physical Medicine and Rehabilitation, Mayo Graduate School of Medicine, University of Minnesota, and Temple University School of Medicine. Formerly Professor of Physical Medicine and Rehabilitation, Tufts University School of Medicine.

MATHEW H. M. LEE, M.D., M.P.H., F.A.C.P.
Associate Professor of Rehabilitation Medicine, School of Medicine, Clinical Associate Professor of Preventive Dentistry and Community Health, College of Dentistry, New York University. Director of Department of Rehabilitation Medicine, Goldwater Memorial Hospital, New York University Medical Center.

JUSTUS F. LEHMANN, M.D.
Professor and Chairman, Department of Rehabilitation Medicine, University of Washington School of Medicine. Attending Physician, University Hospital, Harborview Medical Center, Veterans Administration Hospital, Children's Orthopedic Hospital and U.S. Public Health Service Hospital.

CARL LEVENSON, B.A., M.D., F.A.C.P.
Clinical Professor, Temple University Medical School. Senior Attending Physician, Albert Einstein Medical Center, Philadelphia. Consultant, Philadelphia General Hospital; Philadelphia Geriatric Center; Veterans Administration Hospital, Coatesville, Pennsylvania.

CHARLES LONG, II, M.D.
Associate Professor of Physical Medicine and Rehabilitation, Case Western Reserve University. Acting Director, Department of Physical Medicine and Rehabilitation, Highland View Hospital, Cleveland, Ohio.

EDWARD W. LOWMAN, M.D., M.S. (MED.), F.A.C.P.
Professor, Rehabilitation Medicine, New York University School of Medicine. Clinical Director, Institute of Rehabilitation Medicine, N.Y.U. Medical Center. Attending Physician in Physical Medicine and Rehabilitation, New York University Hospital, N.Y.U. Medical Center.

RICHARD A. MANNING, M.D., M.S.
Director of Children's Services, Montgomery County Mental Health Clinic, Norristown, Pennsylvania. Formerly Child Psychiatric Consultant to the Elwyn Institute, Media, Pennsylvania, and Coordinator of Mental Retardation, Department of Child Psychiatry, Albert Einstein Medical Center, Philadelphia.

GORDON M. MARTIN, M.D., M.S. (PHYSICAL MEDICINE)
Associate Professor of Physical Medicine and Rehabilitation, Mayo Graduate School of Medicine, University of Minnesota. Chairman, Department of Physical Medicine and Rehabilitation, Mayo Clinic, Rochester, Minnesota.

LEONARD D. POLICOFF, B.S., M.D.,
F.A.C.P.
Professor of Physical Medicine and
Rehabilitation, University of Penn-
sylvania School of Medicine. Chief of
Rehabilitation Medicine and Medical
Director of the Merwick Rehabilitation
Center, Princeton Hospital, Princeton,
New Jersey.

HERSCH L. SACHS, M.D.
Former Assistant Clinical Professor of
Physical Medicine and Rehabilitation,
Temple University School of Med-
icine. Attending Physician, Kingsbrook
Jewish Medical Center and La Guardia
Hospital, Queens, New York. Associate
Physician, Jewish Hospital and Brook-
dale Hospital, Brooklyn.

BERNARD SANDLER, M.D.
Clinical Professor of Rehabilitation
Medicine, Downstate Medical Center,
Brooklyn, New York. Director and
Attending Physician, Rehabilitation
Medicine, Kingsbrook Jewish Medical
Center. Consultant, Veterans Admin-
istration Hospital, Brooklyn, New
York.

ALAN DAVIES SESSLER, M.D.
Assistant Professor of Anesthesiology,
Mayo Graduate School of Medicine,
University of Minnesota, Rochester,
Minnesota.

HAROLD M. STERLING, M.D.
Professor of Physical Medicine and
Rehabilitation and Professor of Pediatrics, University of California School
of Medicine, Davis, California. Consultant, Sacramento Medical Center,
Sacramento, California.

G. KEITH STILLWELL, M.D., PH.D., C.M.
Associate Professor of Clinical Physical Medicine and Rehabilitation, Mayo
Graduate School of Medicine, University of Minnesota. Consultant, Department of Physical Medicine and Rehabilitation, Mayo Clinic, Rochester,
Minnesota.

WALTER C. STOLOV, M.A., M.D.
Professor, Department of Rehabilita-
tion Medicine, University of Washing-
ton School of Medicine. Attending
Physician, University Hospital, Seattle
Veterans Administration Hospital,
Harborview Medical Center. Chief, Re-
habilitation Medicine Service, United
States Public Health Service Hospital,
Seattle, Washington.

EMERY KAUFMANN STONER, M.D., M.MED.
SCI. (PHYSICAL MEDICINE), F.A.C.P.
Associate Professor of Physical Medi-
cine and Rehabilitation, School of Med-
icine, University of Pennsylvania. Clin-
ical Director, Department of Physical
Medicine and Rehabilitation, Hospital
of the University of Pennsylvania.
Assistant Visting Physician in Physical
Medicine and Rehabilitation, Phila-
delphia General Hospital. Consultant,
Bryn Mawr Hospital.

HERBERT S. TALBOT, A.B., M.D.
Regional Coordinator for Spinal Cord
Injury, Veterans Administration Hos-
pital, West Roxbury, Massachusetts.

DONALD R. TAYLOR, JR., B.S.E.E.
Engineer and Senior Research Scientist, Temple University School of Medicine — Moss Rehabilitation Hospital.

EDWARD TEITELMAN, M.D.
Instructor in Psychiatry, University of
Pennsylvania School of Medicine.
Teaching Consultant, Graduate School
of Nursing, University of Delaware.
Consulting Psychiatrist, Horizon
House, Philadelphia. Attending Psy-
chiatrist, Friends Hospital and Penn-
sylvania Hospital, Philadelphia, and
Cooper Hospital, Camden, New Jersey.

JEROME S. TOBIS, M.D.
Professor and Chairman, Department
of Physical Medicine and Rehabilitation, California College of Medicine,
University of California at Irvine. Director, Department of Physical Medicine and Rehabilitation, Orange
County Medical Center, Orange, California.

ROBERT A. WALKER, M.A.
President, Walker and Associates, Inc., St. Paul, Minnesota.

ROY W. WIRTA, B.S., P.E.
Engineer and Senior Research Scientist, Temple University School of Medicine—Moss Rehabilitation Hospital.

HELEN J. YESNER, M.S.W., A.C.S.W.
Professor, School of Social Work, University of Minnesota. Coordinator, Graduate Fieldwork for Social Work.

JACK M. ZISLIS, M.D.
Associate Professor of Physical Medicine and Rehabilitation, Temple University School of Medicine, Director, Department of Physical Medicine and Rehabilitation, Albert Einstein Medical Center, Philadelphia. Director, Department of Physical Medicine and Rehabilitation, Philadelphia Geriatric Center. Attending Physiatrist, Moss Rehabilitation Hospital. Consultant, Physical Medicine and Rehabilitation, Lutheran Home for Orphans and Aged.

PREFACE TO THE SECOND EDITION

It will be noted that, in the preface to the first edition of this book, it was explained that an organized group of professors of Physical Medicine and Rehabilitation (the Expert Medical Advisory Committee of the American Rehabilitation Foundation) from medical schools scattered across the United States had carefully planned the structuring, contents and arrangement of this volume.

In this second edition, which is appearing approximately six years after publication of the first edition, the same general plan has been followed. Extensive revisions have been made, however; and there has been careful expansion into important new phases of the growing specialty of Physical Medicine and Rehabilitation.

Fourteen new contributors have added material to that revised by the twenty-four authors retained from the first edition. So, the number of contributors has increased from twenty-five for the first edition to thirty-eight for the second edition.

The contributors to this edition are associated with thirteen different university medical centers, from California and Washington State, in the West, to Pennsylvania and Massachusetts, in the East. A high percentage of the contributors come from the medical centers with which I, as senior editor, have been associated. There are seven from the University of Minnesota Medical School, six from the University of Minnesota, Mayo Graduate School of Medicine, seven from Temple University School of Medicine and two from Tufts University School of Medicine.

Readers of and contributors to the first edition have suggested expansion of the discussion of certain topics. After careful analysis, many such additions, and a few deletions, have been made.

Both physicians and allied health workers concerned with various phases of rehabilitation have been contributors. To the four allied health professionals who contributed to the first edition (a clinical psychologist, a speech pathologist, a vocational counsellor, and a social worker) have been added four more allied health professionals (a speech and hearing specialist, a master of engineering directing industries for the blind, a mechanical engineer and an electrical engineer).

The physicians who are new contributors include a urologist, an anesthesiologist, three psychiatrists, two physiatrist clinicians, two physiatrist epidemiologists, and one physiatrist educator.

In this second edition, the number of pages, exclusive of index pages, has been increased from 702 to 897, the number of chapters from 36 to 42; and the number of Parts from 3 to 4, as follows: Part I, Principles of Evaluation and Management; Part II, Techniques of Management; Part III, Evaluation and Management of Specific Disorders, and Part IV (new), Basic Considerations of Importance in Total Rehabilitation.

The number of illustrations has been increased from 357 to 448.

Only a few chapters carried over from the first edition required little or no revision. Most chapters have been revised, many of them extensively.

I have modified Chapter 1 slightly to indicate the expansion in the scope of physical medicine and rehabilitation.

In Part I, Principles of Evaluation and Management, Chapter 2 has been expanded extensively and greater clarification has been achieved. Three authors, Drs. Stolov, Cole and Tobis, have developed three sections of this chapter: Evaluation of the Patient; Goniometry; and Muscle Testing.

Dr. Stoner has made extensive additions to Chapters 3 and 4 on amputees: Chapter 3 now deals with Evaluation of the Amputee; and Chapter 4 is concerned with Care of the Amputee.

Dr. Fordyce has completely rewritten his Chapter 6 on Psychologic Assessment and Management, adding a discussion of the timely subject of operant conditioning in rehabilitating the handicapped.

Under Part II, Techniques of Management, Dr. Stillwell has expanded his Chapter 10 on therapeutic heat to include a discussion on cold therapy, with the new title Therapeutic Heat and Cold.

Dr. Lehmann has brought his Chapter 11 on Diathermy right up to date and has discussed, for example, such recent problems as the contraindications to employing diathermy when a patient has been provided with an implanted cardiac pacemaker.

Dr. Zislis has expanded his Chapter 12 on Hydrotherapy to include a discussion of cryotherapy. Other authors have brought their chapters up to date without having to make extensive changes in their contributions to the first edition.

In Part III, Evaluation and Management of Specific Disorders, these authors, also, have brought their chapters up to date. Dr. Knapp has added to his Chapter 26 on the Aftercare of Fractures a helpful discussion of special problems, and of the prevention of serious complications.

Chapter 31, prepared by a new contributor, Dr. Talbot, brings the reader the latest information concerning the Management of Neurogenic Dysfunction of the Bladder and Bowel.

To Chapter 34 on Disorders of Respiration (Pulmonary Function), has been added a new section by Dr. Sessler on Chest Physical Therapy. This section will be helpful to the physician and therapist in the management of obstructive lung diseases, such as asthma, bronchitis, emphysema, bronchiectasis, and cystic fibrosis.

A new Chapter 37 by Dr. Gerstman, Auditory Disorders: Evaluation and Management, adds to this second edition a comprehensive discussion of the diagnosis and treatment of the deaf, which I had predicted in 1965 would soon be absorbing the attention of health workers concerned with the total rehabilitation of handicapped persons.

It has been apparent also that those who work with rehabilitation of the physically handicapped must always recognize and deal with the intertwining psychiatric problems. To this end we have added another new chapter (Chapter 38) dealing with the psychiatric aspects of rehabilitation. Three psychiatrists, Drs. Herman, Manning, and Teitelman, have presented in this chapter three aspects of this subject. Dr. Herman has discussed Psychiatric Rehabilitation of the Physically Disabled. Dr. Manning has presented a consideration of the Management of Psychiatric Complications of Mental Retardation; and Dr. Teitelman has discussed the Rehabilitation of the Psychiatrically Impaired.

We have added to this second edition an entirely new Part IV, Basic Considerations of Importance in Total Rehabilitation. This part, I believe, rounds out a most comprehensive, one-volume presentation of the field of physical medicine and rehabilitation.

Chapter 39 indicates the relationships between the rehabilitation of the blind and the rehabilitation of persons having other disabilities. I believe that there should be closer relationships between the rehabilitators of the blind and the rehabilitation workers serving persons having other disabilities. Mr. Goodpasture has painted the picture clearly in his concise and extremely informative chapter.

The comprehensive centers for rehabilitation of the disabled have recently become deeply interested in the development of sections on engineering, in which a team of highly qualified engineers collaborates with the other members of the rehabilitation team in developing the engineering tools and technics to assist the handicapped patient achieve maximal function. Chapter 40 is a meticulously prepared presentation of the basic engineering principles with which the modern rehabilitation worker should become familiar. Engineers Wirta and Taylor have titled their new chapter Engineering Principles in Rehabilitation Medicine. More and more devices and engineering procedures to aid disabled persons will be developed in the future by engineers like Wirta and Taylor. Ever more frequently other members of the rehabilitation team will lean on engineers for assistance in restoring disabled persons to the fullest possible effectiveness.

As it is revised, a text like this, which has become a reference work for many rehabilitation centers, must keep its readers informed about changing relationships, variations in educational practices, and modifications in clinical procedures. In the new Chapter 41, Dr. Policoff, distinguished educator, has described the changing philosophies in education of rehabilitation professionals. This chapter presents the modern educational approaches for the members of the rehabilitation team.

Finally, the specialists in physical medicine and rehabilitation have become concerned recently with the epidemiology of disability. So, a concluding Chapter 42 by Drs. Itoh and Lee deals effectively with this topic. There was a time when the average physician thought of epidemiology as dealing only with the problems of the so-called "epidemic diseases." Today, concepts have broadened greatly. Those health workers interested in rehabilitation of the handicapped now study, under epidemiology, factors which influence the distribution of various disabilities, both physical and mental. Itoh and Lee describe the "practical application of an epidemiologic approach to the daily practice of rehabilitation medicine." These concepts should be helpful indeed to all rehabilitation professionals.

As editor I wish to thank all the contributors for their cooperation. Also, I thank my associate editors, Dr. Frederic J. Kottke and Dr. Paul M. Ellwood, Jr., for their excellent revisions of their several chapters and for their constant support.

Lastly I extend, once again, my sincere thanks to the staff of the W. B. Saunders Company for their continuing skillful handling of my editorial and publishing needs.

Frank H. Krusen, M.D.

PREFACE TO THE FIRST EDITION

In 1943, when I was serving as director of the Baruch Committee on Physical Medicine and Rehabilitation, I conferred with the late Dr. Alan Gregg, of the Rockefeller Foundation, regarding the efforts of the Baruch Committee to develop a good program of practice, teaching and research in the field of physical medicine and rehabilitation in the medical schools of the United States.

Dr. Gregg told me that in the early part of this century, the Rockefeller Foundation had been interested in supporting the development of practice, teaching and research in psychiatry in the medical schools of this country. He said that in order to accomplish this development, he had established a group known as the G.A.P., the Group for Advancement of Psychiatry. What the Rockefeller Foundation had done was to select a group of leading professors of psychiatry from various medical schools throughout the nation to think and plan for the future of their specialty and to develop adequate programs in the medical schools of the nation. This group was extremely successful in advancing the whole field of psychiatry and in the development of adequate teaching programs in our medical schools.

In 1957, the American Rehabilitation Foundation decided to take a leaf from Alan Gregg's book and established, under my chairmanship, a Medical Advisory Committee, consisting of leading professors of physical medicine and rehabilitation from various medical schools throughout the nation. This group became known as the A.R.F. group, the American Rehabilitation Foundation Medical Committee. Like the G.A.P. group, the A.R.F. group has been extremely diligent in advancing practice, teaching and research in its field of medical interest in our American medical schools.

As the American Rehabilitation Foundation Medical Committee studied various developments, it seemed apparent to its members that we needed a well organized Handbook of Physical Medicine and Rehabilitation, and plans for the publication of this textbook were developed.

The Committee, at this time, consisted of the following physicians: Dr. Robert L. Bennett, Emory University; Dr. Ernest W. Johnson, Ohio State

University; Dr. Robcliff V. Jones, Jr., Yale University; Dr. Miland E. Knapp, University of Minnesota; Dr. Frederic J. Kottke, University of Minnesota; Dr. Edward M. Krusen, Jr., Southwestern University; Dr. Justus F. Lehmann, University of Washington; Dr. Edward W. Lowman, New York University; Dr. James W. Rae, Jr., University of Michigan; Dr. Oscar O. Selke, Jr., Houston Methodist Hospital; Dr. Charles D. Shields, Georgetown University; Dr. G. Keith Stillwell, Mayo Graduate School of Medicine; Dr. Jerome S. Tobis, New York Montefiore Hospital; the late Dr. Frederick E. Vultee, Medical College of Virginia; Dr. Ralph E. Worden, University of California at Los Angeles; and Dr. Walter J. Zeiter, Cleveland Clinic.

A group of the members of this Committee then held a series of conferences to plan the structuring of this volume, to discuss its contents and arrangement and to make suggestions as to contributors of the various chapters. I assumed the role of editor and Dr. Kottke and Dr. Ellwood served as associate editors. It will be noted that many of the members of the Committee have contributed chapters.

As this volume goes to press, in my capacity as editor, I should like to thank the members of the Committee for their assistance in planning this textbook, and I should like to thank, especially, those members who have contributed chapters. My particular thanks go to Dr. Kottke and Dr. Ellwood for their assistance as associate editors.

Appreciation is extended to our colleagues from various medical schools who, because of special knowledge, have contributed chapters to this volume. These include: Dr. Kosiak and Dr. Schoening of the University of Minnesota, Dr. Long of Western Reserve University, Dr. Sterling of Tufts University and Dr. Stoner of the University of Pennsylvania. I am grateful to Dr. Stoner who stepped into the breach, following the death of our lamented colleague, Dr. Vultee, and at the last moment prepared, so effectively, his chapters which were originally assigned to Dr. Vultee.

As editor, I wish to thank our colleagues who have contributed very important chapters on allied health topics, which must be included in a modern textbook on physical medicine and rehabilitation, including Dr. Fordyce of the University of Washington, Dr. Goehl of Temple University, Mr. Walker of the University of Minnesota and Mrs. Yesner of the University of Minnesota.

My thanks go out, also, to my former associates at the Mayo Graduate School of Medicine who have contributed chapters, including Drs. Elkins, Helmholtz, Martin and Stillwell, and finally, among the contributors, I wish to thank my associates in the Department of Physical Medicine and Rehabilitation at Temple University School of Medicine, Drs. Sandler, Levenson, Sachs and Zislis, for their significant contributions to this volume.

These acknowledgements would not be complete without my expression of sincere thanks, for assistance with the editing, to my secretaries, Romayne Curran, Mavin Fredd and Marcy Leonard.

Lastly, I am especially desirous of expressing grateful appreciation to the staff of the W. B. Saunders Company for their extremely efficient collaboration, prompt support in attending to details in editing and constant encouragement.

FRANK H. KRUSEN, M.D.
Editor
Temple University
School of Medicine

CONTENTS

PART II TECHNIQUES OF MANAGEMENT

Chapter 22

PART III EVALUATION AND MANAGEMENT OF SPECIFIC DISORDERS

Chapter 23

Chapter 24

Chapter 25

PART IV   BASIC CONSIDERATIONS OF IMPORTANCE IN TOTAL REHABILITATION

Chapter 1

THE SCOPE OF PHYSICAL MEDICINE AND REHABILITATION

by Frank H. Krusen

DEFINITION

Physical medicine has been defined as that branch of medicine using physical agents, such as light, heat, water and electricity, and mechanical agents in the management of disease. Rehabilitation involves treatment and training of the patient to the end that he may attain his maximal potential for normal living physically, psychologically, socially and vocationally. Another definition commonly employed states that rehabilitation is "the restoration through personal health services of handicapped individuals to the fullest physical, mental, social, and economic usefulness of which they are capable, including ordinary treatment and treatment in special rehabilitation centers."

Rehabilitation is a creative procedure which includes the cooperative efforts of various medical specialists and their associates in other health fields to improve the physical, mental, social and vocational aptitudes of persons who are handicapped, with the objective of preserving their ability to live happily and productively on the same level and with the same opportunities as their neighbors.

The Community Health Services of San Francisco have defined rehabilitation as "the process of decreasing dependence of the handicapped or disabled person by developing to the greatest extent possible the abilities needed for adequate functioning in his individual situation."[7]

In this handbook Yesner has defined rehabilitation as "a treatment process designed to help physically handicapped individuals make maximal use of residual capacities and to enable them to obtain optimal satisfaction and usefulness in terms of themselves, their families and their community." Likewise, Fordyce has defined rehabilitation in this handbook as being "concerned typically with people who have disabilities with enduring and pervasive effects. The essence of the rehabilitation process is recognition that what has happened to the patient affects, and will continue to affect, many aspects of his life extending beyond the limits of bodily function."

A physician who specializes in physical medicine and rehabilitation combines his skills in the application of physical agents in the restoration of the handicapped with a concern for the evaluation and treatment of the physical, mental, social and vocational problems of his patient. The designation *physiatrist* is now commonly applied to the specialist in this field. This term derives from the Greek words *physikos* (physical) and *iatros* (physician). The term signifies that the specialist is a physician who employs physical agents for the evaluation of the extent of disability and for the rehabilitation of his patients.

The practice of physical medicine and rehabilitation involves the medical examination and evaluation of the disabilities of handicapped patients, the prescription and medical supervision of physical and occupational therapy and other forms of therapy, the training of the handicapped person in ambulation and self-care and medical supervision and coordination of other rehabilitation procedures. Frequently the supervision of the use of devices for artificial respiration is provided by the physiatrist and many physiatrists are concerned with the electrical tests for the study of neuromuscular disorders. Oscillometry, skin temperature studies, oximetry, fever therapy and a wide variety of miscellaneous uses of physical agents for diagnosis and therapy are usually considered to be the specific responsibility of the physiatrist.

In this chapter the term "scope" will be used according to that portion of the definition of scope appearing in the Oxford Universal Dictionary,[20] which designates it as "the sphere or area over which any activity operates or is effective."

It now becomes ever more apparent that the team providing physical medicine and rehabilitation is operating in a continually widening sphere and is becoming increasingly effective in the evaluation and management of a growing number of problems of disadvantaged persons.

THE INCREASING IMPORTANCE OF PHYSICAL MEDICINE AND REHABILITATION

The practice of physical medicine and rehabilitation is growing rapidly in importance because of the changing concepts with regard to the approach that the modern physician should take toward the management of his patients. We know today that in the care of the sick and the disabled we should go beyond the antiquated approach in which the physician concerned himself simply with the diagnosis of a static pathologic process, provided the necessary surgical procedures for elimination of the pathologic lesion, or administered the necessary drugs to cure a specific disease, and then dismissed his patient with the conclusion that his responsibilities to the patient had ended. Today the physician realizes that he must take a dynamic approach to the study of disorders of physiologic processes which are constantly changing and that he must concern himself not only with the physical disability but also with the psychologic, social and vocational problems of his patient. Instead of providing episodic care for specific diseases, the modern physician should take a holistic approach in which he makes every effort to maintain his patient in the best possible health physically and mentally even though the patient may have extensive disability. It is a dynamic rather than a passive approach to the health needs of each patient.

Recently Dr. John B. Youmans, Professor Emeritus of Medicine at Vanderbilt University School of Medicine, stated, "To the public, the doctor has become a super-scientist. To the doctor, the patient is too often a biological unit that he manipulates objectively but with little subjective feeling."[28] The modern physician must strive at all costs to avoid this impersonal approach and he must make every effort to take the broad approach with a deep personal interest, not so much in the specific disease as in the patient as a person with emotional, social and vocational problems as well as physical disease or disability.

In *World Health* (the magazine of the World Health Organization), which deals with hospitals throughout the world, in December, 1970, two leading health authorities, Dr. F. Bauhofer, Director-General of Public Health, Austrian Ministry for Social Affairs, and Dr. R. F. Bridgman, Inspector General, Ministry of Health, France, stressed the importance of rehabilitation medicine in the newer hospitals.

Dr. Bauhofer stated: "Rehabilitation in hospitals will play a more important role, and will be associated not only with the treatment of the physically handicapped but with all branches of medicine."[4]

Dr. Bridgman wrote: "The basic hospital of the type we are considering is something entirely different from the traditional general hospital. The inclusion of dispensaries providing preventive, curative and rehabilitation services . . . are all features which give it a new character. . . ."[5]

THE DEVELOPMENT OF MEDICINE AS A SOCIAL SCIENCE

Some years ago the distinguished medical educator, Dr. Raymond B. Allen, said, "Medicine is coming of age as a social science in the service of society."[1] And shortly thereafter, the president of the Rockefeller Foundation, Chester I. Barnard, in discussing medical care, commented: "The old idea that biophysics and biochemistry would eventually unravel all the problems of health and disease is less tenable today than was the case 40 or 50 years ago. There is a growing realization that interrelated social factors outside the physics and chemistry of the body also are involved. When research has accumulated and systematized the data into a scientific discipline, biosocial medicine may become an indispensable part of the school curriculum. We may expect medical schools then to introduce students to the practice of community medicine, with an emphasis on social diagnosis comparable to that on physical diagnosis."[3]

Today the physiatrist working with his associates in the allied health professions and with community health agencies is achieving the kind of practice of community medicine and emphasis on social diagnosis predicted by Dr. Barnard two decades ago.

THE IMPORTANCE OF THE PSYCHOLOGIC, SOCIAL AND VOCATIONAL ASPECTS OF DISABILITY

In a book entitled *When Doctors Are Patients,* edited by two physicians, Max Pinner and Benjamin Miller, a group of physicians have described their own personal experiences with various serious diseases. It is perhaps a revelation to some physicians to discover that almost every one of these seriously ill physicians, as he recited the problems that he faced in dealing with his own illness, stressed almost invariably the psychologic and social aspects of his disease. This led the late Dr. Pinner to conclude in his preface that "This collection of case reports can only emphasize again and, I believe, in a peculiarly urgent and moving way, how essential it is to treat the whole patient." Pinner added, "The need is not, in my opinion, diagnosis and specific treatment of so-called psychosomatic diseases, but the recognition—which is not new, but so frequently forgotten and ignored—that every disease is psycho-somatic, that is, that it affects both body and soul."[22]

Growing understanding of the ways in which the rehabilitation team in a comprehensive center for physical medicine and rehabilitation operates has led to an increasing awareness of the fact that the team must consider routinely the physical, psychologic, social and vocational problems of each handicapped patient or client.

Furthermore, it has become increasingly apparent that the development of *evaulation procedures* (other than the usual diagnostic techniques) is an essential part of the routine practice of the physiatrist. Such evaluation lays the ground work for the provision of proper therapeutic management.

Finally the rehabilitation teams are becoming continually more expert in the skillful management of disabling conditions and of the reaction of their patients toward disability. Thus, Fordyce (Chapter 6) and his associates have found that *operant conditioning* is a very useful tool in expediting the management of the disabilities of certain patients.

AGING OF THE POPULATION AND ADVANCE IN THE NUMBER OF SERIOUSLY DISABLING INJURIES IS INCREASING THE NEED FOR PHYSICAL MEDICINE AND REHABILITATION

The amount of chronic illness among aging and aged persons is constantly increasing. The medical problem of chronic illness is, therefore, a major one, and, because it is increasing, it deserves as much consideration as the problem of acute illness, if not more. Until recently, and to a certain extent even now, physicians have devoted their major attention to the causes, diagnosis and cure of acute diseases. Efforts in this direction have been outstandingly successful and the life span of the average person has been extended from 49 years in 1900 to approximately 70 years today. In 1950 there were 11.27 million people over the age of 65 and by 1980 it is estimated that there will be 22 million. Because of the magnitude of this problem, we must abandon the traditional attitude of passive acceptance and neglect of chronic diseases of the aged and place the physical, psychologic, social and vocational rehabilitation of the chronically ill on the same level with medicine and surgery for the acutely ill.

Because of the increased tempo of modern living more and more persons are becoming disabled by accidents in the home, on the highways, in industry and on the farm. Each time the surgeon saves the life of a person having such extensive and seriously crippling injuries and each time the medical practitioner prevents the death of an extensively paralyzed patient, a triumph over death is achieved; but at the same time these physicians have created for themselves a new problem in management of chronic disability and in providing facilities for the rehabilitation of a living, but extensively disabled, chronically ill and often aged, patient. One of the major responsibilities of the modern physician is to restore such persons to self-respecting citizenship.[15]

THE TEAM APPROACH EMPLOYED IN PHYSICAL MEDICINE AND REHABILITATION

It is estimated that there are approximately three million persons in the United States who could be rehabilitated and returned to useful lives provided we had the facilities and the personnel to serve them properly. Over the past three decades there has been an enormous expansion in the number of departments of physical medicine and rehabilitation or rehabilitation medicine in the hospitals of the United States, and these departments have learned to develop under the direction of the specialist in physical medicine and rehabilitation a multispecialty and multidisciplinary approach to the management of serious disabilities.

In a monograph on *Concepts in Rehabilitation of the Handicapped*, I have indicated that "Rehabilitation as practiced in modern institutions has become very much a multidisciplinary effort directed by the specialist in physical medicine and rehabilitation, assisted by physicians in other specialties such as internal medicine, pediatrics, orthopedic surgery, neurology, neurosurgery, and plastic surgery. These physicians in turn are assisted in various aspects of the rehabilitation effort by a team of associates" in the allied health professions, "including physical therapists, occupational therapists, rehabilitation nurses, social workers, vocational counselors, clinical psychologists, and speech therapists."[12]

In the modern department of physical medicine and rehabilitation, when a handicapped person is admitted, he is first evaluated by each member of the team in order to determine his physical, mental, social and vocational abilities. The team takes a dynamic approach and concerns itself not so much with the negative aspects of the patient's disabilities as with the positive aspects of the patient's remaining abilities. When the evaluation has been made by the various members of the team, they join in a group conference to develop a comprehensive program to assist the patient in making the most of his remaining abilities.

Such a team working in a fully equipped department or institute of physical medicine and rehabilitation can provide services that it would be impossible to obtain in the hospital that has services only for the acutely ill. This team of experts in the various phases of rehabilitation and physical treatment not only employs all the skills of its own group but also seeks the collaboration of various voluntary and governmental health agencies in an effort to restore the handicapped person to the fullest possible self-sufficiency and self-respect. They take as their slogan that it is the responsibility of the modern health worker "not only to add years to life, but also to add life to years."

It is true that, as this growing field of medical practice develops, its perimeters are somewhat blurred without too sharp a definition of the limits of practice. This is true, however, of all medical specialties, especially the younger ones. For example, if we compare the surgeon, the internist and the physiatrist, we find that from the standpoint of the tools that are employed, in general the surgeon uses the scalpel and other surgical instruments; the internist uses drugs; and the physiatrist uses physical agents and procedures in the care of the sick and disabled. From the standpoint of the diseases with which we are concerned, in general the surgeon deals primarily with acute and chronic diseases in which surgical excision, surgical repair or some similar use of the instruments he employs may be helpful; the internist is concerned primarily with those diseases, acute and chronic, that will respond to the pharmaceutic and biologic agents that he commonly employs; and the physiatrist is concerned primarily with the acute and chronic diseases in which physical agents and procedures employed frequently by a team of medical and allied health workers will be of benefit.

As I have indicated, the perimeters of each of these specialties are somewhat blurred, and the surgeon may use physical agents or drugs in his practice; the internist may employ physical procedures and some surgical techniques in his work; and the physiatrist may use certain surgical or manipulative procedures and prescribe certain drugs in his practice. As "licensed physicians and surgeons" all three groups are privileged to utilize all of these procedures; but if there is a major surgical problem, such as an intercurrent acute appendicitis or the need for surgical revision of an amputation stump, the physiatrist will call in the surgeon; and if there is a major medical problem the physiatrist will call the internist in consultation. Conversely, the surgeon or the internist may call on the physiatrist to manage the problems in rehabilitation of an amputee or a hemiplegic.

There has been an unfortunate slogan which has great appeal but which at the same time is in serious error. This is the slogan that "Rehabilitation is everybody's business." My point is that rehabilitation can only be the "business" of highly skilled workers who have made it their business. I agree that "rehabilitation is everybody's *interest,*" and everyone who has an interest in the welfare of his less fortunate neighbors should be interested in the rehabilitation of the handicapped. Not long ago I made the following statement:

> Because of the tremendous national and international interest in rehabilitation as a mass humanitarian endeavor, there has been an unfortunate tendency for professional groups, and for many individuals, to assume that they know all there is to know about rehabilitation, to set themselves up as experts in rehabilitation, and to assume that the very small segment of rehabilitation with which they are concerned is the whole of rehabilitation.
>
> Actually, however, each group which is really qualified to handle any one of the four major phases of rehabilitation—physical, psychological, social, or vocational—has developed a body of knowledge and programs for employing such knowledge, and has trained experts who have obtained such knowledge and can apply it properly. These are the qualified specialists who can carry on the *business* of rehabilitation in truly effective fashion. Good rehabilitation is not a field for tyros. While rehabilitation should be everybody's interest, it cannot be everybody's business.
>
> Qualified teachers and well structured departments in our schools of medicine, and in our departments of psychology, social sciences, and education must first provide the training and develop the research in each of the four phases of rehabilitation. Once this has been accomplished, the personnel trained in such departments must carry on the business of rehabilitation in the physical, psychological, social, and vocational fields.[16]

This handbook deals with the special evaluation techniques used in physical medicine and rehabilitation, with the management techniques employed by the physiatrist and his associates and with the disorders commonly treated in physical medicine and rehabilitation, including hemiplegia, connective tissue disease, lesions of the spinal cord, fractures, lower motor neuron disorders, lesions of the central and peripheral nervous system, back disorders, respiratory disorders and cardiovascular diseases.

In the first edition of this handbook, published in 1965, I predicted that in future editions discussions of the rehabilitation of "the psychiatrically impaired, the mentally retarded, the blind and the deaf" might well be included.

It is interesting to note that as I write this, six years later, in 1971 we do have, in this second edition, new chapters on all of these conditions. There is also a discussion of the psychiatric problems of the physically disabled and their management.

Furthermore, there are new chapters dealing with engineering principles in rehabilitation medicine, with the general philosophy of education of physicians and allied health professionals in physical medicine and rehabilitation and with the newly developing field of the epidemiology of disability.

Psychiatric Rehabilitation

With regard to psychiatry as related to rehabilitation, it is to be expected that every patient who has developed a serious physical disability will have associated psychiatric disturbances. Herman discusses these in Chapter 38. Then too there are patients who are primarily psychiatrically impaired and to whom rehabilitative procedures may be applied. These patients are also discussed in Chapter 38. Finally a special type of psychiatric management has been developed for the extensive group of patients who are mentally retarded. This subject is likewise discussed in Chapter 38.

As Herman has indicated: "It is not enough to be satisfied with symptom relief, emotional balance or insight into one's mental mechanisms. Rather, the ultimate goal of effective assimilation into the family and community becomes of equal prominence."

Rehabilitation of the Blind

Even though centers for rehabilitation of the blind are usually organized as separate units, independent of the centers for the rehabilitation of a wide variety of other disabilities, all workers with the handicapped should know certain basic facts concerning special techniques employed in the rehabilitation of blind persons. Surprisingly, a study made by ophthalmologist consultants to the Federal Vocational Rehabilitation Administration several years ago revealed that the one group of physicians who knew the least about rehabilitation of the blind was the ophthalmologists! It was concluded that, since preservation of sight was a major objective of ophthalmologists, when sight was lost there was a tendency toward subconscious rejection of the patient who had lost his sight. A course dealing with travel training and other rehabilitative procedures for the blind was then offered for residents in ophthalmology at Georgetown University School of Medicine. A new chapter describing the essential developments in rehabilitation of the blind (Chapter 39) by Goodpasture will provide workers for the handicapped with basic general information concerning rehabilitation of blind persons.

Rehabilitation of the Deaf

The rehabilitation of deaf persons is usually accomplished in special separate centers directed by otologists, specialists in speech and hearing and audiologists. The evaluation and management of auditory disorders is discussed by Gerstman in a new chapter (Chapter 37).

It is my opinion that in large medical centers it is often advisable to have the units for rehabilitation of the blind and the deaf combined with the units for rehabilitation of other types of physical disabilities and psychiatric illnesses. Although there must be special kinds of workers for each of these handicaps, still there are many advantages in having a large center where a variety of experts (social workers, counselors and engineers, for example) can be provided.

Engineering Principles in Rehabilitation Medicine

I have long been convinced of the need for electronic, mechanical and design engineers as full-time members of the hospital rehabilitation center team. Such experts can be of tremendous assistance in designing, developing and providing the devices or equipment which will assist handicapped persons to make the most of their remaining but impaired abilities. While I was serving as senior consultant to the Moss Rehabilitation Hospital we were able to organize, right in the hospital, a center for research and engineering. Wirta and Taylor from that center have prepared a new chapter (Chapter 40) dealing with the engineering principles in rehabilitation with which all workers for the handicapped should be familiar. Further growth of these engineering activities can be expected to improve substantially the quality of medical rehabilitation.

The Epidemiology of Disability

Epidemiology deals with the distribution of disease or disability and the factors which influence this distribution. It is concerned with various degrees of health, from minimal to optimal. Since an understanding of the modern principles of epidemiology is valuable to the health workers in rehabilitation, Itoh and Lee have provided a new chapter on this subject (Chapter 42).

Education of Physicians and Allied Health Professionals in Physical Medicine and Rehabilitation

It is desirable, in a textbook of this sort, to present a broad philosophical discussion of the teaching of the subject which is being considered. Such a dissertation is within the scope of this presentation. No one is better qualified than Dr. Leonard Policoff, teacher, clinician and administrator, to discuss this subject, so he has prepared a new chapter (Chapter 41) which deals effectively with education.

Broadening Scope of Physical Medicine and Rehabilitation

It has been necessary for me to expand, somewhat, this chapter on scope because (as indicated by the new chapters in this edition) the scope is rapidly increasing. Even after nearly a half century since its birth, the practice of physical medicine and rehabilitation is still in the developmental stages of its growth. I venture then to predict that in subsequent editions additional chapters will be added, indicating still further broadening of the scope.

THE ROLE OF THE PHYSICIAN IN PHYSICAL REHABILITATION OF THE HANDICAPPED

Because of the fact that in most of our medical schools today major emphasis is placed on the diagnosis and treatment of specific diseases with specific remedies, the graduates of our medical schools are for the most part woefully unprepared to evaluate and to manage the problems of the chronically ill and seriously disabled. This situation led Sedgwick Mead to comment: "If the cause, prevention, and treatment is unknown; if the person is senile . . . today's young physician feels completely unprepared to deal with the problem and is somewhat annoyed that society places any responsibility on him for such a patient's care."[17]

The need for better teaching of physical medicine and rehabilitation in our medical schools is demonstrated significantly in a study made by Charles M. Wylie of Baltimore on "The Participation of General Practitioners in a Rehabilitation Program." Wylie compared the utilization of a rehabilitation program by the general practitioners of Baltimore who had graduated from two Maryland schools of medicine. It became apparent that the graduates of School A, which had no physiatrists on its teaching staff, were not sufficiently familiar with rehabilitation to give their patients the benefits that could be derived from the rehabilitation program. The graduates of School B, which did have physiatrists on its teaching staff, comprehended the advantages of the rehabilitation program for their patients and did participate in bringing these rehabilitation services to their patients. Wylie stated, "a significantly higher proportion of non-participants were graduates from Maryland School A." He added, "For example, of 2069 graduates of School A who have specialized, none had entered the field of physical medicine and rehabilitation; in contrast the 1844 specialist graduates of School B include 9 physiatrists. At the present time, School A has no full-time physiatrists on its staff; the staff of School B includes two full-time physiatrists."[27]

Recently I pointed out that only half of the nation's medical schools have physiatrists on their staffs. There is still a shortage of teachers in our medical schools and we need many more in order to keep the concept of rehabilitation in the foreground of medical education and general medical practice. The problem is the same now as it was in 1943 when I became director of the Baruch Committee on Physical Medicine and Rehabilitation. At that time Bernard Baruch listened patiently to a series of lengthy reports covering the needs of all areas of physical medicine and rehabilitation and then he turned to me and said: "Dr. Krusen, the whole problem is very simple — we have got to train teachers to teach!"

Since 1943, thanks largely to the efforts of the Baruch Committee, great gains have been made. Unfortunately, however, too few practitioners in other medical specialties are familiar with the advances constantly being made in physical medicine and rehabilitation. To solve this problem we must place sufficient emphasis on physical medicine and rehabilitation during the medical student's undergraduate and graduate years to familiarize him with the role of this specialized field.

CONCLUSIONS

Sandler,[24] has pointed out that physical medicine and rehabilitation is a specialty still in its infancy. Owing to its youth and its lack of clearly delimited boundaries, many physicians are still relatively ignorant of its philosophy and scope. In fact, however, it is the breadth of this new specialty that sets it apart from other specialties. This breadth gives it strength and points the way to a shift in emphasis in medical school curricula.

There is hardly any demur to the argument that undergraduate training emphasizes diagnosis. The patient is thought of as a pathologic organ system — a diseased heart or kidney or lung. No one questions the importance of diagnosis. We submit, however, that today medical management (as opposed to pharmacotherapy alone) of the total individual having acute or chronic disease or permanent disability in relation to his normal environment including family, community and vocational milieu is necessary.

The term "medical management" here refers to any and all types of medical care necessary to restore patients having disability to optimal function. This implies more than diagnosis and assessment of the pathologic processes involved. It implies in addition enhancement of physiologic and psychologic adaptation to disability by every possible means — pharmacologic, physical, psychologic (psychiatric), substitution of mechanical devices and alteration of the environment.

Atchley has pointed out that "The goal of medical education is to produce a scholar in the science of human biology who will practice his profession as a perceptive humanist."[2]

If this goal is to be realized, we must impart to the medical student, as my co-editor, Dr. Frederic Kottke, has said, "an understanding of the whole individual as he functions in his normal environment, of the mechanisms by which disease and disabilities impair functional performance, and of the mechanisms available for compensatory adaptation to minimize dysfunction."[11]

Recent advances in medical science have had the effect of reducing mortality owing to acute disease and increasing the number of patients having chronic disease or permanent disability. In a survey of physical disability in Minnesota, England and Lofquist[9] found that one person in 10 had a disability severe enough to interfere with self-care or with employment. There is every reason to believe that the problem is equally great nationwide. Kottke[11] pointed out that this group "although constituting only 10 per cent of the population requires more than 10 per cent of the entire medical effort." Since many medical students will become general practitioners, it is extremely important that they be taught proper management of chronic diseases in conjunction with their medical practice.

The role of the physician is to maintain his patient at an optimal level of performance. Unfortunately it is still the case that in most medical schools the student is not taught to fill this role. A study made by Payson, Gaenslen and Stargardter[21] indicates that even during the internship minimal time and attention are given to medical management in the sense previously described. Generally speaking, the medical student and intern are led to believe that medical management is not very important since it is not taught, or is barely taught, during the undergraduate years or during the internship. Problems of medical management differ from those of diagnosis. They are not made a part of the student's experience and when he is confronted with them, he avoids or tries to avoid them.

It is not surprising then that medical students believe that professors rate diagnostic ability higher than skill in comprehensive medical management.[10] They suffer from a lack of balance between their knowledge of medicine and their knowledge of diseased people. "They are inclined to relish cases of clear-cut organic disease and to fight shy from the more difficult problems of dysfunction."[8] In short the medical student is often frightened away from consideration of the problems of the "whole man." He will tend to seek out instead cases of clear-cut organic disease so that he can practice what he considers to be "scientific medicine."

To summarize then, physical medicine and rehabilitation has an important place to fill in the practice of medicine. The medical student must be trained to evaluate patients in new ways and he must learn new skills in the management of chronic illness and serious disability. He must be taught to differentiate between those problems that he can manage himself and those that require the services of a specialist. More important, he should obtain experience in the management of patients having multiple diseases or chronic disabilities requiring continuing need for medical services. We cannot expect him to develop a comprehensive synthesis of medical care from bits and pieces of experience with single diseases or acute episodes of diseases alone. It is to be hoped that this handbook will aid the undergraduate medical student, the intern, the resident and the practitioner of medicine to achieve these goals.

A short time ago, Howard Rusk concluded, "Rehabilitation of the chronically ill and the chronically disabled is not just a series of restorative techniques: It is a philosophy of medical responsibility. Failure to assume this responsibility means to guarantee the continued deterioration of many less-severely disabled persons until they, too, reach the severely disabled and totally dependent category. The neglect of disability in its early stages is far more costly than an early aggressive program of rehabilitation which will restore the individual to the highest level of physical, economic, social, and emotional self-sufficiency."[23]

The Broadening Scope of Physical Medicine and Rehabilitation in the Future

I predict now that rehabilitation teams, in increasing numbers of rehabilitation centers, will lead the way in modern methods of medical care. In 1969 I wrote: "The representatives of our medical specialty are now in a position to make extremely significant contributions toward the provision of increasingly effective medical care in the future."[13] The Commission on Education in Physical Medicine and Rehabilitation has stated, "The dominant problems that have produced the widespread demand for change throughout the medical community relate directly to needs which rehabilitation medicine is uniquely fitted to fulfill."[6]

But if our scope is to expand, as mentioned by Dr. Stanley Olson, formerly Dean of Baylor University College of Medicine, "We must be in a position to furnish leadership to the rest of the medical faculty in development of broadly based programs of medical care."

Another trend in broadening our scope is the move toward providing "total rehabilitation" including the development of rehabilitation programs for persons who are primarily "socially disadvantaged" or "culturally deprived." Nearly all such persons also have secondary physical, psychologic, and vocational problems. Despite this fact some physicians and health workers view with alarm this development because it seems to lead into fields which they believe are too remote from direct medical care.[19]

Nevertheless I have pointed out that "Even though our rehabilitation centers have been oriented toward the physically and mentally disabled, we must now strive to apply our collective skills to the socially and culturally deprived if we are to achieve the ultimate in adequate service."[14]

Other persons who are recognized authorities have come to similar conclusions. Dr. Dwight Wilbur, when he retired from the presidency of the American Medical Association, made the following statements in his Farewell Address, entitled "Clinical Sense, Social Sense, Common Sense": "The need was never greater for physicians with compassion for those who suffer and are less fortunate. . . . Medicine and society have become so intertwined they are inseparable. . . . Our problem as physicians . . . is to develop a social sense that matches our clinical sense. . . . Much can be done through participating by increasing numbers of people on the health team."[26]

Adrian Towne, Administrator, Division of Vocational Rehabilitation, State of Wisconsin, directed a long-term study in which "total rehabilitation" was provided for the citizens of Wood County. This included rehabilitation of the "culturally deprived" as well as the physically and psychiatrically handicapped. He reported that the project "sought to demonstrate the feasibility . . . of extending vocational rehabilitation services to all handicapped persons, including both medically and socially handicapped." He added that "this million dollar . . . project came up with extraordinary findings. Not only did it prove that the culturally disadvantaged can benefit from rehabilitation services, but research disclosed that they profited the most of any group."[25]

Finally Dr. Edward Newman, Commissioner, U.S. Rehabilitation Services Administration, reported recently that the vocational rehabilitation act "allows for the provision of vocational evaluation and work adjustment services to the disadvantaged whether disabled or not." He spoke of this as a "vital new program direction for rehabilitation," and then he predicted that this "fledgling specialty in the rehabilitation movement . . . will soon blossom into a large and full grown area of the program."[18]

I do not expect that physiatrists and other medical rehabilitation workers, concerned with the management of physical and psychologic disabilities, will become involved primarily with the rehabilitation of the culturally deprived or the socially disadvantaged. But I do believe that they should seek to develop social rehabilitation units—units that are either associated with the medical rehabilitation centers or that are independent centers for the socially deprived. I think the programs for the medically and socially handicapped should strive to become mutually supportive.

Increasing support of the rapidly expanding number of centers of physical medicine and rehabilitation for the restoration of the chronically ill and seriously disabled and now also the culturally deprived to self-sufficiency is a triumphant affirmation of our society's belief in the intrinsic dignity and worth of the individual. The person's right to such services is not measured by his potential ability to bear arms for the state or to fill his established production quota or to become a useful servant of the community according to purely utilitarian standards. These programs in physical medicine and rehabilitation seek to restore the patient to his maximal degree of self-sufficiency even if this means that he will merely be able to lift a fork to his lips, hoist himself from his bed into a wheel chair or write with a pencil clutched in a clawlike device. The fact that he is a human being in need is sufficient justification for exerting every effort to help him use whatever abilities remain, however slight they may be. It is our hope that this handbook will aid physicians and other health workers concerned with the handicapped and the disabled to understand their problems, to learn how to evaluate their disabilities and to provide the modern techniques of management so that they can achieve the fullest degree of self-sufficiency, productivity and happiness of which they are capable.

REFERENCES

1. Allen, R. B.: Medical Education and the Changing Order. New York, The Commonwealth Fund, 1946.
2. Atchley, D. W.: The Clinical Clerkship in Medicine, Keystone of the Arch of Undergraduate Medical Education. J.A.M.A., *174:*1413-1416, 1960.
3. Barnard, C. I.: The Rockefeller Foundation: a Review for 1950 and 1951. New York, Rockefeller Foundation, 1952.
4. Bauhofer, F.: Old and New. World Health, December, 1970, pp. 4-11.
5. Bridgman, R. F.: Basic Hospitals. World Health, December, 1970, pp. 12-17.
6. Commission on Education in Physical Medicine and Rehabilitation. Bulletin 8. Recommendations for Teaching Programs. Minneapolis. Privately printed, 1968.
7. Community Health Services, Community Health Council of the United Community Fund of San Francisco: Report on Rehabilitation of Chronically Ill and Disabled Persons in San Francisco. Apr., 1960, p. 4.
8. Ellis, J. R.: The Medical Student. J. Med. Educ., *31:*42, 1956.
9. England, G. W., and Lofquist, L. H.: Minnesota Studies in Vocational Rehabilitation. VI. A Survey of the Physically Handicapped in Minnesota. Bulletin 26, Industrial Relations Center, University of Minnesota, Dec. 1958.
10. Karman, M., and Stubblefield, R. L.: Role Perceptions in Freshman and Senior Medical Students. J.A.M.A., *184:*287-289, 1963.
11. Kottke, F.: Contemporary Concepts in the Teaching of Physical Medicine and Rehabilitation to the Medical Student. J. Med. Educ., *39:*935-945, 1964.
12. Krusen, F. H.: Concepts in Rehabilitation of the Handicapped. Philadelphia, W. B. Saunders Co., 1964.
13. Krusen, F. H.: Historical Development in Physical Medicine and Rehabilitation. Arch. Phys. Med., *50:*1-5, 1969.
14. Krusen, F. H.: The New Philosophy in Rehabilitation of the Handicapped. The Deaver Award Lecture, No. 42 in the Rehabilitation Series. Institute for the Crippled and Disabled. New York, N.Y., 1968.
15. Krusen, F. H.: Rehabilitation of the Aging. Southern Med. J., *53:*1375-1381, 1960.
16. Krusen, F. H.: Relationships Between the Medical and Vocational Aspects of Rehabilitation. Rehab. Record, *1:*30-32, 1960.
17. Mead, S.: Rehabilitation. In Cowdry, E. V.: The Care of the Geriatric Patient. St. Louis, The C. V. Mosby Co., 1963, pp. 451-483.
18. Newman, E.: Vocational Evaluation and Work Adjustment, A Future Thrust of the Rehabilitation Movement. Rehab. Rec., *12:*13-15, 1971.
19. Olson, S. W.: Position Paper Submitted to the Commission on Education in Physical Medicine and Rehabilitation. (Cited in Reference 6.)
20. Oxford Universal Dictionary, Third Edition, Oxford, Clarendon Press, 1955.
21. Payson, H. F., Gaenslen, E. C., and Stargardter, F. L.: Time Study of an Internship on a University Medical Service. New Eng. J. Med., *264:*439-443, 1961.
22. Pinner, M., and Miller, B. F.: When Doctors Are Patients. New York, W. W. Norton and Co., 1952.
23. Rusk, H. A.: Preventive Medicine, Curative Medicine — Then Rehabilitation. New Physician, *13:*165-167, 1964.
24. Sandler, B.: Unpublished communication.
25. Towne, A.: Wood County Project — Total Rehabilitation. Brochure, p. 32. Division of Vocational Rehabilitation. Madison, Wisconsin, 1969.
26. Wilbur, D. L.: Clinical Sense, Social Sense, Common Sense. Farewell Address. J.A.M.A., *209:*680-684, 1969.
27. Wylie, C. M.: Participation of General Practitioners in a Rehabilitation Program. J. Chronic Dis., *17:*359-369, 1964.
28. Youmans, J. B.: Address to the Graduates of the University of Minnesota Medical School. Cited by Medical World News, *5:*34, 1964.

Part I

PRINCIPLES OF EVALUATION AND MANAGEMENT

Chapter 2

EVALUATION OF THE PATIENT; GONIOMETRY; MUSCLE TESTING

by Walter C. Stolov, Theodore M. Cole and Jerome S. Tobis

EVALUATION OF THE PATIENT

by Walter C. Stolov

The reader might ask why the need for a chapter on patient evaluation in a textbook on physical medicine and rehabilitation. He has, after all, learned and gained experience on how to elicit symptoms and signs from the history and physical examination of a patient. He already knows how to use these data for the establishment of a diagnosis of a patient's disease. Why not get on with the special therapeutics?

The reason is simple. *The symptoms and signs required for the diagnosis of disability are not synonymous with those required for the diagnosis of disease.*

Consider the following example:

A 22 year old medical student in a skiing accident fractures his left humerus. As the history is being taken, he complains, "I can't raise my hand." "I can't straighten my fingers." "My grip is weak." Examination reveals paralysis of the wrist and finger extensors, and hypesthesia over the dorsum of the first digit.

The diagnosis of the *disease* is clear. The patient has, in addition to a fracture, a radial nerve palsy. The *disability*, however, is not clear and has not yet been diagnosed. One question must yet be asked: "With which hand do you

17

usually write?" If the answer is "The left," one additional examination finding must be elicited. After the fracture is reduced and the arm placed in a cast, the patient's writing skill must be assessed. If he is unable to write, then at least part of his disability diagnosis (there may be other functions interrupted) includes the *inability to write*.

Neither the question, "With which hand do you usually write?" nor the examination of his writing skill after casting was necessary to make the diagnosis of the disease, but both were necessary to diagnose the disability. The history and physical examination required for the two diagnoses were different.

Consider further the possibility that the patient may have answered, "I write with my right hand." The writing disability would therefore not be present, yet the disease is still the same. This illustrates:

There is no one-to-one correlation between a disease and the spectrum of disability problems that may be associated with it. The disability is dependent on the patient's total requirements.

Consider further that our patient with the writing disability is advised that his radial nerve will not regrow successfully. As a result, he enters a deliberate systematic training program to develop writing ability with his normal right arm, and succeeds. He then has removed his disability, although the radial nerve palsy which caused it in the first place is still present. This illustrates:

There is no one-to-one relationship between a disease and the amount of residual disability. Disability problems can be removed even though the disease is unchanged.

This principle further points out a second important reason for a chapter on patient evaluation in a textbook on rehabilitation.

The ability of a patient and his physician to remove disability in the face of chronic disease is dependent on the residual capacity of the patient for physiological and psychological adaptation. His residual strengths must be evaluated and built upon to "work around" impairment in order to remove disability.

Disability means lost function. Our initial example dealt with the loss of a physical function, writing. Other kinds of functional losses can occur:

A 55 year old male outdoor construction worker complained of "shortness of breath" and "weakness." History and physical examination along with laboratory data confirmed the diagnosis of chronic obstructive pulmonary disease.

What, however, of his disability! Inquiry about employment revealed he was fired from his job because of a gradual reduction in work output. The patient confirmed that he no longer had the energy for the work. His physician indicated that response to treatment of the lung disease would not be sufficient to allow for a return to outdoor construction work. The disability diagnosis will then include the problem of *unemployment*.

Were the same patient engaged in a minimum energy white-collar job, unemployment would not be a problem. On the other hand, a white-collar worker with chronic obstructive pulmonary disease, while not disabled from work, may have the disability problem of loss of his major avocational pursuit (e.g., hunting) because of his disease.

The examples indicate the character of those diseases that produce disability. They are either diseases in which part or all of the pathologic process is irreversible and hence are always present, i.e., chronic diseases, or they are diseases in which a significant period of time must elapse before the pathologic process can be reversed. In either class, they may produce problems of dependency on others in activities of basic *physical* function. They may produce problems that relate to *social* functions in the home and with the family unit. They may produce problems in *vocational* functions and in the ability to engage in *avocational* pursuits. And finally, they may produce chronic emotional stresses which may produce *psychological* problems requiring adjustments not only by the patient but by his family unit as well.

A host of conditions exist for which diagnosis of disease alone without also the diagnosis of disability will lead to insufficient treatment. The disabilities must first be identified. The spectrum of disability problems that occur depends upon the interaction of the patient with his environment. This interaction is shown schematically in the diagram below (Fig. 2–1A). It indicates that the total disability (i.e., the disability diagnosis – the total list of disability problems) derives from factors specific to the patient and specific to the environment.

Weed's problem-oriented approach[6] to the process of patient care is particularly suited to the evaluation of a patient with chronic illness and disability. The reader will profit by reviewing his monograph. He divides the patient treatment process into four phases. *Phase 1* includes the history, physical examination and the initial laboratory studies as a data base. *Phase 2* identifies a specific problem list from the data base. *Phase 3* identifies a specific treatment plan for each of the problems. *Phase 4* describes the effectiveness of each of the plans and describes subsequent alterations in each of the plans, depending on progress.

The data base, therefore, goes beyond diagnosis determination. While a problem list will include known diagnoses, it will also include physiological syndromes, symptoms, signs and laboratory abnormalities for which a disease diagnosis is as yet undetermined. The problem list also includes the specific impairments of function in the basic physical self-care skills, and those specific problems in social, vocational and psychological function either secondary to or concurrent with the diseases. The individual identification of these functional problems leads to a plan for their solution, and hence for the removal of disability.

In this chapter are discussed specific methods of patient evaluation that will create the appropriate data base necessary to allow the physician to achieve

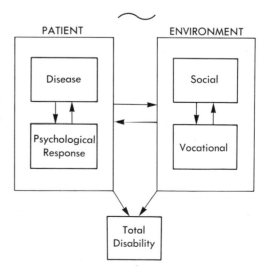

Figure 2–1A Schematic representation of the interaction of the patient with his environment. On the left, disease factors are reciprocally influenced by psychological factors. On the right, social factors are mutually influenced by vocational factors. The patient and his environment mutually influence each other. The Total Disability is fed by all areas.

a diagnosis of disability. History and physical examination data pertinent to an evaluation of lost function are described.

HISTORY

Historical data of prime importance in diagnosing disability are obtained from the *Chief Complaint, Present Illness*, and *Social and Vocational History* sections of the usual patient work-up. The nature of the *Chief Complaint* may provide a hint to the existence of disability. The *Present Illness* data can determine the extent of lost function in basic self-care activities. The *Social and Vocational History* evaluates the environment, and provides insight into the psychological makeup of the patient. The *Review of Systems* and *Past Medical History* contribute to the assessment of residual capacity.

Chief Complaint

All chief complaints or main reasons a patient may seek the assistance of a physician derive from changes in health or in well-being. These changes create within the patient either (1) fear or anxiety, (2) discomfort or (3) an inability to function. Chief complaints which include information on inability to function are the ones most apt to be associated with chronic illness and are those most likely to indicate that disability is present. The class of diseases most likely to produce complaints of loss of function are those which involve either the *musculoskeletal system*, the *neurologic system*, or the *cardiovascular system*.[2]

The accompanying list of chief complaints and final discharge diagnoses

Chief Complaint	Discharge Diagnosis
"Pain in calves after *walking* several blocks"	Peripheral vascular disease
"Can't *control* right leg"	Stroke
"Right-sided *clumsiness*, trouble with *balance*"	Multiple sclerosis
"Inability to *use legs* well"	Multiple sclerosis
"Can't *walk* or *talk* well"	Parkinsonism
"Leg weakness, unable to *stand* alone"	Transverse myelitis
"Pain in back and left leg. The more I *do physically*, the more I hurt"	Herniated disc
"*Walking* and *bladder* trouble"	Parkinsonism
"Low back pain increased by *walking* and *sitting*"	Lumbar disc disease
"Difficulty *walking*"	Musculoskeletal trauma
"Unable to *stand* up"	Stroke
"Aching wrist aggravated by *activity*"	Degenerative joint disease
"Difficulty with *ambulation* control"	Brain trauma

extracted from a series of charts is illustrative.* In this list, the statements referring to function are in italics.

While the majority of chief complaints related to loss of function are associated with chronic diseases of the musculoskeletal, neurologic, or cardiovascular systems, diseases in other systems also may yield statements related to loss of function.

Chief Complaint	Discharge Diagnosis
"Severe chest pain while *driving car*"	Chronic lung disease
"Pain after *eating*"	Peptic esophagitis
"Trouble *breathing* after *exercise*"	Obstructive pulmonary disease
"*Weakness*"	Carcinoma of the lung

In these illustrations, the chronic diseases were in the pulmonary and gastrointestinal systems.

Complaints related to loss of function are presented also by patients with psychiatric disease and without organic pathologic changes, as in the following examples extracted from charts of patients hospitalized on a psychiatric ward:

"Unable to *take care of myself*"

"*Fear of going* places"

"*Incapable of doing* job"

"Continuous ache in neck made worse by *movement and exercise*"

"I just can't *work, eat or sleep*"

"I have had a *terrible family life*"

These examples illustrate that psychological responses to the stress of chronic disease may aggravate disability from organic pathologic changes.

When, therefore, chief complaints contain statements related to loss of function, the physician is alerted to pursue carefully a search for disability. He must search for the dependency of the patient on others to carry out his basic self-care skills. He must search for problems in social functions in the home and family unit, problems of employment and problems secondary to chronic psychological stress. He is further alerted to the need for careful study of the musculoskeletal, neurologic and cardiovascular systems.

Present Illness

One of the hallmarks of disability is a dependency on others for the performance of basic self-care activities, sometimes termed activities of daily

---

*The charts from which the statements have been abstracted are those of 50 patients consecutively discharged from a Veterans Administration hospital in 1967—ten each from a Medical, Surgical, Neurologic, Psychiatric, and Rehabilitation Medicine Service.

living. Historical information about this dependency is best included under the category of *Present Illness*. Such data are really part of the symptom complex of the disease and are the essence of the disability the disease is producing. For example, it is not so much weakness that a patient is concerned about but the reduced ambulation that results. It is not the tremor that worries a patient, but the lost ability to hold a cup of coffee. Similarly, it is not so much the reduction in shoulder and elbow range of motion that a patient wishes to correct, but rather the lost ability to comb his hair or attend to his perineal hygiene after defecation.

The basic activities for which inquiry should be made as part of the *Present Illness* review can be divided into five categories: (1) Ambulation, (2) Transfer activities, (3) Dressing activities, (4) Eating skills, and (5) Personal hygiene activities. The quantification of dependency in the performance of any of these activities of daily living is achieved by determining from the patient who in the family unit provides the assistance and the nature of the assistance provided. Assistance is in one of the following categories:

1. *Standby Assistance.* As the activity is being performed by the patient, he may not always do it safely or correctly. The assistant then is "standing by" to guard against the occurrence of accidents and to ensure the correctness and completeness of performance by pointing out errors or omissions.

2. *Partial Physical Assistance.* As the activity is being performed, the patient is able to do a good part but not all of it by himself. The assistant then provides partial physical assistance. For example, the assistant may buckle the patient's belt after the patient himself puts on his pants, or he may hold the wheelchair stationary while the patient is himself transferring into bed.

3. *Total Physical Assistance.* For the activity to be accomplished, the assistant has to do all of it because the patient can contribute little or nothing toward its execution. He is, therefore, totally dependent.

Ambulation History.   Ambulation may be defined in the broadest sense as *travel from one place to another over a finite distance.* Ambulation thus includes not only walking but also wheelchair travel, and even crawling. To assess the extent of disability with regard to ambulation, the patient's capacity for ambulation in different environments must be obtained.

The environments of significance are his home, its immediate vicinity and the community at large. A patient may, for example, be totally independent in walking within and around his house but not in the community. The environments found in theaters, restaurants, subways or downtown stores may require that he have partial physical assistance in order to negotiate them safely. The disability diagnosis for such a patient will therefore include the problem of *decreased community ambulation.*

If a patient is not walking but uses a wheelchair, the extent of his independence in its use needs to be known. For example, the examiner should determine whether the patient is able to maneuver it independently within the home, whether he is also independent in its use outside his home, and if he can take it successfully into the community at large without assistance.

Sample questions in an exploration of ambulation skill are:
1. Can you walk without assistance?
2. Do you use equipment (i.e., canes, crutches, braces)?
3. Do you use a wheelchair?
4. Is there a limit to how far you can walk (or use your wheelchair) outside the home?

5. Can and do you go out visiting friends, or to restaurants, theaters or stores?
6. Do you have falls?
7. Do you drive a car?
8. Can you climb stairs?

Transfer History.   Transfers are movements which involve *changes of position in place.* They include such activities as going from a bed to a wheelchair or regular chair; going from a wheelchair to a toilet, bathtub, shower or car; and going from a wheelchair, regular chair or toilet seat to a standing position. These activities are more basic than ambulation. For example, while a patient may be independent in walking, he may be physically dependent on others to get out of his chair into a standing posture. His independent ambulation therefore is not always available to him if the assistance for the transfer into the upright posture is not always present.

Sample questions to begin an assessment of disability in transfer abilities are:
1. Can you get in and out of bed unaided?
2. Can you get on and off a toilet unaided?
3. Can you get in and out of the tub unaided?

Dressing History.   A disabled patient's ability to put on and take off his clothes must be carefully assessed. If a patient is not independent in dressing, he is less likely to leave his home and is less likely to receive guests other than his immediate family. Dressing dependency therefore greatly restricts the environments available to the patient.

In obtaining a history of performance in dressing skills, it is not sufficient merely to ask, "Do you dress yourself?" An untrained disabled patient may have for some time abandoned the use of those garments more difficult to put on. Typically abandoned are shoes, socks, pants, clothes with buttons, and close fitting undergarments. A patient therefore may answer "Yes" to such a question without realizing how few clothes he still wears. A more complete probe is therefore necessary to gain insight into his performance.

Sample questions that may be asked to explore competence in dressing are:
1. Do you dress in street clothes daily?
2. Can you put on without assistance your shirt, pants, dress, undergarments and so forth?
3. Do you need help with shoes and socks?

Eating History.   The loss of independence in a patient's ability to feed himself can be most devastating to his self-image. Unlike the activities already discussed, it is the one activity that *must* still go on even if total physical assistance is necessary. A patient who is dependent on others to feed him is literally reduced to the level of a two- to three-year-old.

Eating skills include the use of a fork, spoon and knife, and the handling of cups and glasses.

Sample questions in an exploration of this area include:
1. Can you feed yourself unassisted?
2. Can you cut meat?
3. Do you have trouble holding glasses and cups?

Personal Hygiene History.   Personal hygiene activities include the spectrum of skills concerned with cleaning and grooming: toothbrushing, hair combing, shaving, the use of tub and shower, perineal care and the successful handling of bowel and bladder elimination. Loss of independence in the performance of these skills is severely disabling to the patient. This is particularly so when the patient cannot handle bowel and bladder elimination in a socially acceptable manner. If a patient has to concern himself with the possibility that he may soil his trousers or the bed or someone's car with feces or urine, the emotional stresses to him and his family can be quite severe. The adult who requires that his spouse clean him after defecation may soon deal with a strained marriage. Efforts at increasing social functioning and directed toward vocational rehabilitation will be unsuccessful until the patient can develop a system of elimination that is consistently successful.

Socially acceptable elimination does not necessarily require that the systems be physiologically normal. Patients with catheters can develop a successful system if they can handle the emptying of collecting bags and can satisfactorily hide the collecting system under trousers.

Sample questions to explore the personal hygiene area include:
1. Can you shave (use makeup) and comb your hair unaided?
2. Can you shower or bathe without assistance?
3. Can you use a toilet unaided?
4. Do you need help in cleaning up after a bowel movement?
5. Are bladder and bowel accidents a problem for you?

General Principles in Determining Disability in Basic Functions.   In exploring for disability in the five basic functions of ambulation, transfers, dressing, eating and personal hygiene, several principles should be kept in mind:

1. When the patient reports he is not independent, determine the type of assistance: standby, partial physical or total physical.

2. Determine who is supplying the assistance.

3. Separately interview the people (usually family members) who are supplying the assistance. The assistant may indicate that the degree of assistance is actually greater than reported by the patient. The two may not interpret in the same way what is actually occurring. A significant difference in the context of their remarks may indicate neither is satisfied with what is going on.

4. When it is expected or anticipated that the patient may be dependent, questions of the "Can you . . ." or "Do you . . ." type should be rephrased to "Who helps you . . . ." Questions asked this way may yield more information. Patients may wish initially to appear more independent than they actually are.

5. When the disability is of acute onset, the inquiry should also include the pre-morbid level of independence. This is particularly important in the older patient. Earlier disease or trauma may have left some residual dependency. Therapeutics brought to bear on the new problems are not likely to result in a degree of independence greater than pre-morbid levels.

6. If dependency is present and the disease is of a chronic progressive type, determine the time course of the loss of independence. Therapeutics are more likely to remove disability in more recently lost functions rather than in those lost many years previously.

7. For some patients, the answers to certain of the preceding sample questions may be obvious and hence need not be asked. It is best, however, to assume less and inquire more, thereby avoiding omissions of significant data.

When an inquiry into the basic self-care functions of ambulation, transfers, dressing, eating and personal hygiene is complete, specific disability problems become identified. They need to be identified separately in the patient's list of problems even though they are secondary to a specific disease. Since the pathologic condition may be irreversible in part or in whole, these functional problems will not be eliminated by reversal of the disease process and will have to be attacked individually. Before therapeutics can be applied, however, problems must be identified.

Review of Systems

As already indicated, the ability of a patient and his physician to remove disability is dependent on the patient's residual capacity. Often, specific exercise and training activities are required to remove disability and restore function. The status of four systems in particular must be evaluated to assess the patient's capacity for this training. The *Review of Systems* inquiry, therefore, requires careful study of the cardiovascular, respiratory, neurologic and musculoskeletal systems. The cardinal symptoms in each of these systems are:

Cardiovascular. Dyspnea, orthopnea, chest pain, limb claudication, palpitation and cough.

Respiratory. Cough, sputum, hemoptysis, chest pain and dyspnea.

Neurologic. Numbness, weakness, fainting or loss of consciousness, dizziness, pain, headache and defective memory or thinking.

Musculoskeletal. Pain, deformity, weakness, limitation of movement and stiffness.

Past Medical History

Like the *Review of Systems,* the *Past Medical History* provides information on the residual capacity of the patient. Concurrent disease or previous trauma and surgery may have produced residual impairments. Although these impairments no longer produce disability themselves, they may compound the disability of the present illness when added to the new impairments.

A few examples may help clarify this principle:

A patient suffered a severe left brachial plexus injury, which resulted in paralysis of the triceps and the muscles of the wrist and hand. His past medical history revealed an earlier right hip fracture. Although the hip fracture had healed well, residual hip abductor muscle weakness required the use of a cane in his left hand for safe ambulation. Prior to the brachial plexus injury, the patient had not been disabled, since he could then handle all his ambulation needs with his cane.

The profound paralysis of the left arm, as a result of the brachial plexus injury, has now disabled the patient for ambulation.

Loss of ambulation is never a consequence of a brachial plexus injury alone. The past medical problem has compounded the disability.

A patient in an automobile accident suffered a complete paraplegia as a result of injury at the level of the tenth thoracic vertebra. His past medical history revealed a problem of recurrent shoulder dislocation, which was successfully repaired by surgery. The patient, after paraplegia occurred, began a heavy exercise program for his upper extremities in preparation for training in transfer activities. During a bout of exercise, shoulder dislocation occurred. After reduction, immobilization of the arm for six weeks was recommended.

The patient, therefore, became disabled for transfer activities not as a result of his paraplegia but because of the compounding effect of his previously dormant past medical problem.

A careful *Past Medical History* review is therefore an essential component of the evaluation of a patient with disability. A simple recitation of past or concurrent disease or trauma may not be enough. The inquiry requires an understanding of residuals, however slight they may seem.

Social and Vocational History

The social and vocational history of the patient is the source for the necessary data about the environment with which the patient must interact. A careful review will identify environmental problems secondary to or concurrent with the disease. It also provides insight into the personality of the patient. Information on his ability to adjust to the stress of chronic disability can be obtained, and the psychological problems that may need to be dealt with can therefore be identified early.

It is convenient to divide the personal history data of the patient into three categories: *social, vocational* and *psychological.*

Social History.   When dependency on others for the performance of basic self-care skills occurs, or if a job is lost because of disease, the patient's family unit is compromised. The need to help the disabled person perform his activities of daily living and the loss of income may force some family members to alter their own plans greatly. A major disability of one member of a family unit will create problems of adjustment for all and even threaten the integrity of the unit. Superimposition of a major disability on a family unit already beset with social problems is particularly threatening. Identification of secondary and concurrent social issues as *patient problems* and inclusion of them in the patient's problem list allows the physician to begin to attack the environmental problems at the same time that he attacks problems directly related to organic pathologic processes.

The assessment of social impairment is obtained from inquiries into the stability of the family unit, the history of the unit, the resources within the unit, the responsibilities of the patient within the unit, and the physical environment of the home and the community.

The physical environments are important because independence or dependence in the performance of an activity is directly related to where the activity is being carried out. The following examples illustrate the influence of physical environments on independence:

A patient who is independent in wheelchair travel may require physical assistance to transfer from toilet to wheelchair if the toilet seat is too low. Similarly, a patient may be dependent in bed transfers if the bed is too high. On the other hand, a patient who is independent in wheelchair travel and in transfers, regardless of the toilet seat height, may still be dependent on others for bathroom activities if the door to the bathroom is too narrow to allow for entrance of the wheelchair.

A patient who lives in a large city may be totally confined to his home and be unable to go downtown or to a store because such a trip may require the use of the subway and hence the ability to negotiate three flights of stairs. If he is not independent in such stair-climbing skills, subway travel will be beyond his reach and downtown inaccessible. On the other hand, a patient with identical skills who lives in a smaller city or in a suburban or rural community and who can perform autombile transfers and knows how to drive or has someone who can drive for him will have downtown accessible to him.

Sample questions to begin a search for problems in social functioning can include:
1. Where do you live? (Urban? Suburban? Rural?)
2. Do you rent or own?
3. Are the bedroom, bathroom, kitchen on the same floor?
4. Are there entrance stairs or stairs within the home or apartment?
5. Who else is at home? (Wife, husband, children (ages) and friends?) Do any of them go to work or school? Are they in good health? Are the children having trouble in school?
6. Do your parents, brothers and sisters live in the area? Do you maintain any contact with them?
7. Are you (how long have you been) married? Is this your first marriage?
8. What activities and functions did you do at home for the family that you no longer can do? (i.e., discipline, financial management, chores, sexual functions, avocational activities.) How are these functions now handled?
9. Where were you born?
10. Where else have you lived?
11. What did (or do) your father and siblings do for a living?
12. When did you leave your parents' home?
13. What was your family life as a child like?

The answers to these questions will provide the social background and current resources, as well as suggest current or potential problems. "Abnormal" responses to these questions should be pursued. For example, if a patient has been married before, inquiry into the number of previous marriages, their lengths, reasons for break up, other children, and financial obligations will yield further insight.

Vocational History.   A patient's disease may also produce the disability of unemployment. Whether there is or will be a problem in this area requires an understanding of the physical, intellectual and interpersonal requirements of the patient's job.

Sample questions to determine if the disease and the lost function in the activities of daily living will be compatible with employment are:
1. When did you last work?
2. For whom did (do) you work?
3. How long have you worked for them?
4. Describe what you did (do) on the job. Be specific. Start with what you do when you first arrive.
5. Was (is) your income sufficient to support your family or do you have other sources? Do you have debts?

If job instability is suspected—for example, if the last (current) job was held for less than two years, or if the last (current) job seems to be incompatible with the current illness even after rehabilitation treatment—then further inquire:
1. What kind of work do you plan to do in the future?
2. Obtain chronological history of employment, job requirements and reasons for change.

3. Inquire about special skills, licenses, union memberships and ratings received.

4. Inquire about highest attained educational level, age at time left school, and level of school performance.

These additional data will indicate whether there have been work adjustment problems. The strengths in the patient's vocational background on which one can build will also become clear. If the patient has not been working, inquire into his current sources of financial support and their sufficiency.

For the housewife who is not employed outside the home, inquire:

1. When did you last do the cooking? Shopping? Light housekeeping? Heavy cleaning?

2. Who does these things now?

3. Is this arrangement satisfactory for you and your family?

Avocational activities are also an important aspect of a patient's function. Many patients derive more of their enjoyment from life from their avocational pursuits rather than from vocational activities. *To seek for problems in this area, the following sample questions are useful:*

1. What do you do with your leisure time after work and on weekends by yourself? With your family?

2. What organizations or church groups are you active in?

3. When did you last participate in these activities?

Psychological History. Psychological function needs to be assessed in patients with a chronic illness or physical disability for several reasons: (1) Since the organic pathologic changes may be incompletely reversible, the stress of the disease is always present. This stress may be of great magnitude. For example, a patient who loses his leg has to adjust not only to this loss but also perhaps to the secondary stress of loss of his job. The physical requirements of the job may be incompatible with activity limits of an artificial limb. (2) The patient and his family may have to relinquish established goals and old ways of doing things. The patient may have to learn new ways to protect his health that are not at all consistent with his personality. These new modes of behavior are usually not his preferred way of doing things, and often not society's preferred way. (3) The patient's psychological makeup needs to be understood, for if new learning is to be facilitated in treatment an understanding of what is likely to motivate the patient and reinforce new learning is necessary. (4) For patients with brain damage from trauma or disease, an understanding of intellectual function will be required if they are to be trained successfully in the removal of disability in the basic functions.

Psychological problems should be included in the patient's problem list when the reaction to the stress of the disease is inappropriate or insufficient and when new learning is not occurring during treatment. While the *Mental Status* examination can assess current function, the social and vocational history data will yield a great deal of information about the patient's basic personality.

Interpretation of social and vocational data to yield psychological characteristics is a relatively simple matter when organized into four categories:

1. The patient's previous life style;

2. The patient's past history or response to ordinary life stresses;

3. The patient's current response to the stress of his disease;

4. The activities likely to motivate the patient to "train around" his disability.

Life Style.   Characterization of a patient's life style is an attempt to identify a common thread in his social, vocational and avocational activities. A *symbol-oriented* person is concerned predominantly with the world of ideas, abstract concepts, words and numbers. A *motor-oriented* person is concerned with the world of objects or physical movement. An *interpersonally oriented* person's life is dominated by activities involving close personal contact with others.

For many people, their usual style is heavily invested in only one of these areas. If such a person suffers a loss of function which interferes in his ability to maintain his mode of living, the psychological burden his disease produces will be great. For example, a professional athlete whose illness produces lower limb paralysis will have a greater psychological burden to adjust to than will a bookkeeper with identical paralysis. If, however, the bookkeeper's major source of enjoyment of life was derived from his hunting, fishing and camping activities, his burden may be as great as the athlete's. Those whose life style is well balanced among these three areas will be more likely to adjust to disability that affects only one of the areas.

Knowledge of the patient's usual life style and the effect of his disease will yield insight into the psychological response and the problems the patient may have.

The following sample groupings of vocational and avocational data obtained from the history will assist in this determination:

Symbol-Oriented
> *Vocations:* Law, accounting, science, clerical fields.
> *Avocations:* Reading, conversation, theater, museums.

Motor-Oriented
> *Vocations:* Manual labor, tools, machinery, athletics.
> *Avocations:* Active sports, hobby shop, hiking, camping.

Interpersonally Oriented
> *Vocations:* Sales, service, teaching.
> *Avocations:* Church groups, clubs, meetings, parties.

Past Response to "Ordinary" Life Stresses.   For some people the simple business of living produces stresses that they are unable to handle successfully. For these it can be anticipated that the superimposition of the stress of disability may be overwhelming. Such patients may actually be more psychologically comfortable with the state of dependency the disability creates. To achieve success in the removal of disability for such patients may be a difficult task.

The physician is alerted to this potential problem when the social and vocational data reveal such things as multiple marriages, multiple vocational and business failures, alcoholism, psychiatric hospitalization, police involvement, delinquent children and excessive debts.

When, however, the history is devoid of such social and vocational events, the patient may be more likely to be successful in removing his disability and regaining independence.

Current Response to the Disease Stress.   If a patient is being evaluated some time after the onset of the disability-producing disease, insight into his ability to handle stress can be obtained from what has transpired. If the social history and present illness data reveal that the patient has been getting his prescriptions filled, taking his medicine, making his appointments, altering his habits, monitoring his diet and avoiding preventable secondary complications, then he is exhibiting a satisfactory adjustment. Such a patient is more likely to be able to remove disability and achieve independence.

Motivational Factors.   The same social and vocational data that identify the patient's life style will also identify the type of activities that can be used as goals toward which the patient works as he strives to remove dependency during treatment. The likelihood of success in an activity consistent with his pre-morbid life style will serve as a motivational factor, even if the work the patient must perform to achieve his goals includes activities which are in themselves alien to his usual style.

For example, an interpersonally oriented individual may be motivated to perform certain heavy exercises important for his health if, on achieving a required level of strength, increased visitation with others is permitted. Similarly, a symbol-oriented individual may be motivated to develop transfer skill independence (a motor-oriented task) if, on success, the opportunity to attend a play or concert is made available.

Thus, the social and vocational data provide information that will allow the physician to build on the patient's strengths as he attempts to assist the patient in the removal of disability.

Summary

When the classic approach to the history is elaborated in certain key areas, a patient's total disability can be properly diagnosed.

If the *Present Illness* is studied with regard to the patient's status in ambulation, transfers, eating, dressing and personal hygiene, the spectrum of problems in self-care functions can be identified.

Study of the *Review of Systems* and the *Past Medical History* provides information on the residual capacity of the patient.

If the *Personal History* is elaborated to include careful study of the *Social and Vocational History*, then the problems within the environment can be identified. When such data are also scrutinized with regard to the psychology of the disabled patient, then problems of his reaction to the stress of the incompletely reversible pathologic condition can also be identified.

Not until these four classes of problems are identified (*physical, social, vocational* and *psychological*) can the rehabilitation treatment process begin.

THE PHYSICAL EXAMINATION

The information obtained from the physical examination of a patient whose history reveals the presence of disability serves three functions. First of all, the examination searches for the signs that signify deviations from normal structure and function. Correlation of these signs with the patient's history and laboratory data will yield the disease diagnoses. Secondly, in the examination of a disabled patient the physician searches for those signs that signify secondary problems which are not a necessary direct consequence of the disease. Such secondary problems may occur either as a result of treatment of the disease or as a result of lack of institution of appropriate preventive measures. Finally, the third main function of the physical examination is to assess the residual strengths in the systems or parts of systems unaffected by the disease. It is on these strengths that the patient and his physician build to remove the disability and reestablish the lost functional skills. These residual abilities are what the patient uses to "train around" the impairment induced by his chronic disease.

Some examples of secondary problems that occur as a result of treatment are as follows:

The arm of a patient with a Colles' fracture of the wrist is placed in a cast. To prevent motion of the proximal fragment the elbow is incorporated into the cast in a position of flexion. When the cast is finally removed, elbow flexion contracture is observed. Such a contracture is not a natural consequence of the wrist fracture but is secondary to correct treatment.

An elderly patient receives a severely comminuted hip fracture for which operative reduction and internal immobilization is not feasible. A hip spica cast is applied. As a result of total bed immobilization, the secondary problems of generalized disuse weakness, urinary retention and postural hypotension develop. These problems are natural direct consequences not of the fracture but of the appropriate treatment.

Examples of secondary problems which result from inappropriate preventive measures are:

A patient develops a partial radial nerve palsy secondary to trauma. The strength of the wrist dorsiflexors is insufficient to produce a full active range of wrist dorsiflexion. The patient is later found to have a wrist flexion contracture with shortening of wrist and finger flexor muscles. These contractures are not natural consequences of radial nerve palsy but are secondary to the omission of the preventive measure of regularly performed passive range of motion exercises of the wrist and fingers.

A patient suffers a fracture-dislocation of the seventh thoracic vertebra with resultant total paraplegia. During his hospitalization, a decubitus ulcer develops over his sacrum. Such an ulcer is not a direct natural consequence of the paraplegia. While the anesthesia over the sacrum is a direct consequence, the ulcer itself is secondary to omission of the preventive measure of periodic relief of pressure over the sacrum.

The major importance of secondary problems, whether treatment-induced or secondary to omission of prevention measures, is that they add to the patient's disability and they lengthen the treatment time necessary to remove the disabilities induced by the primary disease process. For example, the elbow flexion contracture will need to be treated before the patient can get full use of his healed fractured wrist and hand. Disuse weakness and postural hypotension will need to be treated before the patient with the healed hip fracture can achieve meaningful ambulation. The sacral ulcer has to heal before the paraplegic patient can begin to learn dressing skills or begin to sit for long periods.

The particular areas of the physical examination that need close consideration in the search for secondary problems and for the evaluation of residual strengths are *skin, eyes, ears, mouth and throat, cardiovascular, respiratory, genitalia and rectum, neurologic, musculoskeletal, functional neuromuscular* and *mental status.*

What follows is not an exhaustive description of the examination of these areas. Pertinent highlights only are given.

Skin

Examine the skin over bony prominences in patients with anesthetic areas or those who have been on prolonged bed rest. Look for vasomotor changes in the skin of the hands and the feet in patients with arm and leg weakness, joint contractures, or pain.

Eyes

Carefully assess for near and far visual acuity, for visual field defects, diplopia, and adequacy of glasses. Since the patient may need to relearn new motor acts to eliminate disability in basic self-care skills or may require vocational alterations, visual skills may need to be maximized.

Ears

Assess hearing acuity. Impaired acuity will impair relearning.

Mouth and Throat

In order to insure adequate nutrition, disabling factors that interfere with mastication and swallowing will need attention. Status of teeth, gums and dentures should be made optimal.

Cardiovascular System

Retraining to restore basic self-care skills that are lost as a result of musculoskeletal and neurologic disease usually requires specific therapeutic exercise regimes. An adequate cardiovascular reserve and optimized cardiovascular function are therefore essential.

Examination of the blood pressure (supine, sitting and standing), liver size, peripheral pulses, carotid pulses, venous return systems, peripheral skin temperature, peripheral skin hair and peripheral edema should therefore be done. Cardiac size, cardiac rhythms and cardiac sounds will need correct interpretations. All treatable abnormalities will need identification.

Respiratory System

Much like the cardiovascular system, the respiratory reserve needs assessment in the evaluation of exercise tolerance.

Examination of the respiratory rate and rhythm, the chest shape, the fingers for clubbing, the facies for cyanosis, and the lungs for congestion and obstruction are essential. Pulmonary function laboratory tests may also be needed to supplement the physical examination of the respiratory system.

Genitalia and Rectum

Particularly critical for patients with diseases affecting functions of micturition and defecation are examinations for cystocele and rectocele, prostate size, sphincter tone, anal wink reflexes, perineal sensation, the presence of orchitis and epididymitis and the presence of the bulbocavernosus reflex.

The bulbocavernosus reflex, if present, means that the sacral conus of the spinal cord at the level of S2 to S4 is intact. The afferent sensory stimulus is elicited by pressure on the clitoris or glans. For patients with catheters, a tug on the catheter will stimulate the afferent response. The efferent response is contraction of the external sphincter. A finger in the anus will detect this response.

Neurologic Examination

This exam should be performed with the same care as is exercised by the neurologist searching for signs in a difficult diagnostic problem.[3] All twelve cranial nerves must be reviewed. Sensory examination should include superficial touch and pain, deep pain, position sense (large joints as well as small), vibration sense, stereognosis, two-point discrimination, hot and cold perception and the presence or absence of extinction to bilateral confrontation. Cerebellar and coordination functions need careful review as do the deep tendon and pathological reflexes. Language functions will need to be evaluated with regard to articulation, visual and auditory reception and verbal and written expression.

Musculoskeletal System

The functional unit of the musculoskeletal system is the joint and its associated structures: synovial membrane, the capsule, ligaments and muscles which cross it. Examination of this complex anywhere in the body cannot be completed unless the underlying anatomy is known. A screening examination is useful in localizing abnormalities when the disability problems are minor.[4] For conditions that may result in major disability, individual joint examinations are necessary. Such examinations include *Inspection, Palpation, Passive Range of Motion, Stability, Active Range of Motion,* and *Muscle Strength.*

Inspection.   The two sides should be observed for symmetry in contour and size and differences measured. Atrophy, masses, swellings and skin color changes must be noted.

Palpation.   The origin of a pain symptom may be localized by palpation of the various anatomic structures about the joint. Palpation of the bones can determine their continuity in fracture assessment. Palpation of masses and swellings for consistency can distinguish between bony masses, edema and joint effusions. To determine the presence of muscle spasm, muscle palpation when the patient is at rest can detect a sustained involuntary reflex contraction usually secondary to pain.

Passive Range of Motion.   These tests are performed by the examiner while the patient is relaxed. When range of motion is limited, the examiner must determine if the limitation is due to joint surface incongruities, joint fluid excess or loose bodies, or capsule, ligament or muscle contractures. Methods of measurement of passive range of motion and normal values for all of the various joints are described later in this chapter.

Stability.   These tests assess whether a pathologic condition of the bone, capsule or ligament is causing abnormal movement (subluxations or dislocations). The joint should be moved under stress in the direction it is not supposed to move by virtue of its contour, ligaments and capsule, with the patient at rest. Tears in ligaments or laxity of capsule will result in abnormal mobility. During movement, joint stability is also supported by active muscle contraction.

Active Range of Motion. These tests should be performed prior to strength tests in the event pain is a problem. Muscle tension and joint compressions induced by an active movement are less than in a strength test. If pain is minimal in an active range of motion, the examiner can more easily proceed with a strength test. When active range of motion is less than passive range of motion, the examiner must decide between true weakness, hysterical weakness, joint stability, pain or malingering as possible causes.

Muscle Strength. Muscle strength can be tested if the prime action of a muscle is known. The body part can then be positioned to allow this prime action to occur. Grading systems are based on the ability of the muscle to move, against the force of gravity, the part to which it is attached.

GRADE 5. *Normal Strength.* The muscle can move the joint it crosses through a full range of motion against gravity and against "full" resistance applied by the examiner.

GRADE 4. *Good Strength.* The muscle can move the joint it crosses through a full range of motion against gravity with only "moderate" resistance applied by the examiner.

GRADE 3. *Fair Strength.* The muscle can move the joint it crosses through a full range of motion against gravity only.

GRADE 2. *Poor Strength.* The muscle can move the joint it crosses through a full range of motion only if the part is positioned so that the force of gravity is not acting to resist the motion.

GRADE 1. *Trace Strength.* Muscle contraction can be seen or palpated but strength is insufficient to produce motion even with gravity eliminated.

GRADE 0. *Zero Strength.* Complete paralysis. No visible or palpable contraction.

The key muscle grade with regard to disability assessment is grade 3. Since any activity a patient may perform is done in a gravity field, if he has at least grade 3 function, then the involved body part can be used. For grades less than 3, external support may be necessary to make the involved part useful to the patient. In addition, joints having muscles across them with less than grade 3 strength are prone to develop contractures.

Different examiners should agree on whether a muscle should be graded 0, 1, 2 or 3. For grades 4 and 5, there may be differences among examiners depending on their expectations of different age groups and the amount of resistance they apply. As an examiner's experience increases, so will his accuracy. For asymmetrical problems, grades 4 and 5 are useful even for inexperienced examiners as the two sides of the body are compared.

For conditions in which weakness is associated with spasticity, the grading system described is not as useful in predicting what use the patient may get out of the muscle for the performance of his basic skill needs.

A subsequent section of this chapter discusses the major muscles in the body, and describes how they are best tested, as well as their innervations.

Functional Neuromuscular Examination

The functional examination is the actual translation of the objective neurologic and musculoskeletal examinations into performance. It defines at a given point in time the skill of the patient in the execution of the activities of daily living. It is the starting point from which improvement can occur through treatment even if the objective neurologic and musculoskeletal signs may not be alterable owing to the nature of the disease.

The functional examination confirms the skill status reported by the patient in the history under *Present Illness* with regard to ambulation, transfers, eating, dressing and personal hygiene. The functions to be tested are as follows:

Sitting Balance.   This is a necessary prerequisite for most transfer skills. Test by placing the patient in the sitting posture, with his feet on the floor, his back unsupported and his hands in his lap. If he can hold this position, then nudge him in various directions and observe his ability to recover.

Transfers.   Abilities to be examined include turning from supine to prone and back, rising to a sitting position, rising from sitting to standing, and moving from a bed or low examining table to a chair.

Standing Balance.   This is a necessary prerequisite for safe ambulation. It should be assessed without support and, if present, nudging from side to side should then be done to assess the patient's ability to recover.

Eating Skills.   These can be assessed by demonstration of hand-to-mouth abilities utilizing various examining room objects or by means of actual observation at mealtime.

Dressing Skills.   These skills are easily assessed in the examining room if the examiner is present at the time the patient removes his clothes prior to the examination and puts them on at the conclusion. If the examiner remains in the examining room while the patient undresses and does not leave before he dresses, much information on patient skill and patient family interaction can be gained.

Personal Hygiene Skills.   The motions necessary for face, perineal and back care can usually be mimicked in the examining room. Direct observation of the specific task when actually performed may be necessary if personal hygiene functions are significant disability problems.

Ambulation.   Walking should be observed if the patient has standing balance. The patient should be essentially unclothed. Walking should be inspected with and without street shoes, and from the front and back, as well as from the side. Abnormalities should be described in relation to the phase of the gait at which they occur. If pain is present, it too should be related to the phase of the gait.

Observation and description should be systematically performed and recorded:

Cadence: Symmetrical? Asymmetrical? Consistent?

Trunk: Fixed abnormal posture? Abnormal movements anterior, posterior or lateral?

Arm Swing: Symmetrical?

Pelvis: Fixed abnormal posture? Abnormal pelvic tilt or drop?

Base: Narrow? Broad?

Stride Length: Short? Asymmetrical?

Heel Strike and Push Off: Present?

Swing Phase: Knee flexion? Circumduction?

Chapters 3 and 4 elaborate on gait evaluation and also discuss braces and artificial limbs.

If walking is not present, *wheelchair ambulation* should be evaluated. The patient's ability to produce straight line travel and to negotiate turns should be observed.

Mental Status

The mental status examination, coupled with the psychological history, provides the data base for understanding the patient's basic personality structure and his current emotional reactions to his disease and disability.

In addition, since removal of disability is a retraining and hence a relearning process for the patient, the mental status examination can be used to assess his learning potential. The examination becomes particularly pertinent in patients whose disease or trauma has produced brain damage.

Mental status examinations as they appear in psychiatric textbooks are oriented specifically toward the patient with psychiatric disease. When performed on the patient with physical disability, some of the areas investigated need to be elaborated upon.

For psychiatric patients, the outline described by Storrow[5] includes:

1. Appearance and General Behavior
2. Intellectual Functions
   a. Orientation
   b. Level of Consciousness
   c. Memory
   d. General Information
   e. Numerical Ability
3. Perception
4. Speech and Thinking
5. Affect
6. Insight
7. Judgment

The reader should consult Storrow's textbook[5] for the specific techniques he recommends to evaluate these areas.

For the disabled patient, additional evaluation beyond these usual techniques are necessary in the areas of *Recent Memory, Perception, Affect* and *Judgment.*

Recent Memory.   An understanding of recent memory function in a disabled patient is necessary because his rehabilitation treatment will require him to learn new ways of performing those functions he has lost. He may, for example, need to learn a specific technique to execute a safe transfer or to coordinate crutch and leg movements for ambulation.

Teaching of these skills requires that the patient assimilate, retain and reproduce new material not previously learned.

Recent memory functions with regard to language information may be assessed by asking the patient to remember, for example, an address that is given him. Retention is then evaluated when he is asked to reproduce the address later and perhaps the next day. With regard to non-language inputs, the patient can be taught a simple new motor task during the examination. Retention of this motor skill can then be assessed by later calling for its performance.

The emphasis should be on memory for totally new information. Asking the patient to recall what he ate for breakfast, although in a sense a recent memory check, is not really new material for him.

When recent memory functions are decreased, the physician is alerted to the fact that much repetition should be used when the patient is in training to remove disability.

Perception.   Perception includes the processes by which the patient organizes sensory inputs into information about the environment. This term, as used in the context of the psychiatric interview, refers to statements by patients which represent either gross misinterpretations of observable stimuli or hallucinations. Disturbances of this nature are gross departures from reality and are easily detected. Interpretation of wallpaper designs as ants crawling on the wall, the hearing of voices in a quiet room and the interpretation of radiator noises as special communication codes are examples of disturbed perception associated with psychiatric disease.

There are more subtle disturbances in perception that are not associated with psychiatric disease, and these must be evaluated when retraining of motor skills is to be considered in a brain-damaged disabled patient. These disturbances deal with the interpretation of visual inputs of form, space and distance. Such visual inputs require correct interpretation for the patient to be able to make a correct motor response based on them. For example, a patient in a wheelchair about to make a transfer onto a bed needs to interpret correctly first that both of his feet are on the floor, that he is close enough to the bed and that nothing is in his way that will interfere with his performance. Similarly, a patient about to put on his shirt needs first to interpret correctly the inside and outside parts of the shirt and that both sleeves are right side out.

Disturbances in perception of this type are more likely to occur in brain damage that affects the right cerebral hemisphere. They can be tested for by asking the patient to copy figures such as a square, a triangle and a maltese cross. He can also be asked to reproduce from memory a clock face. When disturbances in perception of form exist, these reproductions are distorted.[1] Asking a patient to put on a shirt that is presented to him rolled up with one sleeve inside out is also a useful test.

When perception disturbances exist the examiner will recognize that the teaching of basic self-care skills by demonstration will not be as successful as verbal instruction.

Affect.   A reactive depression is common following acute onset of a major disability in a previously normal patient, or following a relatively sudden additional functional loss in a patient with long-standing disease. It is a healthy response and indicates that the patient is at least able to recognize his losses. With such a recognition, he is more likely to be successful in removing disability.

A reactive depression requires remedial action if it is associated with disturbances of vegetative function or interferes with the patient's ability to respond to treatment. Judging whether such interference exists comes from observing patient participation during treatment rather than from what he says he is or will be doing.

The absence of a reactive depression may be a disturbing sign. If the patient is unable to face the loss, his ability to overcome the disability created by the loss may be reduced.

Mood swings are another feature of affect to consider. Rapid transitions from laughter to tears and back can represent the lability of an emotionally ill patient. Organic lability secondary to brain damage may show similar mood changes. Organic lability can, however, be more easily interrupted. Vigorously changing the subject matter of the conversation or sometimes a simple snapping of the fingers more easily curtails a flood of tears when such a lability is of organic origin. The presence of pseudo-bulbar neurologic signs will also suggest that the lability of mood is of organic origin.

Judgment. Judgment factors in brain damage relate to difficulties that the patient may have in monitoring his own behavior. In manner of dress or activities of physical function, he may fail to detect errors and be unaware of mistakes. These problems need to be distinguished from simple apathy, carelessness or sloppiness. If such behavior is observed in the general assessment of the patient's appearance and the various activities he performs during the course of the examination, judgment problems may exist. Insight into judgment can also be obtained during observation of the patient as he performs the various tasks given him as part of the intellectual function inquiry. Family reports of exposure of genitals and other evidences of embarrassing behavior implies poor judgment. When such behavior represents changes in the patient's personality that are associated in time with the disease or the trauma, an organic origin is possible. When judgment problems are present, standby assistance may have to be provided for the patient as he performs his various basic functional activities.

Summary

The physical examination of the disabled patient, as for any patient, combines with the history and the laboratory data to achieve diagnosis of disease. In the disabled patient it also reveals secondary physical problems that are not direct consequences of the disease and indicates the residual strengths on which the physician and patient must build to remove disability and reestablish function. It also verifies the functional self-care historical data discussed in the *Present Illness* part of the history. This section has emphasized the specific features to be considered when an examination is performed on a patient with disability.

CONCLUSION

It is essential for us to stress those parts of the classic history and physical examination on which special emphasis and elaboration is necessary when evaluating the disabled patient. Application of the techniques described will yield the diagnosis of disability.

Diagnosis of disease alone is insufficient for the planning of a comprehensive rehabilitation treatment program. The symptoms and signs required to diagnose disease are *not* synonymous with the symptoms and signs required to diagnose disability. To diagnose the disability—that is, the specific losses in physical, social, vocational and psychological functions—requires investigations not ordinarily considered in the treatment of acute short-term disease.

The techniques described also identify those medical problems that are secondary but not natural consequences of a chronic impairment. To achieve a successful treatment program that removes disability, the physician must understand his patient's residual strengths. The methods to achieve this understanding have also been emphasized.

Following an appropriate evaluation, the physician is able then to list all of his patient's problems. Such a problem list will include disease diagnoses and secondary abnormalities. It must also include the specific losses in *physical* basic self-care functions, *social* functions, *vocational* functions and *psychological* functions.

Once the problem list is established, the rehabilitation treatment process can begin. It begins with a specific plan for each of the problems on the list. It succeeds when each of the problems is solved to the highest degree obtainable by available therapeutic techniques.

Some of the other chapters in this book deal with further elaboration of evaluation methods and the therapeutics that can be brought to bear on the solution of disability problems. The reader will find that the therapeutic techniques described will fall within one of six general areas: (1) methods to prevent or correct secondary problems, (2) methods to enhance the capability of systems unaffected by the disease, (3) methods to enhance the functional capacity of affected systems, (4) methods to promote function through the use of adaptive equipment, (5) methods to modify the social and vocational environment, and (6) methods from psychological theory to enhance patient performance.

REFERENCES

Evaluation of the Patient
1. Heimburger, R. F., and Reitan, R. M.: Easily Administered Written Test for Lateralizing Brain Lesions. J. Neurosurg., *18*:301–312, 1961.
2. Lehmann, J. F.: Patient Care Needs as a Basis for Development of Objectives of Physical Medicine and Rehabilitation Teaching in Undergraduate Medical Schools. J. Chron. Dis., *21*:3–12, 1968.
3. Mayo Clinic: Clinical Examinations in Neurology. 3rd Edition. Philadelphia, W. B. Saunders Company, 1971.
4. Rosse, C., and Clawson, D. K.: Introduction to the Musculoskeletal System. New York, Harper and Row, 1970.
5. Storrow, H. A.: Outline of Clinical Psychiatry. New York, Appleton-Century-Crofts, 1969.
6. Weed, L. L.: Medical Records, Medical Education and Patient Care. Cleveland, The Press of Case Western Reserve University, 1969.

GONIOMETRY: THE MEASUREMENT OF JOINT MOTION

by Theodore M. Cole

Goniometry is the measurement of joint motion. It is an essential step in the evaluation of function in a patient with muscular, neurological or skeletal disability. The diagnosis of the way in which a patient functions in his daily life, how he moves about or how he manipulates his environment physically may depend heavily upon the degree to which the parts of his body can tolerate passive or active motion. The presence of voluntary muscular contraction, the application of a prosthetic or orthotic device, or the preservation of sensation in a part of the body may be of little value to the patient if the joints of that part are unable to be moved through all or part of their normal range of motion. In other cases — for example, where limitation of joint motion may still permit the patient to walk — his endurance may be greatly hampered by the fatiguing effect of muscles exerting their forces at a biomechanical disadvantage.

In addition to helping the physician make a diagnosis of the patient's functional loss, the careful examination of joint motion can reveal the extension of a disease process or provide objective criteria for determining the effectiveness of a treatment program. Without such evaluation, not only is the patient's care impaired but legal determination of disability,[1] which in some cases depends upon joint motion, may be muddled and the extent of feasible rehabilitation misjudged.

An accurate medical record is not possible without accurate measurement. Should there be a change in the patient's therapist, should subsequent follow-up of a patient's disease be necessary, or should a dormant disease become reactivated, correct treatment depends upon accurate clinical measurement. If review of data from a patient's record should become necessary for purposes of research, the study will be meaningful only to the extent that procedures such as goniometry were performed and recorded correctly.

The reader setting out to learn the skillful employment of goniometry may have little interest in the accumulated years of controversy over tools and methods to measure the motion of joints. He will, however, be interested in determining how readily he can acquire the skill and how he can apply it to his patients so that they may benefit. He should also want to learn how he can accurately communicate his findings to his colleagues and how he can understand their records. To that end, he should be acquainted with some of the more commonly used tools and techniques.

TOOLS AND INSTRUMENTS

Although many types of goniometers or arthrometers have been described[2] the instrument most commonly used in the clinic is the universal goniometer, examples of which are shown in Figure 2-1. The two arms of the goniometer, with a pointer on one and a protractor scale on the other, are joined by a pivot which provides enough friction so that the instrument remains stable when picked up and held for reading. Some goniometers are made with full circle scales and others with half circle scales, but all should be

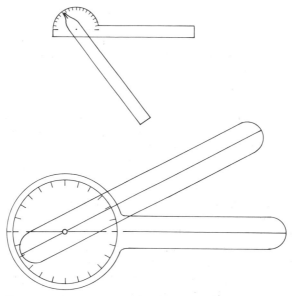

Figure 2–1   Two examples of universal goniometers commonly used by the clinician.

clearly marked in degrees so that the scale may be easily read by the unaided eye at 18 inches. The length of the arms of an easily portable goniometer is usually about six inches. However, if more accurate measurements are required for joints of very large[3] or very small members, then longer or shorter arms may be preferred. The tool should also be lightweight, durable and washable in order to assure that it will be carried in the examiner's pocket or bag often enough to insure its frequent use.

Only rarely will other joint-measuring tools be useful for the bedside examination. The exception to this generalization is the spine: meaningful measurements of joint motion in the spine are confounded by the multiplicity of participating joints, the paucity of reliable landmarks and the bulk of soft tissue overlying the joints being measured. Spinal x-rays in extremes of motion offer more useful, readily available and easily understood information. Bubble goniometers, plumb lines, electronic devices and certain other tools are used only in special settings and will not be discussed here.[4, 5, 6]

SYSTEMS OF MEASUREMENT

Many of the systems suggested for recording measurements of range of motion were reviewed by Moore[7, 8] who argues strongly that, whatever method is selected for use, it would be wise for everyone working in the same hospital, department or clinic to utilize the same system of notation. The method put forth in this chapter is an adaptation of the system used by Knapp and West[9] and is based upon relating the range of motion of a joint to a full circle, or 360°. Since the bones of the body may be considered as levers or systems of levers, they may be thought of as moving in a rotary fashion about an axis of rotation located in the center of their joints. When motion occurs about a joint, every point in the moving bone must describe an arc of a circle, the center of which lies on the axis of rotation.

It is important to locate correctly the axis of rotation of a joint in order to perform accurate goniometry. In almost all joints, the axis of a goniometer can be placed so as to coincide with the axis of rotation of the joint. The angle thus formed by the two arms of the goniometer corresponds to the angle formed by the two members of the joint.

The 0° position of a circle superimposed upon the joint has been arbitrarily assigned. With the patient in the anatomical position, 0° is designated as the point directly over the patient's head, with 180° toward the patient's feet. As shown in Figure 2-2, when the proximal member of a joint is moved from the anatomical position, the 0° position moves accordingly and will no longer lie over the patient's head. In the full circle system, almost all joint motions can be considered as rotating away from or toward the overhead zero point in the frontal or the sagittal planes. Thus, in the sagittal plane flexion is motion which rotates the distal member toward the 0° position on the circle and extension rotates it away from 0°. Abduction is motion toward and adduction motion away from the 0° position in the frontal plane.

The horizontal or transverse plane applies to certain joints which rotate about the longitudinal axis of the body. Neck rotation is an example of such a configuration. The 0° position is designated on the superimposed circle as that point directly in front of the tip of the patient's nose.

Since the 0° position is defined in terms of one of the joint members, expressing the position of a joint in degrees signifies a definite relationship between the two members of the joint. Thus, when two arms of the goniometer are laid along the longitudinal axes of two joint members, and a measurement is made at the two extremes of motion, the examiner at once defines the limits of motion, the range of motion and the many angles which may be formed at that joint.

Other systems of recording joint motion are based upon a different set of numerical figures attached to the zero points or starting points. Some argue for defining the anatomical position as 0° and recording motion as deviation from 0°. Others suggest modifications of this, depending upon the joint and the motion being measured. Still other systems require the joining of positive and negative values to compute a range for the entire motion in question. Some workers argue for the use of small numbers, 180° or less for a single motion, believing that smaller numbers can be more easily visualized.

When used consistently, the method of recording joint motion offered here has been found to be readily understood by therapists, nurses and physi-

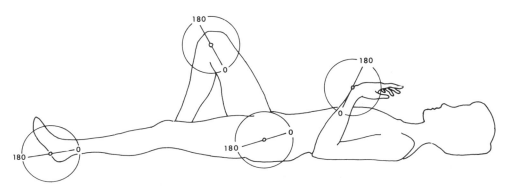

Figure 2-2 The full circle or 360° system of goniometry applied to several joints of the body, illustrating the locations of the zero degree (0°) position.

cians. Examiners have been able to learn quickly where the zero or starting point is located. The notion that large numbers are difficult to visualize has not been borne out by examiners who use this method of recording in their daily work. Indeed, the 360° system was employed years ago by Knapp to facilitate quick learning by persons without medical or anatomical training.[10]

The 360° system has an added advantage. A flexion contracture, which produces an inability to move the part to its normal position of extension, or a recurvatum deformity, which is present when there is an excessive laxness of a joint permitting motion beyond normal extension, can be easily recorded. There is no need for awkward expressions. Further, there is no need to add or subtract numbers to arrive at the limits of motion.

TERMINOLOGY

As in almost all other areas of medical communication, agreement on goniometric terminology has not been universal. The problem of communication is made worse by the insistence of some persons that the nomenclature should not include such terms as dorsiflexion or radial deviation but should utilize the "purer" terms of flexion, extension, abduction, adduction and medial and lateral rotation. However, the choice of words should depend wholly upon whether or not they accurately communicate what the writer intends. The following glossary lists many of the terms commonly used in the language of goniometry.

Glossary of Goniometric Terms

Goniometer: an instrument for measuring angles.
Sagittal plane: the vertical, anterior-posterior plane through the longitudinal axis of the trunk, dividing the body into right and left halves.
Frontal or *coronal plane:* any vertical plane at right angles to the sagittal plane, dividing the body into ventral and dorsal portions.
Horizontal or *transverse plane:* any plane through the body parallel with the horizon.
Flexion: bending of a joint so that the two adjacent segments approach each other and the joint angle is decreased.
Extension: straightening of the joint so that the two adjacent segments are moved apart and the joint angle is increased.
Rotation: turning or moving of a part around its axis.
Supination: rotating the forearm so that the palm is up (anterior in the anatomical position).
Pronation: rotating the forearm so that the palm of the hand is down (posterior in the anatomical position).
Deviation: moving away from a starting position; frequently to denote abduction or adduction relative to the midline, or rotation from a starting point.
Inversion: turning inward; turning the sole of the foot so it tends to face medially.
Eversion: turning outward; turning the sole of the foot so it tends to face laterally.
Abduction: motion at a joint so that segment is moved laterally away from the midline.
Adduction: motion at a joint so that a segment is moved medially toward the midline.
Dorsiflexion: flexing or bending of the foot toward the leg so that the angle between the dorsum of the foot and the leg is decreased.
Plantar flexion: flexing or bending the foot in the direction of the sole so that the angle between the dorsum of the foot and the leg is increased.
Opposition: moving the thumb away from the palm in a direction perpendicular to the plane of the hand.

Axis of rotation: a line at right angles to the plane in which adjacent limb segments move and about which all moving parts of the segments describe circular arcs.

Longitudinal axis: a line passing through a bone or segment, around which the parts are symmetrically arranged, and lying in both frontal and sagittal planes.

ACCURACY

Accuracy is an objective of all measurement techniques. However, like other aspects of the clinical examination, accuracy is a relative term implying careful training and attention to technique, thereby keeping the variability of measurements to an acceptable minimum while making observations and compiling data which closely approximate the true state of affairs. The ultimate test of the data which is recorded is in its interpretation and utilization. Interpretation, in turn, depends upon the level of expectation of the interpreter, who must have a realistic understanding as to just how accurate the data really is. Unless goniometry is carried out by a highly trained examiner using specialized equipment in a time-consuming method, measurement of joint motion cannot be expected to yield figures closer to true value than 3° to 5°.

Hellebrandt[11] found that the mean error for an average trained physical therapist was 4.75°. For a thoroughly experienced physical therapist, it was 3.76°. since the average physician measures joint motion less frequently than the average physical therapist, a 5° error seems reasonable if the equipment is reliable and careful attention is given to technique.

In some cases previous disease or surgical intervention will alter the usual bony landmarks so as to render measurements less reliable. For example, the chronically dislocated hip will make the measurement of hip flexion-extension unreliable, as would the presence of an Austin-Moore prosthesis.

CONDITIONS AFFECTING MEASUREMENT OF JOINT MOTION

The examiner must indicate the conditions under which range of motion was measured. Was it done passively or actively, that is, did the patient move the part himself or did the examiner position the part? Was motion achieved with or without forcing the part through some portion of its total range? Did the patient experience pain during motion? Was motion opposed by voluntary or involuntary resistance? If resistance was detected, did it yield to sustained force exerted by the examiner or was the resistance unyielding? Was the patient able to cooperate with the examiner or was the examination carried out, for example, on a disoriented or confused patient who attempted to oppose the examiner? Was the patient under tension and anxious or was he relaxed? Was the examination encumbered by such things as a restrictive cast, a surgical wound, an appliance or hypertrophied musculature? In addition to all these aspects, the patient's sex and age are known to influence the variability of normal joint motion.

Thus, many factors can influence the results of the examination, and since one or another of them may be present on one day and absent on the next, including such pertinent information is essential to an accurate interpretation of the data. Interpretation, of course, is the basis for decision making.

GENERAL PRINCIPLES IN MEASUREMENT OF JOINT MOTION

All motions which are commonly measured are carried out in one of three geometric planes. In the sagittal plane the following motions take place: flexion-extension and rotation at the shoulders; flexion-extension at the elbows, wrists, and fingers; and flexion-extension at the hips, knees and ankles. Motions in the frontal or coronal plane are abduction and adduction at the shoulders and hips. Rotation of the hips and the cervical spine, which occurs in the horizontal plane of the body, radial and ulnar deviation at the fingers and wrists and pronation-supination of the forearms are exceptions to the full circle, 360° system.

TABLE 2–1 JOINTS AND MOTIONS WHICH CAN BE MEASURED ACCORDING TO FULL CIRCLE OR 360° GONIOMETRY AND EXCEPTIONS TO THE SYSTEM

Joints and Motions Measured on a Full Circle (360°)		Exceptions to the Full Circle System
SAGITTAL PLANE	FRONTAL PLANE	
Shoulder: flexion-extension rotation	Shoulder: abduction-adduction	
Elbow: flexion-extension		
Wrist: flexion-extension		Forearm: supination-pronation (abd.-add.) Wrist: ulnar and radial deviation (abduction-adduction)
Finger: flexion-extension		
Hip: flexion-extension	Hip: abduction-adduction	Hip: rotation
Knee: flexion-extension		
Ankle: dorsiflexion-plantar flexion		Ankle: inversion-eversion

Not all possible joint motions are measured in the usual clinical examination, because not all of the body's possible joint motions are important to the patient's pathological or functional diagnoses or to the treatment plan. Also, some joint motions can be only crudely measured and efforts at accurate representation are not warranted. Instead, motions such as toe flexion-extension or back rotation are recorded descriptively in those cases in which their examination is germane to the patient's problem.

The examiner should become familiar with the normal ranges of motion for each joint. In many cases the patient's unaffected, contralateral extremity can be measured to establish a normal value for that patient.

TECHNIQUE OF JOINT MEASUREMENT

Joint — Shoulder

Motion: Flexion-extension (Fig. 2-3)
Plane of Motion: Sagittal

Positioning the Patient: The arm is at the patient's side.

How to Measure: The goniometer is centered on the shoulder just below the acromion. One arm of the goniometer is placed parallel to the midaxillary line of the trunk; the other arm of the goniometer is placed parallel to the longitudinal axis of the humerus along the lateral side of the patient's arm. The patient's arm moves anteriorly in flexion or posteriorly in extension. Readings are taken at the completion of motion.

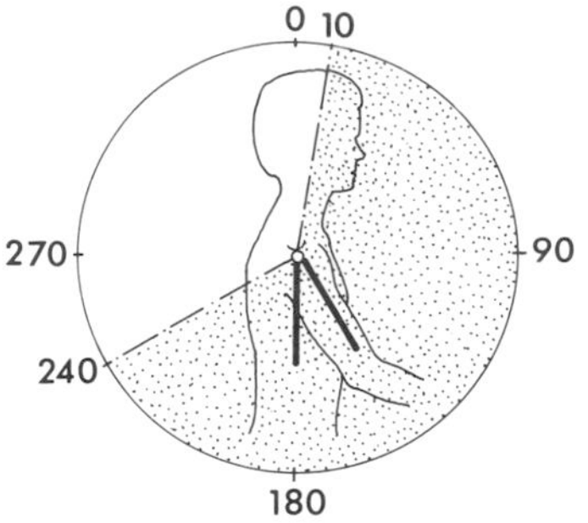

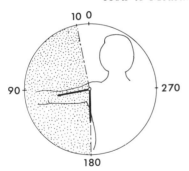

Figure   2–3 Shoulder: flexion-extension.

Normal Limits and Range of Motion: 10° − 240°

Motion: Abduction-adduction (Fig. 2-4)
Plane of Motion: Frontal
Positioning the Patient: The arm is at the patient's side with the palm toward the body. The arm is raised in the frontal plane to 90°. As it continues upward, the arm is externally rotated so that the palm faces the midline at completion of movement. The greater tuberosity of the humerus is a limiting factor in abduction, and by rotating the arm it is partially removed from the line of action.

How to Measure: The goniometer is centered on the posterior aspect of the shoulder joint (on a level with a line projected posteriorly from below the acromion). One arm of the goniometer is aligned parallel to the midline of the body (vertebral column). The other arm of the goniometer is aligned with the longitudinal axis of the humerus, posteriorly, after the patient's arm is moved.

Figure   2–4 Shoulder: abduction-adduction.

Normal Limits and Range of Motion: 10° − 180°

Motion: External and internal rotation (Fig. 2-5)
Plane of Motion: Sagittal
Positioning the Patient: The humerus is abducted to 90°; the elbow is flexed to 90°. The forearm is positioned in pronation with the palm facing the feet.

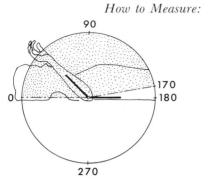

How to Measure: The goniometer is centered on the elbow joint. One arm of the goniometer is held parallel to the midaxillary line of the thorax. The other arm of the goniometer is aligned with the longitudinal axis of the forearm. Measurements are made in extremes of external and internal rotation.

Figure 2–5   Shoulder: external and internal rotation.

Normal Limits and Range of Motion: External rotation,   0°
                                         Internal rotation,   170°

Joint — Elbow

Motion: Flexion-extension (Fig. 2-6)
Plane of Motion: Sagittal
Positioning the Patient: The arm is held at the side in the anatomical position. For the convenience of the sitting patient, the shoulder may be flexed.

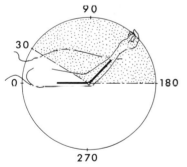

How to Measure: The goniometer is centered over the elbow joint laterally. The forearm is maintained in supination. One arm of the goniometer is parallel to the longitudinal axis of the humerus and the other arm is parallel to the longitudinal axis of the radius. Measurements are made in extremes of flexion and extension.

Figure 2–6   Elbow: flexion-extension.

Normal Limits and Range of Motion: 30° — 180°

Joint — Radio-ulnar Joints

Motion: Pronation-supination (Figs. 2-7, 2-8)
Plane of Motion: This motion is an exception to the full circle or 360° system of measurement. Motion takes place in the frontal plane.
Positioning the Patient: The humerus is adducted to the thorax and the

elbow flexed to 90° with the radial aspect of the forearm directed toward the patient's head. This is the 0° position.

How to Measure:

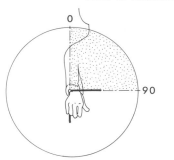

Figure   2–7   Radio-ulnar   joint: pronation.

To measure pronation (see Fig. 2-7), the forearm is first fully pronated. The goniometer is held against the dorsal surface of the wrist and centered over the ulnar styloid; one arm of the goniometer is placed parallel to the longitudinal axis of the humerus. The other arm of the goniometer remains across the dorsum of the wrist.

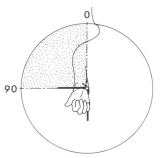

Figure   2–8   Radio-ulnar   joint: supination.

To measure supination (see Fig. 2-8), the forearm is first fully supinated. The goniometer is held against the volar surface of the wrist and centered on the ulnar styloid. One arm of the goniometer remains across the volar surface of the wrist while the other is aligned with the longitudinal axis of the humerus.

Normal Limits and Range of Motion: The 0° reading is as described in *Positioning the Patient.* The normal limits of pronation and supination are 90° in each direction, totaling 180° of range.

Joint — Wrist

Motion: Flexion-extension (Fig. 2-9)
Plane of Motion: Sagittal
Positioning the Patient: The forearm and hand are held in pronation.

How to Measure:

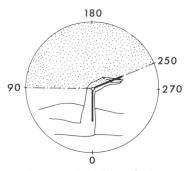

Figure   2–9   Wrist: flexion-extension.

The goniometer is centered on the ulnar styloid; one arm of the goniometer is parallel with the longitudinal axis of the forearm along the ulnar border; the other arm is parallel with the longitudinal axis of the fifth metacarpal and is moved with the fifth metacarpal to measure flexion or extension.

Normal Limits and Range of Motion: 90°–250°

Motion: Radio-ulnar deviation (abduction-adduction) (Fig. 2–10)
Plane of Motion: This motion is an exception to the full circle or 360° system of measurement. Motion takes place in the horizontal plane.
Positioning the Patient: With the elbow at 90° of flexion-extension, the forearm is held in pronation and the wrist at 180° of flexion-extension.

How to Measure: The goniometer is placed over the dorsum of the hand and centered over the proximal portion of the third metacarpal bone; one arm of the goniometer is placed along the midline of the forearm, the other is placed parallel to the longitudinal axis of the third metacarpal bone. Measurements are made when the hand completes maximum deviation to the radial (abduction) and ulnar (adduction) sides.

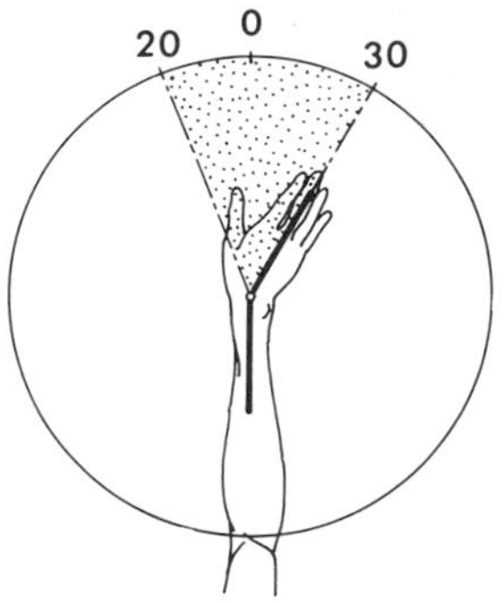

Figure 2–10 Wrist: radio-ulnar deviation.

Normal Limits and Range of Motion: Since this motion is an exception to the full circle or 360° system of measurement, the 0° position is as described in *Positioning the Patient* above. Normal motion is 20° of radial deviation and 30° of ulnar deviation, totaling 50°.

Joint — Metacarpophalangeal Joints

Motion: Flexion-extension (including the thumb) (Fig. 2–11)
Plane of Motion: Sagittal
Positioning the Patient: The hand is held in any restful position and the thumb and fingers are extended.

How to Measure: The patient flexes each finger at the metacarpophalangeal joint. The goniometer is centered over the metacarpophalangeal joint being measured. One arm of the goniometer is placed on the dorsum of the hand and the other arm is placed on the dorsum and parallel to the longitudinal axis of the finger being measured. Measurements are made at maximum flexion and extension.

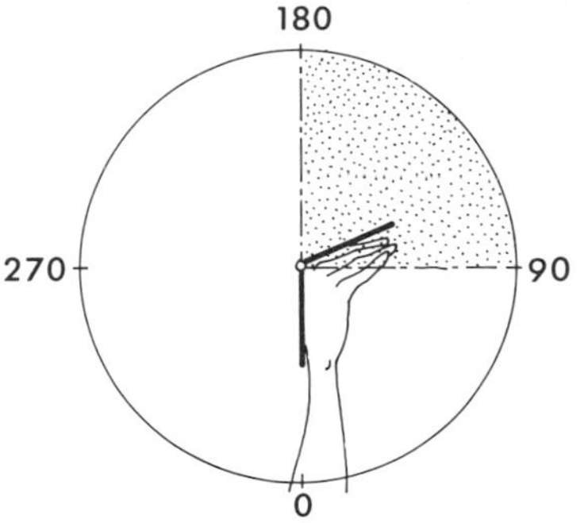

Figure 2–11 Metacarpophalangeal joint: flexion-extension.

Normal Limits and Range of Motion: 90° − 180°

Joint — Interphalangeal Joints (Including Thumb)

Motion: Flexion-extension (Fig. 2-12)
Plane of Motion: Sagittal
Positioning the Patient: The hand is held in any restful position.

How to Measure: The goniometer is centered over the joint to be measured. One arm of the goniometer is placed on the dorsal surface of the proximal phalanx and the other arm is placed over the dorsal surface of the distal phalanx. Readings are taken at positions of maximum flexion and extension.

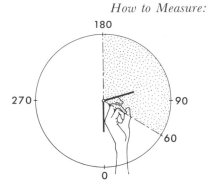

Figure 2–12   Interphalangeal joint: flexion-extension.

Normal Limits and Range of Motion:
    Proximal interphalangeal joints,   60° – 180°
    Distal interphalangeal joints,   110° – 180°

Joint — First Metacarpophalangeal Joint

Motion: Abduction-adduction of the thumb (Fig. 2-13)
Plane of Motion: This joint is an exception to the full circle or 360° system. Motion is in a plane parallel to the palm of the hand.
Positioning the Patient: The hand is in any restful position and the fingers are extended.

How to Measure: The goniometer is centered over the volar aspect of the first carpal-metacarpal joint. One arm of the goniometer is placed parallel to the longitudinal axis of the third metacarpal; the other arm is aligned with the longitudinal axis of the first metacarpal. Readings are made in maximum abduction and adduction of the thumb.

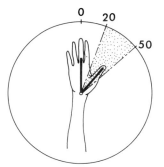

Figure 2–13   First metacarpophalangeal joint: abduction-adduction of the thumb.

Normal Limits and Range of Motion: 20° – 50°

Motion: Opposition of the thumb (Fig. 2-14)
Plane of Motion: This motion is an exception to the full circle or 360° system of measurement. The motion is made in a plane perpendicular to the plane of the palm.

Positioning the Patient: The hand is in any restful position with the fingers extended.

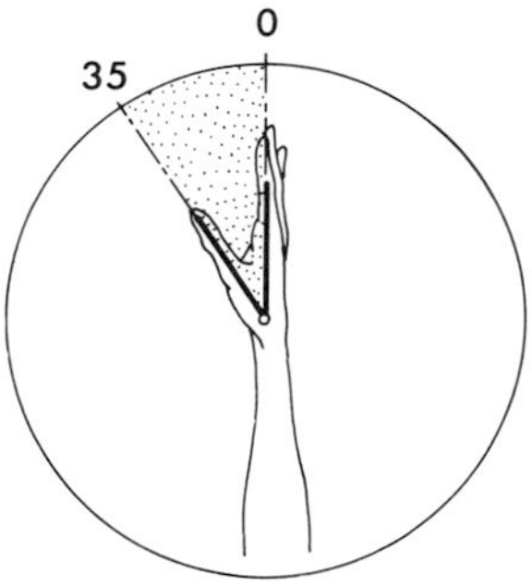

How to Measure: The goniometer is centered over the radial aspect of the first carpal-metacarpal joint. One arm of the goniometer is placed on the radial surface of the hand parallel to the longitudinal axis of the second metacarpal; the other arm is aligned parallel to the longitudinal axis of the first metacarpal. Measurements are made when the thumb is maximally approximated to and opposed from the palm.

Figure 2–14   First metacarpophalangeal joint: opposition of the thumb.

Normal Limits and Range of Motion: 0° – 35°

Joint – Hip

Motion: Flexion-extension (Fig. 2-15)
Plane of Motion: Sagittal
Positioning the Patient: The patient may be supine, lying on his side or standing.

How to Measure: Draw a line on the patient's skin from the anterior-superior iliac spine to the posterior-superior iliac spine. Drop a perpendicular from this line to a point on the skin overlying the anterior-superior aspect of the greater trochanter. One arm of the goniometer is placed on this line with the center of the goniometer placed over the anterior-superior aspect of the greater trochanter. The other arm is placed parallel to the longitudinal axis of the femur on the lateral surface of the thigh. Caution must be taken to assure that the marks drawn on the skin continue to overlie their bony landmarks as the hip is moved into positions of flexion and extension. If they do not, draw new ones.

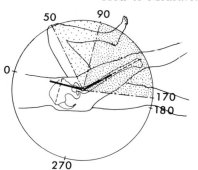

Figure 2–15   Hip: flexion-extension.

Normal Limits and Range of Motion:
  With the knee extended, 90° – 170°
  With the knee flexed, 50° – 170°

Motion: Abduction-adduction (Figs. 2-16, 2-17)
Plane of Motion: Frontal
Positioning the Patient: Patient supine or standing

How to Measure: Draw a line on the skin connecting the anterior-superior iliac spines (see Fig. 2-16). Place one arm of the goniometer on this line. Align the other arm so that it falls on a line parallel to and overlying the midline of the anterior thigh.

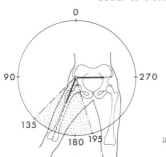

Figure   2–16 Hip: abduction-adduction (Method #1).

An alternate method (see Fig. 2-17) uses the same reference line between the anterior-superior iliac spines, but one arm of the goniometer is placed parallel to and below the reference line rather than on the line, and the goniometer is centered over the trochanter of the hip being measured. The other arm lies parallel to the long axis of the thigh.

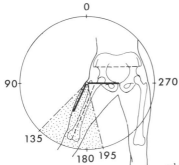

Figure   2–17 Hip: abduction-adduction (Method #2).

Normal Limits and Range of Motion: 135° – 195°

Motion: External and internal rotation (Figs. 2-18, 2-19)

Plane of Motion: This joint is an exception to the full circle or 360° system of measurement. Motion takes place on the horizontal or transverse plane and is measured as deviation in the direction of internal or external rotation from the neutral or anatomical position of the lower extremity.

Positioning the Patient: The patient is supine. To measure motion in the hip-flexed postion (see Fig. 2-18), the hip and knee are flexed to approximately 90° each. To measure motion in the hip-extended position (see Fig. 2-19), the thigh is flat on the table but the lower leg hangs over the end and the knee is flexed to 90°.

How to Measure: The goniometer is centered on the knee joint. Both arms of the goniometer are placed parallel to the longitudinal axis of the tibia on its anterior surface. One arm is moved to overlie the anterior surface of the tibia after it swings laterally or medially, while the other arm remains held in the position where the tibia had been prior to hip rotation.

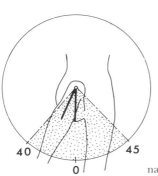

Figure   2–18 Hip: external-internal rotation in the hip (flexed position).

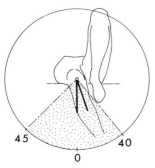

Figure 2–19 Hip: external-internal rotation in the hip (extended position).

Normal Limits and Range of Motion:
   External rotation (hip flexed, 40°)
   External rotation (hip extended, 45°)
   Internal rotation (hip flexed, 45°)
   Internal rotation (hip extended, 40°)

Joint — Knee

Motion: Flexion-extension (Fig. 2-20)
Plane of Motion: Sagittal
Positioning the Patient: The patient may be supine or sitting on the edge of a chair or table.

How to Measure:

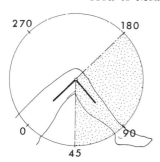

The goniometer is centered over the knee joint laterally; one arm is parallel to the longitudinal axis of the femur on the lateral surface of the thigh; the other arm is parallel to the longitudinal axis of the tibia on the lateral surface of the leg and pointing toward the ankle just anterior to the lateral malleolus.

Figure 2–20 Knee: flexion-extension.

Normal Limits and Range of Motion: 45° – 180°

Joint — Ankle

Motion: Dorsiflexion-plantar flexion (flexion-extension) (Fig. 2-21)
Plane of Motion: Sagittal
Positioning the Patient: The patient may be sitting or supine but the knee should be flexed to permit maximum dorsiflexion of the ankle.

How to Measure: One arm of the goniometer is placed on a line parallel to the longitudinal axis of the fibula on the lateral aspect of the leg. The goniometer is centered on the sole of the foot in line with the longitudinal axis of the fibula. The other arm of the goniometer is placed parallel to the longitudinal axis of the fifth metatarsal. Care should be taken to avoid forced dorsiflexion or plantar flexion of the forefoot.

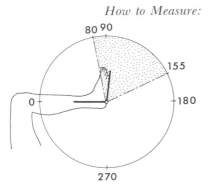

Figure 2–21   Ankle: dorsiflexion—plantar flexion.

Normal Limits and Range of Motion: 80°−155°

Motion: Inversion-eversion (Figs. 2-22, 2-23)
Plane of Motion: This motion is an exception to the full circle or 360° system of measurement. Movement takes place in the frontal plane.
Positioning the Patient: The patient may be sitting or supine. If patient is sitting, the knee should be flexed over the end of the table and the sole parallel to the floor. If patient is supine, the sole of the foot should be perpendicular to the longitudinal axis of the trunk (vertebral column).

How to Measure: The goniometer is set at 90°. This position is considered 0°. One arm is placed parallel to the longitudinal axis of the lower leg. The goniometer is held laterally to measure inversion (Fig. 2-22) and medially to measure eversion (Fig. 2-23). The other arm is held parallel to the plantar surface of the forefoot behind the head of the first metatarsal.

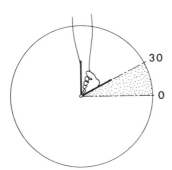

Figure 2–22   Ankle: inversion.

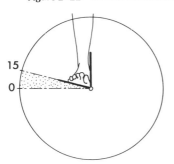

Figure 2–23   Ankle: eversion.

Normal Limits and Range of Motion: Movement is recorded as deviation from the 0° position at which the sole of the foot is either parallel to the

floor or perpendicular to the longitudinal axis of the trunk, depending upon whether the patient is sitting or supine.
Inversion, 30° (see Fig. 2–22)
Eversion, 15° (see Fig. 2–23)

Joint — Cervical Spine

The clinical measurement of motion in the cervical spine is probably the least accurate of all common measurements of the joints of the body because of the paucity of available landmarks and the depth of the soft tissues overlying the bony segments. Kottke and Mundale believe that measurement by x-ray of the specific joints involved, should be made.[11] However, approximations of cervical flexion, extension, internal and external rotation and right and left lateral bending can be made by using the universal goniometer. For more precise measurements, however, roentgenologic examination of the cervical spine will be necessary.

> *Motion:*   Flexion-extension (Figs. 2-24, 2-25)
> *Plane of Motion:*   Sagittal
> *Positioning the Patient:*   The patient should sit erect. (Measurements made in the supine position, with the weight of the head removed from its compressive position, show increased range of motion.) The head is vertical, the eyes forward in a "natural" position, and the shoulder girdle is relaxed. The patient holds the end of a tongue depressor blade firmly between his molars on the same side that the examiner is standing.

How to Measure:

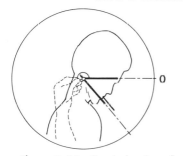

Figure 2–24 Cervical spine: flexion.

The examiner opens the goniometer about 60°. He grasps that corner of the protractor which is at the furthermost end of the goniometer arm. In order to steady the goniometer, the examiner braces his forearm against the patient's shoulder. The goniometer is centered over the angle of the jaw. The protractor arm should be parallel to the long axis of the protruding tongue depressor. The other arm is pointing in the direction of the motion to be measured. During flexion or extension, the pointer arm is adjusted to lie parallel to the new position of the tongue depressor.

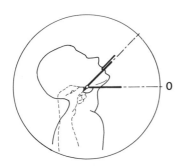

Figure 2–25 Cervical spine: extension.

Motion: Lateral bending (Fig. 2-26)
Plane of Motion: Frontal
Positioning the Patient: The position is the same as for neck flexion-extension except that a tongue depressor is not used.

How to Measure:

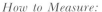
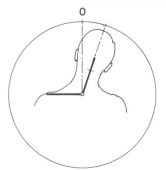

The goniometer is centered at the spinous process of the seventh cervical vetebra; one arm of the goniometer is held in a position parallel with the floor; the other, or moving arm, is aligned with the external occipital protuberance. As the neck flexes from right to left, the moveable arm records right and left lateral bending.

Figure 2–26   Cervical spine: lateral bending.

Motion: Rotation (Fig. 2-27)
Plane of Motion: This motion is an exception to the full circle or 360° measurement. The motion takes place in the transverse or horizontal plane and is recorded as deviation from the zero position, which is achieved when the head is vertical with the eyes forward in a "natural" position. Rotation is recorded as deviation from zero to the right or left.
Positioning the Patient: The position is the same as for neck bending, above.

How to Measure:

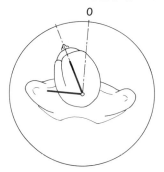

The examiner should stand on a low stool directly behind the patient. The goniometer is set at 90° and is centered over the vertex of the head. One arm of the goniometer is held steady in a line with the acromion process on the side being tested. The other, or moving arm, is in line with the tip of the nose. The moveable arm follows the tip of the nose as the head is rotated from side to side. Readings are taken at the points of maximum rotation.

Figure 2–27   Cervical spine: rotation.

REFERENCES

Goniometry

1. The Committee on Rating of Medical and of Physical Impairment: A Guide to the Evaluation of Permanent Impairment of the Extremities and Back. J.A.M.A. (Special Edition) (Feb. 15), 1958, pp. 1-112.
2. Moore, M. L., in Licht, S.: Therapeutic Exercise (Second Edition, Revised) Clinical Assessment of Joint Motion. Elizabeth Licht, publisher, 1965, p. 128.

3. Clayson, S. J., Mundale, M. O., and Kottke, F. J.: Goniometer Adaptation for Measuring Hip Extension. Arch. Phys. Med., *47:*255, 1966.
4. Defibaugh, J. J.: Measurement of Head Motion, Part I: A Review of Methods of Measuring Joint Motion. J. Amer. Phys. Ther. Assoc., *44:*157, 1964.
5. Defibaugh, J. J.: Measurement of Head Motion, Part II: An Experimental Study of Head Motion in Adult Males. J. Amer. Phys. Ther. Assoc., *44:*163, 1964.
6. Leighton, J. R.: An Instrument and Technic for the Measurement of Range of Joint Motion. Arch. Phys. Med., *36:*571, 1955.
7. Moore, M. L.: The Measurement of Joint Motion, Part I: Introductory Review of the Literature. Phys. Ther. Rev., *29:*195, 1949.
8. Moore, M. L.: The Measurement of Joint Motion, Part II: The Technic of Goniometry. Phys. Ther. Rev., *29:*256, 1949.
9. Knapp, M. E.: Measurement of Joint Motion. Univ. Minn. Med. Bull., *15:*405-412, 1944.
10. Knapp, M. E.: Measuring Range of Motion. Postgrad. Med., *42:*123, 1967.
11. Hellebrandt, F. A., Duvall, E. N., and Moore, M. L.: The Measurement of Joint Motion, Part III: Reliability of Goniometry. Phys. Ther. Rev., *29:*302, 1949.
12. Kottke, F. J., and Mundale, M. O.: Range of Mobility of the Cervical Spine. Arch. Phys. Med., *40:*379, 1959.

MUSCLE TESTING

Manual muscle testing permits one to evaluate the strength of a movement. The strength of an individual muscle cannot be routinely isolated and tested unless it is solely responsible for moving the body part in the performance of a particular movement. For example, the gastrocnemius and soleus are the plantar flexors of the ankle. Since the heads of the gastrocnemius attach to the condyles of the femur, it is possible to reduce the role of that muscle markedly by testing plantar flexion with the knee flexed. In this way the strength of the soleus can be tested. However, the gastrocnemius still makes some contribution in this posture.

It is important that substitution be avoided in evaluating the strength of a muscle responsible for a movement. Thus, in the presence of a paretic muscle or group of muscles, a movement may be performed by a muscle that ordinarily does not serve in that role. For example, the hamstrings flex the knee. In full extension, as in standing, the hamstrings may permit the knee to be fully extended even though the quadriceps—the prime extensor of the knee—is paralyzed.

Manual muscle testing is of value in the peripheral neuropathies and may be helpful in differentiating injury of the peripheral nerves from radicular damage. The peripheral and radicular innervations of skeletal muscles and their actions and tests are shown in Table 2–2 and Figures 2–28 to 2–55 and the following outline which are from the Mayo Clinic's *Clinical Examinations in Neurology.*

Outline of Anatomic Information Required for Tests of Strength of Specific Muscles.   In the following descriptions of the tests, the name of each muscle is followed in parentheses by the peripheral nerve and spinal segmental supply. There is considerable variability in segmental supply, particularly to certain muscles, as given by different authorities. Furthermore, there is some anatomic variation both in the plexuses and in the peripheral nerves. The segments listed cannot, therefore, be regarded as absolute. The principal and usual supply is underlined. Under Action are listed only the principal and important secondary or accessory functions—those particularly useful in testing and those which may cause confusion by substituting for the activity of other muscles. In the description of the test itself the position and movement given first refer to the patient unless otherwise clearly stated. In some instances the movement is adequately indicated by the action of the muscle and, hence, is omitted here. The term "resistance," unless otherwise specifically stated, refers to the pressure applied by the examiner, and this is in the direction opposite to that of the movement. For brevity and uniformity in description of the tests, the method of testing in which the patient initiates action against the resistance of the examiner is given except where the other method is distinctly more applicable. However, *this concession to uniformity and brevity of description is not meant to imply a preference for the method of testing in which the patient initiates action.* The location of the belly of the muscle and its tendon is often given in order to stress the importance of observation and palpation in identifying function of that particular muscle. As participating muscles, only those are listed which have a definite action in the movement being tested and which may substitute at least in part for the muscle being discussed.

Trapezius (Figs. 2–28 and 2–29).   (Spinal accessory N.)

ACTION: Elevation, retraction (adduction) and rotation (lateral angle upward) of scapula, providing fixation of scapula during many movements of arm.

TEST: Elevation (shrugging) of shoulder against resistance tests upper portion, which is readily visible.

Bracing shoulder (backward movement and adduction of scapula) tests chiefly middle portion.

Abduction of arm against resistance intensifies winging of scapula.

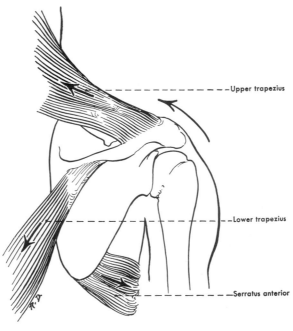

Figure 2–28   Upward rotators of the scapula. (Redrawn from Hollinshead, W. H.: Functional Anatomy of the Limbs and Back.)

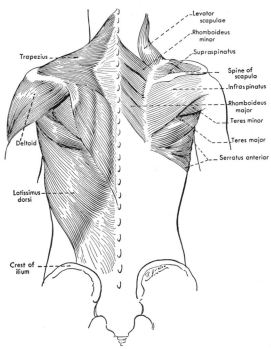

Figure 2–29   Musculature of the shoulder from behind. (From Hollinshead, W. H.: Functional Anatomy of the Limbs and Back.)

Participating Muscles:
   Elevation—Levator scapulae (Cervical N's. 3 and 4 and Dorsal scapular N., C 3 4 5).
   Retraction—Rhomboids.
   Upward rotation—Serratus anterior.
   In isolated trapezius palsy with the shoulder girdle at rest, the scapula is displaced downward and laterally and is rotated so that the superior angle is farther from the spine than the inferior angle. The lateral displacement is due in part to the unopposed action of the serratus anterior. The vertebral border, particularly at the inferior angle, is flared. These changes are accentuated when the arm is abducted from the side against resistance. On flexion (forward elevation) of the arm, however, the flaring of the inferior angle virtually disappears. These features are important in distinguishing trapezius palsy from serratus anterior palsy, which produces an equally characteristic winging of the scapula but in which movement of the arm in these two planes has the opposite effect. Atrophy of the trapezius is evident chiefly in the upper portion.

Rhomboids (Fig. 2–29).   (Dorsal scapular N. from anterior ramus C 5)
   ACTION: Retraction (adduction) of scapula and elevation of its vertebral border.
   TEST: Hand on hip, arm held backward and medially. Examiner attempts to force elbow laterally and forward, observing and palpating muscle bellies medial to scapula.

TABLE 2–2 NEUROLOGIC MUSCLE CHART

Fascicul.	Tone	Size	Strength	R　　　MUSCLES　　　L	Strength	Size	Tone	Fascicul.
				CRANIAL NERVES				
				Temporal　　　　Cr.N. V				
				Masseter　　　　V				
				Pterygoid　　　　V				
				Forehead　　　　VII				
				Orbicularis oc.　　VII				
				Mouth　　　　VII				
				Platysma　　　VII				
				Soft palate　　　X				
				Pharynx　　　　X				
				Sternomastoid　　XI				
				Trapezius　　　XI				
				Tongue　　　　XII				
				Neck, flex.　　　C 1-6				
				Neck, ext.　　　C 1-T1				
				Diaphragm　　C 345				
				Levator scapulae　C 345				
				Rhomboids　　　45				
				Serratus anterior　567				
				Supraspinatus　　456				
				Infraspinatus　　456				
				Pect. maj. (clav.)　567				
				Pect. maj. (stern.)　678 T1				
				Subscapularis　　567				
				Latissimus dorsi　678				
				Teres major　　567				
				Deltoid　　　56				
				Biceps, Brachialis　56				
				RADIAL N.				
				Triceps　　　C 678				
				Brachioradialis　　56				
				Ext. carpi rad. lg.　678				
				Ext. carpi rad. br.　678				
				Supinator　　　567				
				Ext. digitorum　　678				
				Ext. digiti quinti　78				
				Ext. carpi ulnaris　78				
				Abd. pollicis lg.　78				
				Ext. pollicis lg.　78				
				Ext. pollicis br.　78				
				Ext. indicis　　78				

TABLE 2–2 NEUROLOGIC MUSCLE CHART (CONTINUED)

Fascicul.	Tone	Size	Strength	R MUSCLES L	Strength	Size	Tone	Fascicul.
				MEDIAN N.				
				Pronator teres C 67				
				Flex. carpi rad. 67				
				Palmaris longus 7<u>8</u> T1				
				Flex. dig. sublimis 7<u>8</u> 1				
				Flex. dig. prof. II, III 7<u>8</u> 1				
				Flex. pollicis lg. 7<u>8</u> 1				
				Pronator quadratus 7<u>8</u> 1				
				Abd. pollicis br. <u>8</u> 1				
				Opponens pollicis <u>8</u> 1				
				Flex. poll. br. (sup.) <u>8</u> 1				
				ULNAR N.				
				Flex. carpi ulnaris C 7<u>8</u> T1				
				Flex. dig. prof. IV, V 7<u>8</u> 1				
				Hypothenar 8 1				
				Interossei 8 1				
				Flex. poll. br. (deep) 8 1				
				Adductor pollicis 8 1				
				Back				
				Abdomen (upper) T 6-9				
				Abdomen (lower) 10-L1				
				Iliopsoas L 1<u>234</u>				
				Adductors, thigh <u>234</u>				
				Abductors, thi. (Glut. med.) <u>45</u> S<u>1</u>				
				Med. rot., thigh <u>45</u> **1**				
				Lat. rot., thigh <u>45</u> **<u>12</u>**				
				Gluteus maximus 5 **<u>12</u>**				
				Quadriceps 2<u>34</u>				
				Hamstrings, int. <u>45</u> **<u>12</u>**				
				Biceps fem. (ext. hamstr.) 5 **<u>12</u>**				
				PERONEAL N.				
				Tibialis ant. <u>45</u> **1**				
				Ext. digitorum lg. <u>45</u> **1**				
				Ext. hallucis lg. <u>45</u> **1**				
				Peronei <u>45</u> **1**				
				Ext. digitorum br. <u>45</u> **1**				
				TIBIAL N.				
				Gastroc., Soleus 5 **<u>12</u>**				
				Tibialis post. <u>5</u> **1**				
				Toes, flexors <u>5</u> **<u>12</u>**				
				Foot, intrinsic 5 **<u>12</u>**				

Participating Muscles: Trapezius; levator scapulae—elevation of medial border of scapula.

Serratus Anterior (Fig. 2–28).   (Long thoracic N. from anterior rami C 5 6 7)

ACTION: Protraction (lateral and forward movement) of scapula, keeping it closely applied to thorax.

Assistance in upward rotation of scapula.

TEST: Forward thrust of outstretched arm against wall or against resistance by examiner.

Isolated palsy results in comparatively little change in the appearance of the shoulder girdle at rest. There is, however, slight winging of the inferior angle of the scapula and slight shift medially toward the spine. When the outstretched arm is thrust forward, the entire scapula, particularly its inferior angle, shifts backward away from the thorax, producing the characteristic wing effect. Abduction of the arm laterally, however, produces comparatively little winging, demonstrating again an important difference from the manifestations of paralysis of the trapezius.

Supraspinatus (Fig. 2–30).   (Suprascapular N. from upper trunk of brachial plexus, C 4 5 6)

ACTION: Initiation of abduction of arm from side of body.

TEST: Above action against resistance.

Atrophy may be detected just above the spine of the scapula, but the trapezius overlies the supraspinatus and atrophy of either muscle will produce a depression in this area. Scapular fixation is important in this test.

Participating Muscle: Deltoid.

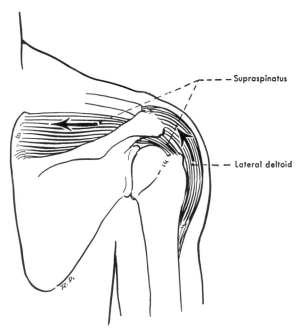

Figure 2–30   Abductors of the humerus. (From Hollinshead, W. H.: Functional Anatomy of the Limbs and Back.)

Infraspinatus (Fig. 2–31). (Suprascapular N. from upper trunk of brachial plexus, C 4 5 6)

ACTION: Lateral (external) rotation of arm at shoulder.

TEST: Elbow at side and flexed 90°. Patient resists examiner's attempt to push the hand medially toward the abdomen.

The muscle is palpable and atrophy may be visible below the spine of the scapula.

Participating Muscles: Teres minor (axillary N.); deltoid — posterior fibers.

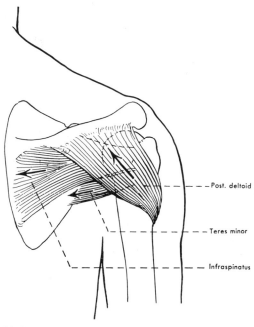

Figure 2–31 The chief external rotators of the humerus. (Redrawn from Hollinshead, W. H.: Functional Anatomy of the Limbs and Back.)

Pectoralis Major (Fig. 2–32). Clavicular portion (Lateral pectoral N. from lateral cord of plexus, C 5 6 7)

Sternal portion (Medial pectoral N. from medial cord of plexus, Lateral pectoral N. C 6 7 8 T 1)

ACTION: Adduction and medial rotation of arm.

Clavicular portion — assistance in flexion of arm.

TEST: Arm in front of body. Patient resists attempt by examiner to force it laterally.

The two portions of the muscle are visible and palpable.

Latissimus Dorsi (Fig. 2–33). (Thoracodorsal N. from posterior cord of plexus, C 6 7 8)

ACTION: Adduction, extension and medial rotation of arm.

TEST: Arm in abduction to horizontal position. Downward and backward movement against resistance applied under elbow.

The muscle should be observed and palpated in and below the

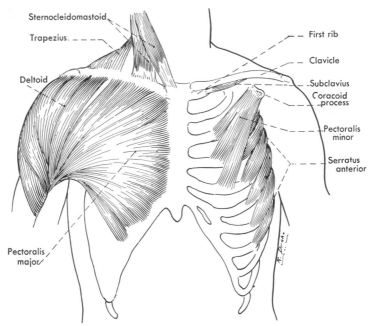

Figure 2–32   Muscles of the pectoral region. (Redrawn from Hollinshead, W. H.: Functional Anatomy of the Limbs and Back.)

posterior axillary fold. When the patient coughs, a brisk contraction of the normal latissimus dorsi can be felt at the inferior angle of the scapula.

Teres Major (Fig. 2–33a).   (Lower subscapular N. from posterior cord plexus, C 5 6 7)
ACTION and TEST are the same as for latissimus dorsi.
The muscle is visible and palpable at the lower lateral border of the scapula.

Deltoid (Figs. 2–32 and 2–33b).   (Axillary N. from posterior cord of plexus, C 5 6)

ACTION: Abduction of arm.
Flexion (forward movement) and medial rotation of arm — anterior fibers.
Extension (backward movement) and lateral rotation of arm — posterior fibers.

TEST: Arm in abduction almost to horizontal. Patient resists effort of examiner to depress elbow.
Paralysis of the deltoid leads to conspicuous atrophy and serious disability, since the other muscles which participate in abduction of the arm (the supraspinatus, trapezius and serratus anterior — the last two by rotating the scapula) cannot compensate for lack of function of the deltoid.
Flexion and extension of the arm against resistance.
Participating Muscles:
Abduction — given above.
Flexion — Pectoralis major — clavicular portion; biceps.
Extension — Latissimus dorsi; teres major.

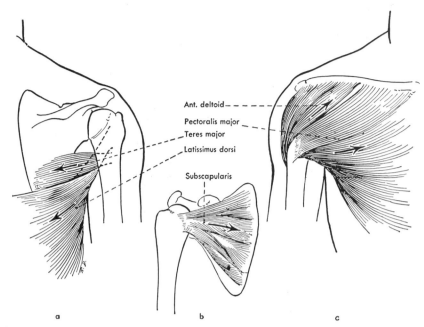

Figure 2–33   The chief internal rotators of the humerus. a. Posterior view. b and c. Anterior views. (From Hollinshead, W. H.: Functional Anatomy of the Limbs and Back.)

Subscapularis (Fig. 2–33b).   (Upper and lower subscapular N's. from posterior cord of plexus, C 5 6 7)

ACTION: Medial (internal) rotation of arm at shoulder.

TEST: Elbow at side and flexed 90°. Patient resists examiner's attempt to pull the hand laterally.

Since this muscle is not accessible to observation or palpation, it is necessary to gauge the activity of other muscles which produce this movement. The pectoralis major is the most powerful medial rotator of the arm; hence, paralysis of the subscapularis alone results in relatively little weakness of this movement.

Participating Muscles: Pectoralis major; deltoid—anterior fibers; teres major; latissimus dorsi.

Biceps; Brachialis (Fig. 2–34).   (Musculocutaneous N. from lateral cord of plexus, C 5 6)

ACTION: Biceps—Flexion and supination of forearm.
           Assistance in flexion of arm at shoulder.
           Brachialis—Flexion of forearm at elbow.

TEST: Flexion of forearm against resistance. Forearm should be in supination to decrease participation of brachioradialis.

Triceps (Fig. 2–35).   (Radial N., which is continuation of posterior cord of plexus, C 6 7 8)

ACTION: Extension of forearm at elbow.

TEST: Forearm in flexion to varying degree. Patient resists effort of examiner to flex forearm further. Slight weakness more easily detected when starting with forearm almost completely flexed.

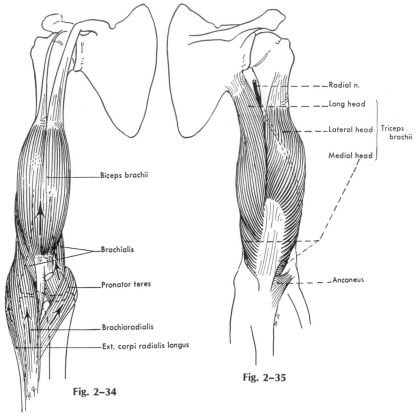

Figure 2–34   The flexors of the elbow. (From Hollinshead, W. H.: Functional Anatomy of the Limbs and Back.)

Figure 2–35   Muscles of the extensor (posterior) surface of the right arm. (From Hollinshead, W. H.: Functional Anatomy of the Limbs and Back.)

Brachioradialis (Fig. 2–36).   (Radial N., C 5 6)

ACTION: Flexion of forearm at elbow.

TEST: Flexion of forearm against resistance with forearm midway between pronation and supination.

The belly of the muscle stands out prominently on the upper surface of the forearm, tending to bridge the angle between the forearm and arm.

Participating Muscles: Biceps; brachialis.

Supinator (Fig. 2–36).   (Posterior interosseous N. from radial N., C 5 6 7)

ACTION: Supination of forearm.

TEST: Forearm in full extension and supination. Patient attempts to maintain supination while examiner attempts to pronate forearm and palpates biceps.

Resistance to pronation by the intact supinator can usually be felt before there is appreciable contraction of the biceps.

Extensor Carpi Radialis Longus (Fig. 2–37).   (Radial N., C 6 7 8)

ACTION: Extension (dorsiflexion) and radial abduction of hand at wrist.

TEST: Forearm in almost complete pronation. Dorsiflexion of wrist against resistance applied to dorsum of hand downward and toward ulnar side.

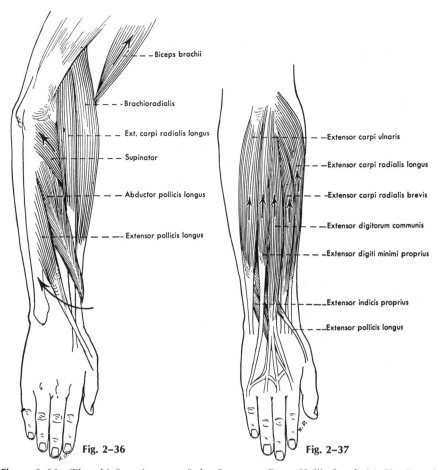

Figure 2–36   The chief supinators of the forearm. (From Hollinshead, W. H.: Functional Anatomy of the Limbs and Back.)

Figure 2–37   The chief extensors of the wrist. (From Hollinshead, W. H.: Functional Anatomy of the Limbs and Back.)

The tendon is palpable just above its insertion into the base of the second metacarpal bone. The fingers and thumb should be relaxed and somewhat flexed to minimize participation of the extensors of the digits.

Extensor Carpi Radialis Brevis (Fig. 2–37).   Posterior interosseous N. from Radial N., C 6 7 8)

ACTION: Extension (dorsiflexion) of hand at wrist.

TEST: Forearm in complete pronation. Dorsiflexion of wrist against resistance applied to dorsum of hand straight downward.

The tendon is palpable just proximal to the base of the third metacarpal bone. The fingers and thumb should be relaxed and somewhat flexed to minimize participation of the extensors of the digits.

Extensor Carpi Ulnaris (Fig. 2–37).   (Posterior interosseous N., from radial N., C 7 8)

ACTION: Extension (dorsiflexion) and ulnar deviation of hand at wrist.

TEST: Forearm in pronation. Dorsiflexion and ulnar deviation of wrist against resistance applied to dorsum of hand downward and toward radial side.

The tendon is palpable just below or above the distal end of the ulna. The fingers should be relaxed and somewhat flexed in order to minimize participation of the extensors of the digits.

Extensor Digitorum (Fig. 2–37). (Posterior interosseous N. from radial N., C 6 7 8)

ACTION: Extension of fingers, principally at metacarpophalangeal joints.
Assistance in extension (dorsiflexion) of wrist.

TEST: Forearm in pronation. Wrist stabilized in straight position. Extension of fingers at metacarpophalangeal joints against resistance applied to proximal phalanges.

The distal portions of the fingers may be somewhat relaxed and in slight flexion. The tendons are visible and palpable over the dorsum of the hand.

Extension at the interphalangeal joints is a function primarily of the interossei (ulnar nerve) and lumbricals (median and ulnar nerves).

The extensor digiti quinti and extensor indicis (posterior interosseous nerve, C 7 8), proper extensors of the little and index fingers respectively, can be tested individually while the other fingers are in flexion to minimize the action of the common extensor. In a thin person's hand the tendons can usually be identified.

Abductor Pollicis Longus (Fig. 2–36). (Posterior interosseous N. from radial N., C 7 8)

ACTION: Radial abduction of thumb (in same plane as that of palm, in contradistinction to palmar abduction, which is movement perpendicular to plane of palm).
Assistance in radial abduction and flexion of hand at wrist.

TEST: Hand on edge (forearm midway between pronation and supination).
Radial abduction of thumb against resistance applied to metacarpal.

The tendon is palpable just above its insertion into the base of the metacarpal bone and forms the anterior (volar) boundary of the "anatomic snuffbox."
Participating Muscle: Extensor pollicis brevis.

Extensor Pollicis Brevis. (Posterior interosseous N. from radial N., C 7 8)

ACTION: Extension of proximal phalanx of thumb.
Assistance in radial abduction and extension of metacarpal of thumb.

TEST: Hand on edge. Wrist and particularly metacarpal of thumb stabilized by examiner. Extension of proximal phalanx against resistance applied to that phalanx, while distal phalanx is in flexion to minimize action of extensor pollicis longus.

At the wrist the tendon lies just posterior (dorsal) to the tendon of the abductor pollicis longus.
Participating Muscle: Extensor pollicis longus.

Extensor Pollicis Longus (Fig. 2–37).   (Posterior interosseous N. from radial
     N., C 7 8)
ACTION: Extension of all parts of thumb but specifically extension of
            distal phalanx.
            Assistance in adduction of thumb.
  TEST: Hand on edge. Wrist, metacarpal and proximal phalanx of
            thumb stabilized by examiner with thumb close to palm at
            its radial border. Extension of distal phalanx against re-
            sistance.
            If the patient is permitted to flex his wrist or abduct his thumb
          away from the palm, some extension of the phalanges results
          simply from lengthening the path of the extensor tendon. At
          the wrist the tendon forms the posterior (dorsal) boundary of
          the "anatomic snuffbox."
The characteristic result of radial nerve palsy is wristdrop. Extension of
the fingers at the interphalangeal joints is still possible by virtue of the action
of the interossei and lumbricals but extension of the thumb is lost.

*   *   *   *   *

The next group of muscles examined is that supplied by the median nerve,
which is formed by the union of its lateral root, from the lateral cord of the
brachial plexus, and its medial root, from the medial cord of the plexus. Then
the muscles supplied by the ulnar nerve (arising from the medial cord of the
brachial plexus) are tested. However, for convenience in order of examination
some of the muscles in the ulnar group are tested with the median group.

Pronator Teres (Fig. 2–38).   (Median N., C 6 7)
  ACTION: Pronation of forearm.
   TEST: Elbow at side of trunk, forearm in flexion to right angle, and
            arm in lateral rotation at shoulder to eliminate effect of
            gravity which, in most positions, favors pronation. Pronation
            of forearm against resistance, starting from a position of
            moderate supination.
            Participating Muscle: Pronator quadratus (Anterior interosseous
            branch of median N., C 7 8 T 1)

Flexor Carpi Radialis (Figs. 2–38 and 2–39).   (Median N., C 6 7)
  ACTION: Flexion (palmar flexion of hand at wrist.
            Assistance in radial abduction of hand.
   TEST: Flexion of hand against resistance applied to palm. Fingers
            should be relaxed to minimize participation of their flexors.
            The tendon is the more lateral (radial) one of the two con-
          spicuous tendons on the volar aspect of the wrist.
            In complete median nerve palsy, flexion of the wrist is con-
          siderably weakened but can still be performed by the flexor
          carpi ulnaris (ulnar nerve) assisted to some extent by the abductor
          pollicis longus (radial nerve). In this event, ulnar deviation of the
          hand usually accompanies flexion.

Palmaris Longus (Figs. 2–38 and 2–39).   (Median N., C 7 8 T 1)
  ACTION: Flexion of hand at wrist.

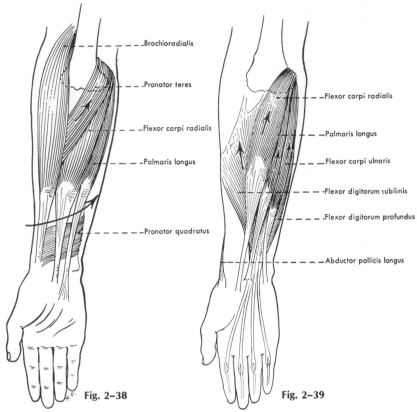

Figure 2–38   Pronators of the forearm. (From Hollinshead, W. H.: Functional Anatomy of the Limbs and Back.)

Figure 2–39   The chief flexors of the wrist. (From Hollinshead, W. H.: Functional Anatomy of the Limbs and Back.)

TEST: Same as for flexor carpi radialis.
The tendon is palpable at the ulnar side of the tendon of the flexor carpi radialis.

Flexor Carpi Ulnaris (Fig. 2–39).   (Ulnar N., C 7 8 T 1)
ACTION: Flexion and ulnar deviation of hand at wrist.
Fixation of pisiform bone during contraction of abductor digiti quinti.
TEST: Flexion and ulnar deviation of hand against resistance applied to ulnar side of palm in direction of extension and radial abduction. Fingers should be relaxed.
The tendon is palpable proximal to the pisiform bone.

Flexor Digitorum Sublimis (Fig. 2–39).   (Median N., C 7 8 T 1)
ACTION: Flexion of middle phalanges of fingers at first interphalangeal joints primarily; flexion of proximal phalanges at metacarpophalangeal joints secondarily.
Assistance in flexion of hand at wrist.
TEST: Wrist in neutral position, proximal phalanges stabilized. Flexion of middle phalanx of each finger against resistance applied to that phalanx, with distal phalanx relaxed.

Flexor Digitorum Profundus (Fig. 2–39).

    Radial portion — usually to digits II and III (Median N. and its anterior interosseous branch, C 7 8 T 1)

    Ulnar portion — usually to digits IV and V (Ulnar N., C 7 8 T 1)

ACTION: Flexion of distal phalanges of fingers specifically; flexion of other phalanges secondarily.

    Assistance in flexion of hand at wrist.

TEST: Flexion of distal phalanges against resistance with proximal and middle phalanges stabilized in extension.

    With middle and distal phalanges folded over edge of examiner's hand, patient resists attempt by examiner to extend distal phalanges.

Flexor Pollicis Longus (Fig. 2–40). (Anterior interosseous branch of median N., C 7 8 T 1)

ACTION: Flexion of thumb, particularly distal phalanx.

    Assistance in ulnar adduction of thumb.

TEST: Flexion of distal phalanx against resistance with thumb in position of palmar adduction and with stabilization of metacarpal and proximal phalanx.

Abductor Pollicis Brevis (Fig. 2–40). (Median N., C 8 T 1)

ACTION: Palmar abduction of thumb (perpendicular to plane of palm).

    Assistance in opposition and in flexion of proximal phalanx of thumb.

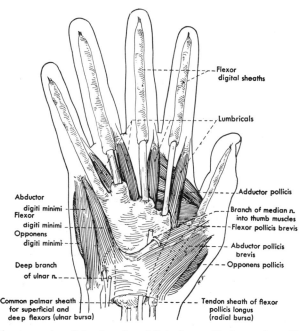

Figure 2–40 Short muscles of the thumb and little finger. (Redrawn from Hollinshead, W. H.: Functional Anatomy of the Limbs and Back.)

TEST: Palmar abduction of thumb against resistance applied at metacarpophalangeal joint.

The muscle is readily visible and palpable in the thenar eminence.

Participating Muscle: Flexor pollicis brevis (superficial head).

Opponens Pollicis (Fig. 2–40).   (Median N., C 8 T 1)

ACTION: Movement of first metacarpal across palm, rotating it into opposition.

TEST: Thumb in opposition. Examiner attempts to rotate and draw thumb back to its usual position.

Participating Muscles: Abductor pollicis brevis; flexor pollicis brevis.

Flexor Pollicis Brevis (Fig. 2–40).   Superficial head (Median N., C 8 T 1)

Deep head (Ulnar N., C 8 T 1)

ACTION: Flexion of proximal phalanx of thumb.

Assistance in opposition, ulnar adduction (entire muscle) and palmar abduction (superficial head) of thumb.

TEST: Thumb in position of palmar adduction with stabilization of metacarpal. Flexion of proximal phalanx against resistance applied to that phalanx while distal phalanx is as relaxed as possible.

Participating Muscles: Flexor pollicis longus; abductor pollicis brevis; adductor pollicis.

Severe median nerve palsy produces the "simian" hand, wherein the thumb tends to lie in the same plane as the palm with the volar surface facing more anteriorly than normal. Atrophy of the muscles of the thenar eminence is usually conspicuous.

Three muscles supplied, at least in part, by the ulnar nerve have already been described: flexor carpi ulnaris; flexor digitorum profundus; flexor pollicis brevis. The remaining muscles supplied by this nerve follow.

Hypothenar Muscles.   (Ulnar N., C 8 T 1)

ACTION: Abductor digiti quinti and

Flexor digiti quinti – abduction and flexion (proximal phalanx) of little finger.

Opponens digiti quinti – opposition of little finger toward thumb.

All three muscles – palmar elevation of head of fifth metacarpal, helping to cup palm.

TEST: Action usually tested is abduction of little finger (against resistance).

The abductor digiti quinti is readily observed and palpated at the ulnar border of the palm. Opposition of the thumb and little finger can be tested together by gauging the force required to separate the tips of the two digits when opposed, or by attempting to withdraw a piece of paper clasped between the tips of the digits.

Interossei (Figs. 2–41 and 2–42).   (Ulnar N., C 8 T 1)

ACTION: Dorsal – abduction of index, middle and ring fingers from middle line of middle finger (double action on middle

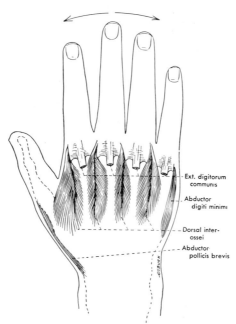

Figure 2–41   Dorsal view of the chief abductors of the digits. (Redrawn from Hollinshead, W. H.: Functional Anatomy of the Limbs and Back.)

finger—both radial and ulnar abduction, radial abduction of index finger, ulnar abduction of ring finger).

First dorsal—adduction (especially palmar adduction) of thumb.

Palmar—adduction of index, ring and little fingers toward middle finger.

Both sets—flexion of metacarpophalangeal joints and simultaneous extension of interphalangeal joints.

TEST: Abduction and adduction of individual fingers against resistance with fingers extended. Adduction can be tested by retention of a slip of paper between fingers, and between thumb and index finger, as examiner attempts to withdraw it.

Ability of patient to flex proximal phalanges and simultaneously extend distal phalanges.

Extension of middle phalanges of fingers against resistance while examiner stabilizes proximal phalanges in hyperextension.

The long extensors of the fingers (radial nerve) and the lumbrical muscles (median and ulnar nerves) assist in extension of the middle and distal phalanges. The first dorsal interosseous is readily observed and palpated in the space between the index finger and the thumb.

Adductor Pollicis.   (Ulnar N., C 8 T 1)

ACTION: Adduction of thumb in both ulnar and palmar directions (in plane of palm and perpendicular to palm respectively).

Assistance in flexion of proximal phalanx.

TEST: Adduction in each plane against resistance.

Retention of slip of paper between thumb and radial border of

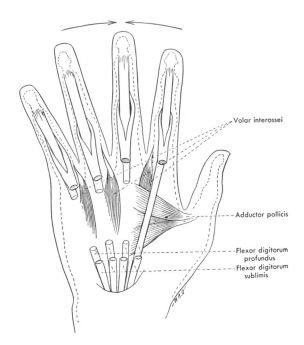

Figure 2–42   The chief adductors of the digits. (From Hollinshead, W. H.: Functional Anatomy of the Limbs and Back.)

hand and between thumb and palm, without flexion of distal phalanx.

It is often possible to palpate the edge of the adductor pollicis just volar to the proximal part of the first dorsal interosseous.

Participating Muscles: Ulnar adduction — First dorsal interosseous; flexor pollicis longus; extensor pollicis longus; flexor pollicis brevis.

Palmar adduction — First dorsal interosseous particularly; extensor pollicis longus.

In severe ulnar nerve palsy, atrophy is evident between the thumb and index finger, between the extensor tendons on the dorsum of the hand and in the hypothenar eminence. The little finger is separated from the ring finger and cannot be brought into contact with it. The little and ring fingers especially are hyperextended at the metacarpophalangeal joints and flexed at the interphalangeal joints. The index and middle fingers are much less affected because of the intact lumbricals of these fingers (supplied by the median nerve). The true "clawhand" (main en griffe) is found only in combined median and ulnar nerve palsy. Attempt at adduction of the thumb is usually accompanied by flexion of the distal phalanx, indicating activity of the flexor pollicis longus (median nerve) in an effort to compensate for paralysis of the adductor. Froment's sign of ulnar palsy is an application of this phenomenon (Fig. 2–43). The patient grasps a piece of cardboard firmly with the thumb and index finger of each hand and pulls vigorously. If flexion of the distal phalanx of the thumb occurs, the test is positive and indicative of ulnar palsy.

Localization of lesions of the brachial plexus (Fig. 2–44) is based on the pattern of muscular weakness (and the distribution of sensory impairment).

Damage to the most proximal elements of the plexus (anterior primary rami) is manifested by weakness or paralysis of one or more of the muscles

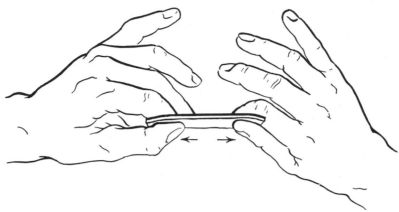

Figure 2–43 Froment's sign of ulnar palsy. Positive in the left hand, as indicated by flexion of the terminal phalanx of the thumb. (From Mayo Clinic: Clinical Examinations in Neurology.)

deriving nerve supply from the rami, such as the rhomboids and the serratus anterior, as well as by segmental distribution of muscular weakness (and sensory deficit) in the more distal portions of the upper extremity. Injury to the anterior ramus T 1 produces Horner's syndrome.

Lesions involving the most distal parts of the plexus spare some of the muscles of the shoulder girdle, and the pattern of muscular weakness (and sensory impairment) is more like that due to peripheral nerve injuries.

Lesions affecting the upper portion of the plexus, such as the upper trunk, impair the function of muscles supplied by segments C 5 and 6 (syndrome of Duchenne-Erb) such as the supraspinatus, infraspinatus, deltoid, biceps, brachialis, brachioradialis and supinator. The arm tends to hang limply at the side, medially rotated and pronated.

Injuries of the lower elements of the plexus, such as the lower trunk, C 8 and T 1 (syndrome of Klumpke), produce disability chiefly of the intrinsic muscles of the hand and flexors of the digits.

These examples illustrate the general principles of localization of lesions on the basis of examination of muscular strength.

*   *   *   *   *

The muscles of the neck and trunk may be examined in groups in most instances.

Flexors of Neck.   (Cervical N's., C 1–6)
TEST: Sitting or supine. Flexion of neck, with chin on chest, against resistance applied to forehead.

Extensors of Neck.   (Cervical N's., C 1–T 1)
TEST: Sitting or prone. Extension of neck against resistance applied to occiput.

Diaphragm.   (Phrenic N's., C 3 4 5)
ACTION: Abdominal respiration (inspiration), as distinguished from thoracic respiration (inspiration) which is produced principally by the intercostal muscles.

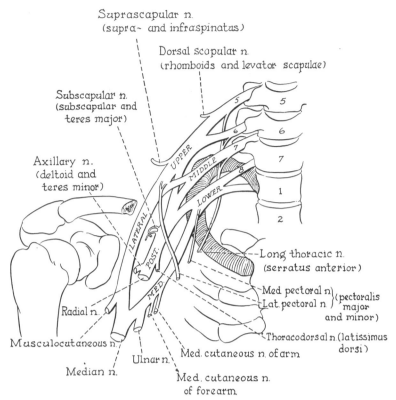

Figure 2–44 The brachial plexus. The muscles supplied by the various nerves are in parentheses. (From Mayo Clinic: Clinical Examinations in Neurology.)

TEST: Observation of patient for protrusion of upper portion of abdomen during deep inspiration when thoracic cage is splinted.

Ability of patient to sniff.

Litten's sign—successive retraction of lower intercostal spaces during inspiration.

Fluoroscopic observation of diaphragmatic movements.

Weakness of the diaphragm should be suspected in diseases of the spinal cord, when the deltoid or biceps is paralyzed, for these muscles are supplied by neurons situated very near those innervating the diaphragm.

Intercostal Muscles. (Intercostal N's., T 1–11)

ACTION: Expansion of thorax anteroposteriorly and transversely, producing thoracic inspiration.

TEST: Observation and palpation of expansion of thoracic cage during deep inspiration while maintaining pressure against thorax.

Observation for asymmetry of movement of thorax, particularly during deep inspiration.

Other more general tests of function of the respiratory muscles are:

Observation of patient for rapid shallow respiration, flaring of alae nasi, and use of accessory muscles of respiration.

Ability of patient to repeat three or four numbers without pausing for breath.

Ability of patient to hold his breath for 15 seconds.

Anterior Abdominal Muscles.   Upper (T 6–9), Lower (T10–L 1)

TEST: Supine – Flexion of neck against resistance applied to fore-head by examiner.

Contraction of the abdominal muscles can be observed and palpated. Upward movement of the umbilicus is associated with weakness of the lower abdominal muscles (Beevor's sign).

Supine – Hands on occiput. Flexion of trunk by anterior abdominal muscles followed by flexion of pelvis on thighs by hip flexors (chiefly iliopsoas) to reach sitting position. Examiner holds legs down.

Completion of this test excludes significant weakness of either the abdominal muscles or the flexors of the hips. Weak abdominal muscles, in the presence of strong hip flexors, result in hyper-extension of the lumbar spine during attempts to elevate the legs or rise to a sitting position.

Extensors of Back.

TEST: Prone with hands clasped over buttocks. Elevation of head and shoulders off table while examiner holds legs down.

The gluteal and hamstring muscles fix the pelvis on the thigh.

The movements of the lower extremities are not as complex as those of the upper extremities. Hence the examination is somewhat simpler. Since the muscles of the pelvic girdle and thigh do not lend themselves as well to a sequence of examination based on the anatomy of the lumbosacral plexus (Fig. 2–45) as the muscles of the upper extremities, the order is determined largely by clinical convenience with some consideration to segmental innervation.

Many of the muscles are so powerful that when little or no weakness is present they can be tested profitably by certain maneuvers performed by the patient on his feet. Observation of the patient's gait will reveal weakness of certain muscles, and atrophy may be visible:

Iliopsoas – difficulty in bringing affected leg forward.

Abductors of thigh (chiefly gluteus medius and gluteus minimus) – sagging opposite side of pelvis and lateral displacement of pelvis to affected side when weight is on that leg.

Quadriceps – keeping knee locked when weight is placed on affected leg.

Tibialis anterior and extensors of toes – varying degrees of "steppage gait" and footdrop.

Gastrocnemius and soleus – limp produced by difficulty in raising heel from floor.

Certain maneuvers by the patient will make muscular weakness more apparent. The principal muscles involved are given:

Stepping up on a step.

Raising leg up to step – Iliopsoas.

Raising body – Gluteus maximus and quadriceps.

Squatting and rising – Quadriceps particularly.

Walking on heels – Tibialis anterior and extensors of toes.

Walking on toes – Gastrocnemius and soleus.

When there is little or no weakness, it is feasible to conduct the more detailed examination of the muscles of the lower extremities with the patient in the sitting posture throughout. However, the action of certain muscles is somewhat different in the sitting posture as compared with the supine or prone position. In particular, some of the lateral rotators of the thigh function also as abductors. Furthermore, the sitting posture interferes seriously with observation and palpation of some muscles—particularly the gluteus maximus and to a lesser extent the hamstrings. The muscles mentioned are therefore more accurately tested in the prone position.

In some instances it is convenient and advantageous to test the corresponding muscles of the two sides simultaneously for comparison. Examples are the adductors and abductors of the thighs and the extensors (dorsiflexors) and flexors (plantar flexors) of the feet and toes.

Iliopsoas (Fig. 2–28). Psoas major (Lumbar plexus [Fig. 2–45], L 1 2 3 4)
Iliacus (Femoral N., L 2 3 4)

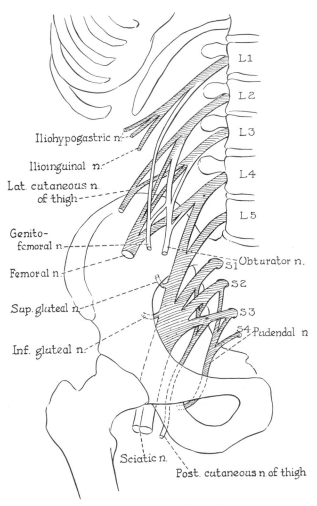

Figure 2–45 The lumbosacral plexus. (From Mayo Clinic: Clinical Examinations in Neurology.)

ACTION: Flexion of thigh at hip.

TEST: Sitting—Flexion of thigh, raising knee against resistance by examiner.

Supine—Raising extended leg off table and maintaining it against downward pressure by examiner applied just above knee.

Participating Muscles: Rectus femoris and sartorius (both—Femoral N., L 2 3 4); Tensor fasciae latae (Superior gluteal N., L 4 5 S 1).

Adductor Magnus, Longus, Brevis (Fig. 2–46).   (Obturator N., L 2 3 4. Part of adductor magnus is supplied by sciatic N., L 5, and functions with hamstrings.)

ACTION: Principally adduction of thigh.

TEST: Sitting or supine—Holding knees together while examiner attempts to separate them.

The two legs can also be tested separately and the muscles palpated.

Participating Muscles: Gluteus maximus; gracilis (Obturator N., L 2 3 4)

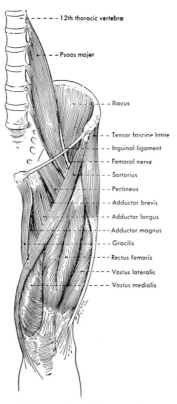

12th thoracic vertebra

Psoas major

Iliacus

Tensor fasciae latae

Inguinal ligament

Femoral nerve

Sartorius

Pectineus

Adductor brevis

Adductor longus

Adductor magnus

Gracilis

Rectus femoris

Vastus lateralis

Vastus medialis

Figure 2–46   The more superficial muscles of the anterior aspect of the thigh. (From Hollinshead, W. H.: Functional Anatomy of the Limbs and Back.)

Abductors of Thigh (Fig. 2–47).   (Superior gluteal N., L $\underline{4}$ $\underline{5}$ S $\underline{1}$)
    Gluteus medius and gluteus minimus principally.
    Tensor fasciae latae to a lesser extent.
    ACTION: Abduction and medial rotation of thigh.
            Tensor fasciae latae assists in flexion of thigh at hip.
            Sitting—Separation of knees against resistance by examiner.
            In this position the gluteus maximus and some of the other lateral rotators of the thigh function as abductors, hence diminishing the accuracy of the test.
            Supine—Same test as above. More exact.
            Lying on opposite side—Abduction of hip (upward movement) while examiner presses downward on lower leg and stabilizes pelvis.
            The tensor fasciae latae and to a lesser extent the gluteus medius can be palpated.

Medial Rotators of Thigh.   Same as abductors.
    TEST: Sitting or prone—Knee flexed to 90°. Medial rotation of thigh against resistance applied by examiner at knee and ankle in attempt to rotate thigh laterally.

Lateral Rotators of Thigh (Fig. 2–48).   (L 4 5 S 1 $\overline{2}$)
    Gluteus maximus (Inferior gluteal N., L 5̄ S 1̄ 2̄) chiefly
    Obturator internus and gemellus superior (N. to obturator internus, L 5 S 1 2)
    Quadratus femoris and gemellus inferior (N. to quadratus femoris, L 4 $\underline{5}$ S $\underline{1}$)

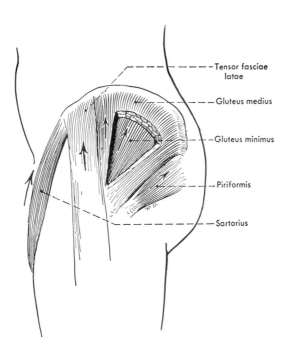

Figure 2–47 The abductors of the thigh. (From Hollinshead, W. H.: Functional Anatomy of the Limbs and Back.)

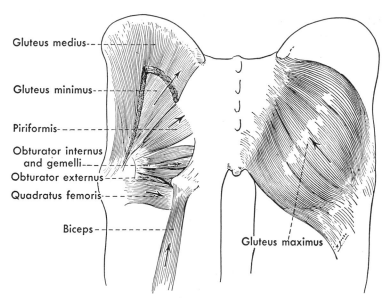

Gluteus medius

Gluteus minimus

Piriformis

Obturator internus and gemelli

Obturator externus

Quadratus femoris

Biceps

Gluteus maximus

Figure 2–48   The posteriorly placed external rotators of the thigh. (From Hollinshead, W. H.: Functional Anatomy of the Limbs and Back.)

TEST: Sitting or prone – Knee flexed to 90°. Lateral rotation of thigh against attempt by examiner to rotate thigh medially.

The gluteus maximus is the muscle principally tested and can be observed and palpated in the prone position.

Gluteus Maximus (Fig. 2–48).   (Inferior gluteal N., L 5 S $\underline{1}$ $\underline{2}$)

ACTION: Extension of thigh at hip.

Lateral rotation of thigh.

Assistance in adduction of thigh.

TEST: Sitting or supine – Starting with thigh slightly raised, extension (downward movement) of thigh against resistance by examiner applied under distal part of thigh.

This is a rather crude test and the muscle cannot be observed or readily palpated.

Prone – Knee well flexed to minimize participation of hamstrings. Extension of thigh, raising knee from table against downward pressure by examiner applied to distal part of thigh.

The muscle is accessible to observation and palpation in this position.

Quadriceps Femoris (Fig. 2–49).   (Femoral N., L 2 $\underline{3}$ $\underline{4}$)

ACTION: Extension of leg at knee.

Rectus femoris assists in flexion of thigh at hip.

TEST: Sitting or supine – Lower leg in moderate extension. Maintenance of extension against effort of examiner to flex leg at knee.

Atrophy is easily noted.

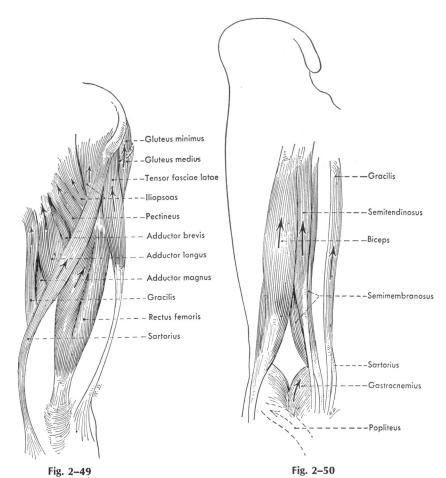

Fig. 2–49   Fig. 2–50

Figure 2–49   Flexors of the thigh. (From Hollinshead, W. H.: Functional Anatomy of the Limbs and Back.)

Figure 2–50   The flexors of the knee. (From Hollinshead, W. H.: Functional Anatomy of the Limbs and Back.)

Hamstrings (Fig. 2–50).   (Sciatic N., L 4 5 S 1 2)

Biceps femoris — external hamstring ($\overline{L}$ 5 S $\underline{1}$ 2)

Semitendinosus   }internal hamstrings
                            {(L 4 $\underline{5}$ S $\underline{1}$ 2)
Semimembranosus

ACTION: Flexion of leg at knee.

All but short head of biceps femoris assist in extension of thigh at hip.

TEST: Sitting — Flexion of lower leg against resistance.

Prone — Knee partly flexed. Further flexion against resistance. Observation and palpation of the muscles and tendons are important for proper interpretation.

Tibialis Anterior (Figs. 2–51, 2–52 and 2–53).   (Deep peroneal N., L 4 5 S 1)

ACTION: Dorsiflexion and inversion (particularly in dorsiflexed position) of foot.

TEST: Dorsiflexion of foot against resistance applied to dorsum of foot downward and toward eversion.

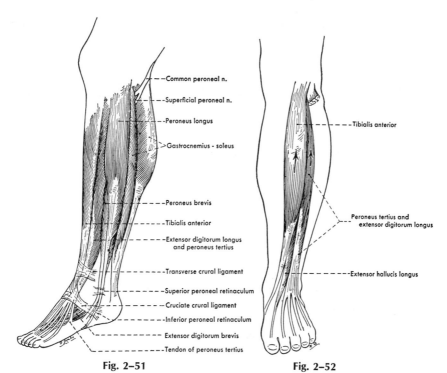

Common peroneal n.

Superficial peroneal n.

Peroneus longus

Gastrocnemius - soleus

Peroneus brevis

Tibialis anterior

Extensor digitorum longus and peroneus tertius

Transverse crural ligament

Superior peroneal retinaculum

Cruciate crural ligament

Inferior peroneal retinaculum

Extensor digitorum brevis

Tendon of peroneus tertius

Tibialis anterior

Peroneus tertius and extensor digitorum longus

Extensor hallucis longus

Fig. 2–51   **Fig. 2–52**

Figure 2–51   The lateral muscles of the leg. (From Hollinshead, W. H.: Functional Anatomy of the Limbs and Back.)

Figure 2–52   The dorsiflexors of the foot. (From Hollinshead, W. H.: Functional Anatomy of the Limbs and Back.)

The belly of the muscle just lateral to the shin, and the tendon medially on the dorsal aspect of the ankle, should be observed and palpated. Atrophy is conspicuous.

Participating Muscles: Dorsiflexion—Extensor hallucis longus; extensor digitorum longus.

Inversion—Tibialis posterior.

Extensor Hallucis Longus (Fig. 2–52).   (Deep peroneal N., L 4 5 S 1)

ACTION: Extension of great toe and dorsiflexion of foot.

TEST: Extension of great toe against resistance while foot is stabilized in neutral position.

The tendon is palpable between those of the tibialis anterior and the extensor digitorum longus.

Extensor Digitorum Longus (Figs. 2–51 and 2–52).   (Deep peroneal N., L 4 5 S 1)

ACTION: Extension of lateral four toes and dorsiflexion of foot.

TEST: Similar to above.

The tendons are visible and palpable on the dorsal aspect of the ankle and foot lateral to that of the extensor hallucis longus.

Extensor Digitorum Brevis (Fig. 2–51).   (Deep peroneal N., L 4 5 S 1)

ACTION: Assists in extension of all toes except little toe.

TEST: Observe and palpate belly of muscle on lateral aspect of dorsum of foot.

Peroneus Longus, Brevis (Fig. 2–53).   (Superficial peroneal N., L 4 5 S 1)

ACTION: Eversion of foot.

Assistance in plantar flexion of foot.

TEST: Foot in plantar flexion. Eversion against resistance applied by examiner to lateral border of foot.

The tendons are palpable just above and behind the external malleolus. Atrophy may be visible over the anterolateral aspect of the lower leg.

Gastrocnemius; Soleus (Fig. 2–54).   (Tibial N., L 5 S 1 2)

ACTION: Plantar flexion of foot.

The gastrocnemius also flexes the knee and cannot act effectively in plantar flexion of the foot when the knee is well flexed.

TEST: Knee extended to test both muscles. Knee flexed to test principally soleus. Plantar flexion of foot against resistance.

The muscles and tendon should be observed and palpated. Atrophy is readily visible. The gastrocnemius and soleus are very strong muscles, and leverage in testing favors the patient rather than the examiner. For this reason slight weakness is difficult to detect by resisting flexion of the ankle or by pressing against the flexed foot in the direction of extension. Consequently, it is advisable to test the strength of these muscles against the weight

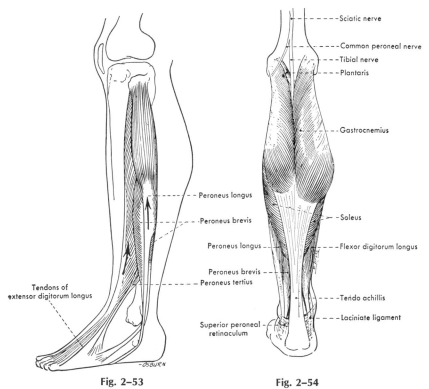

Fig. 2–53   Fig. 2–54

Figure 2–53   Evertors of the foot. (From Hollinshead, W. H.: Functional Anatomy of the Limbs and Back.)

Figure 2–54   The musculature of the calf of the leg, first layer. (From Hollinshead, W. H.: Functional Anatomy of the Limbs and Back.)

of the patient's body. Have the patient stand on one foot and flex the foot so as to lift himself directly and fully upward. Sometimes it is necessary for the examiner to hold the patient steady as he performs this test.

Participating Muscles: Long flexors of toes; tibialis posterior and peroneus longus and brevis (particularly near extreme plantar flexion).

Tibialis Posterior (Fig. 2–55).   (Posterior tibial N., L 5 S 1)
ACTION: Inversion of foot.
Assistance in plantar flexion of foot.
TEST: Foot in complete plantar flexion. Inversion against resistance applied to medial border of foot and directed toward eversion and slightly toward dorsiflexion.

This maneuver virtually eliminates participation of the tibialis anterior in inversion. The toes should be relaxed to prevent participation of the long flexors of the toes.

Long Flexors of Toes.   (Posterior tibial N., L 5 S 1 2)
Flexor digitorum longus
Flexor hallucis longus
ACTION: Plantar flexion of toes, especially at distal interphalangeal joints.
Assistance in plantar flexion and inversion of foot.
TEST: Foot stabilized in neutral position. Plantar flexion of toes against resistance applied particularly to distal phalanges.

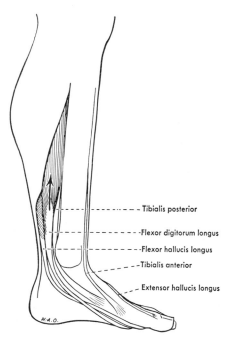

Tibialis posterior
Flexor digitorum longus
Flexor hallucis longus
Tibialis anterior
Extensor hallucis longus

Figure 2–55   Invertors of the foot. (From Hollinshead, W. H.: Functional Anatomy of the Limbs and Back.)

Is patient able to meet the following activity requirements? (Write "N" if not necessary.)

Meal preparation, serving and clean-up _____

Work heights_____ Dominance_____

Marketing_____

Washing and hanging clothes_____

Ironing_____

Bedmaking_____

Light housekeeping (dusting, sweeping, etc.)_____

Heavy household activities (washing floors, windows, etc.)_____

Hobbies and special interests_____

Number of stairs_____ Family members_____

Child care: number of children_____ Ages_____

Will patient be alone for long periods of time?_____

Available help in family and outside_____

Limitations for working and contraindications_____

_____

Budget: Supported_____ Self-sustaining_____ Middle_____ High_____

Ambulation status:_____

Assistive devices:_____

_____

Comments:

Figure 2–56 Household activities information.

Intrinsic Muscles of Foot. Virtually all except extensor digitorum brevis
(Medial and lateral plantar N's. from posterior tibial N., L 5 S 1 2)
ACTION: Somewhat comparable to that of intrinsic muscles of hand.
Many people have very poor individual function of these
muscles.
TEST: Cupping sole of foot is adequate test for most clinical purposes.

If paretic muscles are found which have different peripheral innervations
but similar root innervation, such an observation would tend to support the
localization of the lesion at either the root or the plexus level. This diagnostic
technique can be supplemented by testing for sensory loss and by employing
electrical nerve testing, including electromyography and determination of conduction velocity.

In the presence of an upper motor neuron lesion, manual muscle testing has limited value. It may give the examiner a gross estimate of the severity of the motor loss in a hemiplegic patient. However, spasticity does not permit voluntary movements to be performed with ease and may mask the motor power that the patient possesses for a given movement.

Before obtaining a more detailed evaluation of motor skill, a routine neurologic examination should be performed in order to evaluate the total clinical picture. For example, the presence of a sensory deficit will exaggerate a motor disability. Hemianopia may add to the difficulties of a hemiplegic in receiving adequate visual cues. The presence of spasticity or rigidity will impair motor skill. Thus determination of the neurologic deficits is important not only because of their diagnostic implications but in order to develop an effective program of management.

Motor Skill.   In evaluating the patient's motor performance, one must test not only for range of motion and strength; the patient's capacity to perform various tasks must also be determined. Such testing may consist of an inventory of the activities that are routinely performed in daily life. It may consist of evaluating the transfer activities from bed to wheelchair or chair, the use of a wheelchair, the ability to ambulate and take care of one's personal hygiene and dressing. In Figure 20–1, pages 474–475, is shown a method for recording such an inventory of motor skills.

Since so many of the patients who are treated by physiatric techniques suffer from locomotor disturbances, it is incumbent upon the examiner to study the patient's posture and gait (see page 92).

Figure 2–56 provides a rapid means of analyzing the capacity of the disabled patient to be responsible for his own housekeeping.

REFERENCES

Muscle Testing

1. Chusid, J. G., and McDonald, J. J.: Correlative Neuroanatomy and Functional Neurology. Los Altos, Calif., Lange Medical Publications, 1962.
2. Glathe, J. P., and Achor, R. W. P.: Frequency of Cardiac Disease in Patients with Strokes. Proc. Mayo Clin., *33*:417–422, 1958.
3. Haymaker, W., and Woodhall, B.: Peripheral Nerve Injuries. 2nd Ed. Philadelphia, W. B. Saunders Co., 1953.
4. Mayo Clinic: Clinical Examinations in Neurology. 3rd Ed. Philadelphia, W. B. Saunders Co., 1971.

Chapter 3

EVALUATION OF THE AMPUTEE

by Emery K. Stoner

FUNCTIONAL EVALUATION OF THE UPPER EXTREMITY

NORMAL BIOMECHANICS

The upper extremity is extremely complex as to its anatomy and physiology and its many functions. It is capable of highly versatile and skilled movements. The arm is a compound lever for the hand and the shoulder is a specialized fulcrum for this lever. In addition to its prehension patterns the hand functions in support, striking or pushing actions, and in the clenched fist and the knuckle and digital support postures.

Hand

Gross hand prehension patterns include palmar, tip, lateral, hook or snap, spherical grasp and cylindrical grasp (Fig. 3-1).

Analysis of three of the six prehension patterns by Keller et al.[1] showed that palmar prehension predominates in picking up objects and especially in holding objects for use.

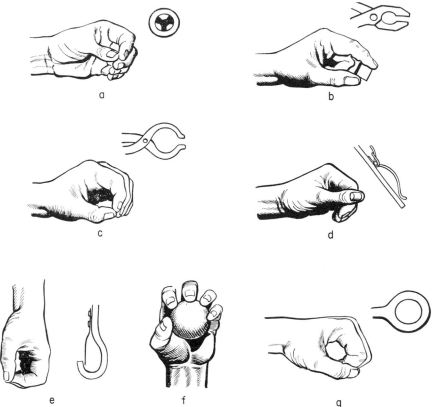

Figure 3–1 Hand prehension patterns. a. Palmar prehension. Opposition of the thumb with the pad of the index and middle fingers gives a three-jawed chuck prehension. b. Palmar prehension. At openings of 1 to 3 inches, opposition between the thumb and digits II and III is in the manner of a pliers grip. c. Tip prehension. The tips of the index and middle fingers are brought into opposition to the tip of the thumb. d. Lateral prehension. The ball of the thumb opposes the lateral surface of the index finger. e. Hook prehension. Load is supported by hooked terminal phalanges, the thumb acting largely to prevent slipping. f. Spherical prehension. In addition to elements of grip prehension, curving across the knuckle line permits conformity to spherical objects. g. Grip prehension. The digits curled about an object, such as a handle; the thumb curves and overlaps the finger tips to close the prehension ring. (From Klopsteg, P. E., and Wilson, P. D.: Human Limbs and Their Substitutes. New York, McGraw-Hill Book Co., 1954. Used by permission of McGraw-Hill Book Company.)

The essential opposing member in all prehension is the thumb. The thumb is capable of moving upon its saddle-shaped carpometacarpal articulation so that it can oppose any other digit. The adductor and opponens muscle groups pull the thumb toward the hand. The adductors act chiefly when the thumb is in the palmar plane; the opponens acts when the thumb is involved in spherical grasp. At all positions over this range the flexor pollicis longus strengthens the opposition by acting on the distal segments of the thumb. Conversely, abduction or extension of the thumb is accomplished by the extensor pollicis longus, the extensor pollicis brevis and the abductor pollicis longus. Thus, the thumb is capable of complex and diverse patterns of actions.

In all types of prehension mentioned the hand assumes a fixed position. If the grasped object is unyielding, reactions to the flexion forces are afforded by the object. If the object is fragile, or the hand empty, the hand is kept in any required posture by cocontractions of the opposing muscle groups.

The normal hand is well supplied with receptors which mediate touch, pressure and muscle joint senses. These receptors make it possible to recognize objects by shape, size, texture, weight and temperature. In addition to the multiplicity of peripheral sense receptors involved are the large areas of cerebral cortex given over to the coordination and sensation of the hand. The cortical area for the hand is almost equal to the total area for the arms, body and legs.

From this brief consideration of hand mechanics it can be noted that normal hand function is the result of a highly complicated structural arrangement plus an elaborate and automatic system of control. Although lost bone and joint mechanisms can be simulated, adequate replacement of the control system is not possible at the present time.

Wrist

The wrist can be simply flexed toward the volar, dorsal, ulnar and radial sides and toward combinations of these sides. The major articulations are radiocarpal and intracarpal. The compound joint actions of the normal wrist permit large angular motion fields approaching a curvature rather than the sharp angularity that would be given by a single joint.

The musculature of wrist flexion is such that for stable grasp the volar and dorsal flexor groups act together to fix the wrist and hand. The line of action of the various muscles contributing to wrist motion is mainly oblique to the major flexion planes. Thus, the desired flexions are accomplished by combined actions of muscle.

Kinematic study of 51 activies of daily living involving wrist motion showed that the maximal volar and dorsal flexions used were somewhat less than those permitted by total range of motion.[1] Ulnar and radial flexion maximums were very close to the measured extreme motion. The modal frequency in the volardorsal plane was zero to 10 degrees, which closely approaches the resting position of 12 degrees of dorsal flexion reported by Steindler.[2]

It is commonly noted that the wrist assumes an angle of 145 degrees when very strong prehension is required.

Forearm and Elbow

The radius, ulna and distal end of the humerus make up the forearm skeleton. The radius can move in flexion and extension as well as in rotation. Distally the radius twists around the ulna. The ulna is limited to the flexion-extension axis of rotation. The forearm bones rotate upon the elbow axis in the manner of a simple hinge. The anatomic center lines of the arm and forearm are not coaxial and the cubital angle thus formed is about 170 degrees.

Shoulder

The action of the shoulder enables us to use our hands to greatest advantage. It does this by suspending the upper extremity, anchoring it to the trunk and providing a fulcrum for movement. Suspension is accomplished by the clavicle which acts as a strut, aided by a powerful group of suspensory muscles—trapezius, deltoid, levator scapula and sternocleidomastoid. Stability is achieved by the broad flat base of the scapula aided by flat muscles piled on top and attached to its surfaces. Mobility is derived from the shallow elongated socket and ball head with systems of rotators such as cuff muscles attached to give varying mechanical advantages.

For practical purposes the action of the shoulder is to lift the arm. Body rotations or trunk actions may then convert single lifts into "flexion" or "abduction."

Lifting the arm from the side of the body over the head is accomplished mainly at the glenohumeral joint. The muscles chiefly concerned are the deltoid, rotator cuff, serratus anterior and trapezius. After the base of the joint is solidly clamped to the chest wall by the actions of the trapezius and serratus, the supraspinatus and infraspinatus snub the head of the humerus. At the same time the deltoid contracts fully and the arm swings up. Elevation starts at the glenohumeral joint and is accompanied by movement at the sternoclavicular joint. The second 90 degrees of elevation is accomplished at the glenohumeral joint aided by contributions from the acromioclavicular and scapulothoracic joints. At 90 degrees the humerus rotates externally allowing the greater tuberosity to slip beneath the bony ligamentous coraco-acromial arch.

ABNORMAL BIOMECHANICS

Loss of the hand by amputation at the wrist or within 2 inches of the distal end of the forearm is the starting point in the analysis of amputee biomechanics. Patients with digital, metacarpal and carpal distarticulations comprise an important, though specialized, segment of the overall amputee problem, but the associated functional losses usually are minor. Design of a corresponding prosthesis, if really necessary, is closely particularized to the individual case. Hand function outweighs in importance any other major function of the arm.

Complete Hand and Wrist Loss. The long below-elbow amputee retains all major functions of shoulder, arm and forearm, but has lost the motions of the wrist and the manifold functions of the hand.

Prosthetic replacement of the wrist and hand is poor at best. Therefore, it is vital to insure maximal utilization of the meager resources remaining. Wrist flexion replacement would require control of motion in four directions and stabilization in two angles about the wrist center. No successful prosthesis has yet been developed that accomplishes even one of these functions. No modern device provides ulnar or radial flexion. Three reasons for the seeming neglect of replacement for wrist motion are: first, usually no controls from a shoulder harness or cineplastic tunnels are available to furnish power; second, the wrist motions, although ideal for fine positioning of the hand, are not absolutely essential to bring the hand into the major action spheres about the body; third, loss of wrist flexions can be compensated for grossly by other arm motions. A pre-position flexion device is a considerable aid to the amputee, especially for manipulation close to the body. The bilateral amputee finds it particularly useful.

The principal motion losses of the below-elbow amputee are those of finger movements, wrist flexion and varying degrees of pronation and supination. Because of the fixed prehension pattern of the prosthetic hand or hook and the fixed wrist nearly all fine orientation movements must be made at levels higher than the forearm, by compensatory movements of the elbow, arm and shoulder. With training in these movements the amputee should be able to carry them out with apparent ease and skill. For the long below-elbow stump the socket can be contoured so that some forearm rotation is preserved. In short below-elbow amputations rotation is abandoned.

The above-elbow amputee retains the functions of arm and shoulder but the shoulder disarticulation amputee has those of the shoulder only. If close adherence to the arm can be achieved in the socket, the amputee regains medial and lateral arm rotation. In the case of disarticulation, only a limited amount of substitutional arm movement can be obtained.

Loss of Elbow Joint.   Forearm flexion-extension is considered as acting at the elbow as a simple hinge joint, and forearm rotation is viewed as torsion about an axis through the center of the forearm. This is an approximation and not accurate in anatomical detail. Elbow flexion-extension that is lost can be substituted for readily by a prosthesis. However, forearm rotation when lost, is difficult to replace mechanically. Substitution for forearm rotation is usually done by shoulder motion.

Loss of Shoulder Motion.   The mobility of shoulder-on-torso and arm-on-shoulder is of great value to the above-elbow amputee. Scapular abduction provides a reliable source for controlled motion in the prosthesis of the shoulder-disarticulation amputee. Loss of shoulder control and shoulder girdle control is a tremendous loss and is difficult to compensate for either prosthetically or orthotically.

EVALUATION OF GAIT

NORMAL BIOMECHANICS

Human locomotion is a complicated process of transformation of a series of controlled and coordinated angular motions occurring simultaneously at the various joints of the lower extremity into a smooth path for the center of gravity of the body.[3]

The basic determinants of locomotion are six: knee-ankle interaction, knee flexion, hip flexion, pelvic rotation about a vertical axis, lateral tilting of the pelvis and lateral displacement of the pelvis. A typical forward step can be divided into two phases: the "stance" phase in which the foot is in contact with the floor and the leg is bearing part or all of the body weight and the "swing" phase in which the foot is not touching the floor and the body weight is being borne by the opposite leg. One foot and leg bear the weight while the opposite foot and leg swing forward and in their turn take over the body weight. For analytic purposes the stance phase may be defined as beginning when the heel strikes the floor and ending when the toe rises at the end of the stride. The stance phase has three parts: heel strike, midstance and push-off. In a similar fashion the swing phase may be defined as beginning when the toe leaves the floor and ending when the forward swing of the leg has ceased. It has three parts: acceleration, swing-through, and deceleration (Fig. 3–2). Both feet are in

STANCE PHASE

Heel-Strike   Mid-Stance   Push-Off

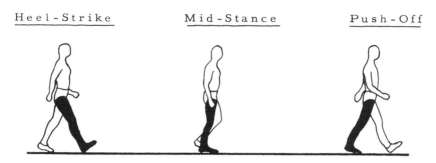

Foot in contact with floor, leg bearing body weight

SWING PHASE

Acceleration   Swing-Through   Deceleration

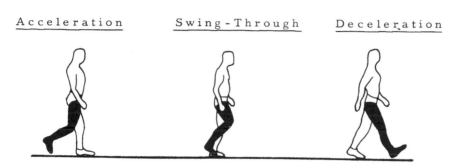

Foot not touching floor; opposite leg bearing body weight

Figure 3-2   Analysis of a single forward step. (From Anderson, M. H., Bechtol, C. O., and Sollars, R. E.: Clinical Prosthetics for Physicians and Therapists. Springfield, Ill., Charles C Thomas, 1959.)

contact with the walking surface simultaneously for approximately 25 per cent of a complete two step cycle. This part of the cycle has been designated as the "double-support" phase.

In Figure 3-2 it can be seen that the knee joint reaches its maximal extension just before heel contact and that a period of knee flexion has then begun, which continues into the stance phase. The decrease in the rate of knee extension at the end of the swing phase, preparatory to foot contact with the floor, is primarily a result of the action of the hamstring muscle group. Because of its attachment posteriorly to the hip joint and to the tibia and fibula below the knee joint, the hamstring group can bring about hip extension, knee flexion or both simultaneously. As the heel prepares to make contact, the hamstring action tends to bring it forcibly backward into contact with the floor. The knee continues to flex rapidly during this phase. The activity in the hamstring group continues, but with decreasing power, while the quadriceps action begins to build up rapidly.

The quadriceps acting anteriorly about the knee joint and the pretibial muscles acting about the ankle joint serve to control the knee-ankle interaction and effect a smooth motion of the fore part of the foot toward the floor. The major function of both knee and ankle during this phase is smooth absorption of the shock of heel contact and maintenance of a smooth path for the center of gravity of the whole body. The function of the knee as a shock absorber is often overlooked. The maximal angle of knee flexion in midstance is about 20 degrees and is reached during the first part of the midstance phase. As the body slides forward over the stabilizing knee, the upward thrust of the floor reaction moving forward in the sole of the foot gradually increases the dorsi-flexion of the ankle causing the knee to begin a period of extension. The knee reaches a position of maximal extension about the time the heel leaves the ground, with the calf group providing the resistance to knee extension and ankle dorsiflexion. The sequence of controlled flexion of the knee at heel contact, release to permit gradual extension in midstance and controlled flexion preparatory to swing is important in accomplishing a smooth and energy-saving gait in normal persons.

During push-off the knee is brought forward by the action of the hip joint and a sensitive balance must be maintained between the interaction of the hip, knee and ankle joints. As the heel leaves the ground and the knee begins to flex, the knee musculature must first resist the effect of the force on the ball of the foot, which passes through space on a line ahead of the knee joint. Then as the knee is brought forward by hip-joint action, the knee must reverse its action to provide controlled resistance to flexion by increasing quadriceps activity.

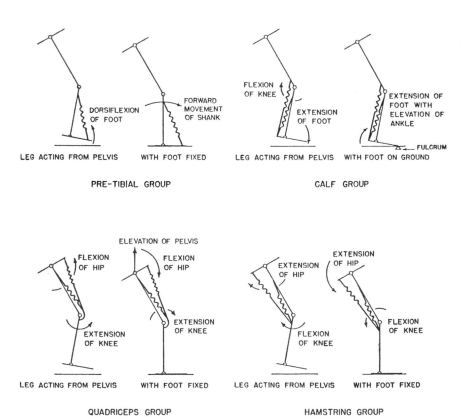

Figure 3–3   Major muscle groups of the lower extremity, demonstrating the major mechanics of the lower extremity in the lateral plane. (From Manual of Below-Knee Prosthetics. Biomechanics Laboratory, Department of Engineering, University of California at Berkeley, 1959.)

The calf group provides active plantar flexion throughout the entire push-off phase (Fig. 3–3). At the time the toe leaves the floor the knee has flexed 40 to 45 degrees of the maximum of 65 degrees it reaches during the swing phase. Knee flexion in the swing phase is not caused by hamstring action in normal persons. The overall objective in the swing phase is to get the foot from one position to the next smoothly, clearing any obstacles in the pathway. The knee continues to flex after toe-off. During rapid walking this momentum would result in excessive knee flexion and heel rise except that the quadriceps limits the angle of knee flexion to approximately 65 degrees and, by controlled action, starts knee extension.

Knee extension proceeds as a result of a continuation of pendulum effect and muscle action. Little quadriceps action is required. During midswing there is a period of minimal muscular activity and the leg accelerates downward and forward similar to a pendulum with forced motion of its pivot joint. Near the end of the swing the rate of knee extension is decelerated in readiness for heel contact. This "terminal deceleration" is primarily due to hamstring activity.

In normal walking the pelvis rotates alternately to the right and left. As the swinging leg moves forward, the pelvis rotates forward on the same side. The total rotation is about 4 degrees on each side of the central axis, or a total of 8 degrees. The rotation actually occurs at each hip joint, which passes from relative internal rotation to relative external rotation during the stance phase. This rotation has the effect of lengthening the stride without increasing the drop of the center of gravity at the instant of heel strike.

The pelvis also tilts during normal walking, listing downward from the weight bearing limb (as in the positive Trendelenburg test). The average amount of pelvic tilt is about 5 degrees reached at the instant of midstance. Pelvic tilt has the effect of reducing the rise of the center of gravity by approximately half. The center of gravity in adults is just anterior to the second sacral vertebra and studies have shown that the pathway followed by the center of gravity of the body is a smooth regular curve in its up and down movement with an average rise and fall of about $1\frac{4}{5}$ inches. A similar curve is followed by the center of gravity in its side to side movement. The total distance traveled is about $1\frac{3}{4}$ inches. The motion is toward the weight bearing leg and the lateral limit is reached at midstance.

ABNORMAL BIOMECHANICS

Two-joint muscles which span both hip and knee are important in coordinating the actions of the two joints. Most of the hip flexors are inserted high above the knee and are not involved by mid-thigh amputation, except for the sartorius and rectus femoris which are involved by amputation at or above the knee. Ordinarily hip flexion power remains strong in the average above-knee stump. The hip extensors, except the gluteus maximus, are two-joint muscles and would be divided during an above-knee amputation. Thus, the extensor power is seriously reduced in the usual above-knee stump. The gluteus maximus does not actually come into play and can yield no appreciable force unless the femur is flexed 15 degrees or more.

The gait pattern is drastically changed in the loss of the knee joint.[4] There is a decrease in the ability to absorb the normal knee moments. Shortened steps are taken by the above-knee amputee to prevent the development of a large moment that would tend to flex the knee. Leaning forward at the hip helps prevent the ground reaction line from passing too far behind the knee. When the heel strikes the ground, forces are developed tending to flex the knee, and the amputee resists these forces by hip extension. Normal knee flexion in early stance is impossible. As a result, the vertical amplitude of the center of gravity is greater than normal, increasing the work done in walking and the energy required. Above-knee amputees utilize approximately twice the energy to walk at the same speeds as normal persons.

The short powerful abductor muscles of the hip are not affected by most above-knee amputations even at high levels. Compared to the abductors, the adductors will be weaker, especially in short stumps, because the action of the gracilis muscle and much of the adductor muscle power will be lost.

During the stance phase when a prosthesis is used, the pelvis is held level by the abductor musculature of the hip. In order that the abductor muscles may exert more force the above-knee socket is adducted. This helps in maintaining a level pelvis and a normal gait base.

The socket is fabricated with a certain amount of initial flexion to assist the hip extensors. If hip flexion contraction is present or if the hip extensors are weak, the prosthetic knee joint is positioned slightly to the rear so that stability is built into the leg and the hip extensors are not necessary to maintain knee extension.

The extent of disability and problems of replacement vary with the level of amputation. When the knee joint is preserved, the problems of stability and of proprioceptive sense are both simplified.

Disarticulation of the hip obviously adds serious problems. The forward swing of the normal leg is started by strong contraction of the plantar flexors of the ankle followed by activity of the hip flexors. Normally the ankle extensors contribute about twice as much energy as the hip flexors. In the absence of a device to produce strong ankle flexion, the amputee must rely on his hip flexors to initiate the forward swing. For this reason, artificial limbs that are lighter than the natural leg have been developed.

The moments of force that are developed about a knee mechanism vary with the speed of walking and with the length of step. When the heel rises and the opposite foot has come into contact with the ground, an extensor force is needed at the knee to provide forward acceleration of the shank to prevent excess heel rise. Heel elevation must be sufficient to provide toe clearance during the swing.

REFERENCES

Functional Evaluation of the Upper Extremity

1. Anderson, M. H., Bechtol, C. O., and Sollars, R. E.: Clinical Prosthetics for Physician and Therapist. Springfield, Ill., Charles C Thomas, 1959.
2. Peizer, E.: Human Locomotion. Bulletin of Prosthetic Research. BPR 10-12. Fall, 1969.

Evaluation of Gait

3. Keller, A. D., Taylor, C. L., and Zahn, V.: Studies to Determine the Functional Requirements for Hand and Arm Prostheses. Department of Engineering, University of California (Los Angeles), 1947.
4. Steindler, A.: Mechanics of Normal and Pathological Locomotion in Man. Springfield, Ill., Charles C Thomas, 1935.

Chapter 4

CARE OF THE AMPUTEE

by Emery K. Stoner

ORTHOTICS

The present division between prosthetics and orthotics is somewhat arbitrary. In practice there is a greater relationship between upper extremity prosthetics and upper extremity orthotics (and lower extremity prosthetics and lower extremity orthotics) than there is between upper and lower prosthetics or orthotics.[4]

The relatively few upper extremity patients are poorly cared for by most facilities and their care, particularly for orthoses, is left for the specialized centers.

Great strides have been made in prosthetics, while in the field of orthotics many things appear to be unchanged. Educational efforts in orthotics have been far less successful than in prosthetics.

Braces are applied to the body for support or immobilization of a part, to correct or prevent deformity and to assist or restore function. Common indications for braces are pain, weakness or a paralysis of a part of the body.

One of the basic principles of design of orthoses is to provide adequate surface area for the distribution of the forces involved. Accurate contouring helps in this regard. If immobilization of a joint is desired, the brace will require long lever arms with maximum pressure distribution to give comfort and to be effective.

Orthoses should be simple and durable. Weight should be minimal and yet have the necessary strength. Cosmetically, these devices should be as inconspicuous as possible.

Prescription for an orthotic device should be specific and should be recorded in the patient's record. The prescription should include the part or

parts to be braced, type of brace, material, type of joints and special considerations. After delivery the physician must check out the brace to see that it
conforms to his prescription, that it fits properly and comfortably and that it is
cosmetically acceptable.

UPPER EXTREMITY ORTHOTICS

A great number of splints plus variations have been described for use on
the upper extremity. Four series of basic splints are the Bunnell series, the
Bennett series, the Engen orthoses and the Ranchos Los Amigos splints. Miles
Anderson[1] has described most of the commonly used upper extremity braces in
his *Functional Bracing of the Upper Extremities.* Many of these splints are commercially available in prefabricated form. An excellent construction guide for the
orthotist is Anderson's *Upper Extremities Orthotics.*[2]

There is not adequate space here to describe each series of braces. The
Engen series will be discussed briefly.

The Engen Plastic Hand Orthotics (EPHO)

Thorkild J. Engen at Baylor University College of Medicine, Houston,
Texas, initiated the development of a plastic hand orthosis.

Based on the premise that preservation of hand posture is best maintained
by support, the device is designed to hold the thumb in the opposed position
and at the same time support the metacarpal arch.

The goal has been to develop a standardized item which could be adopted
to meet the needs of a particular patient. The Engen orthosis is made in four
sizes for both right and left hands—large, medium large, medium and small. It
is currently fabricated using a polyester resin and nylon laminate. The orthotist
molds and modifies the device as needed to provide a custom fit.

Attachments were devised or adapted to provide wrist support and prehension.

Common versions of the EPHO are the short opponens orthosis, the long
opponens orthosis and the reciprocal wrist-extension, finger-flexion unit. Additional modifications are available utilizing external power.

Short Opponens Orthosis.   The short opponens orthosis is the simplest
application of the Engen orthosis. It consists of the basic hand shell with a
retaining strap (Fig. 4–1). The purpose of this device is to hold the thumb in
opposition to the index finger and middle fingers and to support the metacarpal
arch. The functional goal is to accomplish "three jaw chuck" grasp. Patients
benefitting from this orthosis include those with spinal cord injuries at C7, C8
and T1 levels, those with median and ulnar nerve neuropathies and those with
hemiplegia.

Long Opponens Orthosis.   The long opponens orthosis consists of the basic
shell with an attached volar extension arm stabilized on the forearm by straps
(Fig. 4-2). The purpose of this device is the same as that for the short
opponens orthosis in a patient who has lost wrist control. Patients with the
following problems may benefit from this type of orthosis: spinal cord lesions
at C5 and C6 levels, hemiplegia, and neuropathy of the radial, median and
ulnar nerves.

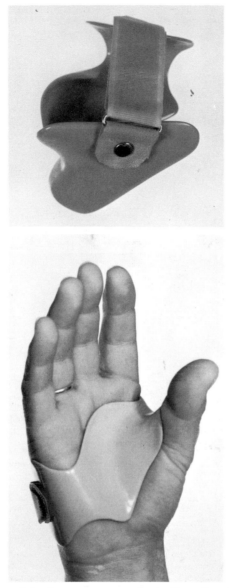

Figure 4–1   Two views of the short opponens orthosis. (From Kay, H. W.: Clinical Evaluation of the Engen Plastic Hand Orthosis. Artificial Limbs, *13(1)*:13–26, Spring, 1969.)

Reciprocal Wrist-Extension Finger-Flexion Orthosis. This device is designed to provide prehension when voluntary wrist extension is available (Fig. 4-3). Quadriplegic patients who have retained power in the wrist extensor muscles may be helped to function by this adaptation. It is more complicated than the other orthoses and an external power source may be used in case wrist extension is weak.

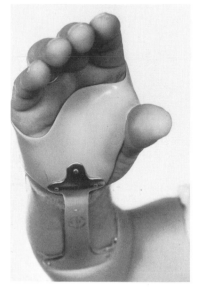

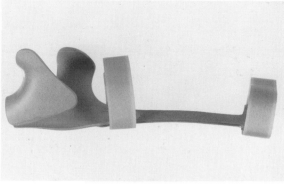

Figure 4–2 Two views of the long opponens orthosis. (From Kay, H. W.: Clinical Evaluation of the Engen Plastic Hand Orthosis. Artificial Limbs, *13(1):* 13–26, Spring, 1969.)

Summary

Orthotists with prior experience in the fabrication of hand splints can learn to apply the EPHO orthoses successfully. The instructional manual and fitting check-out sheets that have been developed are excellent. However, there is no substitute for direct instruction in this field. Important for success in the use of orthoses are proper selection of patients and meticulous care in fitting and follow-up adjusting of these devices.

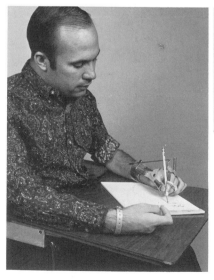

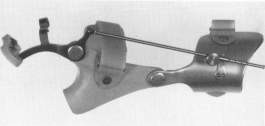

Figure 4–3 Two views of the reciprocal orthosis. (From Kay, H. W.: Clinical Evaluation of the Engen Plastic Hand Orthosis. Artificial Limbs, *13(1):*13–26, Spring, 1969.)

ASSISTIVE DEVICES

Technical aids are an important part of the rehabilitation program. Aids for the handicapped are generally a last resort when medical treatment has failed to restore full function of parts of the body and when other parts of the body have been unable to take over the functions of the injured one. Rehabilitation goals can be set too high. For example, it might be advisable for an elderly bilateral above-knee amputee to use an efficient wheelchair rather than depleting his limited energy by struggling to get out of a chair, walk a few steps and then sit down again in order to accomplish some task.

A major difficulty today is keeping up with technical progress in order to apply it for the handicapped. Therefore, the technician is becoming more and more a member of the rehabilitation team. Technical aids have been divided into five groups: transportation aids, aids for daily living, working tools and household equipment, housing problems and therapeutic aids.[7] One serious need is for some method of collecting information, deciding on the merit of ideas and gadgets and then disseminating this information to the individual who works directly with the handicapped. Today many patients are supplied with wheelchairs that are unsuitable and uncomfortable because of the lack of information and knowledge about which type of chair to order. Proper home designing as well as the planning of public buildings for the use of the disabled are also needed.

Functional Assistive Hand Splints. Functional assistive hand splints and the attachments used with them are designed to prevent or correct deformities of the hand and wrist, to increase the strength of weakened muscles by encouraging their use and by preventing the substitution of stronger opposing muscles and to increase the functional capacity of the hand by providing mechanical assistance to the weakened muscle so that the hand is stabilized in a better position. The basic opponens splint and the long opponens splint are commonly used and many attachments have been developed for use with them. These splints have been used in the treatment of spinal cord injuries, postpoliomyelitis paralysis, hemiplegia, brachial plexus injury, post-traumatic problems, anthrogryposis, muscular atrophies and muscular dystrophies.

Feeders. Feeders are mechanical devices designed to support the hand and forearm on a pivot or suspension strap so that very slight movements of the body or shoulder will result in useful motion of the arms, enabling the patient to reach for objects and bring them to his mouth. These devices are used primarily to permit the patient to feed himself but when they are equipped with special assistive devices, he may be able to comb his hair, shave, brush his teeth and perform other similar activities. There are two basic types of feeders, suspension and supportive. The suspension type supports the arm on an overhead bar which is usually attached to the wheelchair. An adjustable strap and suspension bracket connect the overhead bar and a metal arm trough. The supportive feeder has a similar metal arm trough but it is supported on swivel arms attached to the wheelchair or the trough can be placed on a metal rocker which rests on the table. Parts for feeders may be purchased and installed without difficulty.

Special Assistive Devices. After a patient has learned to perform a few functional acts using splints and feeders he may increase the range of his activities by using special assistive devices. Since ability for self-care is very important to the patient, a variety of devices have been developed to aid him in these activities. These devices are numerous and their utility is limited only by the ingenuity and imagination of those who treat the patient.

FUNCTIONAL ARM BRACES.[1]   Functional arm braces are mechanical devices that provide a limited amount of arm function for the patient who has lost part or all of the use of one or both upper extremities. Because of the many different combinations of functional losses, many different combinations of functional arm braces are necessary. Much work in this field has been done by Dr. Edwin R. Schottstaedt of San Francisco and Mr. George W. Robinson of Vallejo, California. They have worked out components and subassemblies of components that can be put together in different combinations according to the needs of the patient. Subassemblies are available in kit form so that the orthotist can fit and assemble the kits in various combinations as needed. This permits him to spend his time on the important job of brace fitting rather than using his efforts on bench fabrication of parts.

The cable-controlled hook ("Handy Hook") consists of a standard voluntary-opening prosthetic hook mounted on a stainless steel plate that is shaped to fit the patient's hand (Fig. 4-4). The hook is positioned to lie between the patient's thumb and index finger. A loop type harness and a cable assembly are provided so that the hook can be opened by shoulder abduction or, if desired, by shoulder elevation. If the wrist muscles are weak or paralyzed, a wrist splint may be attached to the device. The chief disadvantage of the hook is its lack of sensation and its limited grasp. This device should be used by those patients whose fingers lack sensation or whose finger joints are so badly damaged that they lack mobility.

SHOULDER SUSPENSION CAPS.   The shoulder suspension cap is designed to serve as a foundation for the attachment of various shoulder and arm assistive devices.

In general the purpose of the shoulder suspension is to support the weakened shoulder girdle so that it is held up in its proper position and is not required to withstand the dead weight of the arm. It also serves as a means of attachment for the apparatus required to restore some arm function. Basically these caps are made of plastic impregnated stockinette molded to the contour of the shoulder and held in place by a chest band of plastic covered webbing. A locking elbow unit may be fastened to the cap laterally and at its lower end a hook may be placed for attachment of rubber bands for elbow flexion assistance. In the past, shoulder suspension hoops have been tried to support the shoulder and arm. These consisted of two stainless steel tubes protruding vertically from a padded waist band held in place by a webbing belt. The hoop, which went over, around or under the shoulder, was fitted into the tubes and the forearm was suspended from the hoop. These proved to be too unstable and were rejected by the patients.

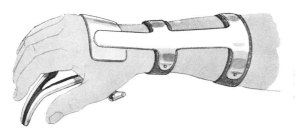

Figure 4-4 The "Handy Hook" as applied to a flail hand. Positioned in the palm by means of a plate passing over the dorsum, it is powered by shoulder harness. Hand sensation is preserved. (Courtesy Robin-Aids Manufacturing Company, Vallejo, Calif.)

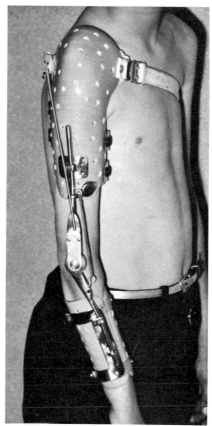

Figure 4–5 Forearm cuff assembly used with a plastic shoulder cap and a locking elbow unit. Rubber bands fastened between the hook on the cap and the hook on the cuff assist in elbow flexion and the lock is controlled by the harness. (Courtesy Dr. M. H. Anderson.)

FOREARM CUFF ASSEMBLY. The forearm cuff assembly is a leather sleeve so shaped that it fits over the forearm of the patient. Forearm cuffs have a variety of applications (Fig. 4-5). When the cuffs are used with the components already mentioned and others not described here, shoulder flexion, abduction and rotation, elbow flexion and forearm rotation can be assisted. In addition, the shoulder may be stabilized and the elbow locked.

LOWER EXTREMITY ORTHOTICS

The objective of bracing is to improve the function of the entire patient. A functionally or structurally deficient extremity that is to be braced must be considered as part of the body as a whole. Special attention must be given to the normal static and dynamic relationships of the hip, knee and subtalar joints. If these normal relationships are not considered during alignment procedures, the brace may hinder performance and may tend to increase further any existing deformities.

A brace may help by decreasing pain, by supporting body weight and by aiding in ambulation. It may be supportive, corrective, protective or dynamic. By supportive bracing is meant the stabilizing of a part such as a painful joint, an area of architectural inadequacy or a joint with paralyzed or unbalanced musculature. Corrective bracing is that used for club feet, metatarsus varus, tibial torsion, congenital hip dislocation or hemophilic arthropathy. Protective bracing is that used in emergency splinting, traction splints, weight relieving devices and fracture bracing. By dynamic bracing is meant the use of a brace to motorize a part or aid weakened muscles. Dynamic braces are usually in the form of springs, cables and elastic bands.

The Ankle Joint.   The natural torsion of the tibia causes the axis of the ankle joint to be rotated externally 20 to 30 degrees with respect to the knee axis (Fig. 4-6). Tibial torsion is a developmental event which increases from a minimum of about 2 degrees in the newborn to a permanent amount of 20 to 30 degrees by the age of seven years. This developmental change places the ankle joint in its best position for walking. During normal walking the center of gravity of the body oscillates from side to side as it moves forward. The axis of rotation of the ankle joint is not perpendicular to the line of progression during the first half of stance phase (Fig. 4-7). Rather, it is apparently perpendicular to the path of the center of gravity of the body, permitting the ankle joint to bend freely in the direction of movement of the center of gravity from heel strike to the midstance phase of walking.

The Subtalar Joint.   The subtalar joint performs three important functions:[9]

1. In standing, it allows medio-lateral shifting so that the center of gravity can be maintained within the base of support, while the foot retains flat heel and sole contact with the floor.
2. It permits the foot to adapt to uneven ground.
3. It helps to compensate for the difference in alignment of the ankle joint and the knee joint during acute knee flexion such as in squatting.

The Knee and Hip Joints.   Since most long leg braces eliminate knee motion by means of a knee lock, alignment considerations at the knee during standing and walking are of little significance. However, the location of the mechanical knee joint must be such that the brace is comfortable both in the extended and flexed positions.

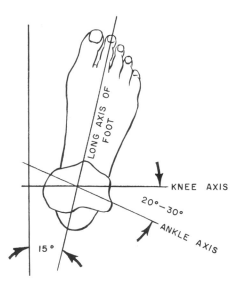

Figure 4–6   (From Lehneis, H. R.: Brace Alignment Considerations. Orthopedic and Appliance J., *18:*110, 1964.)

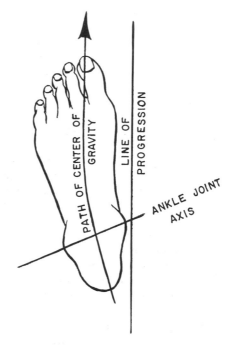

Figure 4–7   (From Lehneis, H. R.: Brace Alignment Considerations. Orthopedic and Appliance J., *18:*110, 1964.)

The mechanical hip joint should be placed approximately ¼ inch anterior to the most prominent part of the greater trochanter. In obese patients the hip joint may be placed farther forward to give more room posteriorly for sitting comfort.

Brace Alignment

In prescribing and fitting braces certain factors of "danger" must be considered. They are areas of anesthesia, decreased circulation to a part, inflammation, progressive disease, general debility and acute pain. These factors may modify the type of brace or even make it inadvisable to recommend bracing.

The alignment of the brace with respect to the frontal plane should be such that (1) the foot is flat on the floor during standing and during the appropriate portions of the stance phase of walking, (2) the mechanical joints are congruous with anatomic joints, (3) the mechanical joints are oriented and horizontal and (4) the side bars conform to the contour of the limb. The midsagittal line is used for reference and the mechanical joints are aligned perpendicular to it. Also, the calf and thigh bands should be horizontal. In the traverse plane alignment, the mechanical ankle joint must be set in accordance with the amount of tibial torsion. This is especially important when free ankle joints are used. Toe-out is normally about 15 degrees and is treated separately by attaching the shoe or foot plate at the proper angle.

Components

Shoes.   A good sturdy shoe is an important prerequisite for a brace. A nonresilient sole material such as oak leather is preferred. There should be a steel shank between the inner and outer sole extending from $\frac{1}{2}$ inch posterior to the plantar aspect of the calcaneus to about $\frac{1}{4}$ inch posterior to the toe break. The counter should extend medially to a point midway between the anterior aspect of the heel and the break of the shoe. The type of shoe depends upon factors such as the amount of the ankle motion, the degree of spasticity, appearance and the ability of the patient to reach down and fasten the shoe. The low quarter Blucher type of shoe is excellent for flaccid conditions and for foot deformities, with or without a brace. Strong spasticity makes it difficult to put on this shoe. A high quarter Blucher shoe may be used in some cases. A high quarter shoe laced to the toe is very useful in spastic conditions. It is called the "surgical" or "pedestrian" type. If necessary, the back of the shoe may be opened to facilitate putting it on and then it is called the "convalescent" type of shoe. It is helpful for an ankylosed or limited motion ankle. For patients with a stiff hip or reduced finger dexterity the shoe may be closed with a strap and buckle, Velcro elastic goring or a clip type fastener.

Various modifications may be added to the basic shoe, including metatarsal pads, metatarsal bars, rockers bars, toe spreaders, sole wedges, heel wedges, scaphoid pads, Thomas heels, medial longitudinal arch supports, Whitman plates, Denver heels or bars and Morton toe extensions.

For reduction of the shock of heel strike for hemiplegics or those with painful heels a so-called "SACH heel" may be made. It absorbs shock, gives pseudoplantar flexion on heel strike and decreases the shock at the calf band and at the top of the brace during ischial weight bearing. This heel may be made up by a shoe repairman using layers of soft and hard (21 and 18 irons) neoprene and ending with $\frac{1}{4}$ inch rubber strapping.

Shoe and Foot Attachments. The solid stirrup type ankle is the most commonly used. It is light and durable and comes in various sizes. It may be used for any type of ankle joint control—free, limited stops or spring loaded. The stirrup may be split at the bottom to permit change of shoes, but this type is heavier, thicker and less durable than the solid stirrup.

The round caliper type is the simplest, easiest to install and lightest. It permits simple shoe exchange and is easy to put on. The main drawback is that the mechanical joint is far inferior to the anatomic joint. This becomes relatively important if there is much range of motion at the ankle.

The foot plate of stainless steel with stirrup attachment gives more control of the foot and better foot support. The joints are well matched and interchange of shoes is simple. On the other hand, it is difficult to get a good comfortable fit and a larger shoe may be needed. The molded sandal with stirrups gives maximal foot control. It, too, is difficult to make and fit for comfort.

Ankle Joints and Controls. A free ankle joint permits full plantar flexion and dorsiflexion but furnishes lateral stability. Limited motion in either plantar flexion or dorsiflexion can be provided. The ankle joint may be spring loaded to assist dorsiflexion, or the assist may be reversed. An example is the Klenzak ankle. It helps in dorsiflexion during the swing phase and decreases the impact load at heel strike. A solid ankle joint can be provided if necessary.

Uprights. The uprights may be of stainless steel, an aluminum alloy (Dural) or carbon steel. The stainless steel upright is about three times as strong as the aluminum but is about three times as heavy. The type of material used depends upon the amount of spasticity present, the weight and strength of the patient and the type of activity in which he engages. The calf bands are 1½ inches wide for adults and ¾ inch wide for children of about four years of age or less.

Knee Joints with Lock. The most commonly used knee joint is the lap joint with a drop ring lock. The lock is simple and sturdy, and is usually placed on the lateral bar. It is difficult to lock and unlock in the presence of spasticity. Cosmetically it is poor and it tends to tear clothing. Unlocking is done manually and a retention button can be used to prevent locking until it is desired. The drop lock may be spring loaded with a thigh level control for unlocking. This reduces the need for bending forward at the hip in order to unlock the knee, but it, too, is difficult to control in presence of severe spasticity.

A cam lock with a bail may be used if there is severe spasticity. It locks and unlocks simultaneously on both bars. It is spring loaded for locking and the bail unlocks the joint when the patient presses it against a chair as he backs up to it. A plunger type of lock with thigh level control that can be unlocked with minimal force is available. Locking is done by a spring. This type is of poor durability and cannot be contoured in the plunger area. In addition, it is difficult to operate when flexion forces are in play. The joint is the clevis (box) type.

Hip Joints and Pelvic Band. The hip joint may be of the lap or clevis type. Motions may be free with a 180 degree stop. Abduction, adduction and rotation control are aided by the hip joint. A drop (ring) lock may be used and this gives control of flexion and extension.

The pelvic band is contoured to the patient and should extend anteriorly to grasp the anterior superior spine and posteriorly to a point just lateral to the post superior spine. When both legs are braced a bilateral pelvic band is necessary. The pelvic band is continuous across the back of the sacrum and is kept low to help control the hips. For maximal hip control a Hessing type of pelvic band is used. This is a double pelvic band with one bar over the iliac crest and the other between the crest and trochanter. It is hinged posteriorly. It is difficult to fit, requiring the making of a body cast.

Ischial Weight Bearing Devices. Ischial weight bearing can be provided in a brace by the use of an ischial ring, an ischial band or a quadrilateral socket. The ischial ring is simplest to fabricate. It is made of ¼ inch steel which is padded and it is easy to adjust but does not give complete weight bearing since the surface for weight bearing is too small.

The ischial band has a greater area for support.

The best solution for full weight relief is a quadrilateral socket which is made of plastic, leather or wood. It may be hinged to facilitate putting the brace in place. The disadvantage of the quadrilateral socket is its expense.

For absolute avoidance of weight bearing on the leg a Patten bottom is necessary so that the foot does not touch the ground but the weight is transmitted directly by the brace to the ischial tuberosity. With such an arrangement the sound leg must be elevated.

Indications for Bracing

Lower Motor Neuron Disorders. Flaccid paralyses and pareses occur in patients with poliomyelitis, nerve root and nerve trunk injury, polyneuropathy and meningomyelocele. Patterns of involvement are usually asymmetric and varied. Fascial tightness is a factor in addition to muscle paralysis or weakness, particularly in poliomyelitis. Areas commonly involved are the plantar fascia, iliotibial band and lumbodorsal fascia. Fixed or functional deformities are common and may be due to muscle imbalance, fascial tightness or prolonged improper positioning. Functional deformities easily become fixed if preventive measures are not taken. Deformities develop more rapidly and are more severe in growing children.

Because of the muscle weakness, often generalized, and the lack of spasticity in these patients the braces must be light in weight. Springloaded ankle joints are frequently advisable. Since the joints retain fairly good range of motion, congruence of the mechanical and anatomic joints is important.

For the common problem of peroneal nerve injury a single posterior spring type brace, a wire spring brace with calf band or a bar brace may be used. The bar brace may be single or double bar with a plantar flexion stop at 90 degrees or a dorsiflexion spring assist. When the gastrocnemius and soleus muscles are weakened, a heel lift may suffice to protect the calf muscles. For combined weaknesses of anterior and posterior leg musculature the type of brace and the components needed depend upon an analysis of the specific foot deformities and the results of a careful manual muscle test.

Bracing for the knee joint may be necessary to prevent recurvatum or flexion contracture. If the quadriceps is strong usually no brace is required. If the quadriceps is weak but the hip extensors are strong, the brace should consist of a double-bar long leg brace with 180 degree knee stop, without lock, to prevent recurvatum. If muscle power is sufficient to lock the knee in extension, a knee cap, an elastic or spring-loaded extension assist, shallow calf and thigh bands and a knee lock are added. This brace is also suitable if recurvatum of less than 20 degrees has already occurred.

For flexion contracture surgical correction should be considered. When hip and knee extensors are strong no brace is required, but if they are weak, knee and pelvic support is needed.

Bracing is not ordinarily used for specific muscle weakness about the hip. However, if the patient is wearing a long leg brace for some other reason, an ischial seat or pelvic band or both may be added. Patients who wear bilateral long leg braces need a pelvic band.

Progressive Muscular Dystrophy.   Children with progressive muscular dystrophy are prone to contractures of the heel cord, iliotibial band and flexors of the hip and knee. Variable and unpredictable muscular weakness increases. A brace that is light in weight is particularly important to help keep the child active. In the early stages of the disease, components such as offset knee joints, spring-loaded ankles or extension assists may be used to encourage motion. In later phases, motor assist at the joints must be replaced by locks. For moderately severe contractures at the hip, knee and ankle, surgical correction followed by bracing as necessary should be considered. For knee flexion contracture of more than 45 degrees and hip flexion contracture of more than 40 degrees, no surgical or bracing treatment is advisable.

Hemophilia.   Braces are used for patients with hemophilia for protection against hemorrhage resulting from excess motion, for stabilization of fixed deformities and traumatized joints and for correction of deformity. The fit of the brace is extremely important and plaster models are used as fabrication guides. Mechanical joint axes must coincide with anatomic joint axes. Joint congruency should be checked by x-ray with the brace in place. The forces involved must be distributed over large areas, thus requiring long molded cuffs. The Lofstrand joint (spring-loaded polycentric joint) is used for knee flexion deformity of less than 25 degrees. For posterior displacement of the proximal tibia, a subluxation hinge or a calf band with anterior-posterior sliding adjustment may be used.

Cerebral Palsy. About 60 per cent of all cerebral palsy patients belong to the spastic (pyramidal) group. A positive Babinski sign, ankle and patellar clonus, hyper-reflexia, the exaggerated stretch reflex, the clasp-knife phemomenon and a tendency for contractures to develop characterize this category. Hemiplegia is frequently a manifestation. In spasticity the deforming factors are the strong or spastic muscles. Bracing may be used to improve function and to prevent deformity. Manual muscle testing is an important aid in assessing the need for bracing.

A good shoe is the basis for a leg brace. A high-top shoe is needed for all of these children who have tight heel cords and who require bracing. The shoe must fit the heel snugly and an extra strap may be added across the dorsum of the foot to hold the forepart of the foot in place. A foot plate in the shoe is needed except for patients who have mild equinus which can be stretched passively to 80 degrees and who can place their heels on the floor when standing. A T-strap is required when valgus or varus is not controlled by the brace.

A short leg brace is used for control and not for support. It may be single or double bar with a split stirrup or a round caliper type shoe attachment. The single upright and round caliper brace has the advantage of permitting the shoe to be put on first and then the brace fitted to the shoe. The caliper may be easily bent to allow for a valgus or varus deformity without changing the alignment of the ankle joint. This Phelps type brace (Fig. 4-8) comes in different sizes so that the orthotist should be able to fit the brace quickly and inexpensively. The offset ankle joint (Pope) has the advantage of being adjustable so that correction of a fixed equinus deformity can be obtained gradually.

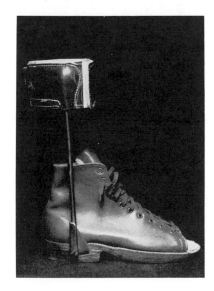

Figure 4–8 Phelps brace used as a night brace. The shoe can be put on first and the brace attached later. Dorsiflexion can be altered by bending the round caliper. It is easy to accommodate for valgus and varus deformity. Note that Velcro replaces the buckler and strap. (From Stamp, W. G.: Bracing in Cerebal Palsy. J. Bone Joint Surg., *44A*:1457–1476, 1962.

Children who walk on their toes in the morning but are able to place their heels on the floor later in the day need night splints, either a brace worn at night (with the toes of the shoe cut out and a large sock worn over the shoe) or a plaster splint.

Long leg braces for the lower extremity are usually double upright braces. This type of brace is necessary for the correction of deformity. However, if the purpose of bracing is merely to control deformity, the single upright brace is adequate. A single-bar brace is easier to fit on the patient; it accommodates flexion and angulation deformities at the knee more easily. In children with flexion deformities of the knees, the dial lock may be used (Fig. 4–9). After the contracture is relieved the mechanical knee joint can be made movable by adjusting the lock.

The type of knee lock used depends upon the manual dexterity of the patient. For many the simple ring lock is adequate. A bail lock is more satisfactory for others. Some patients need a hip level release (Warm Springs type) lock.

Genu valgum can be controlled by a strap or a leather button on the medial upright to apply pressure over the medial femoral condyle. Medial femoral torsion may require the use of a twister in the form of an elastic band or a cable device. The double upright brace can frequently be avoided if the single-bar upright brace is attached to a pelvic band. There are several antiscissoring devices which may be applied to braces if needed.

There is controversy regarding bracing for patients with athetosis. The primary problem is generalized involuntary movement in the trunk and extremities. Secondary problems are weakness and varying degrees of loss of motor

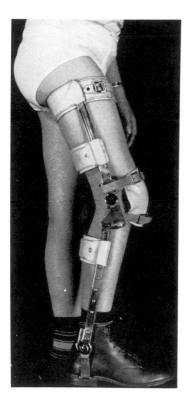

Figure 4–9 Long brace with a dial lock at the knee used to reduce knee-flexion contracture. As the contracture is reduced, tension can easily be altered by changing the position of the bolt in the dial lock. (From Stamp, W. G.: Bracing in Cerebral Palsy. J. Bone Joint Surg., *44A*:1457–1476, 1962.

control. Fixed deformities are not usually found. For young children with moderate or severe athetosis, bilateral double-bar long leg braces with spinal bracing may be used initially. With increased control and maturity the trunk bracing may be removed. For the overall picture, the surgical correction of deformities should be considered so that bracing can be minimized.

Fractures. Bracing may be used for fractures for support and stabilization of nonunion, for control of angular, torsional and compressive stresses, to protect the healing fracture while at the same time permitting joint function or to permit mobilization of the patient without the necessity of a heavy cast. A brace has the advantage of being light in weight, of permitting joints to be mobilized if desirable and of permitting good skin hygiene.

Specific components for the brace depend upon the location of fracture, whether the brace is to transmit the body weight or not and which joints are to be immobilized. Generally a double-bar long leg brace with a free or limited ankle joint, knee joints and locks and calf and thigh bands is required. An ischial band or quadrilateral seat may be added to decrease the weight bearing load on the leg. For patients with Legg-Perthes' disease a Patten bottom, which eliminates any weight transmission through the hip joint, may be added.

Spastic Hemiplegia. In the adult chronic phase of hemiplegia the involved leg is generally spastic. The foot tends to twist into equinovarus when it is not bearing weight and into equinovalgus when it is bearing weight. The hip rotates externally and the thigh adducts.

In cases in which flaccidity persists, a light brace such as those used for footdrop may be employed. When spasticity is present, the equinus may be accommodated with a heel lift. Valgus may be corrected by a long counter in the shoe, a scaphoid pad, a medial heel wedge or a valgus-correcting strap on a short leg brace. A single- or double-bar short leg brace with a plantar flexion stop at 90 degrees is usually indicated. If the knee tends to buckle when it bears weight the foot may be set in slight equinus.

Occasionally a hemiplegic patient requires knee bracing and a double-bar long leg brace with a medial drop lock at the knee is used. Usually the calf and thigh bands are open and a knee cap is provided. Some physicians prefer to use extensive bracing at the beginning and later cut the brace down. Others prescribe limited bracing, usually with a short leg brace. The brace is to be worn until the patient has control of dorsiflexion and eversion of the foot.

Arthritis. In arthritis, joint pain is often the primary factor limiting function. Fixed deformities can cause abnormal pressure distribution which leads to pain and stiffness. In the foot consideration must be given to restriction of motion of the intertarsal joints, by placing a steel shank or a molded rigid foot plate in the shoe. Pressure must be redistributed by the use of pads, supports, wedges and so forth for the relief of pain. In the subtalar joint there may be limited range of motion because of pain, along with the frequent occurrence of pes valgus and peroneal muscle spasm. For most cases a high-top shoe with a low heel is helpful. For severe cases a double-bar short leg brace to restrict subtalar motion is necessary if arthrodesis is contraindicated.

A short leg brace with a fixed or limited motion ankle joint is helpful when arthritic pain causes limited ankle function. Pressures can be reduced at the ankle by using a patellar tendon bearing type of anterior band. Experience has indicated that arthritis patients object to the use of braces even though they provide symptomatic relief.

The knee joint is involved frequently in arthritis. Pain leads to weakness, atrophy and muscle spasm. A feeling of "giving way" is a common complaint. There is swelling, genu varum or genu valgum and flexion deformity. The problem is to stabilize the knee joint and prevent motion during weight bearing, to prevent further deformity and joint instability and, if necessary, to relieve weight from the joint (e.g., during recovery from infectious arthritis) by means of an ischial weight bearing brace. This type is generally a double-bar long leg brace with a knee lock, an ankle joint if there is no ankle involvement, a medial or lateral knee pad for genu varum or valgum and a knee cap if necessary for flexion contracture or for complete stabilization. If the knee is neuropathic, fusion is desirable. The use of a long molded cuff without a knee joint helps to prevent knee motion. Various devices have been used to give some medial-lateral knee support. This may simply be an elastic bandage or a laced elastic knee support with side hinges.

Hip bracing in arthritis is seldom done and rarely effective. The use of canes or crutches is a more effective and more comfortable method for unloading the hip. Weight bearing relief at the hip is difficult to obtain in the adult.

TRUNK BRACING

Spinal braces have been used widely for hundreds of years. They have developed necessarily on an empirical basis. In spite of modifications of fitting and the use of new materials, many back braces are totally useless.

Back braces may be corrective or supportive, and their objectives are relief of pain, protection from further injury, prevention and correction of deformity, and help for muscle weakness. They may be rigid or flexible and are made of a combination of leather, metal, plastic, rubber and cloth.

Biomechanics

The spinal column acts as an elastic vertical rod for maintaining an upright position of the body. Its intrinsic stability is provided by its disc and ligamentous support, while its extrinsic stability depends upon muscular support. The spine is quite flexible primarily because of the intervertebral discs. The combined intrinsic and extrinsic support of the spinal column permits it to withstand the large compression, shearing, twisting and bending forces which are encountered many times each day.

When the annulus fibrosus is intact, the elastic limits by compressive forces cannot be exceeded without vertebral fracture. The endplate is most susceptible, and next to give way is the vertebral body.

The ability of the spine to withstand the numerous forces playing upon it can best be explained by describing the spine as a segmental elastic column supported by the paraspinal muscles, attached to the sides and located within the abdominal and thoracic cavities. The trunk musculature converts these cavities into rigid-walled cylinders capable of transmitting forces developed in loading the spine and thus relieving the pressure on the spine itself.[3]

Morris et al.[8] showed that the larger the weight lifted, the greater the activity of the muscles of the trunk, chest and abdomen. The force on the lumbrosacral disc during lifting was calculated to be 30 per cent less because of the cavitary pressures, and the load on the lower thoracic spine was about 50 per cent less than it would have been without trunk support. A tight corset about the abdomen leads to less thoracic and abdominal muscular activity when lifting. This indicates that the effect of these muscles can be at least partially replaced by external support.

The use of spinal appliances has effects on the gait and on energy expenditure. A patient wearing an appliance that restricts axial rotation of the spine takes shorter steps and a slower pace in order to walk comfortably, keep good balance and to lessen the increased energy requirements. There is the additional tendency in the use of a spinal appliance for spinal motion to be increased in the segments adjacent to the end of the device. This may cause pain and may require extension of the brace well above and below the involved area in order to relieve this discomfort.

Types of Special Appliances

There are confusing numbers of spinal appliances available. It appears that each physician, each clinic and each part of the country has its own favorite brace. With the exception of the hyperextension brace, all the appliances depend partially on compression to accomplish their aim. It can be assumed that abdominal compression in spinal support is the major factor in the relief from back pain. Another factor, which appears to be minor, is decrease in lumbar lordosis.

Corsets. A corset is an encircling garment having vertical or horizontal metal stays. It generally encases the region between the pubis and just above the lower ribs. It is made of woven fabric, such as canvas or duck, combined with rubber, fiberglass or metal.

The physician should prescribe the height of the back of the corset when he desires stiff or rigid stays for added support. The chief indication for a corset is low back pain. The corset should be prescribed and checked by the physician. Corsets may also be prescribed to help support weakened muscles, and to limit joint motion in the spine. A corset should be worn when the patient is out of bed and active. In patients with acute low back pain the corset may give relief if worn day and night.

Generally, women prefer corsets for cosmetic reasons and men prefer braces. In reality, the full-length corset and brace are interchangeable and both can be adapted to provide varying degrees of rigidity.

Rigid Braces. The rigid back brace is commonly used for back pain. It is an efficient method of obtaining abdominal compression with an anterior force and distributing the counterforce over a large area. Properly fitted, the rigid uprights are contoured to follow the lumbar curve.

It is frequently called the "chair-back" brace and has numerous variations. Basically it consists of a pelvic band located at a level between the greater trochanter and the iliac crest and a thoracic band located at the level of the eighth thoracic vertebra. These bands are joined by two posterior and two lateral metal uprights with a corset or apron front. The Knight spinal brace is frequently used but, as mentioned previously, there are many variations.

The long spinal brace is termed a dorsolumbar support. The Taylor brace is the prototype of the dorsolumbar type. It consists of a wide fitted pelvic band and two long posterior paraspinal uprights extending to the shoulders. The uprights are connected by a short transverse bar in the mid-thoracic region. Straps from the uprights pass over the shoulders and under the axillae to the transverse bar. A full-length abdominal apron is attached by straps and buckles.

Belts.   Belts are commonly used by men for conditions in which women usually wear corsets. A trochanteric belt is usually 2 to 3 inches wide and worn around the pelvis between the trochanters and the iliac crests. It may be used for support during healing of pelvic fractures.

Sacroiliac and lumbosacral belts are similar in design and function but differ in width. The sacroiliac belt is from 4 to 6 inches wide, whereas the lumbosacral belt is from 8 to 16 inches wide. These belts are useful for low back pain associated with disc disorders but do not provide sufficient immobilization for use after most spinal procedures.

Molded Jackets.   Molded jackets are made of plaster of paris, plastic or leather. They fit the contour of the body and help distribute pressure evenly. Jackets are particularly useful in providing spinal support for debilitated patients, such as those with severe osteoporosis or malignancy of the spine. Other patients benefitted by a molded jacket include those with severe deformities from congenital anomalies or from longstanding poliomyelitis.

Anterior Hyperextension Braces.   These braces consist of a modified rectangular metal frame which is fitted anteriorly so that pressure is exerted over the pubis and manubrium while counterpressure is maintained over the mid-back by means of a strap attached to the sides of the frame.

MANAGEMENT OF THE AMPUTEE

The "modern" approach to the rehabilitation of the amputee uses the combined efforts of the patient, the physician, the prosthetist and the therapist as a team. No single individual is expected to have expert knowledge in all these areas. Success is achieved by the "team approach" in which each member sees clearly his own function and that of each of the other members. The principal duties of the group are to consider each individual case and to follow through with appropriate measures at the proper times. The steps are prescription, fitting, training, evaluating and follow up. It has been clearly demonstrated that amputees under the care of a clinical team become far better adapted to return to their place in society than those not fortunate enough to receive such guidance and support.

UPPER EXTREMITY PROSTHETICS

In the rehabilitation of the upper extremity amputee, structural replacement poses a relatively easy task. Functional replacement by remote control and by substitute mechanical means is infinitely more difficult.

For the purpose of functional utility, remaining movements of upper arm, shoulder and torso must be harnessed, and use must be made of a variety of mechanical devices. Facility of control is the key to the ultimate value of the upper extremity prosthesis. The best prosthesis presently available is of little or no value to the amputee unless it is prescribed and fitted correctly, unless the patient has been correctly prepared physically and psychologically to receive it and unless he has received adequate training in its use. In order for the patient to return to as full a life as possible he must be trained to use his remaining abilities to the best effect and assisted back to employment.

It is obvious that all these goals cannot be attained by one individual and that a number of workers, each an expert in his own field, must work together in the care of each amputee. The concept of the team approach has evolved and been put into practice. Amputee clinics, consisting of the association of physicians, therapists, prosthetists, social service workers and vocational counselors, have been set up in many parts of our country.

Clinic procedures usually involve the following steps: preclinic examination; detailed prescription including surgical, physical and prosthetics factors; preprosthetic therapy; prosthetic fabrication; initial checkout to determine whether the fit, alignment and mechanical functions are such that training can be instituted; prosthetic training; final check-out to assure that the fit, alignment and appearance of the prosthesis are acceptable and that the amputee's use of the limb is satisfactory; and follow-up examination. Prescription, initial check-out and final check-out are the steps that require full clinic team participation.

Preparation for Amputation

When the decision for amputation has been made, it is the physician's duty to explain to the patient the necessity for operation, the extent of surgery and the deficit that will remain postoperatively. It is well to describe the plan for postoperative care, preprosthetic conditioning, fitting with a prosthesis and training in its use. In addition, the phenomenon of phantom sensation should be discussed.

Sites of Amputation

The trend has been toward more conservative surgery in amputations. Improved surgical techniques, use of antibiotics and the development of new prosthetic materials and devices have made this possible. With minor exceptions in the hand, every bit of length should be preserved in amputation of the upper extremity. In the phalanges, it is better to shorten the finger slightly rather than preserve the bulbous, tender distal expansions of these bones. In most cases the distal two-thirds of the second and fifth metacarpals should be excised when the corresponding finger must be amputated.

As a result of developments in prosthetics, patients with wrist disarticulations (preferably with resection of radial and ulnar styloid processes) can be fitted so that good function is obtained without there being extreme length of the prosthetic extremity. The Krukenberg amputation is one in which clawlike grasp is obtained by fashioning fingerlike appendages out of the forearm by separating the radius and ulna. It is seldom done in this country, but it offers the opportunity for preservation of sensation to the blind hand amputee. Cosmetically it is very poor.

Today there are no sites of election in upper extremity amputation. With the few exceptions mentioned, all possible length should be retained. The aim of the surgeon is to produce a firm tapered or cylindrical stump, free of sensitive scarring, with the bone well padded along its length and covered at its tip by nonadherent fascia and skin.

Postoperative Care

Prevention of joint contracture is of prime importance. The stump should be positioned in good posture and mobilized as soon as possible. Compression bandaging, which is started early to prevent hemorrhage or edema and to promote shrinkage, is continued until the prosthesis is fitted. All joints proximal to the amputation should be moved through their full ranges of motion at least three times a day as soon after amputation as possible. After the stump has healed, the patient is instructed and encouraged to exercise the residual muscles of the stump. Since the upper extremity amputee uses both shoulders for prosthesis operations the exercise program should involve the muscles of both shoulders. As soon as possible the exercise should be of the progressive resistive type. Some attention must be paid to posture since short above-elbow and shoulder disarticulation amputees are likely to have postural deviations which may be caused by loss of weight of the member.

The stump should be washed daily with soap and water and dried thoroughly. For normal stumps the application of alcohol or any other agent to "toughen" the skin is not recommended.

Prescription of Upper Extremity Prostheses

The artificial arm is but poor compensation for the living arm and sensitive hand. The arm prosthesis must therefore favor one or several capacities, depending on whether the chief concern is for cosmesis, heavy duty labor or skilled function. For this reason the prescription must be based upon a consideration of the patient's background, his physical and mental capacities and his future vocational needs.

Surgical reconstruction of the hand has advanced greatly the past few years. The fundamental difference between a reconstructed hand and any present-day hand prosthesis is that the former retains direct sensation. A hand prosthesis is of little use in the dark. Hence, it is generally desirable to preserve all hand structure that can reasonably be expected to have adequate nerve and blood supply (Fig. 4–10). Information on prostheses for partial hands is sparse and a resourceful, ingenious prosthetist is invaluable in fitting and adapting them to the patient's needs. The main points to remember are to keep the device simple and to apply it in such a way that it does not interfere appreciably with sensation (Figs. 4–11 and 4–12).

Terminal Device. Attempts to replace hand function have resulted in the fabrication of the prosthetic hand and the split hook. Because of the complex problems involved in even the simplest hand design, the split hook was developed as a simple substitute. There are two types of prehension control available. In one, called "voluntary-opening," power remaining in a controlling member opens the finger of the device (Fig. 4–13 A); when the force is released, a spring or its equivalent in rubber bands closes the fingers on objects to be grasped. In the other, called "voluntary-closing," the prosthesis is held open by a spring when the amputee is relaxed (Fig. 4–13 B). Application of a positive control force closes the fingers against the spring tension.

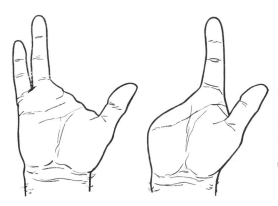

Figure 4–10 Examples of partial hands that require no prosthesis. When the thumb can work against one or more fingers, function is usually better than that obtained with a hand substitute. (From Bunnell, S.: The Management of the Non-Functional Hand — Reconstruction vs. Prosthesis. Artif. Limbs, 1957.)

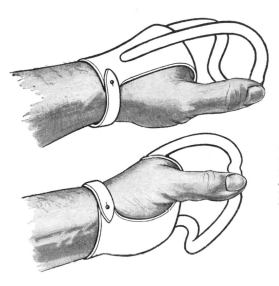

Figure 4–11 Prosthesis for transmetacarpal amputation. The socket may be of leather, molded plastic or hammered stainless steel. A metal ring covered with plastic is shaped to furnish one large hook representing the index finger and a small one representing the little finger. (Courtesy Robin-Aids Manufacturing Company, Vallejo, Calif.)

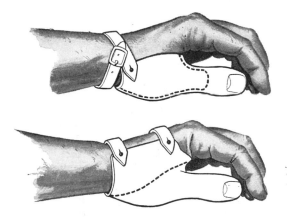

Figure 4–12 Prostheses for partial or complete loss of the thumb. The fingers work in opposition to fixed member. Above, prosthesis for amputation of thumb at metacarpophalangeal joint, with the thumb web deepened surgically to provide a cylindrical stump proximal to site of amputation. Below, variation suitable for amputation of thumb at carpometacarpal joint. (From Bunnell, S.: The Management of the Non-Functional Hand — Reconstruction vs. Prosthesis. Artif. Limbs, 1958.)

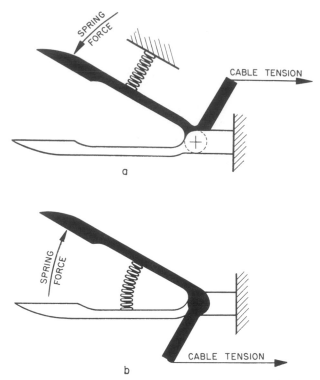

Figure 4–13 *a*. Voluntary-opening and *b*. voluntary-closing terminal devices. (From Klopsteg, P. E., and Wilson, P. D.: Human Limbs and Their Substitutes. New York, McGraw-Hill Book Co., 1954. Used by permission of McGraw-Hill Book Company.)

Voluntary-opening devices are the simplest form of prehension mechanism since they involve nothing more than a spring clamp, but they have several disadvantages. The amputee is just as unable to handle delicate objects as he is incapable of manipulating heavy ones. In addition, voluntary-opening is the opposite of the normal actions of prehension to which the amputee was accustomed with his natural arm and hand.

Much effort has been made to provide voluntary-closing devices that provide palmar prehension. This has resulted in the APRL (Army Prosthetics Research Laboratories) hand. In addition, a plastic glove has been developed that gives good cosmesis (Fig. 4–14).

Prehension in this device is of the three-jawed chuck type between the adjustable thumb and the movable index and middle fingers. The fingers adduct as they close. The ring finger and little finger are passive and flexible and so positioned as to look natural whether the active fingers are opened or closed. Although it is quite durable, the hand is not recommended for hard manual labor or for use under conditions that might damage its fine precision mechanisms. It should be used only with its mating cosmetic glove which not only gives it a natural appearance but also protects the mechanism from dust.

The APRL voluntary-closing hook (Fig. 4–15) consists of a camquadrant type of clutch, with an alternator type automatic lock operating one lyre-shaped finger against a fixed mating lyre-shaped finger. The operating cycle for the APRL hook is: pull to grasp; relax to lock; pull to release; relax to open.

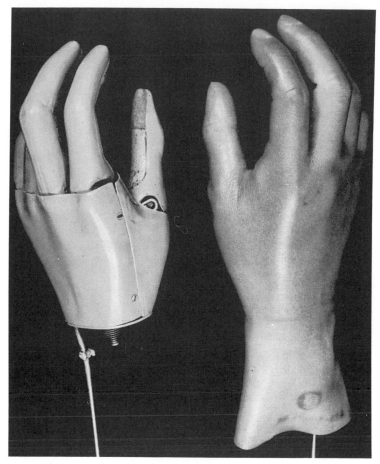

Figure 4–14 The APRL No. 4 C voluntary-closing artificial hand, with and without cosmetic glove. (Courtesy Armed Forces Institute of Pathology.)

To open the lock, the cable pull must be greater than the pull that closed the hook.

There are numerous voluntary-opening (VO) hooks in a variety of sizes, weights and shapes. The most common shapes are lyre or canted. The hooks are usually made of stainless steel or aluminum and are simple and strong. The prehension force is generally supplied by heavy rubber bands.

Wrist Units. Wrist units are needed to attach terminal devices to prostheses and, in addition, to provide terminal device rotation for manual positioning. They are made as manual friction, manual lock or active rotation units. The most commonly used is the manual friction type in which a metal washer bears against a rubber washer as the terminal device is screwed into place. It is not fully satisfactory but has the advantages of simplicity and easy maintenance.

Wrist Flexion Units. Wrist flexion units provide partial replacement of lost volar and dorsal flexion of the wrist. They increase the utility of prostheses, particularly for the bilateral amputee who must operate the terminal device close to the body. So far these units have been suitable only for light duty.

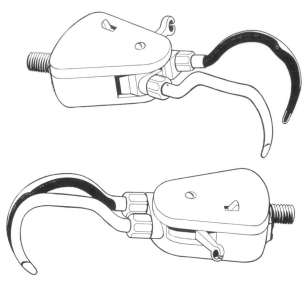

Figure 4–15   The APRL voluntary-closing hook. (From Klopsteg, P. E., and Wilson, P. D.: Human Limbs and Their Substitutes. New York, McGraw-Hill Book Co., 1954. Used by permission of McGraw-Hill Book Company.)

Elbow Hinges.   Flexion of below-elbow prostheses is provided by hinges of various types. The main classes are rigid, semirigid and flexible hinges (Fig. 4–16). They are made of metal, leather or metal cable. Some are step-up in type to provide greater range of motion for a short below-elbow amputee. In the case of a very short below-elbow stump a stump-actuated locking hinge may be used.

Prosthetic Elbow.   Elbow disarticulation, above-elbow and shoulder amputation prostheses usually provide forearm flexion by some type of joint that permits locking at various positions (Fig. 4–17). External elbows are used for elbow disarticulation prostheses and internal elbows are used for above-elbow and shoulder prostheses. The external elbows have five or seven locking positions; the internal type have 11 locking positions.

Shoulder Units.   Many joints for the shoulder have been tried in the past to provide flexion, abduction or elevation. These joints have been relatively unsuccessful. Passive abduction can be provided at the shoulder to facilitate dressing activities. A passive friction shoulder joint has been developed which permits about 60 degrees of angular rotation and has enabled test wearers to perform independent toileting which they were unable to do previously (Fig. 4–18).

Cable Control System.   Nearly all upper extremity prostheses are now controlled by stranded steel cables that glide inside a cable housing which frequently has a nylon liner. The figure-of-eight-shaped harness made of Dacron webbing is used frequently. However, the harness, suspension and kind of control used depend upon the type of amputation, the musculature and mobility of the amputee and his ability to use the system. Trial and error is necessary to achieve the goal of maximal efficiency with a minimum of equipment.

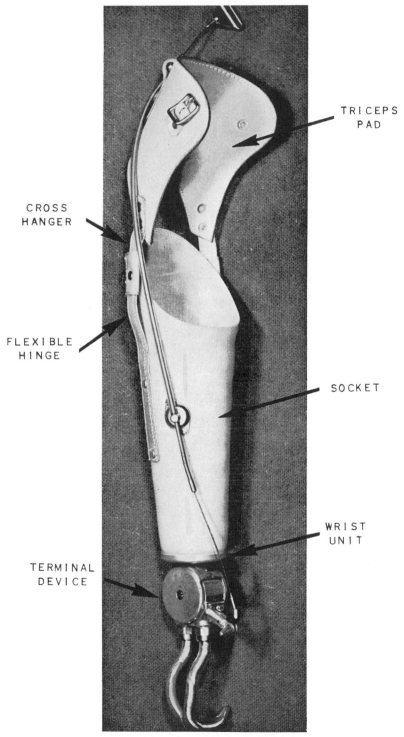

Figure 4–16 Long below-elbow prosthesis. (From Santschi, W. R.: Manual of Upper Extremity Prosthetics. 2nd Ed. Department of Engineering, University of California at Los Angeles, 1958.)

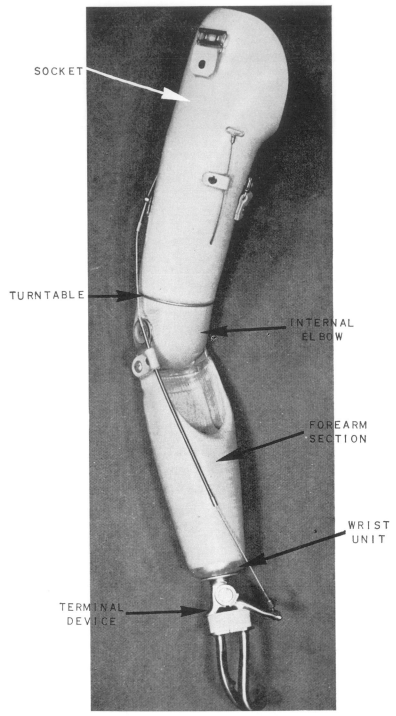

Figure 4–17   Standard above-elbow prosthesis. (From Santschi, W. R.: Manual of Upper Extremity Prosthetics. 2nd Ed. Department of Engineering, University of California at Los Angeles, 1958.)

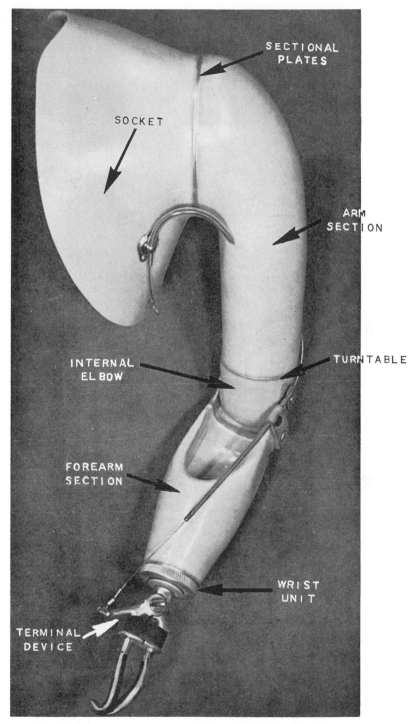

Figure 4–18 Shoulder disarticulation prosthesis. (From Taylor, C. L., In Santschi, W. R.: Manual of Upper Extremity Prosthetics. 2nd Ed. Department of Engineering, University of California at Los Angeles, 1958.)

Training

The unilateral arm amputee who retains complete function in the arm represents the majority of the upper extremity amputee population. The method or procedure of training must be designed to fit the type of amputation. The overall aim is to enable the amputee to become as self-sufficient as possible in all activities of daily living. The recommended "practical" approach is to train the unilateral amputee to use his prosthesis as a helper in two-handed activities.

The amputee is first taught how to put on and take off his prosthesis and how to adjust the harness. A stump sock of cotton, nylon or wool may or may not be worn depending upon amputee preference considering such factors as sweating, padding and warmth. The male amputee generally wears a T-shirt under the harness and some female amputees prefer to wear the harness over the blouse or dress. The amputee is taught correct prosthetic terminology and the characteristics of the prosthetic components. Next, the amputee is trained in the use of controls—terminal device, wrist unit, forearm, elbow lock, elbow motion and arm rotation.

Training in use follows. It involves pre-positioning and drills in approach, grasp and release. The final phase of training is the application of the procedures to useful tasks such as dressing, eating, toilet care, writing, household routines, driving and vocational activities.

It is difficult to select a length of time to use as a criterion for completion of training. Some amputees learn quickly, but others require more time because of differences in neuromuscular coordination, harness design, body configuration and other factors. At present, it is most practical to leave the decision as to when the amputee has had sufficient instruction to the individual conducting the training program.

Cineplasty

Cineplasty is the surgical procedure of providing a "muscle tunnel." It involves the construction of a skin-lined tube through a muscle in which, after healing has taken place, a pin can be inserted that can be linked to a terminal device. The use of cineplasty has been controversial since its inception. According to its advocates, it has the advantages of permitting reduction in harness and providing greater dexterity and sensibility, physiologic use of stump muscles rather than depending on remote sources of energy, and adequate grasping force on objects of varying sizes. Critics have emphasized inadequate force or excursion from many tunnels, frequent irritation or infection, fitting difficulties and the high percentage of unilateral amputees who have rejected cineplastic prostheses. The general consensus at present is that construction of a biceps tunnel for below-elbow amputees is a successful procedure, and it is recommended for carefully selected amputees in the care of a qualified prosthetic team.

LOWER EXTREMITY PROSTHETICS

Today the physician can "diagnose and prescribe" for the eventual welfare of the amputee in just the same way he would for any other patient. He can write a prescription that specifies all of the important factors decided upon as proper for the individual. He knows there is no single device or set of devices best for all patients and that a good prosthesis is one that will provide optimal function, comfort and cosmesis based on the patient's condition, vocation and desires.

Components

Foot and Ankle. The prosthetic foot has generally been a solid block to which the ankle joint and toe section are attached. Conventional models of ankle joints provide flexion and dorsal flexion only, with rubber bumpers to restrain and restore these motions. The axis consists of a horizontal shaft the outer ends of which rotate on plain bushings. Many variations have been tried. Lateral and transverse rotations are provided by rubber blocks or coil springs.

The SACH (Solid Ankle, Cushion Heel) foot is widely used at present. Rubber is molded or laminated over a "keel" of wood or metal. The foot permits inversion-eversion and plantar-dorsiflexion by compression of part of the foot. No ankle joint is used with it. The heel is made of layers of rubber of varying degrees of hardness. When the heel strikes, the rubber compresses and gives the appearance of ankle motion. The SACH foot is excellent cosmetically and it is the foot of choice for the wearing of high heels. The main disadvantage is the gradual loss of elasticity in the material used (Figs. 4-19 and 4-20).

Knee joints. Many prosthetic knees are available that partially satisfy the basic requirements of stability, gait, durability, comfort and cosmesis.

Stability for weight bearing is provided by the backward force the stump exerts within the socket. The prosthesis may be aligned so that the knee is placed in slight hyperextension during weight bearing or auxiliary mechanical aids, manual or automatic, may be added to stabilize the knee by locking it.

The types of prosthetic knees commercially available may be classified as constant friction, constant friction with friction lock, hydraulic and polycentric. The "conventional single axis" knee is low in initial cost and maintenance is simple. The friction or braking action does not vary during the swing phase of locomotion. The amount of friction may be increased or decreased by a simple adjustment.

If the amputee has impaired stump musculature, poor balance or generalized weakness, a knee joint that provides constant friction with a friction lock may be used. In this type the ends of the knee bolt are not fixed but are allowed to slide in a short slot. When the leg bears weight the shank comes closer to the socket and a braking surface of each segment makes contact and a "friction lock" has been formed. During the swing phase a spring holds the two braking surfaces apart. The primary advantage of this type of knee is its stability. It is commonly used by elderly amputees.

The other types of knees are not often used. The hydraulic knee, of which there are several models, permits an excellent gait, but it is highly complex and very expensive.

Knee Extension Stops and Extension Aids. Limitation of extension of the prosthetic knee is usually accomplished by a radial arm or projection fitted around the knee bolt and to the shank which stops the extension movements when the knee strikes it. The impact is usually lessened by a compressible bumper or cushion placed between the two parts. If the arm is made of spring

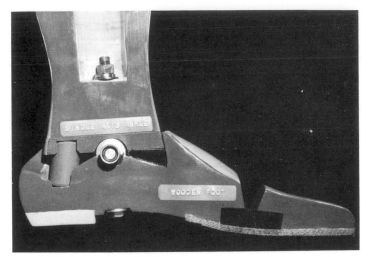

Figure 4–19   Conventional prosthetic foot. (Courtesy Dr. M. H. Anderson.)

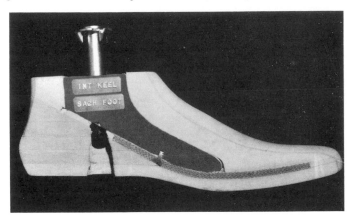

Figure 4–20   The solid ankle, cushion heel (SACH) foot. (Courtesy Dr. M. H. Anderson.)

steel it may also provide assistance in initiating knee flexion. When this principle is used the device is commonly referred to as a "hickory stick" kicker. It may also be designed to provide assistance in bringing the leg into full extension. An elastic strap in the back of the knee will assist in initiating knee flexion. An elastic strap in front of the knee will aid in extension, prevent excessive heel rise and aid slightly in maintaining knee stability during weight bearing.

Above-knee Sockets.   Sockets for above-knee prostheses are generally made of willow wood. Until recently the socket was shaped to the contour of the stump and called a "plug-fit" socket, and the body weight was borne on the tissues of the upper thigh over its entire circumference. With the development of the so-called "suction socket" the shape of the socket was changed to that of a "pressure" contour of the upper thigh and became roughly quadrilateral in shape.[10] The weight is borne more on the ischial tuberosity and gluteal muscle group. Most prescriptions now call for a quadrilateral-shaped wooden socket.

A recent development has been the "total contact socket" for above-knee amputees. In this type the stump is in complete contact with the socket even though the bulk of the weight is carried on the ischial tuberosity and the gluteal tissues. The socket is suspended by suction and the valve is flush with the inner wall of the socket. Claims are made that the amputee has better control of this socket, that he gets more "feedback" from it so that he knows more confidently the position of his artificial limb and that edema of the stump tends to disappear in a short time. Experience has proved the value of these sockets and they are used routinely today.

Suspension for Above-knee Prosthesis. Suspension may be provided by suction, the Silesian bandage, the pelvic belt, shoulder suspenders or a combination of methods. A Silesian bandage is a light webbing band with one end attached by a swivel connector to the lateral aspect of the socket in the region of the greater trochanter. The other end is attached to the socket anteriorly in the midline at a point level with the ischial seat. The belt rests between the crest of the ilium and the trochanter on the sound side. This device is a valuable aid in stabilizing the prosthesis against rotation and lateral instability. The Silesian bandage is sometimes used concurrently with suction.

The pelvic belt may be used with a rigid or flexible pelvic band. It has the advantage of being easy to put on and it gives the new amputee a greater feeling of security and allows him to use one or more stump socks, which in turn permits longer tolerable socket fit.

Prosthetic Prescription

Hip Disarticulation. This classification includes the true hip disarticulation and amputations as far as about 2 inches below the level of the perineum. In a hip disarticulation prosthesis, socket stability must be obtained at the pelvic level, energy for use of the limb must come from pelvic movement and weight must be borne by the pelvic area. This requires a prosthesis that can be suspended from the pelvis and that possesses hip and knee joints that are reasonably stable during standing and capable of permitting the amputee to walk, sit or stand with minimal discomfort, minimal energy cost and maximal cosmesis. The Canadian type hip disarticulation prosthesis (Fig. 4-21) comes nearest to meeting these requirements.

Short Above-knee Stump. This division includes stumps from 2 inches below the perineum to the upper border of the middle third of the thigh. Socket stability and energy must come mainly from the pelvic area and the optimal weight bearing area is the ischial tuberosity and the gluteal fold. Some stumps may permit suction suspension. The prosthesis used is an ischial weight bearing socket, auxiliary suspension plus suction, if possible, with adequate knee stability.

Mid-thigh Stump. A mid-thigh stump results from amputation at any point within the middle third of the thigh. Socket stability is usually obtained from the femoral area, with the use of suction suspension. Power comes from flexion-extension of the hip. Weight is borne on the ischial tuberosity and the gluteal fold. Prescription calls for an ischial weight bearing socket with suspension by suction or auxiliary suspension. Moderate knee stability is needed.

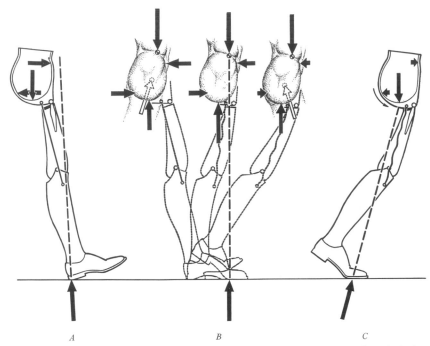

Figure 4–21 Anteroposterior force diagram of the Canadian type hip disarticulation prosthesis. A. Forces acting on prosthesis at heel contact. B. Forces acting on stump at heel contact, mid-stance and push-off. C. Force acting on prosthesis at push-off. (From Radcliffe, C. W.: The Biomechanics of the Canadian Type Hip Disarticulation Prosthesis. Artif. Limbs, 1957.)

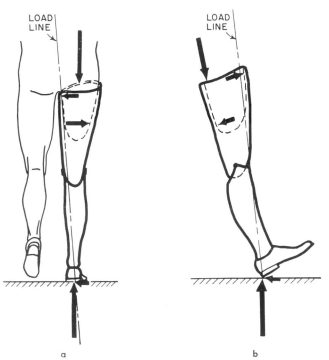

Figure 4–22 Forces acting upon typical above-knee prosthesis during the stance phase. (From Klopsteg, P. E., and Wilson, P. L.: Human Limbs and Their Substitutes. New York, McGraw-Hill Book Co., Inc., 1954. Used by permission of McGraw-Hill Book Company.)

Long Above-knee Stump. This stump ends below the middle of the thigh but it is not capable of end bearing. Socket stability is obtained in the femoral area with suction suspension and power comes from flexion-extension of the hip and has the advantage of the longer lever arm and longer muscles. Weight is borne on the ischial tuberosity and the gluteal fold (Fig. 4–22). An ischial weight bearing socket with suspension by suction (or auxiliary) suspension is prescribed. Minimal knee stability is necessary.

End Bearing Above-knee Stump. This group includes the various amputations at and above the knee which yield an end bearing stump: the Gritti, Kirk, Callander, epicondylar, supracondylar and others. Socket stability is supplied by both the femoral area and the end bearing stump. Weight is divided between the stump end and the ischial-gluteal area. This stump yields the maximum of power for use of an above-knee prosthesis. Prescription of this prosthesis includes an ischial weight bearing socket with provision for partial end bearing suction (or auxiliary) suspension and minimal knee stability.

Short Below-knee Stump. This includes stumps with not more than 2 inches of the tibia remaining. Stability of the socket is dependent on accurate fitting of the stump plus side hinges and a thigh corset if necessary. Weight bearing surfaces are the patellar ligament, the flares of the tibial condyles and the anteromedial wall of the tibia. If necessary a thigh corset can support part of the weight load and, if needed, ischial weight bearing can be provided. Power is provided by the quadriceps and hamstring muscles.

Standard Below-knee Stump. These stumps end at any point from 2 inches below the top of the tibia to the muscle-tendinous juncture of the

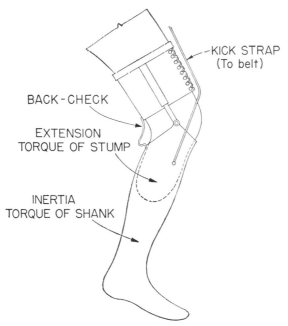

Figure 4–23 Conventional below-knee prosthesis with back check and kick strap, side joint and thigh corset. (From Klopsteg, P. E., and Wilson, P. D.: Human Limbs and Their Substitutes. New York, McGraw-Hill Book Co., Inc., 1954. Used by permission of McGraw-Hill Book Company.)

gastrocnemius. Stability, power and weight bearing are derived from the knee area. The patellar-tendon bearing (PTB) prosthesis appears to be the best below-knee prosthesis at this time (Figs. 4-23 and 4-24).

Below-knee Sockets.   The conventional below-knee prosthesis, in which the socket was a plug fit and weight bearing and suspension were provided by side joints and a thigh lacer, was used almost universally for over 200 years. The development of the patellar-tendon bearing prosthesis (PTB) was the result of a conference of leading prosthetists at the University of California at Berkeley in 1957. The original description of the PTB prosthesis was for a plastic laminate socket formed over a modified plaster-of-paris model of the stump. It contained a soft inner lining that contacted the entire surface of the stump. The weight was borne mainly by the medial flare of the tibia and the patellar tendon. Suspension was provided by a fabric strap around the thigh just above the femoral condyles.

The PTB concept has gained widespread acceptance and today the PTB socket is considered standard for below-knee amputations. Recently, modifications have been introduced as improvements to the basic concept.[18]

The Hard Socket.   The original PTB socket had a liner of leather or plastic backed by sponge rubber. The plastic did not allow the moisture to escape and

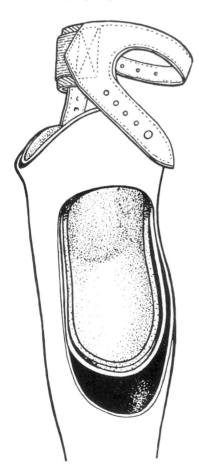

Figure 4-24   Cutaway view of the patellar-tendon bearing socket incorporated in a thin-walled plastic shank. Note especially the cuff-suspension strap, the high lateral and medial wall, and the total contact features. (From Murphy, E. F., and Wilson, A. B., Jr.: Anatomical and Physiological Considerations in Below-knee Prosthetics. Artif. Limbs, 6:4–15, 1962.)

the leather quickly rotted from perspiration. A trial of elimination of the liner proved to be successful and now the hard PTB socket is widely used.

THE PTS SOCKET.   The suspension strap was satisfactory in most cases but improved suspension was desired. The proximal border of the socket was extended above the femoral condyles and the patella and this was found to suspend the limb adequately. This is known as the PTS socket. It may be used with or without a liner.

WEDGE SUSPENSION SOCKET.   A small wedge inserted between the proximal area of the socket and the area of the stump along the medial condyle of the femur proved to suspend the limb satisfactorily. It is known as the supra-condylar-wedge suspension and is normally used with a hard socket.

AIR CUSHION SOCKET.   The air cushion PTB consists of an elastic inner sleeve suspended from the level of the tibial tubercle in a rigid outer sheet that is closed distally. Tension of the sleeve and compression of the air in the chamber between the inner and outer layers produce stump support. This socket has been found to be particularly helpful in patients with very tender stumps. More time is required to make this socket and little modification can be made after fabrication.

POROUS SOCKET.   Problems of perspiration have led to much effort to develop a satisfactory porous plastic laminate. Early porous laminates were too weak for lower extremity application. However, with the use of epoxy resins, a porous laminate socket can be made suitable for below-knee sockets. Problems with perspiration are minimized and the socket is lighter in weight.

CASTING METHODS.   For fabricating the PTB socket the stump is wrapped with plaster and shaped by hand. The male mold is further modified and the socket is cast over the mold. A number of attempts have been made to simplify this procedure.

In the suspension-casting technique, the stump is wrapped while it is held in a vertical position that simulates weight bearing during standing. Felt pads to provide relief for sensitive area of the stump are applied directly to the stump. A synthetic rubber, Polysar X414* has been found to have properties that make it suitable for forming a socket directly over the stump. Temporary or provisional below-knee prostheses made of this material are proving to be useful. Polysar X414 becomes pliable at temperatures tolerated by the skin and can be applied directly over the stump.

Ankle Disarticulation.   The Syme's amputee has lost the foot and ankle but retains essentially the full length of the shank and weight bearing characteristics that approach those of the normal heel. The problem is to restore the equivalent of foot and ankle function, to extend the stump to accommodate the loss of the tarsus and of the calcaneus, to furnish adequate body support during walking and standing, to provide suitable suspension for the prosthesis during the swing phase and to do all these things so that the final result is acceptable to the wearer.

The Canadian type Syme prosthesis ("Plastic Syme") is a vast improvement over the older type because it is lighter in weight, is stronger, requires less maintenance, is less expensive and is much improved in appearance (Fig. 4-25). The socket is made from laminated fiber glass or plastic-impregnated nylon stockinet; there is no ankle joint and the foot is of the SACH type. This

*Registered trademark of Polysar Corp. Ltd.

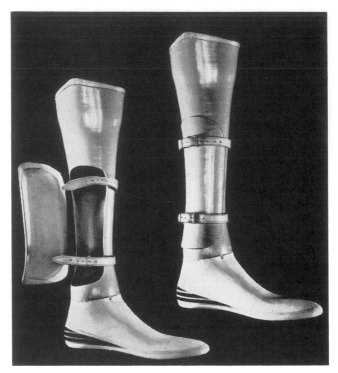

Figure 4–25 Syme prosthesis developed by the Veterans Administration Prosthetics Center, New York. The nylon-Dacron-polyester socket is provided with an opening in the medial wall. Weight bearing may be divided in any proportion between the proximal rim and the distal portions of the socket. (From Wilson, A. B., Jr.: Prosthetics for Syme's Amputation. Artif. Limbs, 6:52–75, 1961.)

prosthesis permits full or partial end bearing, depending upon the tolerance of the stump.

It must be emphasized here that Syme's amputation is indicated for all destructive, infective or other disabling lesions of the foot that cannot be dealt with by a transmetatarsal amputation. Lisfranc's and Chopart's amputations are apt to be unsatisfactory.

Transtarsal Amputation.   Transtarsal amputations are to be avoided.

Transmetatarsal Amputation.   No prosthesis is necessary for transmetatarsal amputees. There is an excellent surface for weight bearing and a regular shoe can be worn. The front of the shoe may be stuffed with lambs wool or some other material and covered with leather. To aid in toe-off a plate of spring metal is placed between the inner and outer sole.

Toe Amputation.   Loss of the small toes leads to no particular gait difficulty. Absence of the great toe, however, prevents a good gait in rapid walking because of loss of toe-off. Here again the front of the shoe can be stuffed and a spring metal plate placed between the soles of the shoe.

Treatment of the Lower-extremity Amputee

Preoperative Care of the Leg Amputee. Before surgery the patient should be prepared psychologically as well as physically for the procedure to guard against needless anxieties and to help him withstand the psychologic trauma of amputation. The patient wants to know the level of amputation, how he will look and how disabled he will be. Before or soon after surgery he should be told about phantom limb sensation. The steps in his rehabilitation program should be outlined to him and he should be given an estimate of the time it will require.

Early Postoperative Care. The first three postoperative days are often uncomfortable ones for the amputee. By the fourth day steps should be taken to prevent contractures. The aim is to prevent abduction, flexion and external rotation at the hip and flexion deformity at the knee. The amputee is taught to lie flat with no pillow under the stump, to lie face down part of the day and to keep his pelvis level. Prolonged sitting in a wheelchair especially during the first 10 days after surgery should be avoided. The same care must be taken even though the amputee is not considered to be a candidate for a prosthesis.

Preprosthetic Training. General conditioning exercises may be started three to five days after surgery. Crutch walking is begun as soon as feasible. After the sutures are removed the patient is taught stump bandaging, a program of specific exercises for the stump and stump hygiene.

Fitting of the Prosthesis. The clinic team—physician, prosthetist, therapist and vocational counselor—decide on the limb for the amputee. Each in his own field can point out factors that should be considered in prosthesis selection. The patient's readiness for fitting is determined by many factors, such as the rapidity of healing, the presence of complications, his general condition and his ability to use crutches.

Experience has shown that the amputee who can swing through in crutch walking and can negotiate stairs on crutches will use an artificial limb satisfactorily. If the economic factors were eliminated these patients could be fitted and trained very early. However, in three to six months a new socket would be needed. The amputee is usually measured by the prosthetist 8 to 10 weeks after surgery. By this time most of the stump shrinkage will have taken place and only minor changes will be necessary to keep the socket well fitted.

At the Hospital of the University of Pennsylvania we have found a number of patients who, although they never learned to use crutches, learned to use an artificial leg in a satisfactory fashion. The energy cost of using a prosthesis, with or without the assistance of crutches or canes, is less than that required for using crutches alone.

Prosthetic Training. Training in the use of his prosthetic limb is an important aspect of the rehabilitation of an amputee. Occasionally an individual is able to learn on his own but certainly this is not to be recommended. A set of parallel bars and a full length mirror are needed for training. Stairs and ramps can usually be found nearby although it is handy to have them in the gymnasium. An exercise mat is helpful for exercising and for practicing falling and getting up.

Training begins with instruction in how to put on the limb. Because an elderly person may have difficulty in putting on a limb with a socket suspended by suction, we rarely prescribe suction suspension for individuals over 50 years of age with recent amputations but prefer to use a pelvic band and belt.

Standing is started in the parallel bars and weight shifting is done forward, backward and sideways. The patient learns to balance on one leg and steps are begun by putting the "best foot" forward and letting the momentum of the body help swing the prosthesis forward. Emphasis is placed upon keeping the steps even in length and keeping the trunk moving forward steadily. Side stepping is practiced, as is the act of getting up and down from chairs—wheelchairs, armchairs and straight back chairs. Negotiation of steps, ramps, curbs and finally rough ground is taught. Falling and getting up is practiced in suitable cases, as is running, pivoting and overcoming obstacles.

Ordinarily training requires about 12 sessions for a below-knee amputee and 18 periods for an above-knee amputee. Training can be done on an outpatient basis, and it is my opinion that training three times a week is sufficient for the elderly amputee. The bilateral above-knee amputee requires prolonged inpatient training (six to eight weeks).

From various reports it seems that walking with a unilateral above-knee prosthesis requires an expenditure of 20 to 25 per cent more energy than walking on two normal legs.[13, 17] Although many geriatric amputees are successfully fitted and trained, the metabolic cost of using their prosthesis may be 10 to 15 per cent more than for the younger amputee and 25 to 35 per cent higher than the energy cost to a younger unimpaired person. Studies by Peizer[17] indicate that a general increase in efficiency of performing standard exercises can be expected with time and practice.

Many amputees can walk with a good gait but fail to do so in daily practice, adopting a more comfortable, less costly in energy, but less esthetic, gait. Walking very slowly is uneconomical because of the partial loss of momentum and the resulting necessity of overcoming inertia at each step. Fast walking is uneconomical because of increased internal friction within the body tissues as well as increased movement of the arms, shoulders and trunk. The tension in postural muscles is increased. All of these adjustments require extra energy. It appears that each person has an optimal rate of walking for which the least energy is required. Normally this rate is the one that feels comfortable or "natural" to the individual.

Stump Bandaging.   After the sutures are removed, elastic compression bandages are used to shrink and shape the stump. This is continued until the patient receives his prosthetic limb. If for any reason he is unable to wear his prosthesis, bandaging should be reinstituted until he again wears the limb.

The elastic bandages may be plain woven cotton or the elastic reinforced type. The above-knee stump usually requires a 6 inch bandage, the below-knee stump, a 4 inch bandage and other stumps, appropriate widths. Wrapping should be done at least twice daily and continued all day.

Bandages should be applied so that the pressure is greatest at the tip of the stump and decreases from the distal to the proximal end. The bandage turns should be diagonal rather than horizontal. The above-knee bandage should be carried high into the groin and the below-knee bandage should reach to the lower pole of the patella.

Swelling.   During healing after amputation there is usually some swelling in the stump. This may be minimized by elevating the stump and by wrapping it with elastic bandages. A poorly fitting socket can also cause edema of the stump.

Stump Hygiene.   By following a simple routine of stump care consistently, the amputee can avoid many problems. Stump hygiene includes skin cleansing and care of the socket, socks and bandages.

The stump should be cleansed with soap and water daily, preferably at night. A liquid antiseptic solution or cake soap containing hexachlorophene (e.g., pHisoHex, Dial, Gamophen) may be used. The skin must be rinsed and dried thoroughly.

The stump sock should be changed daily. It should be washed in warm water with a mild soap, rinsed thoroughly and allowed to dry completely. Elastic bandages should be washed in the same way and allowed to dry on a flat surface.

The socket is washed with warm water and mild soap, wiped with a cloth, and permitted to dry thoroughly before limb is worn. This is to be done at night and should be done on a daily basis in hot weather.

Phantom Pain.   After loss of an arm or leg the missing part may leave its phantom to cause much mental and physical suffering. Phantoms usually include only distal portions of the missing members.[4] An amputation of the lower extremity is most likely to be represented by a phantom foot; an upper extremity by a phantom hand. If the phantom is painless it is known as "phantom sensation" but if there is any unpleasant feeling or pain it is known as "phantom pain."

When phantom pain develops it is usually immediately after surgery and it characteristically persists. It has been described as cramping, squeezing, burning, sharp, shooting or lancinating. Some patients describe the phenomenon in terms of numbness, pins and needles sensations and variations in temperature, position and pressure.

Various theories have attributed the cause of phantom pain to the peripheral and central nervous systems and to psychogenic factors. According to the peripheral theory, painful sensation originates from excitation of nerve endings in the scar, neuroma or infected stump. Impulses from cut nerves set up a reverberating circuit which forms a self-perpetuating vicious cycle between the thalamus and the cerebral cortex. Removal of the neuroma or further local surgery usually fails to relieve phantom pain however. Occasional success with sympathetic block or anterolateral chordotomy has provided a strong argument against the psychogenic theory.

The central nervous system (body image) theory holds that during growth from childhood to adulthood multiple sensory impressions traveling to the cerebral cortex and its association center make us increasingly aware of parts of our body. Subsequently this image shows resistance to change and provides the basis for phantom. In favor of this theory is the complete absence of phantom sensation in children with agenesis of limbs and in those who have had amputations before the age of five years.

Treatment of phantom pain is as controversial as the theories of etiology. Positive findings such as a neuroma, painful scar and tender spur call for treatment, but it is often unsuccessful in relieving the phantom pain.

Phantom pain and sensation have not been explained satisfactorily in terms upon which appropriate treatment may be founded. Methods such as firm bandaging day and night, ultraviolet radiation, diathermy, galvanism, ultrasound, paraffin baths and repeated percussion of palpable tender neuromas have satisfactory transient effects which can be prolonged indefinitely by providing and maintaining function with a prosthesis. An artificial limb that functions like the missing part greatly lessens the pain. Restoration of function as soon as possible after amputation, together with psychotherapy and removal of local irritants, has been used as an efficient means of relieving phantom pain. A psychologic approach has been to "excercise the phantom" through carrying out motions which were formerly done by the missing extremity.

Employment of Amputees

After the amputee has completed training in the use of his prosthesis, the next step is reemployment. The handicapped have much less difficulty in finding employment now than they did a few years ago. If the amputee is unable to return to the same type of work he did formerly, provision is made for retraining for some other job.

The unilateral below-knee amputee has minimal disability. If he has a well fitted prosthesis and has been properly trained in its use he can do almost everything he did before amputation, except for running. This type of amputee usually returns to his former employment.

The unilateral above-knee amputee cannot perform a job that will require carrying heavy objects and it must be understood that he will walk more slowly than the normal person.

The bilateral above-knee amputee has an extreme disability. He cannot be expected to stand for long periods or do much walking although he can stand for short periods and ambulate for short distances. He should be employed where he can sit down for most of the day or, if it is necessary to move, he can use a wheelchair.

The bilateral below-knee amputee can walk and stand well but he should be employed where he can be seated much of the day.

The arm amputee, whether bilateral or unilateral, above-elbow or below-elbow, also has special problems. He has no sense of touch in the terminal device and must look carefully at everything he does. Often an arm amputee can return to his former job or a similar one if changes are made in the equipment he uses. This may require the cooperation of the prosthetist, engineer, amputee and employer.

IMMEDIATE POSTSURGICAL FITTING OF PROSTHESES

Excellent results are being obtained worldwide with the use of immediate postsurgical fitting of prostheses. Sufficient experience has been gained so that it is now safe to form and train new teams in its use. The concept of fitting patients with prostheses immediately after surgery and initiating ambulation training the next day was first carried out by Berlemont in 1958, and reported on in 1961 at the Congress of Physical Medicine at Nancy. Weiss, in Warsaw, is given credit for the worldwide acceptance of this method. Burgess perfected the technique of the immediate prosthesis.

A number of benefits result from the use of immediate fitting: less pain for the patient, more rapid healing of the wound, psychological benefits, early weight bearing with maintenance of postural reflexes, quicker maturation of the stump and earlier fitting with the definitive prosthesis.

Every effort should be made to preserve the knee joint, even if it means a very short stump. As the surgeon gains experience he will be operating more frequently at the limits of viability and the chances of primary wound healing will correspondingly decrease. Techniques of amputation that provide for secure fixation of the muscle at the end of the stump at physiologic tension result in a firm well-shaped stump.

Wound hematoma is the main complication in amputation surgery and usually it is advantageous to use a drain.

The plaster cast using elastic plaster is applied at the completion of the operation and it prevents swelling of the stump. Because of change in the shape of the stump, such as that induced by changing position from bed rest to weight bearing, some resilient material needs to be placed between the plaster and the soft tissue. Zettl et al.[21] studied various types of "interface" materials and found that reticulated polyurethane foam, 20 pores per inch, is ideal for use. It is available in preformed pads of suitable sizes.

The general principles of management have been spelled out by Burgess et al.[11] They are:

1. A "team" approach which includes all relevant disciplines.
2. Definitive surgery is carried out at the lowest suitable level. The amputation is essentially a plastic-surgery procedure with conservation of dynamic stump function.
3. The immediate postsurgical prosthesis is applied as a rigid supportive pressure dressing designed to accept a temporary prosthesis.
4. Early ambulation is permitted consistent with the patient's condition.
5. A progressive program from amputation to definitive prosthesis involves continuous wound support and progressive ambulation with controlled weight bearing. Serial socket changes are made as needed.

Postoperative Management.   The goals of immediate postsurgical fitting of a prosthesis are prompt primary wound healing, early ambulation and rapid maximum rehabilitation of the patient. A patient who is unable to ambulate still benefits from the rigid dressing.

The initial period of standing on the prosthesis is limited to minimal, involving no more than 10 pounds of measured weight. The prosthesis unit must be aligned accurately with the patient standing. Usually the patient stands on the first or second postoperative day from 1 to 5 minutes. When endurance has increased to allow standing for several 5 minute periods twice daily, then ambulation is begun in the parallel bars. Weight on the amputation side should not exceed 20 pounds until primary wound healing is assured.

The patient begins and ends each training session by standing on paired scales to get the "feel" of the permitted weight bearing.

On the first postoperative day the therapist goes to the patient's room with a Walkerette and assists him to stand with minimal weight bearing on the prosthesis for 5 minutes or less. The pylon and foot are removed after the patient is returned to bed. On the second postoperative day the patient usually starts going to the physical medicine department in a wheelchair twice daily for periods of standing and exercises for the arms. From then until two weeks postoperatively, the patient gradually begins ambulation in the parallel bars. Approximately 20 to 30 pounds is the maximum weight permitted on the amputation side.

In the second two weeks after surgery the patient can usually progress to crutch walking. Forearm crutches are used if appropriate. They permit a more normal gait. Continue to limit weight bearing to 30 pounds.

Measurement for the definite prosthesis can be taken about one week following the second cast change if the sutures are removed and the wound well healed. It is well to avoid any interruption that would leave the stump without support. Elastic bandaging is commonly used for several weeks after the definite prosthesis is delivered. At times a night cast may be necessary if the patient is not skillful in bandaging.

Upper Extremity Immediate Postsurgical Fitting

Immediate postsurgical fitting is as applicable to upper extremity amputation as it is to leg amputation. Experience with myoelectric immediate postsurgical fitting has been very encouraging.[12] The scarcity of severe painful vascular disease in the upper extremities and the absence of the factor of weight bearing should enhance the likelihood of successful immediate fitting.[19]

THE GERIATRIC AMPUTEE

Amputees in the older age group are beset with additional problems. Whereas in the child amputee factors such as growth, development, coordination and muscular strength present problems, in the elderly amputee there are a multitude of medical complications and degenerative changes. Although the geriatric amputee is by far the most common patient seen in the amputee clinic of a general hospital, most efforts in the field of prosthetics have been for the young adult amputee.

Aged people walk with a significantly slower cadence. There is a decrease in the average speed of walking as age increases. In addition, aged people walk in a less vigorous fashion. There is a less dynamic transfer of the body weight onto and off the stance leg.

In the adult population peak aft shear stresses occur before double support begins, while in the elderly maximum aft shear stresses are generated after double support begins.[17] Apparently older poeple attempt to improve stability by increasing the period of double support.

Some biological aging becomes symptomatic between 50 and 55 years of age. Biological and chronological aging are frequently not identical. It seems logical to use age 55 as a guide for classifying an amputee as a "new amputee" or an "old amputee"—it is clear that a patient whose limb was amputated earlier in life and attains age 55 presents different problems from the individual who loses a limb after the age of 55 years.

In the geriatric amputee about one third of the amputations are done because of the factor of atherosclerosis. About 39 per cent are secondary to atherosclerosis associated with diabetes mellitus. Thus, over 70 per cent of geriatric amputees have loss of limb directly attributable to vascular disease.

Care of the Amputation Stump

Stump care of the geriatric patient is similar to that for other amputees. Generally the sutures remain in place longer (10 to 14 days) since wound dehiscence is more frequent in this group. Prevention of contractures is of primary importance in the geriatric patient. Supervised active resistive exercise is the best means of preventing contractures.

Criteria for Prosthetic Fitting

Most geriatric amputees should be fitted with limbs. Many will not function at a very high level, but this is not to be considered reason for denying the patient an artificial limb and training in its use. This is not true for the elderly bilateral above-knee amputee. It is difficult to set up clearly defined criteria for fitting, but certainly if the amputee can use crutches satisfactorily he will make good progress with a prosthesis.

Somewhat easier to list are factors which absolutely contraindicate limb fitting. These include (1) lack of motivation, (2) threatened gangrene of the remaining leg, (3) class IV heart disease, (4) severe neurological problems, (5) unyielding stump problems and (6) multiple major physical impairments.

Except in the case of absolute contraindications there is seldom justification for failing to recommend prosthetic fitting for the elderly amputee.

Prosthetic Factors

Comfort, fit, alignment and appearance are criteria for an acceptable prosthesis for all amputees. Additional factors are important in fitting the elderly amputee. These include (1) minimum weight of prosthesis, (2) a stable knee joint and (3) easily applied and effective suspension.

All means should be used to minimize the weight of the prosthesis while still retaining sufficient structural strength. Lightweight woods, reinforced duralumin ankle, knee and hip joints with Teflon washers in areas of metal-to-metal contact, and rawhide finishing help in keeping the total weight very low. The socket thickness need not be as great as that for a young vigorous amputee. Lightweight knee units are available. A new type of molded SACH foot is now made which is about half the weight of the laminated type.

There is a definite need for a knee unit which has a positive lock during the stance phase and which permits motion during the swing phase. The Otto Bock safety knee is used frequently for the elderly amputee. A manual knee lock may be used for severely unstable knee conditions. It is true that a knee lock is associated with a circumducted gait with or without vaulting on the remaining foot. It is preferable to have a poor gait than not to walk at all. At times softening of the SACH foot will aid in stability.

Initial flexion for the above-knee amputee should be built into the socket so that the amputee can stand erect without unlocking the knee. Hip flexion contractures in the elderly are prevalent and very resistive to correction.

Suspension of the prosthesis can present a difficult problem. The amputee must be comfortable while sitting for long periods, and the prosthesis must also be easy to put on and give effective suspension. Suction would be ideal except that it is difficult for an elderly person to put the limb on. It is seldom indicated in an older amputee. A pelvic band and belt with hip joint is easier to put on and adjust and gives effective suspension but is not comfortable on prolonged sitting. A good compromise is a pelvic belt (without the pelvic band) and a single axis metal hip joint. A Silesian bandage is quite comfortable and easy to apply, but many amputees feel that the suspension is ineffective.

Because of weakness of hip musculature the elderly above-knee amputee may have difficulty in clearing the floor with his prosthesis. During the training period the artificial limb may be about one half inch shorter than his remaining leg. As training progresses the limb is lengthened until leg lengths are equal and the iliac crests level.

Energy Costs

Walking speed is greatly limited in the above-knee amputee. Even at low speeds a high metabolic effort is needed. This amounts to about 700 cc. of oxygen per minute—roughly the same as maximum effort in older people. The energy costs for the elderly bilateral above-knee amputee are overwhelming. Wheelchair locomotion has been shown to require the least effort and energy expenditure.

Psychosocial Aspects

The process of aging has a detrimental effect on physical and psychological function. The trauma of amputation is added disaster. Thus, the older amputee must struggle with two negative forces which make it difficult for him to adjust—amputation and aging.

Self-image is constantly being adjusted. Slow changes permit gradual modification in self-image. A person losing a limb must drastically revise his body image. This reorganization of self-image is a major and at times an overwhelming task.

Prosthetic restoration plus the activity necessary to learn to use the limb should help with this adaptation or modification in self-image. For this reason alone, to institute training in the use of a prosthetic device might be considered a proper decision even though the chance of ultimate success is very slim.

THE JUVENILE AMPUTEE

Amputation in children is usually traumatic, congenital or secondary to the treatment of malignancy. The prosthetic management of the child amputee is essentially the same as that of adults. For the most part nearly all the prosthetic components are scaled-down versions of adult models.[30] This is not an ideal approach but this is the way it has evolved.

The flexibility of the child, with his greater reserve of all tissues, permits him to adapt quickly to prostheses. The young amputee grows up with his appliance and accepts it as a necessary item for his daily life.

Amputation done on an individual in whom bone growth is not complete leads to certain alterations in form and internal structure of the long bones and the axial skeleton. Below-knee amputation occurring before the age of 10 years will show bowing and kyphosis of the stump after some time. Medium or long below-elbow stumps at times develop overgrowth of the radius compared to the ulna, resulting in bowing inward of the stump. Above-knee amputation is accompanied by hemiatrophy of the pelvis on the same side as the amputation. Complications of amputation seen in adults, such as painful spurs, symptomatic neuromata, bursitis and phantom pain, are relatively rare in children. However, stump overgrowth is a complication seen only in the child amputee.

Between the ages of six and ten there is a disproportionate growth between the skin and bone, as shown by a long thin spindle of bone growing from the end of the amputation stump. Clinically the stump becomes red, swollen and tender, and unless surgery is done the bony end protrudes from the stump. This occurs most commonly with the fibula and less frequently with the tibia and humerus. Surgical revision relieves this complication promptly. This phenomenon has not been observed in the true congenital amputee unless the periosteum has been altered by surgery.

Age for Prosthetic Fitting

Children with lower extremity defects should be fitted with their first prosthesis when they start making efforts to stand. The average age for children to stand and attempt walking is between 10 and 18 months. When this stage of development is reached, a prosthesis should be fitted even if it is quite simple. As balance is developed a conventional type of limb is indicated.

The upper extremity pattern of development is more complex. Index finger-thumb prehension is developed at 40 weeks of age. By two years the child is doing more complex tasks. At the four-year level he is usually willing to accept verbal instruction and to take pride in accomplishment. Actually the patient should be fitted as early as possible with passive prostheses, preferably before eight months. This encourages bilateral function, improves balance, helps the child and parents to accept the prosthesis and gets the child familiar with the normal length of the limb. It is hoped that scoliosis will be minimized by early fitting.

Purposeful grasp and release of an active terminal device can seldom be developed under 24 months of age — usually not well developed until 30 months of age.

A variety of components are available for prescription by the clinic team for the child amputee. In uncomplicated cases satisfactory functional results are obtained, but many problems remain for the more complicated, severely disabled children. Special devices may need to be designed and fabricated for a particular case. Constant efforts are being made to improve the prostheses available for children.

Upper Extremity Components

For the most part terminal devices are scaled-down models of adult designs. The Dorrance 10P and 12P hooks are commonly used terminal devices for children up to about three years of age. These are covered with Plastisol. For the older child Dorrance voluntary-opening hooks are available in a variety of sizes. Several hands for children have been built (APRL, Dorrance, Robin-Aids) and others are in the process of development. Wrist units generally used are the threaded friction type. A wrist flexion unit is available and used mainly for bilateral and shoulder-disarticulation cases. Elbow joints are available in child sizes for below-elbow, above-elbow and elbow disarticulation.

The Canadian-type hip-disarticulation prosthesis is used almost exclusively in hip-disarticulation cases in adults and children. Components in child sizes are readily available.

Upper Extremity Congenital Defects.   Congenital defects of the upper extremity are difficult problems. A short, unilateral below-elbow absence is one of the commonest congenital defects. The short fleshy stump is difficult to fit. The Munster type of socket has been designed to give stability. The socket is fitted intimately to the stump and olecranon. It fits snugly above the epicondyles. The socket is set in about 35 degrees of initial flexion. This prevents full range of motion but does provide excellent stability. When the range of motion of the stump is limited, a split socket with step-up hinge may be needed so that the terminal device can be brought to the mouth. When the child is at the age of sitting up he may be fitted with a simple prosthesis. It is important to start early so that bimanual function is developed.

The thalidomide syndrome is a fascinating problem. Involvement is typically symmetrical and the upper extremities are affected more commonly than the lower extremities. Sometimes both are involved. For the most part the deformities are amelia, vestigial phocomelias or longer phocomelias. Less severely involved children may show tibial or radial loss. The proximal joint is defective in any affected limb. An adjustable shoulder unit (Wilson-Riblett wedges) permitting change in the alignment of the prosthesis with the socket is available.

In congenital cases in which power and excursion are quite limited, harnessing of the upper extremity prosthesis is a most difficult problem. The ring type of harness is usually more comfortable and is simple to make and adjust. Perineal straps have been used as reaction points for the control cables, but they are uncomfortable and unsatisfactory. Some success has followed the use of a quadrilateral plastic brim to serve as a reaction point for control cables.

Lower Extremity Components

Most lower extremity components are copied after adult models. The SACH (solid ankle/cushioned heel) foot is used routinely for children and is quite satisfactory. The Syme type of prosthesis is like that of the adult. The PTB (patellar-tendon bearing) socket is used routinely in many clinics for the below-knee child amputee. There are still unanswered questions as to the effects of wearing a PTB socket on the knee joint in a growing child. When the PTB socket is not used, the conventional open-end socket and laced leather thigh corset are applied. A single axis knee with constant-friction is used for the above-knee patient. Additional stigmata are seen in these children—saddle nose, coloboma or other eye defects, microtia, nevi of the forehead and face and sometimes atresia of the external meatus. When there is upper extremity amelia or functionless phocomelia, the feet must be trained as prehensile organs. When the legs are involved and the child is unable to sit, a sitting socket must be furnished at the age the child would normally sit. When the child is able to sit independently, functionless upper extremities should be fitted. These may be simple devices or the Heidelberg pneumatic arm may be used. Further functional components can be added as the child develops more skill. The child with severe upper and lower extremity deformities will probably not walk and a motorized chair will be needed.

Lower Extremity Congenital Defects.   Absence of the forefoot is seen at times. A modified shoe can be used but the tendency for the development of equino-varus position may require a Syme amputation. Absence of the fibula is relatively common. This is associated with a valgus ankle and frequently with absence of the lateral two digital rays and bowing of the lower tibia. A strong shoe constructed to correct the valgus ankle is often all that is needed. A modified Syme amputation gives better cosmetic results and may be preferable if a plantigrade foot cannot be attained. Amputation for cosmetic reasons should not be done until the child is old enough to share in the decision.[11] However, when amputation is necessary to improve or promote function it should be done promptly. Absence of the tibia is manifested by total instability at the knee and ankle. The legs are unsatisfactory in an extension prosthesis and surgery is necessary. Disarticulation at the knee may be the most functional procedure. Femoral defects may range from simple coxa-vara to complete absence of the femur. Numerous surgical procedures have been tried for these cases but often the only gain has been in cosmesis, with some decrease of function. These patients usually learn to use an extension prosthesis quite satisfactorily.

Complete bilateral lower limb amelia (with normal upper extremities) has been managed by the use of stubbies of increasing height. Finally a pair of Canadian-type hip-disarticulation prostheses is fitted and the patient walks with a four-point gait.

Conversions

In the case of a severely deformed extremity, amputation or ablation, correcting it to a more functional and cosmetically acceptable stump is termed conversion. This is used basically for congenital deformities. Conversion may simply be amputation at the required level or may be associated with proximal joint fusions to increase the remaining skeletal stability and length. Disarticulation in the lower extremity usually results in full weight bearing.

Training

The training of a child amputee is done with the playing of games. The child is shown how the prosthesis can help him accomplish something that he wants to do. Then he becomes willing to learn. When a child first receives an active device he is given in-patient training sessions for a time, with further training as an out-patient if feasible. Active participation by the parents is of great benefit in the child's learning to make use of a prosthesis.

Since children are generally very active and have periods of rapid growth, frequent adjustments and replacement of the prosthesis are required.

Psychosocial Problems[16]

Parental reaction to a deformed child may vary from complete rejection to overprotection. When possible the mother should be involved in the prosthetic "team." The feeling of guilt and inadequency of the parents may lead to emotional problems in the congenital amputee.

The adolescent period is particularly painful for the congenital amputee. Appearance becomes important—for the first time the amputee realizes the various reactions that his disability brings forth in other people. He questions whether he is accepted as a person or because of his deformity. Reaction of the amputee may vary from withdrawal to denial of his difference. In either extreme there is the tendency to make neurotic use of the disability. However, child amputees as a group do not appear to show more emotional disturbances than those seen in other severely handicapped children.

REFERENCES

Orthotics

1. Anderson, M. H.: Functional Bracing of the Upper Extremities. Springfield, Ill., Charles C Thomas, 1958.
2. Anderson, M. H.: Upper Extremities Orthotics. Springfield, Ill., Charles C Thomas, 1965.
3. Bartelink, D. L.: The Role of Abdominal Pressure in Relieving the Pressure on the Lumbar Intervertebral Discs. J. Bone Joint Surg. *39B:*718, 1957.
4. Fishman, S.: Prosthetics and Orthotics U.S.A. 1969. Artificial Limbs, *13*(1)iii, Spring, 1969.
5. Kay, H. W.: Clinical Evaluation of the Engen Plastic Hand Orthosis. Artificial Limbs, *13*(1):13-26, Spring, 1969.
6. Lehneis, H. R.: Brace Alignment Considerations. Orthopedic and Appliance J. *18:*110, 1964.
7. Montan, K.: Technical Aids — An Important Part of the Rehabilitation Scheme. Prosthetics International. Proceedings of the Second International Prosthetics Course. Copenhagen, Printing Office of the Society and Home for Cripples in Denmark, 1960.
8. Morris, J. M., Lucas, D. B., and Bressler, B.: Role of the Trunk in Stability of the Spine. J. Bone Joint Surg., *43A:*327, 1961.
9. Steindler, A.: Mechanics of Normal and Pathological Locomotion in Man. Springfield, Ill., Charles C Thomas, 1935.

Management of the Amputee

10. Anderson, M. H., and Sollars, R. E.: Manual of Above-Knee Prosthetics for Physicians and Therapists. University of California (Los Angeles), 1959.
11. Burgess, E. M., Romano, R. L., Zettl, J. H.: The Management of Lower Extremity Amputation. TR 10-6, August, 1969.
12. Childress, D. S., Hampton, F. L., Lambert, C. N., Thompson, R. G., Schrodt, G. R.: Myoelectric Immediate Postsurgical Procedure: A Concept for Fitting the Upper Extremity Amputee. Artificial Limbs, *13*(2):55-60, Autumn, 1969.
13. Erdman, W. J., II, Hettinger, T., and Saez, F.: Comparative Work Stress for Above-knee Amputee Using Artificial Legs or Crutches. Amer. J. Phys. Med., *39:*225-232, 1960.
14. Klopsteg, P. E., and Wilson, P. D.: Human Limbs and Their Substitutes. New York, McGraw-Hill Book Co., Inc., 1964.
15. Lehneis, H. R.: Brace Alignment Considerations. Orthopedic and Appliance J., *18:*110, 1964.
16. McKenzie, D. S.: Children — Medical and Psychosocial Consideration. Prosthetics International, *2*(1):7, 1964.
17. Peizer, E.: On the Energy Requirements for Prosthesis Use by Geriatric Amputees. The Geriatric Amputee. Washington, National Academy of Sciences, National Research Council Bulletin 919, 1961.
18. Wilson, A. B., Jr.: Recent Advances in Below-knee Prosthetics. Artificial Limbs. *13*(2):1-12, Autumn, 1969.
19. Wilson, A. B., Jr.: A Material for Direct Forming of Prosthetic Sockets. Artificial Limbs. *14*(1):53-56, Spring, 1970.
20. Wilson, A. B., Jr.: Limb Prosthesis for Children. Prosthetics International, *2*(1):2, 1964.
21. Zettl, J. H., Burgess, E. M., Romano, R. L.: The Interface in the Immediate Postsurgical Prosthesis. Orthotics and Prosthetics, *24*(1):1-7, March, 1970.

Chapter 5

SPEECH AND LANGUAGE DISORDERS

by Henry Goehl

Language may be considered man's finest accomplishment. The use of linguistic symbols to reconstruct the past, characterize the present and hypothesize about the future has been and continues to be a requirement in the entire range of human behavior from the most simple to the most complex. Without speech, it becomes extremely difficult to get directions to the local post office or to solve the problem of putting man on the moon. We accept the "gift" of speech, if we think of it at all, as an inevitable part of us. It takes only a little study, however, to discover that the child needs years to master the complexities of language and that the process by which language is learned continues to be in many respects as mysterious as the human mind itself. The reader may not recall learning to speak, but he appreciates the difficulties of learning a complete linguistic system if he has attempted the conscious study of a foreign language.

The significance of intact communication is immediately apparent when we are confronted with the patient with cleft palate whose inability to direct voice through the oral cavity renders his speech all but unintelligible or the patient with brain damage who gropes ineffectually for the pattern of sounds that represent his own name. The effects of such disturbances are felt in every aspect of the individual's life and critically touch the lives of those around him.

In his practice and in his hospital the physician will encounter individuals representing all types and degrees of speech and language disorders. He will recognize them and want to join in their appraisal and management. Successful rehabilitation requires the concerted attention of many of the specialties represented in this text as well as the specialized attention of the speech pathologist audiologist.

This chapter presents concepts fundamental to an understanding of those disorders typically seen in the physical medicine and rehabilitation situation. The writer attempts to blend his knowledge of the literature with the results of his own experience. The research and ideas of others is not documented and no topic is considered in detail. The reader is encouraged to pursue the items of the annotated bibliography for more exhaustive treatments and other points of view.

DEFINING SPEECH AND LANGUAGE

Language is the general name for a system that includes the expressive operations of speaking and writing and the receptive operations of understanding the spoken and written word. The expressive and receptive are not difficult to observe but the mental-linguistic operations that go on in between remain in the realm of private experience about which we can only infer. This chapter is mainly concerned with oral language (speech) but we will need to consider it against its complex background as well as describe its more obvious features.

The smallest units of speech are speech sounds. Combinations of these sounds can result in words and combinations of words can become sentences. This process is possible only when the speaker knows what sounds are speech sounds and in what ways they may be combined to deserve the designation of word and sentence. Normal speakers are understood because they have learned the underlying principles of speech more or less unconsciously in growing up. Abnormal speakers have not learned or are somehow unable to follow these principles. It is important to note that the dictionary and book of grammar, as records of certain linguistic rules, are determined by normal language usage rather than determiners of that usage. The linguist has had to study us to discover the rules and how they are learned. The speech pathologist–audiologist must make a comparable study of the abnormal speaker.

CLASSIFYING SPEECH AND LANGUAGE DISORDERS

Speech Sounds.   We can produce a great variety of sounds but only a few of them function as speech sounds. English has about 45 such consonant and vowel elements. Vowels and diphthongs are partially represented by the English letters a, e, i, o and u. Their different qualities come from the modification of voice by changes in the resonance characteristics of the pharyngeal, oral and nasal cavities. Consonants are partially represented by such letters as t, p, g and r. They may be voiced or unvoiced and their distinctive acoustic shape results from the obstruction of the breath or voice by the teeth, tongue, lips and palate.

Isolated speech sounds are meaningless, but when they are properly combined to form recognizable words, their communicative weight is great. Consider for example, the two groups of words: "bit," "fit" and "lit;" "load," "lead" and "lad." Any item in the first group is easily distinguished from any item in the second because of broadly different combinations. Items within the two groups, however, differ on the basis of only one consonant or vowel element.

Speakers are not exactly the same and each produces the sounds of English in a slightly different way. In fact, acoustic analysis has shown that the same speaker shows some variation in the production of the same sound from time to time. These variations go unnoticed until they become great enough to change the word so that it is either no longer recognizable or it is confused with another word. We say that speakers who mispronounce or misuse speech sounds to the point where their speech is confusing to the listener have *articulation disorders.*

Words and Grammar. In contrast to speech sounds, many words have definite meaning in isolation. Upon hearing the words "toy," "brick" and "ship," the listener automatically thinks of some specific things to which the words refer. But the reference changes depending on the relation of these words to others. The use of "ship" in the sentence, "Ship the toy ship," illustrates the change in meaning for one word as a function of its position in a word sequence. This particular sentence also has a form that is repeated in other sentences and contributes to our understanding of them. The sentences, "Feed the black dog," and "Bring the gray hat," are of the same form class and many words may be substituted into the verb and adjective-noun slots without changing the imperative meaning of the sentence form. There are some words that have little meaning except as they refer to other words. The word "the" in the preceding sentences symbolizes very little alone but the sequences would be nearly nonsensical if it were omitted.

The selection of the proper words for arrangement into appropriate sequences follows complex rules, many of which are not yet known. The normal speaker has a "built in" understanding of them. He could not state many of the rules, yet implicitly he knows what is nonsense and what is not. The patient who cannot properly understand the spoken words of others and cannot select the right words and arrange them appropriately shows a *language disorder.*

Prosody. The prosodic aspects of speech are not classifiable as sounds or words but they play an essential part in the act of speech. They are voice, stress, intonation and rhythm. We will consider them briefly in the order mentioned.

Voice. Voice production requires a column of air under pressure beneath the vocal folds which is produced by the concerted actions of the chest and abdomen in compressing the thoracic cavity and the approximation of the vocal folds in closing the glottal opening. The rapid opening and closing of the vocal folds "vibrates" the air and the vibrations are heard as voice. Vocal pitch (the characteristic highness or lowness of voice) depends on the frequency of vocal fold movement. The loudness of voice is determined by the amount of pressure built up under the vocal folds before it is released. Voice quality is that dimension that helps us tell who is doing the speaking and also the aspect that we may judge as hoarse, breathy, hypernasal or strident. Voice quality is generally a joint product of vocal fold action and the resonance characteristics of the cavities of the head. *Voice disorders* are those abnormalities of pitch, loudness and quality that are so gross that they distract the listener from what is being said.

Stress and Intonation. We mentioned the role voice plays in the production of vowels and voiced consonants. Patterns of vocal stress and intonation also provide the listener with important cues for interpreting the utterance. The sentences, "I am going out," "I *am* going out!" and "I am going out?" when read aloud indicate that changes in meaning are occasioned by changes in vocal stress and intonation. These patterns are a function of varying loudness and pitch. Abnormalities have their basis in a combination of voice, rhythm or language disturbance.

RHYTHM.   The rhythm of speech refers to its overall flow, particularly its rate, pause pattern and repetition. Rhythm also has communicative significance. Pauses, for example, have grammatical importance for, like written punctuation, they signal the end of one phrase and the beginning of another. The rate of speech affects the precision of speech sound production and the degree to which the listener can assimilate what is said. Repetition is of value for purposes of emphasis. When pause pattern, rate and repetition are consistently inappropriate, they disrupt the flow of speech and we classify this disruption as a *disorder of rhythm.*

General Criterion for a Speech and Language Disorder.   We have classified various disorders of speech and language under the headings of articulation, language, voice and rhythm. We have also suggested that all speakers differ one from the other to some extent. How different must the speech be to be considered a significant problem? The following statement is a general answer to this question and implies that the speech must be different enough to make a real difference:

We will say that the speech and language is truly disordered if it is so different that it interferes with communication, calls attention to itself and contributes to maladjustment on the part of the speaker or listener.

SPEECH DEVELOPMENT AND RELATED VARIABLES

Speech and language are to some extent learned. We have only to watch our children grow to become aware of their progressive acquisition of linguistic skills. Although we do not know exactly how we learn to speak, we have been able to identify some stages of language development and some variables important to the development and maintenance of linguistic skills.

Developmental Summary

The first 9 to 12 months of life may appear to be prelinguistic because the child does not talk per se. We note, however, that he shows awareness of sound by the second month and will turn to the source of familiar sounds before many more months have passed. He seems interested in the speech of others by six months of age and will reveal an understanding of simple, familiar words by age nine months (before he says his own first words). By the end of the first year, he may follow simple commands and in another month or two responds appropriately to "no" and "don't." He comprehends simple questions by about two years and recognizes pronoun usage before he is three years old. Receptive abilities always take the lead and are basic to the development of the expressive function.

Expressively, the child's early months are filled with crying and sound "play." By eight months, he may seem to be imitating environmental sounds and even the vocal intonations of the speakers around him. In contrast to his receptive abilities, his expressive behavior does not strictly begin to follow linguistic rules until the appearance of the first words at about nine months of age. By age two, he will be combining words in phrases and his expressive vocabulary will be growing rapidly. His sentences grow longer and more complex until by age three years, his remarks may average five words in length and may include subordinate clauses. He will make grammatical errors for many years and his articulation of speech sounds may not be fully mature until he is about eight years of age.

Most children follow this general schedule of receptive and expressive development but we cannot expect all children to mature at the same rate. There is considerable normal variation. Experience suggests, however, that a delay of a year or more in the appearance of the behaviors mentioned should be regarded with concern. The first three years of life are crucial for we believe that during this period the child learns the basic rules of the language and that what follows is mainly refinement and elaboration. Disturbance during this period may have irreversible effects if it is not caught early; therefore, even the slightest suspicion of delay should be followed by referral for language evaluation.

Related Variables

The Role of Environment. The child learns from others and if others are absent he will not learn. When the speech of others is present, the nature and amount of language stimulation becomes important. Children raised in institutions develop speech more slowly and show more speech disorders than children raised at home. We think a crucial variable in these instances is the fact that the institutionalized child does not have enough contact with mature speech models but gets proportionately more reinforcing stimulation from the immature speech performance of his peers. Twins and children of large families may show a similar picture. We not only acquire our general linguistic system from parents and close associates but tend to adopt the peculiarities of their speech as well. The child who has taken on the errors of the parent or older sibling is seen fairly often in the clinic. Sufficient and adequate stimulation is an important condition for the development of acceptable speech.

The Role of Hearing. Although all the senses are used to some extent in language development, the most important is hearing. Language that is not heard will not be learned, and language imperfectly heard will be imperfectly learned. The task of the ear is to receive and transmit faithfully to the brain the rapidly fluctuating spectra of sound that are the basic material upon which the recognition of speech depends. The ear not only monitors the listener's environment but his own speech as well, thus providing a mechanism for self-correction and self-control of speech behavior.

The Role of Mental Abilities. Our discussion thus far has suggested some of the complexities of verbal rules and therefore we must recognize that it "takes brains" to learn them. The exact correlation between intelligence and aspects of language is not clear but that there is a strong relationship is apparent from studies of the retarded in whom slower development of language and a significantly greater number of speech disorders are observed. It may be more accurate to expect mental deficiency to have its greatest effects on such matters as vocabulary, grammar and symbolic behavior in general. Programs designed to improve the language status of the retarded have not been popular because the reduced ability to learn of these patients suggested a poor prognosis. Recently workers have recognized that the performance of the retarded is not exclusively a function of limited mental ability and that environmental variables are also important. They have reported that programs of broad stimulation have resulted in limited but practical progress.

Verbal behavior may also be influenced by so-called perceptual abilities. The ability to follow and recall sequences of sound and the ability to attend to one sound stimulus (for example, voice) in the presence of others seem important to the development and maintenance of verbal performance. Although these abilities may be directly related to central nervous system function, they are also to some extent learned.

We must suppose that language itself is both a mental function and a mental ability. Thinking involves language. The act of recognizing and interpreting what is said and the act of formulating something to be said and then selecting and arranging the units to say it in are most certainly functions of the mind. The central nervous system is involved to a great degree in the growth and maintenance of language and damage to it is likely to have profound effects on language growth and performance.

The Role of Muscular and Structural Factors. We have suggested that talking is something more than a specialized function of the oral area. Yet speech is also very definitely a motor act. It is in fact a very intricate motor act requiring the coordinated innervation of a multitude of muscles and the movement of a variety of structures, all of which serve the life functions of feeding and breathing as well. We think of the motor aspect of speech as an "overlaid" or learned function of the organism. The development of articulatory skills depends in part on the maturity of the organism, and voice changes perceptably with the growth of structures. Neuromotor disorganization and structural deficiencies can disturb speech. This is obvious in cleft palate and cerebral palsy but it may be more subtle in cases of mild muscle weakness and malocclusion.

The Role of Personality. The child must want to speak in order to learn speech. The desire to communicate is probably dependent on the existence of a warm familial relationship. This does not mean over-solicitousness toward the child, for such treatment seems to have the effect of inhibiting growth. We mean that the child should feel that he and his attempts to communicate are accepted. The theory that speech is an expression of personality has some validity. Voice quality and patterns of hesitation, to name two aspects of speech, have been shown to be closely related to emotional status. We have treated, in cooperation with psychiatric programs, children whose bizarre speech is thought to be symptomatic of their general need to withdraw from painful emotional relationships. Speech is an essential part of the child's psychosocial development and when that development is disturbed, we should not be surprised to see a reflection of the disturbance in the speech and language behavior. If we can separate them at all, speech and personality may be said to have a reciprocal relationship. Whether the basis for a patient's problem is emotional or not, his speech will often stimulate negative reactions by others. These reactions cannot help but effect his personal adjustment.

INCIDENCE OF SPEECH AND LANGUAGE DISORDERS

How many of what types of speech disorders can the physician expect to see in the physical medicine and rehabilitation setting? The answer will vary from clinic to clinic, but perhaps a study of incidence in the total population will be more helpful. Even in the total population, the findings vary from survey to survey so rather than reproducing various tables, we will borrow a summary statement from Van Riper:[16]

Six per cent of the total population has some variety of speech defect. Four per cent of the total population has an articulation disorder. Seven individuals in each thousand are stutterers. Five out of every thousand have a voice disorder; five more have delayed speech; two more have speech disorders due to brain injuries; and one in each thousand has a cleft-palate speech problem.

Our experience suggests that these figures are conservative and probably more accurately represent the population treated in the typical university speech and hearing center. The results of an informal survey of two prominent rehabilitation centers in Philadelphia may be more useful. We found that about one quarter of all inpatients and about one third of all outpatients were being treated in the speech and hearing department. The great majority of these patients were adults, mostly aphasic. Others types of disorders in order from more frequent to less frequent were: articulation (primarily dysarthria), stuttering, voice, cerebral palsy, hearing loss and cleft palate.

We do not expect these incidence estimates to stand for all time. Programs of research and prevention should reduce the natural occurrence of these disorders. In the areas of cleft palate and hearing loss the results of ever more refined surgical and prosthetic procedures indicate that the numbers of these children growing up with significant speech problems is becoming less each year. In addition, more knowledge is being gained about the dynamics of functional disorders, and applications of this information have been made in various situations to prevent the development of these disorders.

EVALUATION AND MANAGEMENT

The general objectives of the evaluation are (1) to determine whether a problem exists, (2) to define the nature of the problem and (3) to make appropriate recommendations regarding treatment. Although most of the patients referred to the speech pathologist show significant communication disorders, not all are candidates for therapy. For some, the prognosis is prohibitively poor and for others, attention from other specialists may take precedence. The concentration, type and duration of treatment is determined by the nature of the problem and may range from short-term diagnostic study through long-term daily work on a group or individual basis.

Articulation Problems

Misarticulation of speech sounds is the most common of the speech disorders and is found in one form or another among individuals with hearing loss, cleft palate, cerebral palsy and aphasia.

Evaluation. The patient's speech sound production should receive detailed examination in a variety of sound contexts and in running speech. The patient's ability to make positive changes following brief experimental stimulation has prognostic value and should be assessed. This testing will produce an inventory of articulatory abilities and disabilities. Hearing is tested audiometric-

ally and the speech mechanism examined in relation to speech sound production. A paralytic condition or gross structural deviation may be apparent but it
would be unwise to assume a connection to the speech sound errors without
examination. In the case of true dysarthria, the oral examination should seek to
assess the capacity of the patient to improve on present performance and make
compensatory movements.

In the absence of related organic conditions, serious mental retardation or
contributing factors of an environmental or emotional nature, age becomes an
important criterion in the judgment of articulatory performance. The child
with speech sound errors does not necessarily have a speech disorder. We know
that the normal maturation of articulatory skills requires about eight years.
Speech sound errors are to be expected during the child's early years and, if
there is no evidence to the contrary, the child may be expected to develop
competence without special treatment.

Management. The main task of the patient is to learn to identify his
sound errors and to distinguish them from the correct form of articulation.
The process involves learning both to hear and feel the important differences
between the sounds in question. As he learns to produce the sound correctly in
a variety of sound contexts and in more complex utterances, he must also learn
to monitor himself. Eventually, he will have to engage in a conscious program
of transferring what he has learned in the clinic to everyday speech. Others
who come in daily contact with the patient can be of considerable help at this
stage in providing structural practice situations. The dysarthric patient (with
paralysis, parkinsonism or multiple sclerosis) may learn the proper discriminations with ease but he is likely to have great difficulty in executing the movements necessary for improvement of speech sound production. Exercise of the
involved musculature and the use of compensatory patterns involving changes
in rate and phrasing may help, but, without some improvement of physical
condition, the prognosis for dysarthria can be poor. This is not to suggest that
functional disorders of articulation always respond to direct treatment. Sometimes they do not and in these cases reevaluation, particularly of psychologic
status, is in order.

Stuttering

The broken, hesitant, repetitious speech so characteristic of stuttering
behavior marks it as a type of rhythm disorder. Stuttering is special, however,
because it seems always to have a significant component involving heightened
anxiety about speech that may not show up as speech dysfluency per se. We
know that some stutterers will be judged more fluent than some nonstutterers.
Fluency, then, is not the only, nor always the best, criterion for a diagnosis of
stuttering.

Witness to the complexity of the problem of stuttering is the large amount
of divergent theory, research and clinical advice available on the subject. In this
chapter, the evaluation and management of stuttering will be presented in
terms of the writer's view that stuttering is primarily a functional disorder.

Evaluation. Stuttering is a "disease" of childhood; its onset is almost invariably noted during the preschool and early school years. Sudden onset during
the teens or later is quite likely to be related to profound psychic difficulty.

In the appraisal of children, it is important to keep in mind that dysfluency is a *natural* state of affairs. This is especially true of the child during the years when stuttering tends to have its beginnings. The ages three through eight are filled with dysfluency and this is understandable since those years are a time of rapid growth, change and adjustment to the demands of the environment. The child is in the midst of mastering his complex language and has a great deal to say but does not have the precise skills with which to say it. His mind probably does race ahead of his speech. Normally, such dysfluency is developmental and will fall out with maturity. The parent who brings such a child to us has, at best, misevaluated a developmental stage. At worst, the parent may have a need to diagnose normal dysfluency as pathologic stuttering, either because he has set too high standards for the child or perhaps in morbid expectation arising from a history of stuttering in the family. In either case, it does not seem enough to dismiss the parent with the advice that the child will outgrow it. The parent needs an improved understanding of speech development together with a recognition of the significance of parental attitude. Prolonged counseling may be required.

The reason for careful attention to parental reaction is that we may be able to prevent the development of true stuttering. We believe that stuttering often starts and continues to develop in tune with parental rejection of the child's speech or rejection of the child himself. When the child becomes anxious about his personal adequacy and his speech, he is likely to try harder to do well without really knowing how. The effortless repetitions of childhood may become tense conscious struggles with speech and the act of trying not to "stutter" or not to be "bad" becomes the stuttering behavior. Anxiety and tension are fluency disrupters. The sources of these feelings must be identified in the evaluation and dealt with in treatment.

The older stutterer comes to us with a fully developed system of distorted communication. Strong emotions are securely attached to his stuttering behavior. He fears certain words and situations, so he attempts to cut them from his repertoire of experience. He has learned to avoid rejection by avoiding speech. His speech is full of false starts, postponements and bizarre devices which he uses to distract himself from anticipated stuttering. He may now even find stuttering a useful excuse for failure. The uses of stuttering are varied and include the expression of unconscious hostility and unresolved emotional conflicts. The prognosis can be poor and the evaluation must seek to determine the depth to which the roots of stuttering go. This evaluation will be based on a detailed description of behavior and a sensitive interpretation of its implications.

Management.   Children who are beginning to stutter or whose parents are beginning to "see" stuttering are best treated indirectly. The parents require the lion's share of treatment. Through counseling, they must analyze their feelings and behavior in relation to the child; they must learn that their emotional acceptance of him will help decrease his anxiety and the accompanying tension that shows up as stuttering. This objective is rarely accomplished by direct advice. A frontal attack on attitudes usually has the same negative effect as the well-intentioned advice offered the stutterer himself. He is told to "slow down," "think before you speak" and "take it easy." Many stutterers in therapy have informed us how noxious this advice has been for them. They would "take it easy" if they could! Similarly, a confrontation of parents with their errors is likely to stir up the guilt they already feel and spur them to defensive denial. The counseling requires the same sort of acceptance and understanding on the part of the counselor that we are seeking to promote in the counselees.

The child who is not mature enough to "talk out" stuttering may be seen in a play therapy setting that is free from penalty and where he may be able to express and resolve some of his tension by symbolic activity with puppets, clay and a responsive clinician. The older stutterer also has difficulty considering his problem directly. He often behaves as if it is a topic filled with horror and best avoided. He usually needs to approach the feelings around stuttering before he can consider the speech pattern itself. This requires considerable self-exposure and is difficult. The patterns of stuttering eventually need direct analysis and modification. The patient needs to be able to study his responses scientifically and experiment with modifications that are more acceptable than the former automatisms of struggle and avoidance. The therapeutic process requires a clinician who has many of the attributes of the clinical psychologist. Regression and therapeutic failure are not uncommon. Psychiatric consultation should always be considered, hopefully at the time of evaluation rather than after a period of unsuccessful treatment.

Deafness and Hearing Difficulty

The speech and language problems of those patients with peripheral hearing loss are usually classified according to degree of loss and age of onset. We define deafness as a condition of no useful hearing for understanding or learning speech. The hard of hearing have useful hearing but they have difficulty understanding and learning under ordinary conditions. The congenitally deaf and hard of hearing need special attention from infancy. Those who incur hearing loss after developing speech and language will need help in compensating for the impaired modality.

Evaluation.   The study of the hearing handicapped involves a sequence of overlapping evaluations in the following order: medical, audiologic, educational. We will be concerned here with the latter two. The purpose of audiologic evaluation is to determine the type and degree of loss for tonal and speech stimuli. These measures help predict the amount of difficulty the individual will have in hearing and understanding speech. They also are used as a basis for recommending amplification and in the educational evaluation for recommending placement in special classes for the deaf, auditory training or training in speech-reading (lip reading). The educational evaluation should probably include psychologic appraisal. Severe hearing loss of long standing typically has distorting effects on the individual's outlook and sudden onset can be understandably disturbing. In the case of those with adventitious loss, study of speech and language abilities is in order to determine needs.

Management.   The congenitally deaf child needs preschool training through a program designed for use by the parents or a special nursery. He will eventually need the special educational program offered in schools for the deaf. The hard of hearing child can attend regular school but often needs supplementary academic tutoring, auditory training, speechreading and speech therapy. Auditory training is the process by which the individual learns to make the best use of the sound he can hear. Training may be offered on a short-term basis to help the client adjust to a hearing aid or it may go on for a longer period when it is judged that the child can learn to make more effective use of his residual hearing. Speechreading is a skill by which the hearing handicapped use visible aspects of the speaker's behavior and of the total situation to help in the recognition of what the speaker is saying. The deaf and those with severely distorting types of hearing loss must depend almost exclusively on speechreading to understand the speaker. The speech of the deaf and hard of hearing is often distorted in proportion to the hearing loss and the clinician attempts to teach the patient a kinesthetic understanding of speech sounds, pitch, voice quality, and loudness. In cases of progressive hearing loss, the various procedures are started to help the individual maintain his expressive skills and to provide him with compensatory measures for the time when he can no longer depend on hearing for speech recognition.

Delayed Language Development

There is a group of children, usually of preschool age, who have such limited language that they may be considered essentially nonverbal. These children seem almost totally unable to cope with the language of their environment. Frequently the diagnosis and management of their problems are difficult. Their behavior has been etiologically related to mental deficiency, hearing loss, emotional disturbance or childhood aphasia. Aphasia is probably less readily identified than the other conditions, however; we are thinking here of children who are difficult to understand because they do not conform to the clinical picture expected of *any* of the conditions listed. Clinical experience suggests that the language disorder is frequently a product of a combination of etiologic conditions.

Evaluation. One of the barriers to uncomplicated diagnosis is that these children are usually unable to cooperate fully with formal test procedures. Modification of standard approaches is necessary; therefore, clinical findings are often less reliable and more tentative than usual. Repetition of examination and study in a diagnostic training program is often indicated. The etiologic possibilities require psychologic, audiologic and linguistic appraisal.

The psychologic examination searches for evidence of mental deficiency, emotional disturbance and aphasia. The child whose main problem is low intelligence shows a history of overall slow development and present behavior that is responsive and consistent but generally retarded commensurate with mental age. When emotional disturbance is the primary difficulty, the history may show development and then discontinuation of speech, tendency to withdraw from the environment and, presently, behavior that is stereotyped, bizarre and characterized by rejection of contact with others. Evidence for aphasia includes a history suggestive of damage to the central nervous system and some developmental retardation. Present behavior often shows hyperactivity, perceptual disturbance and inconsistent responses to mental test items. The deaf and emotionally disturbed tend to show intelligence within the normal range.

The audiologic evaluation seeks to establish the presence or absence of significant hearing loss and to record other characteristic responses to auditory stimuli that will contribute to diagnosis. Estimates of hearing level in these cases are often based on "play audiometry" techniques, electrodermal response audiometry and EEG audiometry. These methods are all attempts to establish hearing levels for children who are unable to learn to give voluntary responses to specified auditory stimuli. The auditory responses of the deaf and mentally deficient tend to be consistent but, in the case of the former, indicative of hearing impairment. The emotionally disturbed may show fear of sound or an unwillingness to hear. The aphasic is more inconsistent in his response, appears unable to attend and shows problems in recognizing sound. Difficulty in auditory discrimination is also characteristic of children with peripheral hearing loss based on a history of deprived auditory experience as well as of those with types of hearing loss that distort sound even when sound is intense enough to be heard. The differential diagnosis of auditory perceptual disturbance is difficult in itself and the contribution of peripheral hearing loss should not be ruled out without detailed audiologic study.

The purpose of the language examination is to observe the child's symbolic behavior systematically. The examiner is interested in the child's use of vocalization, his response to sound and speech and his play activity as they contribute to a judgment of his linguistic status. The deaf can be expected to respond consistently and appropriately to those sounds they can hear and have learned are meaningful. They tend to show a high degree of visual attentiveness and use of visual clues as a means of understanding the environment. The play of the deaf is appropriate and indicates that they have good inner understanding of the functional relations between things and people. They use voice projectively and at an early age develop an intricate system of gesture for communicative purposes. The mentally deficient child shows retardation in expressive and receptive language that tends to correspond with his mental ability. His responses tend to be appropriate to those situations he understands. The pattern of withdrawal from interpersonal contact shown by the emotionally disturbed is reflected in language behavior. This child tends to ignore the speech of others and when tricked or forced into response may show intensified anxiety. His vocalization tends to be bizarre or he may be mute. His play suggests good inner abilities but his activity tends to serve autistic purposes. There is an ever present feeling that the child *could* talk if he wanted to. The aphasic child's language functioning is characterized by confusion. He hears but does not understand. His comprehension of the relationships among things is often as poor as his overt attempts at language. An occasional appropriate response that cannot be repeated conforms to the pattern of inconsistency. Frustration is inevitable and may lead the child to reject communication but he is seldom bizarre and he does try to relate effectively.

Management.   The profound severity of these disorders leads to recommendations of comprehensive full-time programs in almost every case. The deaf and mentally deficient are candidates for the familiar special educational settings. The emotionally disturbed require psychiatric attention and eventually special education that may include speech and language training. Programs designed for the aphasic are still in the early stages of development. Private schools and schools for the deaf have led the way in designing such programs. Some classes for school-age children whose language disorder does not render them totally unable to handle normal routine have been set up in public schools. Some children are treated in university and hospital speech centers on a part-time basis but this therapy is inadequate except for diagnostic purposes or for problems that are relatively mild.

Voice Disorders

There are several prominent organic pathologic conditions that can result in disturbed voice production. Some of these can be eliminated or minimized by medical treatment. Blockages of the nasal passages and growths on the vocal folds are examples. Some pathologic conditions such as contact ulcer on the vocal folds may be aggravated by attempts of voice training. In postsurgical cases involving subsequent paralysis or destruction of portions of the vocal apparatus, medical opinion concerning residual capabilities of structure is essential. The first step in the evaluation of *any* voice disorder, then, is medical study. Sudden total loss of voice without organic justification should lead to referral for psychiatric evaluation. The competent speech pathologist does not begin therapy without such consultation.

Evaluation. The objectives are (1) detailed description of present performance, (2) identification of aspects of voice and modes of voice production primarily responsible for the judgment of disturbed voice and (3) determination of the degree to which the patient appears capable of making positive changes. The first objective requires judgment of vocal attributes such as pitch, quality and loudness in the range of speaking situations common to the patient. The examiner elicits samples of conversation and oral reading at the time of evaluation but probably will have to depend on the patient or a member of the family for an estimate of performance in daily speaking situations. Knowledge of variations in the adequacy of voice from time to time is important. Voice changes corresponding to tension and stressful circumstances are cues to functional components. The amount of talking and type of frequent vocal performance (singing, public speaking) may bear on a judgment of vocal abuse and may in turn be etiologically related to pathologic states of the vocal folds.

The specific vocal attribute that gives rise to the global judgment of defective voice is identified during the clinical examination. A judgment of inappropriate pitch, hypernasality or insufficient loudness is made by the speech pathologist and this aspect is tested in detail to determine the range of performance of which the patient is capable. It may be possible to say, for instance, that a change in habitual pitch to another level within the patient's range of useful pitch will greatly improve the overall effect. Pitch, quality and loudness are closely related. A change in one will produce a change in the other. The examiner seeks to learn, for example, whether a desired change in quality (less strident or less harsh) results from stimulating a reduction in loudness.

Although no particular pattern of breathing has been conclusively shown to be best, high-chest or clavicular breathing may accompany the tense, weak, high-pitched voice. Evidence of extraordinary tension, particularly in the laryngeal area, may be significantly related to pitch, quality and loudness disturbance. Excessive tension in vocal behavior seems to be a frequent finding in cases of vocal abuse and other disorders of functional origin. Often the tension goes deeper than the laryngeal musculature to the personality of the patient.

In organic problems, the potential of the musculature is an important determiner of success but it is difficult to evaluate. Paralytic conditions of the soft palate and larynx are cases in point. Gross, severe inadequacy suggests a poor prognosis but the degree to which the individual can learn to compensate in the presence of less profound muscular deficiency may require a period of training to define.

Management. The interdependence of aspects of voice indicates that treatment directed at a fraction of behavior is likely to be discouraging. Furthermore, the patient's motivation is crucial, particularly in functional problems. We have known many patients with intact vocal mechanism who verbalize a desire for change but who make only minimal gains and eventually drift away from therapy. In these instances it is apparent that we misevaluated, concentrating on the voice rather than the person. In this connection, the frequent observation of muscular tension has led to the prescription of relaxation. Some patients have learned systematic conscious relaxation of the muscles with good effect on voice, but in the writer's experience these patients have been rare. More often the personal sources of the tension must be worked out before the patient can respond to voice training.

As in therapy for articulatory errors, the patient must attain a good understanding of his habitual production and how it differs from a more acceptable form. He may need literally to discover his voice and its range of variation in order to consider change. The clinician presents the patient with models of voice for the patient to match and suggests movements and kinesthetic sensations associated with the quality that is sought. The patient is taught to detect changes in his own production and drills and practice in application outside the clinic are prescribed when indicated. Supplementary nonverbal exercises like blowing, sustaining exhalation, rapid alternation of oronasal pressure and others may be employed to strengthen weak musculature. But the clinician avoids all activities that lead to excessive strain and disturbance of one vocal attribute at the expense of another. For patients with functional deficiencies, the training is directed toward better use of intact structures; when the problem is organic, training is directed toward maximal compensation for structural deficiencies.

Laryngectomy

The absence of a natural mechanism for producing voice leaves the laryngectomized patient with a number of alternatives: (1) he can carry a pad and write notes to others, (2) he can whisper, depending upon the state of the laryngeal area, (3) he can apply a mechanical source of vibration to the outer surface of the throat and articulate the vibrations as they pass through the oral cavity or (4) he can learn esophageal speech. Although each of these alternatives has been adopted by some patients, the last, esophageal speech, is thought to be the most satisfactory. Esophageal speech tends to be more intelligible, more natural sounding and generally more efficient in comparison with its closest competitor, the artificial vibrator. Esophageal voice is similar in its production and acoustic effect to the sound of a "belch." The patient learns in training, however, consciously to inject or swallow a bolus of air into the esophagus and immediately release it in a controlled manner. The tissues of the esophagus act on the ejected air, resulting in sound which is in turn altered by the oronasal structures to produce respectable speech sounds. Some patients learn very quickly to become good speakers, others require many months of work and guidance and still others do not learn at all. Aside from rare organic barriers to esophageal voice production, it seems that here again, the patient's attitude is significant. The loss of communication with its social and vocational implications can be psychologically traumatic to the patient. His inability to adjust may be expressed in a lack of acceptance of any substitute for his natural voice. Sensitive counseling is needed and may be initiated before surgery to help prepare the patient and his family. Some surgeons and consulting speech pathologists have found it valuable to introduce the candidate for laryngectomy to a good esophageal speaker who may be a teacher of esophageal voice himself and a representative of a Lost Chord Club. This experience requires careful staging and is not indicated for all patients. Certainly nothing should be done to lead the patient to reject surgery.

Cleft Palate

Of all the structural defects associated with disturbed speech, cleft palate conditions are most prominent. In addition to the palatal defect, lip and dental relationships are often affected. Maladaptive postures of the tongue and movements of the nares are common. Since individuals with cleft palate are susceptible to middle ear infection, hearing loss is not uncommon. The disturbance of the oronasal structures is always of consequence, yet with regard to speech, our investigations have made two important points relevant to both evaluation and management. First, in a significant number of cases not all of the speech problem can be attributed to the cleft palate condition. Second, some patients whose structural defect would predict serious speech disturbance show only minimal speech effects, sometimes none at all. These observations as well as our clinical experience with other structural and muscular defects that coexist with speech impairment have taught us that the relations between these conditions are rarely one to one. As with most of the disorders discussed in this chapter, the matter of personal adjustment plays a part. The strong sensitivities shown by many cleft palate individuals in relation to appearance, mouth, speech, and self are not unexpected and we find that they can produce behavior that aggravates the problem in addition to raising barriers to direct therapy on speech.

The speech pathologist spends most of his time with those individuals for whom surgical or prosthetic treatment has not been entirely effective in preventing or eliminating speech disturbance. We note, however, that he may make a significant contribution in decisions as to whether or not certain surgical, prosthetic and dental steps should be taken for purposes of speech. He is, of course, in an excellent position to evaluate the speech effects of these procedures when they have been done.

Evaluation.   If there is a distinguishing feature of "cleft palate speech," it is likely to be isolated in the pattern of hypernasal voice quality and the nasal distortion of consonants. An inventory of speech sound production is made and the errors that appear to be unrelated to the organic condition are noted. The pattern of hypernasality is most often caused by inadequate velopharyngeal closure which in turn is caused by cleft or insufficient velum. The patient's use of the oral mechanism may also show a tendency to carry the back of the tongue high in the mouth, minimal mouth opening during speech and "pinching" of the nares. These practices are learned and have the effect of increasing nasal resonance in the wrong places. For purposes of speech therapy, it is important to estimate the potential of the velopharyngeal port but estimation is difficult and may not be possible until after training has begun. Direct observation of velopharyngeal action is rarely possible although visualization of velar and pharyngeal action is rarely possible although visualization of velar and pharyngeal action during sustained vocalization and fluoroscopic films are helpful. The best estimates probably come from indirect observations such as relative measures of the amount of air pressure that can be developed in the mouth and from speech performance itself. The possibility of encouraging more effective velopharyngeal closure by direct stimulation of the involved areas may also be examined. Periodic hearing measurement is always indicated.

Management.   With the advent of cleft palate teams, the speech pathologist–audiologist has been able to enter the picture during the child's earliest years. He may contribute to the counseling of parents with respect to the child's speech potential, procedures for home stimulation and the importance of developing positive attitudes toward the condition. Later, if the child comes to speech therapy, the speech clinician is likely to have the most frequent and prolonged contact with both child and parents. He needs the support of the rest of the team in his work for he will be in a position to field many of the expressions of guilt and frustration that come from parent and child. In direct speech work, the interrelationship of articulation, voice quality and intelligibility leads us to expect that improvement in one dimension will be accompanied by improvement in the others. Since speech sound errors unrelated to the structural defect as well as the overall precision of articulation tend to respond most readily, these problems are usually considered first. With positive change, improvement in intelligibility and judged voice quality is often noticed. Methods for decreasing hypernasality may include variations on the familiar blowing exercises, not so much for the purpose of teaching velopharyngeal closure per se, but rather to promote in the patient a sense of oral air flow. Direct stimulation of velar and pharyngeal movement through light touch and massage may promote an increase in voluntary movement by the patient. Helping the patient to a conscious sense of the velopharyngeal musculature through mirror visualization, repeated swallowing and sudden sucking may also be first steps in achieving more effective control of the mechanism. The object of all of this work is to teach the patient to increase the flow of air through the mouth, and this is a difficult job. Another approach is to have him invite more air into the oral cavity by using wider mouth openings on vowel elements. Instead of trying to increase the oral air pressure (an increase in effort by the patient is just as likely to result in a louder nasal "snort") the patient may be able to use the available air more efficiently by making lighter articulatory contacts on the short explosive sounds and soft prolongation of the sounds that require deflection of the air stream through the narrow construction of the oral opening. As a result, consonant sounds like "p," "t," "s" and "sh" may not be as intense as we like but they may be more intelligible.

The patient must be willing to learn a heightened consciousness of speech movements and their acoustic results. He needs to engage in much exploration of a variety of alternative behaviors that may lead to an improved speech pattern. This means that he must have a certain objectivity concerning that part of himself that constitutes the essential difference between himself and his fellows. The task in any of its aspects is usually a long-term proposition.

Cerebral Palsy

Neuromotor disturbance has long been considered the distinctive feature of cerebral palsy. This condition alone would be enough to make it difficult for the child to develop competent speech. In addition, however, the chances are good that the individual with cerebral palsy will show mental retardation, psychomotor disturbance and significant hearing loss. As if this were not enough, his childhood environment is often characterized by overprotection and insufficient stimulation. It is no wonder that the majority of these patients show some sort of speech and language disturbance. Although the total picture occasionally is bright, more often it is rather pessimistic. Speech and language are part of that picture.

Evaluation. It is assumed that the individual will have had comprehensive physical and psychologic study. If the child is young, the speech pathologist is interested in the home situation and the pattern of care, particularly with respect to verbal stimulation and feeding practices. In the older individuals, these areas are included in the history. The patient's speech and language are examined in detail. Disorders of articulation, language, voice and rhythm are usually found. Speech muscle ability is tested, including the patient's ability to make movements basic to speech sound and voice production. The older patient is likely to have been through many of these procedures before. Knowledge of his reaction to previous therapy and his motivation for continued work will bear on recommendations.

Management. Generally the most important work on speech and language is done early in the life of the child with cerebral palsy. The object is to promote psychologic and physical readiness for speech and language learning. Muscle activity basic to speech production should be encouraged by direct stimulation and manipulation. This work should be correlated with the total physical therapy program and may best be accomplished in short informal periods throughout the day by the parent.

Although the movements of feeding are not those of speech, there is a common musculature and its strength, range of movement and coordination are important. Perhaps the best early speech muscle training is done by feeding. Food is a compelling source of motivation and the child will make considerable effort to get a dab of peanut butter that has been put in the corner of his mouth. This is not to suggest that the child will be deprived of food or of the peanut butter lure, for instance, if he fails to reach it by moving his tongue in a lateral direction. He should be rewarded for any and all efforts and the particular task set for him should amount to a healthy but enjoyable challenge without threat and as nearly within his capacity as possible.

Communicative effort should invariably be encouraged and approved. However, the conditions that lead to such effort are likely to be months of considerable language stimulation and exposure to those aspects of the environment that interest any child. The child with cerebral palsy is restricted in mobility and needs help in getting around to make contact with his environment. A psychologic readiness to talk and to learn talking develops best from a background of experience that has helped the child have something to say and has indicated that what he says, no matter how distorted it is, will be valued by those important to him. With the older patient, we may employ a variety of specialized techniques to improve voice control and the precision of articulation but our experience suggests that without a feeling of personal value and a need to communicate effectively on the part of the patient, much of our effort will be to no end. There is little doubt that the patient's degree of muscular involvement, mental ability, perceptual skills and hearing status also condition the outcome of treatment but we think that sometimes the clinician's frequent cry of lack of motivation on the part of the patient has some validity. The present degree of motivation has its origin in the nature of the early management.

Aphasia

Disturbance of expressive and receptive language is a frequent sequel to brain damage in the adult, particularly when the lesion is in the left side of the brain. Unfortunately, aphasia is not well understood and when some patients make good recovery of language, we are uncertain of how and why the recovery took place. The study of aphasia as a phenomenon has a long history, but concentrated clinical treatment in this country was rare until World War II when the large number of GI's with head wounds stimulated the development of language retraining programs in military hospitals. Since that time the literature and experience with aphasia have grown.

Although the problem of aphasia (and language itself for that matter) remains poorly defined, some of its outlines are clearer and some promising clues to its study and management are available. The asphasic patient typically shows a number of other problems, such as right hemiplegia, hemianopia, convulsions, increased emotional lability and heightened fatiguability. These conditions are related to the language disturbance in important ways. Their individual and cumulative effect on the patient's total disposition and capabilities is also reflected in his language behavior. The language status in turn has varying effects on other aspects. The almost inevitable presence of multiple problems in the patient predicts the involvement of many specialists in the evaluation and management.

Evaluation.   To state that a person changes after brain injury may appear elementary and unnecessary. The simple idea of change, however, seems more accurate than the tendency to view the aphasic as a transformation from the familiar to the unfamiliar. He has not automatically become a new person because of brain damage even though his behavior is often unpredictable and bizarre by ordinary standards. Study of the patient with as few a priori assumptions as possible will show that he continues to function according to what he was (and still is): an individual with many years of experience during which he has developed a complex repertoire of attitudes, abilities and disabilities. The patient's behavior today cannot be described as a simple function of brain injury and it is more clearly understood if it is viewed as a joint product of pretraumatic experience interacting with the injury and with the experience since the injury. This position is an attempt to "normalize" our way of looking at aphasia, without minimizing the profound changes that do in fact take place. The objectives of the evaluation are to determine the amount of change, the mechanisms of change and the chances for reinstatement of that which has changed.

Knowledge of the patient's pretraumatic educational, intellectual and language status is essential to the assessment of change. We would not want to assign reading disabilities to aphasia in a patient with a history of illiteracy or similarly interpret difficulty in understanding speech in a patient who had habitually used a language other than English.

Information about the patient's pretraumatic intellectual and educational level also has prognostic significance. Generally speaking, more intelligent and better educated patients will make the best linguistic recovery. Post-traumatic measures of mental ability and educational achievement can be used to estimate the degree to which the expression of these areas has been disturbed and may also be employed as indicators of recovery for they will tend to improve as language improves. The disturbance of intelligence or, more importantly, of the aphasic's ability to learn is difficult to determine. Traditional tests are highly verbal and it has not been easy to ascertain whether performance was conditioned by the language disability or a true intellectual deficit or perhaps a combination of both. That the aphasic tends to show a definite problem in learning is supported by the widespread difficulties encountered in language therapy. But language and mental processes such as thinking and problem solving are so intricately interrelated that to assign poor performance to one or the other aspect is rarely possible.

Special tests of aphasic language behavior are useful in the examination. The form of these tests tends to follow the test constructor's system of classifying aspects of language performance. The classification system may in turn be based on a theory concerning the organization of language. The different theories and classifications have produced a rash of terminology variously defined and often confusing. Nevertheless, the main objective of the clinical tests is the same: to describe levels of language ability and disability for the purposes of making predictions about the patient's recovery and planning an appropriate program of language training.

The patient's performance is usually divided into two general categories: expressive and receptive (more recently, encoding and decoding). Within each category, modality-bound functions are tested. Auditory comprehension and visual-word recognition are examples. Classes of skills such as spelling and reading are examined. A useful profile of language performance should emerge. As a result, patients can usually be reliably classified as showing predominantly receptive aphasia, predominantly expressive aphasia, or global aphasia (extreme disability in all areas of language). The writer believes that the predominantly receptive aphasic always has at least as great an involvement on the expressive side; after all, one must understand language in order to use it. In addition, patients with disabilities strictly localized to only some modalities with others intact are rare. Aphasia tends to be present to some degree in all areas. All things being equal, the prognosis for significant recovery from global aphasia is poor. The expressive aphasic with reasonably intact receptive abilities has the best chance for recovery.

The reliability and validity of language estimates are dependent on a number of considerations. Aphasics, for example, generally show a slower response time. If the examiner does not give the aphasic more time than normal for each item, he may miss a correct response. It is widely held that the first six months after injury is a period of "spontaneous" recovery. That is, each patient will show varying amounts of spontaneous return of abilities during the first six months; further gains will probably be a function of treatment. Detailed language testing during this period may be of questionable value except for charting change. Permanent residuals are best assessed after the first half year. It goes without saying that the examiner must try to create an atmosphere that is conducive to optimal performance from the patient. This requires considerable skill and may take some time, perhaps examination over a period of days in a quiet and private setting. We suggest that approaching the patient with a group of interested students and asking for performance in a noisy ward may not be the best approach to evaluating the patient who already is confused and has difficulty in understanding.

The first post-traumatic months deserve further consideration because they may be highly correlated with later performance. One of the things our language appraisal usually shows, in addition to disturbed language, is that the aphasic has a simple but significantly reduced verbal output. As a rule, he just does not talk much. The writer is inclined to believe that the patient has learned this aspect of his disability during the early months after injury. During this time, he becomes aware of his condition and feels natural anxiety and depression. He also becomes aware of his environment and perhaps painfully aware of the reactions of others to him. His nurses, physicians, family and friends often speak to him with language he cannot understand or to which he cannot appropriately respond. They test him often and he fails frequently. His spontaneous attempts at communication are labored and distorted and are met with reactions of pity, embarrassment and sometimes outright impatience. Often enough, those who come in regular contact with him stop talking to him or talk to him in such a manner that no response is required. It is as if others have entered into an unstated agreement that the patient should be treated as if he cannot or should not talk and certainly the patient is affected by such an attitude. Even in speech therapy, clinicians sometimes avoid activities in which the patient is likely to make errors, particularly the activity that is most important—spontaneous, realistic conversation. In most instances, analysis of therapy will show that the *clinician's* verbal behavior predominates even though he knows that it is the patient who has the problem and should be doing the talking.

Not all patients show this tendency toward muteness. Some learn to try and to profit from their errors. Others speak a great deal, using unorganized, seemingly random language. We call these patients "jargon" aphasics and think either that they have lost their ability to monitor their speech critically or that they have been so psychologically traumatized that their blithe jargon is evidence of an inability to accept their problem.

We have suggested that the evaluation must seek to differentiate that aspect of aphasia that is a direct function of brain damage from that part that is acquired. Formal language examination helps to tell us about current language performance but it takes sensitive study to tell us what the patient can do but is unwilling to attempt. Overdependence, withdrawal and unwillingness to make mistakes are thought to be contributors to present functioning and factors that tend to maintain aphasia. Personality is important and some knowledge of pretraumatic characteristics should contribute to the understanding of the patient's handling of post-traumatic experience.

Management.   The rather reliable clinical observation that the aphasic understands and uses elements of the language correctly at certain times but not at others provides the basis for the following interpretation of aphasic behavior: words have not been lost; they have become less available. Our research concentrates on defining the conditions under which language becomes more or less available and our therapy attempts to reestablish conditions that make language more available to the patient.

What conditions need to be reestablished? In line with impressions presented earlier, it is thought that a kind of speech therapy should begin when the patient first returns to consciousness of himself and others. The patient begins to learn the facts of his condition and develops important attitudes toward them. Some of these attitudes were described earlier. If we want to help him acquire a reasonably realistic and accepting view of his disabilities, we must show the way by behavior that indicates we hold those attitudes ourselves. This is not easy; the sense of tragedy in such cases remains with most of us no matter how much previous experience we have had in these situations. The patient's family will be responding to overwhelming personal and economic pressures and cannot help communicating these concerns to him. Environmental conditions that will promote the proper atmosphere must be worked out with the family. The speech pathologist should be present early in this process even when it is uncertain that the language problem will be permanent. He can contribute specific information concerning language stimulation appropriate to the situation.

Speech therapy should begin early both in terms of structuring attitudes and in starting regularly scheduled sessions of direct treatment. Clinical study strongly suggests that the earlier treatment is begun, the better the chances of recovery. Again, the main objective is to establish conditions that will make language more available. The patient must talk and attempt to talk. Verbal output, appropriate and inappropriate, must be stimulated, reinforced and used to advantage by the clinician. It is the patient who must do the learning and to do so he must be active in providing the material (speech) to be examined and manipulated in cooperation with the clinician. The patient must feel free to expose himself and his disability. Routine application of drills, exercises and correction without recognition of the patient as a person does not seem to encourage such behavior; rather it appears to facilitate passive dependence, frustration and forms of resistance. Several recovered patients who have written of their experience report that not until they felt more secure as individuals could they begin to make progress in language. Relevant to some extent are our preliminary experiments at Temple University which suggest that simple, unrestricted reinforcement of all aphasic verbal efforts leads to increased verbal output and improved patient objectivity. In addition, clinicians have reported that group sessions have facilitated increased spontaneity, expression of feelings and appearance of language ability unknown in individual therapy.

Several other treatment concepts should be mentioned. When some modalities show less involvement than others, clinicians attempt to obtain a transfer from one to the other. For example, if writing is more intact than speaking, simultaneous speaking-writing may make language elements more available in speech. Patients often retain automatic, over-learned speech such as rote counting and this material may be used to build a bridge to more voluntary elements. The principle of association is used extensively. Presentation of words is often accompanied by supporting pictures or by the activities the words represent. Some small groups of words have strong associative bonds and practice in making completions like "hot and – – –" or "black and – – –" is often helpful. The patient will probably come closer to recovering linguistic rules if he repeatedly hears short, familiar sentence forms unmistakably related to certain real situations and designed to have only a few highly probable interpretations.

Whatever the specific treatment procedures, and they vary considerably, it has been observed that attempts at teaching the aphasic one word at a time are not rewarding. Single words often have too many meanings out of context. Procedures that help the aphasic rediscover ways of finding words are more successful. Even when therapy goes well, it typically involves daily treatment over periods of months and sometimes years.

THE PHYSICAL MEDICINE AND REHABILITATION SPEECH AND HEARING SECTION

Staff. Some speech and hearing sections have only one full-time staff member; others have as many as fifteen. One of these should serve as section director and he should be a speech pathologist–audiologist with a doctorate degree who also holds the certificate of clinical competence awarded by the American Speech and Hearing Association.* Other staff members should also meet the academic and experience requirements for clinical certification.

Activities. The work of the speech and hearing section is largely consultative, diagnostic and therapeutic. Some sections are also active in teaching and research activity. The director frequently has a teaching appointment in an affiliated medical school or in a university program offering a professional degree in the speech and hearing sciences.

Equipment. Diagnostic equipment includes various test batteries peculiar to speech and language evaluation. Minimal equipment for audiologic screening includes a diagnostic audiometer and a consistently quiet area for testing. Complete audiologic evaluation requires a number of instruments designed for the total range of auditory assessment in addition to test rooms specifically designed to eliminate ambient noise.

Therapeutic equipment includes tape recorders and auditory training units as well as a range of consumable stimulus materials.

Space. Aside from the usual offices, rooms should be set aside for both diagnostic and therapeutic activity. Room size should vary to accommodate both individual and group therapy. A waiting area for patients is also advisable.

---

*Details of A.S.H.A. clinical certificates procedures may be obtained from the Executive Secretary, American Speech and Hearing Association, 1001 Connecticut Avenue, N.W., Washington, D. C. 20036.

REFERENCES

1. Barbara, D. A.: Psychological and Psychiatric Aspects of Speech and Hearing. Springfield, Ill., Charles C Thomas, 1960. Research, theory and therapy mainly from a psychodynamic point of view. Basic material on communication as a function of personality.
2. Berry, M. F.: Language Disorders in Children. New York, Appleton-Century-Crofts, Inc., 1969. An excellent up-to-date integration of theory, research, and diagnostic practice relative to children with serious language disturbance.
3. Cruickshank, W. M., and Raus, G. M.: Cerebral Palsy: Its Individual and Community Problems. Syracuse, Syracuse University Press, 1955. A comprehensive text covering the range of diagnostic and management aspects from the point of view of various specialties.
4. Davis, H., and Silverman, S. R.: Hearing and Deafness. Revised Edition, New York, Holt, Rinehart and Winston, 1947. General survey of hearing problems, measurement of hearing, medical aspects and habilitation procedures.
5. deReuck, A. V. S., and O'Conner, M.: Disorders of Language, Boston, Little, Brown and Co., 1964. Report of a symposium on language disorders, mainly adult aphasia. Many of the current research approaches are represented.
6. Diehl, C. F.: Stuttering: A Compendium of Research and Theory. Springfield, Ill., Charles C Thomas, 1958. Contains abstracts of 193 articles plus relevant bibliography organized according to history, symptomatology, etiology and therapy.
7. Eisenson, J.: Stuttering: A Symposium. New York, Harper and Bros., 1958. Seven authorities discuss the nature and treatment of stuttering. Psychoanalytic through organic points of view are represented.

8. Johnson, W., Darley, F. L., and Spriestersbach, D. C.: Diagnostic Methods in Speech Pathology. New York, Harper and Row, 1963. Under one cover, most of the objective and subjective techniques used to describe and define disturbed speech and language behavior. Includes relevant norms for a variety of speech and language performances.
9. Myklebust, H. R.: The Psychology of Deafness. New York, Grune and Stratton, Inc., 1960. The effects of deafness on learning and adjustment.
10. Myklebust, H. R.: Auditory Disorders in Children: A Manual for Differential Diagnosis. New York, Grune and Stratton, Inc., 1954. A unique integration of theory, research and clinical experience. For use in the diagnosis of language disorders associated with hearing loss, emotional disturbance, mental retardation and aphasia in children.
11. Olmstead, R. W.: Symposium on Disorders of Speech. J. Pediat., 62:1–24, 1963. An introduction to speech and language problems in children written as a series of articles for the pediatrician. Of particular interest is the article by Halfond and Olmstead on the relationship between pediatrics and nonmedical specialties and the article by Lillywhite on concepts of communication.
12. Osgood, C. E., and Miron, M. S.: Approaches to the Study of Aphasia. Urbana, University of Illinois Press, 1963. A report of a conference on theoretical, research and clinical problems which is notable for its clear statement of questions that need answers and the introduction of psycholinguistic modes of study.
13. Penfield, W., and Roberts, L.: Speech and Brain Mechanisms. Princeton, Princeton University Press, 1959. A report of the clinical experiments in electrical stimulation of the cortex. Results are applied to the perennial questions of dominance and localization of function in the brain.
14. Schuell, H., Jenkins, J. J., Jiménez-Pabón, E.: Aphasia in Adults. New York, Harper and Row, 1964. A comprehensive review of neurological and psychological positions and a statement of the author's own findings from research and clinical experience.
15. Travis, L. E.: Handbook of Speech Pathology. New York, Appleton-Century-Crofts, Inc., 1957. A definitive work covering the fields of speech and hearing science, speech pathology and audiology. Revised edition is in press.
16. Van Riper, C.: Speech Correction: Principles and Methods. 4th Ed. Englewood Cliffs, N. J., Prentice-Hall, Inc., 1963. The standard introductory text to the diagnosis and treatment of speech disorders, written by an authority who is at the same time probably the most successful clinician in the field.

Chapter 6

PSYCHOLOGICAL ASSESSMENT AND MANAGEMENT

by Wilbert E. Fordyce

The purpose of this chapter is to analyze the medical rehabilitation process in behavioral terms in order to provide a basis for developing appropriate courses of action when so-called psychological or motivational problems occur in patient management. Major objectives are to provide the physician with an appreciation of the implications for intervention strategies and to examine and analyze the rehabilitation processes from a learning point of view.

The clientele of medical rehabilitation are primarily people who, as a consequence of physical disability, are at a functional disadvantage in the performance of life tasks. Medical rehabilitation is concerned with containing or limiting this functional impairment; with slowing its progression; or with reducing or eliminating the functional impairment, as may be indicated by the nature of the medical problem. Whatever the ultimate course of the medical aspects of the disability, rehabilitation is concerned with optimizing functional performance in the face of impairment. Finally, rehabilitation is also concerned with assisting the individual with the impairment to become re-engaged in the affairs of society and daily living at an optimal level commensurate with the state of his disability. In a sense it might be said that rehabilitation is trying to do something about the patient's medical or physical status, whatever that status may be, and also trying to do something about how effectively the patient performs. The former of those two areas of concern focuses primarily on medical problems, broadly defined. The latter sector of interest clearly involves problems of learning and performance. This chapter will be primarily concerned with this latter sector.

There are several reasons why rehabilitation properly emphasizes learning. In the first place, learning is behavior change. When a person incurs a physical disability, there is some immediate change in his behavior potential or response repertoire. The patient, for example, who sustains injury to the spinal cord undergoes significant change in a host of behaviors, e.g., ambulation. His disability will change what he needs to do as well as what he can do. But he will not do the new things he needs to do and is potentially capable of doing until he learns how. Moreover, as will later be developed in more detail, effective learning consists both of acquiring the skill or ability to do something and of developing the probability that the necessary actions will occur as often as needed. Using again the example of a paraplegic patient, such a patient needs to acquire skill at transferring from bed to wheelchair, but he also needs to perform those transfers at appropriate times and in appropriate places. Both skill acquisition and increasing probability of performance are behavior change processes and therefore learning problems.

Another way in which learning concepts become important in rehabilitation is in the assimilation of disability or adjustment to disability. Traditionally, problems of adjustment have been viewed from a disease-oriented conceptual model. That is, those behaviors the individual engages in which cause others to identify him as either adjusted or maladjusted are seen as under the control of intrapsychic factors within the organism. This approach and logical alternatives are discussed further in Sarason and Ganzer,[42] Ullmann and Krasner,[53] and Szasz.[49] It has evolved from traditional disease concepts in which symptoms are identified as under the control of underlying pathologic conditions. The disease model frame of reference (Fig. 6–1) has been applied by analogy to problems of adjustment. Unfortunately, it has often been the case that people fail to recognize it as an analogy and not a statement of facts. There are alternative descriptive systems one may use to organize phenomena associated with questions about adjustment to disability. The descriptive system or conceptual model used here (Fig. 6-2) views those behaviors defined as indicative of adjustment or maladjustment as subject to the influence of learning processes. Use of a learning model leads one's effort toward applying appropriate learning principles directly to the behavior to be changed rather than trying to change inferred underlying attitude or feeling states in order that an ensuing behavior change may occur.

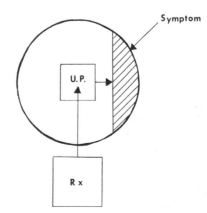

1. Observe sign or symptom of illness.

   ("Illness Behavior")

2. Pursue, identify (or infer) underlying

   pathology "causing" symptom.

3. Treat by attacking underlying pathology.

Figure 6–1 The disease-medical model.

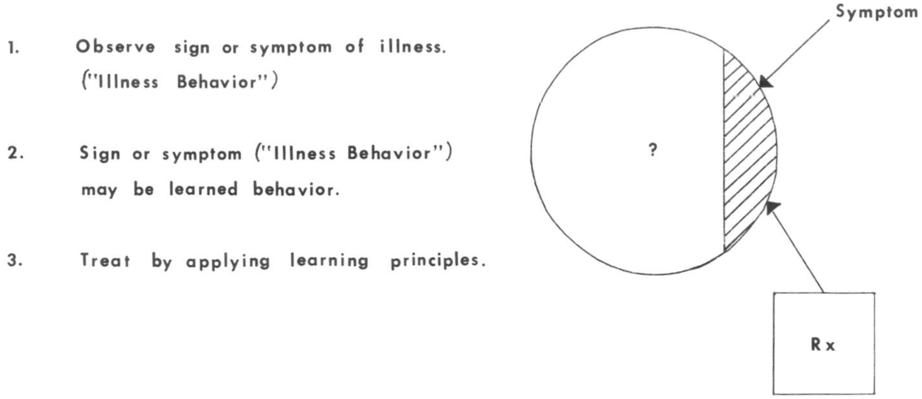

1.   Observe sign or symptom of illness.

      ("Illness Behavior")

2.   Sign or symptom ("Illness Behavior")

      may be learned behavior.

3.   Treat by applying learning principles.

Symptom

?

Rx

Figure 6–2   The learning model.

When a person incurs a disability, certain behaviors he engaged in prior to the onset of disability are no longer appropriate. Those behaviors need to be reduced or eliminated. In addition, the patient needs to acquire new disability-appropriate behaviors. The identification of behaviors to be changed (decreased, eliminated, increased) and efforts to develop conditions favorable for these behavior changes need not await changes in underlying attitudes or feeling states. In essence, the major distinction between the disease model and the learning model, in the context of assimilation of disability, is that the disease model approach emphasizes changing underlying attitudes and feeling states so that new behaviors may occur. In contrast, the learning model aims directly at changing these behaviors, with the expectation that adjustments in underlying feelings and attitudes, insofar as they are crucial or relevant, will follow.

There is yet another way in which learning concepts are important in medical rehabilitation. One of the major differences between rehabilitation medicine and most other medical fields is the emphasis in rehabilitation medicine on medical problems of a chronic nature. Disabilities usually cannot be totally eliminated or resolved. Residual impairments persist. Medical problems relating to disability are chronic and recurring. This difference has a number of implications for the patient, the family unit, the patient's environment, and for professionals dealing with the patient. Acute, time-limited medical problems ordinarily do not require the patient to make a lasting behavior change. Chronic disease problems, as with physical disability, usually require major and permanent behavior changes. Moreover, as will be developed further in a discussion of motivation, many of the behavior changes dictated by the disability are low-frequency, low-strength, low-value behaviors having little attractiveness to the patient or his family, thereby complicating the learning process. Finally, it is generally the case in rehabilitation that rate of progress is relatively slow in comparison to the patient's prior experiences with acute illness. As a consequence, the learning process may be further burdened by a dearth of the rewards of rapid progress.

Psychological interventions have for the most part been derived from various personality theories, though claiming some allegiance to learning theory. Only in approximately the last decade, however, has there emerged meaningful and practical remedial technology derived from learning principles. These new, learning-based therapies may be applied directly to a number of facets of the rehabilitation process. Gendlin and Rychlak,[16] (p. 156), in reviewing the current state of psychotherapy and problems of maladjustment, say, "The new therapies written about tend to reject the older conception of maladjustment as a long-term illness needing long-term treatment and substitute instead a much briefer intervention . . . instead of deep dynamics, the therapies now tend to make the difficulty a mode of interaction, game, or behavior pattern which is to be knocked out not by years of treatment but simply by taking up some other mode of interaction 'game' or 'behavior' pattern."

The learning principles underlying these new therapies can be described rather briefly. It will not be possible to develop mastery over their application by study of the summary statements and illustrations provided here. It should be possible, however, to develop an adequate understanding of the general princples involved, an appreciation of the basic methods sufficient to participate with others in their application, and a grasp of what the adequately trained behavioral engineer is up to when he works out detailed applications.

The principles underlying operant conditioning or contingency management methods derive from the work of B. F. Skinner.[45, 46] Concise treatment of operant principles and illustrations of applications are found, for example, in Krasner and Ullman,[25] Meacham and Wiesen,[29] Michael,[31] Patterson and Guillion,[35] and Reese.[39] The brief statement of these principles given here draws heavily on the work of Michael[32] and of Lindsley and Skinner.[28]

LEARNING PRINCIPLES

A distinction is drawn between respondent and operant behavior. Respondents are responses of the organism involving glandular, smooth-muscle or reflex phenomena. They are under the control of antecedent stimuli—that is to say, upon occurrence of an adequate stimulus, the respondent follows automatically. Operants are behaviors involving striated muscles or voluntary actions. Operants may be elicited by an antecedent stimulus. However, the strength of an operant response (i.e., the probability that it will occur in a given situation) is subject to influence by consequences. Manipulation of consequences is the critical operation in operant conditioning. When an operant is followed by a positive consequence (reinforcer), its frequency tends to increase. When an operant is followed by a negative or aversive reinforcer (punisher), its rate tends to decrease. When positive reinforcers are withdrawn from an operant, its rate will diminish and ultimately disappear, a process termed extinction.

The effectiveness of a reinforcer on an operant is related to the stimulus situation in which the operant has occurred in the past contiguous to that reinforcer. A reinforcer will have more effect on an operant when it is delivered or withheld in the same stimulus setting as has occurred previously. The more the stimulus setting has changed, the less the effect of the reinforcer. As behavior occurs and is reinforced or punished in changing stimulus situations, the new stimuli will tend to act as reinforcers, i.e., they become conditioned reinforcers or conditioned punishers.

A given consequence can be identified as a reinforcer or punisher only by observation of its effects on the behavior it follows. One cannot assume a given consequence is a positive reinforcer. One may hypothesize that it is and try it out. Having done so, if the behavior it follows in fact increases in rate, it may be inferred that that consequence is a positive reinforcer for that person.

In order to be effective, reinforcers must be delivered as soon as possible following the behavior they are designed to influence. The longer the delay, the less likely the reinforcer will be effective.

Schedules of reinforcement play an important role. When starting a new behavior or increasing the rate of a behavior which previously rarely occurred, it is advantageous to reinforce as many occurrences of the behavior as possible (continuous reinforcement), i.e., one approaches a 1:1 response-reinforcement ratio. When a behavior becomes established, it will become more durable if the reinforcement schedule is reduced (intermittent reinforcement), i.e., a decreasing proportion of occurrences of the response receives reinforcement.

New and complex responses are acquired by shaping. In shaping, successive approximations of the desired response are reinforced. Systematically varying the stimulus situations for an established response (stimulus fading) helps bring the response under control of increasingly complex or remote stimuli, thereby making it more durable.

The sequence for setting up operant-based behavior change projects is as follows: (1) Pinpoint the behavior to be increased or decreased. (2) Define measurable units of that behavior, i.e., the beginning and end of the cycle of movements constituting the behavior. A movement cycle may be said to have occurred when the organism is in a position to repeat. (3) Record the rate at which the behavior is occurring. Rate is always defined as the number of movement cycles over a unit of time. (4) Identify reinforcers anticipated to be effective. Reinforcers should not be used unless they can be made contingent upon the behavior to be influenced. If there is incomplete control over a reinforcer's availability to a patient, it should not be used. Reinforcers which occur naturally in the treatment environment ordinarily are to be preferred. Rest, attention, and "time out" from treatment are examples of frequently effective reinforcers in a medical rehabilitation setting. (5) Specify a schedule of reinforcement. (6) Try out the program. If the rate of the behavior in question does not change following a reasonable number of trials, each of the preceding steps needs to be re-examined. As progress occurs, it is usually desirable to decrease the rate of reinforcement, i.e., to expect increasing amounts of performance for each unit of reinforcement.

The foregoing outline is not sufficient in itself to prepare a professional who is otherwise untrained in the application of these methods to set up and carry out behavior change projects. The purpose of the outline is to make the physician familiar with the major dimensions of the process. In later portions of this chapter, examples will be given of applications of these methods to specific problems in patient management.

The behavioral analysis and contingency management systems described here for modifying behavior represent a departure from more traditional approaches. These new methods can be very effective in bringing about behavior change, but their use requires appropriate training and experience. Their use also raises a number of ethical questions which deserve at least brief consideration here. Further discussion of ethical issues can be found in Ulrich, Stachnik and Mabry.[55]

Contingency management methods involve the manipulation of behavior-consequence relationships. When these manipulations are handled with technical correctness, behavior change probably will ensue. The question rightfully should be raised as to whether one is arbitrarily manipulating a patient when these techniques are being applied. Concern about manipulation of patients should be directed toward any treatment approach which fails to specify methods and goals and which fails to provide opportunity for the patient to decide if he will participate.

There is every reason to explain to the patient in detail the design and objectives of a contingency management program. It is sometimes mistakenly inferred that telling the patient about a contingency management program will somehow compromise its effectiveness. Quite to the contrary, a well-planned program involves the patient to much greater degree than frequently is true of more traditional approaches. There should be specification of what behaviors are expected by the end of the program, i.e., the program's goals. Those goals should be formulated with the patient. The patient should also participate, where possible, in selection of reinforcers. Exceptions to this are only those situations in which the patient is not able to participate because he is too young (preschool) or because he suffers intellectual impairment from cortical deficit.

ADJUSTMENT TO DISABILITY

This section will deal with the process of assimilation of disability and some of the more common patient management problems relating to it. These problems will be grouped arbitrarily into three subheadings: crisis management, assimilation of disability, and participation in rehabilitation. Figure 6-3 portrays graphically the conceptualization used here.

Efforts to identify a personality pattern or style of response specific to a given kind of disability have not proved fruitful. The subsequent behavior of a person who has incurred a particular disability will be some function of the behavioral repertoire he had prior to onset, the behaviors left to him by the disability, the meaning or value of the disability to him (i.e., the anticipated loss of reinforcers), and the way those around him behave in relationship to his

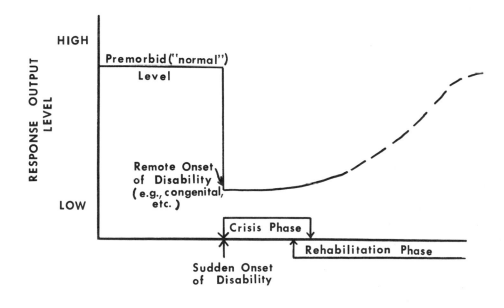

TIME

Figure 6–3   Assimilation of disability – a behavioral approach.

disability. Most of the efforts to develop a typology of personality according to type of disability are but another example of the disease model conceptual system applied by analogy to human behavior. That is, since some diseases have fairly fixed patterns of symptoms or manifestations, some people expect that fixed sequences or patterns of physical disability and emotional state or behavioral expressions will also occur. Such a position assumes that the emotional states and behavioral manifestations are under the control of underlying pathologic conditions. Where the evidence is clear that behavior is under the control of an underlying pathologic condition (e.g., aphasic signs in a right hemiplegic), there is every reason to expect that behavior will accompany the disability at an appropriate base rate. It should be evident, however, that feelings, attitudes, and general styles of behavior are learned and are not ordinarily under the control of pathologic conditions.

There appear to be only three conditions under which one might expect a systematic relationship between behavior, on the one hand, and a particular kind of disability, on the other. One such condition occurs when the disability itself appears only in people who have certain behavioral characteristics. For example, people who consume large amounts of liquor are more likely to develop cirrhosis of the liver. Perhaps also, diabetics who take poor care of themselves are more likely to sustain loss of vision. In both instances, however, there has been very little specification as to exactly what kinds of behavior the individual will display other than consumption of alcohol in the first example and careless diet control or insulin management in the second. Little has been said about a wide range of other behaviors of interest in the rehabilitation process.

A second condition in which behavior and disability may have a significant relationship is that in which the disability has a direct causal relationship to certain behavior changes. The example cited earlier of the signs of aphasia in a right hemiplegic is an illustration, as is the increase in physically sedentary behavior in an advanced case of chronic obstructive pulmonary emphysema. Another example of such a relationship is seen in the changes in recreational patterns of a person with significantly limited ambulation resulting from disability. In each of these examples, it is easy to identify a causal relationship between functional impairment and the ensuing behavior.

A third condition in which behavior-disability relationships might occur is that in which the disability has a consistent effect on the behavior of others toward the person with the disability. Facial disfigurement, athetoid movement in a cerebral palsy patient, and obvious blindness in a retrolental fibroplasia patient are illustrations. When the disability has a consistent effect on the behavior of others, their responses in turn are likely to influence the behavior of the person with the disability. The causal relationships in this example are between the behavior of the disabled person and the behavior of others toward him. There is no need for recourse to postulating an underlying mechanism which has produced the behavior observed.

Once it is recognized that there is no need for recourse to a personality typology when considering problems of adjustment to disability, the direct path of observing behavior-consequence relationships becomes more evident.

Crisis Management

When the human organism is placed suddenly in a situation in which a radical alteration in sensory input occurs or in which previously effective behavior is no longer possible, a period of confusion and disorganization is likely to occur. Those are the conditions surrounding onset of insignificant physical disability. The person who suddenly sustains a transected spinal cord, head injury or blindness, for example, immediately enters a state of relative sensory deprivation in at least two different ways. Sensory input to the cortex is likely to be altered. Impairment in sensory modalities from the disability immediately alters the sensations he receives. At the same time, medical management is likely to include immobilization in a hospital bed, a state of relative sensory deprivation. Instead of visitors, movement and the sensory enrichment of environmental variability, there is immobilization, isolation and the stimulus constancy of a hospital room. It has been shown (Hebb[19]) that when marked reduction in sensory input occurs, people commonly respond with confusion and disorganization. Grieving and depression may accompany such a response.

In discussing adjustment to disability, Michael[32] says, "The ordinary adult's social and verbal history is sufficiently well-developed that it can be affected emotionally by his own and other descriptions of his future somewhat as he will be affected by the future itself . . . he is fully capable of reacting to his own immediate (disability) in a manner somewhat appropriate to the future loss of reinforcers that he will experience . . . the human . . . because of his verbal skills can react to the situation all at once, as soon as the verbal stimuli are appropriate. Furthermore, he can react to it over and over again as he and others provide further stimuli related to the irreversible change."

The ability of the patient symbolically to project himself into the future tends to make all of the deprivations he thinks he is going to experience immediately accessible to him. At the same time, he probably does not know enough about rehabilitation to be able to judge accurately what reinforcers will become available to him as functional performance improves. Informing him about things he is going to be able to do in the future which will provide access to reinforcers tends to have little influence on his feelings and behavior because the information is an unexperienced abstraction. Moreover, because of his relative immobilization, he receives limited opportunity to confirm future possibilities by exercise or rehearsal of behaviors leading toward an effective repertoire in the future.

It would be a mistake to assume that the crisis period following sudden onset of significant disability inevitably produces confusion and disorganization. In our society crisis has tended to be viewed as harmful and disadvantageous, but, as Hanford[18] has pointed out, some people may not respond to crisis with disorganized behavior. What the individual does in a crisis state will depend upon what techniques he has in his repertoire for dealing with crisis situations and the manner and extent to which his behavioral repertoire has been altered by the crisis itself. The more radical the alterations in his repertoire produced by the disability and the greater the changes in his environment, the greater the chance of a period of disorganized behavior.

Caplan[8] (p. 48) has pointed out that ". . . during crisis, the individual is more susceptible to influence by others than at times of stable functioning. . . . This means that the help offered him by significant others may have a major effect in determining his choices of . . . [ways of] . . . coping." That observation leads to one of the major characteristics of an effective crisis management program. Guidelines for developing a crisis management program to help the patient and his family through the crisis phase and to lay the groundwork for an effective treatment relationship to enhance subsequent rehabilitation efforts may be summarized as follows:

1. *Provide calm, stable models for the patient and family to emulate.* Because people in crisis are more suggestible, they are more subject to influence by the behavior of people around them. It is important and therapeutically useful to engender a calm, confident, matter-of-fact style in each of the members of the rehabilitation team interacting with patient and family.

2. *Promote performance mastery.* Provide the patient with tasks chosen carefully to optimize chances of success. Tasks should be oriented to rehabilitation goals as much as possible and devised so that brief periods of effort can produce tangible results. This approach helps to fill the sensory void, thereby reducing confusion. It may help to reaffirm a sense of mastery and give the patient access to the reinforcers of attention and approval by the professional staff for having engaged in effective performance.

Finally, this approach helps the patient experience success at the first approximation of entry into the rehabilitation process. For example, the newly paraplegic patient can be given a bedside occupational therapy task, such as knot-tying, as a way of working toward upper extremity strengthening. Another task might be for a social worker, to work with the patient on details of a relatively simple family problem, such as bus transportation to the hospital. Tact, persistence and a rich schedule of encouragement for early efforts will be important factors in strengthening these approaches to serve the patient.

Members of the patient's family will also be in a crisis state. The same principles may be used in helping them, although tasks may vary.

Assimilation of Disability

Rehabilitation as Punishment. The conditions defining punishment also describe the typical situation for a person who has recently incurred a significant disability. Punishment (Ferster,[9] Michael,[32] Reese,[39] can be defined as any consequence which either weakens the behavior that follows or strengthens behavior designed to avoid or escape the punishing stimulus. Another way of stating it is that punishment may be thought of either as the loss of positive reinforcers or the onset of aversive stimuli. When positive reinforcers are no longer accessible following a behavior, the subsequent rate of that behavior diminishes. Similarly, when an aversive stimulus is applied following some behavior, that behavior's rate diminishes and behavior designed to enable escape from the aversive stimulus increases.

Those conditions characterize what happens with sudden onset of disability. The patient immediately loses access to the positive reinforcers previously sustaining his work and leisure behavior. The patient also immediately begins to experience aversive stimuli. There is likely to be pain and physical distress. As discussed previously, there is likely to be relative sensory deprivation and some disorganization. It is probable the patient will perceive his disability and related functional impairments as very aversive. Finally, those around the patient are likely to attribute negative value to the disability and to communicate that to the patient in one way or another (Siller and Chipman,[43] Siller, Ferguson, Vann, and Holland,[44] Wright.[60, 61])

Punishment, whether in the form of aversive stimuli or loss of positive reinforcers, tends to increase behavior designed to avoid the punishment or escape from it. It follows that the patient is likely to identify disability and the rehabilitation procedures associated with it as stimuli leading to punishment. The patient may avoid what he perceives as punishment by engaging in behavior which keeps him out of the rehabilitation process. Similarly, when he is actively engaged in some rehabilitation activity, escape behavior on his part may serve to terminate the aversive stimuli of disability and rehabilitation. There are many ways in which the patient may engage in avoidance or escape behaviors in the medical rehabilitation setting. He may refuse treatment appointments or be consistently late for them. He may lose himself in a passive withdrawal into fantasy. He may provoke arguments or encourage rejection by angry and rebellious behavior. He may depart precipitously by signing out of the hospital against medical advice. Remedial action for these problems will be discussed later in this section.

Ferster[9] has observed that ". . . it is problematical whether a repertoire consisting entirely of escape and avoidance behavior can be maintained." The disabled patient who engages in escape or avoidance behavior gains "time out" from a noxious situation, but what he escapes to is not likely to be effectively reinforcing for long. There are several reasons why that is the case. The act of withdrawing or escaping from rehabilitation does not re-establish access to reinforcers which maintained functioning prior to onset of disability. Similarly, daydreaming about what one used to be able to do does not provide access to the reinforcers to those behaviors. Fantasy provides only momentary relief. Finally, avoidance or escape from rehabilitation limits access to certain other reinforcers. Specifically, the attention and regard of professionals working with the patient will no longer be available. Reinforcers which become accessible only upon completion of an effective rehabilitation program will also be lost.

In the natural course of events, then, the chances of the patient engaging in escape or withdrawal behavior when confronted with significant disability will tend to diminish across time. Exceptions may result if the rehabilitation program has failed to handle the escape or avoidance behavior in effective fashion or the non-treatment environment of the patient reinforces avoidance behavior excessively.

To this point in considering onset of disability relative to the concept of punishment, the focus has been on people with recent and sudden onset. Under certain conditions persons who have had a disability for a long period of time and who then enter a rehabilitation program may present similar problems. The person of remote onset who enters rehabilitation probably does so because of some medical complication or because some change in his functional performance is contemplated. The home environment of such a patient likely will have evolved relationships between his disability and his family's behavior toward it which serve to maintain or reinforce the ways in which he has been doing things. When he enters the rehabilitation program, he will be cut off from those reinforcers. If rehabilitation plans for such a patient involve major changes in how the patient performs, he may perceive the program as the functional equivalent of punishment.

The work of Azrin, Hake and Hutchinson,[2] Ulrich and Crane,[54] Ulrich, Wolfe and Dulaney,[56] and others has shown that punishment may produce aggressive behavior in animals. The studies cited show that aggressive behavior in response to punishment is more likely to occur when there is an available target to attack.

Experience in medical settings with persons who have suddenly become disabled indicates that man, too, may respond to punishing circumstances with aggressive behavior. When viewed in the context of the concept of punishment, some of the arbitrary and rebellious behavior of recently disabled patients may become more understandable. The patient who lashes out, verbally or otherwise, at therapists working with him may interrupt activities which remind him of his disability or which directly produce pain or discomfort. Temper outbursts and rebellious recalcitrance about engaging in treatment procedures sometimes are viewed as loss of emotional control in an impulse-dominated or emotionally labile personality. Sometimes these behaviors are identified as self-destructive. Such behaviors may be responses to what is perceived as a punishing situation.

Psychological interventions for problems of withdrawal or aggression should be directed toward decreasing the aversive qualities of rehabilitation and decreasing the positive consequences to avoidance or escape behavior. A critical first step in this process is to establish an effective therapeutic relationship. Conceptually, during the initial phases of rehabilitation, the emphasis should be on substituting the interim reinforcer of positive interaction with an interested and attentive therapist for the natural reinforcers to effective behavior which become accessible to the client when he gains more mobility and functional capacity and re-engages in home and work activities. If those working with the patient are not effective social reinforcers, the reinforcers left to sustain rehabilitation efforts are mainly relief from pain, relief from sensory deprivation, interruption of disturbing ruminative fantasies about disability, and awareness by the patient that he is progressing toward those reinforcers which will become available upon completion of the program. How effective those reinforcers are will vary from patient to patient, depending upon the patient's prior experiences. It is well to remember, however, that reinforcers are more effective if they are delivered immediately following the behavior they are designed to influence. Some of the reinforcers just cited are delayed. The rehabilitation program which fails to establish an effective treatment relationship with the patient will be proceeding under what may well be seriously comprimised circumstances.

At the outset of rehabilitation the attention and positive regard of the therapist should be directed to each increment of engagement in the rehabilitation process. This may be seen as a process of shaping participation in rehabilitation (Goodkin,[17] Ince,[21] Meacham and Wiesen,[29] Meyerson, Kerr and Michael,[30] Michael,[31, 32] Reese.[39] Tactically, the objectives are: to delineate graded increments of the treatment task scaled to maximize chances of success; to identify and deliver positive reinforcers, initially on an almost continuous (1:1) schedule; and, as progress occurs, to increase performance expectations by adding components to the task while maintaining or lowering the amount of reinforcement. The goal of this approach is to make involvement in rehabilitation as reinforcing as possible rather than aversive. If it is effective, the patient's positive experiences in treatment are accompanied by reduction of isolation and sensory deprivation, thereby adding a further reinforcement.

The steps just described may decrease the aversive qualities of rehabilitation or increase its positive value. At the same time, when confronted with withdrawal or aggressive behavior, efforts should be made to decrease their reinforcement. In the hospital setting a number of steps can be taken to influence responses of hospital personnel to withdrawal or aggressive behavior (Ayllon and Michael,[1] Fowler, Fordyce and Berni.[15]

It is easy for hospital personnel to fall into the trap of paying attention to the patient only when something is going wrong. The patient's long-range objectives are better served if professional attention is contingent upon productive activity. For example, upon observing a disabled patient in what appears to be a withdrawal reverie, a nurse might encourage him to work on a previously prescribed bedside occupational therapy task. If he beings to work at the task, the nurse may then remain to interact with him. If he works for a time and then stops, she may then prepare to leave and say to him something like, "That's fine. Let me know when you feel like doing some more and I'll come join you." If a nurse socializes with a patient on a non-contingent basis, she thereby dissipates her effectiveness as a therapeutic agent. If she socializes only when the patient is not working, she may encourage the very behavior the program is trying to reduce. If her attention is contingent upon his engaging in rehabilitation-appropriate behavior, she contributes directly to treatment objectives.

Family members should be helped to perceive how their interactions with the patient can make a direct contribution to progress. Families are at particular risk in socially reinforcing withdrawal behavior. Two relatively simple steps can be taken to help with this problem. One is to establish contact and communication with the family to help them understand how they can contribute to progress in his rehabilitation program. The second step is to make visible indications of treatment accomplishments. One way of doing this is to draw graphs showing performance in each aspect of the program and affix them to the wall at the patient's bedside. The graphs provide visible evidence of increments in performance, remind the family about the importance of selective responsiveness and give them a subject which they can discuss appropriately. Care should be exercised in the construction of graphs to ensure that increments in performance are scaled appropriately to the patient's rate of progress in each activity recorded.

Management of Grieving

In most important respects, both conceptually and tactically, the management of grieving parallels closely that of punishment. The conceptualization of grieving used here draws heavily on the work of Ferster,[9] Lazarus,[26] and Lewinsohn and Atwood.[27] Grieving or depression is seen as a state of deprivation of reinforcers. The sudden shift in life style brought about by onset of disability results in the loss of previously sustaining reinforcers. The result is grieving and depression. This is true of the newly disabled patient. It is true of the person whose spouse has suddenly died. It is true of the patient who, having been in the hospital so long that previously established relationships have faded and a new set of intrahospital relationships have been developed, is suddenly confronted with discharge from the hospital.

The objective of intervention (for problems of grieving) is to help the patient gain access to reinforcers as expeditiously as possible. An analysis should be made of those activities the patient engaged in previously which can be made available readily in the hospital setting. Effort should also be made immediately to provide tasks related to treatment which elicit reinforceable responses from the patient. One way of describing this approach is to note that one does not treat grieving or depression so that the patient can do things; one helps the patient to start doing things as a way of treating the grieving or depression. The essential features of the tactical approaches by which this may be accomplished have already been described in the sections dealing with crisis management and punishment. The steps to follow are to pinpoint units of performance at the highest level of difficulty consistent with guaranteed patient performance, to define movement cycles and their current rate, to identify reinforcers, to schedule reinforcement initially at a near continuous rate and to monitor carefully the program as it is applied.

Chemotherapeutic intervention with mood elevating drugs is sometimes indicated. Some depressive patterns are so severe as to leave the patient virtually incapable of producing reinforceable responses. Psychiatric consultation is certainly indicated in that kind of situation. Chemotherapeutic intervention should not be seen as in any way incompatible with the behavioral approaches just described. Quite to the contrary, when chemotherapy is used, it should be coupled with graded introduction of treatment-related tasks and application of the appropriate reinforcing contingencies.

Extinction of Premorbid, Disability-inappropriate Behavior

As noted in the introductory section, extinction occurs when a behavior is no longer reinforced. Certain behaviors the patient engaged in prior to onset of disability are incompatible with his disability. That is true of specific performance skills in daily activities, in larger complexes of behavior such as vocational or leisure time activities, and in many behaviors subsumed under the terms self-concept, attitudes about one's self and so forth. For a recently disabled patient the concern here is with leisure and vocational behaviors engaged in previously which are no longer feasible. Those behaviors cannot again occur in fact. The patient may, however, daydream about those activities. As noted previously, that kind of withdrawal behavior is intrinsically reinforcing for only a short time.

A problem arises when people around the patient reinforce fantasy behavior by unrealistic statements implying that the disability is only temporary. Remedial action to this kind of problem is based on the same principles as in dealing with punishment and grieving. The rehabilitation program should seek to minimize the direct reinforcement of unrealistic fantasies, i.e., minimize reinforcement of withdrawal. The rehabilitation program should also move as rapidly as possible to shape in alternative, disability-appropriate behaviors under optimal conditions of reinforcement.

The patient's family also needs help with problems relating to extinction of disability-inappropriate behavior. One reason families engage in unrealistic denial and reassuring behavior with the patient is because they lack viable alternatives. Providing families with information about what the patient is going to be able to do at the end of the program and about his progress helps give them alternatives about which they can communicate with the patient. The use of performance graphs at the patient's bedside, as discussed earlier, is one illustration of how this may be accomplished.

Family members, like everyone else, need positive reinforcement for their behavior. Often it is not sufficient to provide them with relevant information. The social worker and others on the rehabilitation team can make important contributions to patient progress by systematic contact with family members. These contacts should be designed to help the family anticipate the reinforcers which will become available to the patient and to themselves as the rehabilitation program progresses. Once communication and working relationship are established, less effort should be spent on feelings and more on working out details of what the patient and family will be doing upon completion of the rehabilitation program.

Most recently disabled patients have not yet learned ineffectual behaviors relative to their disabilities, and their families have not evolved a pattern of reinforcing such behaviors. If the recently disabled patient were to leave the rehabilitation program, in most instances he would not likely long receive effective reinforcement for his withdrawal. The outlook for change in both the patient and the family unit under those conditions is favorable. In contrast, the patient who has long had his difficulty may come from an environment which has evolved effective reinforcement patterns for ineffectual or disability-inappropriate behavior. If ineffectual behavior has been going on at a substantial rate, it must have been receiving reinforcement. If such a patient were to leave the rehabilitation program precipitously, he would return to an environment which would sustain his existing behavioral repertoire. If the patient successfully completes the rehabilitation program, he returns to an environment which may fail to reinforce the new behaviors and which may resume reinforcing the previously ineffectual behaviors reduced by rehabilitation. It should be evident that rehabilitation programs for patients who have had their disabilities for long periods of time need to be particularly concerned with analyzing the home situation. If a program concerns itself only with the patient's behavioral repertoire and ignores that of the family, behavioral changes brought about in rehabilitation may not persist.

The tactical steps for helping family members to change their behavior are the same as those for helping patients to change behavior. Family members need aid to pinpoint their own and the patient's behavior, to be aware of the rate of these behaviors, and to establish patterns of desired behaviors by the use of contingent rewards.

PARTICIPATION IN REHABILITATION

This section will deal with problems relating to motivation, with techniques for enhancing patient acquisition of disability-appropriate behaviors, and with helping the patient to maintain new behavioral repertoires upon completion of rehabilitation.

Motivation

There can be little doubt that the most frequently mentioned psychological problem in the context of disability and rehabilitation concerns patient motivation. Fishman[10] states, "Empirical evidence substantiates the theoretical consideration that the single most important problem facing the rehabilitation worker concerns the ways and means of implementing marginal motivation."

The conceptualization of motivation implicit in the learning model approach and the management techniques derived from that model are quite different from the more traditional view based on a disease model system. Motivation is not an attribute of behavior but an inference about an inner state of the organism derived from observations of behavior. Typically, a patient is held to be "motivated" if he engages in the behaviors of interest at an acceptable rate. If those behaviors do not occur at an acceptable rate, the patient is considered to be "unmotivated" or to be "motivated" for some less desirable goal. Used in that way, the concept of motivation adds nothing to information about the patient or to the clarification of courses of remedial action. All that has happened is that the observer has noted the extent to which the patient has done what the program hoped he would do and has labeled him "motivated" or "unmotivated," as the case may be. Statements about the patient's motivation, though used characteristically as if they described some inner state of the organism, are in fact based on a relationship between what the patient has done and what observers thought he should do.

Approaching the concept of motivation from a learning model point of view leads to a different formulation. Behavior is governed by consequences. If a behavior is occurring at an inadequate rate (i.e., the "unmotivated" patient), some adjustment is needed in the contingencies to that behavior. If a patient is doing too much of something which interferes with performance of rehabilitation-appropriate behaviors at a desired rate (i.e., the "unmotivated" patient or the patient "motivated" for the wrong things), the reinforcers to those undesired behaviors need to be withdrawn. To quote Michael,[32] "From a behavioral point of view, however . . . marginal motivation seems merely to be a case of insufficient or poorly arranged reinforcement. The basic question that should be asked is 'What does the patient get out of his activity?' The problem of motivation is a simple one. One must merely arrange the environment so that its desirable features are only available contingent upon participation and accomplishment in the rehabilitation training activity."

There are several reasons that motivation problems are so prominent in rehabilitation. The earlier discussion of punishment has shown how becoming disabled and entering into rehabilitation may initially be aversive. It is not surprising, therefore, that many patients fail to produce disability-appropriate behaviors at the desired rate. There is another reason for the prominence of motivational problems. Staats[47] points out, "Discussions with therapists in rehabilitation suggest that much of their work, especially with children, involves training new behaviors under circumstances in which the reinforcers are weak. For example, prior to developing skill with the prosthesis the child secures reinforcement more easily for various already learned substitution movements. Thus, some way must be found at first to supply 'prosthetic responses,' in a competitive sense, since these responses are not in themselves 'naturally' reinforcing." It may be said that disability-appropriate behaviors, particularly in the case of physical disability, initially are low-frequency, low-strength, low-value behaviors to the rehabilitation client without experience with those behaviors.

The essential features in the psychological management of motivation problems in rehabilitation consist of establishing treatment relationships which enhance the reinforcing value of interactions with rehabilitation professionals, of enhancing the value of long-term reinforcers for disability-appropriate behavior, and of carrying out the behavioral analysis and contingency management steps which promote acquisition of the new behaviors provided by effective rehabilitation.

Evaluation

The objectives of psychological evaluation in rehabilitation are to predict what the patient is likely to do in rehabilitation and in relevant situations in the future and to identify stimulus situations and reinforcers likely to influence patient behavior. As the picture of the patient's potential functional capabilities emerges from the diagnostic process, it becomes important to specify what behavioral changes the patient will need to make and the way in which these changes can more readily be brought about. As noted in the discussion of motivation, disability is likely to require the patient to engage in some low-frequency, low-strength, low-value behaviors.

The more similar what the patient has done in the past is to what he is functionally capable of doing in the future, the less likely the disability behaviors will be low-frequency, low-strength, and low-value. It is important, therefore, to identify what he has done in the past in order to assess whether special reinforcement is going to be needed to establish new, disability-appropriate behaviors. Identifying reinforcers is itself a procedure specifically related to what the person has done in the past. The best estimate of what activities are reinforcing to a person is derived from the knowledge of what activities he has pursued frequently in the past.

Evaluation can be carried out in part by obtaining current behavior samples from the patient in the form of direct observations or from psychological testing, as will be discussed later. Evaluation also may be carried out by indirect observation of behavior in the form of history taking about the patient and family members.

The kinds of activities the patient has engaged in in the past which are reinforcing to him are mainly to be found in his recreation and leisure-time pursuits. Those data, supplemented by a detailed job history, should tell much about what is likely to be reinforcing to him in the future. There are many reasons why the patient's past may not be an adequate prologue of the future. Youthfulness of the patient, a vague or incomplete picture of what he has done, or radical changes in what is possible in the future all may make additional information essential.

An additional and frequently very rich source of information for providing estimates of future activities likely to be reinforcing is the activities the patient's early models—usually parents or older siblings—have engaged in. Personality or modes of self-expression *are* learned. They are learned by a combination of the influence of consequences in the environment in which behaviors have been practiced and of modeling or social imitation learning (Bandura,[5, 6] Bandura and Walters.[7] The most significant models usually will have been parents and older siblings. Many of their behaviors will have been emulated. In addition, these same models will themselves have been exercising some selectivity as to which behaviors of the patient they will have reinforced, ignored or punished. Their choices in that regard will reflect, in part, what they find reinforcing to themselves. Thus, so long as there has been reasonably effective communication between patient and models, patient behavior will reflect much of the behavior style of the models. It frequently proves fruitful, therefore, to obtain a detailed picture of both the leisure and vocational activities of those in the patient's background who have served as significant models for him.

A system is needed to organize and synthesize the information one might obtain from history material about the patient and his models. The method proposed here considers leisure and vocational activities as differentially falling into three classes. The first class is *symbol-centered.* That refers to activities emphasizing ideas, concepts, numbers and words. Examples of this group in leisure activities are reading, political interest and activity, and gambling. Examples in work are bookkeeping, clerical work and computer programing. A second class is *motor-manipulative-centered.* This category emphasizes manipulation of objects and physical movement. Leisure-time examples are outdoor activities, athletics, gardening, tinkering and making things. Work examples are physical labor and working with tools and machinery. The third class or category is *interpersonal-centered.* Leisure-time examples are visiting, socializing and club or organizational participation. Vocational examples are sales and such relationship-centered services as the ministry, counseling and teaching. Organizing history information about the patient and his models in terms of the relative emphasis on each of these three categories will help reduce the data to more manageable and comprehensible form.

Psychological testing in patient evaluation needs some consideration. Which tests are used and how frequently they are used varies markedly from psychologist to psychologist. That variability and the sometimes seemingly inexplicable relationship between the stimulus materials in a test and the inferential comments made about test responses make it difficult to maintain a clear perspective as to what psychological testing is all about. Psychological tests are one kind of behavior sample designed to provide a basis for predicting what the tested person will do in non-test situations.

Sometimes tests, like x-rays, are seen as revealing underlying characteristics which, when understood, permit rather precise predictions of future behavior. That view, however, is of questionable validity. It implies that personality steers the individual into actions somewhat independently of the context in which he functions. It is more accurate to recognize that human behavior is governed by a combination of the repertoire of the individual and influences from the immediate environment. Psychological test responses are one kind of behavior. What the person will do in some other situation is another kind of behavior. The degree to which these two behaviors are in fact correlated cannot exceed the degree of comparability of test stimuli and future situation. As future situations depart more and more from stimuli surrounding testing and the test itself, the predictive efficiency of the test data will be correspondingly diminished.

The accuracy of predictions which a psychologist may make on the basis of test data will depend in part upon the extent to which the test has been standardized in stimulus situations comparable to those about which the predictions are made. This point is illustrated by the obvious fallacy of trying to predict subsequent academic performance of an English-speaking native of upper Sudan based on scores derived from intelligence tests standardized on middle-class American normative groups. Some tests have normative data based on reference populations about which much is known. When the rehabilitation clients being tested are from comparable reference populations, the normative data are directly relevant and few interpretative problems exist. When standardization is carried out on a quite different population or when very limited standardization is carried out, as frequently is the case in many psychological tests, there must be increasing reliance on the extrapolating acumen of the psychologist.

Rehabilitation programs are confronted with many evaluation problems for which little, if any, standardization data are available. The compromise imposed by necessity is to ask the psychologist to make his estimates or predictions according to his best judgment and experience, based on the test data he accumulates. He must therefore have some latitude in selecting the tests to be used so that he can draw upon the instruments with which he is most experienced. Under these conditions, the utility of the psychological test report will be correspondingly greater as the psychologist becomes better acquainted with the stimulus situations in which the behavior he is trying to predict will occur. The psychologist's contribution will be enhanced if he is helped to become better acquainted with the rehabilitation process and the specific styles of the rehabilitation team. The rehabilitation physician can enhance the contribution of the psychologist by encouraging continuing functional exposure to the rehabilitation team and continuing feedback to the psychologist about the accuracy of his predictions. Further discussions of specific tests pertinent to rehabilitation may be found in Fordyce.[12]

Evaluation should lead to a specification of the behaviors required in the environment toward which the client is headed and an understanding of the behaviors likely to be reinforced or punished by that environment. The rehabilitation team sometimes conceptualizes its goals in broad generalities, e.g., greater independence, more mobility. Eventually, a concept like independence must be translated into terms specifying what operations or behaviors the patient and those about him are to engage in. Failure of the rehabilitation team to arrive at those specifications leads to two kinds of problems. One is that individual therapists may be unclear as to what it is they are to do. What they do may even contradict other aspects of the program. Failure to specify the target behaviors of the program also makes it difficult realistically to identify the extent to which the program has succeeded or failed. The failure to specify goals in operational terms risks fostering the continuation of procedures that are ineffectual or inefficient.

Contingency Management Methods

This section will illustrate the use of consequence manipulation or contingency management systems to bring about behavior change. Evaluation should have yielded specification of the behaviors to be reduced, maintained and shaped or increased. Evaluation should also have indicated at least a general picture of the behaviors likely to be reinforcing to the patient and the behaviors which are likely to be reinforced or punished by the environment toward which he is headed. There are some additional steps which can be taken to identify reinforcers immediately available to help the patient entering the rehabilitation process.

A useful guide to identification of reinforcers is the Premack Principle (Premack[37]), which states that of any two activities, the more probable one will function as a reinforcer for the less probable one. Stated another way, activities which previously have been attractive to a patient are likely, when made available contingent upon completion of specified units of rehabilitation-related efforts, to prove effective positive reinforcers to the rate of those efforts. Reinforcers naturally occurring in the rehabilitation environment offer considerable advantage over more remote reinforcers. History data will tell a lot about what is likely to be reinforcing. In addition, direct observations of what the patient now does should prove helpful.

Two important characteristics of reinforcers are that they be available and that they be contingent upon performance. Rest or periods of time-out from treatment and attention are naturally occurring and readily available reinforcers in rehabilitation. These and other reinforcers will be of little value, however, if they are available to the patient whether or not he performs, i.e., if they are non-contingent upon performance. If a reinforcer is not subject to control, it should not be used.

A third functional characteristic of an effective reinforcer is that delivery of the reinforcer should not interfere with the performance one is trying to improve. To illustrate that point, consider a program designed to increase standing in long-leg braces in a paraplegic patient. If rest is the reinforcer and it is programed so that one minute of standing earns 30 minutes of rest delivered immediately following performance, training sessions would be protracted unduly by reinforcement.

The number of reinforcers which can be used effectively in rehabilitation can be enhanced considerably by the use of token or point systems. When a token economy is used, upon completion of a designated number of movement cycles, the patient receives a token (e.g., poker chip or point) that can be traded

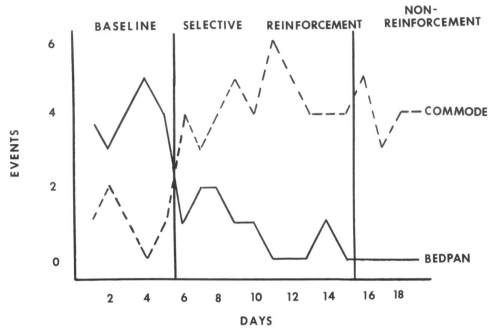

Figure 6–4   Improving self-care performance with social reinforcement. (See text for details.)

in subsequently on some previously designated reinforcer. Token economies make available a range of reinforcers which can be delivered immediately following performance without disrupting the behavior one is trying to strengthen. The use of tokens makes it possible to relate a series of reinforcers to one behavior and, conversely, to make more than one behavior relate to one or more reinforcers.

More detailed discussions of the use of token economies can be found in Meacham and Wiesen,[29] Michael,[31] and Krasner.[23] An annotated bibliography on token economies is found in Krasner and Atthowe;[24] Sand, Trieschmann, Fordyce and Fowler[41] describe an application of these methods to a medical rehabilitation problem.

The following example* illustrates an application of contingency management systems to a problem of patient participation in medical rehabilitation. Figure 6-4 illustrates the results.

Case Example 1

The patient was a 62-year-old female who had had a resection of the left femoral head and neck because of infection. Postoperatively she had hyponatremia, a myocardial infarction, acute tubular necrosis and anemia. Three weeks after the myocardial infarction, she began rehabilitation for ambulation. She was emaciated, weak and had a painful left hip. She rapidly learned transfers and gained strength. However, routinely she requested a bedpan rather than transfer to a commode. *Target behavior:* Increased use of commode. *Movement cycle:* Transfer to commode and return to bed or wheelchair.

REINFORCERS.   It was observed that the patient engaged the staff in conversion at any opportunity and that she seemed to get a great deal of pleasure from these

_____

*The projects in Case Examples 1 and 2 were carried out under the direction of John Kirby, M. D., a resident in Physical Medicine and Rehabilitation.

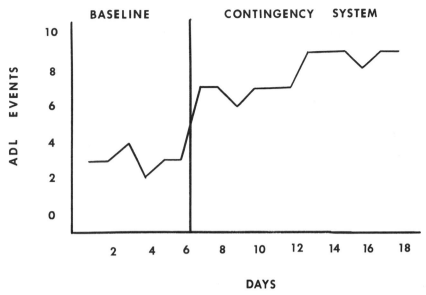

Figure 6–5   Increasing ADL events by using visits as reinforcers. (See text for details.)

conversations. Therefore, chatting and interacting with the staff were chosen as the reinforcers.

PROCEDURE.   (1) *Baseline:* Requests for bedpan or commode were honored without comment and the nursing staff continued to chat with the patient at those times. In general, the patient used the commode once daily and the bedpan the rest of the time. (2) *Selective Reinforcement:* As before, the bedpan or commode was supplied upon request. The nurse would stay to chat only when the commode was used. The patient was not informed of this. Nonetheless, within three days use of the bedpan had fallen essentially to zero. (3) On the 16th day the selective reinforcement program was terminated in order to assess how well the new behavior was established. Use of the bedpan remained at zero, as shown in Figure 6-4.

The second example illustrates use of a simple point or token system with a commonly encountered problem in medical rehabilitation. Results are shown in Figure 6–5.

Case Example 2
The patient was a 57-year-old male with a five-year history of paraplegia secondary to degenerative joint disease. He was admitted to the rehabilitation service because of a decubitus ulcer of the metatarsal head of his right great toe. He had lived independently in an apartment and utilized the help of a practical nurse who lived nearby for transfer and Activities of Daily Living (ADL) assistance. On the ward he refused to do his own ADL and it was done by his friend on her daily visits.

TARGET BEHAVIOR.   Increase ADL tasks performed by the patient. *Movement cycle:* Completion of ADL tasks which were known to be in his repertoire; e.g., groom hair, brush teeth, shave, wash hands and face, wash trunk, eat meals.

REINFORCERS.   Amount of time the patient's friend would be allowed to visit. The contingencies gained full approval of the friend and reluctant approval of the patient.

PROCEDURE.   (1) *Baseline:* At the start of the project, before the contingency system was applied, the patient averaged successful completion of approximately three tasks (of nine) per day. (2) *Point system:* Successful completion of each task earned one point or token. At the end of each day the tokens could be used to "purchase" ten minutes of visiting time by his friend.

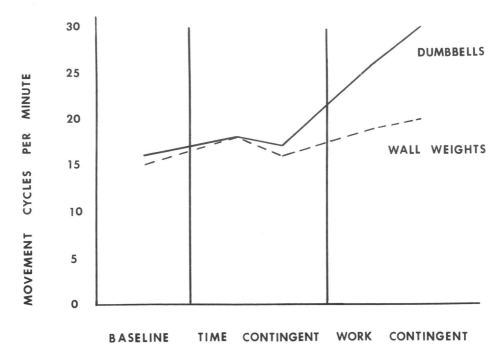

Figure 6–6   Rest as a reinforcer in physical therapy exercise. (See text for details.)

The third example* illustrates an application of rest as a reinforcer. (See Figure 6-6.)

Case Example 3

The patient was a 20-year-old female paraplegic of recent onset, who was on an exercise program for upper extremity strengthening.

TARGET BEHAVIOR.   Increase performance at weightlifting and wall weights. *Movement cycles:* Number of lifts at a fixed weight.

REINFORCER.   Rest.

PROCEDURE.   Purpose of the project was to study effectiveness of rest as a reinforcer by comparing performance when rest was contingent upon the passage of time as compared with rest contingent upon completion of a given amount of work. (1) *Baseline:* Patient instructed to "exercise at your own rate for as long as you can." Patient performed for two minutes. (To allow for effects of fatigue the units performed at each task are shown only for the first minute.) (2) *Time-contingent rest:* "Exercise for one minute and then you may rest for two minutes." (3) *Work-contingent rest:* "As soon as you have completed fifteen cyles you may rest for two minutes."

Figure 6-6 shows improvement of the rate per minute of both tasks when rest was made contingent upon work.

These examples illustrate the influence on patient performance of naturally occurring reinforcers in the rehabilitation setting when they are made contingent upon performance. The examples also illustrate pinpointing target behaviors, identifying movement cycles and recording rate of performance. Further illustrations in the application of these methods to a variety of prob-

*This project was carried out by Miss Nancy Pengra, a Physical Therapy student.

lems in rehabilitation may be found in such references as Fordyce, Fowler, Sand, and Trieschmann;[13] Fowler et al.;[15] Goodkin;[17] Meyerson et al.;[30] Pigott;[36] Sand et al.;[41] Trombly;[51] Trotter and Inman;[52] Walls;[58] and Zimmerman, Stuckey, Miller, and Garlick.[62]

Maintenance of Patient Performance

It is important to distinguish between the ability to do something and the probability that it will be done (Wallace[57]). It is easy to lose sight of the fact that these concepts are not the same. That someone has the ability to do something by no means ensures that he will in fact do it. If a rehabilitation program has given a patient the ability to do something but he subsequently does not do it, the program can hardly be considered a success. The objectives of a rehabilitation program ought to be that the target behaviors occur at an appropriate rate in the environment in which they are supposed to occur and not only in the rehabilitation center. Obviously a rehabilitation program is limited in the extent to which it can influence the extra-treatment environment in order to optimize the probability of adequate patient performance. Nonetheless, the program should consider its efforts incomplete if it has failed to assess the influence of the target environment on the behaviors being developed within rehabilitation and has failed to take whatever actions it can to influence that environment toward the end of optimizing patient performance.

As noted earlier here and by Staats,[47] rehabilitation may require the patient to perform tasks which are not intrinsically reinforcing and which may in fact initially be noxious, cumbersome or unrewarding. The environment outside the rehabilitation program is not likely to reinforce many disability-appropriate behaviors (e.g., ambulating by wheelchair, drinking large amounts of fluids, wearing an upper extremity prosthesis) at the same rate that it does for corresponding non-disability behaviors. That, in turn, means that special effort must be made to provide contingencies in the environment which will maintain disability-appropriate behaviors. If that effort is not made and the natural environment fails to reinforce disability-appropriate behaviors acceptably, those behaviors will fade or be carried out at a lower than desirable rate.

The maintenance of disability-appropriate behaviors following departure from the formal rehabilitation program is essentially a problem of generalization. Generalization in this context refers to the extent to which behavior which occurs in one time or place (e.g., rehabilitation) will also occur in another time and place (e.g., the natural environment).

There are two major strategies to consider in promoting generalization. One is to bring disability-appropriate behaviors under the control of reinforcers naturally occurring in the target environment. Failing that, the alternative strategy is to make a specific effort to re-program the natural environment so that it will deliver appropriate reinforcement contingent upon performance of the disability-appropriate behaviors.

The first of these strategies, that is, relating the disability behaviors to naturally occurring reinforcers, provides the major conceptual basis for the importance of social and vocational programs to physical or medical rehabilitation. When a patient is effectively employed, for example, the reinforcers available in the work situation are likely to maintain behaviors immediately elicited by the job and such work-related behaviors as effective self-care, mobility and fluid intake. The reinforcers provided by work may be money, status and prestige, socialization, sense of accomplishment or others. One or more of those reinforcers may effectively maintain work behavior. For some people they will not maintain work behavior at an adequate rate. For yet other rehabilitation patients, employment may not be a feasible objective. In either case, there may be alternative reinforcers available in the home environment to maintain essential disability-related behaviors. Stimulating recreational and leisure-time activities, for example, may provide sufficient reinforcement to maintain both the behaviors immediately elicited by those kinds of activities and related self-care behaviors.

When it appears likely that the natural environment will fail to provide sufficient reinforcement for essential disability-appropriate behaviors or that it will reinforce disability-inappropriate behaviors, special effort should be made to modify the existing contingency relationships. Earlier discussions about punishment and about family involvement in the rehabilitation process described methods for dealing with these problems.

A rehabilitation program can enhance generalization also by providing for gradual and systematic rehearsal of disability-appropriate behaviors in environments more closely approximating the natural environments in which they are to be carried out following rehabilitation. When a patient is provided the opportunity to exercise his new disability-related skills outside the treatment setting, it is more likely those behaviors will come under the influence of reinforcers available in the non-treatment environment.

Excellent discussion of the principles of generalization and some illustrative applications are found in Baer and Wolf[3] and Baer, Wolf, and Risley.[4]

PSYCHOLOGICAL FACTORS IN BRAIN DAMAGE

The effect of brain damage on behavior is not consistent. Changes in patient behavior following brain damage will vary according to the type, location and amount of cortical deficit. Behavioral effects of brain damage will also be influenced by the patient's premorbid repertoire. Nonetheless, there are certain generalizations which can be made. There are also a number of remedial approaches which can be used in rehabilitation to enhance the progress and ultimate performance of the brain-damaged patient.

The most likely functional consequence of brain damage is some reduction in learning efficiency. Functional impairment in learning resulting from brain damage may occur at any of a number of points in the sequence of mental processes going into learning. Generally, learning impairments can be related to difficulties in receiving and processing incoming information, in assimilating or retaining that information, in associating it with previously acquired information, or in retrieving it as effective memory to influence subsequent behavior. The effects of brain damage on rehabilitation are usually great because of the central role learning plays in the rehabilitation process. It is therefore important to delineate learning impairments which may exist and to design the rehabilitation program accordingly. The following section will describe briefly a system of organizing information relating to brain damage and some implications for rehabilitation planning.

There is much evidence (Fitzhugh, Fitzhugh and Reitan;[11] Hirschenfang;[20] Kimura;[22] Milner;[33] Reed and Reitan;[38] Reitan;[40] Stark;[48] Teuber;[50] Weinstein[59]) to indicate differentiation of intellectual functions between the cerebral hemispheres. The left cerebral hemisphere is concerned primarily with symbol functions such as language, numbers, concepts and ideas.

Performance of symbol-related tasks involves ability to receive, comprehend and respond with language or number systems. These symbol-centered functions are likely to be interfered with when there is a significant amount of cerebral damage in the left hemisphere. In rehabilitation the most commonly encountered example of this is the right hemiplegic who is also aphasic. Deficits in symbol functions may exist even when the patient does not have so much language deficit as to warrant a diagnosis of aphasia.

A second major category of intellectual functioning considered here is termed "perceptual." Perceptual functions refer to mental operations involving discrimination and appreciation of form, position, movement and distance. For the most part these perceptual functions can be carried out with little if any involvement of language or symbol systems. These functions are primarily associated with the right cerebral hemisphere. It is the left hemiplegic patient with right cerebral hemisphere damage who is likely to have poor standing balance, to have difficulty finding his way from one place to another, and to bump the door frame as he steers his wheelchair through a doorway.

The major exceptions to this lateralization differentiation occur in left-handed people (Palmer[34]). Even in left-handed people, perceptual functions are associated mainly with the right cerebral hemisphere. Symbol functions will be impaired in approximately one third of left-handed people when there is damage to the right cerebral hemisphere, but most left-handed people will show symbol deficit when there is left cerebral hemisphere damage.

Patients with symbol or perceptual deficit will tend to have problems in receiving and processing information coming to them in the involved medium. For example, the patient with left cerebral hemisphere damage is more likely to make mistakes in comprehending, learning, and speaking in language or number terms. Similarly, the person with perceptual deficits is more likely to have difficulties in analyzing form, position, and movement signals sent to him (e.g., demonstrations) as well as in associating, remembering and performing in perceptual-based tasks. Unless both hemispheres are involved, or there are problems of arousal or activation, people having significant damage in one hemisphere may be able to perform quite adequately in tasks involving the other hemisphere. For example, some patients with marked aphasia may carry out complex form and position discriminations very accurately. A patient with damage exclusively in the right cerebral hemisphere may seem very unimpaired intellectually because of the absence of problems involving language, but that same patient may display marked difficulty in tasks involving movement and differing body positions.

It has been observed that hemisphere lateralization effects involve signal detection as well as response production. The work of Fordyce and Jones[14] illustrates one practical implication of cerebral lateralization in the brain-damaged patient. The right hemiplegic patient (left cerebral hemisphere damage) is likely to have difficulty receiving or understanding oral instructions, even when he is not formally identified as aphasic. The same patient may process information more accurately if it is delivered in the form of pantomime gestures or visual demonstration rather than in language or number terms. Conversely, the left hemiplegic patient (right cerebral hemisphere damage) with significant perceptual deficits is more likely to profit from instructions presented orally or in written form. Pantomime and demonstration directions may prove confusing to him.

A third major dimension of functional impairment from brain damage relates to memory. Memory is a very complex concept. It is beyond the scope of this chapter to consider it in depth. However, there are a number of dimensions of memory functioning which should be considered at least briefly. In the first place, it is important to discriminate between immediate memory in the sense of the number of units of a signal a person can assimilate (auditory attention span) from memory functions involving the retrieval of information received more remotely than a few moments before. Some patients with auditory attention span problems will be able to handle a short message without difficulty but may have virtually no comprehension of longer messages. Where there are auditory attention span problems, therapists should speak with extremely brief signals.

The content of memory deficits correlates moderately with the distinction between symbolic and perceptual functions. Persons with symbol deficits (left cerebral hemisphere damage) show more memory problems in tasks involving language and numbers. Persons with perceptual deficits (right cerebral hemisphere damage) have greater memory difficulties in tasks involving position, movement and so forth than in tasks involving language and numbers.

It is important to distinguish memory for things learned prior to the cerebral insult from memory for those learned subsequently. Remote or premorbid learning is less likely to be interfered with by brain damage than is the ability to learn. In evaluating memory functioning, it is therefore important to test for current learning rate.

There is some evidence to suggest that interference in learning occurs mainly with the rate of learning rather than the ultimate ability to learn. If a learning situation is programed carefully to provide sufficient rehearsal, clear signals, and adequately paced increments, the brain-damaged patient may well learn. Once he has learned, as measured by demonstrated ability to retain the response he has been taught, his subsequent ability to remember that response may be quite adequate. In short, perhaps it is learning rate rather than learning ability that is impaired.

A fourth major dimension of impairment from brain damage relates to emotional expression. Brain damage patients frequently display an ease of emotional expression. This occurs more commonly in the form of outbursts of crying, though there may also be laughter or expressions of anger or frustration. These expressions seem to occur with little or no provocation from the external environment. These behaviors are sometimes termed "organic" affective lability, disinhibition or inappropriate affect. They seem more likely to occur when there is brain stem involvement. These disinhibited emotional expressions can usually be discriminated from more normal expressions of feeling states by observing how easily they can be interrupted. If outbursts of crying, for example, can be interrupted effectively by the examiner snapping his fingers or by impinging upon the patient's attention with a question, one is probably observing "organic" affective lability.

Brain damage patients frequently are observed to be rather uncritical about their own behavior. They may make mistakes in the performance of some action which ordinarily they are capable of doing. They may seem unaware of their mistakes. These difficulties in exercising quality control over their own behavior seem to be related to deficits in processing informational feedback from their own behavior or in maintaining alertness. Observers sometimes make the mistake of perceiving these quality control problems as the behavior of a careless or indifferent person. In the presence of brain damage, particularly when there are problems of alertness, and activation or sensory discrimination, it should be recognized that these errors may occur because of the brain injury.

There are several approaches therapists may use in working with brain-damaged patients to help circumvent some of the difficulties associated with memory, affective lability and quality control. In nearly every case, a careful analysis of the kinds of information the patient can and cannot handle and corresponding adjustments in the information and feedback he receives will be of help. More specifically, if language is impaired, use pantomime or picture information. If perceptual functions are impaired, use language or numbers. If proprioceptive or kinesthetic sensitivity is impaired, special efforts must be made to encourage the patient to substitute visual observation or other kinds of cues to remind himself of what next to do. If the ability to remember directions is impaired, it is often fruitful to equip the patient with a prosthetic memory in the form of written directions, cue cards and so forth. If sequences of actions are too complex for the patient to recall, training in the use of a check list may be of assistance.

It is of paramount importance to rehabilitation programs with persons having sustained brain damage that there be a detailed analysis of the functional impairments and the residual capacities. It is equally important that there be a detailed analysis of the methods by which the patient is to be taught. Therapeutic retraining programs need to be designed in these cases with great care and precision to maximize learning.

REFERENCES

1. Ayllon, T., and Michael, J.: The Psychiatric Nurse as a Behavioral Engineer. J. Exp. Anal. Behav., *2*:323-334, 1959.
2. Azrin, N., Hake, D., and Hutchinson, R.: Elicitation of Aggression by a Physical Blow. J. Exp. Anal. Behav., *8*(1):55-57, 1965.
3. Baer, D., and Wolf, M.: The Entry into Natural Communities of Reinforcement. *In* Achieving Generality of Behavioral Change. Symposium presented at the meeting of the American Psychological Association, Washington, D.C., September, 1967.
4. Baer, D., Wolf, M., and Risley, T.: Some Current Dimensions of Applied Behavior Analysis. J. Appl. Behav. Anal., *1*(1): 91 97, 1968.
5. Bandura, A.: Behavioral Modification through Modeling Procedures. *In* Krasner, L., and Ullmann, L. (Eds.): Research in Behavior Modification. New York, Holt, Rinehart and Winston, 1966. Pp. 310-340.
6. Bandura, A.: Psychotherapy Conceptualized as a Social-Learning Process. Unpublished manuscript, Stanford University, 1964.
7. Bandura, A., and Walters, R.: Social Learning and Personality Development. New York, Holt, Rinehart and Winston, 1963.
8. Caplan, G.: Principles of Preventive Psychiatry. New York, Basic Books, 1964. P. 48.
9. Ferster, C.: Classification of Behavioral Pathology. *In* Krasner, L. and Ullmann, L. (Eds.): Research in Behavior Modification. New York, Holt, Rinehart and Winston, 1966. Pp. 6-26.
10. Fishman, S.: Amputation. *In* Garret, J., and Levine, E. (Eds.): Psychological Practices with the Physically Disabled. New York, Columbia University Press, 1962. Pp. 1-50.
11. Fitzhugh, K., Fitzhugh, L., and Reitan, R.: Wechsler-Bellevue Comparisons in Groups with "Chronic" and "Current" Lateralized and Diffused Brain Lesions. J. Consult. Psychol., *26*:306-310, 1962.
12. Fordyce, W.: Psychology and Rehabilitation. *In* Licht, S. (Ed.): Rehabilitation and Medicine. New Haven, Elizabeth Licht, 1968. Pp. 129-151.
13. Fordyce, W., Fowler, R., Sand, P., and Trieschmann, R.: Behavior Analysis Systems in Medical Rehabilitation Facilities. J. Rehab., Mar.–Apr., 1971.
14. Fordyce, W., and Jones, R.: The Efficacy of Oral and Pantomime Instructions for Hemiplegic Patients. Arch. Phys. Med. Rehab., *47*:676-680, 1966.
15. Fowler, R., Fordyce, W., and Berni, R.: Operant Conditioning in Chronic Illness. Amer. J. Nurs., *69*:1226-1228, 1969.
16. Gendlin, E., and Rychlak, J.: Psychotherapeutic Processes. Ann. Rev. Psychol., *21*:155-190, 1970.

17. Goodkin, R.: Case Studies in Behavioral Research in Rehabilitation. Percept. Motor Skills, *23:*171–182, 1966.
18. Hanford, D.: Life Crisis Viewed as Opportunity. The Bulletin, Division of Mental Health, State of Washington, *9*(2):87, 1965.
19. Hebb, D.: The Organization of Behavior. New York, John Wiley and Sons, 1949.
20. Hirschenfang, S.: A Comparison of Bender–Gestalt Reproductions of Right and Left Hemiplegic Patients. J. Clin. Psychol., *16:*439–442, 1960.
21. Ince, L.: Behavior Modification in a Rehabilitation Service Setting. Paper presented at the meeting of the American Psychological Association, San Francisco, September, 1968.
22. Kimura, D.: Some Effects of Temporal-Lobe Damage on Auditory Perception. Canad. J. Psychol., *15:*156-165, 1961.
23. Krasner, L.: Applications of Token Economy in Chronic Populations. *In* Token Economies: Current Status—Future Directions. Symposium presented at the meeting of the American Psychological Association, San Francisco, September, 1968.
24. Krasner, L., and Atthowe, J.: Token Economy Bibliography. *In* Token Economies: Current Status—Future Directions. Symposium presented at the meeting of the American Psychological Association, San Francisco, September, 1968.
25. Krasner, L., and Ullmann, L. (Eds.): Research in Behavior Modification. New York, Holt, Rinehart and Winston, 1966.
26. Lazarus, A.: Learning Theory and the Treatment of Depression. Behav. Res. Ther., *6*(1):83–90, 1988.
27. Lewinsohn, P., and Atwood, G.: Depression: A Clinical-Research Approach. Paper presented at the Washington-Oregon Psychological Association's Joint Meeting, Crystal Mountain, Washington, May, 1968.
28. Lindsley, O., and Skinner, B.: A Method for the Experimental Analysis of the Behavior of Psychotic Patients. Amer. Psychol., *9:*419–420, 1954.
29. Meacham, M., and Wiesen, A.: Changing Classroom Behavior: A Manual for Precision Teaching. Scranton, International Textbook Company, 1970.
30. Meyerson, L., Kerr, N., and Michael, J.: Behavior Modification in Rehabilitation. *In* Bijou, S., and Baer, D. (Eds.): Child Development: Readings in Experimental Analysis. New York, Appleton-Century-Crofts, 1967. Pp. 214–239.
31. Michael, J.: Management of Behavioral Consequences in Education. Inglewood, California, Southwest Regional Laboratory for Educational Research and Development, 1967.
32. Michael, J.: Rehabilitation. *In* Neuringer, C., and Michael, J. (Eds.): Behavior Modification in Clinical Psychology. New York, Appleton-Century-Crofts, 1970.
33. Milner, B.: Laterality Effects in Audition. *In* Mountcastle, V. (Ed.): Interhemispheric Relations and Cerebral Dominance. Baltimore, Johns Hopkins Press, 1962. Pp. 177–195.
34. Palmer, R.: Development of a Differentiated Handedness. Psychol. Bull., *62*(4):257–272, 1969.
35. Patterson, G., and Guillion, M.: Living with Children. Champaign, Illinois, Research Press, 1968.
36. Pigott, R.: Behavior Modification and Control in Rehabilitation. J. Rehab., *35*(4):12–15, 1969.
37. Premack, D.: Toward Empirical Behavior Laws: I. Positive Reinforcement. Psychol. Rev., *66:*219–233, 1959.
38. Reed, H., and Reitan, R.: Intelligence Test Performances of Brain Damaged Subjects with Lateralized Motor Deficits. J. Consult. Psychol., *27:*102–106, 1967.
39. Reese, E.: The Analysis of Human Operant Behavior. Dubuque, William C. Brown, 1966.
40. Reitan, R.: The Effects of Brain Lesions on Adaptive Abilities in Human Beings. Indianapolis, Department of Neurology, Indiana University Medical Center, 1959.
41. Sand, P., Trieschmann, R., Fordyce, W., and Fowler, R.: Behavior Modification in the Medical Rehabilitation Setting: Rationale and Some Implications. Rehab. Res. Pract. Rev., *1*(2):11–24, 1970.
42. Sarason, I., and Ganzer, V.: Concerning the Medical Model. Amer. Psychol., *23:*507–510, 1968.
43. Siller, J., and Chipman, A.: Attitudes of the Nondisabled Toward the Physically Disabled. New York, New York University School of Education, 1967.
44. Siller, J., Ferguson, L., Vann, D., and Holland, B.: Studies in Reactions to Disability. Vol. XII. Structure of Attitudes Toward the Physically Disabled. New York, New York University School of Education, 1967.
45. Skinner, B.: The Technology of Teaching. New York, Appleton-Century-Crofts, 1968.
46. Skinner, B.: Verbal Behavior. New York, Appleton-Century-Crofts, 1957.
47. Staats, A.: A case in and a Strategy for the Extension of Learning Principles to Problems of Human Behavior. *In* Krasner, L., and Ullmann, L. (Eds.): Research in Behavior Modification. New York, Holt, Rinehart and Winston, 1966. Pp. 27–55.
48. Stark, R.: An Investigation of Unilateral and Cerebral Pathology with Equated Verbal and Visual-Spatial Tasks. J. Abnorm. Soc. Psychol., *62:*282-287, 1961.

49. Szasz, T.: The Myth of Mental Illness. Amer. Psychol., *15*(2):113-118, 1960.
50. Teuber, H.: Effects of Brain Wounds Implicating Right or Left Hemisphere in Man. *In* Mountcastle, V., (Ed.): Interhemispheric Relations and Cerebral Dominance. Baltimore, Johns Hopkins Press, 1962. Pp. 131-157.
51. Trombly, C.: Principles of Operant Conditioning: Related to Orthotic Training of Quadriplegic Patients. Amer. J. Occup. Ther., *20*(5):217-220, 1966.
52. Trotter, A., and Inman, D.: The Use of Positive Reinforcement in Physical Therapy. Phys. Ther., *48*:347-352, 1968.
53. Ullmann, L., and Krasner, L. (Eds.): Case Studies in Behavior Modification. New York, Holt, Rinehart and Winston, 1965.
54. Ulrich, R., and Crane, W.: Behavior: Persistence of Shock-induced Aggression. Science, *143*(3609):971-973, 1964.
55. Ulrich, R., Stachnik, T., and Mabry, J.: Control of Human Behavior. Glenview, Illinois, Scott, Foresman and Company, 1966.
56. Ulrich, R., Wolfe, M., and Dulaney, S.: Punishment of Shock-induced Aggression. J. Exp. Anal. Behav., *12*:1009-1015, 1969.
57. Wallace, J.: An Abilities Conception of Personality: Some Implications for Personality Measurement. Amer. Psychol., *21*:132-138, 1966.
58. Walls, R.: Behavior Modification and Rehabilitation. Rehab. Counsel. Bull., *13*(2):173-183, 1969.
59. Weinstein, S.: Differences in Effects of Brain Wounds Implicating Right or Left Hemisphere. *In* Mountcastle, V. (Ed.): Interhemispheric Relations and Cerebral Dominance. Baltimore, Johns Hopkins Press, 1962. Pp. 159-176.
60. Wright, B.: Disabling Myths About Disability. Paper presented at the meeting of the National Society for Crippled Children and Adults, Denver, September, 1963.
61. Wright, B.: Physical Disability—A Psychological Approach. New York, Harper and Brothers, 1960.
62. Zimmerman, J., Stuckey, T., Miller, M., and Garlick, B.: Effects of Token Reinforcement on Productivity in Multiple Handicapped Clients in a Sheltered Workshop. Rehab. Lit., *30*(2):34-41, 1969.

Chapter 7

PSYCHOSOCIAL DIAGNOSIS AND SOCIAL SERVICES—ONE ASPECT OF THE REHABILITATION PROCESS

by Helen J. Yesner

RATIONALE FOR PSYCHOSOCIAL CONCERNS IN REHABILITATION

In order to understand the importance of the psychosocial aspects of diagnosis and treatment in rehabilitation, it might be helpful to restate the definition of rehabilitation. For the purposes of this chapter rehabilitation is defined as a treatment process designed to help physically handicapped individuals make maximal use of residual capacities and to enable them to obtain optimal satisfaction and usefulness in terms of themselves, their families and their community. Rehabilitation may result in restoring the patient to complete independence and functioning, or it may mean only partial restoration. In some cases rehabilitation goals may include as the best adjustment for the patient only a life of dependence upon others. In a situation of this kind, helping the patient develop as much self-dependence and self-help as possible would be desirable along with helping him make a constructive adjustment to these extreme limitations.

196

One of the values of our society is that all men should be able to lead satisfying lives. We know that the well-being of a society is related to the well-being of its individual members. A satisfying life is achieved when basic needs are met and when the individual has opportunity for self-realization in a socially constructive way. Needs are universal in all people but are expressed and gratified in various and individual ways depending upon the culture in which the individual lives out his life. Illness and disability interfere with gratification of needs and with self-realization and, therefore, prevent to some extent a satisfying life. Rehabilitation is a means for helping the disabled individual make the most of his capacities for wholesome gratification of needs and self-realization. This means maximal physical restoration, more comfortable acknowledgment of the disability, alteration in goals, a substitution of new satisfactions for old, and possibly the development of new or unused resources in place of the old.

Successful rehabilitation demands a highly individualized treatment process based on a full and complete diagnosis of the physical disability and physical functioning of the patient; moreover, the psychologic and social functioning of a patient along with his environment and life situation cannot be disregarded. The diagnosis, which must go beyond the mere gathering of facts, requires an assessment of facts in order to clarify the interrelationships of the various aspects of the patient's personality, situation and condition. The potential resources of the patient must not be ignored. Indeed, at times, untapped resources must be explored and exploited. Ultimately, it is the patient, his family and the community that must be considered, involved and utilized.

Therefore, the rehabilitation process must use the knowledge and skills of many professional disciplines working together, and it must include the use of community services and resources.

The social worker is one of the professionals who is competent to perform this type of psychosocial assessment.

PSYCHOSOCIAL ASPECTS OF DISABILITY

Approach to the Patient. In keeping with the current comprehensive nature of medical care and of rehabilitation, it is essential to view the patient in terms of his social functioning, past and present. We all recognize the interrelatedness of the physical, psychologic and social aspects of man. Trouble, disease or malfunctioning in one area will have their effects in other areas. Thus it becomes imperative to consider the patient's physical functioning, his feelings about it and about himself, his relationships to others, and the milieu in which he lives and functions. In other words, the physical illness or disability must be viewed not only in terms of its effect upon physical functioning, but also in terms of how it has affected the overall life of the patient. Conversely, it is important to consider how social and psychologic functioning affect adjustment to physical illness and disability. There is a direct relationship between the severity of the disability and the degree to which social functioning is impaired. If the disability is such that extensive residuals remain, one can anticipate an increase in social problems. Further, if the patient has had previous difficulty in social functioning, if his social functioning has been at a rather low level, one can expect him to have greater difficulty in coping with a severe physical disability and in making use of rehabilitation services.

Organizing and Assessing Materials.   Probably one of the most useful ways of organizing and assessing the complex materials involved in determining any individual's well-being is to attempt to assess his functioning as a social being. Social functioning refers to the effectiveness with which the individual fulfills his many life roles. These roles may include that of marital partner, parent, child, worker, community member and, in the case of illness, patient. Werner Boehm states, "Social functioning, then, is the sum of the roles performed by a person. . . . One value in the role concept is that it permits identification of affected areas of social functioning."* In applying this concept to rehabilitation, it is necessary to formulate the psychosocial diagnosis in terms of the social roles the patient has ordinarily carried. Further, it is essential to assess the effectiveness with which he has carried these roles and to clarify the effect of the disability on his usual role-carrying responsibilities. In turn, it is vital to consider the probable impact of the role-carrying responsibilities on the disability and on treatment.[15]

It is the social worker's responsibility to gather this kind of information and to make this kind of assessment so that the rest of the rehabilitation team can be helped to bring into focus the effect of the disability on the patient and his situation, and the effect of the patient and his situation on his disability. This assessment is also the basis for social casework treatment and for all types of social work treatment. The role concept concentrates on areas of difficulty in social functioning and provides direction for the gathering of additional pertinent information.[15]

As was stated previously, health is a basic need. Illness or disability interferes with the gratification of this need. In addition, illness and disability usually produce increased dependence upon others and arouse fear and uncertainty. These internal reactions, these emotions, immediately affect the individual's equilibrium and, in turn, affect social functioning.[1]

Attitude of the Patient.   Many patients are able to use medical treatment effectively. They are well motivated and eager to achieve as much restoration as possible. Other patients find secondary satisfaction in illness and disability because of neurotic and immature attitudes. The first patient will need facilitating help primarily; the second will need help in growing up and finding more appropriate kinds of satisfactions. The amount of help and kind of help needed will in part depend upon how radical the effect of the illness or disability is upon the patient and the situation.[20]

For example, take the case of a patient who has suffered quadriplegia as the result of an accident. The patient soon discovers he is unable to use any of his limbs. He is unable to control elimination. He is almost totally dependent upon others. In some respects he is like an infant. He is frightened, he may be angry, and very likely he is depressed. He is at least subjectively aware that he has lost a large measure of control over his own life. Internally he begins to wonder whether people care enough about him to give him the very intimate and personalized attention he now needs. To a large extent his present insecurities will be either magnified or diminished by his previous life experiences. Knowledge of these previous life experiences can be helpful in understanding his current reactions. Regardless of his past experiences, it can be anticipated

---

*Boehm, Werner: The Social Casework Method in Social Work Education. Vol. X in Social Work Curriculum Study. New York, Council on Social Work Education, 1959. Quoted on p. 374 in Perlman.[15]

that he will not be able to cope immediately with the catastrophic change in his physical functioning. However, his level of maturation, his particular personality organization and his overall situation will in large measure determine the ultimate outcome.

We do know that this patient will not immediately respond to his family as he did formerly, nor will he respond positively, in all cases, to treatment personnel. Because of his fear of death, his fear of almost total dependency, his fear of loss of family role and of possible repudiation by the family, he may withdraw and become extremely passive or extremely hostile.

Attitude of the Patient's Family.   As a result, the family, wishing to cooperate, may feel threatened, confused and even antagonistic. They may be tangibly threatened by income loss, particularly if the patient has been the main source of income. This could increase family tension. Such an antagonistic dialectic could produce an increase of the difficulties. It takes no leap of the imagination to see, from this oversimplified example, that the patient's response to treatment could be affected. Further, with this patient, it is essential to take into account the fact that he will be dependent in some measure upon others the rest of his life. Thus it becomes essential to consider not only the current psychosocial aspects of the patient and his situation but also the long range psychosocial prognosis.

The Social Worker's Approach to the Patient's Problems.   To help this patient involve himself and respond positively to treatment, intervention on several levels must take place. In addition to the medical diagnosis and treatment, the social worker will now have to bring into play both psychosocial assessment and casework treatment. In addition to casework treatment, the social worker may need to use other modes of treatment or involve other social workers with these competencies. These interventive modes include group work treatment and community organization. In other words, treatment must be focused on interrelated medical and psychosocial problems. The social worker will attempt (1) to gather a social history; (2) to compile and assess data about the family situation; (3) to study the patient's current responses and functioning; and (4) to assess and analyze all this material, including information derived from other professional sources, so that a psychosocial diagnosis can be made. Further, the social worker, while engaged in the diagnostic process, will try to help the patient and family resolve their conflicts and their environmental difficulties.

Summary.   In summation, the psychosocial aspects of disability must be considered in terms of the patient, his family and his total life situation. Disability can mean temporary or permanent dependence upon others. It may mean dependence upon others for physical care as well as for economic and social support. It may mean temporary or permanent change in role responsibilities for the patient and for family members. These effects, inasmuch as they are crucial and stressful, must be seriously considered in the treatment of any disabled patient. Finally, any disability has its impact on the psychosocial aspects of the patient and his life situation. The impact may be relatively benign, one that the patient and his family can handle with little outside help; or the disability could cause considerable dislocation. Then more extensive help will be required, particularly in the area of psychosocial functioning.

SOCIAL WORK AND REHABILITATION

The social worker is the professional whose central concern is with the social functioning of people in relation to their life problems. Through training and experience the social worker has developed knowledge and skills in working with people in the solution of their social problems. Social work concepts take into account the interrelatedness of physical, social and emotional factors in the precipitation of social breakdown. Illness and disability come within the purview of physical causes of social breakdown. Since the social worker is committed to helping people lead socially satisfying, useful lives, he fits very logically into the physical rehabilitation effort. As a profession, social work has developed methods for working with individuals, groups and communities in the solution of their social problems. Even though some rehabilitation agencies offer social group work services as well as casework services, for the purposes of this book, we will consider primarily the social casework method and the role and function of the social caseworker in rehabilitation. Social group work, community organization, social policy and administration are all important methods that have been developed by the profession of social work for helping people solve their problems and bring about change in their personal and communal lives. All these methods play a part in the rehabilitation process and all should be considered in greater depth than is possible here.

Social group work should be utilized much more extensively than it is at the present time in rehabilitation facilities. We do know that many individuals move faster and more effectively in treatment when helped through the group process. Groups can be problem-oriented or can be focused on self growth and development. The group process can enhance milieu therapy, can improve the quality of institutional life and can help the patient move more quickly toward return to life in the community, to his family or to a more permanent life situation.

THE FUNCTION OF THE SOCIAL CASEWORKER IN REHABILITATION

The social caseworker has six major functions in rehabilitation: (1) to participate in the psychosocial diagnostic effort; (2) to give social casework services; (3) to offer consultation to treatment staff concerning the psychosocial functioning of the patient; (4) to influence the team as a group regarding their attitudes, feelings and objectives toward and concerning the patient and his family; (5) to influence social policy development and social policy changes within the institution and the community toward a more satisfying quality of life for all; and (6) to function in developing effective liaison between the rehabilitation agency and the larger social welfare community.

Psychosocial Diagnosis

The psychosocial diagnosis serves two purposes. First, it contributes to an overall team diagnosis that becomes the basis for rehabilitation goals and treatment. Second, it serves as the basis for determining casework problems and casework treatment so that the caseworker can fulfill his part in the total rehabilitation service in the achievement of rehabilitation goals.

The psychosocial diagnosis in a rehabilitation setting is threefold. It comprises study, assessment and evaluation. First, a study must be made of the social functioning of the patient, of the family functioning and relationships, and of the pertinent cultural, social and environmental factors that are immediately related to the patient's rehabilitation problem. Then an assessment must be made of the patient's strengths, capacities, motivations and difficulties in functioning. Finally, the diagnostic process demands an evaluation of the interaction of all these factors (cause and effect must be considered) for the purposes of determining the central problem or problems and to establish goals with the patient. Skillful utilization on the part of the social worker of this threefold process—study, assessment and evaluation—can facilitate physical rehabilitation.

Sources of Information.   The social worker draws upon many sources of information to arrive at a psychosocial diagnosis. These sources include social agencies familiar with the patient and his family, records of previous contacts with the rehabilitation agency, medical and other treatment personnel currently working with the patient, the patient himself and the patient's family. In addition, the social worker's own experience with the patient is a valuable source of information. The patient in almost every case is the best source of information about himself and his situation and can provide information that will be most effective in furthering the rehabilitation process. For the most part, diagnosis and evaluation of treatment in social work are based on clinical observations and case by case analytical judgments. This method continues to dominate practice.

However, in the past few years rather extensive research projects have been devoted to finding more objective means for implementing social work diagnosis and evaluation of social work treatment. An example of this is the Family Centered Project sponsored by the Greater St. Paul Community Chest and Councils, Inc. In this project the effort was directed toward developing (1) a method of evaluating family behavior based on the concept of social functioning and (2) ways of measuring changes in function or, to state it another way, measuring movement. Another example is the Hunt Movement Scale which has been developed to assess treatment results in groups of cases. The Minnesota Work Reorientation Project sponsored by the Minnesota Department of Public Welfare in conjunction with Community Research Associates has also been concerned with developing more standardized tools for purposes of making possible a more systematic diagnosis and for measuring the outcome of treatment.

Clarification of the Social Situation.   By utilizing as many of these sources and techniques as possible, the social worker can attempt to clarify the patient's immediate social situation, such as his living arrangements, his family relationships, his financial situation, the effect of the disability on him, his employment history, educational background and achievement, and in general his level of social functioning. The social worker very specifically attempts to comprehend the patient's feelings about his disability and the nature of his motivations in seeking rehabilitation services. It is essential to determine how the patient has coped with his physical limitations, how he has adapted to previous stress situations and what his present condition means to him. It is important to clarify family interaction, including family reaction to the patient and his disability. It is also important to know the resources within the family and the impact of the patient's disability on the family functioning and situation. The diagnostic effort must be geared to understanding the meaning of all the significant details of the patient's situation. This diagnostic effort is a continuous one which begins with the admission of the patient and ends only when the patient is considered rehabilitated.

Diagnosis on the part of the social worker carries with it the responsibility for interpreting and sharing this diagnostic material with the rest of the rehabilitation team and for participating with the team in the establishment of rehabilitation goals and treatment. As a member of the team, it is very important that the social worker draw on his or her knowledge of the small group process to help promote teamwork and to meet his or her responsibilities for contributing to and influencing the team's work with the patient.

Social Casework Services

Social casework is a problem-solving process. It is the professional method that the caseworker uses in helping an individual in some area of social functioning. Helen Perlman, in her book, *Social Casework*, has described social casework as "a process used by certain human welfare agencies to help individuals to cope more effectively with their problems in social functioning." She described the social casework process as "a progressive transaction between the professional helper and the client (patient). It consists of a series of problem-solving operations carried on within a meaningful relationship. The end of the process is contained in its means: to so influence the client-person that he develops effectiveness in coping with his problem and/or to so influence the problem as to resolve it or vitiate its effect."[14] In addition, the social worker may influence not only the problem but also the situation so that, for all practical purposes, the effects of the problem are reduced or made more manageable. Furthermore, help with a particular situation may free the person so that he can cope more effectively with the problem. For example, the placement of a homemaker may relieve the anxiety of a disabled mother to such an extent that she is freer to contemplate what is expected and required of her in the rehabilitation program. Before the placement of the homemaker she may have been extremely anxious about what was happening to her children because of lack of care and supervision. Preoccupation with this concern could reduce her capacity to participate in treatment. Thus, change in situation, or manipulation of environment, may reduce stress and free the patient to cope more effectively with a central problem.

Helping the Patient. The social worker is frequently called upon to help encourage the patient to understand his condition. Sometimes internal stress interferes with this. The caseworker, by supportive measures, may reduce the sense of threat, and this can facilitate the patient's participation in treatment and, therefore, facilitate restoration. If stress arises primarily from external difficulties, the social worker can help deal with these difficulties. For example, if the patient is concerned about the financial status of his family, he may find it too threatening to consider the permanent nature of his disability. The social worker can help the patient and the family consider ways of meeting their financial problem. One of the ways might be to make application for public assistance. The combination of support and tangible help quite often is enough to enable the patient to begin to take appropriate action to improve his condition and, as a result, his situation. Frequently casework help may involve working not only with the patient but also with his family, and often the major help is given to the family. In fact, in every situation in which the patient is a part of a family, the patient and his family should be viewed and worked with as a unit. Much has been written about the value and methods of working with families as units, and, whenever possible, this should be attempted as a part of the rehabilitation process.

Social work help is social in its very process. The help emerges as a result of a professional relationship that is focused on meeting the needs of the patient and on eliciting maximal participation and involvement of the patient in the solution of his problems.

Social casework is the means for providing the social services offered by the rehabilitation agency. These services include direct help to the patient in utilizing the therapeutic services of the agency, help in coping with the immediate situation during rehabilitation and help in planning for the future after discharge. At any point in treatment the caseworker may refer the patient or family to other agencies in the community for help with problems that cannot be dealt with in the rehabilitation setting.

The Interview. Basic to all social casework treatment is the relationship between worker and client (patient). The major tool in treatment is the interview, which presupposes the establishment and development of this relationship. Social casework treatment usually involves a series of interviews that are both diagnostic and therapeutic in their focus. Once the initial diagnosis has been achieved, the social caseworker establishes certain mutual goals with the patient and proceeds with the treatment according to a plan he has developed.

Casework Treatment Methods. Casework treatment usually involves one or both of the following methods: (1) *providing support* and (2) *encouraging change*. The supportive method helps the patient through times of stress so that he can function at maximum while he is engaged in solving crucial life problems. This type of treatment does not envision basic changes in personality functioning but merely seeks improvements in it. Of course, indirectly, this type of treatment could foster maturation and, as a result, could bring about a change in personality functioning. In the supportive method, the caseworker always employs supportive techniques such as *reassurance, logical discussion, advice and guidance* and *intervention*. The supportive method would always be concerned with the patient's troubled feelings about himself, his disability, his situation and anything else that interferes with his use of treatment and his solution of current problems.

The second type of treatment envisions modification in certain areas of personality functioning that interfere with the solution of problems. This type of treatment combines the use of supportive measures with an attempt to clarify with the patient inappropriate patterns of behavior. By clarification of these inappropriate patterns of behavior, the patient may develop enough insight so that a change in functioning can occur. This type of treatment is employed only when personality function seriously impairs problem-solving and when ego strength seems adequate to tolerate insight.[8]

Crisis theory is a useful theory in the early stages of work with the patient and his family, and also at any time additional crises occur during rehabilitation. Social workers have developed effective ways of working and intervening at times of crisis.[12]

Consultation

The social worker shares with all members of the rehabilitation team the responsibility for providing consultation to members of other disciplines. Consultation involves the giving of expert advice, information or insights related to the treatment of the patient. The social worker's advice is sought on the basis of his competence and knowledge about psychosocial aspects of the disability that affect the patient and his situation, or vice versa.

Liaison Between Rehabilitation Agency and Larger Social Welfare Community

The social worker is the professional who probably has the most complete knowledge of community social welfare resources. As such, he should be the team member responsible for referring the patient and family to the appropriate community resources. In helping a patient and family consider community resources it is important for the caseworker to give enough information about these resources so that they can decide which ones they can best use. At this point the caseworker may have to help the patient and his family overcome their feelings of discomfort in making application to a new and different resource.

The caseworker may also have to facilitate the referral by taking appropriate actions. The caseworker's activity depends in part upon the adequacy of the client and the family. In some instances they are able to take a great share of the responsibility in making application to a new resource; in other instances, they may need a great deal of help. This may include such specific aids as a telephone call to the agency, an appointment, a letter of referral and sometimes a conference with the new agency. In general, people have considerable anxiety about asking for assistance. This must always be taken into consideration in helping the patient consider community resources. He must be helped at all times to maintain his sense of worth and of adequacy.

WHEN SHOULD A PATIENT BE REFERRED TO SOCIAL SERVICE?

This question is related in part to the administrative structure and organization of a hospital or rehabilitation facility. In many rehabilitation settings each patient is seen by a member of the social service department at the time of his admission. This policy reinforces the current concept of the interrelatedness of the physical, psychologic and social functioning of man in the rehabilitation process. As a result the caseworker, even though he is not working intensively with all patients, is usually familiar with all the patients' situations and can become involved whenever a patient seems to need assistance. In this kind of setting it is helpful if the non-social work staff will alert the social worker to any current problems of a psychosocial nature that the patient seems to manifest so that the social worker can determine whether his active involvement is necessary.

In most hospitals for the acutely ill the social service department sees patients only upon referral by other staff or upon request of the patient or family members. In this kind of organization the medical and treatment staff must be unusually sensitive to the psychosocial impact of disability and illness and, in turn, the impact of psychosocial problems on illness and disability and on the treatment of these conditions. A referral to social service should be made in any case in which (1) the patient seems to be reacting inappropriately to the illness or disability, (2) the patient seems unable to cope with the illness, disability or treatment, (3) family relationships or family problems impinge upon the patient's use of medical care or (4) the patient's illness and disability create overpowering problems for the family. In general, the social worker can be helpful to the patient in those situations in which the patient's attitude interferes with the use of treatment and in which the actual treatment situation seems to have created conflict for the patient and is, therefore, obstructing treatment. All cases in which there are tangible environmental problems such as a financial need, the need for homemaker service, foster home care or nursing home care should be referred to the social worker.

HOW TO REFER PATIENTS TO SOCIAL SERVICE

When a patient is to be referred to social service for help, it is advisable to discuss the referral with him. It is important that the referring person clarify with the patient the reason for referral so that he has some understanding of why the social service worker has been called in. There may be a few exceptions to this. For instance, it may be impossible to explain the need for referral to a person who is psychotic or mentally incompetent. In the case of children, especially when the social worker will be working more directly with the family, no explanation may be necessary.

COMMUNITY RESOURCES COMMONLY USED IN THE REHABILITATION PROCESS

The community resources can be divided into public and private agencies. Public agencies are supported through tax funds and are under the sanction and auspices of some branch of the government. Private agencies are voluntary in their organization and financing and usually have the sanction of certain groups in the community. The public welfare agencies offer a wide range of services, including financial assistance to certain categorical groups such as the aged, the disabled, the blind, and dependent children whose fathers are disabled, dead, absent from the home or, in some states, unemployed. Most communities provide some form of general assistance that serves to meet the economic needs of all residual problem situations not included in these categorical groups. General assistance could include help to single, unattached individuals under the age of 65, help to families when the head of household is unemployed, or help to any persons or families not covered by categorical aid programs.

Most communities provide for medical care through state or local hospitals and, in some instances, through private facilities.

Public Welfare Agencies. *Departments of public welfare* offer services to dependent and neglected children in the form of guardianship, protection, foster home and adoption programs. Departments of public welfare also provide for care and supervision of the mentally retarded and the mentally ill. *State boards of education* provide special services to children who suffer some type of handicap. Public resources include *vocational rehabilitation programs* that are sponsored jointly by federal and state governments. Also under public agencies are *court services* and *probation offices.* The *Veterans Administration* provides many services for veterans, including medical, psychiatric and rehabilitation care, and also administers disability compensation programs and pension programs. In addition, state and local groups may provide for subsistence needs of veterans and their families. Community mental health centers should also be considered as resources of help to the patient and his family.

Private Agencies.   In most medium-sized or larger urban areas a wide range of social services are available through private agencies, including *social casework counseling* to families who are experiencing parent-child problems, marital difficulty or problems in normal functioning because of either mental or physical illness of one of the parents. Services in this instance might include *homemaker service* or *foster home care,* as well as *counseling services.* In addition, many communities offer mental hygiene and child guidance services. They may offer institutional care for disturbed and delinquent children. Many rehabilitation agencies are sponsored by private groups; we see examples of this in the *curative workshops,* and *out-patient physical rehabilitation services.* Privately sponsored resources include a wide range of health agencies such as the *Cerebral Palsy Association,* the *National Society for Crippled Children and Adults* and the *American Heart Association.*

WHAT IS THE TRAINING FOR THE SOCIAL WORKER?

Professional social work training involves a two year graduate course in an accredited school of social work. Satisfactory completion of this course leads to a Master of Arts or Master of Social Work degree.

Professional training for social work involves theoretical courses in human growth and behavior, community organization, administration, research, social policies and programs, social group work and social casework. The training program provides for heavy concentration in the following areas: dynamics of normal and pathological growth and behavior, social policies and programs and a primary methods course, such as social casework. Throughout the two year training period the student is enrolled in field training for instruction in one of the following primary methods: casework, group work or community organization. The field training instruction is provided for in a social agency or in an allied host agency such as a hospital or rehabilitation setting. Each student has experience in two different types of settings during the two year period. At this point, social work training curricula are undergoing great changes, as are all the helping professions. Instead of being organized around primary methods, the curriculum is frequently organized around concentrations and target populations.

REFERENCES

1. Bartlett, H. M.: Social Work Practice in the Health Field. New York, National Association of Social Workers, 1961.
2. Bartlett, H. M.: The Widening Scope of Hospital Social Work. Social Casework J., *44:*3-10, 1063.

3. Cooper, R.: Social Work in Vocational Rehabilitation. Social Work, National Association of Social Workers, 8:92-98, 1963.
4. Family Service Association of America: Methods and Process in Social Casework. New York, Report of a Staff Committee, Community Service Society of New York, 1958.
5. DeWolfe, A. S., Barrell, R. P., and Spaner, F. E.: Staff Attitudes Toward Patient Care and Treatment-Disposition Behavior. J. Abnorm. Psychol., 74(1):90-94, 1969.
6. Geismar, L. L., and Ayers, B.: Measuring Family Functioning. St. Paul, Minnesota, Family Centered Project, Greater St. Paul Community Chests and Councils, Inc., 1960.
7. Grosser, C. F.: Changing Theory and Changing Practice. Social Work, 5:16-21, 1969.
8. Hollis, F.: Analysis of Casework Treatment Methods and Their Relationship to Change. Smith College Studies in Social Work, 32:97-117, 1962.
9. Hunt, J. McV., and Kagen, L.: Measuring Results in Social Casework. New York, Family Service Association of America, 1950.
10. Ludwig, E. G., and Adams, S. D.: Patient Cooperation in a Rehabilitation Center: Assumption of the Client Role. Journal of Health and Social Behavior, 9:322-336, 1968.
11. National Association of Social Workers, Medical Social Work Section: Report of Subcommittee on the Medical Social Worker in Rehabilitation. New York, Committee on Medical Social Work Practice, 1957.
12. Parad, H. J.: Crisis Intervention: Selected Readings. Family Service Association of America, New York, 1965.
13. Parks, A. H.: Short Term Casework in a Medical Setting. Social Work, National Association of Social Workers, 8:89-94, 1963.
14. Perlman, H. H.: Social Casework: A Problem Solving Process. Chicago, University of Chicago Press, 1957.
15. Perlman, H. H.: The Role Concept and Social Casework: Some Explorations. 1. The "Social" in Social Casework. Social Service Review, 35:370-381, 1961.
16. Rapaport, L.: The State of Crisis: Some Theoretical Considerations. Social Service Review, 36:211-217, 1962.
17. Simon, B. K.: Relationship Theory and Practice in Social Casework. Monograph IV in series, Social Work Practice in Medical Care and Rehabilitation Settings. New York, Medical Social Work Section, National Association of Social Workers, 1960.
18. Specht, H.: Casework Practice and Social Policy Formulation. Social Work, 13:42-52, 1968.
19. Thomas, E. J.: Behavioral Science for Social Workers. Free Press, New York, 1967.
20. Thomas, E. J.: Selected Sociobehavioral Technologies and Principles: An Approach to Interpersonal Helping. Social Work, 13:12-26, 1968.
21. Upham, F.: A Dynamic Approach to Illness. New York, Family Service Association of America, 1960 (reprinting).
22. Vernick, J.: The Use of the Life Space Interview on a Medical Ward. Social Casework J., 44:465-469, 1963.
23. Wright, B. A.: Physical Disability—A Psychological Approach. New York, Harper and Brothers, 1960.

Chapter 8

VOCATIONAL ASSESSMENT AND MANAGEMENT

by Robert A. Walker

Working with a vocational counselor can sometimes be a disappointing experience for physicians. This disappointment arises because the counselor cannot consistently produce the desired result—a job for the physician's handicapped patient. These expectations often develop within the mind of the physician in the following fashion. A patient enters a hospital in a dependent state requiring the services of many rehabilitation personnel. The physician, working with a team of competent professionals and through a great deal of group effort, sees the patient attain a series of rehabilitation goals and ultimately leave the hospital. However, at follow-up, the team's accomplishments are diluted if employment has not been obtained. If and when this unfortunate situation occurs, it would be wise to keep the following issues in mind:

Patients who respond well to medical services may be poor candidates for vocational services. The hemiplegic is a good example.

Successful vocational services are objective and measurable (a job), and when failure occurs, it is clearly visible to the entire team. Unlike other professional goals, there are no degrees of success; outcome is usually a matter of success or failure.

Vocational counseling is not well endowed with an advanced technology. It is the newest field in rehabilitation and suffers from a number of philosophic, personnel and methods deficits.

The professional staff's interest in employment is usually greater than the patient's.

208

Employers are not always receptive toward hiring the disabled, in spite of exhortations to hire the handicapped.

Employment usually involves the entire sum of a person's capacities and abilities to adjust to a very complex and challenging situation. The vocational counselor is usually only a very small part of this adjustment process. In short, his influence as to whether or not the patient returns to the labor market is not necessarily very substantial.

Understanding and acceptance of these points should have some effect on an evaluation of the adequacy of a vocational counseling service. Hopefully this understanding will reduce professional conflicts between the counselor and other team members.

THE PHYSICIAN'S EXPECTATIONS

It should not be inferred that there are not reasonable demands that a physician can make of a vocational counselor. Like other members of the team, he too has a role to play, and he should play it well. Essentially, a vocational counselor should be expected to develop a vocational plan and to assist in its implementation. The vocational plan should cover:

A statement reflecting the problem or the assistance required to help the patient return to the labor market. The plan should be stated in specific terms to facilitate communication between the counselor and the team and permit the center to monitor the effectiveness of the vocational services. An example of a poor problem statement is "patient is not motivated." An example of a good statement of the problem is "lacks occupational skills—needs training in book-keeping."

A plan for the vocational treatments needed for the problem. This goal may be "conseling as an out-patient by vocational counselor and physician" or "referral to the state agency for training in a local business school."

A statement of the counselor's services for the patient which structures more definitively the counselor's role in implementing the plan. This statement may be: "will be seen weekly for counseling interviews and will coordinate plans with physician" or "state agency will follow in business school—can see monthly in out-patient department for surveillance interviewing."

Although the physician may feel some sense of gratification at seeing definitive vocational plans being developed by the counselor, such planning still does not completely resolve the issue of outcome, which is important not just for the patient and physician but for other team members and the community as well. In spite of the many problems involved in establishing expectancies, system accountability requires that reasonable achievement in outcomes be defined. Such expectancies not only offer protection to the consumer of services but they enable the center to define those elements which appear to be sub-optimizing.

THE COUNSELOR'S EXPECTATIONS

Vocational counselors have expectations also. Probably the most important of these is that the other members of the rehabilitation staff should feel that the counselor knows more about vocational rehabilitation than anyone else on the team. When the team fails to feel this way, serious problems will undoubtedly occur. Also, the counselor expects that in the give and take of what often is primarily a medical service the counseling program will be given fair consideration. He expects such things as an organized referral system, free access to information, adequate time in the patient's program for vocational services and, most important, professional recognition. This last has to be earned, but it can be difficult to acquire in a hostile or indifferent climate. Hostility toward counselors sometimes occurs since in many ways the counselor alone reflects what the community will tolerate in a disabled person. Such realities are often not well received by staff members whose professional duties are restricted to the hospital environment where they do not always develop an awareness of the attitude of the community toward the disabled.

THE PATIENT'S INTEREST IN VOCATIONAL REHABILITATION

Most patients will not voluntarily request vocational services. If the physician waits for the patient to express an interest before referral to a counselor, few in-patients will receive vocational services. The primary reason for the lack of interest is that people are in hospitals because they are sick and their chief concern is getting better. Employment goals, while ultimately crucial, are of secondary importance to a patient who is involved in a struggle to resolve the issue of residual physical impairments. Because most sick people do not naturally start thinking about jobs, a most important function of the physician in the vocational rehabilitation process is to create interest in the patient for vocational services. If interest can be developed, a major obstacle to vocational rehabilitation is removed. However, preceding a discussion of motivational techniques, the physician must first be able to identify those patients who need to be referred for vocational services.

Identifying Patients Who Need Vocational Services

Patients who need vocational services are those who say they want to work or those who have to work. The first group consists of patients who voluntarily ask for vocational services. Within this group of potential referrals will be a number of severely physically disabled patients. Because so much decision making in hospitals centers around illness, physicians sometimes rule out employment goals for patients because of limited physical capacities. However, this reason is usually not a major cause of unemployability. Even if the physician feels that a patient cannot work, referral to a vocational counselor is usually advisable since the prediction as to employability is an exceedingly complex one.

Those patients who need vocational services but who do not openly request them constitute the majority of the referrals for vocational services and they are difficult management problems for the physician. The next question to resolve occurs when the patient has not exhibited any interest in vocational planning. When then does the physician begin to discuss with the patient his referral for vocational services? This is an exceedingly difficult question to answer since the variables are so numerous. For example, a psychologically sophisticated physician can develop readiness in the patient for vocational services very early in the patient's program. Some patients have a less disabling psychologic reaction to the disability and can tolerate with minimal anxiety a discussion of vocational goals even though such a discussion often implies to the patient that the disability is permanent. A vocational counselor with a great deal of counseling skill can work through resistance even with a very early referral. Other counselors find late referrals most appropriate since frequently, because of impending discharge from the hospital, the patient is forced to consider vocational alternatives. Since the variables influencing the time to refer are so numerous, the best solution is probably to discuss individual cases in a team meeting with the vocational counselor. The counselor should be able to tell whether or not the patient is ready for referral and how to prepare the client for vocational services. Staff members who have communication with the patient in other treatment areas should also have valuable opinions regarding this question. Such a meeting also enables the counselor to ask pertinent questions about the patient and thus prepare himself better for the first interview.

Developing an Interest in Vocational Services

The first step in developing an interest in vocational services is to establish in the patient's mind the fact that he has a vocational future. A physician who is willing to discuss such matters brings with him a necessary accompanying ingredient: his own personal concern for the vocational success of his patient. As indicated in previous sections, the issue of the patient's interest in working is vital to the outcome, and is frequently absent among the patients themselves.

The most useful and probably the most consistently successful technique in stimulating an interest in the patient for vocational services is confrontation. A few questions such as "What vocational plans have you been making?", "Do you have a job lined up?" or "How do you plan to earn your living?" are usually good starting points. Such questions tend to focus the attention of the patient on an experience which is often not enjoyable: discharge from the hospital and the severance of certain dependency ties. However, the questions will often force the patient to face the need for vocational planning. Rather commonly, patients respond to such questions with a vague plan or no plan whatsoever.

Once it has been established and accepted that a vocational problem does exist, it is essential next to commit the patient to taking an active part in obtaining vocational services by having him take the initiative in seeing the vocational counselor. When the patient does this it tends to place maximal responsibility for services on him and not on the counselor. Such procedures commit the patient to active participation in vocational rehabilitation. This is important because the process of employment usually involves more personal and physical resources from the patient than does any other rehabilitation goal.

Interpreting Vocational Services

To facilitate the patient's realistic participation in vocational services a good deal of care should be given to the manner in which vocational services are described. One step has already been discussed—that of getting the patient interested in such a service. The second step, a realistic description of the services, is of equal importance. The focal point of the interpretation of vocational services should be the *process* of vocational rehabilitation rather than the outcome. It is unwise to make a referral for vocational services with a statement such as "they can get you a job." Such statements commit the patient to a conclusion as to the end result rather than to an understanding that vocational services are part of the process of preparing him for the labor market. It holds the promise of a reward but fails to relate it to effort. Patients who are so advised fail to see that the essential ingredient is not merely the existence of the service but his active involvement in the process.

A description of the process need not be complex. The vocational counselor can do that in considerable detail. A reasonable referral statement by the physician might be, "Our counselor will talk with you about the kinds of jobs you feel you would like and can do and perhaps he can help you make some suitable plans by discharge time." Avoid answers to questions from the patient like "Can he send me to school?" or "Will he get me a job?" by referring them to the counselor.

The patient entering vocational services with unrealistic vocational aspirations is another major problem faced by the counselor. The physician should never suggest vocational goals to the patient or reinforce vocational plans offered by the patient unless he is sure the vocational counselor thinks they are realistic.

VOCATIONAL EVALUATION METHODS

There are three basic methods or services used in the diagnosis of a vocational problem: the counseling interview, psychologic testing and pre-vocational units.

To a greater extent than is the case with other rehabilitation disciplines, the vocational counselor must consider the assets and liabilities of the patient's past, present and future activities. These concerns are not just in the vocational area but also in the medical, social and psychologic areas in ways that may seem peculiar to other staff members. The physician may focus on the adolescent's paraplegia, but the counselor may feel that his long hair is a greater problem in job placement. The psychologist may justifiably be concerned with the dynamics of the patient's depression, but the counselor's vocational rehabilitation goals are affected because the patient presents a poor impression by not bathing. The occupational therapist may be amused by the patient's inability to discriminate between colored yarns, but the counselor's anxiety is increased by the knowledge that hundreds of potential jobs are eliminated because of color blindness. The complexities of our industrial society demand that the counselor understand a great many things about his patient. The counselor's grasp of the problem must be complete and thorough if employment goals are to be realized.

The Counseling Interview

The counseling interview is the most effective evaluative tool of the vocational counselor. There does not appear to be much disagreement as to its ultimate purpose, to determine the necessary services which will enable the patient to enter the labor market. Counseling is a highly individualized skill and considerable differences exist among counselors regarding the many important variables of the counseling interview. Again, the physician should expect some pertinent and insightful diagnostic statements and he should not be too concerned with the particular style of interviewing used by the counselor.

The material covered in a counseling interview can be broadly classified as dealing either with feelings or with facts. As the profession of vocational counseling matures, it becomes obvious that vocational counselors are now less concerned with labor market information and more concerned with attitudes and feelings as the most important factors in vocational rehabilitation. Because of the importance that counselors attach to attitudes a brief description of the counselor's typical approach to such issues follows.

It is rather common for patients to present to the counselor a picture of their disability which is not in keeping with the facts. The physician may respond to this with annoyance or the psychologist with a diagnosis of denial, but for the counselor, vocational planning is often halted. This halt occurs with the counselor because vocational planning is structured within the confines of physical capacities. When the vocational counselor is faced with the realization that the patient still believes that his completely severed spinal cord will regenerate, a discussion of sedentary occupations becomes academic. This particular attitude of non-acceptance of reality is usually, but not always, a danger signal. Dealing with such a case will require a great deal of finesse by several team members.

Of all the various attitudes toward employment held by patients the worst is indifference. Unfortunately, it is a rather common one. This problem of apathy can manifest itself in a veritable syndrome of problems, such as occupational choice indecision, poor scores on vocational tests or chronic difficulty in looking for jobs when job placement activities begin. Just why patients react this way is a moot point. It depends somewhat upon the patient, his problems and the professional frame of reference of the person giving the opinion. One observation that might be made is that many patients needing vocational services did not function well before they became disabled and the additional burden of physical limitations is simply too much for whatever personal resources they may possess. Hospital routines that reward the compliant and docile patient tend to perpetuate apathetic attitudes and make life difficult for the counselor and ultimately for the patient. In any event, indifference to vocational planning is a challenging and difficult problem to solve and requires considerable skill for even a well trained counselor.

The patient's vocational plans do not rest solely on attitudes; facts also contribute heavily to vocational rehabilitation. A significant area for the vocational counselor is the patient's educational and work history. The educational record can be quite misleading, and superficial generalizations can lead to serious errors. Grade averages are especially deceptive since absolute grading standards rarely exist. Schools have rather unique grading standards whose true meaning is known only within the school setting. Achievement tests probably offer a more accurate indication of school success than grades.

The work history is usually a profitable area for the vocational counselor to explore and considerable time is devoted to it, especially in the initial series of interviews. Many job titles given by patients reflect what they thought they were or what they wanted to be, rather than what they actually were. The well qualified counselor will obtain a job history which includes a description of duties rather than just titles. This particular aspect of the interview usually leads to a better understanding of the patient's skills. Salary level is also an important area for exploration and a number of inferences can be made from it. A reasonable correlation exists between salary and skills, and the salary level gives the counselor a clue as to what salary expectations the patient will have. Few patients seem to be willing to take a pay cut regardless of the diminution of employability created by a physical handicap.

The work history can also reveal such occurrences as long periods of unemployment between jobs. There are occupational groups, such as seasonal workers, whose employment gaps can be considered "normal," but in some patients they can reflect such things as borderline skills, poor community reputation or lack of persistence in job hunting.

Psychologic Tests

Tests are one of the most frequently discussed but least favored assessment techniques. Unfortunately, many of the tests commonly used in vocational rehabilitation cannot consistently isolate the skills of many patients now receiving vocational rehabilitation services. Some of the general areas of tests are:

Aptitude Tests.   Theoretically, aptitude tests measure capacity to perform certain tasks. Three of the most common types of tests used in rehabilitation are mechanical, clerical and motor speed tests. These tests are often closely timed and usually require that the patient be well motivated to score well. Patients with severe depression often fail to do well and it is usually best to defer testing until the depression has lifted. Older and less well educated patients frequently fail to involve themselves enough in testing to obtain optimal results. The vocational counselor has a large number of tests to choose from but some of the most commonly used tests of mechanical abilities are Minnesota Paper Form Board and Bennett Test of Mechanical Comprehension; of clerical abilities, General Clerical Test and Minnesota Clerical Test, and of motor speed, Purdue Pegboard and Minnesota Rate of Manipulation.

Interest Tests.   These tests usually require the patient to respond to a series of questions in such a way as to indicate their interest in terms of occupations, general activities or school subjects. From them one can obtain some measure of interests in specific occupations or broad occupational categories. Patients with a reading ability on or below the sixth grade level often will have difficulty in taking such tests and the counselor of necessity will determine interest by other methods. Two commonly used tests are the Kuder Preference Record and the Strong Vocational Interest Blank (SVIB) usually referred to as "the Strong."

Proficiency or Achievement Tests.   These tests measure knowledge in a particular field or area. Examples are tests measuring knowledge of algebra, general science or plumbing. They are indicators of past attainments. Because high school graduation does not necessarily reflect what a person has learned, tests of this type are often used as a measure. Two rather widely used educational achievement batteries are the California Achievement Tests and the Iowa Tests of Educational Development. Proficiency tests for specific industrial skills have not been well developed. Knowledge of the patient's industrial skills are usually evaluated by a review of past work and educational histories as well as using work samples within prevocational units.

Personality and Intelligence Tests.   Tests of these types are generally given by a clinical psychologist although many vocational counselors do administer them. In any event, the vocational counselor finds these types of tests indispensable in vocational planning.

Prevocational Units

Prevocational units as discussed in this chapter are defined as units which are contained in an in-patient setting where the patient performs simulated job tasks which represent work performed in industry. The primary reason for the development of such units was to facilitate the rehabilitation of patients having severe physical disabilities. It was hoped that such units would be helpful to the counselor in developing vocational objectives not possible through more formal diagnostic methods.

The two most significant variables within such units leading to better diagnosis are the duplication of certain industrial jobs and skilled observations on the part of the staff. The tasks, commonly called work samples, represent the essential duties of a specific job found in industry. Some of the more common jobs usually duplicated are machine operation (drill press or punch press), clerical work (typing, bookkeeping and office machines) and occupations such as printing, drafting, negative retouching or watchmaking. The professional staff within this unit are usually from professional fields such as occupational therapy, industrial arts and psychology. With careful observation it is possible to gain information regarding such things as the patient's general approach to work, his interest in a particular task, his work habits and his ability to get along with others in a work situation. Although such data are quite subjective, they nevertheless provide a wealth of information not easily obtainable in any other way.

The units can offer a great many evaluative experiences for the well trained and imaginative counselor. For example, it is possible to verify work skills claimed by the patient and to measure the physical ability of the patient to tolerate an eight hour work day. Such units can assist in the measurement of the patient's ability to learn, which is especially significant in the brain injured. It is also possible to evaluate a wide variety of personality factors thought to be important in employment.

Although prevocational units have undoubtedly increased the counselor's ability to provide sound vocational services, certain problems detract from their usefulness. First, it is difficult to reproduce industrial jobs accurately and to obtain industrial information which can be used to judge a patient's productivity in comparison with that of industrial workers. Second, the units can reproduce only a small number of occupations and some danger exists that the patients will be forced into a limited number of occupations because of the size limitations of such units. Third, to vocationally experienced and sophisticated patients such units do not represent the world of work and no amount of persuasion can convince them otherwise. Because of their lack of involvement such patients often perform minimally and unjustifiably they are classified as "poorly motivated" or they are given other such uncomplimentary designations. Conversely, many dependent patients perform well in protected atmospheres but disintegrate rather rapidly in competitive industrial jobs after discharge. Although many units have these shortcomings, and others as well, they can make a significant contribution to vocational planning when used in conjunction with other information. Although prevocational units were developed to aid in vocational diagnosis, in recent years there has been a noticeable trend to develop a more therapeutic atmosphere in order to provide services for a wide variety of residual behavior problems such as poor work habits, lack of consistency of production, inability to get along with others and lack of other work personality factors essential in employment. The changing emphasis from diagnosis to treatment will have considerable effect on the professional development and structure of such units and ultimately should make prevocational units an even more important tool in vocational rehabilitation.

Referral to a Prevocational Unit.   Prevocational units facilitate vocational rehabilitation rather than medical rehabilitation. If this statement can be accepted as being generally true, a possible source of ill will between the counselor and the physician can be removed. The problem arises at the time when the patient should be referred to the unit — a prerogative some physicians are unwilling to delegate without some reluctance. Physicians argue, with some validity, that the patient is their ultimate responsibility. Counselors state, with equal fervor, that it is hardly appropriate to delegate vocational responsibility to the counselor without granting responsible authority. Both disciplines are correct, since the physician does have an overall responsibility to the patient, and, on the other hand, it is a questionable procedure to expect a vocational counselor to produce results without considerable control over the process. Both sides should be able to agree that the vocational counselor has the responsibility to "prescribe" a prevocational program but that he should routinely discuss the use of the unit with the physician. Apart from the need for the physician to have a grasp of the patient's total program, the physician would then be in a position to assess the wisdom of the action from the point of view of the patient's physical capacities, and perhaps to contribute other ideas as well.

It is generally a poor policy for a physician, regardless of his level of sophistication, to write an order for a patient to engage in prevocational activities without consulting the counselor. Referrals to such a unit even with a prescription such as "evaluate physical capacities on a drill press" may provide a wealth of data on the client's standing tolerance, but at the same time suggest erroneously to the patient that this is a suitable occupation. Such thoughts are often more wrong than right and because of the patient's vulnerability to his physician's suggestions, they can be exceedingly difficult to dislodge.

THE PROCESS OF VOCATIONAL REHABILITATION

At the completion of the counselor's assembling of his diagnostic impressions and as discharge of the patient from the hospital nears, the counselor has three basic choices to make regarding additional vocational services. First, he can decide that referral to a separate vocational agency is not necessary and that the hospital counselor will provide all needed services. Usually, the core service required in these instances will be counseling or job placement or both. A significant factor in the decision to provide these services is the demand for his diagnostic skills within the hospital setting. Second, he can refer the patient to the state agency that provides vocational rehabilitation services. A referral to the state agency is often necessary since that agency has not only technical skills but also funds to pay for services such as skill training work adjustment services in a vocationally oriented rehabilitation center. Third, the counselor may decide that no hospital counseling services are necessary and that it is not even necessary to refer the patient to an outside agency. Such a plan can be dignified by classifying it as skillful neglect. It is not used very frequently, but it has originated because there are some patients who achieve more without any professional help. There are also patients who cannot use help effectively and only take up professional time better spent on other patients. Skillful neglect should not be the refuge of the ineffectual counselor but rather a decision reached only after careful consideration of the patient's problems and of his ability or inability to use professional services.

The types of services commonly used by vocational counselors are counseling services, training, referral to centers and workshops, referral to the state agency, job placement and follow-up.

Counseling Services

These services can be provided by the state agency or by the hospital counselor. Typically the counseling interviews involve issues such as the development of interest in employment, establishment of a vocational goal and the planning of a procedure for entering the labor market. Most vocational counselors are not concerned with a major restructuring of a patient's personality. Their aim, apart from the vocational planning element, is to provide a situation in which selected behavioral changes can take place. The counselor typically provides the patient with a great deal of information regarding his capacities, skills and interests, as well as about the labor market. Like the workers in other rehabilitation disciplines he tends to talk more of assets than liabilities. As a therapeutic technique, counseling is the most commonly used method.

Training

The use of training as a solution of a disabled person's employment problem has historically been seen as a panacea for unemployment. It has been justified as being necessary in order to give the disabled a competitive edge in obtaining employment. The use of this technique appears to be in decline because of the changing nature of the handicapped population. Instead of caring only for the mildly disabled, eager and bright young patient, rehabilitation, in an effort to expand its services, has encouraged the referral of a population group which is not nearly so trainable. In the place of the bright young patients, a steady stream of elderly, more severely disabled patients is entering the rehabilitation market possessed with alarming educational and personal deficits which often make training programs more difficult to attain than employment. As the technologic demands of our industrial society increase, many schools respond by increasing the complexity of the curriculum to the point where persons of average intelligence are considered mediocre training risks. In recent years the field of vocational education has made a considerable effort to develop training programs for the marginally unemployed. More effective institutional training programs, use of on-the-job training and various combinations of innovating services may, in the future, open up new training opportunities for the disabled. When the opportunities for skill training decline, counselors often find themselves hard pressed to discover assets that are salable in a competitive labor market and they often use other techniques to attack the problem of employment.

Referral to Vocationally Oriented Centers and Sheltered Workshops

A number of patients discharged from hospitals will need additional vocational services beyond those provided by a counselor or an educational training program. These patients usually have one or more of the following three kinds of residual problems necessitating more extensive vocational services.

Vocational Evaluation Problems.   In these instances the counselor has difficulty in establishing a vocational objective. Some of the reasons for this difficulty are a severe disability (such as cerebral palsy, mental retardation, mental illness or quadriplegia) or such problems as old age or limited education. The essential problem, from the counselor's standpoint, is that he cannot develop an appropriate vocational goal using traditional counseling techniques. Such patients are usually referred to a vocationally oriented facility which is able to simulate a large number of occupations and thereby facilitate an appropriate vocational choice.

Multiple Treatment Problem.   The referral of these patients is usually prompted by the counselor's perception that the patient has problems in addition to his medical and vocational problems that interfere with his vocational rehabilitation. They are usually in the psychologic and social areas. Furthermore, these problems must be treated in a coordinated fashion since the patient is not able to profit from discrete services provided by several different agencies. Referrals of this type further suggest that vocational counseling alone will not be sufficient to enable the client to return to the labor market. Agencies providing such services must have comprehensive staffing patterns to produce results.

Behavioral Problems.   Many patients who are discharged from medical centers have residual behavior problems which cannot be ameliorated through counseling techniques. The problems may be concerned with such things as poor work habits (getting to work late, failure to obey shop rules, inconsistency of production, or verbal statements on the part of the patient that he cannot work. Well staffed vocational centers and sheltered workshops are surprisingly effective in the treatment of these types of problems and others as well.

The last few years have seen a substantial growth of rehabilitation centers and facilities whose purpose is not physical restoration but vocational rehabilitation. These centers recognize that the physical disability is only one problem in a person's vocational rehabilitation and that a single professional service is often not sufficient to deal with a problem as complex as that of achieving employment. Unfortunately, although these centers are theoretically of great value, they often are understaffed and do not always consistently provide the services that they claim.

Referral to the State Agency

The primary source of vocational services in most states is the State Division or Department of Vocational Rehabilitation. This state agency, through the use of federal and state funds, provides a wide variety of services to the physically, emotionally and mentally disabled. The services are usually provided through a vocational counselor and cover such areas as physical restoration, vocational counseling, vocational or professional training, job placement, and tools, licenses and equipment for self-employment. Some services are provided directly by the state agency while others are purchased from private resources. Patients receiving services must have a vocational handicap resulting from the disability (eligibility) and the counselor must feel he can provide services which have a reasonable chance of assisting the patient to obtain employment (feasibility).

Because many patients need these services, the state agency counselor should become an integral part of the hospital rehabilitation team. Some medical treatment centers have found it helpful to have a state agency counselor assigned to the hospital for liaison purposes. This enables the counselor to become personally acquainted with hospital personnel and policies, and it facilitates referrals.

Certain aspects of the program of the state agency can be a potential source of conflict with hospital personnel. The central problem will often involve the question of feasibility. It is not uncommon for hospital personnel to become involved in the rehabilitation of a severely disabled person (a quadriplegic, for example) only to find the state agency counselor somewhat reluctant to accept the patient for services because he considers the patient a poor candidate for employment. The state counselor may feel that the expectations of the hospital staff are unrealistic because in their isolated existence the members of the hospital staff do not understand the demands of the labor market. On the other hand the hospital staff may sometimes feel that the state counselor lacks skills, resourcefulness and energy. The hospital counselor is often caught in the middle; he owes allegiance both to the hospital and to his professional colleague who he knows has to produce a number of "closures" each year to satisfy administrative requirements. Frequently the state agency counselor will have a long list of clients waiting for services whose chances of rehabilitation are much more promising than those of a wheelchair-bound quadriplegic. Such conflicts are not always easy to resolve but basically each resource must be able to accept and understand the other's point of view and service limitations. The state agencies have, over a period of several years, gradually modified their feasibility requirements until now they seem to feel that to fail in rehabilitation is less of a problem than not to have tried at all. As society changes its conception of the duties of the state agency, the justification for rehabilitation may be based more on humanitarian objectives than economic ones. If this occurs it is to be hoped that the philosophic disagreements between referring agencies and the state agency will disappear.

Job Placement

Employment is the culmination of a series of very complex and expensive services and deserves some attention. A number of counselors look upon job placement activities as an undesirable part of their duties. In these instances, it is seen as an accepted function, often necessary, but unpleasant. Some counselors seem to thrive on the fast-moving give and take of employer contacts, but many seem to find it difficult to leave the comfortable surroundings of their offices and the companionship of professional colleagues to wander like missionaries among industrial personnel. Their glibness, so noticeable in team meetings, dissolves in the presence of the indifferent glances of the personnel manager. The counselor's fears are not groundless. Employer contacts are anxiety-producing and difficult. They require personal stamina and toughness not found in many counselors. Some counselors prefer to place maximal responsibility on the patient to obtain a job. These patients, in the inevitable process of changing jobs, will often be able to find a second job without returning to a public agency. However, some patients simply cannot find their own jobs. In these instances the counselor should be expected to take an aggressive role in job finding.

The striking changes undergone by state-affiliated programs of the Department of Labor's Manpower Administration are a major force influencing the employment of the disabled. The past few years have seen a dramatic change in the operations of state employment agencies. Historically, the services were focused on meeting the needs of employers and the system's core program involved providing a matching service between the unemployed and community job openings. However, spurred by recent legislation, the employment service is now the nation's major source of employability development programs for the severely unemployed. With the exception of not being able to purchase comprehensive physical restoration programs, the employment service can arrange or directly provide virtually any service which can develop the employability of severely unemployed persons. It is probable that within the next few years increasing numbers of physically disabled will enter the employment service system. As their skills improve in serving this type of population it is hoped that hospitals will find them to be an effective ally in enabling larger numbers of the disabled to enter the competitive labor market.

The state rehabilitation agency also offers placement services to the handicapped, but the problem of counselor resistance and the large caseloads of most of these counselors make it difficult to provide concentrated placement services to a single person.

Job placement services are a necessary ingredient in the process of vocational rehabilitation. Unfortunately, the professional community has found it difficult to program such services to the point that the marginally employable can always be guaranteed an opportunity to demonstrate their productivity.

SUMMARY

Vocational counselors represent the newest addition to the hospital rehabilitation team. Their presence reflects the realization that the complexities of a patient's employment problem require additional specialized help. The counselor's role is not an easy one to perform. Not only must he develop his program in a service which is essentially medical, but he must also be able to assist his patient into community life which lacks a climate of acceptance equal to that of his professional colleagues. The newness of his profession, with the resulting deficiencies in skills, contributes to the difficulty of his task. His ability to perform suitable services will in large measure be the result of the team's willingness to provide an atmosphere in which he can function to his maximum so that the disabled will have the opportunity to avail themselves of vocational rehabilitation services.

REFERENCES

1. Borow, H.: Man in a World at Work. Boston, Houghton Mifflin Company, 1964.
2. Cronbach, L.: Essentials of Psychological Testing. 2nd Ed. New York, Harper and Brothers, 1960.
3. Hochhauser, E.: Objectives of Sheltered Workshops. The Jewish Social Service Quarterly, 25:533–545, 1949.
4. McGowan, J. F., and Schmidt, L. D.: Counseling: Readings in Theory and Practice. New York, Holt, Rinehart and Winston, 1962.
5. McGowan, J. F., and Porter, T. L.: An Introduction to the Vocational Rehabilitation Process. U.S. Government Printing Office, 1967.

6. Lofquist, L. H.: Vocational Counseling with the Physically Handicapped. New York, Appleton-Century-Crofts, 1957.
7. Nyquist, R. H., Manson, M. P., and Romiti, A. S.: Vocational Counseling Services within a Physical Medicine Program of Total Rehabilitation. Amer. J. Phys. Med., 31:393–399, 1952.
8. Patterson, C. H.: Counseling and Psychotherapy: Theory and Practice. New York, Harper and Brothers, 1959.
9. Roe, A.: The Psychology of Occupations. New York, John Wiley and Sons, Inc., 1956.
10. Super, D. E.: The Psychology of Careers. New York, Harper and Brothers, 1957.
11. Sheppard, H. L., and Belitsky, A. H.: The Job Hunt. Baltimore, Maryland, The Johns Hopkins Press, 1966.
12. Thomason, B., and Barnett, A. M.: The Placement Process in Vocational Rehabilitation Counseling. GTP. Bulletin No. 2, Rehabilitation Service Series, No. 545, September, 1960.
13. Tyler, L. E.: The Work of the Counselor. 2nd. Ed. New York, Appleton-Century-Crofts, 1961.
14. Usdane, W. M.: Vocational Counseling with the Severely Handicapped. Arch. Phys. Med., 34:607–616, 1953.
15. Vroom, V. H.: Work and Motivation. New York, John Wiley and Sons, 1964.
16. Zytowski, D. G.: Vocational Behavior. New York, Holt, Rinehart and Winston, Inc., 1968.

Chapter 9

ELECTRODIAGNOSIS

by Ernest W. Johnson

ELECTROMYOGRAPHY AND NERVE STIMULATION TECHNIQUES

Neurophysiology

Electrodiagnostic techniques are dependent on the activation and display of the electrical activity of the motor unit. This is the physiologic unit of the nervous system comprised of the anterior horn cell, its axon and terminal branchings and all the muscle fibers which it innervates. The number of muscle fibers per motor unit varies from a few in an extrinsic eye muscle to several hundred or more in a large limb muscle.

The motor unit is activated in an all or none manner, the activation consisting of an electrical disturbance passing from the anterior horn cell, down the axon and its twigs to the myoneural junctions where the liberation of a chemical mediator initiates a wave of excitation along each muscle fiber. The muscle fiber contraction occurs approximately 1 millisecond after the action potential. The summated muscle fiber action potentials represent the motor unit action potential and thus, the electrical activity displayed by the electromyograph.

Each motor neuron, that is, the cell body and axon, has a threshold of stimulation; the reciprocal of this threshold is its excitability. The speed with which the wave of excitation passes down the axon is its impulse propagation rate or conduction velocity. This velocity varies almost directly with the diameter of the axon and is influenced favorably by the presence of a myelin sheath. The fastest conducting nerve fibers in humans are the "A" fibers, the large myelinated motor fibers to skeletal muscle. Their conduction velocity varies from 45 to 90 meters per second in adults. The thresholds of various "A" fibers

222

in a motor nerve vary; therefore in clinical application one must insure a supramaximal stimulus to activate all the axons to a particular muscle.

The action potential of a muscle fiber, examined in detail, represents a change from a potential of 100 millivolts positive to a potential of 15 millivolts negative outside the cell membrane. Recovery to the resting states proceeds immediately following the wave of excitation. The short delay immediately prior to this recovery is termed the refractory period. The first 0.2 millisecond of this delay is termed the absolute refractory period because no stimulus, no matter how intense, will excite the cell. A longer period following this is the relative refractory period since a stronger stimulus than normal is necessary to cause excitation.

If an exploring electrode is placed in the vicinity of the cell membrane undergoing change in polarization, the resultant electrical disturbance can be picked up, amplified and displayed by the electromyograph.

Since living tissue is dispersed in three dimensions, electrical activity is dispersed in three dimensions also. We speak of tissue as a volume conductor; thus the resultant wave form will depend on the location of the electrode tip with respect to the wave of excitation (Fig. 9-1). It is possible for the action potentials to be monophasic, biphasic or triphasic depending on this relationship. The structural distribution of the muscle fibers of one particular motor unit within the muscle as a whole makes more complex the shape of the action potential. Usually the motor unit action potentials are diphasic or triphasic with fewer than 10 per cent polyphasic in normal individuals.

The excitation disturbance sweeps along the cell membrane of the muscle at 4 to 5 meters per second. Electrical characteristics of the tissue as well as those of the electromyograph influence the amplitude, duration and shape of the displayed action potentials.

Instrumentation

The basic components for electromyography and nerve stimulation include a set of electrodes, a pre-amplifier, an audio-amplifier and a loudspeaker, an oscilloscope and a physiologic stimulator (Fig. 9-2). Provisions for storing the displayed electrical activity include a magnetic tape recorder and a camera.

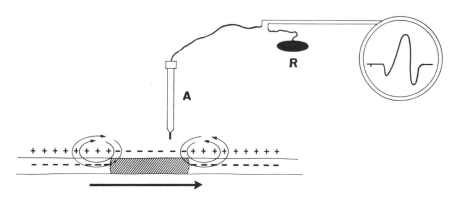

WAVE OF EXCITATION PASSING ALONG A MUSCLE FIBER

Figure 9-1   Diagram of the activation of a muscle fiber with the exploring electrode (A) in proximity. Note that tissue is a volume conductor; therefore the shape of the visualized potential will depend on the relationship of the electrode tip to the electrical disturbance.

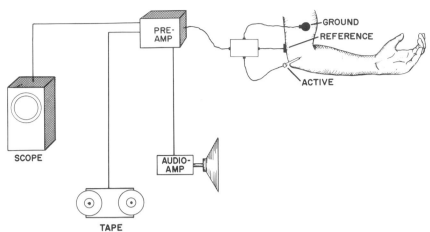

Figure 9–2   Schematic representation of an electromyograph. The reference electrode should be placed on the skin near the exploring or active electrode (monopolar).

Electrodes.   SURFACE.   These vary from 0.5 to several centimeters in diameter. They are useful for kinesiologic electromyographic studies and also for recording the muscle action potential during nerve stimulation techniques. One, the active electrode, is placed over the middle of the muscle and another, the reference electrode, over the tendon.

MONOPOLAR.   These are sharpened pieces of stainless steel wire coated, except for a fraction of a millimeter at the tip, with insulating material such as Tygon or Teflon (Figs. 9-3 and 9-4). A surface electrode on the skin over the muscle is necessary as a reference electrode.

COAXIAL.   This is a hollow needle with a wire, insulated except at the tip, in the barrel to act as the exploring or active electrode. The barrel serves as the reference electrode. This electrode has a sharp beveled tip and thus is less painful to insert through the skin than the monopolar needle (Fig. 9-3). There is some reduction in amplitude of the motor unit action potentials with the coaxial electrode and it responds to a smaller sphere of influence, which is directional as related to the bevel.

All of the above electrodes require a ground electrode placed centrally to the muscle examined. Contact between skin and surface electrodes is enhanced by electrolytic paste, sparingly used.

BIPOLAR.   Two insulated wires are inserted in a hypodermic needle to serve as active and reference electrodes and the barrel serves as a ground (Fig. 9-3). Bipolar electrodes permit very restricted areas to be investigated.

Pre-amplifier.   The pre-amplifier should have a uniform response for frequencies from 16 to 16,000 cycles per second with an input impedance of several megohms. It should be a differential or "push-pull" amplifier so that the "common mode" signal will be rejected. The rejection ratio of the common mode signal should be at least 100,000:1 for use in general hospital surroundings. Provision should be made for stepwise adjustment of the gain and for the optional insertion of high and low frequency filters. These filters may appreciably distort the displayed electrical activity.

Some commercially available electromyographs have features which eliminate or minimize certain interference, for example, a narrow band elimination filter for 60 cycles, and a filter at the input to remove radio frequency interference.

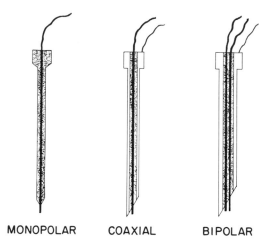

Figure 9–3 Three types of E.M.G. electrodes.

MONOPOLAR COAXIAL BIPOLAR

TYPES OF ELECTRODES

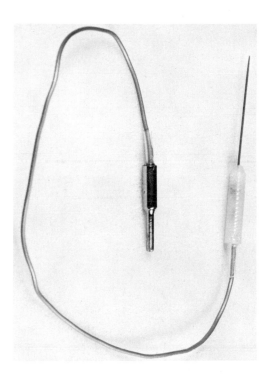

Figure 9–4 Closeup view of a monopolar E.M.G. electrode, coated with Teflon and with a nylon handle.

Oscilloscope. The oscilloscope provides a visual display of the electrical signal so that the amplitude, duration and shape of the potentials can be observed. Sweep speeds used for electromyography vary from 5 to 10 milliseconds per centimeter. For determination of motor and sensory nerve conduction velocities sweep speeds should range from 2 to 30 milliseconds per centimeter.

Stimulator. The physiologic stimulator should have sufficient output to insure a supramaximal stimulus under all clinical conditions. Stepwise and vernier adjustments for intensity and duration of stimulating voltage as well as step adjustments for frequency and delay of the stimulus are necessary. The stimulating electrodes are usually bipolar with the cathode placed distally; however, a monopolar electrode, with either a needle or surface electrode placed over the nerve and with the large indifferent plate electrode placed over another part of the body, may be used. The stimulator must be isolated from ground with an isolation transformer. The stimulator triggers the sweep for nerve conduction velocity measurements and may be coupled to a one or two kilocycle oscillator so that the time base is "locked" to the start of the sweep.

Time Base.   Crosshatching on the oscilloscope face corresponding with the known sweep speed will usually give a satisfactory time base for clinical nerve conduction velocities. It may be desirable to make the time base independent of the sweep speed by introducing a one or two kilocycle signal on a second oscillographic channel or superimposing the oscillator signal on the tracing.

Intramuscular Thermometer.   Since changes in temperature may alter the conduction velocity, it is helpful to have a needle thermistor to indicate the temperature of the tissue. The thermistor is inserted in the muscle near the middle third of the peripheral nerve being investigated. Several studies suggest that a drop in temperature of 1° C. may reduce the conduction velocity 5 per cent.

Precautions.   It is important to take the following precautions: Clean the skin thoroughly. Place electrodes securely. Use electrode jelly sparingly. Use firm pressure on stimulating electrodes. To insure supramaximal stimulus, increase the stimulus intensity by at least 30 per cent after the "M" response amplitude no longer increases. If peak stimulation voltage has been reached, double the duration of stimulus.

The Normal Electromyogram

Figure 9-5 shows an electromyographic examination in progress. The patient should be recumbent and comfortable, and the procedure should be thoroughly explained before starting. A brief history and a short but systematic neurologic examination is absolutely necessary to plan the electromyogram.

First the needle electrode is inserted and the patient is asked to contract the desired muscle to insure that the electrode is in the proper muscle. Adequate exploration of each muscle examined may require 5 to 10 needle advancements at several locations in the muscle.

There are five steps to the electromyographic examination. Sweep speeds vary from 5 to 10 milliseconds per centimeter, the faster sweeps for detailed examination of the individual action potentials. The gain is usually 50 microvolts per centimeter, except during maximal contraction when it is 200 to 500 microvolts per centimeter.

Muscle at Rest.   When normal muscle at rest is examined, there is electrical silence (Fig. 9-6).

Insertional Activity.   When the needle is moved briskly, a burst of electrical activity occurs which stops abruptly when the movement stops. The duration of this burst is dependent somewhat on the character of the needle

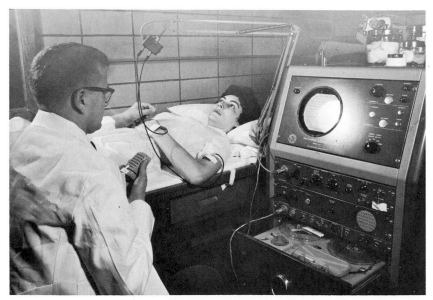

Figure 9–5   Electromyograph with examiner dictating notes while recording motor unit action potentials from the first dorsal interosseous muscle in the hand.

insertion but is usually 10 to 30 milliseconds in duration. This results from the activation of muscle fibers with the mechanical stimulus of electrode movement. The absence of insertional activity indicates that there are no functioning muscle fibers or that the electrode is not in muscle tissue.

If the tip of the needle is in the vicinity of motor end plates, a sputtering burst of electrical activity occurs on the background of a high frequency, low amplitude electrical disturbance which has been likened to a sea shell murmur. These potentials are diphasic with amplitudes of 50 to 200 microvolts and duration of 1 to 2 milliseconds. The initial phase is negative and the rhythm of firing is irregular. Their clinical significance is, first, that functioning end plates are present, and second, that these potentials may be confused with fibrillation potentials since they are of similar amplitude and duration. The initial phase of the fibrillation potential is positive, however and the rhythm of firing is regular.

The patient usually complains of pain as end plate potentials are elicited (Fig. 9-7). These potentials are more likely to be encountered in the middle third of the muscle and particularly in the small muscles of the hands and feet.

Minimal Muscle Contraction.   A single motor unit action potential is elicited by asking the patient to just think of contracting the desired muscle and

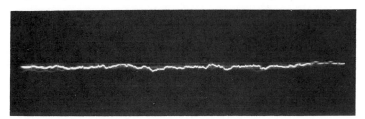

Figure 9–6   Normal muscle at rest. Note that there is no electrical activity.

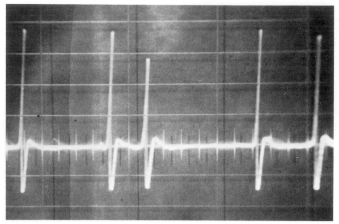

Figure 9–7   Calibration: 30 milliseconds per major horizontal division; 100 microvolts per vertical division. Negativity indicated by upward deflection.

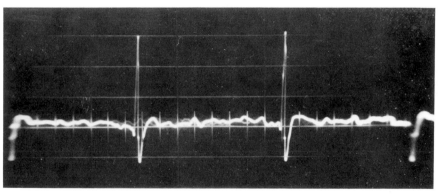

Figure 9–8   Minimal contraction. Calibration: 6 milliseconds per horizontal division; 100 microvolts per vertical division. Negative polarity is upward deflection.

then carefully moving the needle electrode as close to the firing unit as possible. The sound becomes louder and amplitude increases as the tip of the exploring electrode nears the activated motor unit (Fig. 9-8).

It is important to observe the amplitude (usually 200 to 2000 microvolts), the duration (4 to 12 milliseconds), the wave forms (most are diphasic or triphasic), the number of motor units recruited as compared to the strength of contraction and the rhythm and frequency of firing (voluntary motor units begin firing at five per second).

Maximal Muscle Contraction.   To demonstrate maximal muscle contraction the patient is asked to control the muscle against maximal resistance by the examiner. Placing the needle electrode superficially will reduce the discomfort.

The *interference pattern* is normal when the face of the oscilloscope is blotted out with motor unit action potentials. It is estimated that there are five to six motor units in the vicinity of the exploring electrode and contributing to the interference pattern.

Normal motor units begin activating at five per second and increase their rate of firing with increasing force of contraction effort. Simultaneously additional motor units are recruited. Maximal rates of firing are from 30 to 50 per second. *The patient's contraction effort is estimated from the rate of firing.*

The amplitude is 200 to 2000 microvolts. Sound is more important in determining the duration. Fine crackling sounds indicate shorter duration; thuds suggest increased duration. The number of action potentials should be compared to strength of contraction.

Distribution of Abnormality.   If abnormal potentials are observed, it is necessary to identify the anatomic distribution of the abnormality. Is it a branch of a nerve, a peripheral nerve, a portion of a plexus, a root or cord segment, or is it diffuse?

Children and Electromyograms.   Always separate children from their parents. Explain the procedure to all above the age of four. Often a few words such as "you're going to see your muscles on television" will put the youngster at ease. Always refer to the electrode as a pin or mosquito bite. Avoid showing the needle electrode if possible and use the smallest possible diameters ($\frac{1}{2}$ to $\frac{3}{4}$ inch in length). The needle electrode (pin) should be inserted concomitantly with a slap or pinch on the thigh or arm, particularly if the room is semidarkened.

Careful physical examination and planning are necessary to insure that the minimal number of muscles are examined to make a proper diagnosis.

Anesthesia is rarely necessary, but for children under the age of four, the electromyographer will need assistance to immobilize the child.

Obtaining muscle relaxation is the difficult part of the examination, but it may be done by forcibly positioning the muscle at its shortest length. For example, to investigate the anterior tibial muscle in an uncooperative child, the foot should be dorsiflexed as much as possible.

Caution.   *It is imperative that the electromyogram be performed by a physician since a neurologic history and examination is necessary to plan the electromyogram; the plan must usually be modified as the electromyographic findings unfold; the displayed electrical activity depends on the actions of the electromyographer at a particular moment as well as on the location of the electrode and therefore taping of the electromyogram by a technician for later interpretation by the physician is unsatisfactory; the E.M.G. findings can then be interpreted in the light or orderliness of the history and neurologic examination.*

Normal Motor Nerve Stimulation

Almost any nerve that has motor fibers and is placed superficially along a portion of its course can be stimulated with a surface electrode on, or a needle electrode in, distal muscles. A reference electrode is placed over the tendon and the ground electrode is placed between the active and stimulating electrodes (Fig. 9-9).

The conduction velocity is determined by stimulating a motor nerve supramaximally at two points along its course and photographing or observing the delay between the stimulation artifact and the muscle action potential. The distance between the points of stimulation is measured on the skin and divided by the conduction latency between the points of stimulation. Results are expressed as meters per second (Fig. 9-10). Figures 9-11 through 9-18 show sample records of conduction velocities.

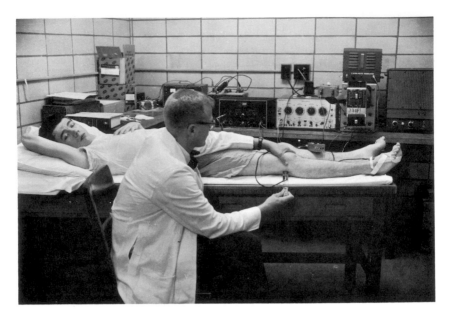

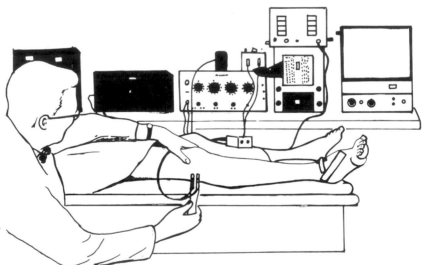

Figure 9–9 Assembled components for motor nerve conduction velocity determination. From left to right: pre-amplifier, stimulator, oscilloscope with camera attached in front and timing fork oscillator on top, audio-amplifier and loud speaker. Note the bipolar stimulating electrodes over the fibular head, the active electrode over the extensor digitorum brevis, the reference electrode on the little toe and the ground electrode on the dorsum of the ankle.

If a peripheral motor nerve is stimulated at its most distal point, that is, where it enters the muscle, there is a conduction delay of several milliseconds. This latency represents the delay at the myoneural junction (0.5 millisecond) and the prolonged conductivity along the terminal axon twigs which are small in diameter and unmyelinated at their endings. This delay is referred to as the terminal conduction delay. The difference between this delay and the expected delay, i.e., calculated from the observed velocity along the more proximal nerve trunk (which is shorter), is referred to as residual latency.

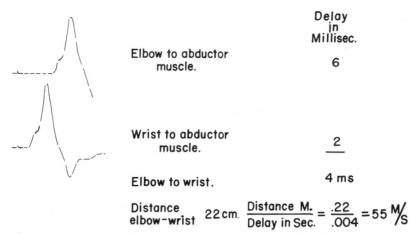

	Delay in Millisec.
Elbow to abductor muscle.	6
Wrist to abductor muscle.	2
Elbow to wrist.	4 ms

Distance elbow-wrist 22 cm. $\dfrac{\text{Distance M.}}{\text{Delay in Sec.}} = \dfrac{.22}{.004} = 55 \text{ M/s}$

Figure 9–10   Sample of calculation of the conduction velocity of the ulnar nerve.

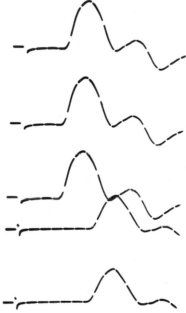

Figure 9–11   Record of the conduction velocity of median nerve (56 m/s) with assembled components. Stimulus artifact is to the left of the trace after 1 millisecond delay. Time base is 1 millisecond intervals. The top three traces are stimulations at the wrist and the bottom two are at the elbow. Note the normal delay in the median nerve at the wrist (less than 5 m/s).

There is no clinically significant difference in the conduction velocity between the segments from axilla to elbow, and from elbow to wrist. A measurement error of 1 centimeter will result in errors of 1 part in 25, or 4 per cent in the adult arm. Inspection of photographs or determination of the conduction latency permits an accuracy of at best 1 part in 20 if one uses 0.5 millisecond as the time base and a latency of 10 milliseconds.

(Text continued on page 236)

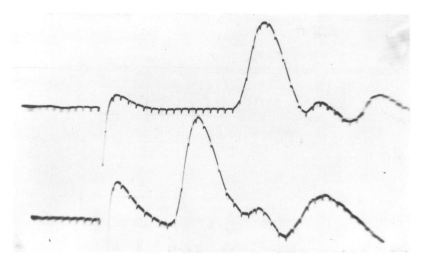

Figure 9–12 Record of peroneal nerve conduction velocity (48 m/s) with the TECA electro-myograph. Time base is 0.5 millisecond intervals.

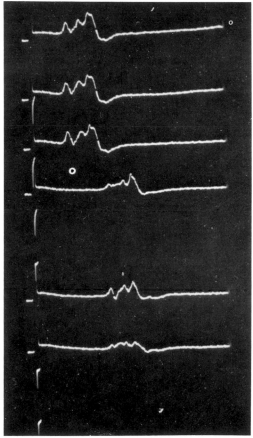

Figure 9–13 Actual photograph of peroneal nerve conduction velocity in patient with muscular dystrophy (58 m/s). Note the ragged and low amplitude "M" response, although the velocity is normal.

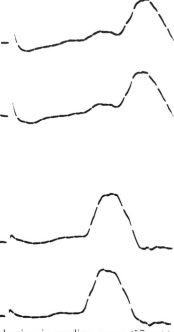

Figure 9–14   Normal conduction in median nerve (57 m/s) but prolonged (9 milliseconds) delay at the wrist in a patient with carpal tunnel syndrome.

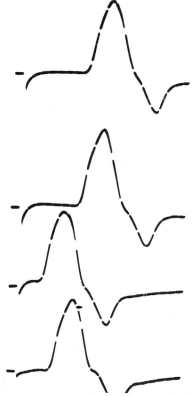

Figure 9–15   Neuroma of the ulnar nerve in the proximal wrist. The top trace is stimulation above the elbow; the next is stimulation below the elbow; the next is stimulation distal to the neuroma at the wrist; the bottom trace is stimulation at the wrist proximal to the neuroma. Note the 4 millisecond (prolonged) delay proximal to the neuroma. The conduction velocity calculated to the distal wrist is 42 m/s. The conduction velocity calculated to the proximal wrist is 60 m/s.   **233**

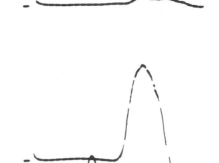

Figure 9–16 Block of the peroneal nerve at the fibular head in a patient with "crossed leg palsy." The top trace is stimulation above the fibular head; the middle trace is stimulation below the fibular head; the bottom trace is stimulation at the ankle. Note the temporal dispersion and reduced amplitude of the "M" response when the peroneal nerve is stimulated above the fibular head. The time base is 1 millisecond intervals. The stimulus artifact is to the left, the "M" response is to the right.

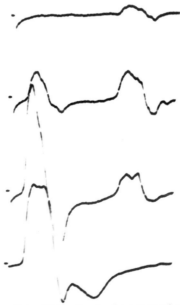

Figure 9–17 Demonstration of the "H" reflex in the peroneal nerve and recording over the anterior tibial muscle in a multiple sclerosis patient. The trace is interrupted at 1 millisecond intervals. In the top trace the reflex "H" response is to the right; the next shows the "M" response and "H" response as stimulation voltage is increased; in the next the "H" response has almost disappeared as stimulation voltage was increased; the bottom trace shows only the "M" response with supramaximal stimulus.

234

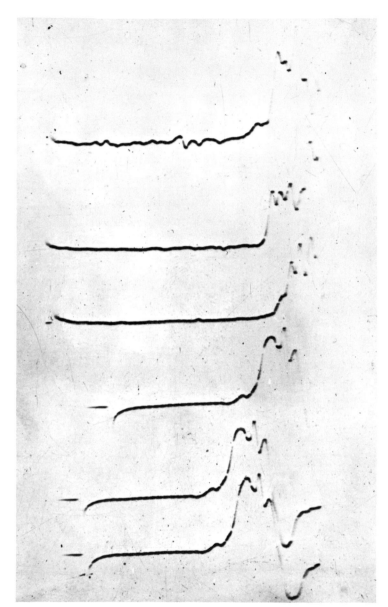

Figure 9–18 Marked slowing of conduction velocity of the peroneal nerve in a 6 month old child with idiopathic polyneuritis (1 m/s). The trace is interrupted at 1 millisecond intervals. Note the ragged and temporarily dispersed "M" response particularly when the nerve is stimulated proximally.

Surface electrodes permit comparisons of the amplitude of the "M" response to be made between different locations of stimulations along the nerve and repetitive stimulations at one site. The hand or foot should be firmly immobilized when attempting repetitive stimulations. However, surface electrodes may not isolate the proper muscle response.

Needle electrodes move when the muscle contracts and thus cannot be used to compare amplitudes. They do, however, isolate the response more precisely.

"M" response varies from 5 to 20 millivolts in normal subjects when recorded with surface electrodes.

"H" Reflex.   If the tibial nerve is stimulated with a low voltage (10 to 20 volts) and active reference electrodes are placed over the gastrocnemius, a muscle action potential may be observed after a latency of 30 to 40 milliseconds, a delay presumably necessary for the afferent and then the efferent limbs of the two neuron muscle stretch reflex arcs to conduct the impulse. The "H" reflex is facilitated by placing the cathode of the stimulating electrodes proximally rather than distally and a rate of 1 per 2 to 3 seconds. It may also be demonstrated in the femoral nerve and in any peripheral nerve of infants under one year of age.

If found in relaxed muscles of human adults by stimulating the median, ulnar or peroneal nerves, the "H" reflex may indicate upper motor neuron disease or injury below the midbrain. However, it has been demonstrated in apparently normal adults by having the individuals contract the muscle slightly, a maneuver that results in facilitation of the muscle stretch reflex. The "H" reflex was named after Hoffmann, who first described it (Fig. 9–17).

	Sites of Stimulation			Conduction Velocity	Terminal Conduction Delay
Nerve	Proximal	Distal	Pick Up	M/Sec.	ms.
Ulnar	Posterior elbow or axilla	Wrist (Lateral to flexor carpi ulnaris tendon)	Abductor digiti quinti	45–70	2–4
Median	Antecubital area or axilla	Between tendons of palmaris long-us and flexor carpi radialis	Opponens	45–70	3–5
Deep Peroneal	Knee Fibular head or sciatic notch	Ankle (Anterior lateral aspect)	Extensor* Digitorum brevis	40–65	3–5
Tibial	Lateral popliteal area or sciatic notch	Posterior to medial malleolus	Abductor digiti quinti pedis	40–65	4–6
Facial		Under ear lobe	Frontalis	—	4
Radial	Spiral groove	Lateral antecubital space	Extensor indicis proprius	50–70	—
Femoral	Proximal and distal to inquinal ligament	Vastus medialis		—	6–8

*In 20 per cent of individuals an anomalous branch separates from the peroneal nerve and courses below the lateral malleolus to the extensor digitorum brevis.

Effect of Age on Motor Nerve Conduction Velocity.   At birth, the conduction velocity in the motor fibers of the ulnar nerve averages 28 meters per second. By age two to three it reaches low adult values and by age four or five it averages adult values.

In premature infants the conduction velocity correlates well with the weight and may serve as an index of the degree of prematurity. In a group of premature infants of approximately eight months gestation, the conduction velocity in the peroneal nerve averaged 19 meters per second.[4]

The conduction velocity of motor nerves in adults beyond the fifth decade is gradually reduced up to 10 per cent per decade, perhaps as result of metabolic or circulatory disturbances.

Effect of Changes in Temperature.   Reduced temperature in an extremity may result in lowered conduction velocities. Estimates for this in the conduction velocity, varying from 1.8 to 4 meters per second per degree Centigrade, should precede clinical interpretation of a reduced velocity. Increase in the temperature of the body can raise the conduction velocity in motor nerves in a similar manner.

Pathophysiology

The lower motor neuron (anterior horn cell and its axon) responds in three ways to an insult.

Wallerian Degeneration.   If it is injured or diseased severely, the entire neuron (if it is anterior horn cell) or the axon distal to the injury undergoes wallerian degeneration. This is, first, a dissolution of the myelin sheath and then a disintegration of the axis cylinder. This process ordinarily takes 18 to 21 days in human axons. When the degeneration is complete, the electromyogram shows fibrillation potentials.

Injured axons that will undergo wallerian degeneration are excitable and will conduct distal to the injury for about 72 hours, after which time they are no longer excitable.

Neurapraxia.   A segment of an axon or an anterior horn cell may temporarily lose its excitability and yet not undergo wallerian degeneration. In this situation, stimulation proximal to the site of compromise will not result in muscle contraction (assuming that all fibers are neurapraxic), but stimulation distal to the compromise will cause contraction (Erb's paradoxical palsy). This is called neurapraxia. If not all of the axons in a motor nerve are neurapraxic, then stimulation proximal to the injury will result in a smaller "M" response than distal stimulation (Figs. 9–15 and 9–16).

Axonstenosis or Axonocachexia.   If a localized compromise is prolonged or more severe, the axon may retain its excitability, but at a reduced level. This may necessitate an increased intensity of stimulus for excitation and it also results in reduced conductivity across the involved segment. This is termed axonstenosis. Altered excitability and conductivity extending throughout the entire distal axon is called axonocachexia. If some of the axons are normal, the amplitude of the "M" response will be roughly proportional to those when stimulating proximal to a segment of axonstenosis. Axonocachexia will result in temporal dispersion of the "M" response as the axons conduct at different velocities proportional to their altered physiology.

Combinations of all three may exist with coexistent electromyographic and nerve stimulation abnormalities.

Abnormal Potentials in Electromyography

Fibrillation Potentials.   The amplitude of fibrillation potentials is 50 to 300 microvolts; the duration 0.5 to 2 milliseconds with a regular rhythm and a frequency of 2 to 10 per second (Fig. 9-19). They are usually diphasic or triphasic, with the initial phase positive. Their sound resembles that of eggs frying or cellophane paper being crumpled. This is the electrical activity associated with a single muscle fiber, presumably activated by mechanical or chemical stimuli when the muscle fiber is denervated, "sick" or injured. Single muscle fiber contractions are not visible grossly through intact skin or mucous membrane. Their appearance is enhanced by heat, cholinergic drugs and mechanical stimulation.

Fasciculation Potentials.   The amplitude and duration of fasciculation potentials vary. They may be simple or polyphasic. Fasciculation potentials are identified by the *irregular* rhythm and a rate of firing less than 3 or 4 per second. These may be visible through intact mucous membrane or skin. They represent spontaneous discharges of part or all of a motor unit. They are thought to originate in the peripheral part of the motor unit, probably at the myoneural junction (Fig. 9-20). These discharges may be simple or complex in shape. Complex fasciculation potentials include the polyphasic type as well as grouped or iterative discharges.

Iterative or grouped discharge fasciculation potentials result when the excitability of the motor unit is heightened so that the relative refractory period is shortened, permitting repetitive activation. Thus the motor unit may fire two or three or more times (Fig. 9-21).

Polyphasic Potentials.   Polyphasic potentials are usually motor unit action potentials having more than four phases (i.e., crossing the isoelectric line more

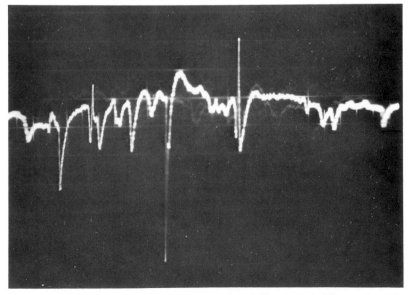

Figure 9–19   Positive waves and fibrillation potentials. Calibration: 6 milliseconds per horizontal division; 50 microvolts per vertical division. Negative polarity is indicated by upward deflection.

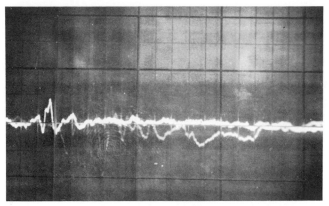

Figure 9–20 A fasciculation potential. Calibration is 1000 microvolts per major vertical division and 30 milliseconds per major horizontal division.

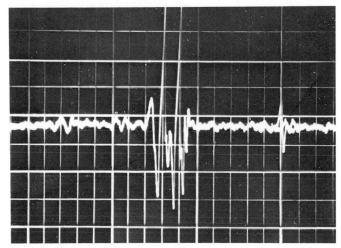

Figure 9–21 Repetitive or iterative potential. Calibration: 6 milliseconds per horizontal division, 100 microvolts per vertical division.

than three times) (Fig. 9–22). Fewer than 10 per cent of motor unit action potentials in normal individuals are polyphasic. Motor units with heightened excitability may fire repetitively and result in a polyphasic potential.

Possible origins of these potentials are differences in conduction times over the terminal axon branches; synchronous but not simultaneou firing of multiple motor units; repetitive discharge of part or all of a motor unit; or loss of some muscle fibers in a motor unit so that the anatomic dispersion of the remaining fibers does not permit smooth summation.

A special type of polyphasic potential is the previously mentioned repetitive discharge or iterative potential.

Positive Waves. Positive waves are potentials having a sharp positive deflection associated with a long-duration negative phase. They occur when one or a group of "sick" muscle fibers are activated by the tip of the exploring electrode, when the tip is in the injured or diseased area of the muscle fiber with the depolarization wave moving away from the electrode tip. These are induced by mechanical stimulation, either by tapping the muscle in the vicinity

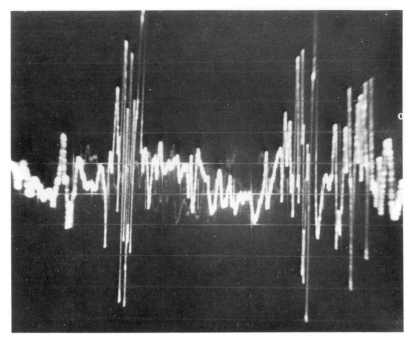

Figure 9–22   Polyphasic fasciculation potentials recorded from patient with amyotrophic lateral sclerosis. Calibration: 6 milliseconds per horizontal division; 100 microvolts per vertical division. Note the raggedness and complexity.

of the needle or advancing the needles abruptly. They are abnormal only if they persist after the electrode movement stops.

The amplitude and duration vary considerably, as does the frequency. These potentials may appear as trains of discharges at the rate of 50 to 100 per second.

Giant Potentials.   Giant potentials are voluntary motor unit action potentials of 10 millivolts in amplitude or greater and 12 to 15 milliseconds in duration (Fig. 9-23). They are frequently seen in anterior horn cell disease such as amyotrophic lateral sclerosis and poliomyelitis. Their possible origins

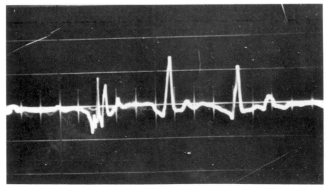

Figure 9–23   Large amplitude potentials recorded from a poliomyelitis patient. Calibration: 5000 microvolts per vertical division. Note the complexity of the potential to the left.

are selective destruction of small motor units so that large ones are the only ones remaining; sprouting from intact neuron branches to neighboring denervated muscle fibers, thus enlarging each motor unit; and simultaneous discharge of two or more motor units. Preferred terminology employs a description of the amplitude, the duration and the number of phases rather than imprecise terms such as "giant" potentials.

Bizarre High Frequency Discharges. High frequency, usually polyphasic, discharges, up to 200 per second, are seen in a variety of motor unit diseases (Fig. 9-24). It is likely that these represent discharges from the muscle spindles now relatively isolated by muscle atrophy.

Myotonic Discharges. Myotonic discharges are trains of positive waves which vary in frequency and amplitude. Audibly they have been likened to a diving airplane as they wax and wane. They are seen only in myotonic dystrophy and myotonia congenita (Fig. 9-25)

Cramp. In cramp there is synchronous, high frequency discharge of a group of motor units.

Reinnervation Potentials (Nascent). Reinnervation potentials are low amplitude (50 to 200 microvolts), highly polyphasic potentials which appear early in the process of reinnervation. Initially, they do not appear to be under voluntary control but may be elicited by mechanical stimuli over the muscle.

Myopathic Potentials. Myopathic potentials are motor unit action potentials under voluntary control which are of reduced amplitude and duration (Fig. 9-26). They average 50 to 200 microvolts in amplitude and 5 milliseconds in duration. They result from destruction of muscle fibers with a consequent reduction of the number of muscle fibers comprising the motor unit.

As mentioned previously, it is recommended that descriptive jargon such as "giant," "myopathic," "reinnervation" and "myotonic" potentials not be used in electromyographic reports but rather that the electrical discharges be described by specifically identifying the amplitude, duration, shape, rate and rhythm of firing.

Clinical Application

Anterior Horn Cell Disease. Examples of anterior horn cell disease include acute paralytic poliomyelitis (Fig. 9-27), amyotrophic lateral sclerosis, Werdnig-Hoffmann disease, myelopathies (such as syringomyelia) and intramedullary spinal cord tumors.

Fibrillation potentials appear 18 to 21 days following the death of the anterior horn cell. Voluntary potentials are increased in amplitude (up to 8 to 10 millivolts) and in duration (showing a mean of 13 milliseconds) and are so-called "giant potentials." The number of motor unit action potentials is reduced and they fire rapidly. Unless the motor units are firing rapidly, it is not possible to evaluate the number of units present.

A myelopathic electromyogram shows a reduced number of motor unit action potentials and an increase in amplitude and duration ("giant potentials") and in fibrillation potentials.

Fasciculation potentials are very frequently seen in anterior horn cell disease, probably as a result of the "sick" neuron. They may be simple or

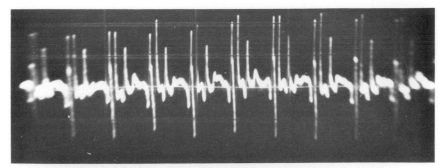

Fig. 9–24

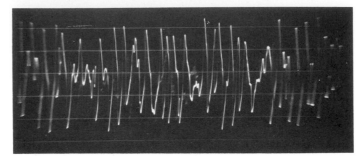

Fig. 9–25

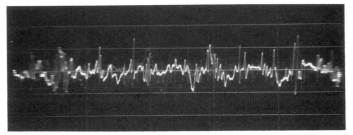

Fig. 9–26

Figure 9–24 Bizarre high frequency discharge recorded from a 6 year old muscular dystrophy patient. This electrical activity is probably from a muscle spindle. Calibration: 30 milliseconds per major horizontal division; 100 microvolts per vertical division.

Figure 9–25 Myotonic discharge recorded from a patient with myotonic dystrophy, elicited by moving the electrode. Calibration: 30 milliseconds per major division; 100 microvolts per vertical division.

Figure 9–26 Electromyogram from a patient with polymyositis. Note the short duration, small amplitude potentials. Calibration: 30 milliseconds per horizontal division; 50 microvolts per vertical division.

polyphasic. In amyotrophic lateral sclerosis they are quite common and generally are of low amplitude and of short duration. These are the so-called "malignant" fasciculations.

Synchronous discharge of motor units in different locations in the muscle frequently occurs early in acute paralytic poliomyelitis.

The motor nerve conduction velocity is normal or low normal in anterior horn cell disease. If it is reduced, the temperature of the extremity should be checked.

Axonal Disease. Conditions affecting the axon as a whole or in segments include idiopathic polyneuritis (Guillain-Barré syndrome), diabetic neuropathy, Charcot-Marie-Tooth disease and toxic neuropathy. Examples of localized

242

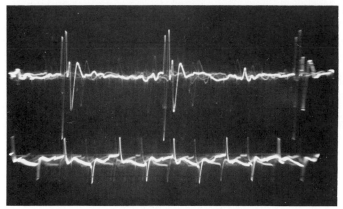

Figure 9–27   Neuropathic electromyogram from a 16 year old girl who had poliomyelitis for seven years. Note the large amplitude, long duration potentials. The bottom tracing is a 60 cycle per second calibration signal with 1000 microvolts per vertical deflection.

problems are tardy ulnar nerve palsy and median nerve neuritis (or carpal tunnel syndrome).

If the segment of axon has undergone wallerian degeneration distal to the injury, the electromyogram will show neuropathy. This type of electromyogram exhibits a reduced number of motor unit action potentials, fibrillation potentials and perhaps an increased proportion of polyphasic potentials and fasciculation potentials.

Axonal disease is differentiated from anterior horn cell disease by the reduced motor nerve conduction velocity. In acute disease the reduction may appear after one to two weeks, and after three to four weeks conduction velocity may be markedly reduced. The reduced conductivity is probably the result of the myelin sheath alteration. In chronic polyneuropathies the reduced caliber of the axis cylinder may be a factor. The conduction velocity reduction is heralded at 7 to 10 days by a raggedness and temporal dispersion of the stimulated muscle action potential. The amplitude of the muscle action potential may be lower and the duration increased when the nerve is stimulated proximally than when it is stimulated distally.

Velocities may be reduced 50 to 75 per cent in idiopathic polyneuritis, and in chronic polyneuropathies, such as Charcot-Marie-Tooth disease, they may be even lower. In chronic peripheral neuropathies, fibrillation potentials are rare and insertional activity is reduced.

Localized areas of compromise may be identified by stimulating proximally and distally to the site of compromise and noting prolonged latency across the diseased segment or reduced amplitude of the muscle action potential when stimulation is proximal to the compromise (Figs. 9–14 to 9–16). In chronic compressive (ischemic) compromise of motor nerve, a single stimulation frequently results in a repetitive discharge polyphasic motor unit action potential as recorded by a needle electrode.

Peripheral nerve injury and motor root compression produce neuropathic electromyograms. The distribution of abnormalities permits the localization of the compromise. For example, fibrillation or fasciculation potentials or an increased proportion of polyphasic potentials in the anterior tibial, peroneal and gastrocnemius muscles as well as in the sacrospinalis muscle at L-5 level indicates a compromise at or proximal to the root level. The motor and sensory root join and leave the spinal canal via the intervertebral foramen as a mixed nerve, then split into the posterior primary ramus which goes to the muscles and skin of the back and the anterior primary ramus which is distributed to the plexus and then to the extremity. Thus, an electromyographic abnormality in the muscles of the extremity as well as in the paraspinal muscles at the appropriate level indicates a compromise of the spinal nerve before it divides into the anterior and posterior primary rami.

Myoneural Junction Disease.   Myasthenia gravis is a disease affecting this part of the motor unit.

Electromyographically, the motor unit action potentials are reduced in amplitude and duration as the muscle contraction is sustained. This occurs as more and more of the myoneural junctions, and thus muscle fibers, drop out of the firing effort. There is a normal number of motor units but each unit grows progressively smaller. The E.M.G. will show an increase in the number of motor unit action potentials as compared with the strength of contraction.

To obviate the necessity for cooperation by the patient, repetitive nerve stimulation can demonstrate the myasthenic reaction objectively. With surface recording electrodes the motor nerve is stimulated at the distal site two or three times per second for one series. The muscle action potential will show a reduction as the fatigued myoneural junctions fail to contribute when the second or third shock comes along. To make this test more sensitive, the myoneural junction can be sensitized with exercise or curare. If the defect of transmission appears, it may be repaired with Tensilon.

In certain malignancies—particularly small cell carcinoma of the lung—a myasthenic-like syndrome may be present. Here, repetitive stimulation will increase the amplitude of the muscle action potential corresponding to the clinical finding of initial weakness and then subsequent muscle contractions will increase the muscle strength.

Muscle Disease.   Diseases affecting this portion of the motor unit present "myopathic" electromyograms. Examples are muscular dystrophy, polymyositis, thyrotoxic myopathy and potassium alteration. Here the motor unit is functioning with the exception that it loses the muscle fibers which are involved in the myopathic disease. Thus the motor unit action potentials are reduced in amplitude and duration (50 to 200 microvolts and 4 to 6 milliseconds). Each contraction results in an increase in the number of motor unit action potentials activated with respect to the strength of contraction. Polyphasic potentials are common and are usually of short duration and of low amplitude as one would expect with the fewer and anatomically dispersed muscle fibers and resultant ragged summation.

Generally the first recruited potentials are affected early in the disease. In this early stage the only electromyographic abnormality may be action potentials of short duration. As muscle fibers degenerate, spontaneous single muscle fiber action potentials appear, so that fibrillation potentials are commonly seen in muscular dystrophy. There are showers of fibrillation potentials in polymyositis, and prolonged insertional activity. Fibrillation potentials indicate active degeneration of muscle fibers. Positive waves are found often in both muscular dystrophy and polymyositis as well as in other types of myopathies. Again, these represent hyperirritable muscle cell membranes depolarizing away from the electrode tip. Motor nerve conduction velocity is normal in myopathic disease.

Myotonic dystrophy is characterized by a unique electromyographic pattern (Fig. 9-25). When the needle electrode is inserted or moved, prolonged trains of positive waves that vary in frequency and amplitude appear. The sound is similar to that of a diving airplane. The myotonic potentials are seen only in myotonic dystrophy or myotonia congenita (Thomsen's disease). Also, following volitional contraction, an after discharge persists as the voluntary effort triggers cycling depolarization and repolarization.

Specific Applications

Diabetic Neuropathy. Typically the motor nerve conduction velocity is reduced earliest in the peroneal nerve, then in the facial nerve and finally in the ulnar and median nerves. Usually when onset of diabetic neuropathy is insidious, electromyographic abnormalities are minimal, if present at all, while the velocity is reduced 20 to 30 per cent. In a few severe neuropathies, a classic neuropathic electromyogram, with progressively reduced conduction velocities, can be demonstrated. We assume, and preliminary studies suggest, that the conduction velocity may be reduced earlier in the sensory fibers than the motor fibers in some patients.

Diabetes mellitus apparently alters the metabolism of the peripheral nerve so that the nerve becomes more susceptible to local traumata. Tardy ulnar nerve palsy, carpal tunnel syndrome, and other mononeuritides may be frequent manifestations of diabetic neuropathy.

The so-called "femoral neuralgia" seen in diabetic patients has been shown electromyographically to be multiple lumbar radiculopathies rather than a peripheral mononeuropathy as was suggested clinically.

Carpal Tunnel Syndrome. The median nerve is anatomically located within a rigid tunnel at the wrist. Any disease or injury which increases the volume of the tunnel's contents or distorts its structure may thus compromise the median nerve with resultant axonstenosis. The conduction delay from proximal wrist crease to thenar eminence is less than 5 milliseconds normally; in carpal tunnel syndrome the delay is greater than 5 milliseconds and averaged 8.5 milliseconds in a recently published series. If compromise is severe, the electromyogram will be neuropathic, but fibrillation potentials are rare. The sensory delay is usually prolonged before the motor delay and after operation returns to normal later (see Fig. 9-14).

Tardy Ulnar Nerve Palsy. Stimulation of the ulnar nerve above the elbow will show prolonged delay and reduced muscle action potential of the abductor digiti quinti; stimulation below the elbow may show normal conduction velocity and increased "M" response. The electromyogram will be neuropathic with a paucity of fibrillation potentials and reduced insertional activity.

Amyotrophic Lateral Sclerosis. Normal conduction velocity is found but the electromyogram is neuropathic. Fasciculation potentials are numerous and may be polyphasic or simple short-duration potentials (the so-called "malignant" fasciculation potentials). Voluntary motor unit action potentials are increased in amplitude (to 10 or more millivolts) and duration (9 to 18 milliseconds). Fibrillation potentials are present but may be difficult to demonstrate. Positive waves and prolonged insertional activity are invariably present. The abnormalities shown with the electromyograph are generalized even though in the clinical findings the weakness is apparently localized.

Acute Idiopathic Polyneuritis.   Reduced motor nerve conduction velocity is present together with a neuropathic electromyogram. The motor unit action potentials are usually of normal amplitude. There are fasciculation potentials, fibrillation potentials and a reduced number of voluntary potentials, of which there is an increased proportion of polyphasic potentials. The reduction in conductivity may appear as early as 10 to 14 days and may drop 75 to 80 per cent of normal (Fig. 9-18). Early in the disease (during the first two weeks) there is usually a temporal dispersion of the "M" response when the nerve is stimulated proximally and an increase in the amplitude in the "M" response when the nerve is stimulated distally or near the muscle. The rise in the conduction velocity follows but lags behind the clinical recovery.

Root Compression Syndrome.   Early compromise of the motor root may result in an increased proportion of polyphasic potentials, fasciculation potentials or only positive waves in the muscle innervated by the root. These would include muscles innervated by the anterior primary ramus (extremity) and the posterior primary ramus (paraspinal). More severe compromise causes a neuropathic electromyogram with fibrillation potentials (after 18 days). Ordinarily, fibrillation potentials appear earlier, often after 14 days, in the paraspinal muscles.

When the diagnostic problem includes differentiating an intraspinal tumor from a root compression syndrome, it is helpful to attempt to elicit the sensory fiber action potential in a peripheral nerve having sensory fibers chiefly from that level. If the root is compromised severely, sensory axons will of course have undergone wallerian degeneration and will not conduct. Conversely, if the compromise is within the cord, sparing the dorsal ganglion, then the intact afferent (sensory) axon will conduct. In these conditions the electromyographic findings would probably be quite similar.

Peripheral Nerve Injury.   The distal segment of the injured nerve will conduct for about 72 hours; then if wallerian degeneration is taking place, no conduction will occur. After 72 hours the amplitude of the "M" response will be proportional to the number of motor fibers that were not injured severely enough to undergo wallerian degeneration. From the time of injury to 18 to 21 days, there will be a reduced number of motor unit action potentials or none, depending on the degree of injury (Fig. 9-28). At about 12 to 16 days positive

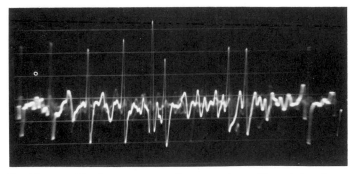

Figure 9–28   Neuropathic electromyogram from a patient with peripheral nerve injury. Note the reduced number of potentials with normal amplitude and duration. Calibration: 30 milliseconds per major horizontal division; 200 microvolts per vertical division. Negativity is indicated by upward deflection.

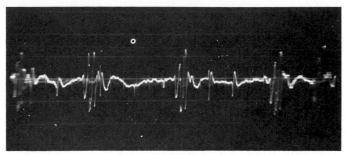

Figure 9–29 Polyphasic potentials recorded from a patient with regenerating radial nerve. Note the positive waves and fibrillation also. Negative polarity is indicated by upward deflection. Calibration: 30 milliseconds per major horizontal division; 50 microvolts per vertical division.

waves may appear during insertional activity and at 18 to 21 days fibrillation potentials will appear.

The earliest indications of reinnervation are: the disappearance of fibrillation potentials; the appearance of low amplitude highly polyphasic "reinnervation potentials" or "nascent potentials" (Fig. 9-29), which in the early period are not under voluntary control but appear when the needle is moved or the muscle is tapped; a supramaximal stimulus proximal to the injured site resulting in a temporally dispersed muscle action potential with the surface electrode or a complex motor unit action potential with the needle electrode (conduction velocity of the motor nerve fibers which are regenerating is markedly slowed, by 50 per cent or more, since the diameter of regrowing fibers is considerably reduced).

After prolonged periods of denervation, muscle fibers may be replaced by fibrous tissue, a condition which reduces the number of fibrillation potentials as well as the amount of insertional activity.

Myasthenia Gravis. With surface electrodes over the abductor digiti quinti and bipolar stimulating electrodes over the ulnar nerve at the wrist, repetitive stimulation at 2 or 3 stimulations per second is done. The hand is held securely to avoid movement.

Reduction in "M" response of abductor digiti quinti during supramaximal repetitive stimulation indicates a "myasthenic reaction." This may be confirmed by the repair of the transmission defect with Tensilon. Other tests using curare-like agents or depolarizing drugs may be even more sensitive in detection of a myasthenic reaction.

Muscular Dystrophy. PROGRESSIVE OF LITTLE BOYS. (Duchenne, X-linked recessive) The electromyogram is myopathic and shows fibrillation potentials (because of disintegrating muscle fibers) and positive waves. The increased proportion of polyphasic potentials are low in amplitude and of normal or short duration; some are disintegrated potentials. Insertional activity is reduced and there is increased resistance to needle advancement late in the disease as fibrosis and fat infiltration occur.

RESTRICTIVE (e.g., fascioscapulohumeral, autosomal dominant). There is a myopathic electromyogram but fewer, often rarely demonstrable, fibrillation potentials since this has a slower, more insidious course. As muscles fibrose, insertional activity is reduced.

MYOTONIC DYSTROPHY (autosomal dominant). The myopathic electromyogram shows trains of positive waves varying in amplitude and frequency.

These are elicited by tapping the muscle near the needle or by moving the needle. The myotonic reaction is specific for myotonic dystrophy and myotonia congenita. Conduction velocity is normal.

Polymyositis (Dermatomyositis). There is a myopathic electromyogram with showers of fibrillation potentials and prolonged insertional activity. Fibrillation potentials parallel the activity of the disease and may be suppressed with steroids. Bizarre high frequency discharges, positive waves and polyphasic potentials are found (Fig. 9-26). There is normal conduction velocity.

Metabolic Myopathies. The myopathic electromyogram shows many frequent trains of positive waves. Insertional activity is prolonged. Hyperthyroidism, familial periodic paralysis and other electrolyte imbalances may be causes.

Tetany. Incipient tetany may be manifested first by volitional repetitive discharge polyphasic potentials (iterative discharges) as the heightened irritability shortens the relative refractory period. Progressively increased motor unit hyperirritability results in spontaneous appearance of these repetitive discharges, which are grouped fasciculations. Hyperventilation may also produce these abnormal potentials.

Facial Paralysis. It is helpful in prognosticating the outcome of facial paralysis to stimulate the facial nerve under the tip of the ear lobe and record over the frontalis above the center of the brow. In the first 72 hours the excitability should be normal; after this time, if the distal axons are undergoing wallerian degeneration, excitability will disappear. With the use of surface electrodes, the amplitude of the "M" response should be proportional to the number of conducting fibers, those which presumably are neurapraxic in a segment of compromise. If the facial delay is greatly prolonged, the prognosis is less favorable. The contralateral facial nerve should be stimulated for comparison.

Sprouting may occur from the normal side of the face across the midline so that interpretation of active potentials under voluntary control as recorded near the midline after prolonged time may lead mistakenly to a report that reinnervation is occurring. Here, stimulation of both facial nerves can give the answer.

Anomalous Innervation. Interpretation of a variety of clinical conditions depends on a knowledge of innervation patterns. Since anomalous patterns occur frequently, it is necessary to identify these variations in order to avoid erroneous conclusions regarding electrodiagnostic findings. Isolation of the muscle response, with a needle electrode if necessary, then stimulation of the motor fibers of the involved nerve proximally and distally will indicate the correct pathway. Examples include ulnar nerve fibers communicating with the median nerve in the forearm so that the ulnar nerve of the wrist contains median nerve fibers going to the thenar eminence. Similar anomalous connections may occur between the peroneal and tibial nerves in the leg. In 20 percent of individuals an anomalous branch separates from the peroneal nerve to innervate a portion of the extensor digitorum brevis muscle. It runs beneath the lateral malleolus, so will not be stimulated by the usual distal placement of stimulating electrodes on the anterior ankle.

Sensory Nerve Conduction Velocity. When surface electrodes are placed over a mixed nerve trunk and sensory nerve fibers are excited, nerve action

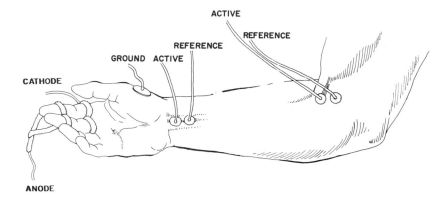

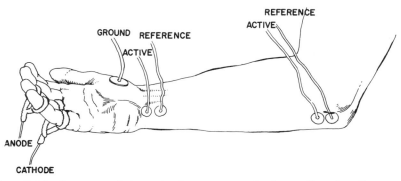

Figure 9–30 Placement of electrodes for sensory conduction studies of median nerve (upper) and ulnar nerve (lower). Clinically only the delay from fingers to wrist is obtained. Antidromic technique is done by recording on the fingers and stimulating at the wrist.

potentials may be recorded (Fig. 9-30). Since the desired signal is usually only 15 to 30 microvolts, it may be obscured by the noise level of the oscilloscope tracing. This can be obviated by lowering the trace intensity and repeating the stimulation 10 to 20 times. Since noise is random and the signal is constant, the latter will appear in the same place during each trace and thus appear on the photograph as a deflection. Needle electrodes placed in the vicinity of the nerve trunk are more sensitive for recording the nerve action potential than are surface electrodes.

Median nerve sensory fibers can be stimulated over the index finger and the orthodromic nerve action potential recorded over the nerve trunk at the wrist between the tendons of the palmaris longus and the flexor carpi radialis. The ulnar nerve is stimulated at the little finger with the action potential recorded over the nerve trunk at the medial aspect of the wrist. Antidromic sensory delay may be obtained by reversing the stimulating and recording electrodes. Values are similar. Conduction velocity of sensory fibers may be determined by recording the action potential at the wrist and elbow, and dividing the latency difference into the distance. The peroneal sensory fibers are difficult to activate at the dorsum of the foot but recording can be done over the nerve trunk at the head of the fibula. A delay rather than conduction velocity is observed and compared with the normal.

In the median nerve from the base of the index finger to the wrist (14 cm.) the average delay from a stimulus artifact to the peak of the action potential in

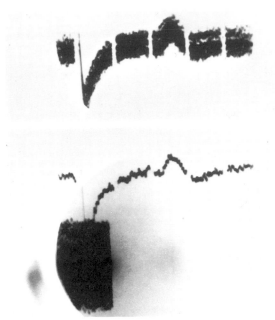

Figure 9–31   Sensory nerve conduction delay (2.5 milliseconds) in the median nerve fibers obtained orthodromically with the assembled components. The trace is interrupted at 1 millisecond intervals. The top recording represents 20 sweeps superimposed and the bottom trace is single. Calibration voltage is 50 microvolts.

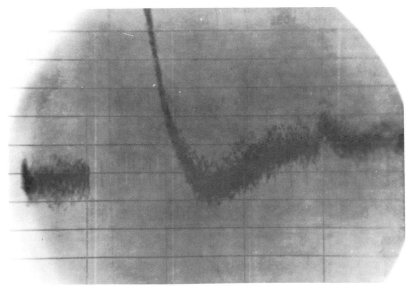

Figure 9–32   Long conduction delay (15 milliseconds) in median sensory fibers. This probably represents "C" fibers. Orthodromic technique was used; 20 traces superimposed.

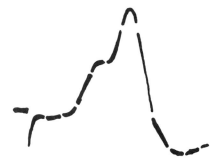

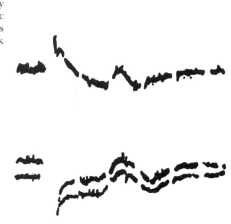

Figure 9–33 The top trace is the motor delay in the ulnar nerve. The next trace is the orthodromic delay in the sensory fibers and the bottom two traces are antidromic sensory delays. Note the sharper peak in the orthodromically elicited action potential.

healthy adults is 3.0 milliseconds (Figs. 9–31 and 9–32). The takeoff of the deflection is too gradual for satisfactory measurement. Orthodromic delay in sensory fibers of the ulnar nerve from the little finger to the wrist is similar in magnitude (Fig. 9–33). Insufficient data have been published for normal values in the sensory fibers of the peroneal nerve.

Antidromic stimulation of the sural nerve may be accomplished at the midposterior calf, then recording over the distal sural nerve just under the lateral malleolus. This is a frequently and early involved sensory nerve in many peripheral neuropathies.

Reporting the Electromyogram

Many different forms are used to report the electromyographic findings (Fig. 9–34). They are based on the necessity of recording the muscles examined, the electrical activity observed and the interpretation of the findings. (Fig. 9–35)

Muscles Examined. In addition to listing the muscles examined, it is often helpful to record locations of needle insertions (proximal, central or distal) within the muscle. The peripheral nerve and the cord level of innervation should be noted routinely. If differential diagnosis involves a branch of a plexus or a peripheral nerve, more specific identification of the nerve supply is indicated.

THE OHIO STATE UNIVERSITY HEALTH CENTER
UNIVERSITY HOSPITAL
COLUMBUS, OHIO

Division of Physical Medicine and Rehabilitation

ELECTROMYOGRAPHIC EXAMINATION

DATE 1/1/63

PATIENT JOHN SMITH   REFERRING PHYSICIAN JOHN ADAMS MD.
ADDRESS 100 LANE   AGE 42   STATUS OUT PATIENT
PROBLEM WEAKNESS ® FOOT

MUSCLE	INNERVATION	INSERTIONAL ACTIVITY	SPONTANEOUS FIBRILLATION	FASCICU-LATION	MOTOR UNIT ACTION POTENTIALS
® QUADS	L2,3,4 FEM	NORMAL	0	0	NORMAL INTERFERENCE PATTERN
® BICEPS FEM.	L5S1 Sc.	positive waves	+	0	MIN. ↓ in # ; ↑ PROP. POLYPHASICS
® ANT. TIB.	L5S1 PER.		0	0	↑ POLYPHASIC POT.
® GASTROC	S1,2 TIB.		+	+	MINIMAL ↓↓ IN #, ↑ PROPORTION OF POLYPHASIC
® ABD. DIG. Q. ped.	L5S1 TIB.	↓	0	occas	POTENTIALS
® SACROSPINALIS					NORMAL INTERFERENCE PATTERN
L4		NORMAL	0	0	
L5	POSTERIOR PRIMARY	↓	0		; ↓
S1		POSITIVE WAVES	+		↑↑ POLYPHASIC POTENTIALS
Ⓛ S1	RAMI	NORMAL	0		NORMAL
Ⓛ GASTROC	S1,2 TIB	↓	0	↓	↓

CONDUCTION VELOCITY ®PER. N 54 M/S

COMMENT: EMG EVIDENCE OF PARTIAL DENERVATION IN MUSCLES SUPPLIED BY ® S1 ROOT. NORMAL CONDUCTION VELOCITY. (OR PROXIMAL TO ROOT)

IMP: PARTIAL COMPROMISE ® S-1

(HOSPITAL CHART OR REFERRING PHYSICIAN)

Figure 9–34 Sample E.M.G. report.

Insertional Activity. The report should include: the duration, listed as normal, reduced or prolonged (fibrosis may be the cause of reduced duration and hyperirritable muscle fibers result in prolonged insertional activity with a sound similar to a musical tone like that of the cello); the mechanical resistance to needle advancement (fibrosis and myositis produce increased resistance); the positive waves, noting whether there are few or many or trains, the frequency of which may be constant or variable; end plate potentials; and bizarre high frequency discharges.

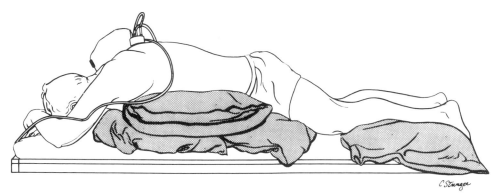

Figure 9–35 Position of patient for needle electromyography for suspected cervical radiculopathy. Needle electrode is in posterior cervical muscles.

Spontaneous Activity. FIBRILLATION POTENTIALS. These are graded according to the number present, on a scale from 1 to 4. Grade 1 usually indicates that fibrillation is difficult to find, and is present only when the muscle is stimulated mechanically. Grade 2 represents the presence of a few fibrillation potentials without mechanical stimulation of the muscle. Grade 4 indicates that the oscilloscope screen is filled horizontally with fibrillation potentials. Grade 3 is between 2 and 4. Some electromyographers use simply minimal, moderate and considerable number of fibrillation potentials.

FASCICULATION POTENTIALS. These should be reported as simple, polyphasic, disintegrated or iterative type. Quiet muscle should be observed for at least one minute. The number of fasciculation potentials present is usually recorded as rare, occasional, few or many.

Motor Unit Action Potentials. The amplitude, duration, shape, rate and rhythm of firing and the number activated with respect to the strength of contraction should be described.

Nerve Stimulation Studies. The motor or sensory conduction velocity of the stimulated nerves should be indicated as well as the terminal latency. Normal values should be included for comparison. Any variation in "M" response at the proximal and distal stimulation sites and during repetitive stimulations should be reported. Presence or absence of "H" reflex should be noted.

Comment. *The electromyographic findings should be summarized and then translated into a clinical diagnosis. An electromyogram without a clinical impression is of little value to the practicing physician.*

TRADITIONAL ELECTRODIAGNOSTIC TECHNIQUES

Rheobase. When a current is allowed to flow for an infinite period, the minimal amount or intensity of current which will stimulate the muscle is termed the *rheobase.* For practical purpose infinite time is 300 milliseconds of current.

Chronaxie. The duration of flow of a current twice the intensity of the rheobase required to stimulate a muscle is termed the *chronaxie.*

Strength-Duration Curve. It is apparent that the intensity of current and its duration of flow are nerve-exciting parameters which are inversely related. Plotting the duration of current flow against the intensity of current applied results in the strength-duration curve. Instruments are available which give a constant current or a constant voltage so that either the voltage or current may be plotted as the intensity of stimulus. The chronaxie is one point on the strength-duration curve.

Reaction of Degeneration. When an electrical stimulus is applied to a muscle which has an intact nerve supply, the muscle is activated by impulses arriving from the motor nerve since nerve tissue is inherently more excitable (has a lower threshold of stimulation) than muscle tissue. Thus if a current which is two times the rheobase is applied to an innervated muscle, the duration of flow needed to produce a contraction could be very short. One current which has an extremely short duration is induced or faradic current.

Conversely, if the muscle has lost its nerve supply, then the muscle fibers must be stimulated directly, and since they are less excitable (have a higher threshold of stimulation) than nerve tissue, the flow of current must be longer at similar intensities to produce a contraction of muscle. A galvanic or direct current permits current flow of prolonged duration.

Reaction of degeneration (R.D.) is the reaction of a muscle responding to galvanic but not faradic stimulation (i.e., current flow of less than one millisecond). Innervated muscle also responds best when stimulated at its middle third or at the *motor point*, which is the point where the nerve enters the muscle. Conversely, denervated muscle responds equally to the stimulus applied anywhere over the muscle. The muscle twitch is quite brisk in intact muscle since the stimulus is conducted throughout the muscle by fast conducting nerve fibers while in denervated muscle the twitch is quite slow and "worm-like" since the non-nervous tissue is the conducting medium. The cathode closing current is the most effective in exciting nerve tissue, while for denervated muscle it has no such property. This has led to Erb's law for the effectiveness of stimulation of normal muscle CCC>ACC>AOC>COC (cathode, anode, opening, closing and current).

When alternating current is used, the quarter cycles of the sinusoidal wave compare to CC, COC, ACC, and AOC. Thus one fourth of the wave corresponds to the exciting stimulus, and an alternating current with a frequency of 1000 cycles per second would compare to an induced current having a duration of 0.25 millisecond, a duration too short to activate denervated muscle. However, an alternating current of 100 cycles per second would have a quarter cycle of 2.5 milliseconds, a duration of flow sufficient to excite denervated muscle.

Partial Reaction of Degeneration.   When the muscle is only partially denervated, the muscle twitch in response to faradic or other current flowing for short duration would be diminished in proportion to the number of denervated muscle fibers since they would be unable to respond.

Tetanus Twitch Ratio.   In order to excite denervated muscle it requires a high intensity of current. A very slight further increase of intensity will tetanize the muscle (ratio almost 1:1).

However, very little current is required to excite normal nerve, but considerable more to tetanize it, so that the tetanus twitch ratio is 5:1 (i.e., five times the current intensity is needed to tetanize rather than to cause a twitch).

Summary

These traditional electrodiagnostic techniques require interpretation through several variables: the location of the underlying muscle, the resistance of the skin, the thickness of the subcutaneous layer and then the visible recognition of a minimal twitch. All compound the variability of the tests and cloud their significance.

Electromyography and efferent and afferent fiber stimulation techniques are considerably more sensitive and objective than these obsolescent and less reliable techniques, and thus should supplant them.

REFERENCES

1. Bauwens, P.: Electrodiagnostic Definition of the Site and Nature of Peripheral Lesions. Ann. Phys. Med., 5:149-152, 1960.

1a. Bonsett, C., and Abreu, B.: Skeletal Muscle Studies by Means of Combined Electromyography and Needle Biopsy. II. The Muscle Spindle. Neurology, 13:328-330, 1963.

2. Carpendale, M. T. F.: Conduction Time in Terminal Portion of Motor Fibers of Ulnar, Median, and Peroneal Nerves in Healthy Subjects and Patients with Neuronopathy. Thesis, University of Minnesota, 1956.

3. Cerra, D., and Johnson, E. W.: Motor Nerve Conduction Velocity in "Idiopathic" Polyneuritis. Arch. Phys. Med., 42:159-163, 1961.

4. Cerra, D., and Johnson, E. W.: Motor Nerve Conduction Velocity in Premature Infants. Arch. Phys. Med., 43:160-164, 1962.

5. Dawson, G. D., and Scott, J. W.: The Recording of Nerve Action Potentials Through the Skin in Man. J. Neurol., Neurosurg. and Psychiat., 12:259-267, 1949.

6. Denny-Brown, D., and Pennybacker, J. B.: Fibrillation and Fasciculation in Voluntary Muscle. Brain, 61:311-332, 1938.

7. Eaton, L. M., and Lambert, E. H.: Electromyography and Electrical Stimulation of Nerves in Diseases of the Motor Unit. J.A.M.A., 163:1117-1124, 1957.

8. Erlanger, J.: Interpretation of Action Potential in Cutaneous and Muscle Nerves. Amer. J. Physiol., 82:644-655, 1927.

9. Gasser, H. S., and Grundfest, H.: Axon Diameters in Relation to Spike Dimensions and Conduction Velocity in Mammalian Fibers. Amer. J. Physiol. 127:393-414, 1939.

10. Gilliatt, R. W., and Sears, T. A.: Sensory Nerve Action Potentials in Patients with Peripheral Nerve Lesions. J. Neurol., Neurosurg. and Psychiat., 21:109, 1958.

11. Gilliatt, R. W., et al.: The Recording of Lateral Popliteal Nerve Action Potentials in Man. J. Neurol., Neurosurg. and Psychiat., 24:305-318, 1961.

12. Harvey, A. M., and Kuffler, S. W.: Motor Nerve Function with Lesions of Peripheral Nerves; Quantitative Study. Arch. Neurol, and Psychiat., 52:317-322, 1944.

13. Hendriksen, J. D.: Conduction Velocity of Motor Nerves in Normal Subjects and Patients with Neuromuscular Disorders. Thesis, University of Minnesota, 1956.

14. Hodes, R., Larrabee, M. G., and German, W. U.: Human Electromyogram in Response to Nerve Stimulation and Conduction Velocity of Motor Axons; Studies on Normal and on Injured Peripheral Nerves. Arch. Neurol. and Psychiat., 60:340-365, 1948.

15. Hursh, J. B.: Conduction Velocity and Diameter of Nerve Fibers. Amer. J. Physiol., 127:131-139, 1939.

16. Johnson, E. W.: Examination for Muscle Weakness in Infants and Small Children. J.A.M.A., 168:1306-1313, 1958.

17. Johnson, E. W., and Olsen, K. J.: Clinical Value of Motor Nerve Conduction Velocity Determination. J.A.M.A., 172:2030-2035, 1960.

18. Johnson, E. W., and Waylonis, G. W.: Facial Nerve Conduction Latency in Diabetes. Arch. Phys. Med., 45:131-139, 1964.

19. Johnson, E. W., Wells, R. M., and Duran, R. J.: Diagnosis of Carpal Tunnel Syndrome. Arch. Phys. Med., 43:414-419, 1962.

20. Johnson, E. W., et al.: Femoral Nerve Conduction Studies. Arch. Phys. Med., 49:528-532, 1968.

21. Kugelberg, E.: Electromyogram in Muscular Disorders. J. Neurol., Neurosurg. and Psychiat., 10:122-129, 1947.

22. Lambert, E.: The Accessory Deep Peroneal Nerve. Neurology, 19:1169-1176, 1969.

23. Lambert, E., and McMorris, R.: Size of Motor Unit Action Potentials in Neuromuscular Diseases. Fed. Proc., 12:263, 1953.

24. Lambert, E., et al.: Unipolar Electromyograms of Patients with Dermatomyositis. Fed. Proc., 9:73, 1950.

25. Lambert, E., et al.: Information Concerning the Formulation of Minimal Requirements for Electromyographs for Clinical Use. Report by Committee on Instrumentation, American Association of Electromyography and Electrodiagnosis, 1955.

26. Mavor, H., and Libman, I.: Motor Nerve Conduction Measurement as a Diagnostic Tool. Neurology, 12:733-744, 1962.

27. Ruppert, E., and Johnson, E.: Motor Nerve Conduction Velocities in Low Weight Infants. Pediatrics, 42:255-260, 1968.

28. Skillman, T. G., Johnson, E. W., Hamwi, G. J., and Driskill, H. J.: Motor Nerve Conduction Velocity in Diabetes Mellitus. Diabetes, 10:46-51, 1961.

29. Tajima, T.: Comparison of Conduction Velocity of Sensory and Motor Fibers in Ulnar Nerve in Man. Thesis, Ohio State University, 1959.

30. Thomas, J. E., and Lambert, E. H.: Ulnar Nerve Conduction Velocity and H-Reflex in Infants and Children. J. Appl. Physiol., 15:1-9, 1960.

31. Wagman, I. H., and Lesse, H.: Maximum Conduction Velocities of Motor Fibers of Ulnar Nerve in Human Subjects of Various Ages and Sizes. J. Neurophysiol., 15:235-244, 1952.

32. Weddell, G.: The Electrical Activity of Voluntary Muscle in Man Under Normal and Pathologic Conditions. Brain, 67:178-257, 1944.

Part II

TECHNIQUES OF MANAGEMENT

Chapter 10

THERAPEUTIC HEAT AND COLD

by G. Keith Stillwell

RATIONALE OF THE USE OF LOCAL HEATING

The indications and contraindications for the use of local heating are based on the physiologic effects of this procedure. In certain situations, particular benefits may be gained by a particular type of heating. Generally, however, it is satisfactory to use whichever type of heating is most readily available.

Physiologic Effects. The physiologic effects of local heating are shown in Figure 10-1. The primary effect is to cause a local increase in temperature. This leads to an increase in local metabolic rate with the production of an increased quantity of metabolites and more heat. The metabolites in turn cause an arteriolar dilatation with an increase in capillary blood flow and an increase in capillary hydrostatic pressure. These are beneficial effects. Note, however, that the increase in capillary hydrostatic pressure leads to an increased tendency to formation of edema. In persons who have a particular tendency to edema formation, this effect of heating may require subsequent measures to reduce the edema caused by the heat.

The increase in blood flow also leads to a convective dissipation of heat from the area being heated. If the vascular system of the patient is unable to respond adequately in this respect, the heat will tend to accumulate. Such a patient will be burned by dosages of heat which would normally be well tolerated.

On the left-hand side of the figure are indicated some local effects that probably are not directly attributable to an increase in local metabolic rate. The mechanism underlying the analgesic effect of local heating is not understood; it may be related to a reduction in the thermal gradient through the skin.

259

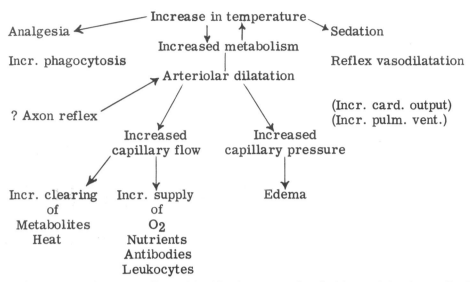

Figure 10–1 Physiologic effects of local heating. (Reproduced with permission from Stillwell, G. K.: The Use of Physical Medicine in Office Practice With Particular Emphasis on the Aftercare of Fractures. J. Iowa Med. Soc., *53:*12–18, 1963.)

On the right-hand side of the figure are noted some systemic effects that may occur with local heating. Heat is sometimes used to cause reflex vasodilatation in areas remote from that being heated, in an attempt to improve the cutaneous circulation in an area where this circulation is not adequate to permit direct heating.

The sedative effect is poorly understood. Its importance lies in the danger to the patient who may go to sleep during the heat treatment. Precautions should be taken that the patient will not come to harm should he do so, as, for example, by being burned or by falling off the treatment table.

Indications for Local Heating.   Local heating is indicated for analgesia (this is the most frequent indication), to increase cutaneous blood flow either locally or remotely, to accelerate the suppurative process, for sedation, and for hyperthermia.

Contraindications to Local Heating.   Most of the contraindications to local heating are relative. It is a matter of clinical judgment whether to use local heating and, if it is used, which method of heating to apply and in what dosage. In this sense, the indications for local heating are also relative. One is less likely to be considered negligent in failing to use heat when there was an indication for it than in producing burns when there was a contraindication.

Impaired Circulation.   With impairment of circulation to the skin, burns are likely to be produced whether superficial or deep methods of heating are being used. With defective circulation to deeper structures, even when the skin is relatively well supplied with blood, there is a theoretic risk involved in the use of procedures for deep heating. With proximal obstruction limiting blood flow into the limb, little benefit is likely to be gained by shunting from the deep to the superficial structures the little blood that does enter the limb.

Impaired Sensation for Temperature or Pain.   In these cases, extra precautions must be taken, such as reduction in the intensity of the heat below that usually used and frequent visual inspection of the heated area while it is being heated. Areas of skin denervated by lesions of the peripheral nerves may have less tolerance for heating than does adjacent innervated skin. This could conceivably be due to the loss of the protective mechanism of the axon reflex indicated in Figure 10-1.

With shortwave and microwave diathermy, in which there is no precise measurement of the amount of energy being delivered to the tissues, the only gauge of the adequacy or tolerability of the dosage is the sensation of the patient. It is generally safer, therefore, not to use these types of heating in the patient with deficient sensation.

Noninflammatory Edema.   Because edema is aggravated by the use of either local or remote heating, heat is best avoided in the presence of noninflammatory edema unless there is some strong indication for its use.

Very Young Patients.   Infants tolerate heat poorly, largely because of the inadequacy of the function of their thermoregulatory mechanisms. Furthermore, because of lack of communication from infants, it may be difficult to evaluate the dosage being used.

The restless child may be burned if radiant heating devices are being used, and shortwave and microwave diathermy generally cannot be satisfactorily applied to the child who will not lie still.

Elderly Patients.   In addition to the frequent presence of impaired peripheral circulation and sensation in the elderly, their cardiac and respiratory reserves may also be diminished, causing them to have a poor tolerance for more than minimal heating.

METHODS OF THERAPEUTIC HEATING

Conductive Heating

Physics of Heat Exchange by Conduction.   When two objects are in contact and are not at the same temperature, heat is transferred, by conduction, from the warmer object to the cooler one. The rate of heat exchange is dependent mainly on the difference in temperature. The quantity of heat exchanged will depend in addition on the length of time the process continues.

In Figure 10-2, the temperature of surface 1 (T_{s1}) will be affected by the quantity of heat available in the heat source, and this depends on the temperature of the heat source, the generation of heat (if any) within the heat source, and the specific heat of the heat source.

T_{s1} will also be affected by the rate of delivery of this heat to the surface, which depends on the thermal conductivity of the substance and the magnitude of the thermal gradient between the interior of the substance and the surface.

The temperature of the skin (T_{s2}) will be affected by the rate at which heat is dispersed, and this depends on the following: the specific heats of the dispersing substances; the thermal conductivity of the tissues (about 0.0005 gm.-cal./cm.^{2}/°C./sec.; cf. linen, 0.0002; silver, 0.99); the quantity of blood flow; and the temperature gradients between T_{s2} and the various thermal "sinks"

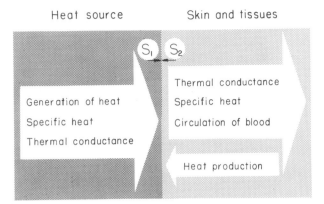

Figure 10–2 Heat exchange by conduction.

into which the heat is being drained (this factor is influenced somewhat by the production of heat locally in the region).

If heat is transferred more rapidly than it can be dissipated, T_{s2} will increase. This decreases the difference between T_{s1} and T_{s2} and increases the difference between T_{s2} and the thermal sinks. T_{s2}, therefore, will tend to stabilize at some level below T_{s1}. It is important that this level not be so high as to cause destruction of tissue which occurs, generally, above 47.0° C. (116.6° F.) if the duration is more than a few minutes (Fig. 10-3).

The figure shows that the temperature and the time through which it acts are both factors of the threshold for thermal injury. Temperatures at the dermal-epidermal interface as low as 42.0° C. (107.6° F.) sustained for several hours can cause thermal damage (surface temperature about 44.0° C. or 111.2° F.). Damage to mammalian cells in tissue culture has been induced by a temperature of 43.0° C. (109.4° F.) maintained for an hour. There may be large differences between the temperature of the surface of a heating device and that of the dermal-epidermal interface. The temperature of the interface is the critical one with regard to the production of damage. Stinging pain of a severity that is easily tolerated and easily suppressed by analgesic drugs may or may not precede or accompany the burning process. An occult thermal injury takes time for recovery, and a summation of such injuries close enough together may produce an overt injury.

The rule of thumb that exposure with close contact to a surface with a temperature of 45.0° C. (113.0° F.) for 30 minutes is the maximum safe exposure is a reliable one. It is not, however, a rigid rule, because burns may occur after half an hour at lower temperatures and may not occur at higher temperatures, presumably because of individual differences in the temperature at the dermal-epidermal interface.

Therapeutic Devices. ELECTRIC HEATING PAD. This device maintains its temperature as it is being used. Most heating pads have three levels of intensity. Because the temperature is maintained during use, patients are more likely to be burned by this than by the other conductive heating devices, particularly if the patient lies *on* the heating pad rather than *under* it. The weight of the body reduces the flow of blood through the skin adjacent to the pad (more so with the muscular relaxation that occurs when the patient falls asleep), and the temperature of the skin may increase to damaging levels.

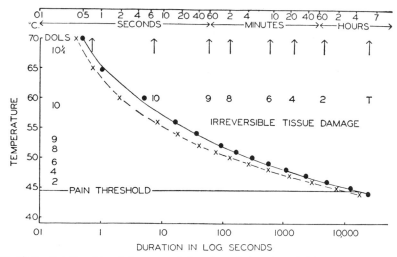

Figure 10–3 Relationship of degree and duration of elevation of skin temperature to production of transient erythema (broken line) and irreversible tissue damage (solid line). Relationship between temperature and pain (in dols) is also shown. Scale of abscissa is shown at top of figure in seconds, minutes and hours; it is shown at bottom of figure as logarithm of time in seconds. (Reproduced with permission from Hardy, J. D.: Thermal Radiation, Pain and Injury. In Licht, S.: Physical Medicine Library. Vol. 2. Therapeutic Heat. New Haven, Conn., Elizabeth Licht, 1958, pp. 157–178.)

Excessive elevation of temperature rather frequently occurs even with heating pads turned on "low." The electrical insulation should, of course, be in good condition.

HOT-WATER BOTTLE. A hot-water bottle holds about a liter of water at 65.0° C. (149.0° F.) or less and so can deliver about 30,000 gm.-cal. to its environment (including the patient) by the time heat transfer to the patient ceases. Considerable insulation is needed between the water at 65.0° C. (149.0° F.) and the skin, since elevation of the temperature of the skin to 65.0° C. (149.0° F.) for as brief a time as 1 second causes irreversible damage (Fig. 10–3). A hot-water bottle that can be tolerated next to the skin for several minutes is probably not warmer than 48.0° C. (118.4° F.) and can deliver only 13,000 gm.-cal., of which probably less than half will go to the patient.

The principal advantage of the hot-water bottle as a home heating device is that it can do double service as an enema bag. Because it can deliver only a limited amount of heat to the patient and must periodically be refilled with hot water, there is a tendency to fill it with water that is dangerously hot.

HOT PACK. Wet hot packs are often used in the home. Their heat content is principally in the water they hold. Evaporation of the water consumes much of this energy so that relatively little heat is delivered to the subject; moreover, this heat is delivered over a brief period (a few minutes). Towels soaked in hot water and lightly wrung out by hand must be resoaked every 5 to 12 minutes. This procedure is sometimes advantageous in keeping someone busy. Attempting to keep hot wet packs hot by radiant heating of the hot packs is inefficient, even if evaporation is obstructed. Wrapping an electric heating pad around a hot pack creates a shock hazard.

Kenny hot packs are made of wool or wool-like blanket material from which the water has been removed by a centrifugal extractor or by repeated mechanical wringing. Although they are steamy, the packs contain no liquid water, and the heat content is low. They can be applied at higher temperatures than can other conductive heating devices because this temperature persists only a few seconds. The temperature of the Kenny pack may be in the neighborhood of 60.0° C. (140.0° F.) at the instant of application, but it falls 22.0° C. (39.6° F.) in the first few minutes. It has been suggested that this brief, strong thermal stimulus may have special value in relaxing muscular spasm. If the water is not adequately removed from packs applied at such high temperatures, burns will result.

Kenny packs are generally left in place for 10 to 20 minutes and then replaced once or twice, the duration of the treatment being 30 to 60 minutes altogether.

PARAFFIN.   By the addition of one part of mineral oil to seven parts of paraffin, the melting point of the wax is lowered to about 52.0° C. (125.6° F.). Because its specific heat is only 0.5, the paraffin may be applied directly to the skin at this temperature if the circulation is normal. When a light scum forms on the surface of the cooling paraffin bath, the temperature of the paraffin is near the melting point. This temperature should be measured with a thermometer so that it will be known. Scum should form regularly at this temperature unless the mixture of paraffin and mineral oil is changed. If the mixture is changed, the temperature at which a scum forms should be determined anew with a thermometer. Most waxes that are not thinned with mineral oil melt at temperatures that are too hot for therapeutic use.

The paraffin may be applied by means of a brush or by dipping the part into the wax. It may be preferable first to paint the part with paraffin until a thin insulating layer of paraffin is accumulated and then to dip it for progressively longer periods until the layer of paraffin is built up. When it is known that the patient tolerates paraffin well, the part can be dipped from the beginning. The coating of paraffin may be left on for 15 to 20 minutes and then removed and dropped back into the bath.

Paraffin is used most often to heat hands and wrists but can be used for other areas. The heat is transferred from the paraffin to the skin principally by conduction. In changing state from liquid to solid, the paraffin may well be emitting some long infrared rays capable of deep penetration of tissue.[14] This is presumably of brief duration, although measurements have not been reported.

Advantages of the use of paraffin are principally that it softens the skin, that it may be applied with the part elevated, and that many patients prefer it to other types of heating. The factor of deep heating is probably inconsequential. The disadvantages of the use of paraffin are that it is messy and somewhat malodorous, that it tends to accumulate dirt and debris from the skin, and that it is difficult to keep in a state of readiness for use in the home (small units are commercially available for home or office use, however).

Advantages of Conductive Heating.   Conductive heating devices are easy to use in the home (except paraffin), can be applied with the part elevated to diminish production of edema, and can be applied to a patient confined to bed.

Disadvantages of Conductive Heating.   The part cannot be observed during the heating, it is difficult to apply the devices to irregularly shaped parts of the body such as the shoulder, only the area in contact with the heater is heated, the method is not usually suitable for open wounds, it may help spread superficial skin infections, and the heating is superficial.

Infrared Heating

Physics of Infrared Heating. SPECTRAL ENERGY. In the electromagnetic spectrum (Fig. 10-4), wavelengths from about 4000 to 7700 Angstroms have the appropriate quantum energy to produce photochemical reactions in the retina that will cause the perception of light. The adjacent band at the red end of the visible spectrum—from 7700 to 14,000 Angstroms—is the "near" infrared region (being near to the visible spectrum); that extending to about 400,000 Angstroms is the "far" infrared. The terms "radiant heat" and "infrared radiation" are essentially synonymous.

Adjacent to the visible spectrum at its violet end is the ultraviolet portion of the electromagnetic spectrum. Note from Figure 10-4 that as the wavelengths become shorter (and the frequency correspondingly higher) the energy of the quantum increases. The quantum energy in the infrared spectrum is sufficient only to increase the molecular and atomic motion ("thermal agitation"), which is heat. The shorter wavelengths can dislocate orbiting electrons of the atoms and thus bring about chemical changes. The energy required to shift an electron from its orbit to another one is highly specific, and the quantum that, when absorbed, accomplishes this shift must provide specifically this amount of energy. There is thus considerable specificity of wavelength for the effects produced by visible and ultraviolet wavelengths. An "action spectrum" may be measured, which shows wavelengths that are associated with a particular reaction. The effect of practically all of the wide infrared spectrum, however, is the same.

With wavelengths that are shorter than those of the ultraviolet spectrum, more extreme changes are produced by the higher quantum energies, including changes in the atomic nucleus.

ABSORPTION AND PENETRATION.   All of the radiant energy incident upon a substance must be reflected, absorbed, or transmitted. In the infrared region to 200,000 Angstroms, human skin absorbs more than 95 per cent of the energy, and there is almost no reflection (of rays perpendicular to the surface) or transmission. The maximal penetration (wavelength 12,000 Angstroms) is about 3 mm., and only a small part of the energy penetrates that far. It is well known that the red end of the visible spectrum can be transmitted through the full thickness of an adult hand, but this property does not extend to the

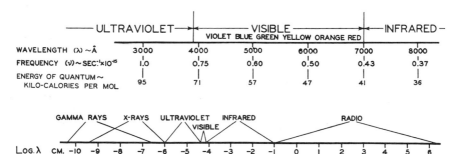

Figure 10–4 Electromagnetic spectrum showing the relationship of quantum energy to wavelength (in Angstrom units on upper scale; in centimeters on lower scale) and frequency. (Reproduced with permission from Blum, H. F.: Photodynamic Action and Diseases Caused by Light. New York, Reinhold Publishing Corp., 1941.)

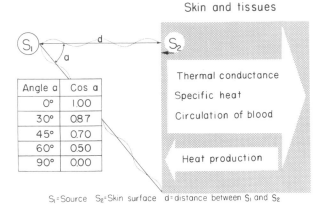

Figure 10–5   Energy exchange by radiation.

infrared region of the spectrum. The "far infrared" penetrates even less than does the "near infrared," being nearly totally absorbed in the superficial 0.1 mm. of the skin. Wavelengths longer than 30,000 Angstroms are absorbed by the moisture on the surface of the skin, except that very long waves (100,000 to 400,000 Angstroms) may penetrate several centimeters of tissue. Skin color does not materially affect these properties of the infrared.

For the same intensity of radiant heating, emissions of the far infrared may feel warmer to the recipient because of greater warming of the nerve endings in the superficial portion of the skin. Transfer of the heat (with either near or far infrared) to deeper tissues is by conduction or by the convective action of the circulation.

ENERGY EXCHANGE BY RADIATION (FIG. 10–5).   The intensity of radiation falling on S_2 from S_1 is inversely proportional to d^2 (inverse square law) and directly proportional to the cosine of the angle "a" (Lambert's law).

The wavelength of maximal emission (Wien's law) is inversely proportional to the absolute temperature of the source. For a tungsten filament lamp (at about 3000° K.), this wavelength is 9620 Angstroms in the near infrared (S_1), while for the skin (S_2) at about 300° K. (81° F.) it would be 96,167 Angstroms in the far infrared.

SOURCES OF INFRARED.   As a source of radiant energy becomes warmer, the maximal spectral emission will be in progressively shorter wavelengths. Thus, the emitter may change from black to "red hot" to "white hot." Glowing red heating units (1000° K.), even though they are emitting some energy in the red portion of the visible spectrum, still emit the major portion of their energy in the far infrared region, with maximal emittance at 29,000 Angstroms. The incandescent bulb with its extremely hot (3000° K.) filament units emits much of its energy in the near infrared region with a maximal emittance at 9600 Angstroms. The glass envelope is also hot and secondarily emits infrared energy. Although the filament is emitting through the whole visible spectrum and into the ultraviolet, the ultraviolet rays are unable to penetrate the glass.

Therapeutic Devices for Infrared Heating.   FAR INFRARED.   Considerably less use is made of these devices currently than of the near infrared sources. Heated carborundum rods or glowing wire coils are backed by suitable reflectors.

Near Infrared.   Incandescent bulbs of various strengths are available. Some have a built-in aluminized reflector and, most commonly, are of 250 watt strength, with a clear glass lens. A similar bulb with a lens of red glass has a less glaring visible emanation, but the lens is more likely to have imperfections which produce "hot spots" in the area being heated.

If the bulb does not have a built-in reflector, it will heat more efficiently if the socket is mounted in a reflector. The reflector will, of course, have a secondary emanation of heat more in the far infrared.

The pattern of heating will be markedly influenced by the geometric characteristics of the reflector. With some reflectors, a spotlight effect will be produced, with others, a floodlight effect. The use of several ordinary incandescent bulbs under a cradle-type canopy throws a fairly even intensity of heat over a relatively large area.

A relatively long, thin, quartz-contained infrared source in a rectangular reflector has also been found to provide fairly even heating over a large surface.

Dosage Factors.   *Duration* is usually 30 to 45 minutes. The maximal effect on arterial circulation is not attained in less than 20 minutes.

Intensity should be such that the heat is easily tolerated by the patient. The intensity can readily be controlled by varying the distance from the heat source to the skin (bearing in mind that the intensity of heating from a point source will vary inversely with the square of this distance). If the heat is too intense, blotchy areas of vasoconstriction may appear against a background of vasodilation. A subject with white skin will show blotchy white areas on a pink background (erythema ab igne), and this area may later have a blotchy pigmentation.

Draping of the device with towels to decrease *air movement* across the heated area is often employed. Care must be taken that the draping material does not ignite. Deliberate cooling of the surface by an electric fan at the same time that heating is going on has been suggested. The objective is to heat the deeper part of the skin (and subsequently deeper tissues) without heating the surface. This practice is rarely followed in the United States.

The *distances* usually employed with incandescent sources are from 15 to 24 inches, depending on the size of the source and the tolerance of the subject.

Advantages of Use of Infrared.   This method has the advantage of being clean, of permitting observation of the part being heated any time during the heating, of permitting elevation of the part being heated, of easy modification of the intensity of heating, and of ease of use in the home.

Disadvantages of Use of Infrared.   The disadvantages are that it may cause undesirable drying of surface, the incandescent bulb may break (rarely), with hot glass falling on the patient (when possible, it is preferable to heat the patient from the side rather than from directly above), the heating is superficial (but elevation of temperature of the deeper tissues does occur), and the field of maximal intensity of heating may be circumscribed with some devices.

Convective Heating

Physics of Convective Heating.   Convection involves the exchange of heat between a surface and a fluid moving past the surface. The transfer of heat is by conduction to the molecular layer of the fluid immediately adjacent to the surface and thence through consecutive molecular layers that are moving progressively more rapidly with respect to the surface.

Convective heat exchange can be considered mathematically as a special case of conduction in which, in addition to the thermal gradient, the factors of area and time are involved. Other factors that are pertinent include the velocity of movement of the fluid, the viscosity of the fluid, the density of the fluid, the specific heat of the fluid, and the thermal conductivity of the fluid.

Therapeutic Devices. AGITATED-WATER BATHS. Heat exchanged in a whirlpool bath or any other stirred-water bath is exchanged by convection. The water temperatures employed will vary with the state of the peripheral circulation and the amount of the body to be immersed. Immersion of one or two limbs for 30 minutes is usually done at temperatures from 40.0° to 43.0° C. (104.0° to 109.4° F.). A normal person would experience burning at 47.0° C. (116.6° F.).

Immersion of the trunk and all four extremities in water at 38.8° C. (102.0° F.) will induce a mild fever in most persons. Total-immersion baths that are warmer than this are used for persons able to tolerate the induction of fever (see also Chapter 12, Hydrotherapy).

MOIST-AIR BATHS. Hot air at about 40.0° to 45.0° C. (104.0° to 113.0° F.) that is saturated with water vapor is circulated by a blower. It may be applied to part of the body or to most of it. To the extent that it interferes with loss of heat from the body, it will tend to induce fever, but as applied to the average-sized adult, no fever is induced. The patient must be dried well immediately after treatment to minimize chilling due to evaporation.

HOT-AIR BATHS. Various devices have been employed to produce forced convection of hot air about parts or all of the body. The low heat content of the air and the cooling by evaporation of sweat render these methods relatively inefficient for therapeutic heating or induction of fever.

THERAPEUTIC COLD

Physiologic Effects. In many respects, the physiologic effects of cold are the opposite of the effects of heat. Cooling the tissues is associated with a decrease in their metabolism. Arteriolar vasoconstriction probably occurs because of the decreased formation of metabolites and the local action of cold on the minute vessels; in addition, in the skin, the vasoconstriction acts reflexly as a component of the thermoregulatory response of the organism. Cooling during ischemia reduces the subsequent reactive hyperemia in both skin and skeletal muscle.

The vasoconstriction is associated with a decreased tendency to edema formation and decreased lymph production. This is so even though cold also induces venous constriction with some elevation of venous pressure. The delivery of nutrients and phagocytes to the region is decreased, and the phagocytic action of the latter is diminished. The convective heat exchange associated with blood flow is concomitantly reduced so that the lowering of the temperature of deeper tissues is less impeded. Thus, cold is more penetrating than heat. Furthermore, because of the countercurrent heat exchange between the blood in the arteries and that in the venae comitantes, the arterial blood that reaches the acral parts is several degrees cooler than the core temperature.

With extreme degrees of cooling, as by immersion in a mixture of ice and water, periodic bursts of vasodilatation occur; this was named the "hunting reaction" by the late Sir Thomas Lewis. Vasodilatation is believed to occur principally in the arteriovenous anastomoses, possibly by the axon reflex mechanism.[5] The ease with which it occurs is modified by the ambient temperature which, when lower, tends to inhibit the vasodilating episodes. Failure of the vasodilatation to occur may lead to injury to the local tissues by cold.

Chilling a sufficient area of the surface of the skin or lowering the core temperature of the body (more specifically of the hypothalamus) induces shivering, which tends to raise the core temperature by increasing heat production. Such a threat to the constancy of the core temperature also causes a reflex constriction in the cutaneous vascular beds of other parts of the body. In some persons, the arterial blood pressure may increase.

Over a relatively narrow range, the conduction velocities in human peripheral nerves are reduced by 2.4m./sec./°C. of cooling.[8] Local cooling of the saphenous nerve in cats showed that the small unmyelinated fibers were more resistant to blocking by cooling than were the larger myelinated fibers.[3] However, within the "A" group of fibers, the smaller fibers were more sensitive to cooling than were the larger fibers. Gamma-motor fibers were more easily blocked than were alpha-motor fibers. If the length of nerve blocked is too short (for example, 2 mm.), saltatory conduction across the block may occur, but this was not observed when a length of 20 mm. was cooled. The order of susceptibility to blockage by cold was greatest in the small medullated fibers (22.0° C., 71.6° F.), least in unmedullated fibers (5.0° to 10.0° C., 41.0° to 50.0° F.), and intermediate in the large medullated fibers (12.0° C., 53.6° F.).

Largely because cooling at the cathode was effective whereas cooling at the anode was ineffective, Schoepfle and Erlanger decided that these effects of cooling in the axon are due to reduction of the local membrane excitability.[18] The ascent and descent of the spike potential were both considerably prolonged, and the absolute refractory period was increased.

In man, the order of loss of function is first the senses of light touch and cold, secondly motor power, thirdly vasoconstriction, and finally pain and gross pressure.[5] The sensations experienced by the subject to whom ice is applied were said by Grant to be successively an appreciation of cooling, a sensation of burning or aching, and finally, and after 5 to 7 minutes, relative cutaneous anesthesia.[6]

Not particularly relevant to the present discussion is the effect of localized cooling in the central nervous system in the cat. Siegfried and associates noted, between 20.0° C. (68.0° F.) and 5.0° C. (41.0° F.), a reduction of evoked potentials in the optic chiasm to 50 per cent of normal and abolition at 0.0° C. (32.0° F.).[19] Evoked activity of the temporalis muscle was abolished by cooling the internal capsule to 5.0° C. (41.0° F.).

Neuromuscular transmission was impaired in the rat with cooling at 15.0° C. (59.0° F.), and was blocked at 5.0° C. (41.0° F.)[10] At 5.0° C., nerve conduction had not yet failed, and miniature end-plate potentials were still recorded. After neuromuscular transmission was blocked by cooling, the muscle still responded to direct stimulation. In the frog, neuromuscular transmission was impaired by temperatures below 5.0° C. (41.0° F.) and blocked completely at −1.0° C. (30.2° F.).[11]

The cooling of muscle may reduce its efficiency by increasing its viscosity. There is some possibility that contraction of the superficial fibers may not occur.[5] Clinically, persons with moderate weakness may be temporarily weaker when cooled.

Chatfield noted that the twitch tension in the rat gastrocnemius in response to single shocks was greatest at 18.0° to 26.0° C. (64.4° to 78.8° F.).[1] The twitch duration was prolonged at the lower temperatures, enabling better fusion of tetanic contraction with a stronger tetanic tension.

Eldred and associates have reported on the effects of cooling the muscle spindles of the cat gastrocnemius.[4] With the "de-efferented" spindle, the frequency of firing of the primary and secondary endings varied linearly with temperature from 38.0° C. (100.4° F.) to 28.0° C. (82.4° F.) when the frequency was reduced by 50 to 80 per cent. Below 25.0° C. (77.0° F.) the firing became irregular, and below 20.0° C. (68.0° F.) the firing stopped. The primary ending was a little more sensitive than the secondary ending. Because the Golgi tendon apparatus was also rendered less sensitive by cooling, they reasoned that these changes were brought about by changes in membrane stability in the sensory terminals themselves.

Spindles with efferents intact also showed a decrease in firing when cooled. The monosynaptic reflex was nearly abolished by cooling the muscle 10.0° C. (18.0° F.), as was decerebrate rigidity. Lippold and associates noted the beginning of spontaneous firing of the primary spindle afferents of the cat at 32.0° C. (89.6° F.), and a decrease in firing commencing at 28.0° C. (82.4° F.).[12] Firing ceased at 15.0° C. (59.0° F.). Newton and Lehmkuhl,[15] observing that elevation of the temperature of the body increased the frequency in firing of the spindle afferents while cooling of the muscle decreased it, suggested that the technique of DonTigny and Sheldon[2] has merit. In this technique, sufficient heating is applied to prevent shivering, while local cooling of the muscle is used to reduce spasm or spasticity. Petajan and Watts observed that the relaxation phase of the myotatic reflex was increased in man and spasticity was reduced, often for several hours, after 15 or 30 minutes of cooling.[16] The mechanism of this reduction is not clear, but they believed that it is not a result of direct cooling of the muscle spindle and that it is more likely related to blocking of the efferents to the spindle or to the slowing of the contraction and relaxation processes in the extrafusal fibers. In man, Miglietta observed a reduction in clonus for several hours after immersion of the part in a whirlpool bath at 18.3° C. (65.0° F.).[13] The cooling of connective tissue around joints may diminish the ease and precision of movement, again, probably because of increased viscosity.

Indications for Local Cooling. Local cooling is used to reduce extravasation of blood and fluid into the tissues after trauma, to reduce pain and the reflex muscle spasm accompanying it, to reduce spasticity, to preserve the viability of parts when their circulation is temporarily inadequate, and to retard the development of gangrene in an ischemic limb. Plechas pointed out that in the last instance "withdrawal of refrigeration without amputation produces disastrous effects; therefore, permission to amputate should precede refrigeration."[17]

Contraindications to Local Cooling. Some patients react excessively to the application of cold, with an abrupt increase in arterial blood pressure. Those who suffer from the Raynaud phenomenon usually do not tolerate cooling either of the affected digits or of other parts of the body. The fibrositic stiffness of rheumatoid disease is usually aggravated by cooling. With efficient methods of cooling, particularly in patients whose cutaneous circulation cannot respond with the "hunting reaction," frostbite is a hazard. Horton and associates reported the rather uncommon hypersensitivity to cold characterized by the development of wheals, flushing of the face, and a tendency to syncope.[9]

About 25 per cent of these persons experienced syncope after swimming, and a few needed to be rescued from the water. The reaction could be induced by immersion of one hand in water at 8.0° C. (46.4° F.) for 6 minutes, a practice which is currently not rare in athletic training rooms.

METHODS OF THERAPEUTIC COOLING

Immersion. Immersion is usually begun in cold water, to which ice is added. The total immersion lasts for 10 to 20 minutes. Less vigorous cooling at 10.0° to 18.0° C. (50.0° to 64.4° F.) may serve to reduce spasticity.

Cold Packs. These may be made of ice wrapped in wet toweling or of ice-filled plastic or rubber bags. Commercially available reusable cold packs can be kept refrigerated until ready to be used. If kept in a "zero freezer" (−17.7° C., 0.0° F.) in a household variety of refrigerator, the pack will be below the freezing temperature when applied and should not be placed in direct contact with the skin.

Cryokinetics. This term was coined by Hayden[7] for a treatment concept described by her and by Grant[6] in which local cooling of the part is followed by active exercise to mobilize the parts. Cooling is accomplished either by immersion in cold water with added ice for 10 to 20 minutes or by rubbing the surface of the skin for 5 to 7 minutes with ice ("ice massage"). This produces a mild analgesia, which permits the active exercise to be done. The method is considered to be particularly effective in recent acute strains. Most of their subjects returned to duty the same day that the treatment began.

Combined Local Cooling and Remote Heating. This has been suggested by DonTigny and Sheldon as a method to reduce muscle spasm or spasticity.[2] The remote heating maintains the core temperature and thus inhibits shivering and the central augmentation of muscle spindle activity. Reports on the clinical efficacy of this technique are sparse.

REFERENCES

1. Chatfield, P. O.: Hypothermia and Its Effects on the Sensory and Peripheral Motor Systems. Ann. N. Y. Acad. Sci., *80:*445-448, 1959.
2. DonTigny, R. L., and Sheldon, K. W.: Simultaneous Use of Heat and Cold in Treatment of Muscle Spasm. Arch. Phys. Med., *43:*235-237, 1962.
3. Douglas, W. W., and Malcolm, J. L.: The Effect of Localized Cooling on Conduction in Cat Nerves. J. Physiol. (London), *130:*53-71, 1955.
4. Eldred, E., Lindsley, D. F., and Buchwald, J. S.: The Effect of Cooling on Mammalian Muscle Spindles. Exp. Neurol., *2:*144-157, 1960.
5. Fox, R. H.: Local Cooling in Man. Brit. Med. Bull., *17:*14-18, 1961.
6. Grant, A. E.: Massage With Ice (Cryokinetics) in the Treatment of Painful Conditions of the Musculoskeletal System. Arch. Phys. Med., *45:*233-238, 1964.
7. Hayden, C. A.: Cryokinetics in an Early Treatment Program. J. Amer. Phys. Ther. Ass., *44:*990-993, 1964.
8. Henriksen, J. D.: Conduction Velocity of Motor Nerves in Normal Subjects and Patients With Neuromuscular Disorders. Thesis, Mayo Graduate School of Medicine (University of Minnesota), Rochester, 1956.
9. Horton, B. T., Brown, G. E., and Roth, G. M.: Hypersensitiveness to Cold: With Local and Systemic Manifestations of a Histamine-Like Character; Its Amenability to Treatment. J.A.M.A., *107:*1263-1268, 1936.

10. Li, C.-L.: Effect of Cooling on Neuromuscular Transmission in the Rat. Amer. J. Physiol., *194*:200–206, 1958.
11. Li, C.-L., and Gouras, P.: Effect of Cooling on Neuromuscular Transmission in the Frog. Amer. J. Physiol., *192*:464–470, 1958.
12. Lippold, O. C. J., Nicholls, J. G., and Redfearn, J. W. T.: Study of the Afferent Discharge Produced by Cooling a Mammalian Muscle Spindle. J. Physiol. (London), *153*:218-231, 1960.
13. Miglietta, O.: Electromyographic Characteristics of Clonus and the Influence of Cold. Arch. Phys. Med., *45*:508–512, 1964.
14. Mills, C. A.: Infra-red Heat Transfer Principles: Application to Man. In Glasser, O.: Medical Physics. Chicago, Year Book Medical Publishers, Inc., 1960, Vol. 3, pp. 299–302.
15. Newton, M. J., and Lehmkuhl, D.: Muscle Spindle Response to Body Heating and Localized Muscle Cooling: Implications for Relief of Spasticity. J. Amer. Phys. Ther. Ass., *45*:91–105, 1965.
16. Petajan, J. H., and Watts, N.: Effects of Cooling on the Triceps Surae Reflex. Amer. J. Phys. Med., *41*:240–251, 1962.
17. Plechas, N. P.: Refrigeration in Surgery. Ann. West. Med. Surg., *2*:552–557, 1948.
18. Schoepfle, G. M., and Erlanger, J.: The Action of Temperature on the Excitability, Spike Height and Configuration, and the Refractory Period Observed in the Responses of Single Medullated Nerve Fibers. Amer. J. Physiol., *134*:694-704, 1941.
19. Siegfried, J., Ervin, F. R., Miyazaki, Y., and Mark, V. H.: Localized Cooling of the Central Nervous System. I. Neurophysiological Studies in Experimental Animals. J. Neurosurg., *19*:840-852, 1962.

SUPPLEMENTAL READING

Benzinger, T. H.: Heat Regulation: Homeostasis of Central Temperature in Man. Physiol. Rev., *49*:671–759, 1969.
Coulter, J. S.: Physical Therapy: Heat and Cold. In Glasser, O.: Medical Physics. Chicago, Year Book Medical Publishers, Inc., 1944, Vol. 1, pp. 1043–1054.
Erickson, D. J.: Physical Medicine: Light. In Glasser, O.: Medical Physics. Chicago, Year Book Medical Publishers, Inc., 1960, Vol. 3, pp. 455–456.
Krusen, F. H., and Elkins, E. C.: Physical Therapy: Light. In Glasser, O.: Medical Physics. Chicago, Year Book Medical Publishers, Inc., 1944, Vol. 1, pp. 1054–1068.
Krusen, F. H., and Elkins, E. C.: Physical Medicine: Light. In Glasser, O.: Medical Physics. Chicago, Year Book Medical Publishers, Inc., 1950, Vol. 2, pp. 715–717.
Licht, S.: Therapeutic Heat and Cold. Ed. 2, New Haven, Connecticut, Elizabeth Licht, 1965.
Murphy, A. J.: The Physiological Effects of Cold Application. Phys. Ther. Rev., *40*:112–115, 1960.

Chapter 11

DIATHERMY

by Justus F. Lehmann

Definition. For therapeutic purposes, diathermy is defined as deep heating.

Rationale for Selection of Diathermy Modalities

Heating of the superficial tissues produces only a few mild physiologic and therapeutic reactions, mostly reflex in nature, while on the other hand, many desired biologic and therapeutic effects can be obtained readily by employing diathermy for heating the deep tissues directly. The practical complication to avoid is that of burning the intervening tissues while raising the temperatures in deeper structures to a therapeutic range. This indicates the need for the highest temperature produced throughout the tissues to be at the area being treated. By varying the dosage, the temperature developed can be varied within the therapeutic range. Thus, when the temperature distribution produced by any given diathermy modality is known, the physician is in a position to select the most effective modality for a specific problem. This information, together with other physiologic and pathophysiologic data related to the specific effects of heat on tissues, would allow the clinician to be more discriminating in the selection of the appropriate procedure. Beyond the heating effects of a modality, an additional factor of importance that should be included in this consideration is the possibility of producing certain still little understood nonthermal biologic reactions.

Three types of diathermy modalities are used for therapeutic purposes: shortwave, ultrasound and microwave. The energy of shortwave diathermy is transferred into the deeper tissue layers by a high frequency current; ultrasound utilizes a high frequency acoustic vibration which penetrates into the deeper tissue layers; microwave diathermy is propagated by means of electromagnetic radiation. The type of heating produced by these diathermy modalities is called heating by conversion, since the various types of energy penetrating the deeper tissue layers are finally converted into heat.

Physiologic Effects of Therapeutic Significance

Local Effects. These are produced locally, partly through a direct effect of the elevated temperature on the cellular functions and partly through axon and other reflexes. The temperature receptors may play an important role.[1]

The blood flow is increased owing to arteriolar and capillary dilatation. The rate of filtration and of diffusion across biologic membranes is increased. There may be a greater capillary membrane permeability with a resulting escape of plasma proteins. Vigorous heating may result in cellular responses associated with an inflammatory reaction, ranging from mild to severe degrees.[2, 3] The tissue metabolism is initially increased, as a result of the temperature elevation. If temperatures are elevated extensively for a prolonged period of time, tissue metabolism may be decreased.[4-6]

Associated with the changes in metabolic rate are changes in enzyme reactions. These may be speeded up by moderate tissue temperature elevation and may be gradually abolished at higher temperatures. This may be explained by the fact that the rate of the chemical reaction is increased by temperature elevation while the protein component of the enzyme system is destroyed at higher temperatures. Proteins may be denatured and the resulting products, such as polypeptides and histamine-like substances, in turn may become biologically effective.

There is marked alteration of the physical properties of fibrous tissues as found in tendons, joint capsules, and scars.[7] These tissues yield much more readily to stretch when heated.[8] This effect is illustrated in Figure 11-1. In this experiment the tendon was loaded at 73 grams in a 25° C. bath. The length of the tendon was maintained, and the tension decreased slightly. When the temperature of the bath was changed from 25° to 45° the tension deteriorated rapidly. Figure 11-2 shows the increase in length if various loads were applied at 45° C. It shows clearly that at 45° a marked increase in length could be

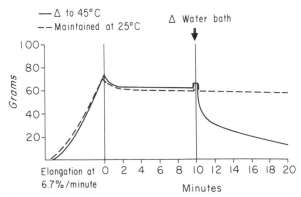

Figure 11–1 The effect of temperature elevation on tendon extensibility. (From Lehmann et al.: Effects of Therapeutic Temperatures on Tendon Extensibility. Arch. Phys. Med., *51*:481–487, 1970.)

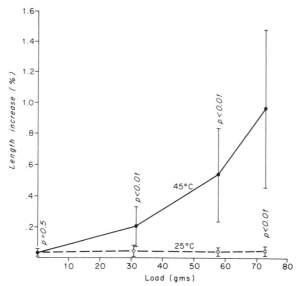

Figure 11–2 Residual tendon length as measured after loading at the indicated levels of 45° C. and 25° C. baths. (From Lehmann et al.: Effects of Therapeutic Temperatures on Tendon Extensibility. Arch. Phys. Med., *51*:481–487, 1970.)

obtained, which increased in proportion to the load. In contrast to this, the controls at 25° C. did not show such an elongation. It can be concluded that heating produces a greater extensibility of fibrous collagen tissues. The optimal condition for obtaining this effect is the combination of heat and stretch application, with cooling before release of stretch. Long steady stretch is more effective than intermittent or short-term stretch. This obviously is of great significance in the management of joint contractures, such as those due to tightness of the joint capsule, fibrosis of muscle and scarring.

Heating of tissues has been shown to affect the gamma fiber activity in muscle.[1] The resulting decrease in the sensitivity of the muscle spindle to stretch, as well as reflexes triggered through temperature receptors, may be the physiologic basis for the clinically observed relaxation of muscle spasm following the use of heat.

Recent investigations by Backlund and Tiselius have shown that the subjective complaints of stiffness on the part of the rheumatoid patient coincide with changes in the measurements of the visco-elastic properties of joints.[9] The joint stiffness could be influenced both subjectively and objectively by measurement, by treatment with drugs such as cortisone, as well as by physical therapy, such as the application of heat and cold. Heat application markedly decreased the stiffness and the patient's discomfort. Cold application increased the stiffness and the patient's discomfort.

Application of heat to a peripheral nerve causes an increase in the pain threshold in the area supplied by the nerve. Also, by heating other tissues such as skin, the pain threshold, as measured with the Wolff-Hardy-Goodell method, is elevated in the area treated.[10]

This brief review of the most significant local reactions to heat application indicates not only that a large number of physiologic responses can be elicited, but also that many of them can be produced to any desired degree.

Reactions Occurring Distant From the Site of Tissue Temperature Elevation.
These reactions are usually produced by elevating the surface temperature of
the body.

If the skin of one part of the body, e.g., over one extremity, is heated, a
consensual response is observed in other parts of the body, e.g., the opposite
extremity. The consensual reaction is always less pronounced than the local
response to heat application, and its degree of intensity is dependent on the
size of the area treated.[1]

If the skin is heated, the vessels of the musculature beneath show no
increase in diameter or may even show a vasoconstriction.[1]

If the skin of the abdominal wall is heated, it has been observed that a
blanching of the gastric mucosa occurs.

Relaxation of the smooth musculature of the gastrointestinal tract during
superficial heat application has also been observed. This is evidenced by the
decrease in peristalsis.[1]

Heating of the superficial tissues produces marked relaxation of the
striated skeletal muscles, and even protective muscle spasms may be resolved.
The reaction may be reflex in nature and be triggered by the effect on the
temperature receptors in the skin. Or this effect may have a strong psychologic
component.

Some reactions may be produced by an elevation of the core temperature
of the body which in turn produces all those reactions which are commonly
found as a part of the mechanism regulating the body temperature.

In summary, the reactions occurring distant from the site of temperature
elevation resulting from heating are limited as to their numbers, as to the site
where they occur and as to the degree to which they may be produced. They
are always less pronounced than the corresponding reactions occurring locally
at the site of temperature elevation.

Factors Determining the Extent of Biologic Reactions

The temperature of the tissues is a most important factor which rather
critically determines the extent of the physiologic response to heat.

Figure 11-3 shows the percentage of hyperemia occurring in a series of
560 experimental animals plotted against the tissue temperature.[3] The duration of the tissue temperature elevation was kept constant. Below a certain
temperature threshold no reactions are observed. The curve of reactions is S
shaped with the most rapid increase in the percentage of reactions in the
midrange. In the upper portion of the curve destructive changes are inevitably
associated with the therapeutically desirable hyperemia. Thus the therapeutic
temperature range is a rather narrow one and extends in this particular
reaction between approximately 43° C. (109.4° F.) and 45° C. (113° F.). It is
apparent that any minor change in tissue temperature produces a major
change in the degree of the physiologic response and that the margin of
effectiveness and safety is narrow.

In a similar type of experiment it was found that the duration of the tissue
temperature elevation was important in determining the extent of the biologic
reaction (Fig. 11-4).[3] It seems that a minimal effective duration of exposure is
three to five minutes, whereas complete reactions were obtained after exposure
of approximately 30 minutes. The tissue temperature was kept constant
throughout the experiment.

The rate of the rise of temperature also played a role in determining the
extent of the biologic response. This is owing in part to the fact that of the total

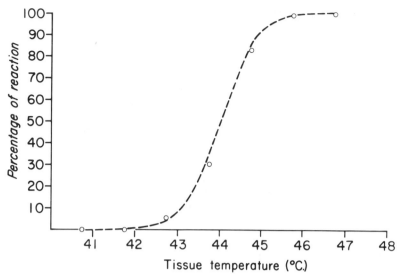

Figure 11–3 Dependence of hyperemia on tissue temperature. (From Lehmann. The Bio-physical Basis of Biologic Ultrasonic Reactions with Special Reference to Ultrasonic Therapy. Arch. Phys. Med., vol. 34, 1953.)

period of heat application, only that limited portion will be biologically effective during which an effective temperature level is obtained in the tissues. Thus a modality which will rapidly raise the temperature to biologically effective levels will produce a more pronounced effect than a modality which raises the tissue temperature more slowly, provided that both modalities are applied over the same period of time.

In addition, it has been noted that some physiologic responses of tempera-

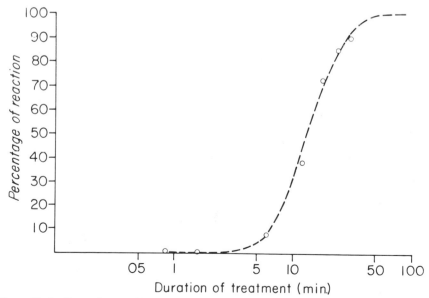

Figure 11–4 Dependence of hyperemia on duration of treatment. (From Lehmann. The Bio-physical Basis of Biologic Ultrasonic Reactions with Special Reference to Ultrasonic Therapy. Arch. Phys. Med., vol. 34, 1953.)

ture receptors seem to be more pronounced when the rate of the tissue temperature elevation is rapid.[10-14]

The degree to which some reactions induced by reflexes occur may depend on the size of the area treated.[1]

In summary, the major factors determining the number and intensity of the physiologic reactions to heat are:

1. The level of tissue temperature. The approximate therapeutic range extends between 40 and 45.5° C. (104 and 113.9° F.).

2. The duration of the tissue temperature elevation. The approximate therapeutic range is 3 to 30 minutes.

3. The rate of temperature rise in the tissues.

4. The size of the area treated.

For practical heat therapy the physiologic responses can be grouped into two categories: vigorous heating and mild heating.

Vigorous Heating.   With vigorous heating the highest temperature is produced at the site of the pathologic lesion or where the therapeutic response is desired; the tissue temperature is elevated close to the tolerance level; the effective elevation of the tissue temperature is maintained for a relatively long period of time and the rate of rise of the tissue temperature is rapid.

Vigorous heating is most often used in chronic disease processes, as for treatment of joint contractures when scarring and tightening of the joint capsule and the periarticular structures have occurred. It will increase the temperature in the scar tissues to a level where they become more extensible and thus more amenable to therapy designed to increase the range of motion. Chronic pelvic inflammatory disease represents another indication for vigorous heating. A marked increase in vascularity is produced which may assist in the resolution of the pathologic process or may render antibiotic therapy more effective.

On the other hand, vigorous heating is contraindicated in an acute inflammatory process since it will superimpose another severe inflammatory reaction which ultimately may lead to undesirable tissue necrosis.[15] An acute protruded intervertebral disk impinging upon a nerve root in the intervertebral foramen represents a contraindication since any marked temperature elevation at the site of the encroachment will produce an increase in vascularity and edema, which are space-occupying processes and may aggravate the symptoms.

Mild Heating.   With mild heating a relatively low temperature is obtained in the tissues at the site of the pathologic lesion or the highest temperature is produced in a superficial tissue distant from the site of the lesion; effective tissue temperature is usually maintained for a relatively short period of time; the rate of the rise of temperature in the tissues is often slow. Mild heating is often used in more subacute disease processes.

Selection of Modality

In order to produce vigorous heating the tissue temperature must be elevated close to tolerance levels at the site of the pathologic lesion. This means that one must select the modality which will produce the highest temperature at the site of the lesion without exceeding tolerance levels either in the overlying or underlying tissues. In order to select the proper modality for this purpose it is important to know the temperature distribution produced by the various deep heating devices, the factors which will predetermine this tissue temperature distribution and the absolute temperature obtained within the distribution.

If mild heating is desired, there is a choice between superficial heating agents, such as infrared, hot packs, hot soaks, paraffin baths and others, and a deep heating modality which is applied in such a way as to limit the rise of the tissue temperature to moderate levels at the site of the lesion. However, if small parts of the body are treated, such as the fingers, even a superficial heating agent if injudiciously applied may produce a marked elevation of the temperature in the deeper tissues, thus producing vigorous heating effects which might be contraindicated.

Factors Determining Tissue Temperature Distribution

The relative amount of energy converted into heat at any given point throughout the tissues is of importance. This is called the pattern of "relative heating." The amount of energy converted into heat at the level of the interface between the subcutaneous fat and the musculature is customarily set as one. The pattern of relative heating depends on factors which will be discussed for the individual diathermy modalities since these factors vary from one deep heating agent to another.

The tissue temperature distribution in turn depends on the pattern of "relative heating" and on the properties of the tissues, i.e., the specific heat and specific weight. The temperature change is determined by the following formula:

$$\Delta T = H \cdot \text{specific heat} \cdot \text{specific weight}$$

where ΔT is the change in temperature and H is the amount of energy converted into heat. The temperature distribution is also modified by the thermal conductivity of the tissues if heating extends over a period of time long enough to allow for heat exchange to occur.

A temperature distribution thus produced in the live tissues will finally be modified by physiologic factors such as the temperature distribution in the tissues prior to the diathermy exposure and blood flow changes. Usually the skin surface is relatively cool, the core temperature relatively high. Any temperature elevation produced by diathermy application is superimposed upon the pre-existing physiologic temperature distribution. As the diathermy is applied an increase in the blood flow may occur locally as a result of the tissue temperature elevation and since the blood temperature is usually cooler than that of the heated tissue it may act as a cooling agent. A modification of the temperature distribution can be produced in this fashion.

SHORTWAVE DIATHERMY

Equipment

Shortwave diathermy is the therapeutic application of high frequency currents. In spite of many variations, shortwave diathermy machines have three basic components of the circuitry which are common to all. They are power supply, oscillating circuit and the patient circuit. The frequency of the oscillating circuit, and thus of the patient circuit, is rigorously controlled to comply with the tolerances specified by the Federal Communications Commission. The frequencies which are allowed for shortwave diathermy operations are

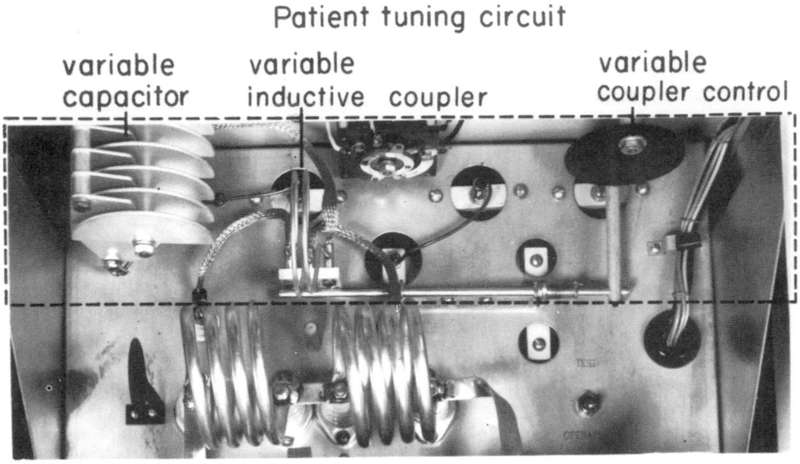

Patient tuning circuit
variable capacitor
variable inductive coupler
variable coupler control

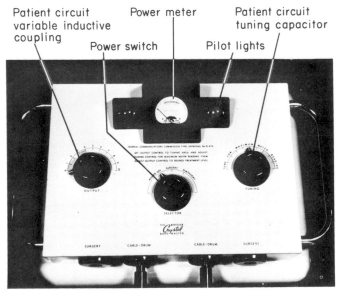

Figure 11–5 Patient tuning circuit of a typical shortwave diathermy machine. (Courtesy of the Birtcher Corporation.)

Patient circuit variable inductive coupling
Power meter
Patient circuit tuning capacitor
Power switch
Pilot lights
OUTPUT
SELECTOR
TUNING
SURGERY
CABLE-DRUM
CABLE-DRUM
SURGERY

Figure 11–6 Typical control panel of a shortwave diathermy machine. (Courtesy of the Birtcher Corporation.)

13.66, 27.33 and 40.98 megacycles (Public Notice 7722, Federal Communications Commission). Wavelength is determined by the formula:

$$\lambda = \frac{V}{N}$$

where λ is the wavelength, N is the frequency of oscillation and V is velocity of light. The wavelengths corresponding to the allowed frequencies are 22, 11 and 7.5 meters respectively. Most of the commercially available diathermy machines operate at a frequency of 27.33 megacycles and hence a wavelength of 11 meters.

It is worth noting that in all machines, regardless of the technique of application, the patient's electrical impedance becomes part of the impedance of the patient circuit. It is necessary for any given therapeutic application to retune the patient circuit to resonance after the patient has been inserted into the circuit. Thus the frequency of the patient circuit is made equal to the frequency of the oscillating circuit of the machine. Tuning is often accomplished by adjusting a variable capacitor (Figs. 11–5 and 11–6). The power meter on the panel of the machine will indicate maximal flow of current when the resonance frequency is obtained in the patient circuit. Some machines have eliminated the need for tuning by an automatic tuning device or by designing the patient circuit such that the patient's electrical impedance has a negligible effect on the overall impedance of the patient circuit.

After the machine has been tuned, the current flow through the patient circuit can be regulated. One way of doing this is to change the inductive coupling of the patient and high frequency oscillating circuits. This can be done by varying the coupling of a coil of the patient circuit with another coil of the high frequency oscillating circuit (Figs. 11–5 and 11–6).

Dosimetry

At present it is not possible to measure the high frequency current flow through the body of the patient. The meter on the panel does not give this information. The dosimetry still depends largely on biologic factors—the therapist is guided by the feeling of warmth on the part of the patient. When the dose applied is high the patient's feeling of warmth goes up to tolerance, when the dose is medium he feels comfortably warm and when minimal he just barely feels warmth. Although these are guide lines, it is obvious that they are unreliable for accurate dosimetry and depend on intact sensation and alertness on the part of the patient. However, in the application of pelvic diathermy with an internal electrode it is possible to obtain accurate measurement of the biologically effective dose. Since the electrode is placed in the area of highest temperature elevation in the body, it rapidly assumes the tissue temperature due to the high conductivity of the metal. Therefore, if a thermometer is inserted into the electrode, a direct reading of the tissue temperature can be obtained. The duration of the tissue temperature elevation can be readily controlled by a timing device.

Technique of Application[16]

Condenser Technique. The part of the patient to be treated is placed between two condenser plates. Four modifications of this technique are used. (1) Space plates are condenser plates enclosed in rigid plastic material. A plastic ring surrounding the condenser plate is adjustable and provides for proper spacing between body surface and condenser plates (Fig. 11–7). (2) The condenser plates are covered by a glass envelope. The position of the condenser plate within the glass envelope, and thus the distances between the body surface and the condenser plates are adjustable. (3) The condenser plates are flexible and are enclosed in rubber or plastic materials called condenser pads.

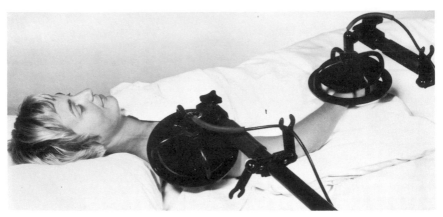

Figure 11–7 Shortwave diathermy application to the arm with condenser plates. Spacing is provided by space plates. (Courtesy of the Burdick Corporation.)

Proper spacing between the skin and the electrode is provided for by a 1 to 2 inch layer of terry cloth between the skin and the pads (Fig. 11-8). (4) Internal metal electrodes are inserted into the vagina or the rectum. The vaginal electrode is inserted with the large diameter fitting the large diameter of the vulva (sagittal plane), then the electrode is turned around by 90 degrees so that the concave part comes to rest under the cervix and the upper portion in the posterior fornix of the vagina. The rectal electrode is inserted to fit the slightly concave part over the prostate. A large belt-like electrode is applied over the abdomen, thus producing a high current density around the internal electrode (Fig. 11-9). The largest internal electrodes that fit should be used, to provide for complete contact with the surrounding tissues. If the contact is partial, current concentrations may occur and lead to burns.

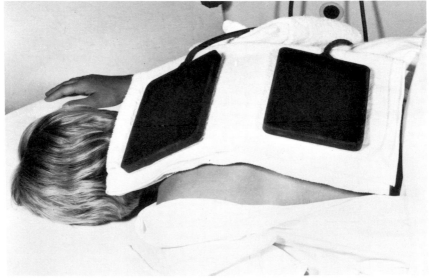

Figure 11–8 Shortwave diathermy application with condenser pads to back, with spacing between skin and electrodes provided by layers of terry cloth. (Courtesy of the Birtcher Corporation.)

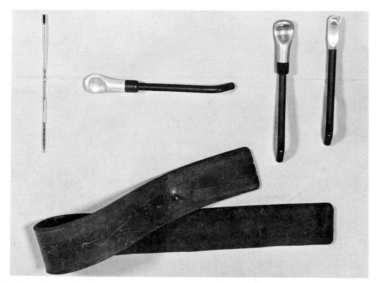

Figure 11–9 Internal vaginal and rectal electrodes with external belt and alcohol thermometer. (Courtesy of the Burdick Corporation.)

Induction Coil Application. Another mode of application is with the induction coil which also requires tuning of the patient circuit to resonance. The induction coil may be applied with the so-called "drum" (Fig. 11-10). The coil is enclosed in a plastic container which is flexible at hinges and can be molded to fit the body. This plastic housing provides for proper spacing between the skin and loops of the cable. Another applicator of this type is the "Monode" which operates on the same basic principle but is not flexible (Fig. 11-11).[17]

A heavily insulated cable can be shaped to any desired form of applicator, such as a "pancake" coil (Fig. 11-12), or it may be wrapped around a joint (Fig. 11-13). Spacers are used to keep the loops apart. Special precautions must be taken to insure that the cable turns do not cross each other, or if this is inevitable, a special separator must be inserted between the turns of the cable. In all these cases of cable application the proper spacing between the skin and the loops of the cable is provided by an insertion of a 1 to 2 inch thickness of terry cloth between the skin and the cable.

Special Techniques of Application to Specific Parts of the Body

To the Shoulder. Condenser plates, pads or the drum are usually used (Figs. 11-7, 11-8, 11-10).

To the Elbows. Condenser plates, pads or wraparound coils are commonly used (Figs. 11-7, 11-8, 11-13).

To the Hands. The method of choice is usually the application of condenser plates either in the form of pads or space plates (Figs. 11-7, 11-8).

To the Back. Condenser plates, the pancake coil or the drum are used (Figs. 11-7, 11-8, 11-10, 11-12). The depth of penetration is relatively poor with this type of application.

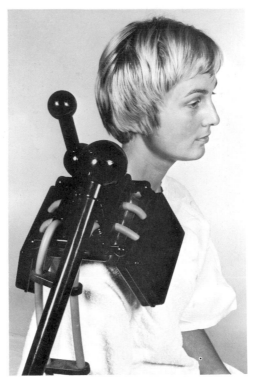

Figure 11–10 Shortwave diathermy application with induction coil (drum applicator). (Courtesy of the Birtcher Corporation.)

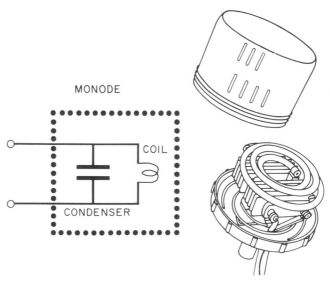

Figure 11–11 Monode applicator with wiring diagram. (Courtesy of Siemens-Reiniger Werke Ag.)

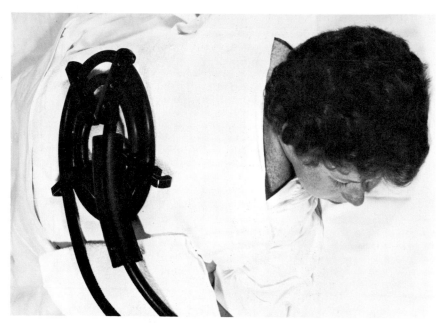

Figure 11–12 Shortwave diathermy application to back with induction coil (pancake coil). Spacing between coil and skin is provided by layers of terry cloth. (Courtesy of the Burdick Corporation.)

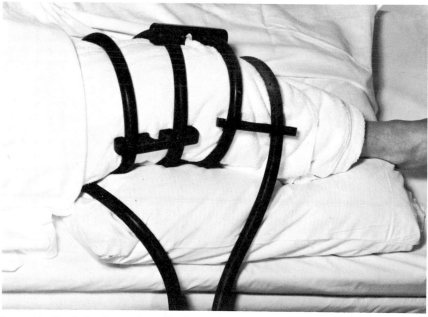

Figure 11–13 Induction coil application to knee, with spacing provided by layers of terry cloth. (Courtesy of the Burdick Corporation.)

To the Neck. Condenser plates, pads, the drum and the pancake coil are used (Figs. 11-7, 11-8, 11-10, 11-12).

To the Head. Application to the eyes and to the paranasal sinuses is shown in Figures 11–14 and 11–15.

To the Hip.[18] The usual method is with pads, the drum or pancake coil, or using coil and pad (Figs. 11-8, 11-10, 11-12, 11-13).

To the Knees and Ankles. Condenser plates, pads and wraparound coil are used (Figs. 11-7, 11-8, 11-13).

To the Pelvic Organs. The method of choice is application with internal electrodes. The temperature elevation is measured with an alcohol thermometer inside the electrodes. Temperatures up to 45° C. (113° F.) have been recom-

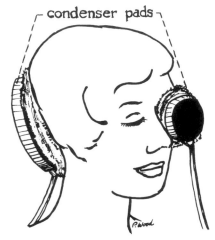

Figure 11–14 Condenser pad application of shortwave to the eye, with spacing provided by layers of terry cloth.

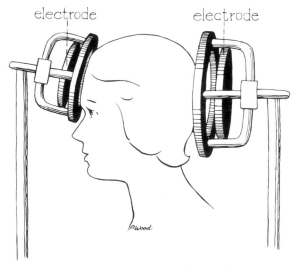

Figure 11–15 Condenser plate application to the frontal sinuses, with spacing provided by space plates.

mended and duration of application varies from 5 to 30 minutes. Often it is advisable to start with a lower temperature and shorter durations and observe the tolerance of the patient. Actually, it is most important to realize that the more acute the process to be treated, the less the tissue temperature elevation should be and the shorter the duration of the treatment.

Precautions. Special precautions must be taken with all techniques of application. The patient should be undressed for the application. All metallic objects, such as watches or jewelry, should be removed. Patient should be positioned on a wooden plinth or chair. These precautions are necessary since selective heating of metal parts could occur because of current concentration. For this same reason the accumulation of sweat beads should be prevented by using terry cloth. Tuning of the patient circuit should always be done at the low output level to prevent excessive heating from an uncontrolled surge of current through the patient. The tuning of the patient circuit should be optimal. Then the output of the machine should be adjusted to the desired level. If this procedure is not followed, small movements of the patient may change the impedance of the circuit in such a fashion that resonance occurs and the current flow may be greatly increased without the therapist's being aware of it. An increase in dose and possibly burns may result.

The fluid media of the eye should be treated with low dosage since selective heating may take place.

CARDIAC PACEMAKERS. Physicians and therapists using shortwave diathermy should be cognizant of the high potential for hazardous interference with electronic cardiac pacemakers.

These devices are very susceptible to dysfunction in patients treated with shortwave diathermy or in persons who might operate the shortwave apparatus or be in its very close proximity. The greatest danger exists for the person wearing a pacemaker of the noncompetitive type, which provides a pulsed output to the heart through one electrode based on information received from the heart through a second electrode. The shortwave energy can produce a signal in the second electrode which mimics the feedback signal from the heart, thereby causing changes in the pacemaker's output. The fixed rate pacemaker is less susceptible to interference since it does not require a feedback signal from the heart. Shortwave diathermy can provide sufficient energy, however, to cause a change in its pulse frequency. A direct application of the shortwave energy to implanted pacemakers can induce currents in the electrode wires of sufficient magnitude to cause burns in the heart tissue or disable the pacemaker permanently. Shortwave diathermy *should not* be used on patients with implanted pacemakers without full recognition of these hazards and should in no circumstances be used to treat the area containing the device or electrode wires.

Biophysics[19]

The temperature distribution produced by the various techniques of shortwave diathermy application varies widely in the tissues. Therefore, it is most important to understand how this temperature distribution is altered by change in the technique of application, since the temperature distribution and the location of the highest temperature elevation in the tissues will determine the selection of the technique of application and of the modality for a given case treated. It is for this reason that biophysical considerations which identify the variation of the temperature distribution resulting from technique of application are important for the clinician.

According to Kirchhoff's law, the greatest amount of heat is developed in the area of greatest current density.

$$H = 0.24 \ I^2RT$$

H is the amount of heat developed, I is the electrical current, R the resistance and T the time. The current distribution depends on the properties of the tissues such as geometry (anatomy), conductivity (specific resistance) and dielectric constant. Tissues can be considered to be in series or in parallel as they are traversed by the high frequency current. If they are in parallel it can be assumed that the greatest current flow will occur in the tissue with the least resistance, that is, the tissue with the highest conductivity. If they are in series the tissue with the greatest resistance will be heated most. The conductivity of tissues is closely related to their water content. The higher the water content, the better the conductivity.[20] Since the water content of musculature is relatively high, muscle tissue is selectively heated. As noted earlier, sweat droplets that accumulate on the skin are selectively heated. Care must be taken to prevent sweat accumulation in order to prevent burns. High current densities are produced in and around metallic surgical implants and may lead to undesirable selective heating of the area. Therefore shortwave treatment is contraindicated in such cases.

In addition, consideration must be given to the technique of application, which is a more important factor for determining the current densities in the tissues than the current distribution in the tissues that results from differences in their conductivities.

If the application is done with condenser plates, the patient is inserted between the plates and the current produced in the tissues will be in proportion to the intensity of the field. The field between the plates shows its greatest intensity close to the plates and rapidly decreases to minimal intensities equidistant between the two plates (Fig. 11-16). Therefore, current densities produced at the surface of the body are usually greater than those at the depths of the tissues in the core of the treated part. Since the most rapid decrease in the

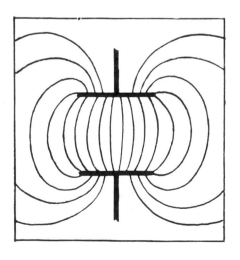

Figure 11–16 Field pattern between two parallel electrodes of equal size. (From Scott: Short Wave Diathermy. In Licht, S.: Therapeutic Heat. New Haven, Conn., Elizabeth Licht, 1958.)

intensity of the field occurs close to the condenser plates, it is important to leave a space of 1 to 2 inches between plates and body surface (Fig. 11–17). This will provide for relatively less heating in the superficial tissues. Even though the surface concentration of the current can be minimized by proper spacing of the electrodes, there will always be a greater field intensity and current density in the superficial tissues than in the deeper tissues when the electrodes are applied to the body surface.

Complete information about the temperature distribution produced throughout the tissues under therapeutic conditions is not available at present.[21] It is important to recognize that the location of the highest tissue temperature in the area treated will depend largely upon the technique of application (Fig. 11–17). Modification of the heat distribution in the body can be provided by variation of the size of the condenser plates and of their application in relation to the body (Figs. 11–8, 11–17B and 11–18). In case of pelvic diathermy application with internal electrodes, special use is made of the

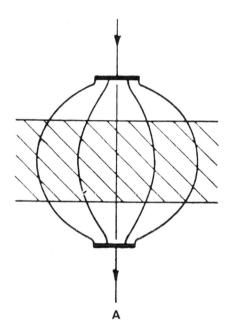

Figure 11–17 *A,* Schematic field pattern that might be expected with proper spacing between tissue and electrodes. (From Schwan: Biophysics of Diathermy. In Licht, S.: Therapeutic Heat. New Haven, Conn., Elizabeth Licht, 1958.) *B,* Schematic field pattern between electrodes of different size.

A

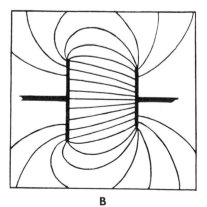

B

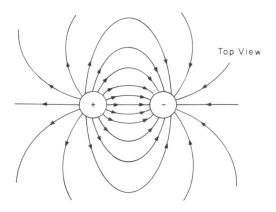

A   Current density proportional
to current flow line density

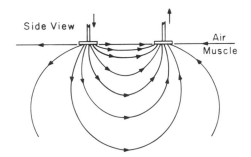

Current density proportional
B   to current flow line density

Figure 11–18   *A*, Schematic drawing of current flow lines in uniform tissues when shortwaves are applied with condenser plates (current density proportional to the current flow line density), top view. *B*, Schematic drawing of current flow lines in uniform tissue when shortwaves are applied with condenser plates, side view. *C*, Schematic drawing of current flow lines in tissue layers when shortwaves are applied with condenser plates in one plane to fat-muscle-tissue layers, side view.

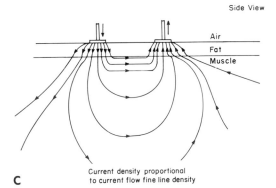

C   Current density proportional
to current flow fine line density

concentration of the field around the small internal electrode (Fig. 11–19). A large pad-like electrode applied over the lower abdomen produces a very low field of concentration in the superficial tissues and the result is that the maximal temperature is obtained in the pelvic organs. Such an effect cannot be duplicated by any other form of deep heating (Fig. 11–20).[22, 23]

     With the use of the induction coil technique there is the production of an alternating magnetic field around the coil which in turn induces a current in

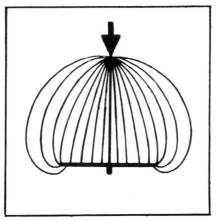

Figure 11–19 Field pattern which might be expected with the use of an internal electrode. (From Scott: Short Wave Diathermy. In Licht, S.: Therapeutic Heat. New Haven, Conn., Elizabeth Licht, 1958.)

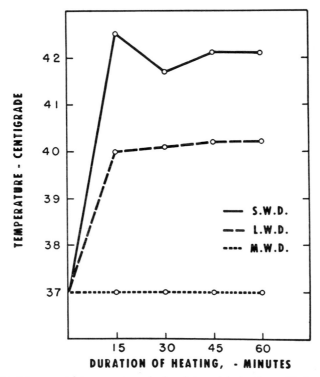

Figure 11–20 Mean rectal temperature during intrapelvic heating with long wave or short-wave diathermy or low abdominal heating with microwave diathermy. (From Kottke: Heat in Pelvic Disease. In Licht, S.: Therapeutic Heat. New Haven, Conn., Elizabeth Licht, 1958.)

the tissues. The current will be strongest where the magnetic field is strongest (Figs. 11-12, 11-13 and 11-21). The field strength, again, is greatest close to the loops of the coil and it rapidly diminishes with increasing distance. Thus there is a tendency to induce a greater current density in the superficial tissues than in the deeper tissues but this can be modified by the technique of application.

It has been demonstrated that if the monode, a helical induction coil applicator, is used the peak temperatures reached in the live human volunteer

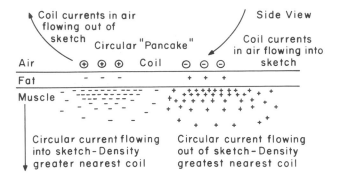

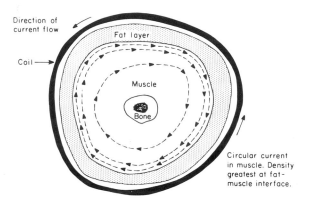

A Horizontal cross section of thigh showing current flow at 27 mc. induced by a solenoidal coil enclosing a limb.

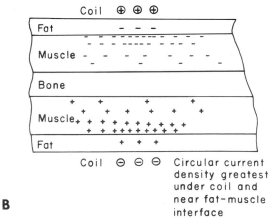

B

Figure 11–21   *A*, Horizontal cross section of thigh showing flow at 27 mc. induced by a Solenoidal coil enclosing a limb (wraparound coil).

B, Longitudinal cross section of thigh with wraparound coil showing current flow at coil and near fat-muscle interface.

are located in the superficial musculature. Thus it is an efficient agent to heat musculature up to a depth of 1 or 2 centimeters.[24, 25]

Physiologic Reactions

Most of the physiologic effects which have been demonstrated to occur as a result of shortwave diathermy applications are due to heating.[26-33]

Clinical Application

General Indications.   All therapeutic effects investigated so far are related to the temperature elevation in the tissues. The temperature distribution in the organism produced by shortwave diathermy application may depend greatly on the technique of application. When applied to joints, such as the hip, that are covered with a *thick soft* tissue layer, shortwave diathermy will not appreciably elevate the temperature in the joint itself.[34] In most such applications, as well as in the applications to the back and the neck, it can be assumed that the highest temperatures will be reached in the subcutaneous tissues and the superficial musculature.[35] Conversely, the highest temperatures are obtained in joints that are covered with a minimal amount of soft tissue. The depth of heating obtained with this modality is between that produced by superficial heating agents such as infrared on the one hand, and low frequency microwave or ultrasound application on the other hand. Thus shortwave diathermy often will produce the highest temperature elevation distant from the site of the pathologic lesion if a joint lesion is being treated and will produce a rather mild, therapeutic reaction which may be mainly reflex in nature and may produce beneficial relief of muscle spasm and pain.

Shortwave diathermy as applied to the musculoskeletal system is usually used to relieve secondary muscle spasm and pain when it occurs as a result of protruded intervertebral disks, degenerative joint disease, sacroiliac strains, bursitis,[36] rheumatoid spondylitis, or in any disease process where a subacute or chronic inflammatory reaction is present in the joint.[37] On the other hand, in joints with minimal soft tissue coverage shortwave diathermy should be considered as a potentially vigorous deep heating agent. In treatment of conditions resulting from trauma, such as sprains and bruises, pain may be relieved and the rate of resolution of the pathologic process may be increased. If the site of lesion is in the more superficial tissues, shortwave diathermy applied with high dosage could be considered a vigorous heating agent and indications and contraindications should be observed correspondingly. If joints that are not covered with a heavy soft tissue mass, such as the knee, elbow and ankle, are treated, better depth of heating is obtained. It is most likely that in these cases the highest temperatures are produced in the joint itself. Also, if small parts, such as the fingers, are treated, very effective deep heating may be obtained.

Shortwave diathermy is the ideal deep heating agent for application to the pelvic organs with internal electrodes.[22, 38] The typical indication for this type of treatment is a chronic pelvic inflammatory disease. The highest temperature is obtained in the tissues to be heated and the problem of dosimetry is solved since the tissue temperature can be measured and controlled. The elevation of the effective tissue temperature can be readily determined. The vascularity in the area is greatly increased. Not only will the resolution of the inflammatory process be speeded up but also antibiotic therapy may become more successful since scarring associated with a lack of vascularity often does not permit establishment of adequate antibiotic levels in the area of the chronic inflammatory process. Sensitive organisms may even be directly affected by the high temperature elevations which can be obtained in the pelvic organs.

Similarly, selective heating can be obtained in the fluid media of the eye. However, the application of the proper dosage is not as well controlled as in pelvic diathermy and must depend on the feeling of warmth on the part of the patient.[39, 40]

Because of its relatively poor depth of penetration, shortwave diathermy has not proved to be more effective than superficial heating for the treatment of pathologic lesions in the abdominal or chest organs. It is rarely used any more in these conditions although such treatment was highly advocated in the past.[41, 42] The clinical claims, however, have not been substantiated on an objective basis.

Treatment of the lower part of the abdomen and back with shortwaves has been recommended to produce a reflex vasodilation in the lower extremities,[43] an effect which is used in peripheral arterial insufficiency and in reflex dystrophies associated with a decrease in blood flow through the extremity.

Contraindications.   Shortwave diathermy should be used only with caution over areas with sensory impairment. Special care is necessary in debilitated patients who are not fully alert, since dosimetry depends to a large degree on the feeling of warmth on the part of the patient. Pain is a warning that excessive heating is occurring.

Shortwave should not be used when it is expected that high current densities could reach surgical metal implants in the tissues.[44, 45] Selective heating of the area of the implant may lead to localized burning, an undesirable side effect.

Scott[46] pointed out that localized heating could occur if the eye is exposed to shortwave while the patient is wearing contact lenses.

Shortwave diathermy should not be applied over ischemic tissues since an increase in the metabolic demand cannot be satisfied by the corresponding vascular response. Pain and tissue necrosis may result.

Pelvic diathermy applied with internal electrodes may produce such an increase in the blood flow to the pelvic organs that the cardiac output is increased markedly. Therefore, pelvic diathermy should be applied only with caution in patients with cardiac disease and borderline decompensation.[22]

Diathermy application over the lower back allegedly has resulted in increase in menstrual flow. Pregnancy is considered a contraindication to shortwave diathermy application.[47, 48] The fetus could be directly affected by pelvic diathermy application; however, it seems doubtful that the high frequency current applied to the back or the abdomen would reach the pregnant uterus. Nevertheless, pregnancy remains a contraindication until evidence to the contrary is available.

Furthermore, the general contraindications to heat therapy should be observed. It is inadvisable to apply shortwave diathermy to malignancies and to patients with hemorrhagic diathesis or thrombophlebitis.

It remains to be investigated whether fluid accumulations in the body cavities, such as the joints and pleural cavity, represent an indication for decreasing the dosage since selective heating of these areas may occur.

Application of Pulsed High Frequency Currents.   Recently the application of pulsed high frequency currents of high intensity has been advocated. The equipment operates at a frequency of 27.12 megacycles. The duration of the pulse is 65 microseconds; the rate of the pulse is adjustable from 80 to 600 per second. The instantaneous energy level of the pulse is adjustable up to 1025 watts. At a pulse rate of 600 per second, the duty cycle is 3.9 per cent. The average radiated power under these conditions is 40 watts. This power is applied by an applicator containing an induction coil. It is claimed that pulsed energy penetrates deeper into the tissues than continuous output. From our present knowledge of the physics or biophysics of high frequency currents there is no evidence suggesting that this is true.[19]

EXPERIMENTAL RESULTS.   Since Muth,[49] Liebesny[50] and Krasny-Ergen[51] discovered that shortwave diathermy application could produce nonthermal effects such as pearl chain formation, the interest in the search for nonthermal effects of the application of high frequency currents has been stimulated in the hope of finding specific clinical indications. The pearl chain formation has been observed when shortwave diathermy was applied to blood or milk samples. The blood cells and the fat globules in the milk aligned in the form of "pearl chains." This phenomenon is probably related to the development of surface charges on the particles. There is no evidence so far that this type of reaction is of therapeutic significance.

The pulsed diathermy application has been developed to produce the nonthermal effects selectively and to minimize the heating effect. If the rate of pulsing is rapid, the heating effect will be in proportion to the average output of the machine, whereas it is conceivable that nonthermal reactions would be produced during the high intensity pulses which require intensity levels above those of the average output.

Thus, nonthermal reactions, as well as thermal ones, that are in proportion to the average intensity can be obtained equally well by continuous wave output. Reactions which require a threshold intensity above that of the average output could be produced by pulsed shortwave application, which would minimize the heating effect and permit the application of high instantaneous intensities during the pulses without burning.

Unfortunately, only the conditions under which pearl chain formation occurs have been investigated in detail. Gersten and co-workers[52] found that the pearl chain formation could be obtained as easily by continuous wave application as with pulsed energy, suggesting that this nonthermal reaction is in proportion to the average output and does not require a high intensity threshold that would provide excessive heating if applied with continuous output. As could be expected, the absorption of the pulsed energy also produced an appreciable rise of temperature in the media exposed.

Cameron[53] applied pulsed shortwaves to experimental wounds in dogs. He found that the transverse alignment of the fibroblasts, the collagen formation, the white cell infiltration, phagocytosis and histiocytic activities, hematoma canalization and fat activity all were speeded up by the application of pulsed shortwaves. Animals that did not receive any shortwave application served as controls. With this type of experimental approach, the question cannot be answered as to whether the observed effects are related to the average output and can be produced as well by low intensity continuous wave application, or whether those effects require the high intensity thresholds as produced during the pulses. Nor can the question be answered as to whether or not these effects are due to the heating effect which inevitably occurs when outputs up to 40 watts are absorbed in the tissues.[52] Only the investigations of Witte and associates[54, 55] used pulsed and continuous wave application of the same average output in order to kill larvae of Drosophila and found the pulsed application to be more effective. They concluded that this resulted either from selective heating or from nonthermal effects. Nadasdi[56] observed that experimental arthritis in rats was less pronounced when they were treated with pulsed shortwave diathermy. Because the controls were animals that were not treated, no conclusions as to the value of the pulsed shortwave application can be drawn. In addition, the joint temperature was not measured during irradiation. It is likely that the tail and limbs are selectively heated since the field will concentrate in these areas.

Erdman[57] applied the pulsed shortwave to the epigastric area and found an increase in the skin temperature of 1.5° C. in the area treated. He also found an increase in the skin temperature of 2.0° C. in the foot and no change in rectal temperature. There was an increase in peripheral pulses of 1.75% of the resting state. Silverman compared the effect of pulsed and continuous shortwave application with the same average power output. He found no differences in the effects on the circulation when these two applications were compared.[58, 59] Other claims are made that the body's defense mechanism to bacterial infection and other disease processes can be stimulated with the application of pulsed shortwave.[54] Bach et al.[61] concluded that one can alter the electrophoretic pattern and the antigenic reactivity of human gamma globulin by exposing it in vitro to pulsed shortwave energy of the proper frequency. The authors stressed that frequency was the prime critical factor in the reaction, whereas mass heating under widely varied conditions of voltage, power, pulse width or pulse repetition rate were unimportant when the frequency was not suitable.

Effective frequencies were 13.1, 13.2, 13.3, 13.5, 13.6 and 14.4 megacycles for a 2.2 per cent solution of gamma globulin in normal saline at 37.5° C. (99.5° F.) with a phosphate buffer at pH 7.6. None of the commercially available machines for pulsed therapy operate at any of these frequencies. Heller,[62] in preliminary experiments in which rats were exposed to pulsed shortwave, found that small amounts of energy could stimulate phagocytosis, while somewhat larger amounts could inhibit phagocytosis. To date no effort has been made to discriminate between effects which are related to average output and those which may result from the high intensity energy during pulses. Thus the experimental results do not answer the question as to whether the pulsing of the shortwave equipment is of any specific advantage in producing physiologic or therapeutic reactions.

CLINICAL USE. Ginsberg[63] treated calcific bursitis with pulsed shortwave diathermy and found improvement in a large number of cases as well as a resolution of the calcium deposit in the subdeltoid bursa in some of the patients. However, an objective evaluation of the improvement as well as statistical evidence for the efficacy of this modality or its superiority over ordinary shortwave diathermy application could not be furnished. A resolution of the calcium deposits may also occur spontaneously and, again, evidence is lacking that it occurred more often than could be expected from the natural course of the disease or from the application of shortwave with a corresponding continuous wave output. Levi[64] treated sinusitis, lymphadenosis, recurrent otitis media and sinobronchitis.

These clinical evaluations have been made in an effort to assess potential indications for pulsed shortwave diathermy. So far clinical evidence has not been accumulated to show that pulsed shortwaves are superior in the clinical application to continuous wave application.

In summary then, neither the experimental evidence nor the clinical evaluations have been performed as yet to furnish definite evidence for the efficacy of pulsed shortwave applications in clinical practice.

ULTRASONIC DIATHERMY

Physics[65, 66]

Ultrasound is defined as a form of acoustic vibration occurring at frequencies too high to be perceived by the human ear. Thus, frequencies under 17,000 cycles per second are usually called sound while those above this level are designated as ultrasound. With the exception of the differences in frequencies, the physics of ultrasound is in no way different from that of audible sound. Sound and ultrasound are propagated in the form of longitudinal compressional waves. The movement of the particles in the medium occurs parallel to the direction of the wave propagation. In the case of a cylindric ultrasound beam, the propagation also occurs parallel to the axis of the beam. Hence, the propagation of sound depends on the presence of a medium capable of being compressed. It follows that sound cannot be transmitted through a vacuum.

Ultrasonic frequencies used for therapeutic purposes range between 0.8 and 1 megacycle. The sound velocity in water and in tissues is approximately $1.5 \cdot 10^5$ cm./sec. The wavelength is approximately 0.15 cm. Thus, many tissue structures are large as compared with the wavelength, although they are small as compared with the wavelength of audible sound. The result is that biologic interfaces and structures which are transparent to audible sound waves may reflect or scatter ultrasound.

The sound beams produced by therapeutic applicators are almost cylindric in shape. The beaming properties of the sound applicator depend on its diameter and the wavelength. The angle of divergence, γ, is in proportion to the ratio of the wavelength to the diameter of the applicator. Thus, a transducer operating at therapeutic frequencies will produce a beam with a greater angle of divergence if the diameter of the transducer is small than if it is large (Fig. 11-22).[67]

The sound intensity across the beam produced by a therapeutic transducer is not uniform. If measurements are made of the sound intensity along the central axis of the beam produced by a therapeutic applicator, the intensity distribution shows maxima and minima near the applicator and then a gradual decline beyond the last maximum of intensity[68] (Fig. 11-23). The "interference" or "near field" is the area in the ultrasound beam extending from the applicator surface to the location of the most distant intensity maximum. In this area, maxima and minima of intensity are located close to each other (Fig. 11-24). Beyond this point, the beam has a more uniform intensity and is called the "far" or "distant field"[67] (Fig. 11-25). Figure 11-26 shows the distance between transducer surface and last intensity maximum, dependent on the diameter of the radiating surface of the applicator.

The primary reactions occurring within an ultrasonic beam at therapeutic intensities of the order of 1 to 4 watts/cm.^{2} are directly related to the particle movement as a result of the wave propagation. It is possible to assess quantitatively the amplitude of the displacement of the particles in the medium as rarefaction and compression occur alternately. The amplitude of displacement

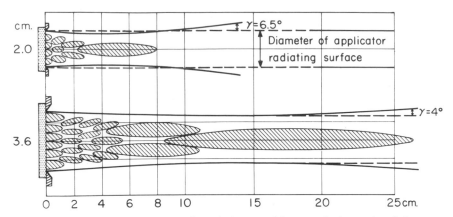

Figure 11–22 Schematic representation of ultrasound beam; γ is the angle of divergence of the beam; shaded areas are zones of high ultrasound intensity. (From Pohlman. Die Ultraschall Therapie. Stuttgart, Georg Theime, 1951.)

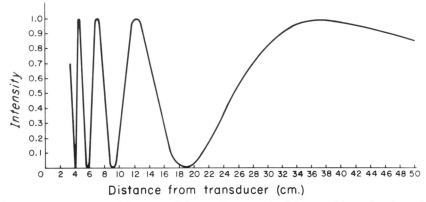

Figure 11–23 Calculated location of the maximum and minimum of intensity along the axis of the sound beam produced by a transducer with a diameter of 8 cm. operating at a frequency of 0.35 mc. in water. (From Born. Zur Frage der Absorptions messungen im Ultraschall gebeit. Z. Phys. Bd., *120:*383, 1943.)

is of the order of $1 \cdot 10^{-6}$ to $6 \cdot 10^{-6}$ cm. The maximum velocity of the particles is approximately 10 to 26 cm./sec. The accelerations to which the particles are subjected are about $5 \cdot 10^7$ to $16 \cdot 10^7$ cm./sec.^{2} This represents an acceleration which is approximately 100,000 times that of gravity. The pressure amplitude in the waves is approximately 1 to 4 atmospheres (Fig. 11-27). It should be noted that the area of maximal pressure in the medium is separated by just one-half wavelength from the area of the maximal rarefaction. Thus a great difference in pressure occurs over a relatively short distance.

These powerful mechanical forces can create secondary reactions in the tissues. Since dissolved gases are always present in biologic media, the phenomenon called gaseous cavitation may occur. Gas-filled cavities may be produced in the fluid medium during the phase of rarefaction in the sound waves. During the following phase of compression, these cavities may collapse, creating a high energy concentration in the form of shock waves. Or the gas bubbles may become larger. The growth of the bubbles can be explained by the following mechanism. During the phase of compression when the surface of the gas bubble is relatively small, the gas moves out of the bubble into the surrounding fluid. During the following phase of rarefaction when the bubble

INTENSITY DISTRIBUTION ALONG THE CENTRAL AXIS
OF THE ULTRASONIC BEAM

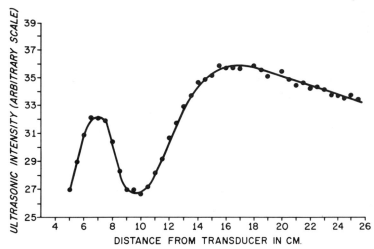

Figure 11-24 Measured intensity distribution along the central axis of the ultrasonic beam. (From Lehmann and Johnson: Some Factors Influencing the Temperature Distribution in Thighs Exposed to Ultrasound. Arch. Phys. Med., Vol. 39, 1958.)

INTENSITY DISTRIBUTION IN THE VERTICAL DIAMETER OF THE
ULTRASONIC FAR FIELD

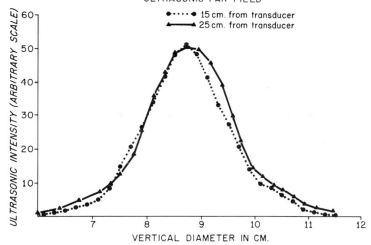

Figure 11-25 Intensity distribution in the vertical diameter of the ultrasonic far field. (From Lehmann and Johnson: Some Factors Influencing the Temperature Distribution in Thighs Exposed to Ultrasound. Arch. Phys. Med., Vol. 39, 1958.)

is expanded and its surface is relatively large the gas moves out of the fluid into the cavity. The amount of gas passing into or out of the bubble is in proportion to the bubble surface; thus, there is a net gain of gas moving into the bubbles. Electrical as well as chemical phenomena have been described as results of cavitation. Mechanical destruction also may be produced when the cavities collapse or when gas bubbles grow large enough to vibrate in resonance with the sound waves.[69] The occurrence of gaseous cavitation can be prevented by application of external pressure of a sufficient magnitude.

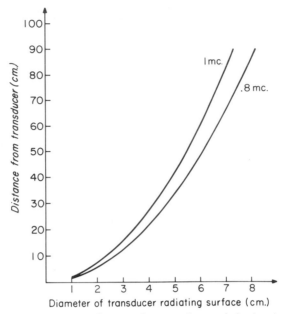

Figure 11–26   Distance between the transducer surface and the last interference maximum dependent on the diameter of the radiating surface of the applicator for the therapeutic frequency of 0.8 and 1 mc. (From Pohlman: Die Ultraschall Therapie. Stuttgart, Georg Theime, 1951.)

   As sound is propagated through the tissues, it is gradually absorbed and converted into heat. The surface intensity is gradually attenuated in an exponential fashion. The depth of penetration is commonly defined as that depth of the tissues where the surface intensity drops to one half of its value.

   Carstenson et al.[70] and Piersol et al.[71] have demonstrated that ultrasonic absorption occurs primarily in the tissue proteins, although such structural elements as cellular membranes are responsible for a minor degree of absorption. Hüter[72, 73] has shown that attenuation of ultrasound in muscle tissue

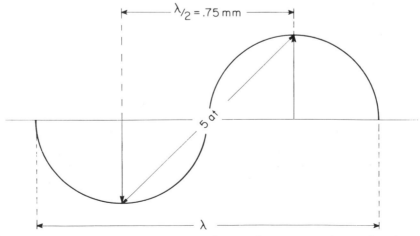

Figure 11–27   Pressure distribution in the ultrasound wave; λ equals wave length, pressure given in atmospheres (at).

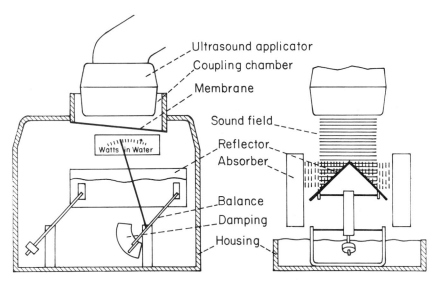

Figure 11-28 Schematic arrangement of a so-called sound-pressure balance. (From Pohlman: Die Ultraschall Therapie. Stuttgart, Georg Theime, 1951.)

depends on whether or not the ultrasonic beam is parallel to myofascial interfaces, thus demonstrating a selective absorption at interfaces, which can be explained on the basis of scattering which in turn results in an increased absorption at irregular surfaces. It is also possible that the longitudinal ultrasound waves may be converted into transverse, i.e., shear waves, which are quickly attenuated.

Measurement of Ultrasound. If ultrasound is incident on a totally reflecting surface, a pressure is exerted on the surface.[67] Figure 11-28 shows a schematic arrangement of the so-called sound-pressure balance. The balance is usually calibrated in watts. Also, small probes have been developed to determine sound intensities in small areas of the field.[65-67]

Therapeutic Equipment

The therapeutic ultrasound machine consists of a generator which produces a high frequency alternating current of about 0.8 to 1 megacycle. The high frequency electric current is then converted by a transducer into mechanical, i.e., acoustic, vibration. The transducer consists basically of a crystal inserted between two electrodes. The conversion of the high frequency alternating voltage into mechanical vibration is accomplished by reversal of the piezoelectric effect as shown in Figure 11-29.[65] If an alternating electrical charge is supplied to the surfaces of the crystal, the crystal will be deformed, depending on the sign of the charges. The three basic components of the electrical generator usually found in the therapeutic machines are the power supply, the oscillating circuit (radio frequency generator) producing the high frequency current and the transducer circuit. The power supply of therapeutically acceptable machines has full wave rectification and filtering to provide for a steady output not appreciably modified by the 60 cycle alternating line current. The capacitance and inductance of the oscillating circuit are selected to produce an

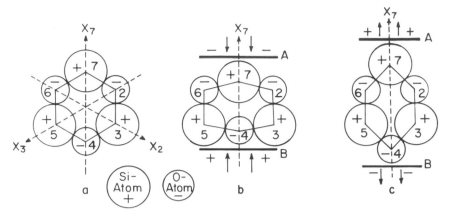

Figure 11–29   Quartz crystal lattice demonstrating the piezo-electric effect. (From Bergmann: Der Ultraschall. Stuttgart, S. Hirzel Verlag, 1949.)

alternating current of the same frequency as the mechanical resonance frequency of the quartz crystal in the transducer. Adjustment of the frequency is made possible by tuning, usually by adjusting a variable capacitor. Some manufacturers have eliminated tuning by controlling the oscillating frequency.

The sound applicators produce an ultrasonic field in the vicinity of the applicator which shows a characteristic interference pattern. In the far field, the intensity distribution across the beam shows a bell-shaped distribution curve.[68] (See Fig. 11–25.) The intensity of the sound field drops gradually to zero at the edge of the distribution. A commonly used procedure to determine the radiating surface of the applicator is that of inserting baffles of decreasing diameter in front of the applicator to cut out the sound at the edge of the beam. The total output of the applicator is then measured beyond the baffle. When the output value is decreased to an arbitrary level, the corresponding opening of the baffle is called the radiating surface of the applicator. Customarily, the decrease of the output is set at about 10 per cent. A preferable applicator for therapeutic purposes has a radiating surface area which is only slightly smaller than the total applicator surface. This minimizes the problem of maintaining full contact between the skin and the applicator surface, at the same time utilizing the total surface of the applicator, for therapeutic irradiation. The ultrasonic intensity is expressed in watts/cm.^{2}, referring to the average intensity of the field. This average intensity is obtained by measuring the total output of the applicator (watts) and then dividing it by the size of the radiating surface of the applicator (cm.^{2}). The peak intensity, in the bell-shaped distribution curve, should be not more than approximately three times the average intensity. This means that a therapeutically acceptable transducer has a broad-based, bell-shaped intensity distribution curve, in contrast to an undesirable applicator which produces a pencil-shaped type of beam with either one or several high intensity peaks in the field distribution. Such machines may be dangerous because undesirable side effects may be produced by the high intensities in the peaks of the distribution curve.

The losses in the therapeutic applicator should be kept to a minimum in order to avoid excessive heating during application which may modify the therapeutic results dependent on temperature. Since the total output of an applicator is a product of average intensity (watts/cm.^{2}) and the total radiating surface area (cm.^{2}), it is desirable to have larger applicators. The angle of divergence of the beam is less if an applicator with a large diameter is used. It is for this reason that applicators smaller than 5 cm.[2] are not acceptable for therapeutic purposes. It is also difficult to treat the deep tissues in an area of limited size with a beam of small diameter. On the other hand, if the radiating surface of the applicator is too large, it may be difficult to maintain contact with the surface of the body at all times. Therefore an applicator with a radiating surface of 7 to 13 cm.[2] is most convenient and effective for therapeutic application.

Physiologic Effects of Ultrasound

A large number of biologic and therapeutic responses have been investigated.[66] In this chapter the results of an extensive research effort in this area will be reviewed briefly. Reactions due to heating of the tissues and nonthermal reactions will be discussed.

Reactions Due to Heating. Since physiologically effective temperature elevations can be produced in the tissues, it is logical to assume that all those reactions which are known to occur as a result of temperature elevation in the tissues will also be produced by ultrasound. Three groups of researchers[75-77] found that the peripheral arterial blood flow is increased as a result of ultrasound application. The tissue metabolism can be changed, according to Lehmann and co-workers[78, 79] and Pauly and Hug.[80] Experimental evidence has been furnished that these reactions are quantitatively due to the heating effect of ultrasonic energy.[81, 82] It has been observed that reactions such as hyperemia and inflammatory responses characterized by an increase in vascularity, edema and tissue necrosis all can be quantitatively explained on the basis of the heating effect of ultrasonic energy. It was also found experimentally that a marked increase in permeability of biologic membranes and change of membrane potentials can be produced and is to a large degree the result of the temperature elevation in the tissues during exposure to ultrasound.[81-83] However, part of the effect is also due to nonthermal mechanisms. The effects of ultrasonic energy on nerve tissues have been studied extensively and most of them have been found to be due entirely to the heating effect.[84-87]

It is of interest for therapeutic purposes to note that conduction velocity in peripheral nerves can be altered and temporary blocks can be produced. Different types of fibers show differences in sensitivity to ultrasound; the smallest, C fibers, are most sensitive. An increase or decrease of spinal reflexes can also be produced, depending on dosage.[88-90] Some of these effects on the spinal cord function are nonthermal in nature.[90] The pain threshold can be elevated by application of ultrasonic energy to the peripheral nerve or to the area of the free nerve endings.[91] "Muscle spasm" as found in poliomyelitis can be relieved by ultrasonic application.[92, 93] An increase in vascularity and skin temperature can be produced by ultrasonic radiation applied to the sympathetic nerves.[94, 95] Careful investigations of the action of ultrasonic energy on bone showed that if therapeutic dosage is applied, no detrimental effects are observed in either the growing or the adult bone.[96, 97] On the other hand, no beneficial influence on the healing of fractures or callus formation could be demonstrated.[98, 99] Excessive dosage led to pathologic fractures.[100]

Nonthermal Reactions. A review of the biologic reactions indicates that most of these reactions clearly are due to the temperature elevation resulting from exposure to ultrasound.[101] In some instances, however, the entire reaction could not be explained on the basis of the heating effect of ultrasonic energy. The reaction was due in part to nonthermal effects. In only a few instances have nonthermal effects been studied in detail. It has been found that the permeability of biologic membranes is altered not only by the heating effect of ultrasonic energy, but also by nonthermal effects occurring during exposure to ultrasound which speed up the rate of diffusion of ions across the membrane.[102] Lehmann[81, 82] and Lehmann and Biegler[83] showed that this nonthermal reaction can be explained on the basis of streaming of fluids in the ultrasonic field and a resultant stirring effect, i.e., an increase in the gradient of concentration of ions across the biologic membrane which accelerates the rate of diffusion. Quantitatively, the thermal effect was definitely the dominant one. The stirring effect could also be demonstrated in living cells. Membrane potentials were similarly affected by the mechanical effect of ultrasonic energy. Gersten[90, 103, 104] pointed out that neither the effect on tendon extensibility produced by ultrasound nor the effects on musculature or the spinal cord could be explained entirely on the basis of thermal reactions alone.

There are numerous reactions to gaseous cavitation; most of them, however, occur in the test tube only.[105] Typically destructive reactions such as hemolysis occur only if there is a low concentration of cells and the viscosity of the medium is low as compared with therapeutic conditions.[81, 82] Cavitation also was studied in the live organism.[106] The histologic appearance of the cavitation reaction was characteristic: the destruction of cells was spotty and led to petechial hemorrhages. This appearance could be explained by the spotty occurrence of gas bubbles in the tissues (Fig. 11–30). Intensity thresholds of 1 to 2 watts/cm.^{2} were required to produce these lesions. The reactions could be prevented by the application of external pressure, proving that they were due to cavitation. It was noted that under conditions similar to those in therapy

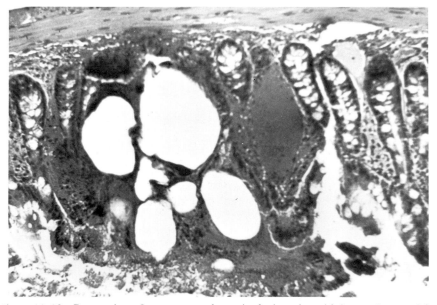

Figure 11–30   Destruction of mucous membrane in the intestine with hemorrhage and formation of gas bubbles. (From Lehmann and Herrick: Biologic Reaction to Cavitation—A Consideration for Ultrasonic Therapy. Arch. Phys. Med., Vol. 34, 1953.)

(i.e., at intensities of 1 watt/cm.^{2} or below applied with stationary technique), the destructive effects of cavitation did not occur. It was observed that when stroking technique commonly used in therapy was simulated, intensities up to 4 watts/cm.^{2} were tolerated without the appearance of destructive effects of cavitation. It also could be demonstrated that the potential danger of producing cavitation under therapeutic conditions is increased if unsuitable equipment is used. Animals were irradiated with the stationary applicator with an ultrasonic intensity of 1.5 watts/cm.^{2} and a total output of the applicator of 15 watts. The machine had a power supply with full wave rectification. In one series of irradiations, filters were used to produce a steady ultrasonic output; in another series, the filters were removed, producing a greatly modulated ultrasonic output. In the animals treated with the steady output, a few reactions to cavitation were observed, whereas when ultrasound was applied with the same machine with the same average output but with the filtering removed, cavitation effects were observed in 55 per cent of the animals. These experiments demonstrate that peak ultrasonic intensities resulting from the lack of filtering of the rectified line voltage may be potentially dangerous.

Also, the effects of the application of pulsed ultrasonic energy were investigated. With the exception of cavitation, the heating effect of ultrasonic energy as well as some of the nonthermal effects such as the acceleration of diffusion processes could be produced equally well by continuous wave output of the same average intensity. There is no evidence available so far that indicates that it is advantageous to utilize pulsed ultrasonic energy to produce biologic reactions of therapeutic significance. Pulsing does not accomplish anything beyond reducing the average output and those reactions which are in proportion to it, including the heating effect. This can be accomplished if desired by a simple reduction of the continuous wave output.

In conclusion, this brief review of the physiologic reactions to ultrasound indicates that those reactions of potential therapeutic significance are due primarily to the temperature elevation resulting from absorption of ultrasonic energy. In addition, a few effects have been demonstrated, such as the acceleration of diffusion processes across biologic membranes which may be therapeutically useful and are nonthermal in nature. These effects are also dependent on temperature and occur at a faster rate if they are associated with temperature elevation. Fortunately the destructive effects due to cavitation have not been observed under therapeutic conditions if the proper equipment is used and a therapeutic dosage is applied. A more detailed investigation of the nonthermal effects would be most desirable since they could potentially lead to new specific indications to ultrasonic therapy. Investigation has also shown that there are marked differences between thermal reactions produced by ultrasound and those produced by other heating modalities. These discrepancies have been attributed mainly to the variation in temperature distribution throughout the live organism, and they are produced by ultrasound and other heating modalities. Therefore, it is important to obtain information on those reactions which ultimately produce the temperature distribution characteristic of ulstrasound application.

Biophysics

The propagation of ultrasonic energy in tissues depends mainly on two factors, absorption characteristics of the biologic media and reflection of ultrasonic energy at tissue interfaces.

TABLE 11–1   ULTRASONIC ATTENUATION IN PIG TISSUES

TISSUE	NUMBER OF SAMPLES	ATTENUATION IN DB./CM.	STANDARD DEVIATION
Whole bone	13	8.4	±1.2
Skeletal muscle	30	0.8	±0.1
Subcutaneous fat	28	1.8	±0.1

Absorption.   It has been demonstrated that ultrasonic absorption is direct-ly related to the protein content of the tissues.[70, 71, 107] These studies also showed that cellular structures may contribute to absorption and Hüter[72] showed that macroscopic tissue interfaces may contribute significantly to the attenuation of ultrasound. The selective absorption occurring at interfaces could be related to scattering of ultrasonic energy as a result of reflection and to the production of transverse or shear waves which are quickly attenuated. The absorption of ultrasound in uniform tissue has been investigated by Hüter,[72] Hüter and Bolt,[73] Dussick et al.[108] and Lehmann and Johnson.[68] From the data in Table 11–1 it is evident that bone absorbs ten times more ultrasonic energy than soft tissues.

Selective absorption at interfaces can produce selective rise of temperature in these areas.

Reflection.   Reflection can occur at interfaces between tissues of different acoustic impedance. The impedance was measured and reflection at tissue interfaces determined by Lehmann and Johnson.[68] The results shown in Table 11–2 indicate that very little reflection occurs between soft tissues but a great deal occurs at the surface of the bone where up to 30 per cent of energy may be reflected. Surgical metallic implants constitute artificial interfaces. Acoustic impedance of stainless steel, vitallium and titanium was found to be greatly different from that of bone or soft tissues. Thus, it could be anticipated that the major problem encountered with surgical metallic implants in the ultrason-ic field might be that of reflection leading to an intense increase in ultrasonic energy due to the production of a pattern of standing waves and focusing.

Therapeutic Application of Biologic and Biophysical Research

Heating of the Tissues.   Once the absorption coefficient of the tissues and reflection at tissue interfaces are known, it is possible to calculate the so-called pattern of relative heating. This was done for therapeutic ultrasonic frequen-

TABLE 11–2   EXPERIMENTAL AND CALCULATED REFLECTION OF ULTRASONIC ENERGY AT TISSUE INTERFACES

INTERFACE	OBSERVED REFLECTION % OF INCIDENT ENERGY	CALCULATED REFLECTION % OF INCIDENT ENERGY
Water-fat (pig)	0	0.2
Water-muscle (pig)	0	0.3
Fat-muscle (pig)	—	1.1
Water-bone (pig)	30	30
Muscle-bone (pig)	—	26.8

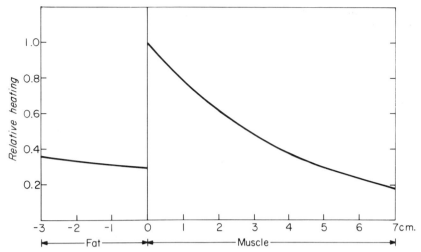

Figure 11-31 Patterns of relative heating produced by ultrasound in fat and muscle tissue. (From Schwan: Biophysics of Diathermy. In Licht, S.: Therapeutic Heat. New Haven, Conn., Elizabeth Licht, 1958.)

cies by Schwan[109] (Figure 11–31). The data indicate that relatively little energy is converted into heat in the subcutaneous fat but that much more energy is converted into heat in the musculature. Also, the depth of penetration of the ultrasonic energy in the musculature is very satisfactory. One-half of the intensity at the muscle surface is still available at a depth of 3 cm., indicating that ultrasound is an effective deep heating agent, probably better than either shortwave or microwave diathermy. In addition to the energy available for heating at any given depth of the tissues as expressed in a pattern of relative heating, the actual temperature obtained in the tissues depends also on other characteristic properties of the tissue such as specific heat and specific weight.

If heating extends over a relatively long period of time, thermal conductivity of the tissues will also modify the temperature rise. Other factors that would influence the ultimate temperature distribution are the pre-existing temperature distribution in the live subject and the selective cooling of areas which may occur as a result of changes in blood flow.

The temperature distribution produced by ultrasound is unique among deep heating modalities. Ultrasound causes comparatively little temperature elevation in the superficial tissues and has a greater depth penetration in the musculature and other soft tissues than shortwave and microwave diathermy. Biophysical research suggests that ultrasound is the most effective deep heating agent. The temperature in joints covered by heavy masses of soft tissues can be raised to therapeutic and even tolerance levels without any deleterious effects elsewhere in the tissues.[110] It was found by comparison that neither shortwave nor microwave diathermy produced any therapeutic rise of temperature in the hip joint, even though a first degree burn was obtained in the superficial tissues with either modality (Figs. 11-32A and 11-32B). The high degree of reflection of ultrasound on the surface of the bone, as well as the high coefficient of absorption of bone tissue, eliminates the possibility of heating the distant side of the bone or joint, for the major amount of the energy

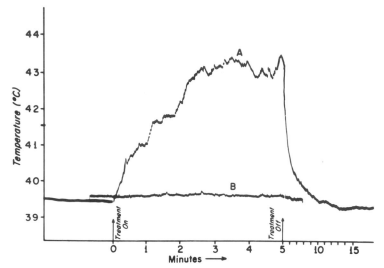

Figure 11–32A Change in temperature inside hip joint during exposure to A, ultrasound, and B, microwave. (From Lehmann et al.: Comparative Study of the Efficiency of Shortwave, Microwave, and Ultrasonic Diathermy in Heating the Hip Joint. Arch. Phys. Med., Vol. 40, 1959.)

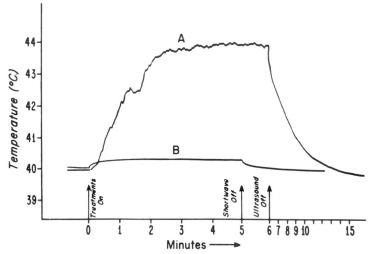

Figure 11–32B Change in temperature inside hip joint during exposure to A, ultrasound, and B, shortwave. (From Lehmann et al.: Comparative Study of the Efficiency of Shortwave, Microwave, and Ultrasonic Diathermy in Heating the Hip Joint. Arch. Phys. Med., Vol. 40, 1959.)

penetrating into the bone would be absorbed and would not be available for this purpose.[110] A practical conclusion evolving from this research is that when treating an entire joint, one should utilize a multiple field technique exposing all joint surfaces directly to the ultrasonic beam if the joint is to be heated uniformly throughout.

Experiments in pigs have shown that the structures of the knee joint can be selectively heated. As shown in Figure 11-33 the temperature was measured through the capsular tissues and bone just above the knee joint and at the level of the joint space through the capsular tissues and meniscus. The resulting temperature distributions are shown in Figures 11-34 and 11-35.[111]

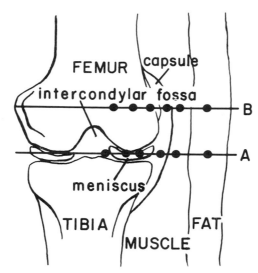

Figure 11–33   Needle location in the knee joint (*A*) and 2 cm. proximal (*B*).

It is characteristic of ultrasound that a selective rise of temperature may occur at the interface between tissues of different acoustic impedance. Such a selective rise of temperature occurs in the human being as shown in Figure 11-36.[112] In addition, it has been documented that the temperature distribution in the human largely depends on the type and temperature of the coupling medium used.[112] For instance, if water, which has a high thermoconductivity and high thermal heat carrying capacity, is used as a coupling medium, an adequate selective rise of temperature in front of the bone still can be obtained

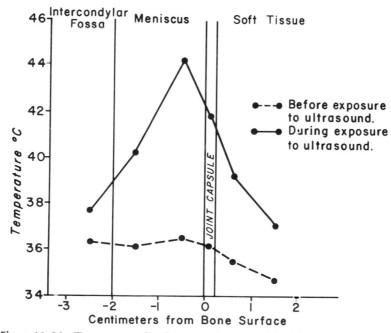

Figure 11–34   Temperature distribution at the level of the joint space.

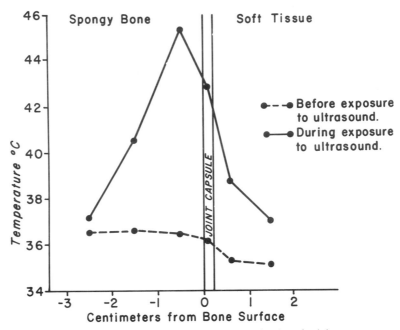

Figure 11–35   Temperature distribution 2 cm. proximal to the joint space.

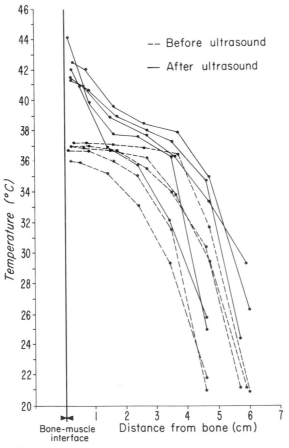

Figure 11–36 Comparison of temperature distributions in five human thighs before and after exposure to ultrasound, using a mineral oil coupling medium at 18° C.

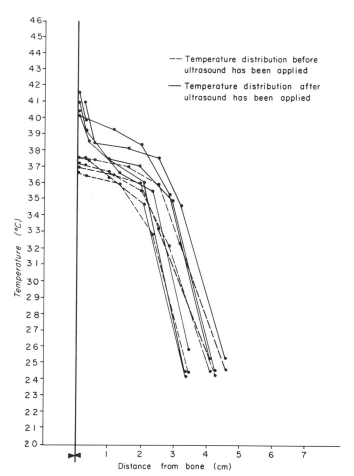

Figure 11-37 Comparison of temperature distribution in five human thighs before and after exposure to ultrasound, using degassed water coupling medium at 24° C.

at a temperature of 24° C. (Figure 11-37). This is not so with the use of mineral oil (Figure 11-38). Also, for practical purposes, the temperature of the applicator itself should be kept low. These studies, both in animals and in humans, indicate clearly that it is possible to heat joint structures, such as capsules, synovia and others, selectively with ultrasound. However, it must also be recognized that the temperatures obtained in the superficial bone would be slightly higher than those in the capsular tissues in front of the bone.[113]

If the therapeutic objective is to heat the capsular synovial tissues of the joint, the technique of application should be modified so as to minimize the difference between the peak temperature in the superficial bone and the temperature in the adjacent soft tissue structures.[114] This is illustrated in Figure 11-39 where the temperature was measured in front of the bone when the first pain was perceived. It should be noted that in individuals with less than 8 cm. soft tissue cover of the bone higher temperatures were obtained at lower wattage. Also, at higher wattage the temperature in front of the bone, at pain, was markedly higher in the individual with thick absorbing tissue cover of the bone as compared to the thin individual. This discrepancy was explained on

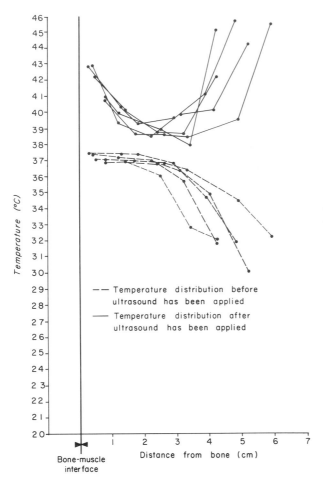

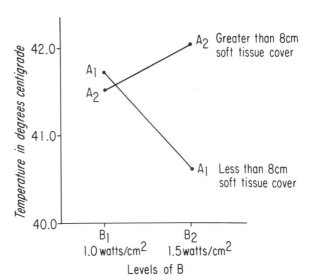

Figure 11–38 Comparison of temperature distribution in human thighs before and after exposure to ultrasound, using a mineral oil coupling medium at 24° C.

Figure 11–39 Interaction of ultrasonic intensity and soft tissue cover.

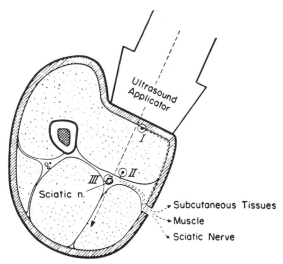

Figure 11–40 A cross section through the thigh exposed to ultrasound with thermocouples in I, subcutaneous tissues; II, muscle tissue; III, sciatic nerve. (From Rosenberger: Über den Wirkungs mechanismus der Ultraschall behandlung, insbesondere bei Ischias und Neuralgien. Chirurg, Vol. 21, 1950.)

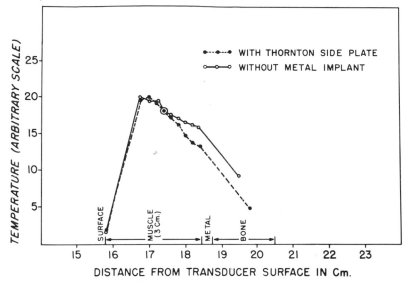

Figure 11–41 Temperature distribution in a specimen consisting of muscle and bones with and without a Thornton side plate inserted in front of the bones. (From Lehmann et al.: The Influence of Surgical Metal Implants on the Temperature Distribution in Thigh Specimens Exposed to Ultrasound. Arch. Phys. Med., Vol. 39, 1958.)

the basis that if higher wattage were used in the thin individual the temperature rose very rapidly and selectively, and thus no time interval was available for a temperature conduction to take place which would minimize the temperature difference between superficial bone and the site of measurement. Thus, pain occurred earlier in these cases, whereas in the slim individual with lower dosage the treatment was tolerated longer without pain; therefore, heat conduction from the superficial bone into the soft tissues in front of the bone substantially elevated the tissue temperature in front of the bone at the site of measurement. Similarly, at high wattages temperature rose rapidly to the pain threshold in the superficial bone in the thin individual, and it took a longer period of time in the more obese individual.

The therapeutic application of these findings is that one should treat over a longer period of time, at least over 5 to 10 minutes per field, to obtain optimal heating of tissues, such as a joint capsule, which are located right in front of the bone.

There is also evidence that other biologic interfaces are selectively heated by ultrasound.[115-119] Pätzold and Born[117] demonstrated that myofascial interfaces, as they occur in the musculature, are selectively heated. Rosenberger[118] found a selective rise of temperature in the sciatic nerve of experimental animals (Fig. 11-40) and Herrick[119] and associates were able to destroy experimentally the sciatic nerve in dogs without affecting the histologic structure of surrounding musculature or the tissues.

On the other hand, ultrasound can be utilized safely in the presence of surgical metallic implants. Marked reflection occurs resulting in the development of patterns of standing waves, or the production of focal concentrations of energy may occur in the vicinity of the implant. This causes a large increase in ultrasonic intensity close to the metal. Lehmann, Brunner and McMillan[120] studied the distribution of temperature throughout specimens with metal implants and found that, when exposed to ultrasound, no selective rise of temperature occurred in these areas (Fig. 11-41). Often the temperature in the specimen close to metal was lower than the temperatures measured in the same place without metal present. This was explained on the basis that the metal implants have a very high thermal conductivity. Thus the heat energy is removed from the areas of increased intensity more rapidly than it is absorbed. The experimental findings obtained in specimens were later confirmed in live pigs.[121] Temperatures in the focal areas and in the standing waves close to the implants were within the therapeutic range and could be well controlled. In another series, identical implants were inserted bilaterally into live pigs. One side served as a control and the other was exposed to ultrasound. After the pigs were killed, histologic examinations showed no evidence of any retardation of the healing process or callus formation or any other untoward effects on the side treated with ultrasound, when compared with the side serving as controls. In conclusion, ultrasonic energy seems to be the only type of diathermy which can be used with metallic implants in the treatment field, a finding consistent with previous observations of Gersten.[122]

Dosimetry

The factors which determine the biologic response to ultrasound are mainly the temperature obtained in the tissues, the duration of the temperature elevation and the rate of temperature rise. It would be ideal if it were possible to measure and control these factors accurately, permitting a quantitative control of the biologic response. However, the ultrasonic energy entering the tissues and the duration of the treatment can be measured and thus the resulting tissue effect can be estimated if we have information on the temperature distribution and the approximate rate of rise as well as an understanding of how these can be modified by the technique of application. For therapeutic purposes it is necessary to determine the ultrasonic output (watts) and the average intensity (watts/cm.²). Therapeutic machines can be tuned adequately in water and then applied to the patient without retuning. The output of the machine can be preset in a water bath utilizing a meter on the front panel of the machine which indicates total output (watts) and average intensity (watts/cm.²). Some machines do not require tuning. The output indicated on the meter will be transmitted to the tissues, provided that reflection at the skin surface is prevented by proper technique including the insertion of a coupling medium between the sound applicator and the skin.

Some machines are equipped with a protective system. The moment that contact with the body is partially lost and the load of the applicator is therefore changed, a feedback to a control system reduces the output. This is indicated by the meter on the panel and a buzzing device. The system protects the ceramic crystal of the applicator from overheating and warns of faulty technique of application resulting from poor coupling. Its disadvantage is that no ultrasonic energy is applied to the body when poor coupling is inevitable because of uneven body surfaces where full contact cannot be maintained. This type of machine does not require any tuning. The output can be preset by pressing a contact button activating a simulated load. Intensities found useful in therapy range from 0.5 to 4 watts/cm.² usually applied with a moving applicator. If the applicator is kept stationary, intensities less than 1 watt/cm.² are tolerated. The rise in temperature of the tissues is determined by the technique of application. The duration of the treatment is usually 3 to 10 minutes per field. Applications usually are repeated on a daily basis. Sometimes treatment is given twice a day or three times a week.

Technique of Application

Before ultrasound can be applied, the machine must be tuned and the output must be set. Proper coupling between the applicator and the skin surface must be provided for. The coupling media commonly used are mineral oil, a synthetic material called "Aquasonic 100" and water. It is important to remove all gas bubbles that may stick to the skin since they would produce a large amount of uncontrollable reflection. Pätzold and associates[123] have demonstrated that reflection up to 30 per cent can be due to such small gas bubbles. If such gas bubbles present a problem, the application of a wetting agent prior to treatment is indicated. However, it is important to make sure that the detergent is removed completely by rinsing with water before the treatment is begun, to prevent the development of a rash.

Two types of application have been developed. The sound head may be held stationary or it may be moved slowly in a back and forth stroking motion. The stationary technique is rarely used because it produces a rapid rise of temperature in a very small area which is rather difficult to control. "Hot spots" are produced in the interference field and in the far field where the highest intensity is found in the center of the beam. These "hot spots" are liable to heat small areas excessively while the rest of the tissues are not heated adequately for therapeutic purposes.

The stroking technique is most commonly employed. Strokes are comparatively short, of the order of one inch in length, and each stroke partially overlaps the area of another, with the applicator gradually moving in a direction perpendicular to the strokes. Circular strokes may be used, but they are somewhat more difficult to control.

Small areas are treated one at a time in this manner, thus permitting an adequate and relatively steady heating of the tissues. The strokes of the applicator over the area of the temperature recording instrument are indicated only as ripples superimposed on a steady rise of temperature. With the stroking technique, it is possible to distribute the dosage over a much larger area than with the stationary technique and there is smearing of the interference pattern in the near field as well as in the high intensity center portion of the beam, preventing the development of "hot spots." The temperature in the tissues will also be modified by the temperature of the coupling medium or the temperature of the surface of the metal applicator. The cooler the temperature of the coupling medium or the applicator, the greater the heat loss at the skin and the deeper the peak temperatures found in the tissues. These investigations suggest that if ultrasound is applied for deep heating purposes, it is important to state the temperature of the coupling medium if water is used. Also, it is important to use an applicator with minimal electrical and mechanical losses which maintains a fairly constant temperature during the treatment if mineral oil or "Aquasonic 100" are employed.

Clinical Application

The physician who understands the biophysical factors that ultimately determine the particularly important temperature distribution in the tissues and who is acquainted with the possible ways of modifying this temperature distribution by selected techniques of application will be in a position to use ultrasonic energy effectively for specific therapeutic purposes. Usually ultrasound is used as a vigorous deep heating agent which affects specifically those areas where a selective rise of temperature can be produced. Proper diagnostic evaluation of the patient's problem, therefore, is also required to enable the physician to select ultrasound or any other diathermy modality and to adapt the technique of application appropriately. The evaluation must provide detailed information as to the type of pathologic lesion, the acuteness or chronicity of the process and its location in the tissues. Thus, indications have been developed essentially from information on biophysical and physiologic research. At the same time, they have been investigated clinically and developed on an empirical basis. It is gratifying to note that these two approaches have produced essentially the same type of indications and contraindications.[114]

Conditions in which ultrasound treatment is indicated can be divided arbitrarily into three groups: those in which ultrasound is of established value; those in which it is of suggested value; and those in which it is of potential but questionable value.

Conditions in Which Ultrasound Is of Established Value.   Joint contractures resulting from tightness and scarring of the periarticular structures and capsular tissues have been successfully treated irrespective of their cause, be it immobilization, rheumatic processes, degenerative joint disease or trauma. The rationale for this treatment is that those structures can be heated adequately and perhaps selectively. The result is an increase in the extensibility of the tight structures limiting the joint motion. To maximize the effect of heat, it would be most desirable to stretch the tight structures while heat is applied and to maintain the stretch, even for a period of time after heat treatment is discontinued. For practical purposes, however, stretching usually follows the heat application immediately. In this case, manual stretching and range of motion exercises can be utilized. Other factors contributing to the successful application in these indications are the pain and muscle spasm-relieving effect of ultrasound. Only a few statistical studies have been performed comparing the results of ultrasound treatment with those obtained in placebo controls or controls treated with another accepted heating modality. A large number of authors agree that ultrasound can be used in cases of periarthritis of the shoulder, if given in conjunction with other forms of physical therapy.[124] Some authors did not observe statistically significant improvement in the small number of cases treated when ultrasound was used alone and not as an adjunct to other physical therapy.[125] Perhaps this fact stresses the importance of utilizing the effectiveness of ultrasonic therapy in conjunction with a complete and adequate physical therapy program.

On the other hand, a statistical comparison was made between the results after exposure to ultrasound and those obtained with microwave treatment. The ultrasound and microwaves were given in conjunction with a standardized physical therapy program consisting of the diathermy application, massage and exercise. The two groups of patients with periarthritis were comparable for statistical purposes in terms of their disease, age distribution, duration of symptoms prior to therapy and range of motion before treatment. Evaluation after treatment revealed that the gain in the range of motion was significantly greater when the patients were treated with ultrasound than when they were treated with microwave diathermy.[126, 127] The results are shown in Table 11-3.

Another clinical study was designed to evaluate statistically the efficiency of ultrasonic treatment of contractures associated with internal fixation of hip fractures.[128] Geriatric patients were selected as subjects since they almost invariably develop contractures that become problems in treatment. Patients who had sustained hip fractures which were fixed internally with Richard's screws were treated with either ultrasound or infrared. Both groups received in addition a standard range of motion exercise program, since any therapeutic procedures involving stretch cannot be applied without endangering the surgical results. It was found in this study, and is shown in Table 11-4, that all patients treated with ultrasound gained in the range of motion whereas the majority of the patients who were treated with infrared developed further limitations of the range of motion. The difference between the two groups was statistically significant. In addition, there was a general clinical impression that the functional results, such as level of ambulation skills, were more favorable in the group treated with ultrasound. In summary, there is good statistical evidence that ultrasound is an efficient modality when used for the treatment of all types of joint contractures resulting from the development of capsular tightness and scarring. It can be used safely in the presence of surgical metallic implants. It seems to be the treatment modality of choice for joints covered by a

TABLE 11-3 GAIN IN RANGE OF MOTION AFTER ULTRASONIC AND MICROWAVE TREATMENT

GAIN IN:	AFTER TREATMENT WITH:	
	Ultrasound	*Microwaves*
Forward flexion	27.4°; ± 2.3°*	16.1°; ± 1.5°
Abduction	32.6°; ± 2.5°	21.2°; ± 2.1°
Rotation	45.4°; ± 2.8°	17.3°; ± 4.0°

*Standard error of the mean.

TABLE 11–4 COMPARISON ON AMOUNT OF CHANGE IN RANGE OF MOTION AFTER ONE WEEK OF TREATMENT*

| | WITH ULTRASOUND | | | WITH INFRARED | | | | |
	N	Mean	S.D.	N	Mean	S.D.	t	p
Hip								
Flexion	15	21.67	9.7	15	5.40	11.4	4.057	.01
Extension	15	10.40	8.2	15	−3.20†	7.7	4.503	.01
Abduction	15	6.33	7.4	15	−1.67†	5.6	3.225	.01
Adduction	15	9.67	6.6	15	−1.20†	6.0	4.567	.01
External Rotation	14	12.86	7.9	15	0.20	7.9	4.178	.01
Internal Rotation	14	10.93	7.6	15	−1.60†	8.8	3.965	.01
Knee								
Flexion	15	18.33	14.9	15	10.33	13.3	1.498	.20
Extension	15	3.60	3.9	15	−3.47†	4.8	4.259	.01

* Ultrasound and infrared groups compared using independent samples method.
† When the mean is expressed as a negative value, range of motion has been lost during treatment.

thick layer of soft tissues, since neither microwave nor shortwave diathermy can heat such structures to a therapeutic level and produce results comparable to those of ultrasound treatment. Ultrasound certainly should be selected rather than superficial heating modalities such as infrared.

Conditions in Which Ultrasound Is of Suggested Value. Even though it is the belief of many authors that ultrasound is of therapeutic value in the following conditions, evaluations of the efficiency by statistical and objective means are still not available because of difficulties encountered in experimental design. There is, however, an acceptable biophysical and physiologic rationale for treatment of the conditions listed.

Contractures of joints can develop as a result of the shortening and fibrosis of the musculature extending across joints or as a result of scarring of skin and subcutaneous tissues. It is likely that the temperature level in these tissues can be selectively elevated to such a degree that it produces an increase in extensibility that can be utilized by subsequent physical therapy. Therefore, it can be assumed that such fibrosis or scarring, irrespective of its cause, represents an indication for ultrasonic treatment. Conditions that produce these contractures are polymyositis resulting in fibrosis of the musculature, paralysis due to conditions such as polymyositis and scarring of the skin due to trauma, burns or diseases such as scleroderma.[129-131]

Successful ultrasound treatment of calcific bursitis and tendinitis of the shoulder has been reported by various authors.[66] It can be assumed that selective heating of the areas where calcific deposits occur may be produced by application of ultrasound since calcific deposits probably have a high coefficient of absorption. The resulting hyperemia and mild inflammatory reaction may be comparable to the therapeutic effects of needling or other well accepted procedures.[132] Even though several studies suggest that calcific deposits may disappear after the sound treatment, there is no statistical evidence that this occurs more frequently than would be anticipated from the natural course of the disease. Ultrasound has also been used in combination with hydrocortisone injections.[133, 134] The rationale for the treatment is based on experimental evidence that hydrocortisone is more evenly distributed throughout the joint when ultrasound treatment is applied following the injection. On the other hand, in the acute phase of periarthritis, calcific bursitis and tendinitis of the shoulder ultrasound treatment is not always successful. In the acute condition, high ultrasonic intensity applied to the shoulder may increase the discomfort of the patient. If ultrasound is used at all, it should be used at low dosage at first.

Another clinical application is the treatment of pain and painful phantom limbs as they occur in postoperative neurofibromas. The rationale for this treatment is that these fibromas may be selectively heated, especially when they are embedded in scar tissues, and physiologic experimentation has demonstrated that nerve function can be altered temporarily or permanently by ultrasound treatment. Chateau,[135] Tepperberg and Marjey,[136] and Rubin and Kuitert[137] agreed that the marked and sometimes even dramatic improvement may be observed clinically after the sound application. This was true even in cases which had been resistant to most other forms of therapy applied over long periods of time.

Ultrasound treatment of reflex dystrophy such as the shoulder-hand syndrome, Sudeck's atrophy and causalgia has been advocated.[138, 139] The results have been similar to those obtained by repeated sympathetic blocks. Raynaud's phenomenon has been treated by Buchtala.[140] He found an increase in skin temperature of 2.5° C. when the ultrasound was applied locally or to the appropriate sympathetic ganglia. These findings were confirmed by Stuhlfauth.[141]

During the First International Congress of Ultrasonic Medicine, held in 1949, a statistical study was presented on the successful treatment of rheumatoid spondylitis with ultrasound.[142] Evaluation was done on an entirely subjec-

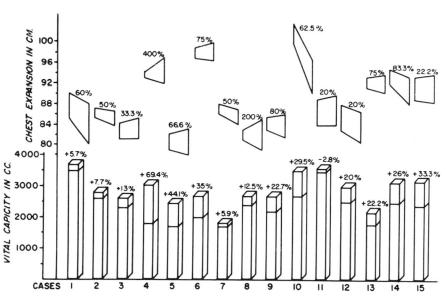

U.S. THERAPY

Figure 11–42 Chest expansion and vital capacity before and after treatment of patients with rheumatoid spondylitis. (From Hintzelmann. Ultraschalltherapie rheumatischer Erkrankungen. Deutsch. Med. Wschr., vol. 72, 1947 and Ultraschalltherapie rheumatischer Erkrankungen. 2. Mitteilung. Deutsch. Med. Wschr., vol. 74, 1949.)

tive basis. No controls were mentioned. Hintzelmann,[143, 144] on the other hand, measured an increased of vital capacity and chest expansion after treatment (Fig. 11–42). Pain relief was also observed after ultrasonic therapy.

Beyond the treatment of joint contractures secondary to scarring associated with rheumatoid arthritis, the treatment of the rheumatoid process itself has been proposed.[66] It seems justifiable to conclude that the treatment of rheumatoid arthritis with ultrasound should be reserved to the more subchronic and chronic processes or applied with great caution and low dosage in the more active cases. Otherwise, an aggravation of the symptoms may occur. The treatment of degenerative joint disease has met with partial success.[66] Not only are the joint contractures relieved, but also the patient may become free of pain for longer periods of time.

It is claimed that pain which sometimes persists following sprains can be relieved by ultrasound in a comparatively short period of time. Relief of pain by ultrasound treatment is probably the reason athletes often go back to competitive sports events shortly after the occurrence of the injury.[145-148] Sound may also accelerate the healing of the injury. The physiologic basis for this treatment is that the pain threshold can be elevated experimentally by application of ultrasound to the peripheral nerve or to the pain receptors.[91] Often the site of the lesion will be adequately and perhaps selectively heated.

Several authors have advocated the treatment of plantar warts with ultrasound.[149] Bender and his associates[150] in a controlled study found supportive evidence which strongly suggested that this is a treatment of value.

Conditions in Which Ultrasound Is of Potential But Questionable Value. Symptoms of sciatica and other forms of radiculitis have been treated extensively in the past in Europe, regardless of etiology, although the percentage of improvement was approximately that which can be expected from spontaneous recovery. Recently treatment of neuritis and radiculitis has again been advocated.[66, 151, 152] Pain relief has been observed after treatment of the persistent pain syndrome occurring as a result of herpes zoster.[153, 154] The rationale for this type of treatment seems to be the relief of pain and muscle spasm. Yet the clinical evidence of the usefulness of ultrasound for these conditions is extremely limited because of lack of uniformity of the conditions treated and largely because some of these conditions show a high rate of spontaneous recovery.

The treatment of peripheral arterial insufficiency has been suggested. Results of experimental research have shown that an increase of blood flow can be obtained in the extremity when either the sympathetic nerves or ganglia are treated.[141] According to Dussick,[108] it is doubtful whether appreciable ultrasonic intensities can penetrate to the area of the sympathetic ganglia. Ultrasound should never be applied to the ischemic area itself.

Recently the treatment of nerve roots, sympathetic ganglia or nerves has been advocated for a large variety of conditions. The so-called segmental treatment has been suggested by Sonnen,[155] Thiele[156] and Sonnenschein[157] and has been recommended for the treatment of rheumatic disease and peripheral vascular disorders. The rationale for this treatment is somewhat doubtful.

Since Bonica[158] developed the management of the "myofascial pain syndrome," ultrasound also has been used to treat the focal irritation or to interrupt the reflexes perpetuating the pain syndrome.[159] Clinical impressions indicate that ultrasound is possibly useful for treatment of this condition. Final proof is not available as yet because of the nonuniformity of the etiology and the variability of the clinical symptomatology.

The combined use of ultrasound and electrical stimulation has been advocated using the sound applicator as the stimulating electrode. "Aquasonic 100" must be used as coupling agent because it transmits both the electric current and ultrasound. There is no clearly established physiologic basis for this type of treatment nor any clinical evidence demonstrating that this type of treatment is superior to either electrical stimulation or ultrasound treatment alone or used consecutively.

Chronic skin ulcerations resulting from various causes such as peripheral venous insufficiency (varicose ulcers) and decubital ulcers have been treated.[160-162] In some of these conditions, general management such as bed rest or a relief of pressure may increase the rate of healing. Since no controlled studies are available, it remains open to question whether these conditions represent indications for ultrasound therapy.

Finally, ultrasound has been used for a large number of clinical conditions in the hope of finding more specific indications.[66]

Contraindications to Ultrasound Therapy

Ultrasound is a very powerful and effective heating agent. Therefore, it must be applied with the proper precautions, in the proper dosage and with the correct technique of application. There are, however, only a very few specific contraindications. Ultrasound should not be applied to the eye in therapeutic dosage range since cavitation will most likely occur in the fluid media and may lead to irreversible damage. There is still a controversy as to whether ultrasound may produce untoward changes when applied to the pregnant uterus. Usually this is not a problem since the uterus is not reached by any appreciable amount of energy in any of the therapeutic applications. Special precautions in adjusting the dosage should be taken when the area of the spinal cord is treated after laminectomy. After the covering tissues have been removed, it is likely that higher energy levels may be obtained in the spinal cord.[108] Ultrasound should be applied with caution over anesthetic areas. Since dosimetry is better developed in ultrasound than in shortwave or microwave diathermy, it is possible to use ultrasound in such cases. Ultrasound should not be used in patients with hemorrhagic diatheses. It should not be applied over malignancies. Tumor growth may be retarded or accelerated, depending on the dosage.[163] Sound should not be applied over areas of vascular insufficiency because the blood supply would be unable to follow the increase in metabolic demand and necrosis may result. Finally, all general contraindications to heat therapy should be observed carefully.

MICROWAVE DIATHERMY

Physics

Microwaves or radar waves are a form of electromagnetic radiation. Therapeutic frequencies of microwaves are higher and the wavelengths shorter than those of radio waves. Like other electromagnetic waves, microwaves travel at the speed of light. They can be propagated through a vacuum and they are similar to light waves in that they can be reflected, scattered, refracted or absorbed. The total amount of microwaves reflected or absorbed is dependent on the characteristics of the material being exposed to the microwave beam as well as on the frequency and power density of the field.

Therapeutic Apparatus

The apparatus used for the production of therapeutic microwave radiation consists of a power supply, a special tube (magnetron) that produces the high frequency oscillation, and the applicator (antenna).

The power supply provides the rectified high voltage to be applied to the anode of the magnetron tube and the various voltages for filaments and relays. Important for clinical application is the fact that the output of the machine is regulated by a variable transformer which alters the input voltage of the power supply and thus the rectified voltage applied to the anode of the magnetron tube. This, in turn, controls the microwave power output. Overloading of the magnetron is avoided by a time delay relay which insures that after the machine is turned on, enough time is allowed for heating the filament before the full voltage is applied to the magnetron. Indicator lights on the panel of the machine show when the apparatus is ready for operation. If therapeutic application is interrupted, it is necessary to turn the power output down to zero before it can be increased again. This action closes a safety switch and insures that the voltage that is applied to the magnetron is gradually increased.

The high frequency oscillations are produced by the multicavity magnetron tube. The power is transmitted through a coaxial cable arrangement into the antenna or director. Three commercially available microwave directors, "A," "B" and "C," are commonly used in therapeutic application. The "A" director consists of an antenna and a hemispheric reflector (diameter approximately 9.3 cm.) which produces a beam having a cross-section field pattern in

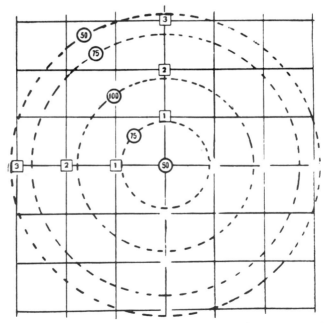

Figure 11–43   Field pattern produced by "A" director at a distance of 2 inches. (Courtesy of the Raytheon Corporation.)

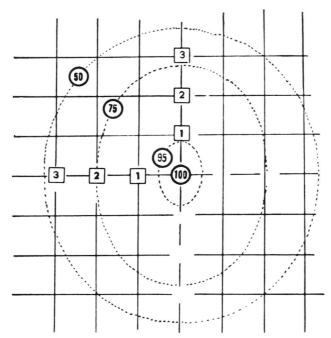

Figure 11–44 Field pattern produced by "C" director at a distance of 3 inches. (Courtesy of the Raytheon Corporation.)

the shape of a ring[164] (Fig. 11-43). The intensity in the center of the field is half the value of the intensity in the ring. However, the field distribution directly under the tip of the antenna rod varies from this pattern in that the highest intensity is found in the center of the field. The construction of the "B" director is similar to that of the "A" director, but the diameter of the reflector is approximately 15.3 cm. and the field pattern is similar to but larger than that of the "A" director. The "C" director consists of a half wave (6.1 cm.) dipole antenna with a corner reflector. It produces a beam with an oval cross section. The area of maximum intensity is found in the center of the field (Fig. 11–44).

Most recently, an "E" director has become available. It consists of a full wave (12.2 cm.) dipole antenna with a corner reflector; however, since it is larger than the "C" director, the pattern is narrower in the plane parallel to the dipole.

As in ultrasound, the beaming properties of an applicator are better (i.e., the divergence will be less) the larger the diameter of the antenna is, compared with the wavelength. Since the wavelength in air is 12.2 cm., it is obvious that the angle of divergence of the beam produced by therapeutic applicators will be significant.[165] Thus, the field intensity decreases rapidly with an increasing distance from the applicator. The total output of the machines when measured is up to 100 watts.[166]

Biophysics

It has been well documented that most, if not all, of the therapeutically desirable physiologic responses to microwave application are due to heating. There are, however, documented non-thermal effects, such as the pearl chain formation. The significance of these effects, however, as far as therapy is concerned, is unknown. There are also claims in the Russian literature as to non-thermal physiologic responses which are not related to direct therapeutic effects and may represent contraindications. Again, very little is known about these effects and the conditions under which they occur.[167-169]

Propagation and Absorption of Microwaves in Tissues.   Even though most therapeutic effects are due to heating, the temperature distribution in the tissues treated is specific for this modality and is influenced by the frequency used. It is on this basis that this modality is selected. The temperature distribution in turn depends on the propagation and absorption characteristics of the tissues traversed by the beam.[170-173]

Several workers have studied the absorption of microwave energy in biologic media.[174-177] It is apparent that the dielectric properties of the medium and the specific resistance or conductivity are responsible for the energy absorp-

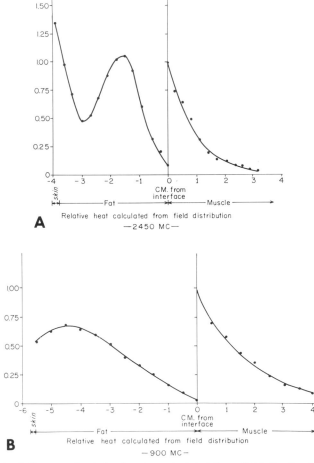

Figure 11–45   *A*, Pattern of relative heating calculated from field distribution at a frequency of 2450 mc. *B*, Pattern of relative heating calculated from field distribution at a frequency of 900 mc. (From Lehmann et al.: Comparison of Relative Heating Patterns Produced in Tissues by Exposure to Microwave Energy at Frequencies of 2,450 and 900 Megacycles. Arch. Phys. Med., Vol. 43, 1962.)

tion. Tissues with high water content, such as musculature, subcutaneous fat and fluid media, such as found in the eye or in sweat beads, are likely to absorb more microwave energy than is bone.

The reflection of microwaves at the body surface and at the tissue interfaces can be calculated if the dielectric properties and the conductivities of the tissues are known. Schwan[165] has pointed out that a large and variable amount of energy may be reflected at the skin surface under therapeutic conditions. It is possible to have variable losses of more than 50 per cent of the energy irradiated from the director and thus it is difficult to reproduce the biologic effects in a reliable fashion.

Schwan[165] calculated a pattern of relative heating for homogeneous tissues with plane and parallel interfaces. Lehmann and associates[178] obtained the pattern of relative heating by actual measurements of the power distribution throughout a specimen consisting of skin, subcutaneous fat and musculature with typical anatomic and biologic interfaces. They concurred with Schwan's calculations that an appreciable reflection of microwave energy occurred at the interface between subcutaneous fat and musculature, with the result that a large amount of energy converted into heat in the subcutaneous tissues (Fig. 11–45 A). Also in agreement with Schwan, they found that the depth of penetration was poor in muscle tissues if the frequency of 2450 megacycles was used. The intensity available at the surface of the muscle dropped to a 50 per cent level at a depth of 1 cm. By contrast, the amount of energy converted into heat

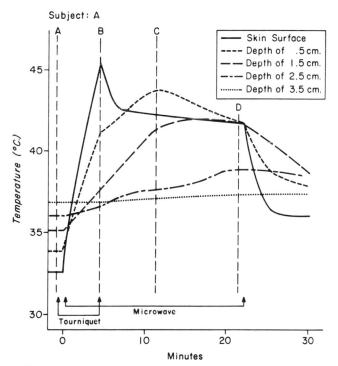

Figure 11–46 Temperatures recorded in the human thigh during exposure to microwaves at 2456 mc. applied with waveguide. (From Lehmann et al.: A Comparative Analysis of Therapeutic Heating Patterns and Blood Flow Changes Produced by the Application of Modern Diathermy Modalities in Human Volunteers. Unpublished data.)

in the subcutaneous tissues was much less and the depth of penetration (3 cm.) in the musculature much better if microwave frequency of 900 megacycles was used (Fig. 11–45 *B*). The resulting temperature distribution in the live human was modified not only by such constants as specific heat, specific weight and thermal conductivity but also by physiologic responses such as change in the blood flow, as illustrated in Figures 11–46 and 11–47.[191] In this case, the temperature distribution shows the peak values in the subcutaneous fat. If a tourniquet was applied to prevent cooling of the most superficial tissues due to the increased blood flow, the highest temperature was obtained in the most superficial subcutaneous tissues. On the other hand, as shown in Figure 11–48, the temperature distribution produced with a new experimental 915 megacycle contact applicator provides simultaneous cooling of the surface temperatures.[179] Even heating of the muscle can be obtained from the most superficial musculature to a depth of approximately 4 centimeters, that is, to the tissues adjacent to the bone. Whereas the temperature distribution of microwaves operating at a frequency of 2456 megacycles in most instances can be duplicated by shortwave diathermy application, the 915 megacycle direct contact applicator is a unique tool for selective heating of the musculature.[180]

The conclusion for therapy was that the application of microwaves at the commercially available frequency of 2456 megacycles would result in a relative-

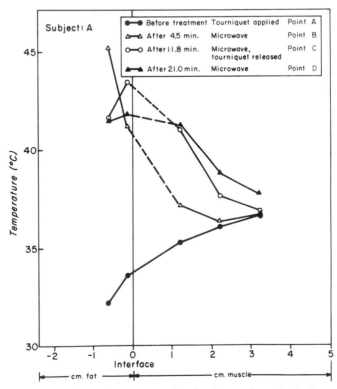

Figure 11–47 A comparison of temperature distribution produced in the human thigh during exposure to microwave at 2456 mc. applied with waveguide. (From Lehmann et al.: A Comparative Analysis of Therapeutic Heating Patterns and Blood Flow Changes Produced by the Application of Modern Diathermy Modalities in Human Volunteers. Unpublished data.)

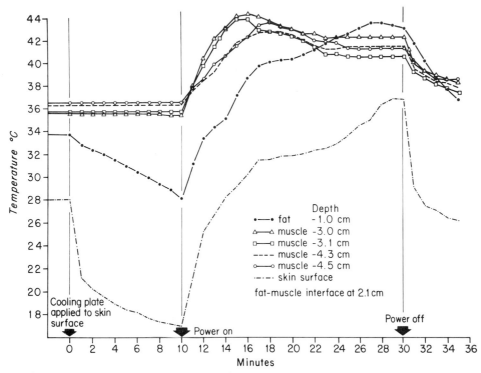

Figure 11–48 Temperatures resulting from application of microwave with a 915 MHz. contact applicator in a typical experiment at various depths of tissue.

ly high if not the highest temperature in the subcutaneous tissues unless they are applied to an area where skin and subcutaneous fat are of minimal thickness as could be demonstrated by Rae and co-workers[181] with dogs. Also, Hollander and Horvath[35] were able to elevate the joint temperature above the skin temperature in elbows and knees, both joints having a minimal soft tissue cover. Their temperature differential was less pronounced in patients with rheumatoid arthritis.

The application of microwaves at or below the frequency of 900 megacycles to a person with a moderate amount of subcutaneous fat would result in a temperature distribution in which the highest temperature would occur in the muscle; also the muscle could be evenly heated down to the bone.

Lehmann and associates[182] later studied a pattern of relative heating and the actual temperature distribution produced in specimens with more complex geometry, similar to that encountered in the treatment of joints for the frequencies of 2456 and 900 megacycles (Fig. 11–49 *A* and *B*). It was found that during exposure to high frequency of 2456 megacycles, a heating pattern indicative of energy reflection and production of a pattern of standing waves at the muscle-bone interface was observed. The development of undesirable "hot spots" can be the result (Fig. 11–50). This possibility seems to be less at or below frequencies of 900 megacycles. The difference between the frequencies with regard to the development of "hot spots" in front of the bone may be explained by the fact that the bone represents a reflecting obstacle for wave propagation

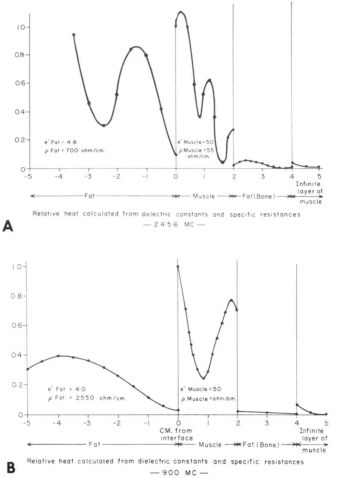

Figure 11–49 *A*, Pattern of relative heating calculated from dielectric constants and specific resistances in a complex specimen at a frequency of 2456 mc. *B*, Pattern of relative heating calculated from dielectric constants and specific resistances in a complex specimen at a frequency of 900 mc. (From Lehmann et al.: A Comparative Evaluation of Temperature Distributions Produced by Microwaves at 2,456 and 900 Megacycles in Geometrically Complex Specimens. Arch. Phys. Med., Vol. 43, 1962.)

at the higher frequency since its diameter is relatively large as compared with the wavelength in muscle tissue. This relation between bone diameter and wavelength is reversed at the low frequency. Thus, the waves of high frequency are reflected to a greater extent than those of the low frequency.

Consistent with these conclusions, Worden and co-workers[183] observed burns over the femurs of dogs (Fig. 11-51), which appeared to be the result of energy reflected at the bone surface. Engel and associates[184] reported that horse flesh was heated to a higher degree if bone was present under the flesh at a depth of 1 cm. Most recently, Addington and others[185] found that the hollow viscera heat differentially and the stomach and liver may be considered as "hot spots." Selective burns in these areas were observed in dogs. Also, the tissues overlying the thoracic cage were selectively burned[186] and the anterior cardiac surface was selectively heated.[187, 188] Selective absorption can also occur

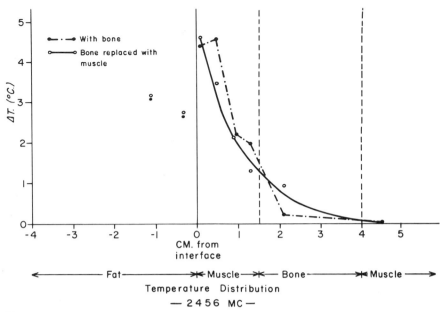

Figure 11–50 Distribution of temperature in complex specimen with and without bone at a frequency of 2456 mc. (From Lehmann et al.: A Comparative Evaluation of Temperature Distributions Produced by Microwaves at 2,456 and 900 Megacycles in Geometrically Complex Specimens. Arch. Phys. Med., Vol. 43, 1962.)

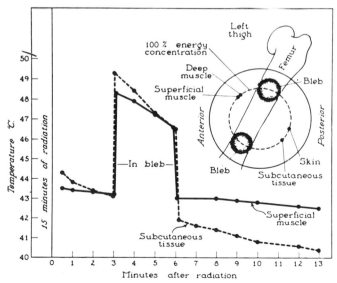

Figure 11–51 Temperature variations after microwave radiation across femur when blebs are present. (From Worden et al.: The Heating Effects of Microwaves With and Without Ischemia. Arch. Phys. Med., Vol. 29, 1948.)

TABLE 11–5 DIFFERENCE IN TEMPERATURES INDICATED BY MEASUREMENTS IN FRONT OF AND BEHIND BONE AFTER EXPOSURE TO MICROWAVES AT FREQUENCIES OF 2456 AND 900 MEGACYCLES

2456 MEGACYCLES	900 MEGACYCLES
6.4° C.	5.1° C.
4.6° C.	1.7° C.
9.2° C.	3.6° C.
6.0° C.	2.4° C.

if metallic implants are present in tissues which can be reached by any appreciable amount of microwave energy.[189] A dramatic illustration of this can be given by igniting steel wool in the microwave field in air.

This review of the investigations using different frequencies strongly suggests that the microwave machines used presently do not operate at the most therapeutically effective frequency. They were introduced into therapy because generators operating at these frequencies were available for medical application after the war and not because 2456 megacycles was considered to be the best frequency for medical use. The data now suggest that the optimal frequency would be at 900 megacycles or below, minimizing the heating effect in the subcutaneous tissues and heating the underlying tissues more adequately. The development of "hot spots" as a result of reflection from bone is prevented to a large degree. These frequencies also have a better depth of penetration.

These investigations also suggest that, because of the large amount of reflection at the bone surface, very little energy reaches the area beyond the bone at either frequency, 2456 or 900 megacycles. This is indicated by the difference in temperature between the area in front of and behind the bone when exposed to microwaves (Table 11-5). Though this difference is less when a frequency of 900 megacycles is used, it is still too great to allow full therapeutic exposure of a joint through bone. If it is the purpose to heat the entire joint, the joint should be exposed from all aspects, as is the case in ultrasonic therapy.[190, 191]

Physiologic Responses

Since microwave diathermy was introduced into physical medicine,[192, 193] extensive studies have been conducted on the physiologic effects produced by this new type of radiation. A large number of physiologic, pathologic and biochemical reactions were studied. In some instances the mechanism by which they were produced was also investigated.[194] The result of these studies indicated that the microwave heating effects was responsible for the vast majority of the reactions of potential therapeutic significance. However, nonthermal reactions could also be demonstrated.

Heating Effects. Since microwave energy is absorbed in the body and is effective in elevating the tissue temperature, it is obvious that all reactions which can be produced by temperature elevation in the tissues can be observed after exposure to microwave energy of adequate power levels.

An increase in blood flow was measured with a bubble flow meter during exposure to microwaves.[195] Other reports[196, 199] demonstrated that the observed increase in blood flow was closely related to the increase in tissue temperature. Kottke et al.[200] observed a decrease of the circulation in organs covered with thick tissue layers, such as the kidneys.

The effects of microwave irradiation on the chick embryo have been investigated by Szarski[201, 202] and by Van Ummersen.[203] The results of these studies suggest that the untoward effect on the growth of the chick embryo is a secondary effect of heat, where a loss of viability of the tissues is not caused by the heat, per se, but results from the accumulation of products of metabolism and lack of oxygen following circulatory failure. Organs of higher metabolic rate succumb sooner.

Cooper and associates[204] studied the effects of adrenalectomy, vagotomy and ganglionic blockade on the circulatory response to hyperthermia produced by microwave application. Hyperthermia of 40.5° C. (72.9° F.) was induced by exposure to microwaves at a power density of 0.8 watt/cm.[2]. They found that these procedures modified the normal circulatory responses to hyperthermia, but that the responses were basically similar to those produced in the presence of any other type of hyperthermia.

A temperature increase of 3 to 5° C. (5.4 to 9° F.) in the tibia of dogs after exposure to microwave diathermy of 65 watts was reported some time ago by Engel and associates.[205]

Other more recent investigations have included the study of the effect of microwaves on bone growth. Wise, Castleman and Watkins[206] found, after the application of a high dosage of microwaves, a decrease in bone growth, probably related to the heating effect. On the other hand, lower dosage applied with shortwave diathermy by Doyle and Smart[207] produced a stimulation of bone growth. Most recent investigation by Granberry and Janes[208] did not reveal any stimulation of bone growth by microwave diathermy in animals with dosage that was not associated with the sensation of pain. The authors concluded that the length of treatment might have been insufficient, that continuous heating of the area might be necessary to stimulate growth, or that external or artificial heating of this type might not represent a stimulus to acceleration of growth.

The physiologic effects of microwave irradiation on peripheral nerves and other neurophysiological responses were studied by McAfee.[209, 210] The author studied the effects on cats, dogs, rabbits and rats and found that nociceptive responses could be obtained when heating the peripheral nerves with warm water, a resistance wire thermode or microwaves of 12.2 and 3 cm. wavelength. Temperatures produced were in the range of 45 to 47° C. (113 to 116.6° F.). Responses elicited included arousal reactions, blood pressure and vascular responses and signs of neurohumoral activity. Thermal stimulation of peripheral nerves occurs independently of a significant increase in skin temperature or of total body heating.[211] Action on the autonomic nervous system was studied by Hauswirth and Kracmar.[212]

The effects of microwaves on the eye have been studied extensively.[213-220] It has been found that it may be possible to heat selectively the fluid media of the eye, including the lens, with microwaves. It is most likely that cataracts of the lens are produced by the heating effect of microwaves. Below a power density of 0.12 watt/cm.[2], opacities have not been observed even after prolonged exposure.[221] It also was found that the cataract-producing effect of microwaves is apparently a cumulative one. If injurious power levels are applied to the eye, the effect is probably additive and the cataracts may appear after a period of latency.

Nonthermal Effects. Searle and associates[222] studied the effect of microwaves on the testes of rats. They monitored the temperature elevation in the tissues and compared the effects with those obtained with infrared. They found significant differences which suggested that the microwave effects were not due entirely to heating of the tissues. On the other hand, when they irradiated larvae of the common fruit fly, they did not find any biologic effects unless the temperature was maintained at an optimal level. These findings are essentially in agreement with those previously obtained by Imig et al.[223] and by other researchers.[224, 225]

A pearl chain formation is observed during microwave exposure of appropriate materials as was observed during exposure to shortwaves. The theoretical aspects of the effects as produced with microwaves have been recently studied in detail by Saita and Schwan.[226] As in shortwave diathermy, the therapeutic significance of this effect is unknown.

In contrast to American authors, a Russian investigator found that the effects of microwaves on nerve tissue, specifically on eye function, were not related to the heating effect since they could be produced at power levels which were too low to produce any appreciable rise of the tissue temperature. The levels used were 5 milliwatts/cm.[2]. He found a change of the optic rheobase, the chronaxie and the area of the blind spot during microwave irradiation. The decrease of the blind spot area suggested a mobilization of the light sensitive elements of the retina.[227]

A number of physiologic responses have been studied recently without elucidating the biophysical mechanisms by which they are produced. Richardson[228] found that blood coagulation changes may be induced by microwave irradiation. He also found that the coagulation time may be significantly increased or decreased depending on the dosage. The author pointed out that when microwaves were applied in relatively high dosage, biologically effective power densities were obtained in the liver tissues. This is a situation which would rarely occur under therapeutic conditions.

In summary, most of the biologic reactions of therapeutic significance are due to the heating effect resulting from microwave absorption in the tissues. There are, however, some effects which are nonthermal in nature. The significance of these effects for therapeutic purposes is still inadequately understood. It is not known how many of these would actually occur in the live organism under therapeutic conditions. Therefore, for therapeutic purposes, this discussion is limited to the heating effect of microwave energy. However, it is possible that some specific reactions may be unveiled in the future which are nonthermal in nature and may add to the specificity of the therapeutic results.

Dosimetry

The dose can be defined as the product of applied energy times duration of action. As in the other diathermics, the actual tissue temperature is more important than the applied energy for determining the biologic results, since most of the reactions to microwaves are thermal in nature. Even though we have information on the relative distribution of temperature in the organism exposed to microwaves, we do not presently have a way to assess the absolute level of the temperatures obtained in the tissue because the meters on the commercially available machines do not give any information on the amount of energy entering the organism, nor, of course, do they give any information on the distribution of the energy throughout the tissues. The development of an adequate dosimetry at 2456 mc. is hardly possible since a variable amount of the energy may be reflected at the surface of the organism.[2] This situation also could be improved by using lower frequencies. In order to apply microwaves of 2456 megacycles in adequate dosage it is necessary to depend on the feeling of warmth on the part of the patient exactly as it was described in the paragraph on shortwaves (p. 281).

Technique of Therapeutic Application

The main advantage of microwave application is the ease with which it can be applied. The technique of application is almost as simple as shining a luminous light on the patient. Proposed outputs and the proposed spacing of the applicators by the manufacturer can at least serve as guide lines. In order to get an adequate therapeutic effect, it is very often necessary to use higher outputs and also to space the director closer to the skin surface than is suggested by the manufacturer. The heating patterns produced in the specimen have been studied by Lehmann and associates.[229] They found that a more vigorous heating effect is produced when the applicator is brought closer to the skin. One inch is probably satisfactory if vigorous application is desired. Because of the danger of developing "hot spots" close to the antenna rod, the applicator should not be brought in contact with the skin. This is especially true for the "A" director.[229] Since the beam produced by the directors is limited in size, it is important to expose the area to be treated. To heat a joint, a multiple field method of application should be used and the joint should be exposed from all sides. If a mild heat application is desired, the dose can be reduced either by increasing the distance of the applicator from the skin or by reducing the output of the machine. By increasing the distance between the director and the skin, a somewhat larger field is treated. Special precaution must be taken that sweat beads do not accumulate on the skin, since these are selectively heated and often lead to small surface burns (see Fig. 11-50). Care should be taken also that the eyes are not exposed to a vigorous treatment. The eyes can be shielded with a fine mesh of copper wire padded with felt to prevent burns. Also, precaution should be taken that other metal parts are not within the microwave field since they can be heated selectively.

The duration of the application is usually 20 to 30 minutes. Recent experiments have confirmed that this duration produces an adequate rise of temperature even in the deeper tissues.[191] The patient always should be undressed and no clothing should cover the area being treated.

Therapeutic Indications

General Indications. Microwave diathermy is the easiest to apply of the forms of deep heating. However, even with the "E" director, the area which can be treated at any given time is limited to a comparatively small field. As far as the depth of the heating effect is concerned, the commercially available frequency of 2456 megacycles presumably produces the highest temperature in the subcutaneous tissues or sometimes in the more superficial musculature[230] (see Figs. 11-46 and 11-47). Microwaves cannot be used for the vigorous heating of joints which are covered by heavy layers of soft tissue. It has been demonstrated that they cannot heat the hip joint to any degree of practical significance.[231] Microwave diathermy has proved to be less effective than ultrasound in treatment of the shoulder joint if vigorous heating is desired.[232] Microwaves also cannot heat the pelvic organs effectively, according to Kottke.[233] Consistent with his observations, Rubin and Erdman[234] observed that neither conception nor pregnancy was disturbed by therapeutic microwave application. Because of their relatively poor depth of penetration, microwaves are often used in subchronic or subacute processes which lend themselves to a mild type of heating and the associated reflex effects.

With the future use of lower frequencies, experimental evidence suggests that microwave might become a very potent modality for heating musculature selectively. What type of therapeutic responses can be expected from such a diathermy modality is a question which remains to be investigated.

Specific Indications.[235, 236]   Most of the specific indications for microwave diathermy are conditions of the musculoskeletal system, such as joint disease ranging from degenerative joint disease to rheumatoid arthritis, calcific bursitis, tendinitis and periarthritis of the shoulder. From the discussion of biophysics, it is apparent that microwave is the modality of choice if mild heating is indicated. In dealing with a chronic condition, e.g., joint contractures, the choice would be ultrasonic diathermy; in treating highly acute inflammatory reactions, such as a joint flare-up, superficial heating agents or sometimes even a cold application should be used.

Even though the application of microwaves has been advocated for the protruded intervertebral disk syndrome, either superficial heat in the acute stage or shortwave diathermy in the chronic stage would be more effective than a heat application which covers only a very small area.

Traumatic conditions, such as sprains, can be treated with microwaves, especially if they are located in superficial tissues.[193, 237, 238]

Superficial inflammatory reactions, such as furuncles, axillary sweat gland abscesses and tenosynovitis, have been treated with microwaves.[239]

Low doses of microwaves have also been applied to various conditions of the eyes like iridocyclitis, scleritis and keratitis. Special precautions should be taken to apply the microwaves in low dosage only.[240, 241]

SUMMARY.   A large number of clinical indications have been developed for microwave therapy which, for the most part, are consistent with the suggested indications developed from biophysical research. Unfortunately, statistical and objective evaluation of the clinical efficacy of microwave therapy is not available as yet. In the case of periarthritis, where microwaves have been compared with ultrasonic diathermy, the microwave diathermy was less effective, as would be anticipated.

Contraindications.   Again, microwave diathermy is biologically effective mainly because it is a deep heating agent. The general contraindications to heat should be observed, including contraindications to radiation of areas of ischemic tissue, hemorrhagic diathesis, regions having malignant tumors, areas of impaired sensation or debilitated patients. Because of the possibility of a selective rise of temperature resulting in burns, microwaves should not be applied in high dosage to edematous tissues, over wet dressings or near metallic implants when it is anticipated that a large amount of energy will reach the area of the surgical implant.[189] Nor should microwaves be applied over adhesive tape. They should be applied with extreme caution over bony prominences because reflection may result in an uncontrolled increase in intensity in these areas.

Special care should be taken to avoid exposing the eye to higher dosage. Since the development of cataracts was observed, this problem has been studied extensively.[215, 242, 243] Opacities of the lens have been produced experimentally in animals.[214, 216, 244, 245] In recent reviews of the problem, the authors found a statistically significant increase in the occurrence of posterior polar defects and early opacification of the lens in personnel exposed to microwaves.[217, 218, 220] Another group of personnel not exposed to the microwave radiation served as controls. It was also found that the frequency of defects may be dependent upon duration and severity of exposure. No impairment of visual acuity, however, was necessarily associated with these findings. Thus, the results of animal experimentation and the clinical observations of personnel exposed to microwave radiation both suggest strongly that comparatively small dosage may produce opacities or cataracts in the crystalline lens which may or may not be associated with visual disturbances. The evidence also suggests that these effects are thermal in nature. However, they are cumulative and may lead to cataract formation after a period of latency. This is of special interest since it is the only cumulative thermal effect which can be demonstrated so far. When microwaves are applied to the eye for therapeutic purposes, it is necessary to lower the dosage. It must also be recognized that a calculated risk is probably taken, especially if long-term repeated exposures are considered. If microwaves are applied in high dosage to areas in the vicinity of the eye, shielding of the eye is required.

The safety of microwaves has been investigated extensively because of the hazards of accidental exposure of military and civilian personnel to high power radar beams.[246-248] The interest in safety was greatly stimulated by the publication of one death of a worker exposed to a high power radar beam. In the article, the question was raised as to whether or not the peritonitis with multiple peforations of the intestinal tract was related to microwave exposure.[249]

It has been shown by Howland and Michaelson[250] that in exposures of the whole body, the possibility of localized burns in animals is a result of the reflection of microwaves at interfaces with production of standing waves, and it may represent a real danger. However, the power densities necessary to produce such burns must exceed 0.165 watt/cm.². Pressman[251] found a rise of skin temperature only at power densities higher than 0.005 watt/cm.² when 11 cm. waves were used. An exposure to a power density of approximately 0.1 watt/cm.² is necessary to produce any effects of biologic significance.[252, 253] Presently, a safety factor of ten is observed by the Air Force; that is, personnel are not exposed to levels of power in excess of 0.01 watt/cm.². At these energy levels cataracts have not been observed since they appear only at power densities of 0.12 watt/cm.² and above and only after prolonged exposures.[221] The effect of microwaves on reproductive organs has been studied in detail and Susskind[254] concluded that sterilization could be produced only at a power level which would be high enough that death would occur from heating.

On the other hand, it must be recognized the power densities used for therapeutic application definitely are of the order of 0.1 or 1.0 watt/cm.², at which level untoward effects have been described. It is for this reason that special precautions should be taken in therapeutic application of microwaves to the eye, and to interfaces, specifically when bony prominences covered by little soft tissue are exposed to the microwave beam. Selective heating may also occur in the fluid accumulations such as sweat beads or in fluid accumulations within the body such as in joint cavities. The exposure of the reproductive organs should be deferred until evidence is accumulated that even low dosage may not produce untoward effects.

Microwave diathermy has the same potential as shortwaves to cause dysfunction of implanted electronic cardiac pacemakers in patients being treated with the modality. The same dangers also exist for other persons who wear pacemakers that may be in the close vicinity of the diathermy applicator. The microwaves can induce changes in pacemaker output while treating any area of the body and could produce burns at the electrode positions when used directly in the implant or heart areas. Again, microwave diathermy *should not* be used on patients with implanted pacemakers without a clear understanding of these hazards and in no circumstances should it be used directly in the areas where the device and interconnecting wires are implanted.

SUMMARY

The introduction of new deep heating modalities such as ultrasound and radar or microwaves and the improvement of the technique of application of older diathermy procedures, such as shortwaves, have made it possible to elevate the tissue temperature level at the site of a pathologic lesion or in the area to be treated to any desired level up to tolerance. Thus, the modalities that before these developments were used more or less indiscriminately and that produced more or less mild heating effects have become really potent with regard to their biologic effects. It is now essential to select the modality specifically for a specific therapeutic purpose. They are not interchangeable as to their therapeutic results. Even though there may be some areas of overlap, each modality has its specific therapeutic indications where it alone can produce therapeutic results. The specificity of the effects is related to the specific temperature distribution produced by each modality. Generally speaking, the indications have been developed by matching the location of the peak temperature within the distribution produced by any given modality in any specific application with the site of the lesion or the area to be treated. Thus a large number of physiologic responses can be elicited, ranging from mild to severe degrees. As with any other therapeutic agent, with an increase in effectiveness there is also an increase in danger. Each modality has its specific contraindications and special precautions which must be observed in order to apply the modality not only effectively but also safely. Thus, only with the knowledge of the biophysics, the physiologic responses and their modification by the technique of application, and the indications and contraindications can the physician utilize these powerful modalities intelligently, effectively and safely.

REFERENCES

1. Fischer, E., and Solomon, S.: Physiological Responses to Heat and Cold. In Licht, S.: Therapeutic Heat. New Haven, Conn. Elizabeth Licht, 1958, pp. 116–156. This chapter contains many literature references.
2. Lehmann, J. F.: Biophysical Mode of Action of Biologic and Therapeutic Ultrasonic Reactions. J. Acoust. Soc. Amer., 25:17–25, 1953. This article contains many literature references.
3. Lehmann, J. F.: The Biophysical Basis of Biologic Ultrasonic Reactions with Special Reference to Ultrasonic Therapy. Arch. Phys. Med., 34:139–152, 1953. This article contains many literature references.
4. Zankel, H. T.: Effect of Ultrasound on Blood Flow. American Institute of Ultrasonics in Medicine, Proc. 7th Ann. Conf., New York, 1962, pp. 7–17.
5. Lehmann, J. F., and Hohlfeld, R.: Der Gewebestoffwechsel nach Ultraschall und Wärmeeinwirkung. Strahlentherapie, 87:544–549, 1952.

6. Pauly, H., and Hug, O.: Untersuchungen über den Einfluss von Ultraschallwellen und von Wärme auf den Staffweschel überlebender Gewebe. Strahlentherapie, *95*:116–130, 1954.

7. Gersten, J. W.: Effect of Ultrasound on Tendon Extensibility. Amer. J. Phys. Med., *34*:362–369, 1955.

8. Lehmann, J. F., Masock, A. J., Warren, C. G., and Koblanski, J. N.: Effects of Therapeutic Temperatures on Tendon Extensibility. Arch. Phys. Med., *51: 8*:481–487, 1970.

9. Backlund, L., and Tiselius, P.: Objective Measurement of Joint Stiffness in Rheumatoid Arthritis. Acta Rheum. Scand., *13*:275–288, 1967.

10. Lehmann, J. F., Brunner, G. D., and Stow, R. W.: Pain Threshold Measurements after Therapeutic Application of Ultrasound Microwaves and Infrared. Arch. Phys. Med., *39*:560–565, 1958.

11. Dodt, E., and Zotterman, Y.: Mode of Action of Warm Receptors. Acta Physiol. Scand., *26*:345–357, 1952.

12. Dodt, E., and Zotterman, Y.: The Discharge of Specific Cold Fibres at High Temperatures (The Paradoxical Cold). Acta Physiol. Scand., *26*:358–365, 1952.

13. Hensel, H.: Temperaturempfindung und intracutane Wärmebewegung. Pflueger Arch. Ges. Physiol., *252*:165–215, 1950.

14. Hensel, H., and Zotterman, Y.: Quantitative Beziehungen zwischen der Entladung einzelner Kältefasern und der Temperatur. Acta Physiol. Scand., *23*:291–319, 1951.

15. Selke, O. O.: Complications of Heat Therapy. Amer. J. Orthop., *4*:168–169, 1962.

16. Scott, B. O.: Short Wave Diathermy. In Licht, S.: Therapeutic Heat. New Haven, Conn., Elizabeth Licht, 1958, pp. 255–283. This chapter contains many literature references.

17. Kebbel, W., and Pätzold, J.: Die Wärmeverteilung in Fett-Muskel-Schichten bei verschiedenen Spulenanordnungen, zugleich ein Beitrag Zur Problematik der Microwellentherapie. Strahlentherapie, *95*:107–115, 1954.

18. Scott, B. O.: An Alternative Technique of Treating the Hip with Short-wave Diathermy. Ann. Phys. Med., *2*:169–173, 1955.

19. Schwan, H. P.: Biophysics of Diathermy. In Licht, S.: Therapeutic Heat. New Haven, Conn., Elizabeth Licht, 1958, pp. 55–115. This chapter contains many literature references.

20. Scott, B. O.: Heating of Fatty Tissues in a Short-Wave Field. Ann. Phys. Med., *2*:48–52, 1954.

21. Whyte, H. M., and Reader, S. R.: Effectiveness of Different Forms of Heating. Ann. Rheum. Dis., *10*:449–452, 1951.

22. Kottke, F. J.: Heat in Pelvic Diseases. In Licht, S.: Therapeutic Heat. New Haven, Conn., Elizabeth Licht, 1958, pp. 402–416. This chapter contains many literature references.

23. Schüly, H., and Volk, H.: Comparative Temperature Measurements after Irradiation with Various Types of Shortwaves, with Special Reference to the Small Pelvis. (Ger.). Geburtsh. Gynaek., *141*:288–294, 1954.

24. Lehmann, J. F., Guy, A. W., DeLateur, B. J., Stonebridge, J. B., and Warren, C. G.: Heating Patterns Produced by Shortwave Diathermy Using Helical Coil Induction Coil Applicators. Arch. Phys. Med., *49*:193–198, 1968.

25. Lehmann, J. F., DeLateur, B. J., and Stonebridge, J. B.: Selective Muscle Heating by Short-wave Diathermy With a Helical Coil. Arch. Phys. Med., *50*:117–132, 1969.

26. Hill, L., and Taylor, H. J.: Supposed Specific Effect of High Frequency Currents on some Physiological Preparations; Reaction of Nerve Muscle Preparation to Stimulation on Isolated Frog's Heart. Arch. Phys. Therapy, *18*:263–269, 1937.

27. Kottke, F. J., Koza, D. W., Kubicek, W. G., and Olson, M.: Studies of Deep Circulatory Response to Short Wave Diathermy and Microwave Diathermy in Man. Arch. Phys. Med., *30*:431–437, 1949.

28. Wise, C. S.: The Effect of Diathermy on Blood Flow. Arch. Phys. Med., *29*:17–21, 1948.

29. Abramson, D. I., Bell, Y., Rejal, H., Tucks, J., Burnett, C., and Fleischer, C. J.: Changes in Blood Flow, Oxygen Uptake and Tissue Temperature Produced by Therapeutic Physical Agents. II. Effect of Short-wave Diathermy. Amer. J. Phys. Med., *39*:87–95, 1960.

30. Barth and Kern: Experimentelle Untersuchungen zur Frage der Durchstörmungsänderung im Muskel unter dem Einflus der Kurzwellenbehandlung im Spulenfeld. Ein Beitra zur Frage der Dosierung der Kurzwelle. Elektromed., *5*:121, 1960.

31. Lasch, F., Mente, W., and Schneider, G.: Clinico-Experimental Studies on the Influencing of Renal Function during Short Wave Diathermy of the Kidneys. Wien. Klin. Wschr., *71*:915–918, 1959.

32. Millard, J. B.: Changes in Tissue Clearance of Radioactive Sodium from Skin and Muscle During Heating with Short-wave Diathermy. A Preliminary Report. Ann. Phys. Med., *2*:248–252, 1955.

33. Adler, E., and Magora, A.: Experiments on the Relation Between Short-Wave Irradiation and the Pituitary-Cortico-Adrenal System. Amer. J. Phys. Med., *34*:521–534, 1955.

34. Lehmann, J. F., McMillan, J. A., Brunner, G. D., and Blumberg, J. B.: Comparative Study of

the Efficiency of Shortwave, Microwave, and Ultrasonic Diathermy in Heating the Hip Joint. Arch. Phys. Med., *40:*510-512, 1959.

35. Hollander, J. L., and Horvath, S. M.: Influence of Physical Therapy Procedures on the Intra-Articular Temperature of Normal and Arthritic Subjects. Amer. J. Med. Sci., *218:*543-548, 1949.

36. Kraut, R. M., and Anderson, T. P.: Trochanteric Bursitis: Management. Arch. Phys. Med., *40:*8-14, 1959.

37. Harris, R.: Effect of Shortwave Diathermy on Radio-Sodium Clearance from the Knee Joint in the Normal and in Rheumatoid Arthritis. Third International Congress of Physical Medicine and Rehabilitation, Washington, D.C., 1960.

38. Bierman, W., and Horowitz, E. A.: A New Vaginal Diathermy Electrode. Arch. Phys. Therapy, *17:*15-16, 1956.

39. Konarska, I., and Michniewicz, L.: Shortwave Therapy of Diseases of the Anterior Portion of the Eye. Klin. Oczna, *25:*185-194, 1955.

40. Klare, V.: Ultra-Short Wave Therapy of Stomach and Duodenal Diseases with Tube Electrodes. Wien. Med. Wschr., *108:*273-275, 1958.

41. Schliephake, E.: Kurzwellentherapie. Jena, G. Fischer, 1935.

42. Yang, T. P.: Effects of Ultra-shortwave Diathermy on Chronic Pneumonia in Children. Chin. Med. J., *81:*109-115, 1962.

43. Wise, C. S.: The Effect of Diathermy on Blood Flow. Arch. Phys. Med., *29:*17-21, 1948.

44. Scott, B. O.: The Effects of Metal on Shortwave Field Distribution. Ann. Phys. Med., *1:*238-244, 1953.

45. Feucht, B. L., Richardson, A. W., and Hines, H. M.: Effects of Implanted Metals on Tissue Hyperthermia Produced by Microwaves. Arch. Phys. Med., *30:*164-169, 1949.

46. Scott, B. O.: Effects of Contact Lenses on Shortwave Field Distribution. Brit. J. Ophthal., *40:*696, 1956.

47. Mussa, B.: Embryopathology Due to Physical Cause (Shortwave in Pregnancy Causing Fetal Malformation). Minerva Nipiol. *5:*69-72, 1955.

48. Ghietti, A.: Embryopathology Caused by Shortwaves, Clinico-Experimental Study. Minerva Nipiol. *5:*7-12, 1955.

49. Muth, E.: String-Formation of the Emulsoid Particles in an Alternating Electric Field. Kolloid-Z, *41:*97-102, 1927.

50. Liebesny, P.: Athermic Short Wave Therapy. Arch. Phys. Therapy, *19:*736-740, 1938.

51. Krasny-Ergen, W.: Nicht-Thermische Wirkungen Elektrischer Schwingungen Auf Kolloide. Hochfreq. Tech. Elektroak, *48:*126-133, 1936.

52. Gersten, J. W., Wakim, K. G., Herrick, J. F., and Krusen, F. H.: The Effect of Microwave Diathermy on the Peripheral Circulation and on Tissue Temperature in Man. Arch. Phys. Med., *30:*7-25, 1949.

53. Cameron, B. M.: Experimental Acceleration of Wound Healing. Amer. J. Orthop., *3:*336-343, 1961.

54. Witte, E.: Impulsdiathermie mit extremen Feldstärken und ihre spezifischen biologischen Effekte. Strahlentherapie, *97:*146-148, 1955.

55. Witte, E., Strathmann, W., and Hertel, A.: Impulsdiathermie. Strahlentherapie, *94:*320-326, 1954.

56. Nadasdi, M.: Inhibition of Experimental Arthritis by Athermic Pulsing SW in Rats. Amer. J. Orthop., *2:*105-107, 1960.

57. Erdman, W. J.: Peripheral Blood Flow Measurements During Application of Pulsed High Frequency Currents. Amer. J. Orthop., *2:*196-197, 1960.

58. Silverman, D. R., and Pendleton, L.: A Comparison of the Effects of Continuous and Pulsed Shortwave Diathermy on Peripheral Circulation. Arch. Phys. Med., *49:*429-436, 1968.

59. Obrosor, A. N., and Jasnogordshi, V. G.: A New Method of Physical Therapy-Pulsed Electric Field by Ultra-High Frequency. Moscow, Academy of Medical Sciences of the USSR, p. 156.

60. Silverman, D. R.: A Comparison of the Effects of Continuous and Pulsed Shortwave Diathermy Resistance to Bacterial Infection of Mice. Arch. Phys. Med., *45:*491-499, 1964.

61. Bach, S. A., et. al.: Biologic Effects of Microwave Radiation. New York, Plenum Press, 1961, p. 117.

62. Heller, J. H.: Reticuloendothelial Structure and Function. New York, The Ronald Press Co., 1960, Chapter 12.

63. Ginsberg, A. J.: Pulsed Short Wave in the Treatment of Bursitis with Calcification. Int. Rec. Med., *174:*71-75, 1961.

64. Levy, H.: Pulsed Shortwaves in Sinus and Allied Conditions in Childhood. Western Med., *2:*246, 1961.

65. Bergmann, L.: Der Ultraschall. Stuttgart, S. Hirzel Verlag, 1949.

66. Lehmann, J. F.: In Licht, S.: Therapeutic Heat and Cold. 2nd Ed. (To be published.)
67. Pohlman, R.: Die Ultraschall Therapie. Stuttgart, Georg Theime, 1951.
68. Lehmann, J. F., and Johnson, E. W.: Some Factors Influencing the Temperature Distribution in Thighs Exposed to Ultrasound. Arch. Phys. Med., 39:347-356, 1958.
69. Lehmann, J.: Beitrag zur Ultraschallhämolyse. Strahlentherapie, 79:533-542, 1949.
70. Carstenson, E. L., Li, K., and Schwan, H. P.: Determination of Acoustic Properties of the Blood and Its Components. J. Acoust. Soc. Amer., 25:286-289, 1953.
71. Piersol, G. M., Schwan, H. P., Pennell, R. B., and Carstenson, E. L.: Mechanism of Absorption of Ultrasonic Energy in Blood. Arch. Phys. Med., 33:327-332, 1952.
72. Hüter, T.: Messung der Ultraschallabsorption in tierischen Geweben und ihre Abhangigkeit von der Frequenz. Naturwissenschafter, 35:285, 1948.
73. Hüter, T. F., and Bolt, R. H.: An Ultrasonic Method for Outlining the Cerebral Ventricles. J. Acoust. Soc. Amer., 23:160, 1951.
74. Fry, W. J., and Fry, H. B.: Determination of Absolute Sound Levels and Acoustic Absorption Coefficients by Thermocouple Probes—Experiment. J. Acoust. Soc. Amer., 26:311, 1954.
75. Paul, W. C., and Imig, C. J.: Temperature and Blood Flow Studies After Ultrasonic Irradiation. American Institute of Ultrasonics in Medicine, 1954; Amer. J. Phys. Med., 34:370-375, 1955.
76. Abramson, D. I., Burnett, C., Bell, Y., Tuck, S., Jr., Rejal, H., and Fleischer, C. J.: Changes in Blood Flow, Oxygen Uptake, and Tissue Temperatures Produced by Therapeutic Physical Agents. Amer. J. Phys. Med., 39:51-62, 1960.
77. Bickford, R. H., and Duff, R. S.: Influences of Ultrasonic Irradiation on Temperature and Blood Flow in the Human Skeletal Muscle. Cir. Res., 1:534-538, 1953.
78. Lehmann, J., and Vorschütz, R.: Die Wirkung von Ultraschallwellen auf die Gewebeatmung als Beitrag zum therapeutischen Wirkungsmechanismus. Strahlentherapie, 82:287-292, 1950.
79. Lehmann, J., and Hohlfeld, R.: Der Gewebestoffwechsel nach Ultraschall und Wärmeeinwirkung. Strahlentherapie, 87:544-549, 1952.
80. Pauly, H., and Hug, O.: Untersuchungen über den Einfluss von Ultraschallwellen und von Wärme auf den Stoffwechsel überlebender Gewebe. Strahlentherapie, 95:116-130, 1954.
81. Lehmann, J. F.: The Biophysical Basis of Biologic Ultrasonic Reactions with Special Reference to Ultrasonic Therapy. Arch. Phys. Med., 34:139-152, 1953.
82. Lehmann, J. F.: Biophysical Mode of Action of Biologic and Therapeutic Ultrasonic Reactions. J. Acoust. Soc. Amer., 25:17-25, 1953.
83. Lehmann, J. F., and Biegler, R.: Changes of Potentials and Temperature Gradients in Membranes Caused by Ultrasound. Arch. Phys. Med., 35:287-295, 1954.
84. Lehmann, J. F.: Über die Temperaturabhangigkeit therapeutischer Ultraschallreaktionen unter besonderer Beruchsichtigung der Wirkung auf Nerven. Strahlentherapie, 79:543, 1950.
85. Lambert, E. H., Treanor, W. J., Herrick, J. F., and Krusen, F. H.: Effect of Heat and Ultrasound on Conduction in Bullfrog Nerve. Fed. Proc., 10:78, 1951.
86. Hüter, T. F., Dyer, J., Ludwig, G. D., and Kyranzia, D.: Thresholds of Damage in Nervous Tissues. Massachusetts Institute of Technology, Quarterly Progress Report, Oct.-Dec., 1950.
87. Madsen, P. W., Jr., and Gersten, J. W.: The Effect of Ultrasound on Conduction Velocity of Peripheral Nerve. Arch. Phys. Med., 42:645-649, 1961.
88. Anderson, T. P., Wakim, K. G., Herrick, J. F., Bennett, W. A., and Krusen, F. H.: Experimental Study of the Effects of Ultrasonic Energy on the Lower Part of the Spinal Cord and Peripheral Nerves. Arch. Phys. Med., 32:71-83, 1951.
89. Shealey, C. N., and Henneman, E.: Reversible Effects of Ultrasound on Spinal Reflexes. Arch. Neurol. (Chic.), 6:374-386, 1962.
90. Gersten, J.: Changes in Spinal Cord Thresholds Following the Application of Ultra-Sound. American Institute of Ultrasonics in Medicine, Proc. 4th Ann. Conf. on Ultrasonic Therapy, Detroit, 1955, pp. 31-39.
91. Lehmann, J. F., Brunner, G. D., and Stow, R. W.: Pain Threshold Measurements after Therapeutic Application of Ultrasound Microwaves and Infrared. Arch. Phys. Med., 39:560-565, 1958.
92. Stillwell, D. M., and Gersten, J. W.: Effect of Ultrasound on Spasticity. American Institute of Ultrasonics in Medicine, Proc. of 4th Ann. Conf. on Ultrasonic Therapy, Detroit, 1955, pp. 124-131.
93. Fountain, F. P., Gersten, J. W., and Sengir, O.: Decrease in Muscle Spasm Produced by Ultrasound, Hot Packs, and Infrared Radiation. Arch. Phys. Med., 41:293-298, 1960.
94. Schroeder, K. P.: Effect of Ultrasound on the Lumbar Sympathetic Nerves. Arch. Phys. Med., 43:182-185, 1962.
95. Stuhlfauth, K.: Neural Effects of Ultrasonic Waves. Brit. J. Phys. Med., 15:10-14, 1952.

96. Janes, J. M., Herrick, J. F., Kelly, P., and Peterson, L. F. A.: Long Term Effect of Ultrasonic Energy on Femora of the Dog. Proc. Mayo Clin., *35*:663-671, 1960.

97. Barth, G., and Bülow, H. A.: Zur Frage der Ultraschallschädigung jugendlicher Knochen. Strahlentherapie, *79*:271-280, 1949.

98. Maintz, G.: Tierexperimentelle Untersuchungen über die Wirkung der Ultraschallwellen auf die Knockenregeneration. Strahlentherapie, *82*:631-638, 1950.

99. Ardan, N. I., Jr., Janes, J. M., and Herrick, J. F.: Ultrasonic Energy and Surgically Produced Defects in Bones. J. Bone Joint Surg., *39A*:394-402, 1957.

100. Ardan, N. I., Jr., Janes, J. M., and Herrick, J. F.: Changes in Bone After Exposure to Ultrasonic Energy. Minnesota Med., *37*:415-420, 1954.

101. Wakim, K. G.: Special Review: Ultrasonic Energy as Applied to Medicine. Amer. J. Phys. Med., *32*:32-46, 1953.

102. Lota, M. J., and Darling, R. C.: Changes in Permeability of the Red Blood Cell Membrane in the Homogeneous Ultrasonic Field. Arch. Phys. Med., *36*:282-287, 1955.

103. Gersten, J. W.: Effect of Ultrasound on Tendon Extensibility. Amer. J. Phys. Med., *34*:362-369, 1955.

104. Gersten, J. W.: Symposium on Ultrasonics; Ultrasonics and Muscle Disease. Amer. J. Phys. Med., *33*:68-74, 1954.

105. Lehmann, J. F.: Die Therapie mit Ultraschall und ihre Grundlagen, Ergebnisse der Physikalisch-diatetischen Therapie. Vol. 4. Dresden und Leipzig, Verlag von Theodor Steinkopff, 1951.

106. Lehmann, J. F., and Herrick, J. F.: Biologic Reactions to Cavitation—A Consideration for Ultrasonic Therapy. Arch. Phys. Med., *34*:86-98, 1953.

107. Smith, A., and Schwan, H. P.: Ultrasonic Absorption and Velocity of Sound of Cell Nuclei. National Biophysics Conf., Columbus, 1957, Abstract p. 66.

108. Dussick, C. T., Fritch, D. J., Kyraizidan, M., and Sear, R. S.: Measurements of Articular Tissues with Ultrasound. Amer. J. Phys. Med., *37*:160-165, 1958.

109. Schwan, H. P.: Biophysics of Diathermy. In Licht, S.: Therapeutic Heat. New Haven, Conn., Elizabeth Licht, 1958, pp. 55-115.

110. Lehmann, J. F., McMillan, J. A., Brunner, G. D., and Blumberg, J. G.: Comparative Study of the Efficiency of Shortwave, Microwave, and Ultrasonic Diathermy in Heating the Hip Joint. Arch. Phys. Med., *40*:510-512, 1959.

111. Lehmann, J. F., DeLateur, B. J., Warren, C. G., and Stonebridge, J. B.: Heating of Joint Structures by Ultrasound. Arch. Phys. Med., *49*:28-30, 1968.

112. Lehmann, J. F., DeLateur, B, J., and Silverman, D. R.: Selective Heating Effects of Ultrasound in the Human Being. Arch. Phys. Med., *47*:331-339, 1966.

113. Lehmann, J. F., DeLateur, B. J., Warren, C. G., Stonebridge, J. B.: Heating Produced by Ultrasound in Bone and Soft Tissue. Arch. Phys. Med., *48*:397-401, 1967.

114. Lehmann, J. F., DeLateur, B. J., Stonebridge, J. B., and Warren, C. G.: Therapeutic Temperature Distribution Produced by Ultrasound as Modified by Dosage and Volume of Tissue Exposed. Arch. Phys. Med., *18*:662-666, 1967.

115. Lehmann, J. F., and Nitsch, W.: Über die Frequenzabhängigkeit biologischer Ultraschall-Reaktionen mit besonderer Berücksichtigung der spezifischen Temperaturverteiling in Organismus. Strahlentherapie, *85*:606-614, 1951.

116. Horvath, J.: Experimentelle Untersuchungen, über die Verteilung der Ultraschallenergie im Menschlichen Gewebe. Arztliche, Forschung, *1*:357, 1947.

117. Pätzold, J., and Born, H.: Behandlung biologischer Gewebe mit gebundeltem Ultraschall. Strahlentherapie, *76*:486, 1947.

118. Rosenberger, H.: Über den Wirkungsmechanismus der Ultraschallbehandlung, insbesondere bei Ischias und Neuralgien. Chirurg, *21*:404-406, 1950.

119. Herrick, J. F.: Temperatures Produced in Tissues by Ultrasound—An Experimental Study Using Various Techniques. J. Acoust. Soc. Amer., *25*:12-16, 1953.

120. Lehmann, J. F., Brunner, G. D., and McMillan, J. A.: The Influence of Surgical Metal Implants on the Temperature Distribution in Thigh Specimens Exposed to Ultrasound. Arch. Phys. Med., *39*:692-695, 1958.

121. Lehmann, J. F., Brunner, G. D., Martinis, A. J., and McMillan, J. A.: Ultrasonic Effects as Demonstrated in Live Pigs with Surgical Metallic Implants. Arch. Phys. Med., *40*:483-488, 1959.

122. Gersten, J. W.: Effect of Metallic Objects on Temperature Rises Produced in Tissues by Ultrasound. Amer. J. Phys. Med., *37*:75, 1958.

123. Päzold, J., Güttner, W., and Bastir, R.: Beitrag zum Dosisproblem in der Ultraschall-Therapie. Strahlentherapie, *86*:298-305, 1951.

124. Lehmann, J. F., and Krusen, F. H.: Therapeutic Application of Ultrasound in Physical Medicine. Amer. J. Phys. Med., *37*:173-183, 1958.

125. Mueller, E. E., Mead, S., Schultz, B. F., and Vaden, M. R.: Symposium on Ultrasonics; A Placebo-controlled Study of Ultrasound Treatment for Periarthritis. Amer. J. Phys. Med., 33:31-35, 1954.
126. Lehmann, J. F., Erickson, D. J., Martin, G. M., and Krusen, F. H.: The Present Value of Ultrasonic Diathermy. J.A.M.A., 147:996-999, 1955.
127. Lehmann, J. F., Erickson, D. J., Martin, G. M., and Krusen, F. H.: Comparison of Ultrasonic and Microwave Diathermy in the Physical Treatment of Periarthritis of the Shoulder. Arch. Phys. Med., 35:627-634, 1954.
128. Lehmann, J. F., Fordyce, W. E., Rathbun, L. A., Larson, R. E., and Wood, D. H.: Clinical Evaluation of a New Approach in the Treatment of Contracture Associated with Hip Fracture after Internal Fixation. Arch. Phys. Med., 42:95-100, 1961.
129. Bierman, W.: Ultrasound in the Treatment of Contractures. American Institute of Ultrasonics in Medicine, Proc. of the 4th Ann. Conf. on Ultrasonic Therapy, Detroit, 1955, p. 100.
130. Bierman, W.: Ultrasound in the Treatment of Scars. Arch. Phys. Med., 35:209-214, 1954.
131. Tuchman, L. S.: Role of Ultrasound in Scleroderma; A Preliminary Report on Two Cases. Amer. J. Phys. Med., 35:118-124, 1956.
132. DePalma, A. F.: Clinical Orthopaedics. Vol. 20. Disorders of the Shoulder Joint. Philadelphia, J. B. Lippincott Co., 1961.
133. Newman, M. K., Kill, M., and Frampton, G.: Effects of Ultrasound Alone and Combined with Hydrocortisone Injections by Needle or Hypospray. Amer. J. Phys. Med., 37:206-209, 1958.
134. Aldes, J. H., and Klaras, T.: The Use of Ultrasonic Radiation in the Treatment of Subdeltoid Bursitis with and without Calcareous Deposits. Western J. Surg., 62:369-376, 1954.
135. Chateau, A.: Quelques Applications Récentes en Ultrasonotherapie. Les Algies des Amputés. J. Radiol. et Electrol., 32:513-514, 1951.
136. Tepperberg, I., and Marjey, E. J.: Ultrasound Therapy of Painful Post-operative Neurofibromas. Amer. J. Phys. Med., 32:27, 1953.
137. Rubin, D., and Kuitert, J. H.: Use of Ultrasonic Vibration in the Treatment of Pain Arising from Phantom Limbs, Scars and Neuromas: A Preliminary Report. Arch. Phys. Med., 36:445-452, 1955.
138. Wachsmuth, W.: Ultraschall bei Sudeckscher Krankheit. Der Ultraschall in der Medizin. Zurich, S. Hirzel Verlag, 1949, pp. 245-248.
139. Woeber, K.: Biological Basis and Application of Ultrasound in Medicine. Ultrasonics in Biology and Medicine, 1:8, 1956.
140. Buchtala, V.: The Present State of Ultrasonic Therapy. Brit. J. Phys. Med., 15:3-6, 18, 1952.
141. Stuhlfauth, K.: Neural Effects of Ultrasonic Waves. Brit. J. Phys. Med., 13:10-14, 1952.
142. Der Ultraschall in Der Medizin. Kongressbericht der Erlanger Ultraschall-Tagung. Zurich, S. Hirzel Verlag, 1949.
143. Hintzelmann, U.: Ultraschalltherapie rheumatischer Erkrankungen. Deutsch. Med. Wschr., 72:350-353, 1947.
144. Hintzelmann, U.: Ultraschalltherapie rheumatischer Erkrankungen. 2. Mitteilung. Deutsch. Med. Wschr., 74:869-870, 1949.
145. Ruiz, Carlos B.: Ultrasonics in Traumatic Conditions. Amer. J. Phys. Med., 37:203-205, 1958.
146. Fry, U.: Behandlung von Sportverletzungne mit Ultraschall. Schweiz. Z. Sportmed., 2:22, 1954.
147. Pöschl, M.: Strahlen- und Ultraschalltherapie in der Sportmedizin. Med. Klin., 48:2, 1953.
148. Weissenberg, E. H.: Ultrasonics In Industrial Accidents. Amer. J. Phys. Med., 37:233, 1958.
149. Kent, H.: Plantar Warts—Treatment with Ultrasound. Arch. Phys. Med., 40:15-18, 1959.
150. Bender, L. F., and Nick, C.: Treatment of Plantar Warts with Ultrasound: Report given at the American Congress of Physical Medicine and Rehabilitation, 40th Ann. Session. Arch. Phys. Med., 43:371, 1962.
151. Kuitert, J. H.: Symposium on Ultrasonics; Ultrasonic Energy as an Adjunct in the Management of Radiculitis and Similar Referred Pain. Amer. J. Phys. Med., 33:61-65, 1954.
152. Aldes, J. H.: Ultrasonic Radiation in the Treatment of Epicondylitis. GP, 13:89-96, 1956.
153. Luzes, F.: Contribution au traitement de l'herpes zoster par les ultrasons. Acta physiother. rheum. belg., 7:354-356, 1952.
154. Aldes, J., Edmundson, F., Agresti, M., and Rhoden, R.: The Use of Ultrasonic Radiation for the Treatment of Herpes Zoster. American Institute of Ultrasonics in Medicine, Proc. 4th Ann. Conf. on Ultrasonic Therapy, Detroit, 1955, pp. 115-123.
155. Sonnen, V. G.: Pathophysiologic Basis of Ultrasonic Treatment of Rheumatoid Disease. American Institute of Ultrasonics in Medicine, Scientific Proc. 3rd Ann. Conf. on Ultrasonic Therapy, Washington, D.C., 1954, p. 93.
156. Thiele, W.: Die Ultraschallbehandlung bei rheumatischen Erkrankungen. Arztl. Wschr., 7:193-197, 1952.

157. Sonnenschein, V.: Die pathophysiologischen Grundlagen der Ultraschalltherapie rheumatischer Erkrankungen. Schweiz. Med. Wschr., *82*:1137-1140, 1161-1163, 1952.

158. Bonica, J. J.: Management of Myofascial Pain Syndromes in General Practice. J.A.M.A., *164*:732-738, 1957.

159. Sola, A. E., and Kuitert, J. H.: Myofascial Trigger Point Pain in Neck and Shoulder Girdle. Northwest Med., *54*:980-984, 1955.

160. Paroni, F.: Tropical Ulcers and Ultrasonic Treatment. Int. J. Phys. Med., *3*:270-272, 1958.

161. Paul, B. J., LaFratta, C. W., Dawson, A. R., Baab, E., and Bullock, F.: Use of Ultrasound in the Treatment of Pressure Sores in Patients with Spinal Cord Injury. Arch. Phys. Med., *41*:438-440, 1960.

162. Jones, A. C.: Ultrasonic Therapy in the Treatment of Circulatory Induration of the Lower Extremities. American Institute Ultrasonics in Medicine, Scientific Proc. 3rd Ann. Conf. on Ultrasonic Therapy, Washington, D.C., 1954.

163. Lehmann, J. F., and Krusen, F. H.: Biophysical Effects of Ultrasonic Energy on Carcinoma and Their Possible Significance. Arch. Phys. Med., *36*:452-459, 1955.

164. Rae, J. W., Jr., Herrick, J. F., Wakim, K. G., and Krusen, F. H. Comparative Study of Temperatures Produced by Microwave and Shortwave Diathermy. Arch. Phys. Med., *30*:199-211, 1949.

165. Schwan, H. P.: Biophysics of Diathermy. In Licht, S.: Therapeutic Heat. New Haven, Conn., Elizabeth Licht, 1958, pp. 55-115.

166. Morgan, W. E.: Microwave Radiation Hazards. A.M.A. Arch. Indust. Health, *21*:570-573, 1960.

167. Tomberg, V. C.: Specific Thermal Effects of High Frequency Fields. Biological Effects of Microwave Radiation. Proc. 4th Ann. Tri-Service Conf. on the Biological Effects of Microwave Radiation, *1*:221-229, 1961, New York, Plenum Press.

168. Livshits, N. N.: The Effect of an Ultra High Frequency Field on the Function of the Nervous System. Biophysics (USSR) *4*:426-437, ATD P 65-68 Libr. Cong., Washington, D.C., 1958.

169. Livshits, N. N.: The Role of the Nervous System in Reactions to UHF Electromagnetic Fields. Biophysics (USSR) *2*:372-384, ATD P 65-68 Libr. Cong., Washington, D.C., 1957.

170. Guy, A. W., and Lehmann, J. F.: Comparative Evaluation of Electromagnetic Diathermy Modalities in 433 MHz. to 2450 MHz. 21st ACEMB—Shamrock Hilton Hotel, Houston, Texas, Nov. 18-21, 1968.

171. Ho, H. D., Guy, A. W., Sigelmann, R. A., and Lehmann, J. F.: Microwave Heating of Simulated Human Limbs by Aperture Sources. Special IEEE Issue of Microwave Theory and Techniques, Biological Effects of Microwaves, Feb., 1971.

172. Guy, A. W.: Electromagnetic Fields and Relative Heating Patterns Due to a Rectangular Aperture Source in Direct Contact with Bi-layered Biological Tissue. Special IEEE Issue of Microwave Theory and Techniques, Biological Effects of Microwaves, Feb., 1971.

173. Guy, A. W.: Analyses of Electromagnetic Fields Induced in Biological Tissues by Thermographic Studies on Equivalent Phantom Models. Special IEEE Issue on Microwave Theory and Techniques, Biological Effects of Microwaves, Feb., 1971.

174. Cook, H. F.: A Comparison of the Dielectric Behaviour of Pure Water and Human Blood at Microwave Frequencies. Brit. J. Appl. Phys., *3*:249, 1952.

175. Schwan, H. P., and Li, K.: Hazards Due to Total Body Irradiation by Radar. Proc. IRE, *44*:1572, 1956.

176. Cole, K. S., and Cole, R. H.: Dispersion and Absorption in Dielectrics. I. Alternating Current Characteristics. J. Chem. Phys., *9*:341, 1941.

177. Schwan, H. P., and Piersol, G. M.: The Absorption of Electromagnetic Energy in Body Tissues; A Review and Critical Analysis. Amer. J. Phys. Med., *34*:425-448, 1955.

178. Lehmann, J. F., Guy, A. W., Johnston, V. C., Brunner, G. D., and Bell, J. W.: Comparison of Relative Heating Patterns Produced in Tissues by Exposure to Microwave Energy at Frequencies of 2,450 and 900 Megacycles. Arch. Phys. Med., *43*:69-76, 1962.

179. DeLateur, B. J., Lehmann, J. F., Stonebridge, J. B., Warren, C. G., and Guy, A. W.: Muscle Heating in Human Subjects with 915 MHz. Microwave Contact Applicator. Arch. Phys. Med., *51*:147-151, 1970.

180. Lehmann, J. F., Guy, A. W., Warren, C. G., DeLateur, B. J., and Stonebridge, J. B.: Evaluation of a Microwave Contact Applicator. Arch. Phys. Med., *51*:143-147, 1970.

181. Rae, J. W., Herrick, J. F., Wakim, K. G., and Krusen, F. H.: A Comparative Study of the Temperatures Produced by Microwave and Shortwave Diathermy. Arch. Phys. Med., *30*:199-211, 1949.

182. Lehmann, J. F., McMillan, J. A., Brunner, G. D., and Guy, A. W.: A Comparative Evaluation of Temperature Distributions Produced by Microwaves at 2,456 and 900 Megacycles in Geometrically Complex Specimens. Arch. Phys. Med., *43*:502-507, 1962.

183. Worden, R. E., Herrick, J. F., Wakim, K. G., and Krusen, F. H.: The Heating Effects of Microwaves with and without Ischemia. Arch. Phys. Med., *29*:751-758, 1948.

184. Engel, J. P., Herrick, J. F., Wakim, K. G., Grindlay, J. H., and Krusen, F. H.: The Effect of Microwaves on Bone and Bone Marrow and on Adjacent Tissues. Arch. Phys. Med., *31*:453-461, 1950.

185. Addington, C. H., Osborn, C., Swartz, G., Fischer, F. P., Neubauer, R. A., and Sarkees, Y. T.: Biological Effects of Microwave Energy at 200 mc. Biological Effects of Microwave Radiation. Proc. 4th Ann. Tri-Service Conf. on the Biological Effects of Microwave Radiation, *1*:177-186, 1961, New York, Plenum Press.

186. Howland, J. W., Thomson, R. A. E., and Michaelson, S. M.: Biomedical Aspects of Microwave Irradiation of Mammals. Biological Effects of Microwave Radiation. Proc. 4th Ann. Tri-Service Conf. on the Biological Effects of Microwave Radiation. *1*:261-285, 1961, New York, Plenum Press.

187. Marks, J., Carter, E. T., Scarpelli, D. G., and Eisen, J.: Microwave Radiation to the Anterior Mediastinum of the Dog (II). Ohio Med. J., *57*:1132-1135, 1961.

188. Linke, C. A., Lounsberry, W., and Goldschmidt, V.: Effects of Microwaves on Normal Tissues. J. Urol., *88*:303-311, 1962.

189. Feucht, B. L., Richardson, A. W., and Hines, H. M.: Effects of Implanted Metal on Tissue Hyperthermia Produced by Microwaves. Arch. Phys. Med., *30*:164-169, 1949.

190. Reinike, A., and Alm, H.: Untersuchungen über die Tiefenwirkung der Mikrowellenbestrahlung im Bereich der Nasennebenhöhlen und des Ohres. Z. Laryn., Rhinol., Otol., *35*(9):556-566, 1956.

191. Lehmann, J. F., Brunner, G. D., McMillan, J. A., and Silverman, D. R.: A Comparative Analysis of Therapeutic Heating Patterns and Blood Flow Changes Produced by the Application of Modern Diathermy Modalities in Human Volunteers. Unpublished data.

192. Krusen, F. H., Herrick, J. F., Leden, U. M., and Wakim, K. G.: Microkymatotherapy; Preliminary Report of Experimental Studies of Heating Effect of Microwaves ("Radar") in Living Tissues. Proc. Mayo Clin., *22*:209-224, 1947.

193. Rae, J. W., Jr., Martin, G. M., Treanor, W. J., and Krusen, F. H.: Clinical Experiences with Microwave Diathermy. Proc. Mayo Clin., *25*:441-446, 1950.

194. Barber, D. E.: The Reaction of Luminous Bacteria to Microwave Radiation Exposures in the Frequency Range of 2608.7-3982.3 Mc. IRE Trans. Biomed. Electronics, p. 77-80. April, 1960.

195. Leden, U. M., Herrick, J. F., Wakim, K. G., and Krusen, F. H.: Preliminary Studies on Heating and Circulatory Effects of Microwaves (Radar). Brit. J. Phys. Med., *10*:177-184, 1947.

196. Kent, C. R., Paul, W. D., and Hines, H. M.: Studies Concerning the Effect of Deep Tissue Heating Upon Blood Flow. Arch. Phys. Med., *29*:12, 1948.

197. Richardson, A. W., Imig, C. J., Feucht, B. L., and Hines, H. M.: The Relationship Between Deep Tissue Temperature and Blood Flow During Electromagnetic Irradiation. Arch. Phys. Med., *31*:19-25, 1950.

198. Richardson, A. W.: Effect of Microwave Induced Heating on the Blood Flow Through Peripheral Skeletal Muscle. Amer. J. Phys. Med., *33*:103-107, 1954.

199. Richardson, A. W.: The Effectiveness of Microwave Diathermy Therapy as a Hyperthermic Agent Upon Vascularized and Avascular Tissue. Brit. J. Phys. Med., *18*:143-149, 1955.

200. Kottke, F. J., Koza, D. W., Kubicek, W. G., and Olson, M.: Studies of Deep Circulatory Response to Short Wave Diathermy and Microwave Diathermy in Man. Arch. Phys. Med., *30*:431-437, 1949.

201. Szarski, H.: Heat Resistance of the Chicken Embryo Tissue in Vitro. Bull. int. Acad. Polon., Cl. Sci. math. nat. Ser. B; Sci. nat. (2) Zool., p. 45, (Nov.-Dec.) 1939.

202. Szarski, H.: Sur la mort thermique de l'embryon de poulet. Bull. int. Acad. Polon., Cl. Sci. math. nat. Ser. B; Sci. nat. (2) Zool., p. 133, (Nov.-Dec.) 1947.

203. Van Ummersen, C. A.: The Effect of 2450 mc Radiation on the Development of the Chick Embryo. Biological Effects of Microwave Radiation. Proc. 4th Ann. Tri-Service Conf. on the Biological Effects of Microwave Radiation, *1*:201-221, 1961, New York, Plenum Press.

204. Cooper, T., Pinakatt, T., Jellinek, M., and Richardson, A. W.: Effects of Adrenalectomy, Vagotomy and Ganglionic Blockade on the Circulatory Response to Microwave Hyperthermia. Aerospace Med., *33*:794-798, 1962.

205. Engel, J. P., Herrick, J. F., Wakim, K. G., Grindlay, J. H., and Krusen, F. H.: Effect of Microwaves on Bone and Bone Marrow and on Adjacent Tissues. Arch. Phys. Med., *31*:453-461, 1950.

206. Wise, C. S., Castleman, B., and Watkins, A. L.: Effect of Diathermy (Short Wave and Microwave) on Bone Growth in the Albino Rat. J. Bone Joint Surg., *31A*:487-500, 1949.

207. Doyle, J. R., and Smart, B. W.: Stimulation of Bone Growth by Short-wave Diathermy. J. Bone Joint Surg., *45A*:15-24, 1963.

208. Granberry, W. M., and Janes, J. M.: The Lack of Effect of Microwave Diathermy on Rate of Growth of Bone of the Growing Dog. J. Bone Joint Surg., *45A*:4:773-777, 1963.

209. McAfee, R. D.: Physiological Effects of Thermode and Microwave Stimulation of Peripheral Nerves. Amer. J. Physiol., *203:*374-378, 1962.

210. McAfee, R. D.: Neurophysiological Effect of 3-cm. Microwave Radiation. Amer. J. Physiol., *200:*192-194, 1961.

211. McAfee, R. D., Berger, C., and Pizzolato, P.: Neurological Effect of 3 cm Microwave Irradiation. Biological Effects of Microwave Radiation. Proc. 4th Ann. Tri-Service Conf. on the Biological Effects of Microwave Radiation. *1:*251-261, 1961, New York, Plenum Press.

212. Hauswirth, O., and Kracmar, F.: Effect of Microwaves on the Autonomic Nervous System. Wien. Med. Wschr., *108:*172-173, 1958.

213. Daily, L., Jr., Wakim, K. G., Herrick, J. F., and Parkhill, E. M.: The Effects of Microwave Diathermy on the Eye. Amer. J. Physiol., *155:*432, 1948.

214. Richardson, A. W., Duane, T. D., and Hines, H. M.: Experimental Lenticular Opacities Produced by Microwave Irradiation. Arch. Phys. Med., *29:*765-769, 1948.

215. Daily, L., Jr., Wakim, K. G., Herrick, J. F., Parkhill, E. M., and Benedict, W. L.: The Effects of Microwave Diathermy on the Eye of the Rabbit. Amer. J. Ophthal., *35:*1001-1017, 1952.

216. Williams, D. B., Monahan, J. P., Nicholson, W. J., and Aldrich, J. J.: Biologic Effects of Microwave Radiation: Time and Power Thresholds for the Production of Lens Opacities by 12.3 cm. Microwaves. USAF School of Aviation Med. Report No. 55-94, Aug., 1955.

217. Carpenter, R. L.: Experimental Radiation Cataracts Induced by Microwave Radiation. Proc. 2nd Tri-Service Conf. on Biologic Effects of Microwave Energy. Rome Air Dev. Center, Air Res. and Dev. Command, Rome, N. Y., ASTIA Doc. AD-131-477, July, 1958, p. 146.

218. Carpenter, R. L., Biddle, D. K., and Van Ummersen, C. A.: Progress Report. Investigator's Conf. on Biol. Effects of Electronic Radiating Equipment, Rome Air Dev. Center, Air Res. and Dev. Command, Rome, N. Y., ASTIA Doc. No. AD-214693, Jan., 1959, p. 12.

219. Merola, L. O., and Kinoshita, J. H.: Changes in the Ascorbic Acid Content in Lenses of Rabbit Eyes Exposed to Microwave Radiation. Biological Effects of Microwave Radiation, Proc. 4th Ann. Tri-Service Conf. on the Biological Effects of Microwave Radiation, *1:*285-291, 1961, New York, Plenum Press.

220. Zaret, M. M., and Eisenbud, M.: Preliminary Results of Studies of the Lenticular Effects of Microwaves Among Exposed Personnel. Biological Effects of Microwave Radiation. Proc. 4th Ann. Tri-Service Conf. on the Biological Effects of Microwave Radiation, *1:*293-308, 1961, New York, Plenum Press.

221. Carpenter, R. L., Biddle, D. K., and Van Ummerson, C. A.: Annual Report of Work and Progress at Tufts University, Jan., 1958.

222. Searle, G. W., Dahlen, R. W., Imig, C. J., Wunder, C. C., Thomson, J. D., Thomas, J. A., and Moressi, W. J.: Effects of 2450 mc Microwaves in Dogs, Rats and Larvae of the Common Fruit Fly. Biological Effects of Microwave Radiation. Proc. 4th Ann. Tri-Service Conf. on the Biological Effects of Microwave Radiation, *1:*187-201, 1961, New York, Plenum Press.

223. Imig, C. J., Thomson, J. D., and Hines, H. M.: Testicular Degeneration as a Result of Microwave Irradiation. Proc. Soc. Exp. Biol. Med., *69:*382-386, 1948.

224. Prausnitz, S. and Susskind, C.: Effects of Chronic Microwave Irradiation on Mice. IRE Trans. Biomed. Electronics, *9:*104-108, 1962.

225. Gunn, S. A., Gould, T. C., and Anderson, W. A. D.: The Effect of Microwave Radiation (24,000 mc) on the Male Endocrine System of the Rat. Biological Effects of Microwave Radiation. Proc. 4th Ann. Tri-Service Conf. of the Biological Effects of Microwave Radiation, *1:*99-117, 1961, New York, Plenum Press.

226. Saita, M., and Schwan, H. P.: The Time Constants of Pearl-Chain Formation. Biological Effects of Microwave Radiation. Proc. 4th Ann. Tri-Service Conf. on the Biological Effects of Microwave Radiation, *1:*85-99, 1961, New York, Plenum Press.

227. Matuzov, N. I.: Effects of Microwaves on Irritability of the Optic Analyzer in Human Subjects. Biull. Eksp. Biol. Med., *48:*27-30, 1959.

228. Richardson, A. W.: Blood Coagulation Changes Due to Electromagnetic Microwave Irradiation. Blood, *14:*1237-1243, 1959.

229. Lehmann, J. F., McMillan, J. A., Brunner, G. D., and Johnston, V. C.: Heating Patterns Produced in Specimens by Microwaves of the Frequency of 2,456 Megacycles When Applied with the "A," "B," and "C" Directors. Arch. Phys. Med., *43:*538-546, 1962.

230. Alm, H. F., and Kuttig, H.: Experimentelle und Klinische Untersuchungen mit hochfrequenten Ströment im oberen Dezimeterwellenbereich. Strahlentherapie, *116:*297-310, 1961.

231. Lehmann, J. F., Brunner, G. D., McMillan, J. A., and Blumberg, J. B.: Comparative Study of the Efficiency of Shortwave, Microwave and Ultrasonic Diathermy in Heating the Hip Joint. Arch. Phys. Med., *40:*510-512, 1959.

232. Lehmann, J. F., Erickson, D. J., Martin, G. M., and Krusen, F. H.: Comparison of Ultrasonic and Microwave Diathermy in the Physical Treatment of Periarthritis of the Shoulder. Arch. Phys. Med., *35:*627-634, 1954.

233. Kottke, F. H.: Heat in Pelvic Diseases. In Licht, S.: Therapeutic Heat. New Haven, Conn., Elizabeth Licht, 1958, pp. 402–417.
234. Rubin, A., and Erdman, W., II: Microwave Exposure of the Human Female Pelvis During Early Pregnancy and Prior to Conception. Case Reports. Amer. J. Phys. Med., *38:*219–220, 1959.
235. Moor, F. B.: Microwave Diathermy. In Licht, S.: Therapeutic Heat. New Haven, Conn., Elizabeth Licht, 1958, pp. 284–294.
236. Kuttig, H.: Die Mikrowellen und ihre Anwendung in der Therapie. Med. Klin., *50:*1262, 1955.
237. Wilson, G. D.: Treatment of Fibrositis in the Neck and Shoulder with Microthermy (Radar). N. Carolina Med. J., *12:*19-22, 1951.
238. Scholtz, H. G.: Klinische Erfahrungen mit Mikrowellen. Arch. Phys. Therapy, *6:*36, 1954.
239. Spiegel, F. G.: Über Kurzwellen- und Mikrowellentherapie. Arch. Phys. Therapy, *8:*215-218, 1956.
240. Clark, W. B.: Microwave Diathermy in Ophthalmology: Clinical Evaluation. Trans. Amer. Acad. Ophthal. Otolaryng., *56:*600-605, 1952.
241. Thorpe, H. E.: Microwave Diathermy in Ophthalmology: Various Diathermy Currents Used in Ophthalmology. Trans. Amer. Acad. Ophthal. Otolaryng., *56:*596-599, 1952.
242. Daily, L., Jr., Wakim, K. G., Herrick, J. F., Parkhill, E. M., and Benedict, W. L.: The Effects of Microwave Diathermy on the Eye. Amer. J. Ophthal., *33:*1241-1254, 1950.
243. Daily, L., Jr., Zeller, E. A., Wakim, K. G., Herrick, J. F., and Benedict, W. L.: Influence of Microwaves on Certain Enzyme Systems in the Lens of the Eye. Amer. J. Ophthal., *34:*1301–1306, 1951.
244. Richardson, A. W., Lomax, D. H., Nichols, J., and Green, H. D.: The Role of Energy, Pupillary Diameter, and Alloxan Diabetes in the Production of Ocular Damage by Microwave Irradiations. Amer. J. Ophthal., *35:*993–1000, 1952.
245. Zaret, M. M., and Eisenbud, M.: Preliminary Results of Studies of the Lenticular Effects of Microwaves Among Exposed Personnel. Biological Effects of Microwave Radiation. Proc. 4th Ann. Tri-Service Conf. on the Biological Effects of Microwave Radiation, *1:*293–308, 1961, New York, Plenum Press.
246. Quan. Kuo-Chiew: Hazards of Microwave Radiations. Industr. Med. Surg., *29:*315–318, 1960.
247. McLaughlin, J. T.: Health Hazards from Microwave Radiation. Western Med., *3:*126–132, 1962.
248. Barron, C. I., and Baraff, A. A.: Medical Considerations of Exposure to Microwaves (Radar). J.A.M.A., *168:*9:1194–1199, 1958.
249. McLaughlin, J. T.: Tissue Destruction and Death from Microwave Radiation (Radar). Calif. Med., *85:*5, 1957.
250. Howland, J. W., and Michaelson, S.: Studies on the Biological Effects of Microwave Irradiation of the Dog and Rabbit. Progress Report, University of Rochester, Jan., 1959.
251. Pressman, A. S.: Temperature Changes of the Human Skin Irradiated with Low Intensity Waves of Several Centimeters in Length. Biull. Eksp. Biol. Med., *43:*180–184, 1957.
252. Knauf, G. M.: The Bio-Effects of Radar Energy. A Research Progress Report. Aerospace Med., *31:*225–228, 1960.
253. Deichmann, W. B., and Stephens, F. H., Jr.: Microwave Radiation of 10mw/cm and Factors that Influence Biological Effects at Various Power Densities. Industr. Med. Surg., *30:*221–228, 1961.
254. Susskind, C.: Cellular and Longevity Effects of Microwave Radiation. Monthly Progress Report, University of California, July, 1958.
255. Born, H.: Zur Frage der Absorptionsmessungen im Ultraschallgebiet. Z. Phys. Bd., *120:*383, 1943.

Chapter 12

HYDROTHERAPY

by Jack M. Zislis

GENERAL PRINCIPLES OF HYDROTHERAPY

Hydrotherapy is the external application of water for therapeutic purposes. The physical properties of water make it a very versatile agent for utilization to this end. Since its specific heat is high, it absorbs and gives up heat slowly and therefore can be used effectively to produce conductive heating and cooling of the body or its parts, and the accompanying general and local physiologic effects. It may be applied in its solid (ice), liquid or vapor (steam) state. Because of its versatility it can be used to heat or cool localized areas as in the application of hot compresses or ice packs, respectively, or on the other hand, it can be used to heat or cool the entire body by totally immersing the trunk and extremities in water of high or low temperature.

Physical Properties of Water

Archimedes' principle states that a body which is fully or partially immersed in a liquid experiences an upward thrust equal to the weight of the liquid which it displaces. This accounts for the buoyancy of water, which buoys up the body with a force equal to the weight of the water displaced. Thus when a patient stands in water up to his chin, the stress through his weight bearing joints is minimal.

This minimal stress through the weight bearing joints is of great value when walking exercises are to be carried out with a patient who is not permitted or cannot tolerate full weight bearing. The aspects of buoyancy also are utilized to resist or assist movement of the limbs by respectively directing them downward to a deeper level or upward toward the water's surface. Pulling the

346

limb vertically downward from the buoyant level uses the upthrust of the water as a resistance. This can be graded in the treatment of a patient with motor weakness and more resistance to movement can be added as muscle power returns.

In addition to these basic progressions, further work can be achieved by increasing the speed of movement, increasing the number of repetitions of the exercise, increasing the range of motion, altering starting positions and fixations, altering leverage or using apparatus.

Other properties of water are cohesion and viscosity. Cohesion in a liquid is the attractive force exerted by each molecule on those surrounding it, which results in a resistance to any object passing through the liquid. Viscosity (internal friction) is the property of a liquid to resist relative motion within it. The greater the cohesion, the greater the viscosity. The degree of resistance will depend on the movement and on the shape of the moving body. The greater the speed, the greater will be the resistance. An exercise in water is first given slowly; progression is accomplished by increasing the speed of exercise performance.

Mechanical stimulation of the skin can be accomplished by agitating the water, as in a whirlpool bath, or by applying jets or sprays of water. The mechanical stimulation achieved by water agitation produces cleansing of the skin surface and débridement in order to aid in combating infection and in the healing of chronic wounds or decubitus ulcers.

Thermal Effects of Water

Water is also applied for its thermal effect. We speak of cold, tepid or hot water but we are often unaware of the temperature ranges involved. Water at 92 to 97° F. gives the sensation of being neither hot nor cold and is called neutral. A general classification is shown in the following table.

	F.	C.
Very cold	34–55	1–13
Cold	55–65	13–18
Cool	65–80	18–27
Tepid	80–92	27–33.5
Neutral	92–96	33.5–35.5
Warm	96–98	35.5–36.5
Hot	98–104	36.5–40
Very hot	104–115	40–46

Factors that affect the results of hydrotherapy include the water temperature itself, the difference between the skin and water temperatures, the methods of application, the suddenness of application, the extent of the surface covered, the duration and frequency of the treatment and the weight, age and general condition of the patient.

Cold Water. Brief application of cold water has a tonic or stimulating effect and results in peripheral vasoconstriction, pallor of the skin, chilliness, increased muscle tone, increased pulse rate, increased respiratory rate, rise in blood pressure and involuntary shivering, which in turn is responsible for more heat production in the body. Removal from the water results in peripheral vasodilatation, redness of the skin, a feeling of warmth, a decrease of blood pressure, relaxation and a decrease in pulse and respiratory rates.

Hot Water.   Local application of mild heat has a sedative effect upon irritative conditions of sensory and motor nerves. It affords relief in painful sensory conditions and in cramps and spasm.

Heat applied to a large portion of the body in sufficient dosage results in an increase in body temperature and general physiologic changes. There is an increase of the circulatory rate and of metabolism, a rise in blood volume and oxygen consumption and a change in the pH of urine, blood and sweat to the alkaline side.

The clinical effects of mild general body heating are increased heat elimination and profuse perspiration; increased circulation, a rise of the pulse rate in the ratio of about 10 beats for every degree Fahrenheit, just as in fever; a lowering of blood pressure in contrast to the effects of cold; increased respiration; and increased elimination through the kidneys. There is a loss of water, salt, urea and other nitrogenous substances with a relative excess of alkali remaining in the blood and in the tissues, and in addition there is a temporary loss of body weight. General nervous sensibility is usually markedly lessened.

Another value of hydrotherapy is psychologic, particularly as applied to the benefits of therapeutic underwater exercises. Even the smallest amount of voluntary motion (not possible in air) helps the patient retain a "body image" of movement and gives him the hope of one day moving the part without the help of water.

METHODS OF APPLICATION OF HYDROTHERAPY

In prescribing hydrotherapy, the physician should specify the type, temperature, duration and frequency of treatments.

Underwater Exercise

Underwater exercise is indicated:

1. When there is muscle weakness of such degree that motion in air is difficult, but in which there is reason to believe that there is the possibility of increasing strength through voluntary motion (e.g., partial peripheral nerve lesions as in poliomyelitis and polyneuritis).
2. After amputation (when strengthening of muscles and stretching of contractures of an amputated stump are desired).
3. Following joint injuries.
4. After abdominal fascial transplants.
5. In paraplegia.
6. In certain cases of cerebral palsy.
7. In extensive skin burns.
8. In rheumatoid arthritis (to promote activity in the convalescent stage).
9. For postsurgical débridement (as in anorectal surgery and amputations).

Therapeutic heating by hydrotherapy can be achieved by hot water bottles, poultices and fomentations. These methods are not efficient because their heating is not constant; they cool quickly and consequently must be reheated and reapplied at frequent intervals.

Hot Packs

Hydrocollator Packs maintain heat for a longer period of time and therefore can conveniently be used for a 20 to 30 minute treatment without reheating. They are canvas-enclosed packs of silica gel that come in several sizes (Fig. 12-1A). They are heated in water to 140 to 160° F. Several layers of towels are applied between the Hydrocollator Pack and the skin of the patient (Fig. 12-1B, C). This device is valuable for the application of moist heat locally to relieve muscle spasm and pain, to aid in the absorption of inflammatory products, to produce relaxation and sedation and to increase perspiration. It is easy to apply to any part of the body, is sanitary to use (that is, the pack itself does not touch the patient), and provides an even distribution of heat.

Other hot packs consist of felt, wool or towels that are wrung out very dry at 55° C. They are used in peripheral nerve disease to relieve muscle spasm and tightness. They are applied to the area in muscle spasm and wrapped around the extremity. Since they cool quickly, it is necessary to reheat and reapply them every five minutes. Duration of treatment is 20 to 30 minutes.

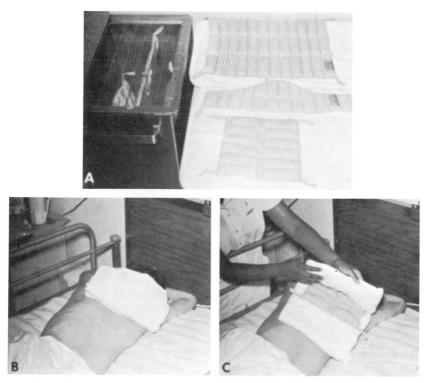

Figure 12–1 Hydrocollator Packs. *A*, Various sizes and shapes of Hydrocollator Packs. At left is hot pack heating and storage cabinet. *B* and *C*, Application of Hydrocollator Pack.

Wet Packs

Wet packs may consist of cloth, gauze, towels or woolen blankets which are wrung out in water of varying temperatures. Small wet packs are applied locally as in a compress. A full wet pack encompasses the entire trunk and limbs. The temperature may be cold, neutral or hot, depending upon the therapeutic response to be achieved. Hot full wet packs are of value in producing a sedative effect in a mentally agitated patient. Hot wet packs are helpful in producing dilatation of cutaneous vessels, relaxing muscles, relieving pain and stimulating perspiration. They are used effectively on strains and sprains, as preparation for exercising stiff joints and in treating low back pain with associated muscle spasm and arthritis. Cold wet packs may also be used locally to reduce swelling after sprains or contusions, by producing local vasoconstriction and reducing bleeding into injured tissues, and to decrease swelling and pain in acute bursitis and fibrositis.

Whirlpool Baths

The whirlpool bath offers water temperature control in combination with the mechanical effects of water in motion (an aerator controls the degree of water agitation). This provides heat, gentle massage, débridement, relief of pain and relaxation of muscles and permits active or assistive exercise of the immersed part. A thermostat keeps the bath temperature at a constant level. Temperature settings are frequently 90 to 100° F. for whole body whirlpool (Fig. 12-2A); 100 to 102° F. for legs (Fig. 12-2B, C); and 105° F. for upper extremities (Fig. 12-2D). Treatment duration is generally 20 minutes. The whirlpool bath is useful in treating chronic traumatic conditions, inflammatory conditions, early joint stiffness, pain, painful scars, adhesions, neuritis, arthritis, tenosynovitis, sprains, strains and painful stumps. In addition, it is used as a preliminary to massage, exercise or electrical stimulation.

Patients with foot or leg lesions which contraindicate weight bearing are often referred to the physical therapy department for whirlpool bath treatments. In some cases there may be considerable difficulty in transferring these patients onto a standard whirlpool chair. A chair with a hydraulic lift may be useful in these cases. The chair in the down position may be no higher than the patient's wheelchair, so that transfer is simplified. Then, when pumped to the high position, the patient's legs are easily placed in the whirlpool bath.

Water Baths

Another form of hydrotherapy is the water bath. It may be applied locally to a small area such as the eye, or the area for treatment may be an extremity where water may be applied by compress, by pouring or by actual immersion of the part in the water. The size of the compress depends upon the area of the body to which it is applied. A cold compress of 60 to 65° F. may be used 10 minutes to one hour twice a day for the relief of pain and swelling by its effects of vascular constriction and analgesia. It should be applied as soon after injury as possible and may be used during the first 24 to 36 hours. The water bath may be cold, neutral, hot or alternately hot and cold (contrast bath).

Cold Baths. Cold baths applied locally, like compresses, are used following acute injury to reduce pain and swelling by the vascular constriction and

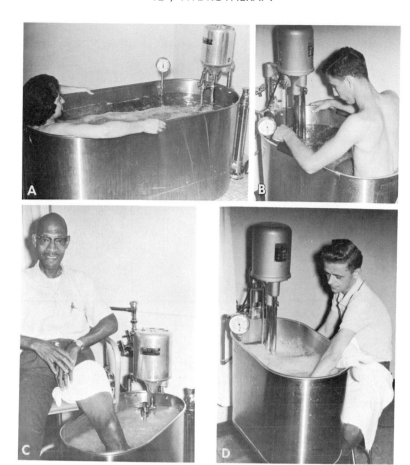

Figure 12–2 Whirlpool bath therapy. *A*, of whole body (temperature dial is at left and water agitator is at right); *B*, of both legs; *C*, of lower leg; *D*, of arm.

analgesic effect of cold. Local cold application has been effective in reducing spasticity in multiple sclerosis and in reducing the knee jerk reflex in hemiplegic patients, but the effect does not endure long beyond the treatment period.

Neutral Baths. The neutral bath is utilized to produce sedation, muscle relaxation and general vasodilatation. Excited patients are benefited by its quieting effect.

Hot Baths. The hot bath is useful in relieving pain and stiffness in chronic arthritic patients with multiple joint involvement and in fibrositis, muscle spasm, chronic myositis and neuritis.

Contrast Baths. Contrast baths are sudden and alternate immersions of the extremities in first hot and then cold water (Fig. 12-3). They greatly stimulate peripheral circulation in limbs without vascular impairment. Two large water containers are used, each large enough to accommodate both arms or legs. One is filled with hot water 38 to 40° C., the other with cold water 10 to 16° C. The extremities are first placed in the hot water for four to six minutes and then are moved quickly to the cold water for one or two minutes. The final immersion is in the hot water.

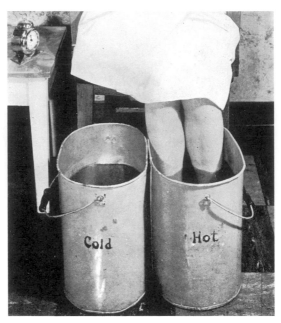

Figure 12–3 Contrast baths. (From Krusen, Physical Medicine. Philadelphia, W. B. Saunders Company.)

Hubbard Tanks

Another form of the full immersion bath is the Hubbard tank (Fig. 12–4). It is designed for underwater exercise and permits full abduction of the patient's arms and legs in the water, as well as enabling the therapist to have access to the patient by standing at the narrow center portion of the tank. An aerator is used to agitate the water for massage effect and débridement while the patient lies immersed on a canvas plinth. Transfer to and from the patient's litter from the Hubbard tank is easily accomplished by means of electrically driven overhead cranes. This form of therapy is very effective in chronic arthritic disorders when there is multiple joint involvement and in burn cases when débridement and active exercise are desirable.

Hydrotherapy not only accomplishes débridement and cleansing of burns but also makes changing of dressings easier, often eliminating the need for anesthesia. It causes the patient little discomfort and saves the patient considerable stress and strain on his general condition. The dressings are gently slit open with bandage scissors before the patient is placed in the tank. The dressings literally float away from the patient, so there is minimal discomfort in pulling them off the burned areas. During this time the patient may also be getting joint range of motion exercise to maintain mobility and prevent contracture as much as possible. This can be accomplished conveniently with a team consisting of one nurse, from the operating room, one physician and one physical therapist. Early hydrotherapy (in saline solutions, with agitation) may result in a greater percentage of successful split-thickness grafts; a delay in hydrotherapy may result in consequent loss of the graft to infection.

Sodium depletion occurring in association with treatment of burn injury by repeated submersion in water has been reported. This may be reversed by

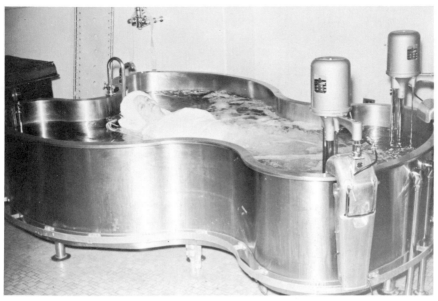

Figure 12–4　Hubbard tank therapy. The patient is supported on a canvas plinth.

appropriate replacement therapy. It has been postulated that a primary loss of electrolyte through the burned surface into the whirlpool may occur. This emphasizes the importance of monitoring fluid and electrolyte levels of patients, not only in early but also in later phases of recovery from serious burns, especially when therapy includes any procedure which may increase fluid or electrolyte losses. Some Hubbard tanks have a grating at the base which can be removed to allow the patient to stand in water at maximum depth (Fig. 12–5). Partial weight bearing and ambulation can be initiated in this way in cases in which walking exercise is indicated but the stress of weight is contraindicated.

The size of water tanks used in underwater exercise varies considerably. Exercise for fingers or hands can be carried out in a small basin, but large stainless steel water tanks are used for one or both arms or legs.

Underwater total body exercises (general or specific), progressive ambulation in water (non-weight bearing and partial weight bearing) and swimming are best performed in a therapeutic pool (Fig. 12–6), but, since they are expensive to install, a less expensive Hubbard tank can be used for all but swimming.

The lining of the therapeutic pool should not be slippery. Mosaic, fire-clay tiles, and fiber glass have all been used. Of these, mosaic seems the most satisfactory but is the most expensive. Pinhead unglazed tiles are also satisfactory and somewhat cheaper. The surroundings of the pool should be nonskid. If steps into the pool are used, the treads should be sufficiently broad and also nonslippery.

Purification of the pool water is essential, preferably accomplished by continuous filtration and chlorination. This system circulates, filters, aerates and chlorinates, while a calorifier maintains the temperature.

Precautions should be taken against *tinea pedis,* and a foot bath for this purpose should be employed, through which the ambulant patient walks after discarding his slippers before entering the water.

Showers should be adjacent to the pool for use before and after treatment.

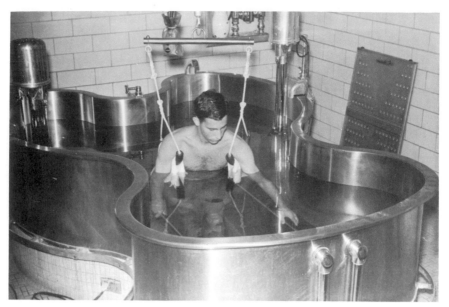

Figure 12–5 Hubbard tank therapy in the walk-in tank. Partial weight-bearing is permitted by buoyancy effect of water and underarm support.

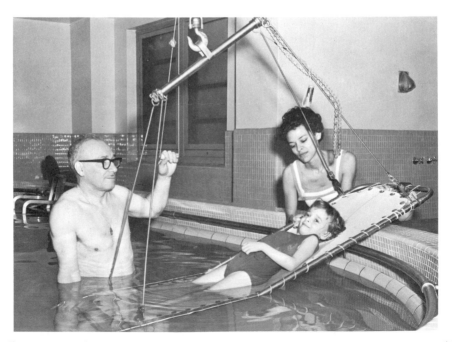

Figure 12–6 Therapeutic pool at Department of Physical Medicine and Rehabilitation, Philadelphia General Hospital. The patient is conveyed to the pool by overhead crane and canvas plinth suspension. (Courtesy Dr. Albert Martucci.)

The temperature of the water should be in the region of 97 to 99° F., so that the patient is warm enough during treatment, but not so warm as to cause exhaustion.

Pool therapy introduces some patients to a new world, and they may anticipate it with voiced or unvoiced anxiety. It is important that from the first moment such patients are made to feel the confidence which full care inspires. If this is achieved they quickly come to look forward to their treatment with great enjoyment.

Douches

Hydrotherapy may be applied by directing one or more streams of water of controlled temperature and pressure against the surface of the entire body or any part of it. This application is called a douche. There are several forms of douche therapy, such as the jet douche, fan douche (Fig. 12-7), Scotch douche (Fig. 12-8), shower douche, hepatic douche, underwater douche, needle shower bath and rain bath, the name being descriptive of the shape of the stream of water utilized, the technique of application or the area of the body to which the douche is applied. The temperature and pressure of the water may be controlled from a hydrotherapy control stand.

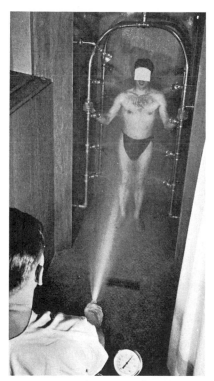 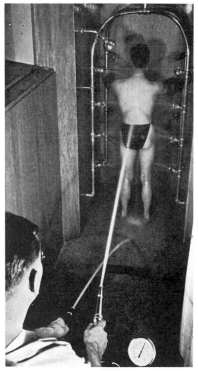

Fig. 12-7   Fig. 12-8

Figure 12-7   Fan douche. (From Krusen, Physical Medicine. Philadelphia, W. B. Saunders Co.)

Figure 12-8   Scotch douche. (From Krusen, Physical Medicine. Philadelphia, W. B. Saunders Co.)

Ablutions

An ablution is a sponge or towel bath. It is most commonly used to reduce temperature in fever. The temperature of the water is usually 22° C., but with successive applications it may gradually be made cooler.

The information included in these few pages has been necessarily limited primarily to the scope and applications of hydrotherapy in general terms. More extensive discussions pertaining to physiologic responses to temperature change, specifications of hydrotherapeutic equipment, techniques of application, indications and contraindications may be found in the references.

CRYOTHERAPY AS A PART OF HYDROTHERAPY

General Principles

Heat for the relief of pain is a universal remedy and methods of application vary from the simple "soak in a hot tub" to the more sophisticated hot packs and diathermy. However, in recent years cold has become increasingly more popular, in the form of baths, packs and ice massage.

Cryotherapy, or the therapeutic use of cold, is being used today by many clinicians for a variety of ailments. An understanding of some of the physiologic effects of cold is helpful in properly employing this modality clinically. A number of references in the literature have indicated that the primary reaction of the circulatory system to cold is vasoconstriction, followed after 3 to 5 minutes by vasodilation. After this period of vasodilation the vessels again become sensitive to the constrictor effect of cold.

If cold is applied to a local area of the skin, the resulting decreased blood flow initially diminishes heat transport from the body core to the skin and enhances the direct cooling effect. The higher the environmental temperature, the higher the blood flow for a given temperature of the local area. Apparently the blood flow rate in the affected area is partially governed by the overall need for heat balance.

The phenomenon of cold-induced vasodilation was first described in 1930. Investigators found that the temperature of the skin of the fingers during continued immersion in ice water fell rapidly for the first few minutes and thereafter spontaneous rewarming took place. Cyclic phases of warming and cooling followed.

There is little likelihood that, in any clinical use of cold or heat, any nerve or muscle will be excited by the thermal change, as a true stimulus. Experimentally, nerve excitation and contraction of skeletal muscles can be elicited only by extremely quick and wide temperature changes.

It has been observed that cold will first diminish the rate of transmission of impulses along a nerve and then, at about 27° C. or lower, nerve conduction will begin to fail.

Assessment of clinical reduction of spasticity produced through cooling is difficult. It is thought that suppression of the myotactic reflex is a result of reduced nerve conduction, decreased muscle spindle excitability and increased tissue and joint viscosity. After removal of ice packs, the skin temperature soon reaches 25° C. and tends to remain at this level for at least an hour.

In their study of the combined effects on muscle of general body temperature and local cold application, Newton and Lehmkuhl found that muscle spindle discharge was most effectively decreased when the body was kept at normal temperature during direct application of cold to muscle.

On pain, Licht believes that the amount of cooling required to relieve or abolish pain does not produce anesthesia but rather counterirritation. The subject often experiences an initial sensation of cold, followed by a burning sensation, aching, and finally numbness.

Nerve and muscle metabolism are decreased with exposure to cold. Since the sensory impulses are decreased with extreme local cold application, this modality can be used effectively to promote muscular relaxation in patients with spasticity and muscular spasm.

Conditions in Which Cryotherapy Has Been Employed

Ice packs have been used by Schaubel after **orthopedic procedures.** Patients treated in this manner responded better in all respects than patients who were not so treated. Some criteria used were postoperative complications, amount of narcotics required, temperatture, white blood count, pulse and respiration. Schaubel believed ice was a valuable adjunct in the treatment of surgical patients.

A wide range of **musculoskeletal disturbances** have been managed successfully by various clinicians with cryotherapy in conjunction with other physical modalities. Some of the conditions treated were acute sprains, chondromalacia of the knee with effusion, acute back strain with splinting, acute bursitis of the shoulder, acute arthritis, herniated nucleus pulposus, functional back pain, cerebrovascular accident, rotator cuff tendinitis, cervical myositis, paralysis agitans, knee sprains and elbow sprains.

An investigation of the effects of cryotherapy in the postsurgical **rheumatoid hand** revealed that cryotherapy produced a trend toward reducing postoperative edema, and that postoperative pain appeared to be reduced also.

Ice massage has been shown to be effective also in the symptomatic relief of **low back pain** and on the basis of some reports may be equally effective as hot packs.

Cryotherapy for several weeks prior to an exercise program appears to have significant and positive implications in eliciting a wider range of motion in joints which exhibit **contractures due to spasticity** from a central nervous system dysfunction. This technique is an effective and practical means of reducing spasticity. Recent literature provides adequate material for further research on the effectiveness of cryotherapy technique on the spastic muscle. However, our present knowledge of spasticity is highly theoretical, and the explanation of the effectiveness of cold applications for the relief of spasticity is speculative.

Hydrotherapeutic Techniques for Applying Cold

Techniques which may be employed include the following:

For spasticity, Turkish towels are plunged into cracked ice and water and, after eliminating as much water as possible, they are placed on the spastic muscles for 8 minutes. Because the towels warm rapidly, a second application of towels is given at the end of the first 4 minutes to effect more rapid cooling of the muscle.

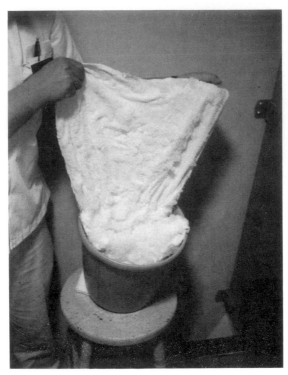

Figure 12–9   *Preparing towel for treatment of spasticity:* (1) Dry towel is immersed in bucket of shaved ice. (2) When ice adheres to towel, withdraw and apply to patient.

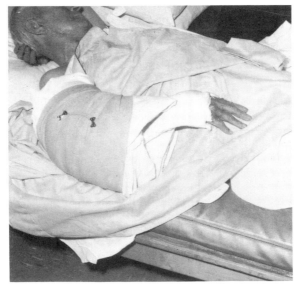

Figure 12–10   *Ice pack application:* (1) Ice bag is wrapped in towel and applied to conform to structure to be treated in order to exclude air. (2) The area is then wrapped with an Ace bandage to fix the ice bag in place.

After orthopedic procedures, immediately postoperatively, cloth-covered ice bags are applied directly to the plaster or soft bandage over the operative site. A sufficient number of ice caps should be used to surround the extremity completely at the operative site. When used on the extremity the bags can be held in place by elastic bandages. For the hip or shoulder, scultetus binders may be used. The ice caps are refilled every four hours and are used for 48 hours postoperatively. The accumulated air in the ice caps should be released at hourly intervals to allow them to hug the cast snugly.

Large cubes of ice are used for ice massage. These are moved slowly over the area to be treated until numbing occurs, usually in 10 to 12 minutes. The cubes may be made by freezing water in empty cans.

The method employed and length of time in administering cryotherapy depend on the part of the body to be treated and the nature of the pathologic condition. If there is a fresh injury, then the purpose of treatment is to control swelling by constricting blood and lymph flow. An example is an **athletic injury,** such as a sprained ankle, which can be treated by immersion in ice water to at least midcalf depth for a period of 10 to 20 minutes. This may be accomplished by using a whirlpool bath or any container suitable for comfortably holding the foot.

Immersion techniques are quite suitable for extremities. However, **ice massage** is a popular form of treatment for flatter areas of the body, such as the low back, shoulder, quadriceps and hamstring areas. Ice massage is more localized and not as uniform in its cooling; thus the treatment time is usually extended to 20 to 30 minutes. Water may be conveniently frozen in 8-ounce paper cups and kept in the freezer section of a refrigerator. The 8-ounce block covers a fairly large area and is easy to hold.

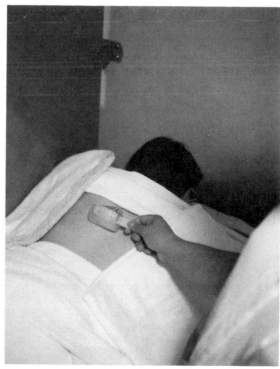

Figure 12–11 *Ice massage:* (1) Cut off one third of tongue depressor; then insert remaining piece in Dixie cup of water and freeze. (2) Patient is positioned and draped. (3) Therapist uses tongue depressor as handle and gently applies ice over area to be treated.

Immersion techniques and ice massage are superior to ice packs because of the ease of application, the resulting uniformity of analgesia, especially in and around bony areas, and the possibility of patient participation. In both methods the application of cold is terminated when the part is sufficiently anesthetized to permit voluntary movement through the desired range.

This level is reached only after some degree of discomfort has been experienced. Initially, only a cold sensation is felt; subsequently, the patient describes a sensation of "burning," "stinging" or "intense aching." This period of discomfort is short-lived, usually lasting one to two minutes, but it is necessary for the patient to submit to it before he can tolerate effective motion. Although pain and discomfort diminish rapidly, tactile sensation remains, indicating that anesthesia in its truest sense is not obtained. The erythema which appears during the cold application usually persists for 5 to 10 minutes following termination of the ice massage. The duration of treatment required to achieve the desired effect varies with the individual and appears to be related to the severity of the injury, the size of the area involved and the individual's response to cold. The period of relief from pain and discomfort varies from 10 minutes in severe trauma to complete and lasting relief in minor injuries or complaints. Exercise is initiated when voluntary movement of the part is possible. The ability to move the part without pain impresses the patient considerably, especially since immobilization previously provided protection against such pain. Following this initial motion, the physical therapist instructs the patient in strengthening, postural, corrective or other types of exercise, as indicated. If discomfort recurs following exercise, the application of ice through submersion or massage is repeated.

Caution.   The danger of freezing tissue, resulting in frostbite, exists if the ice is left directly and continuously on the part. Often an ice pack is made by putting crushed or chipped ice in a towel and attaching it to the part with tape or an elastic wrap. The pack should be shifted and the extremity checked every two minutes to ensure even and safe cooling. Treatment should be given three times a day if possible. Since ice therapy is relatively simple, a patient may treat himself at home under a physician's direction.

In the case of an injury such as sprain, the 20 minute treatment is repeated till internal bleeding has stopped. This varies with the injury. A bruise may take 24 hours, whereas a severe contusion could take as long as 72 to 86 hours. After this period the treatment time is reduced to 5 to 7 minutes. At least 3 to 5 minutes is needed to produce a relaxation of the muscles. This is also enough time for vasodilation to occur and treatment ends before the second vasoconstriction period begins. Injuries may be treated with ice throughout their entire course of recovery. When a plateau of recovery is reached and another modality is indicated, ultrasound can be a valuable adjunct to ice therapy.

General Conclusions Regarding Applications of Cold

Cryotherapy may be considered for some of the conditions usually treated with moist heat. If it proves effective, it is certainly inexpensive and relatively simple to apply, both in the hospital and at home. Contraindications should, however, be considered, such as Raynaud's disease, and the standard contraindications for any thermotherapy.

In summary, cryotherapy can be of benefit to patients with a wide range of neurological and musculoskeletal conditions. Ice packs, immersion techniques and ice massage are usually supplemented with combinations of exercise, bed rest, positioning, traction or analgesics. Results should not be attributed to the use of cryotherapy alone. A need exists for further investigation regarding the therapeutic effects of local cold application. Most of the research reported has been related either to hypothermia or refrigeration in surgery, or to hibernation in space. The available material is inconclusive. More clinical studies, with good controls, are needed in order to accumulate sufficient data on which to formulate sound principles of treatment.

REFERENCES

Hydrotherapy

1. Bierman, W.: Physical Medicine in General Practice. New York, Paul B. Hoeber, Inc., 1947.
2. Bolton, E.: Safety in Relation to Pool Treatment. Physiotherapy, *54:*232, 1968.
3. Coulter, J. S.: Principles and Practice of Physical Therapy. Hagerstown, Md., W. F. Prior Co., Inc., 1937.
4. Goldberg, M. J., Culver, J. V., and Carson, J. F.: Volume Changes in Below-Knee Amputation Stumps As Affected by Type of Whirlpool-Tank Therapy. J. Amer. Geriat. Soc., *16:*101–105, 1968.
5. Gotshall, R. A.: Sodium Depletion Related to Hydrotherapy for Burn Injury. J.A.M.A., *203:*984–986, 1968.
6. Kaplan, C. M.: A Whirlpool Chair. Physical Therapy, Vol. 49, August, 1969.
7. Krusen, F. H.: Physical Medicine. Philadelphia, W. B. Saunders Co., 1941.
8. Licht, S.: Medical Hydrology. New Haven, Conn., Elizabeth Licht, 1963.
9. Lowman, C. L., and Roen, S. G.: Therapeutic Use of Pools and Tanks. Philadelphia, W. B. Saunders Co., 1952.
10. Randall, H. B.: Use of the Whirlpool Bath for Injured Athletes. J. Sch. Health, Vol. 38, November, 1968.
11. Skeversky, N., and Zislis, J. M.: Peripheral Vascular Disorders and the Aged Amputee. Geriatrics, *25:*142–149, 1970.
12. Smith, E. I., and De Weese, H. M. S.: The Topical Therapy of Burns in Children. Arch. Surg., Vol. 98, April, 1969.
13. Watkins, A. L.: A Manual of Electrotherapy. 2nd Ed. Philadelphia, Lea and Febiger, 1962.
14. Whiting, W. B., Welch, T. D., and Kimura, J.: Hydrotherapy at Burn Center. Western Medicine, 7 March 1966.
15. Zislis, J. M.: Rehabilitation of the Cancer Patient. Geriatrics, *25:*150-158, 1970.

Cryotherapy

16. Adams, T., and Smith, R. E.: Effects of Chronic Local Cold Exposures on the Finger Temperature Responses. J. Appl. Physiol., *17:*317–322, 1962.
17. Bing, A. I., Caresten, A., and Christiansen, S.: The Effect on Muscular Temperature Produced by Cooling Normal and Ultraviolet Radiated Skin. Acta Medica Scand., *121:*577–591, 1945.
18. Carlson, L. D.: Physiology of Exposure to Cold, Physiol., *2:*1-7, 1964.
19. Chambers, R.: Clinical Uses of Cryotherapy. Phys. Ther., *49:*245–249, 1969.
20. Chu, D., and Lutt, C. J.: The Rationale of Ice Therapy. J. Nat. Athletic Trainers Assoc., Vol. 4, No. 4, Winter 1969.
21. Clarke, R. S., Hellon, R. F., and Lind, A. R.: Vascular Reactions of the Human Forearm to Cold. Clin. Sci., *17:*165–179, 1958.
22. Fischer, E., and Solomon, S.: Physiological Responses to Heat and Cold. *In* Therapeutic Heat, edited by Sidney Licht. New Haven, Connecticut, Elizabeth Licht, Pub., 1958.
23. Hartviksen, K.: Ice Therapy in Spasticity. Acta Neurol. Scand., 38 Suppl. *3:*79-84, 1962.
24. Hayden, C.: Cryokinetics in an Early Treatment Program. Phys. Ther., *44:*990-993, 1964.
25. Kelly, M.: Effectiveness of a Cryotherapy Technique on Spasticity. Phys. Ther., *49:*349-353, 1969.
26. Landen, B.: Heat or Cold for the Relief of Low Back Pain? Phys. Ther., *47:*1126-1128, 1967.
27. Levine, M. G., Kabot, H., Knott, M., and Voss, D. E.: Effects of Cooling on the Triceps Surae Reflex. Amer. J. Phys. Med., *41:*240-251, 1962.
28. Lewis, T.: Observations Upon the Reactions of Vessels of Human Skin to Cold. Heart, *15:*177-208, 1930.

29. Newton, M. J., and Lehmkuhl, D.: Muscle-spindle Responses to Body Heating and Localized Muscle Cooling. Phys. Ther., *45*:91–105, 1965.
30. Petajan, J. H., and Watts, N.: Effects of Cooling on the Triceps Surae Reflex. J. Appl. Physiol. *19*:877–880, 1964.
31. Rembe, E.: Use of Cryotherapy on the Postsurgical Rheumatoid Hand. Phys. Ther., *50*:19–23, 1970.
32. Schaubel, H. H.: Local Use of Ice After Orthopedic Procedures. Amer. J. Surg., *72*:711–714, 1946.
33. Showman, J., and Wedlick, L. T.: The Use of Cold Instead of Heat for Relief of Muscle Spasm. Med. J. Aust., *2*:612–614, 1963.

Chapter 13

ULTRAVIOLET THERAPY

by G. Keith Stillwell

PHYSICAL PRINCIPLES

Quantum theory states that the energy contained in the individual quanta is greater at higher frequencies of electromagnetic radiation (see Figure 10-4, page 265.) The amount of this energy, q, is expressed (in ergs) by the equation

$$q = h v \qquad (1)$$

in which h = Planck's constant, which is 6.6236×10^{-27} erg seconds, and v = frequency of the wave emanation in waves per second. While lower quantum energies (infrared) are able only to increase the molecular and atomic motion, which is heat, the higher quantum energies can produce changes in the electronic structure of the atoms or molecules. The far ultraviolet energies of radiation (that is, far from the visible spectrum) may be able to separate an electron from the atom, producing an ion. The very high quantum energies of radiation at wavelengths shorter than the ultraviolet (for example, x-rays and gamma rays) may produce more drastic and irreversible effects upon the atoms and molecules.

When an atom absorbs a quantum of energy in the ultraviolet range, it becomes temporarily excited or activated. It then changes to a state of lesser excitation in one or more stages, releasing (emitting) quanta of energy in the process.

The atoms of any particular element can absorb or emit only certain specific quanta of energy (that is, certain specific wavelengths of electromagnetic energy). The energy released in the process of degradation from an excited state may be transferred to another molecule, consumed in a chemical reaction or liberated as ultraviolet energy, visible light (fluorescence) or heat. Ordinarily the emitted quanta are smaller than the absorbed quanta, and some of the energy appears as heat.

Mercury vapor excited by the passage of an electric current will emit energy of several specific wavelengths, which correspond to the wavelengths that mercury vapor can absorb. These have been correlated with the several different levels of excitation that the mercury atom may possess.

The photochemical process of the absorption of a quantum is independent of oxygen and is not influenced much by temperature. Subsequent reactions may require oxygen and have a Q_{10} between 2 and 3. The reactions may be indicated by the following equations,

$$M + h\nu \longrightarrow M_r \qquad\qquad (2)$$
$$M_r + X \longrightarrow X^1 + M \qquad\qquad (3)$$
$$X^1 + O_2 \longrightarrow X_{ox} \qquad\qquad (4)$$

in which M is the substance that absorbs the quantum, $h\nu$, and becomes an activated or excited substance, M_r. M may be some substance normally present in the system or a photosensitizing drug or dye. In equation 3, M_r delivers some or all of this energy of the absorbed quantum to substance X, which becomes excited or activated as X^1. This process may actually be repeated several times through a series of molecules. However, the most that is generally known about these reactions is the absorbing substance M and the final product X_{ox}. The changes represented in equation 3 last for only a few microseconds and are largely unknown. The excited substance X^1 in equation 4 enters into a chemical reaction with oxygen in this example, producing an oxidized compound of X^1 shown as X_{ox}. This reaction is the one that is temperature sensitive. An alternative might be the following,

$$X^1 + Y \longrightarrow XY \qquad\qquad (5)$$

which does not involve oxygen but may be affected by temperature.

Absorption Spectra and Action Spectra

An action spectrum for a particular photochemical reaction is determined by measuring which parts of the spectrum are most effective in energizing the reaction. The action spectrum should correspond with the absorption spectrum of the substance M of equation 2. However, the absorption spectra of many of the proteins present in biologic systems are similar. The precise determination of the substance M by the relationship between action and absorption spectra may not be possible.

It is apparent that the spectrum is not sharply delimited in its photobiologic effects. As one moves from the infrared through the visible spectrum and into the ultraviolet, the quantum energy increases and the potential for photochemical reactions increases. The wavelengths that are effective in the ordinary course of events will be secondarily influenced by the following factors: (1) the wavelengths available (for example, the spectrum of sunlight as modified by passage through the earth's atmosphere); (2) the absorption or reflection of certain wavelengths at the surface of the skin, which in turn may be modified by moisture, ointments or other substances on the skin; and (3) the thickness of the stratum corneum of the skin.

Dosage Factors

Some of the factors discussed under the transfer of energy by radiation in connection with Figure 10–5 in Chapter 10, Therapeutic Heat, are of importance in ultraviolet radiation. This is true of the inverse square law, which states that the intensity of the radiation, I, falling on the surface, S_2, varies inversely with the square of the distance, d, between the source, S_1, and the surface:

$$I \propto \frac{1}{d^2} \tag{6}$$

Lambert's cosine law is also applicable. The intensity of radiation falling on the surface, S_2, varies with the cosine of the angle, a, between the incident beam and the perpendicular to the surface. In addition, the reflection and scatter of radiation are more pronounced with increasingly oblique rays, and this will further decrease their effectiveness.

With the powerful sources of ultraviolet radiation used in some clinical situations, in which erythema may be produced in the skin by exposure at a distance of 30 inches for 15 seconds, *the factors of distance and time are critical and must be governed very closely.* All other factors being equal, the duration of exposure will be determined by the distance from the lamp to the part of the patient that is closest to it.

Minimal Erythema Dose (M.E.D.)

The sensitivity of the human skin to ultraviolet radiation varies considerably because of variation in the thickness of the stratum corneum and in the amount of superficial pigmentation. The dose of ultraviolet radiation that will produce, within a few hours, a minimal erythema in the average Caucasian skin is called the minimal erythema dose. For the high-pressure mercury arc in a quartz burner, this dose is usually in the order of 15 seconds of exposure at a distance of 30 inches. It is determined by observation on several subjects, usually on the volar aspect of the forearm. It is necessary to determine this dose two or three times yearly since the ability of the quartz envelope to transmit ultraviolet emanation deteriorates with age. A very old lamp may be emitting principally heat and visible light.

The minimal erythema dose may be used as a dosage unit in the prescription of ultraviolet irradiation. It is usually possible to increase progressively the number of M.E.D.'s used in each treatment of a given patient as the stratum corneum thickens and the sensitivity to ultraviolet radiation decreases. Pigmentation of the skin also influences the sensitivity to ultraviolet radiation. Brunettes are less sensitive than blondes, and reddish-blondes are more sensitive. The M.E.D. is an *average* quantity, and the dosage for an individual patient in fractions or multiples of the M.E.D. should be prescribed with respect to the probable sensitivity of this individual in relationship to average sensitivity.

Further Degrees of Erythema. The M.E.D. has also been called a first degree erythema. A second degree erythema is caused by a dose of about 2½ M.E.D. It has a latency of four to six hours, may be a little painful and subsides in two to four days. It is followed by desquamation. Third degree erythema is caused by about 5 M.E.D. and has associated edema. The latency may be as brief as two hours. It is followed by marked desquamation. Such a dose cannot of course be safely applied to a large part of the body surface. Fourth degree erythema, which is produced by about 10 M.E.D., is characterized in addition by the development of a superficial blister.

Precautions

Photo-ophthalmia. The eye is highly sensitive to ultraviolet radiation, and therefore the eyes of both the patient and the operator of the lamp *must be shielded* at all times. Shielding can be accomplished by the use of spectacles of ordinary glass or, in the case of the patient, of pledgets of cotton or gauze soaked in water and placed over the eyes.

In addition to conjunctivitis, keratotic changes in the cornea may occur (usually, but not always, reparable). With massive doses of ultraviolet radiation, lenticular opacities may be produced.

Other Susceptible Regions. If there is a significant difference in the distance between the source of the radiation and the various parts of the patient, excessive irradiation of the closer parts may occur. This is most likely to affect the buttocks of the prone patient or the breasts of the supine female patient. In the latter instance, it is often necessary to drape the breasts in order to be able to employ adequate doses of ultraviolet radiation to the face and upper anterior part of the chest, as in the treatment of acne.

Photosensitizing Drugs. Abnormal sensitivity to ultraviolet radiation may occur in some persons when they are taking certain chemicals. As the number and variety of drugs used in medicine increase, the incidence and variety of these cases may be expected to increase also. The sulfonamides may induce an excessive sensitivity to the erythema spectrum. Green soap has also been reported to sensitize the skin to wavelengths shorter than 3200 Angstroms. Tetracyclines have been suspected in this regard.

Photosensitization to wavelengths longer than 3200 Angstroms has been reported with the use of various dyes (eosin, rose bengal, fluorescein), coal tar derivatives and some plant materials. Lipstick cheilitis is probably related to absorption of the fluorescein dye from the lipstick into the skin of the lips.

Protective Factors. The principal protection against erythema (see the next section) is the thickness of the stratum corneum. Pigmentation is located too deeply to provide much protection, except in the Negro skin. Areas of "thin skin," for example, healed indolent ulcers, scars and some skin grafts, are therefore more readily burned than is the rest of the surface. Such areas may be screened from the ultraviolet radiation by wet towels or dressings.

PHYSIOLOGIC EFFECTS

Erythema

The sunburn effect of ultraviolet is well known. The action spectrum for the production of erythema has two maxima, at 2500 Angstroms and at 2970 Angstroms. No erythema is produced by wavelengths longer than 3300 Angstroms. The spectrum of sunlight at the surface of the earth is cut off at 2900 Angstroms, and only a very small fraction of sunlight is erythemogenic. Window glass cuts off all wavelengths shorter than 3200 Angstroms and provides complete protection against sunburn (Fig. 13-1).

The primary phenomenon in the production of erythema is believed to be absorption of the specific quanta by protein(s) in the prickle cell layer of the skin. This denatures the protein and thereby damages the cells. This photochemical reaction is not affected by temperature, and the threshold time of exposure is not affected by temperature. The damaged cells release a vasodilator substance at a rate that *is* sensitive to temperature, and this substance diffuses to the subdermal level, where it causes vasodilatation. The latent period for this process may be several hours. Although the vasodilator substance may be similar to histamine, the absorbing protein is probably not histidine. As a sequel to the erythema the stratum corneum thickens, and this change provides some protection from the erythemogenic effects of subsequent exposure.

Pigmentation

Melanin. As a normal sequel to erythema, melanin granules migrate from the deep layers of the skin toward the surface. The melanin tends to remain too deep in white skin to be of any value in protecting against sunburn. This type of tanning does not require oxygen. The precise origin of the melanin is uncertain.

Other Tanning. A second type of tanning consists of darkening of preformed pigment. The action spectrum extends from 3000 to 4400 Angstroms

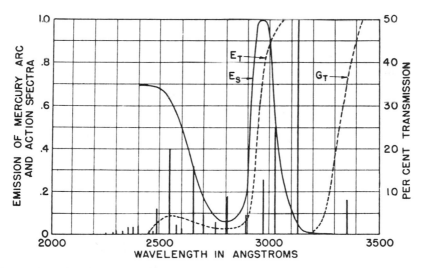

Figure 13-1 Graph of various phenomena in the ultraviolet portion of the electromagnetic spectrum. E_S is the action spectrum of the erythema of sunburn (after Coblentz and Stair, corrected for relative number of quanta). E_T is the curve for transmission of human epidermis 0.08 mm. thick, cleared to diminish scattering (after Lucas). G_T is the transmission through window glass. Vertical lines at the bottom show the position and relatively intensity of lines of "hot quartz" mercury-vapor lamp. Ordinate units for action spectrum and energies of mercury lines arbitrarily chosen. (Reproduced with permission from Blum, H. F.: Radiation: Photophysiologic and Photopathologic Processes. In Glasser, Otto: Medical Physics. Chicago, Year Book Publishers, Inc., 1944, vol. 1, pp. 1145–1157.)

with a maximum at 3400 Angstroms. This is a reversible reaction, requiring oxygen and having a brief latency of an hour or less. Little of the emission of a mercury-vapor arc is in this spectral region. This is the explanation for the fact that a darker tan results from exposure to sunlight or a carbon arc source than from exposure to a mercury-vapor arc.

Antirachitic Effect

The irradiation of ergosterol and some closely related sterols will lead to the formation of antirachitic substances. In human skin this reaction occurs as the conversion of 7-dehydrocholesterol to vitamin D_3. The action spectrum for the antirachitic effect is compatible with the absorption spectrum for 7-dehydrocholesterol, which extends from about 2400 to 3000 Angstroms with a maximum at 2830 Angstroms. This maximum corresponds to a minimum in the action spectrum for erythema. It has been proposed that most of the energy at this wavelength is absorbed in superficial layers of the skin where the vitamin D is produced and that it does not penetrate deeply enough to participate in the production of erythema.

Diseases Caused by Light

Relatively little is known about many of these diseases, and a detailed discussion is beyond the scope of this presentation. Blum[1] divided them into two groups.

1. Abnormal responses to radiation which will cause erythema normally, that is, wavelengths shorter than 3200 Angstroms, which will not pass through ordinary window glass.

    (a) Polymorphic light eruption. The threshold of sensitivity is usually normal, but the response elicited is abnormal.
    (b) Squamous cell and basal cell cancer of the skin.
    (c) Patients with lymphogranuloma venereum may be abnormally sensitive to the sunburn spectrum.

2. Sensitivity to wavelengths longer than 3200 Angstroms, which are transmitted by ordinary window glass.

    (a) Urticaria solaris due to wavelengths of 4000 to 5000 Angstroms. The urticaria appears after a very short latent period and is not dependent on oxygen. The photosensitizing agent may be a carotenoid.
    (b) Urticaria solaris due to wavelengths shorter than 3700 Angstroms. This is the same as (a) except for the different action spectrum and the fact that passive transfer can be demonstrated.

Hydroa aestivale is a rare disease whose action spectrum has not been delineated. It may be that repeated exposure to sunlight makes the skin of these persons more susceptible to trauma and that this disorder has some features in common with epidermolysis bullosa. There may be an associated disorder of porphyrin metabolism, but Blum considers it unlikely that porphyrins act as photosensitizers in this disease.[1]

METHODS OF ULTRAVIOLET IRRADIATION

Therapeutic Devices

Mercury-Vapor Arcs. Mercury vapor enclosed in a quartz envelope is activated by an electric current. The arc emits a continuous spectrum through the visible range into the infrared. In addition, relatively more intense emanations occur at various points in the ultraviolet and the blue end of the visible spectrum, and these are specific for mercury. Most of this portion of the spectrum is not present in sunlight, which has no wavelengths shorter than 2900 Angstroms at the earth's surface. The spectrum emitted is affected by the pressure of the mercury.

"Hot Quartz" Lamps (Fig. 13-2). These lamps operate with a relatively high pressure of mercury and produce a modified mercury emission spectrum with high intensity lines at 2652, 2967, 3025, 3130 and 3660 Angstroms plus some energy on each side of the 2537 Angstrom line. The M.E.D. of a lamp in good condition may be of the order of 15 seconds of exposure at a distance of 30 inches. Smaller lamps of this type may be cooled by a water jacket or an air blower (Kromayer type) so that they can be used close to the surface of the patient without causing thermal burns (Fig. 13-3). They can also be adapted for orificial application. The M.E.D. of such lamps may be of the order of 5 seconds of exposure at a distance of 2 inches.

"Cold Quartz" Lamps (Figs. 13-4 and 13-5). These lamps have a relatively low mercury pressure and contain, in addition, a rare gas such as argon or neon to initiate the arc. Almost all the transmitted ultraviolet emission is at 2537 Angstroms, which is in the lower maximum of the erythema action spectrum. The surface of the envelope is warmed only to about 60° C. The emission at 1849 Angstroms, which generates ozone in air, is not transmitted by the fused quartz burners used in these lamps.

"Sun Lamps." "Sun lamps" contain a tungsten filament with which to heat the lamp and vaporize the mercury so that a mercury arc can be established

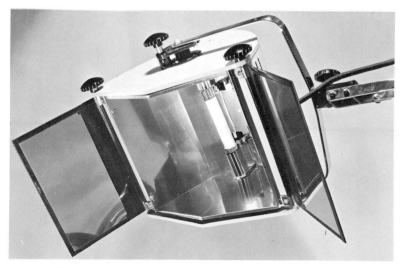

Figure 13–2 "Hot quartz" ultraviolet source, stand lamp, showing the burner and reflector. The wings of the reflector can be folded to close it, but amounts of ultraviolet sufficient to harm the eyes can still escape through the cracks.

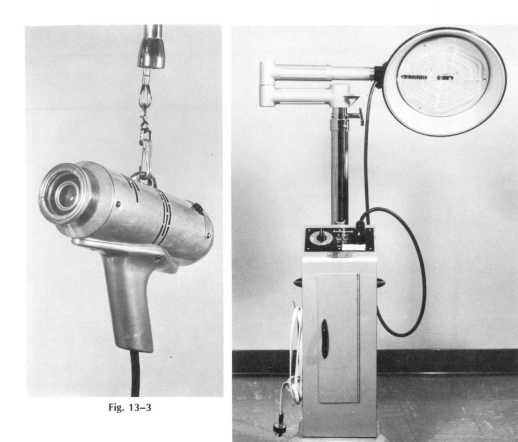

Fig. 13–3

Fig. 13–4

Figure 13–3　"Hot quartz" air-cooled ultraviolet source which may be used with orificial applicators or for small areas.

Figure 13–4　"Cold quartz" ultraviolet source, stand lamp. (Courtesy of Dr. F. J. Kottke.)

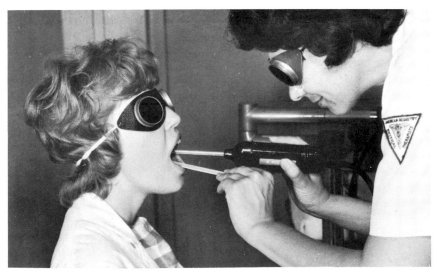

Figure 13–5　"Cold quartz" ultraviolet source, orificial applicator. Note use of protective goggles by patient and therapist. (Courtesy of Dr. F. J. Kottke.)

between tungsten electrodes. The envelope is a glass that will transmit ultraviolet radiation. The M.E.D. is usually measured in minutes.

Carbon Arcs. The carbon arc produces a continuous spectrum ranging from the far ultraviolet to the infrared. The relative intensity in the near or far ultraviolet portion of the spectrum can be modified by the use of carbon rod electrodes having different metallic salt cores. Carbon arcs consume the carbon and must have a reliable automatic feed mechanism to maintain the size of the gap between the electrodes so that sparks and sputtering will be minimized and the spectrum emitted will be reasonably constant.

The production of ozone is slightly annoying, but the concentrations produced are not hazardous in a well ventilated room.

"Black-Light" Lamps. For diagnostic procedures involving the observation of fluorescence, a glass filter may be employed to eliminate the visible emanation from the lamp. With a low-pressure mercury-arc lamp, a black phosphate glass may be used. With a high-pressure mercury-arc lamp, Wood's nickel oxide glass is used.

Technique of Application

The technique of igniting the arc of the burner should be found in the instruction manual for the particular device being employed. The dosage of ultraviolet radiation must be regulated within very narrow limits. In general, the procedure is as follows:

1. Patient and operator must be screened from the ultraviolet source except during the actual time of the therapeutic exposure.

2. The eyes should be shielded at all times by glass or by wet gauze. This applies also to scattered reflected radiation from the walls and other structures.

3. The M.E.D. of the source must be known. If it is not known, it should be determined before the lamp is used on a patient.

4. The timing device used must be capable of accurate measurement of the time units being employed (a good second hand on a watch may be used if the M.E.D. is measured in seconds).

5. The distance from the source to the nearest part of the patient must be measured, not estimated.

6. Draping of the patient to screen some portions of the body from the radiation must be essentially identical in subsequent treatments if the dosage is being increased. It is customary, though perhaps not essential, to drape the genital area.

INDICATIONS FOR ULTRAVIOLET THERAPY

Diseases of the Skin

ACNE VULGARIS. Treatment is generally given three times weekly starting with an initial dose of 1 M.E.D. (or 1½ or 2 M.E.D. if the tolerance of the patient for ultraviolet radiation seems likely to be more than average). The dosage is increased by 1 M.E.D. each treatment until a second degree erythema reaction occurs. The dosage may subsequently be increased if necessary.

PSORIASIS. Aside from the initial acute phase of this disease, it usually is improved by ultraviolet therapy. General irradiation may help to keep the psoriatic patient in better condition. The lesions may be treated with second degree erythema (or even third degree erythema for small areas).

The Goekerman technique, involving the use of a crude coal tar ointment in addition to ultraviolet radiation, may act through a photochemical or photosensitizing mechanism. It is often more effective than the use of either coal tar or ultraviolet radiation alone. Since little or none of the ultraviolet radiation penetrates through the medicament to the skin, relatively large doses of ultraviolet radiation are used. The steps in the technique are as follows:

1. The crude coal tar ointment is applied to the skin in the evening in a thick layer over the psoriatic patches.

2. Before ultraviolet irradiation the next day, the bulk of the coal tar ointment is wiped off with olive oil.

3. Immediately after this, the stained patches are exposed to ultraviolet radiation. The usual initial dosage is 4 M.E.D. with the mercury-vapor lamp, with daily increases by 2 M.E.D. as long as the reaction of the skin is favorable.

4. Following the ultraviolet irradiation, the patient bathes.

DECUBITUS ULCERS AND OTHER INDOLENT ULCERS (Fig. 13-6). It is, of course, most difficult to evaluate the relative merits of various steps one may take to attempt to heal such ulcers. Ultraviolet therapy may be expected to be beneficial because of its bactericidal effects (particularly of the far ultraviolet emanation at 2537 Angstroms from the mercury-vapor arc) and its erythemogenic effect at the margins of the ulcer. Because the usual erythema of ultraviolet radiation is dependent on an initial reaction occurring in skin (see the section on Erythema, p. 366), it cannot be expected to occur in the floor of the ulcer itself. No vasodilating effect of ultraviolet radiation in granulation tissue has been documented.

Ultraviolet radiation has a bactericidal effect as well as a vasodilator effect on superficial ulcers. Two M.E.D. of cold quartz ultraviolet is effective to destroy

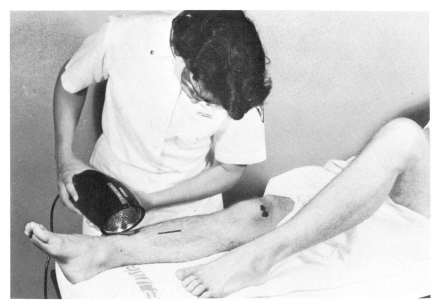

Figure 13–6 "Cold quartz" ultraviolet source being used in treatment of chronic ulcer. (Courtesy of Dr. F. J. Kottke.)

any motile forms of bacteria on the surface of the ulcer.[5] Since the bacteria in a wound are superficial rather than within the tissues, ultraviolet radiation is effective to kill the motile pathogens in the wound. Although the spores of spore-forming bacteria are resistant to ultraviolet, they have no effect until they develop into the motile form. Therefore, daily ultraviolet radiation is effective as a bactericidal agent for superficial wounds. Cold quartz ultraviolet, up to 5 M.E.D. daily by a grid source, or by orificial applicator for fistulas or undermined ulcers, is effective in causing bacteriostasis without tissue destruction. Cold quartz irradiation of more than 5 M.E.D. will delay epithelial formation. Ultraviolet irradiation greater than 10 M.E.D. may cause tissue destruction.

Other diseases of the skin for which ultraviolet therapy is used are pityriasis, atopic dermatitis, nummular eczema, and eczematoid dermatitis.

Tuberculosis. Ultraviolet irradiation may be used, although with caution, in the presence of pulmonary tuberculosis. Its role in the management of tuberculosis, however, has been more particularly directed at the extrapulmonary varieties. In more recent years, the success of chemotherapy in the treatment of tuberculosis has diminished the importance of ultraviolet therapy.

Antirachitic Effect. This is generally an incidental effect of ultraviolet therapy; it is much less expensive to supplement the diet with vitamin D.

Disinfection of Air. The use of ultraviolet radiation for this purpose in operating rooms, nurseries, schools and other areas is variable in its efficacy. There is no doubt of the bactericidal effect, particularly of the 2537 Angstrom band from the "cold quartz" mercury burner, but the application of this phenomenon is difficult.

REFERENCES

1. Blum, H. F.: Photodynamic Action and Diseases Caused by Light. American Chemistry Society Monograph Series. New York, Hafner Publishing Co., 1964.
2. Blum, H. F.: Radiation: Photophysiologic and Photopathologic Processes. In Glasser, O.: Medical Physics. Chicago, Year Book Publishers, Inc., 1944, vol. 1, pp. 1115-1157.
3. Krusen, F. H., and Elkins, E. C.: Physical Therapy: Light. In Glasser, O.: Medical Physics. Chicago, Year Book Publishers, Inc., 1944, vol. 1, pp. 1054-1068.
4. Licht, S.: Therapeutic Electricity and Ultraviolet Radiation. 2nd Ed. New Haven, Conn., Elizabeth Licht, 1967.
5. Koller, L. R.: *Ultraviolet Radiation.* John Wiley and Sons, Inc., New York, 1952.

Chapter 14

ELECTRICAL STIMULATION AND IONTOPHORESIS

by G. Keith Stillwell

ELECTRICAL STIMULATION

Physics

An electric current may be considered to be a flow of electrons. This may be a flow of free electrons, as in a solid conductor, or of electrons carried by ions and delivered at some point, as with the solution of an electrolyte in water. The force which causes the electrons to be moved is the difference in electrical potential between the point at which electrons are being injected into the system and the point at which they are being removed; this is measured in volts. The rate of delivery of the electrons is called the current flow and is measured in amperes. The opposition to the movement of electrons through a conductor is called the resistance of the conductor and is measured in ohms.

The relationship among these three factors is expressed in Ohm's law,

$$E = I R$$

in which E is the electrical potential, I is the amperage, and R is the resistance.

An electric current flowing through a solid conductor causes a magnetic field to be developed around the conductor. The strength of this field varies with the strength of the current. Conversely, changes in a magnetic field around a conductor will induce a flow of electrons in the conductor.

Currents in which the direction of flow of the electrons alternates between two poles are called alternating currents. Many complex concepts are involved in the transfer of energy by alternating currents, but these cannot be adequately considered here and are largely irrelevant as far as electrical stimulation is concerned.

Physiologic Effects

Nature of Stimulus.   Any change in the environment of an irritable tissue may be regarded as a stimulus. If the stimulus fails to elicit a response from the tissue, it is subliminal. If it elicits the maximal response from the tissue, it is said to be a maximal stimulus. Any greater stimulus is supramaximal. Because electric currents are highly effective in stimulating nerve and muscle, and can be accurately measured and finely gradated, they are more suitable than other types of stimulation in producing contraction of muscles directly or by way of nerves for diagnostic or therapeutic purposes.

The factors influencing the effectiveness of a stimulus are the magnitude of the change, the rate of the change and the duration of the altered condition. The relationship between the magnitude of the change and the duration of the change resulting from electrical stimulation is shown in Figure 14-1. Similar curves are obtained whether the strength of the stimulus is measured in volts or in milliamperes. The curve characteristic of muscle is labeled "denervation," while the curve characteristic of nerve is labeled "normal." It will be noted that, in each instance, as the duration of the stimulus decreases, the strength increases. The minimal effective duration for muscle is much longer than that for nerve.

The rate of change of the stimulus is important because of the phenomenon of accommodation. Nerve accommodates relatively well and may not be stimulated by a change of several volts if the change occurs gradually over a

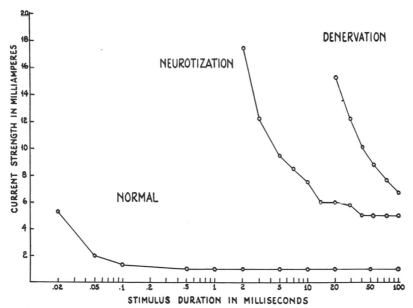

Figure 14–1   Relationship between the strength and the duration of minimal effective stimulus for denervated, neurotized and normally innervated muscle. (From Rose, D. L.: Electrodiagnostic Methods: Evaluation and Interpretation. In Krusen, F. H.: Physical Medicine and Rehabilitation for the Clinician. Philadelphia, W. B. Saunders Company, 1951, pp. 95–108.)

period of 0.2 second or so. Muscle does not accommodate nearly as well and probably loses much of what little accommodation it possesses in the atrophy of denervation.

Types of Electrical Stimulus.   Various electrical changes may be produced by available stimulators. The prototypes are shown in Figure 14–2. From the remarks made earlier about the nature of a stimulus, it follows that the effectiveness of a stimulus, although influenced by the "wave form," is not dependent entirely upon it.

Technique of Electrical Stimulation

The technique of the use of any stimulating device, if unfamiliar to the operator, should be reviewed in the operating manual for the device. Certain points are generally applicable.

1. Good contact should be maintained between the skin and the electrodes. The use of a conductive solution or jelly diminishes the resistance at this point. Sodium chloride solution, soap suds, electrode jelly and other conductive substances may be used. Whatever is employed should not in itself be irritating to the skin.

2. Usually (but not always) "active" and "indifferent" electrodes are employed (monopolar technique), the latter being larger. The density of current flow at the indifferent (larger) electrode is less, and stimulation can be selectively produced at the "active" electrode (Fig. 14–3).

3. In the stimulation of innervated muscle, the active electrode is placed over the motor point of the muscle.

4. Denervated muscle does not have a motor point. The active electrode may be placed at the point giving the best response, or two electrodes of about the same size may be placed one at each end of the muscle so that the current will pass through the muscle and stimulate all of it (bipolar or longitudinal technique).

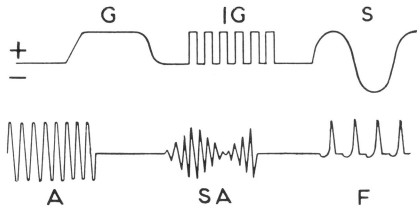

Figure 14–2   Examples of voltage changes in different forms of stimuli. G, galvanic or direct current; I G, interrupted galvanic; S, sinusoidal or alternating current; A, a more rapidly alternating form; S A, surging alternating current; F, faradic or induced current. (From Kovacs, Richard: Physical Therapy: Low-Frequency Currents. In Glasser, Otto: Medical Physics. Chicago, Year Book Publishers, Inc., 1944, vol. 1, pp. 1068–1073.)

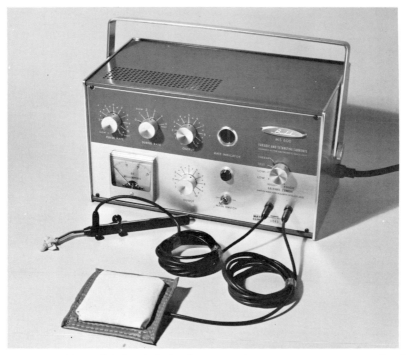

Figure 14–3 Table-model electrical stimulator capable of generating galvanic or faradic types of current. The galvanic current can also be used for ion transfer. Note the milliammeter for measurement of the flow of direct current, the small "active" electrode (with a contact switch on its handle), and the larger "indifferent" electrode pad.

5. The two electrodes should generally be placed on the same side of the body, particularly to avoid passage of the current through the thorax or the genital area.

6. With unidirectional current (direct current, galvanic current), the active electrode may be the cathode or the anode, the choice depending upon which is more effective. Following prolonged stimulation with one pole, adverse cutaneous effects may be noted from the passage of the current. Some believe it is advisable to counteract this by the subsequent passage of a current of reversed polarity for a while, or to reverse the polarity periodically during the treatment.

Clinical Uses of Electrical Stimulation

Stimulation of Denervated Muscle

PURPOSE. One purpose of stimulating denervated muscle is to retard the progression of atrophy. Since the rate of development of denervation atrophy declines exponentially with time, most of the atrophy takes place early. Therefore, steps to prevent it must be taken early if they are to be effective. Another purpose of stimulation is to diminish intrafascicular and interfascicular agglutination and sclerosis of areolar tissue. Stimulation may be of help in this respect even if begun late in the period of denervation. Stimulation is also used to improve the circulation and nutrition of the muscle. Muscular contraction is helpful in moving venous blood out of skeletal muscle and is even more important for the movement of lymph out of the muscle.

TYPE OF CURRENT.   Direct current, either square wave or nearly so, is effective. Sinusoidal alternating current is effective if it is not too high in frequency. The effective frequencies range as high as 7000 cycles per second, but the optimal frequency is in the neighborhood of 25 c.p.s. or less. The slowly increasing stimulus may be able to stimulate denervated muscle without simultaneous stimulation of nerve (or even innervated muscle) in the field.

Impulses briefer than 10 or 20 milliseconds may not be able to cause a contraction of denervated skeletal muscle except at very high intensities. Impulses of a duration of about 100 milliseconds are more satisfactory. The principal spike of a faradic current stimulus has a duration of only about 1 millisecond.

STRENGTH OF CONTRACTION.   Strong contractions should be produced. Denervated muscle may become fatigued rapidly so that only 25 to 50 strong contractions can be obtained at one session. A strong contraction against resistance may be of more benefit, since the development of tension in the muscle seems well correlated with the retardation of atrophy.

SCHEDULE OF TREATMENT.   Work on experimental animals suggests that three or four treatment sessions each day may be required to retard the progress of atrophy. This regimen is generally feasible if the patient has his own stimulator and is taught to use it by himself. A battery stimulator for home use is shown in Figure 14-4.

SUPPLEMENTAL HEAT.   It is helpful but not essential to apply heat before the stimulation. Care must be taken, of course, not to burn insensitive areas.

DURATION OF TREATMENT.   After the patient is able to produce reasonably good active contractions of the muscle, there is no value in continued stimulation.

Stimulation of Innervated Muscle.   Innervated muscle is stimulated by way of its nerve supply. The minimal effective duration of stimulus is about 0.02 millisecond if the voltage is high enough. Innervated muscle is easily stimulated by impulses as brief as 1 millisecond. This method of treatment may be helpful in producing relaxation of muscle in "spasm," for example subsequent to

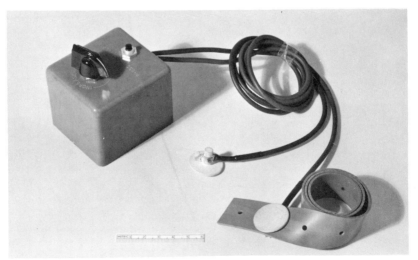

Figure 14-4   Battery stimulator suitable for use in the home. It produces galvanic current only, with no measurement of current flow.

trauma; in preventing atrophy of disuse in a muscle which the patient cannot contract well voluntarily, for example the quadriceps, after injury to the knee; in reeducation of muscles when other methods of reeducation fail; in reducing spasticity in spastic paralysis, particularly that due to injury of the spinal cord; in stimulation of the abdominal wall and diaphragm as an aid to respiration ("electrolung"); in stimulation of the diaphragm by way of the phrenic nerve as a form of artificial respiration ("electrophrenic respiration"); and in stimulation of the calf muscles in the immediate postoperative period to prevent phlebothrombosis.

IONTOPHORESIS

Iontophoresis is the process of transferring ions into the body by an electromotive force. Ions bearing a positive charge may be driven into the skin at the anode and those with a negative charge at the cathode. Positively charged ions, zinc, copper and alkaloids such as the vasodilating drugs, histamine and mecholyl, are introduced into the skin and mucous membranes from the positive pole. Skin anesthesia can be produced by iontophoresis of local anesthetic drugs using the positive pole. Negative ions such as iodine, chlorine and salicylic acid are introduced into the tissues from the negative pole. Other drugs for general metabolic or specific hormonal effects can be driven into the circulating blood by iontophoresis but most physicians employ simpler methods for administering these drugs. The greatest concentration is moved into the skin where the skin is broken, or along sweat glands and hair follicles. Ions transferred through the skin are taken up by the circulation and do not proceed through the tissues to the other electrode. As a rule ions used for medicinal purposes cannot be made to migrate far below the surface of the skin or mucous membranes.

The velocity of movement of the transferred ions is directly proportional to the voltage applied. The quantity transferred is affected by the current flow and the duration of the flow. The usual intensity of current flow is 1 to 3 milliamperes per square inch of surface of the active electrode. The apparatus should include a milliammeter so that the flow can be measured. The duration of treatment is usually 15 minutes or less. The current is turned up slowly to the desired level, maintained as long as desired, *provided that the patient is comfortable and that there are no adverse systemic effects*, and then slowly turned off again (or occasionally reversed for one minute or so).

Any direct current generator may be used for iontophoresis. The electrodes must be connected to the correctly identified positive and negative terminals of the generator. For treatment through the skin the active electrodes should be an absorptive material of sufficient thickness to hold the solution and keep moist during treatment. Gauze 1/4 inch thick, cotton or filter paper may be used. For the introduction of vasodilating drugs, blotting paper or filter paper is employed, covered by a felt pad soaked in saline beneath the metal electrode. There is no advantage in using a solution at a concentration greater than 1 per cent. The pad, saturated in solution at a comfortable temperature, is firmly applied to the area to be treated. A metal plate somewhat smaller than the pad is placed on the pad; no metal edges should touch the skin, since even a minute direct contact between the metal and the skin may lead to a chemical burn. Breaks in the skin may also concentrate ion flow and cause electrical burns.

For treatment of mucous surfaces a metal electrode, solution or packing containing the ions is placed in direct contact with the walls of the cavity and serves as the active electrode.

The dispersive electrode is a pad considerably larger than the active electrode, soaked in warm saline solution and placed in firm contact with a convenient part of the body surface. Alternatively the foot, hand or arm may be placed in saline bath to provide a dispersive electrode of large area.

After treatment the pads should be thoroughly cleaned and rinsed in order to remove secondary chemical products near the metal plate.

The technique has the advantage of concentrating a relatively large amount of a drug in a local area of the skin when this is desired. The drug will not be delivered locally to structures deeper than the skin but may be taken up by the circulation.

Disadvantages include the difficulty of estimating the dosage of the drug and, particularly, of estimating how much of the drug may act systemically. Severe reactions may occur in allergic persons, for example when histamine is administered by iontophoresis.

The method has been of interest to many investigators as a research tool. Its therapeutic value is limited. It has been employed for a multitude of conditions in the past but with a great paucity of evidence to establish its value. Anyone interested in using the method is referred to an excellent critical review of the matter by Harris[1] which also provides more detailed information on technique.[1]

REFERENCES

1. Harris, R.: Iontophoresis. In Licht, S.: Therapeutic Electricity and Ultraviolet Radiation. 2nd Ed. New Haven, Conn., Elizabeth Licht, 1967, pp. 146–168.
2. Licht, S.: Therapeutic Electricity and Ultraviolet Radiation. 2nd Ed. New Haven, Conn., Elizabeth Licht, 1967.

Chapter 15

MASSAGE

by Miland E. Knapp

Definition. Massage is a term used to signify a group of systematic and scientific manipulations of body tissues which are best performed with the hands "for the purpose of affecting the nervous and muscular system and the general circulation."

HISTORY

Massage is probably the oldest of all remedies since it is instinctive, not only in man but in the lower animals as well. The oldest written record of massage was made 3000 years ago by the Chinese. The ancient Hindus, Persians and Egyptians used manipulation in some form and some of the movements of massage for rheumatic ailments. The Greeks recognized gymnastics as an institution which was an auxiliary to the development of the people both socially and politically. Hippocrates wrote important papers on massage, for instance, about the use of friction after sprains and dislocations and about kneading in case of constipation. About two centuries ago the Chinese books on massage were translated into French, which accounts for the French terminology so common in massage texts. At the beginning of the nineteenth century Peter Henry Ling, a fencing master of Stockholm, Sweden, introduced a system of movement which he had not originated but had systematized. It consists of, first, massage (manipulation of the soft tissues) and, second, medical gymnastics (exercise of the joints). During the last century, Lucas-Championnière championed treatment of fractures by mobilization including massage and exercise. And more recently, during the years 1917 to 1940, James B. Mennell of England, systematized massage movements and applied them to the treatment of a great many conditions.

PHYSIOLOGIC EFFECTS OF MASSAGE

Unfortunately, most of the teaching of massage in the past has been done by lay persons who did not understand physiology in the modern sense so that many statements made in massage texts are obviously untrue insofar as physiologic effects of massage are concerned. The effects may be classified as reflex and mechanical.

Reflex Effects. Reflex effects are produced in the skin by stimulation of the peripheral receptors, which then transmit impulses through the spinal cord to the brain and produce sensations of pleasure or relaxation. Peripherally these impulses cause relaxation of muscles and dilatation or constriction of arterioles. Sedation is one of the very important physiologic effects of massage. It is obtained when the massage is given in a monotonously repetitive manner without sharp variations in pressure or irritating changes in the method of application. These pleasant effects result in relaxation of muscle as well as reduction of mental tension.

Mechanical Effects. The mechanical effects consist of (1) measures that assist return flow circulation of blood and lymph because the massage is given with the greatest force in the centripetal direction, and (2) measures that produce intramuscular motion. They may be effective in stretching adhesions between muscle fibers and mobilizing accumulations of fluid.

Massage does *not* develop muscle strength and should *not* be used as a substitute for active exercise.

TECHNIQUE

Proficiency in the performance of massage movements is not easily acquired. It requires long and diligent practice. Massage is an art rather than a science. One individual may learn to administer acceptable massage quickly and after only a minimum of practice while another may never give acceptable massage even after many months of assiduous effort. Natural ability is an important factor. However, as with other arts, improvement will be gained by practice.

I am not in favor of trying to teach the patient or his family to give massage at home except under unusual circumstances because this kind of training is usually inadequate and the resulting treatment may produce harmful effects as easily as helpful results.

Description of technique is difficult but certain principles may be stated:

1. The patient must be relaxed and comfortable. Clothing should not be tight, especially proximal to the area to be treated. Clothing should be removed from the area to be treated but the patient should not be uncovered unnecessarily to avoid embarrassment and needless cooling.

2. The therapist should also be relaxed and comfortable and should stand in a position such that the entire stroke can be performed without change of stance or undue movement.

3. Skill is required rather than strength. Pain and apprehension must not be produced if deep effects are desired. A relaxed muscle has the physical properties of a liquid enclosed in a membrane, and pressure exerted on any portion of it will be transmitted equally in all directions. Pressure is thus transmitted to the deeper muscles. On the other hand, a tense, contracted muscle has the properties of a solid and does not transmit the force evenly.

4. A lubricating oil, powder or cream facilitates good technique. Heavy mineral oil is suitable.

Stroking (Effleurage). Stroking massage is performed by running the hand lightly over the surface of the skin. The force of the stroke starts distally and progresses proximally to assist return flow circulation. The hands may be lifted off the part at the end of the stroke and returned to the point of beginning if the motion is rhythmic and the contact and release are performed gently, without abruptness. It is probably better, however, to return to the point of beginning with the hands in contact with the skin but producing little or no actual pressure.

Stroking may be superficial or deep. In superficial stroking the direction of the force is not important since the pressure is so light that mechanical effects are not produced. In deep stroking the direction of force is important because the usual major objective is to assist return flow circulation. Therefore, the force of the stroke definitely should be centripetal.

Compression (Pétrissage). Compression includes kneading, squeezing and friction. Kneading may be described as a motion in which the soft tissues are picked up between the fingers and manipulated in an alternating fashion so that there is motion within the muscle itself. It does not proceed in any particular direction but is used to mobilize the tissue fluids and create intramuscular motion to stretch adhesions. Squeezing is performed with larger portions of the muscle, squeezing the part either between the two hands or between the hand and a solid object such as the table or bone. Friction is a circular motion performed by placing a small part of the hand on the area. This portion of the hand is usually the thumb, the heel of the hand or the finger tips. The movement is in circular loops and is done fairly rapidly with increasing pressure.

Percussion (Tapôtement). Percussion movements are alternating movements performed to produce stimulation. Hacking is usually done with the outer border of the hand or the relaxed fingers, bouncing the hands alternately off the part to be treated. It may also be used in a kind of whipping motion using the fingers as the flexible portion of the whip. Clapping is done with the palms of the hand in a similar manner. If the hands are cupped the deeper sound produced may be of some psychologic benefit. Beating is performed with the clenched fist by a similar technique. The therapist produces vibration by placing his finger tips in contact with the skin and shaking his entire arm. This transmits a trembling movement to the patient. The therapeutic value of this type of movement is questionable although it is pleasant when performed expertly.

The movements of massage are not done in sequence but are intermingled, using varying techniques for different purposes. The compression techniques are used to mobilize tissue deposits and to stretch adhesions. They may be followed by stroking massage to remove the deposits or edema fluid. Friction is used to treat very limited areas, particularly nodules such as fibrositic nodules, and this again is followed by stroking massage. The percussion movements are ordinarily used at the end of the treatment. It is my opinion that they are used primarily for psychologic effects rather than for any real physical benefit.

Numerous mechanical devices have been invented and manufactured for the application of massage movements. Rollers of various types operated manually or by electric motors have tried to simulate kneading and stroking types of massage. Perhaps the most common machines are those that produce vibration. They are attached to the hand or incorporated in pads of various kinds and on tables. While they may produce pleasurable effects, it is generally conceded that they are not therapeutically effective.

INDICATIONS

Massage is useful in any condition in which relief of pain, reduction of swelling or mobilization of contracted tissues is desired. Probably its greatest single indication is to overcome the swelling and induration which frequently follow trauma (see Chapter 26). Fractures, dislocations, joint injuries, sprains, strains, bruises, and tendon and nerve injuries may be benefited by massage at certain stages of recovery. Arthritis, periarthritis, bursitis, neuritis, fibrositis, low back pain and paralytic conditions such as hemiplegia, paraplegia, quadriplegia, cerebral palsy and multiple sclerosis may present problems that can be relieved by massage.

Psychoneurotic patients and occasionally even patients with psychoses may be helped by massage. However, such treatment should be prescribed only after careful consideration of its psychologic effects because harmful psychologic trends may be intensified by physical treatment.

Abdominal massage has been advocated and described in the past but is not used to any great extent at the present time. It is also ineffective for weight reduction.

Massage is not a substitute for exercise. It does not increase muscle strength. Strength develops in muscles contracting actively, preferably against resistance.

A masseur once told me he was giving an alcoholic patient massage equivalent to a three mile hike. Perhaps he was, but the hike was being performed by the masseur, on his hands. The patient was getting rest in bed.

CONTRAINDICATIONS

The greatest contraindications to massage are: infections, because of the likelihood of spreading the infection through the tissues and breaking down barriers to the spread of infection; malignancies, because tumor tissues similarly may be spread beyond confined limits and promote metastases or extension of the malignancy; and skin diseases (which might be communicated to the masseur), when irritation is contraindicated or when lesions might be spread by contact. Massage should be given with caution in debilitated individuals and in areas where the skin has been damaged by burns or where it is thin for other reasons. In thrombophlebitis massage may be dangerous because thrombi may be broken into emboli.

REFERENCES

1. Beard, G., and Wood, E. C.: Massage: Principles and Techniques. Philadelphia, W. B. Saunders Co., 1964.
2. Krusen, F. H.: Physical Medicine. Philadelphia, W. B. Saunders Co., 1941.
3. Mennell, J. B.: Physical Treatment by Movement, Manipulation and Massage. 4th Ed. Philadelphia, The Blakiston Co., 1940.
4. Tidy, N. M.: Massage and Remedial Exercises in Medical and Surgical Conditions. 3rd Ed. Baltimore, William Wood and Co., 1937.

Chapter 16

THERAPEUTIC EXERCISE

by Frederic J. Kottke

Therapeutic exercise may be defined as the prescription of bodily movement to correct an impairment, improve musculoskeletal function or maintain a state of well-being. Therapeutic exercise may vary from highly selected activities restricted to specific muscles or parts of the body, to general and vigorous activities used to restore a convalescing patient to the peak of physical condition. The prescription for therapeutic exercise will vary with the purpose for which it is used. This, in turn, is directly dependent upon the condition of the patient. An adequate medical evaluation is essential before therapeutic exercise is prescribed. Therapeutic exercise prescribed without competent medical evaluation and supervision may be not only inadequate but actually detrimental to the patient.

Knowledge of the biophysical and physiologic aspects of kinesiology and the basic principles of therapeutic exercise is needed by the physician who plans to prescribe and supervise a program of therapeutic exercise for his patient. Therapeutic exercises have local and general effects on the physiology of the body. These responses occur in the muscular, skeletal, nervous, circulatory and endocrine systems in particular. Metabolism may be altered significantly. The prescription of an exercise to produce a desired response is just as specific as, and often more involved than, the prescription of a pharmaceutical compound. An adequate program of therapeutic exercise requires that the prescription be modified as the condition of the patient changes.

This chapter contains the principles of therapeutic exercise and information concerning the general types of exercises used in medical practice. Because the exercise program for each patient is developed according to his needs on the basis of the medical evaluation of his disability, no attempt is being made here to provide a "cookbook" of exercises since for any part of the body,

385

exercises may be designed in a number of ways depending upon the desired goal and the equipment at hand.

EXERCISES TO INCREASE OR MAINTAIN MOBILITY OF JOINTS AND SOFT TISSUES

Physiology of Fibrous Connective Tissue

There is a continual turnover of the components of connective tissue by breakdown and replacement and by reorganization of the attachments of the various components. The connective tissue of the body provides the connection between all cells and around and between all organs. The fibers are made up of reticulin and collagen, which do not appear to be essentially different in their ultramicroscopic structure, elastic fibers, which differ from collagen in their physical and chemical characteristics as well as their metabolic response, and fibrin, which is a temporary connective tissue element extremely important in the process of repair. In addition, there is the amorphous ground substance which is structureless but which plays an important role in binding the structural elements together. It appears that the attachments between fibers produced by the ground substance can shift as the result of prolonged tension or can develop as the result of prolonged contact.

Although metabolic studies have not clearly defined the rate at which collagen is removed, altered or replaced under ordinary circumstances, there is considerable information regarding the rapid response of fibrous connective tissue in areas where trauma has occurred. Newly formed collagen fibrils are abundant around proliferating fibroblasts within five days.[1, 2] Recent studies indicate that in normal connective tissue, a small percentage of collagen is turned over rapidly while the remainder of the collagen fibers show a very slow rate of metabolic change.[3]

The collagen fibril is an aggregation of tropocollagen rods in staggered array, forming the characteristic 640 Å bands. The most soluble collagen is that most recently formed. Chemical bonding between parallel tropocollagen molecules leads to increasing insolubility and increased tensile strength. However, the process may be reversible and soluble collagen may result from the breakdown of insoluble collagen as well as from the synthesis of collagen.

Connective tissue is usually described in relation to the arrangement of the fibrous elements.

Organized Connective Tissue.   Tendons and ligaments are made up of organized connective tissue composed of dense bundles of coarse collagen between which columns of fibrocytes are interspersed. Collagen fibers are arranged linearly in the long axis of the tendon or ligament and present a uniform appearance (Fig. 16-1). More fibrocytes are present in columnar arrangement in tendons than in ligaments. These fibrocytes are stellate with processes extending between the bundles of collagen fibers. It appears that this organization is a response to the tension produced by muscular contraction.

TENDON HEALING.   Buck[1] sectioned the Achilles tendon of the rat and allowed it to retract without suturing (Fig. 16-2). A fibrin coagulum was laid down in the defect between the cut ends of the tendon, oriented longitudinally with the tendon. Fibroblasts began to grow into the coagulum from the periphery within three days, and reticulin fibers and collagen fibers were laid down

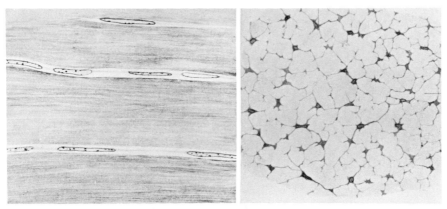

Figure 16–1 Drawing of the histology of a tendon in longitudinal and cross section to show the distribution of fibrocytes between the bundles of collagen fibers. (From Maximow and Bloom.)

within four days. The collagen fibers were oriented parallel to the fibrin threads in the long axis of the tendon. Within two weeks, the entire length of the tendon up to the muscular insertion was invaded by fibroblasts. The reaction as indicated by proliferation of collagen and the persistance of fibroblasts throughout the tendon lasted for four months.

When the muscle was denervated at the time the tendon was cut, the fibrin did not organize in a uniform longitudinal pattern and the collagen fibers, likewise, developed in a random orientation rather than in parallel bundles.

It appears that the regular pattern of fibers produced in the healing

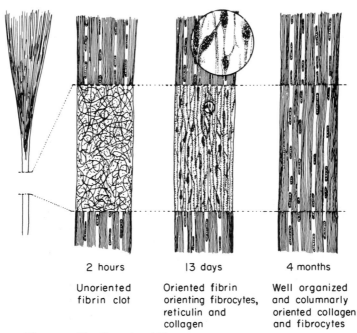

2 hours

13 days

4 months

Unoriented
fibrin clot

Oriented fibrin
orienting fibrocytes,
reticulin and
collagen

Well organized
and columnarly
oriented collagen
and fibrocytes

Figure 16–2 Diagram of healing of Achilles tendon of rat when cut and not sutured. (From data of Buck.[1])

tendon was due to the exertion of tension on the fibrin coagulum to produce a linear pattern and that collagen was organized on this matrix.

ADHESION FORMATION.   The increasing strength of new connective tissue is correlated with the formation and maturation of collagen fibers.[4] After injury collagen fibrils can be detected by using the electron microscope as early as the second day, by biochemical means on the third day, and by use of the light microscope only a day or two later, when molecular accretion has occurred. Within four to five days, collagenous adhesions begin to form between a sutured tendon and the surrounding structures. Watson-Jones[5] observed collagen fibers at fracture sites within five days. Gentle passive or active motion of the sutured tendon begun the day after surgery will prevent adhesions to surrounding structures without producing significant tension on the suture. Motion may be reestablished in this manner before inflammation has weakened the tendon. By two weeks after suture, the inflammatory reaction within a tendon has greatly reduced its tensile strength. This inflammatory reaction lasts for at least four months. Early gentle motion preserves the gliding motion of the tendon without force and shortens the functional recovery time, i.e., the time required for the tendon to be healed and free to move.

Loose Connective Tissue.   Loose or areolar connective tissue forms between organs and other structures, such as joint capsules, fascia, intermuscular layers and subcutaneous tissue, where movement occurs repeatedly. It will allow movement through limited distances, adapt by shortening and fixation if there is no motion, or elongate slowly under prolonged tension.

Histologically, networks of collagen and reticular fibers run in all directions without a regular pattern. These fibers form a loose mesh which allows flexibility for movement. When these fibers are laid down or replaced, their length and mobility between attachments depend upon the motion of the part during the period of formation.

Thousands of reticulin fibers are attached over the entire external surface of the sarcolemma of each muscle fiber so that resistance to motion is provided not only through the heavy fibrous attachments at the ends of each muscle fiber but also through the reticular fibers to the surrounding connective tissue. The proportionate force of the muscular contraction transmitted through these reticular fibers is not known, but in conditions of fibrosis it is increased significantly.

When a part is immobilized, the collagenous and reticular networks become contracted and the distance between attachments in the network is shortened so that the tissue becomes dense and hard and loses the suppleness of normal areolar tissue.

Dense Connective Tissue.   In areas where motion does not occur, such as in fascial planes and the capsules of muscles or organs, collagen is laid down as dense meshworks, sheets or bands. This type of connective tissue is also laid down in scars. If motion is maintained during healing of a wound, connective tissue of the areolar type develops. If the wound is immobilized, dense contracted scar forms. In areas immobilized by edema dense connective tissue will also develop. It is imperative if motion is to be maintained in a part that the motion be initiated early and carried on during the period of healing so that areolar rather than dense collagen networks form. Except in the case of necessary immobilization of a fracture or of an open draining wound, gentle passive or active assistive motion under proper supervision should be begun immediately after surgery or trauma to insure that supple areolar connective tissue rather than dense scar develops in sites in which motion should occur.

Histologic evidence of fibrosis may occur in as short time as four days.[1, 6] Gross evidence of restriction of motion begins to occur in approximately four days and develops progressively from that time. Immobilization of a normal joint for four weeks results in diminution or loss of motion because of formation of dense connective tissue. Immobilization of an injured joint for two weeks results in connective fiber fusion and loss of motion at that joint.

The following indicates the effect of limitation of motion on development of restrictive connective tissue after injury to the shoulder.[7] If the shoulder is not immobilized, recovery occurs in 18 days. If the shoulder is immobilized 7 day, recovery occurs in 52 days. If the shoulder is immobilized 14 days recovery occurs in 121 days. If the shoulder is immobilized 21 days, recovery occurs in 300 days.

Factors promoting the formation of dense fibrosis are immobilization, edema, trauma and impaired circulation. *Immobilization* allows deposition of collagen and reticulin as a dense network instead of a loose areolar network. *Edema* increases the tendency to fibrosis. Whether this is due to increased tissue fluid protein, impaired metabolism, increased metabolites or other causes is not known. Probably all of these factors are important in the formation of both the edema and the fibrosis. *Trauma* causes capillary damage and increases the loss of protein into the tissue. Fibrinogen precipitates as a fibrin meshwork in the tissue spaces forming a matrix on which collagen fibers are laid down. *Impaired circulation* appears to augment the rate of development of fibrosis.

The Normal Maintenance of Mobility

Motion in joints and soft tissues is maintained by the normal movement of the parts of the body, including joint capsules, muscles, subcutaneous tissue and ligaments, through full range of motion many times each day. In the course of the day, these movements traverse the full range of motion. If for any reason the range is restricted, tightness develops and restricts the arc of motion.

It is easier to prevent tightness by frequently repeated activity than to correct it after it has developed.

Limitation of the range of motion is of the greatest importance when it interferes with habitual postures or activities. (For the normal range of motion of various joints see pages 45 to 56 in Chapter 2.

Tightness that prevents normal standing without muscular support is disabling. In the normal relaxed standing posture, extension of the back, the hip and the knee is maintained by positioning the center of gravity of the body above these joints so that the weight of the body holds the joints extended against restricting ligaments and the extensor muscles are relaxed. Muscular activity is used for balance or motion rather than to support the weight of the body. Electromyographic studies of patients during normal quiet standing reveal no continuously active contraction of the muscles in the back, the extensors of the hip or the extensors of the knee.[8] Maintenance of balance is provided mainly by activity of the soleus muscles and intermittent counterbalancing activity of the anterior tibial muscles. During relaxed standing, the center of gravity of the head, arms and trunk falls slightly posterior (0.5 to 1.0 cm.) to the center of motion of the acetabulum, far anterior (3 to 5 cm.) to the

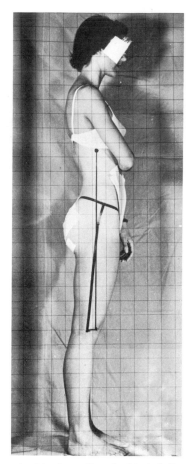

Figure 16–3   During normal relaxed standing the hip is fully extended. The center of gravity falls just posterior to the center of the acetabulum, well in front of the knee and through the tarsal arch. The longitudinal and transverse axes of the pelvis and the longitudinal axis of the femur are marked. The subject is standing behind a two-inch grid. (From Kottke and Kubicek.[9])

center of motion of the knee and through the center of the tarsal arch approximately midway between the points of contact of the heel and heads of the metatarsals[9] (Fig. 16-3).

During relaxed standing, the hip and the knee are fully extended. There is no free extension of the hip or knee beyond this standing position. Further extension is possible only to the extent that connective tissues can be stretched.[10]

Methods purporting to measure hyperextension of the hip beyond the standing position are erroneous because of inaccurate evaluation of the orientation of the innominate bone.

If tightness prevents complete extension of these weight bearing joints, relaxed standing cannot occur. When the joints are not fully extended, muscles must support a part of the weight of the body during quiet standing. Therefore, the patient fatigues more rapidly and has less endurance for standing or ambulatory activity than does a person with normal mobility. The contraction of muscles to hold the body erect places more compressive stress on the joint surfaces resulting in more rapid wear and more likelihood of joint pain.

Mechanics of Ambulation

HIP.   During relaxed standing the hip is fully extended, forming an angle of 160 to 175 degrees between the long axis of the pelvis and the femur[10] (Fig. 16-4). Maximal forced extension may add approximately 5 degrees to this angle. Therefore, it should be remembered that no free range of extension of the hip can occur beyond the position assumed during normal standing. The hyperextension which appears to occur is due to forward rotation of the pelvis with simultaneous extension of the lumbar spine and flexion of the opposite hip.

The act of walking exerts repeated stretch on the ligaments, fascia, muscles and connective tissue across the flexor aspect of the hip. Unless a person is standing and walking frequently each day, the normal reaction of fibrous connective tissue to shorten and fuse together results in a progressive limitation of extension. As extension of the hip becomes more limited, the extension of the lumbar trunk usually increases in a compensatory manner. Because of this compensatory extension in the trunk, the limitation of motion of the hip may develop insidiously until suddenly the patient is observed to stand and walk

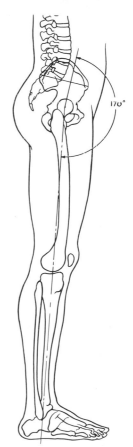

Figure 16–4   Diagram of the relationships of the lumbar spine, pelvis and lower extremity in normal relaxed stance. The transverse axis of the pelvis is defined by a line drawn between the anterior and the posterior superior iliac spines. The longitudinal axis of the pelvis is a perpendicular to this line dropped through the center of the acetabulum. The longitudinal axis of the femur is defined by a line from the center of the head of the femur to the center of weight-bearing at the knee. The pelvifemoral angle is formed by the longitudinal axes of the pelvis and the femur. (From Kottke and Kubicek.)

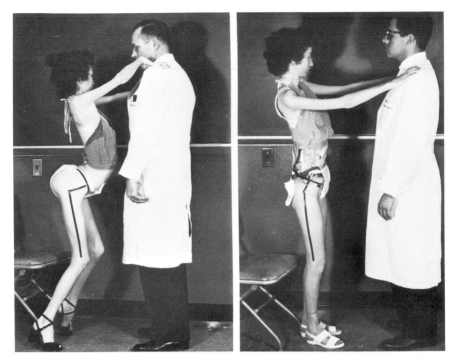

Figure 16–5 A patient with severe contractures of the hip flexors secondary to muscular dystrophy. Pelvifemoral angles have been marked as defined in Figure 16–4. Lumbar extension partially compensates for fixed hip flexion. Release of the contracted connective tissues and prolonged stretching increased the extension of the hips from 95° to 150° and made it possible for the patient to balance on her lower extremities again.

with an excessive lumbar lordosis or he loses the ability to stand (Fig. 16-5). Compensatory lordosis does not exceed the range of extension of the lumbar spine (Fig. 16–6). In children, who normally have lumbar extension of 80 to 90 degrees, compensatory lordosis may be that great. The range of lumbar extension is decreased in adulthood, and adults who develop flexion contractures of the hips do not develop as marked compensatory lumbar lordosis as is seen in children.

Habitual sitting makes flexion contractures of the hips likely unless they are prevented by appropriate stretching exercises. The difficulty in visualizing the change in position of the short innominate bone buried beneath thick soft tissues makes it possible for contractures of the flexors of the hips to develop to a severe degree before they are recognized.

During walking, in addition to full extension of the ipsilateral hip, the pelvis is tilted anteriorly and the lumbar spine is extended in order to bring the leg into the trailing position (Fig. 16-7). If the lumbar spine cannot extend enough to compensate for the anterior tilting of the pelvis, the center of gravity of the torso is shifted forward with the tilt of the pelvis and greater muscular work is required to support the weight of the body. The farther the center of gravity of the head, arms and trunk is ahead of the acetabulum, the greater the muscular work required to support the torso.

Since the center of gravity falls ahead of the acetabulum during walking, weight can be borne on the trailing leg only if the extensor muscles of the hip are contracted. If the hip extensors are weak, the trailing leg may not be able to support the weight of the body. The amount of muscular strength needed to

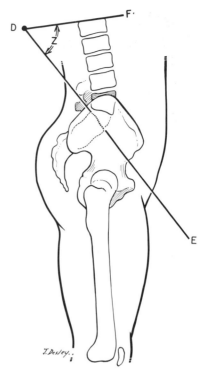

Figure 16–6 Lumbar lordosis is measured as the angle between the plane of the superior surface of the first sacral segment and the plane of the superior surface of the first lumbar vertebra.

DE = PLANE OF SUPERIOR SURFACE OF S_1.
DF = PLANE OF SUPERIOR SURFACE OF L_1.
Z   = ANGLE OF LUMBAR LORDOSIS.

support the body on the trailing leg may be lessened by several compensatory mechanisms. The stride may be shortened. The lumbar spine may be extended further to keep the center of gravity over the acetabulum. The knee may be flexed to allow the foot to trail farther behind the pelvis at the expense of a stronger contraction of the quadriceps femoris.

When there is a flexion contracture of the hip, one or more of the compensatory mechanisms must be utilized to allow stable walking. If lumbar extension is limited and the quadriceps femoris or hip extensors or both are weak, the hip becomes unstable in the trailing position. As the weight of the body moves ahead of the acetabulum, the knee flexes and collapses because the femur cannot extend further at the hip. Patients with a flexion contracture of the hip often can stand successfully when the leg on the side of the contracture is forward or in a mid-position but are unable to maintain the knee extended when the leg is trailing during walking (Fig. 16-8). Consequently, the attention is directed to the knee and the conclusion may be drawn that the major problem is weakness of the quadriceps femoris or abnormality of the knee when, in fact, the primary problem is the flexion contracture of the hip.

When a flexion contracture develops at the hip, the iliotibial band becomes progressively tighter, producing a flexion, abduction, external rotation deformity (Fig. 16-9). This progressive contracture may produce a pelvic obliquity and a secondary scoliosis.

When a patient lies on a flat, hard surface, extension of the hip is not as great as when he stands erect. The average extension when a patient is lying

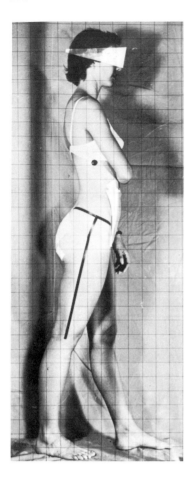

Figure 16–7 During walking, as the leg trails, the pelvis is tilted forward and the center of gravity of the head, arms and trunk falls in front of the acetabulum. (From Kottke and Kubicek.[9])

prone or supine on a hard surface is 155 degrees, (Fig. 16-10), while the average extension during relaxed standing is 170 degrees. The extension of the hip when the patient is lying in bed varies from 135 to 150 degrees. The greater extension when standing is due to the greater extensor torque created by the weight of the torso centered slightly posterior to the hip joint. Patients who must remain in bed, even though they are positioned properly, will develop progressive hip flexion contractures unless they receive daily stretching of the hip flexors (Fig. 16-11).

KNEE. Tightness causing flexion of the knees develops in the hamstring and gastrocnemius muscles and the posterior capsule of the joint if the knees are not stretched to full extension by standing and walking each day. When a patient has a paretic or painful disability and habitually sits or lies with the knees flexed, contractures develop rapidly with progressive limitation of extension of the knees. For arthritis patients or patients with neurologic diseases, the placing of pillows under the knees results in the rapid development of contractures of the knees. The compressive force which must be exerted on the flexed knee during walking is considerably greater than the force exerted when the knee is extended and, consequently, patients with arthritis in the knees have

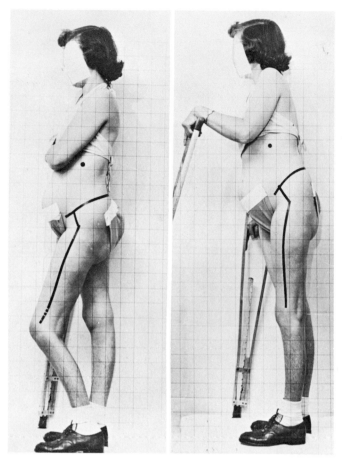

Figure 16–8   The combination of tightness of the flexor structures of the hip and weakness of the extensor muscles of the hip produces instability of both the hip and knee. During relaxed standing the left thigh is flexed forward because tightness of the flexor ligaments and fascia prevents further extension of the left hip. The center of gravity is over the pelvis but all weight is borne on the right lower extremity. If the left knee is forced into extension, the fixed flexion contracture of the left hip causes the pelvis to tilt forward and the center of gravity of the body is shifted ahead of the acetabulum. Since the extensor muscles of the hip are weak, the hip will collapse if anterior support is not provided. Attempts to center the weight of the body behind the acetabulum so that the hip becomes stable result in flexion of the knee because of the limitation of extension of the hip. Consequently either the hip or the knee is always in a position of instability. (From Kottke and Kubicek.[9])

far less tolerance for standing and walking when there are flexion contractures than when the knees can extend fully (Fig. 16–12).

ANKLE.   When a patient lies in bed without the support of a footboard or sits with the feet plantar-flexed much of the time, progressive tightness develops in the muscles of the calf and may become great enough so that the sole of the foot cannot assume a position perpendicular to the long axis of the tibia. Thus the patient cannot bear weight on the heel when standing. Even before this degree of tightness has been reached, tightness in the gastrocnemius increases stress on the longitudinal arch of the foot and the heads of the metatarsal bones when the patient walks. For patients who are chronically ill

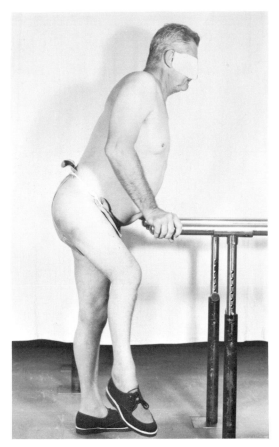

Figure 16–9 Typical postural deformity of flexion, abduction and external rotation of the hip due to paresis and flexion contractures of the hip.

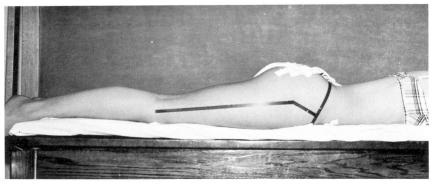

Figure 16–10 Normal hip extension when lying prone or supine on a flat surface is 10 to 20 degrees less than when standing.

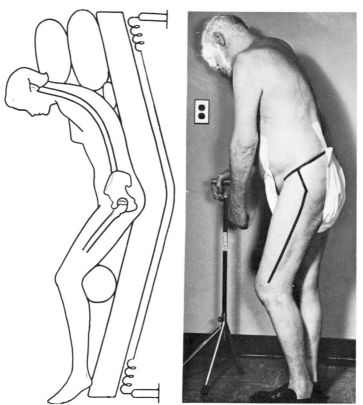

Figure 16–11 The prolonged bedfast position without maintenance of the normal range of motion results in a kyphosis of the spine and flexion contractures of the hips, knees and ankles.

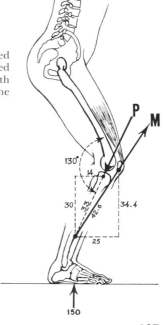

Figure 16–12 The compressive force, P, exerted on the flexed knee is a combination of the weight of the body and tension exerted by the quadriceps, M. If a patient weighing 150 pounds walks with the knee extended to 130°, the calculated compressive force on the knee is:

$$\Sigma F_x = 0$$

$$P \cdot \frac{14}{33} \, M \cdot \frac{25}{42.6} = 0$$

$$P = 1.38M$$

$$\Sigma F_y = 0$$

$$150 + P \cdot \frac{30}{33} - M \cdot \frac{34.4}{42.6} = 0$$

$$150 + \frac{30}{33} \cdot 1.38M - \frac{34.4}{42.6} \, M = 0$$

$$M = 342 \text{ lb.}$$

$$P = 472 \text{ lb.}$$

with painful or paretic disease, tightness in the triceps surae is accentuated by lack of a footboard on the bed, lack of foot support when sitting, and lying prone with the feet plantar-flexed.

Mobility Exercises to Maintain the Range of Motion

Twice daily all joints should be carried through the full range of motion three times. (See the normal ranges of motion on pages 00 to 00 in Chapter 2.) The patient should perform mobility exercises actively after he has been taught the proper procedures. Exercises must be carried on with assistance to the patient if he is weak or has pain.

The greater the inflammation and pain, the more gentle the exercise must be. For cases of acute rheumatoid arthritis, passive motion should be carried out with the patient completely relaxed. Joint inflammation requires more gentle motion than does muscular tightness. The therapist, nurse or member of the family should gently move the part through the full range of free motion but not force motion or cause pain. The joint must be moved very slowly and gently. For patients with acute joint involvement it is highly desirable to have a skilled therapist carry out the passive motions. As the patient improves the range can be increased slowly with gradual progression to active assistive exercise and then to active exercise. Improper exercise or over-exercise may impede rather than help recovery in the acute stage. If motion is not maintained in the presence of inflammation, contractures occur rapidly and may become irreversible.

The therapists, nurses or family should be taught any stretching procedures that are desired. Repeated examinations and supervision of the procedures are essential to assure that the proper motions are obtained. The difference between properly supervised and unsupervised exercise is usually the difference between adequate and inadequate care.

Stretching to Increase Range of Motion

A tight muscle can be stretched vigorously unless there is inflammation, when the stretching must be much more mild. For conditions such as poliomyelitis or Guillain-Barré syndrome, stretching should be past the point of pain, but there should be no residual pain when the stretching is discontinued. When performing manual stretching, hold momentarily at the point of maximal stretch. This type of stretching should be done by a trained therapist. The therapist must use caution in cases of prolonged disuse, paralysis or anesthesia, because osteoporosis may have occurred and vigorous stretching may cause fractures. In the presence of paralysis or hypesthesia, overstretching commonly occurs, causing bleeding into the disrupted connective tissue and subsequent ectopic calcification and ossification. In quadriplegic patients this is seen most frequently in the flexor muscles of the hips and the elbows.

Stretching of tight joints must be less vigorous than stretching of muscles. The motion should be slow and gentle with the patient completely relaxed, and it should stop short of the point which produces pain in the joint, although the patient may experience discomfort from stretch of the soft tissues. Inflamed joints tolerate vigorous stretching less well than joints which are not acutely inflamed. Edematous tissue is more likely to be torn than normal tissue, resulting in residual pain, swelling and soreness. Inflammation in any joint may reduce the tensile strength of the capsule and collateral ligaments to as little as 50 per cent of the normal tensile strength.[11]

Certain principles apply to all techniques of stretching. The body segments on each side of the joint to be stretched must be properly stabilized so that the maneuver is under complete control. The force must be applied in the precise direction that produces tension in the appropriate connective tissues. Prolonged moderate stretching is more effective than momentary vigorous stretching; connective tissue shows the plastic property of "creeping" in response to prolonged tension, although it will resist a much greater momentary force.

Stretching must be held within the pain tolerance of the patient; during brief manual stretching there may be pain when the stretch is applied, with relief of pain as soon as stretch ceases; prolonged stretching should remain within the patient's pain threshold to avoid tearing of blood vessels. Stretching should be repeated in less time than is required for connective tissue to "set" in a shortened position, daily or oftener. Inflammation indicates decreased tensile strength of connective tissue, which must be stretched cautiously. Special procedures are used for prolonged stretching of joints that do not respond well to a manual stretch (Fig. 16-13).

Hip Flexors. The patient, lying prone, is strapped snugly to a padded plinth by a strap run through C-clamps on either side of the hips and across the ischial tuberosities. A sling under the distal end of the thigh is attached by a rope through overhead pulleys to a weight which provides a constant tension. A stretching weight of 30 to 50 pounds ia added to the weight necessary to counterbalance the lower extremity. Only one hip is stretched at a time because it is not possible to immobilize the pelvis adequately to stretch both hip flexors

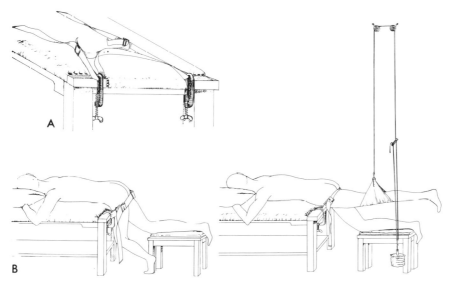

Figure 16–13 Counterbalanced stretching of the hip flexors. a. Two C-clamps fastened to the end of a padded table at hip width provide attachment for a double-ended stretching strap. b. The pelvis is immobilized by a strap fastened over the ischial tuberosities while the hips are flexed. A sling under the distal end of the thigh is attached by rope and overhead pulley to counterbalanced weights, which exert a continuous force on the hip flexors. Thirty to 50 pounds plus the weight counterbalancing the lower extremity are applied for 20 minutes.

simultaneously. The contralateral hip and knee are flexed and the leg is supported on the seat of a chair or cushion of appropriate height. This stretch is maintained for 20 minutes each day.

Knee Flexors. Contractures of the knees can be stretched by placing the patient prone on a firm surface with a pad under the knee and the leg extending unsupported. A 5 to 15 pound sandbag or weight is placed across the heel for 20 minutes (Fig. 16-14).

Alternatively, the patient sits with the knee extended, the heel supported at seat level, and the thigh and leg unsupported, and a sandbag weighing 10 to 15 pounds is placed across the knee for 20 minutes.

Triceps Surae. The patient sits on an Elgin table or other apparatus to which an exercise boot with a toe extension may be attached. The foot is strapped to the exercise boot and 10 to 30 pounds of tension is exerted at the end of the toe extension bar for 20 minutes (Fig. 16-15).

Alternatively, to dorsiflex the ankle, the patient stands at arm's length from a wall with the feet on a wedgeboard that elevates the front of the foot 20 degrees above the horizontal. He leans forward against the wall for one to five minutes three to five times each day. This exercise is the most convenient to do at home. To be effective, the knees must be kept extended and the heels kept in contact with the floor. The same stretch may be obtained by placing the patient on a tilt table (Fig. 16-16).

Elbows. Only active motion is used for mobilizing the elbow because stretch applied through the long lever of the forearm to the relatively weak ginglymus joint results in overstretching and tearing of connective tissue, which increases the contracture rather than relieving it. It has been reported that mild, prolonged spring tension, which allows frequent motion but maintains tension during the intervals of relaxation, is effective to stretch flexion contractures of the elbows.

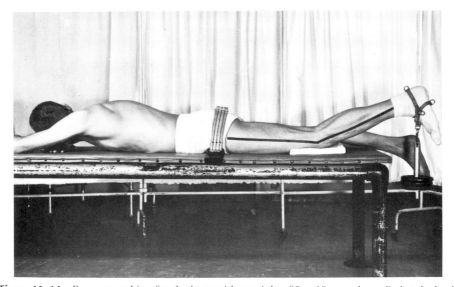

Figure 16–14 Prone stretching for the knee with a weight of 5 to 15 pounds applied at the heel.

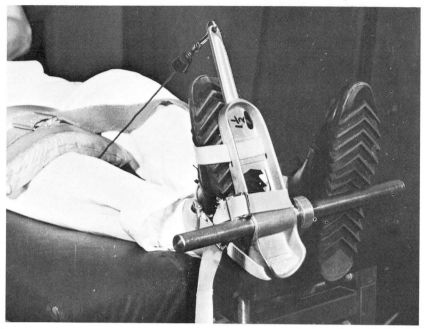

Figure 16–15 Stretching of the triceps surae on an exercise table using a toe extension boot. A weight of 10 to 30 pounds is applied for 20 minutes.

Figure 16–16 Prolonged stretching of the triceps surae using a tilt table and wedge board.

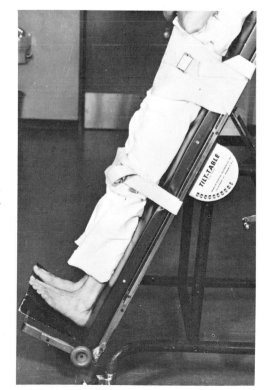

Fingers.   Stretching of fingers in flexion and extension without first mobilizing the soft tissues around the joint is inadequate. These joints have limited motion in other directions, including rotation, anteroposterior sliding, lateral sliding and lateral bending, as well as flexion and extension.[12] General mobility of these joints must be reestablished by gentle manipulatory stretching before full flexion and full extension are possible. All motions are carried out gently a number of times daily. The connective tissue around the joints of the fingers tends to gel rapidly if there is no motion. Splinting devices which hold the hand in one position are not entirely effective because they do not provide the repeated motion necessary to restore suppleness to the connective tissues around the joints. Joint capsules of immobilized hands quickly become edematous and sclerotic. Effective manipulation of fingers is difficult and is best carried out by a skilled therapist.

EXERCISES TO DEVELOP COORDINATION

Teaching Control of Individual Muscles

If a muscle is of major importance in performing a motion of a joint, it is called a prime mover or agonist. Other muscles that assist that motion are called synergists. Muscles that oppose the motion are called antagonists. Muscles of the same or adjacent joints that maintain position to allow the motion and are used synchronously with the prime mover are called stabilizers. Neuromuscular reeducation means the teaching of discrete control of the prime movers of a given motion under the direct consciousness of the patient.

When a muscle is contracting against a load which is very light relative to the total strength of that muscle, it is possible to limit activity to that muscle, or even to a single motor unit, voluntarily.[13] If the load is heavier, the stabilizer muscles must contract to stabilize the proximal joints. As the load becomes still heavier, synergists as well as the prime mover must contract, and with even heavier loading, antagonists participate in the motion to act as stabilizing and regulating forces. Prolonged activity causes fatigue of any muscle and increases the proportionate resistance of a constant load relative to the available strength of the prime mover.

When a prime mover is so weak that the patient does not use it normally and it is desired to retrain him in the use of that muscle to improve its strength and to coordinate it into the normal motor patterns, the patient must learn precise control of the muscle. If heavy exercise is attempted, the spread of excitation to the surrounding synergists, stabilizers and antagonists results in a confused motor pattern or incoordination which results in failure to regain control of the prime mover. For patients with neuromuscular disease, development of precise control of prime movers is an essential step in the development of optimally coordinated motion.

Requirements for Neuromuscular Reeducation.   The patient must be rational, old enough to comprehend and follow instruction and able to learn, cooperate and concentrate on the muscular training during the exercise period.

He must be relaxed, comfortable and securely supported. A patient who is unsteady or insecure cannot concentrate on the activity of an isolated muscle. If he has generalized weakness or a problem of balance, he should be fully supported in the recumbent position. Patients with cerebral palsy cannot relax fully on a high or narrow table or in an erect postion.

The training exercise should be carried on in a quiet room so that the patient will not be distracted.

The patient should be alert and emotionally calm. There should be frequent short rest periods. As soon as he begins to tire or become inattentive, the training session should be discontinued.

The patient must have intact proprioceptors or telereceptors to monitor activity. If proprioception is normal, as is the case with poliomyelitis patients, the patient is taught while lying supine and relaxed and the emphasis is on proprioception because proprioceptive sensation is more rapid and precise. If proprioception is impaired, the patient must be positioned in such a way that he can watch the activity in order to monitor it. Patients without perception of position or muscular activity cannot be taught precise control.

The patient must have a pain-free arc of motion of the joint across which the muscle is working. The sense of position and movement is derived primarily from joint receptors stimulated by motion of that joint.[14] In the presence of pain, inhibition of activity occurs and incoordination results. Usually, neuromuscular reeducation can be begun as soon as the patient has a pain-free arc of motion of about 30 degrees.

There must be competent direction from a trained therapist who provides clear-cut commands for precise performance, is alert to monitor and confirm that performance, rules out any substitution or incoordination and encourages the patient to continue working at the maximum of his ability.

Neuromuscular reeducation should begin with minimal activities and be increased by small increments of intensity or complexity as the patient develops control. These standard requirements for neuromuscular education of patients have been confirmed by Simard and Basmajian to be necessary in order to develop conscious control of individual motor units.[13]

Technique of Establishing Control of Individual Muscles

STIMULATION.   The proprioceptive stretch reflex is stimulated by repeated lengthening and relaxation of the muscle. A single stretch with a slow return toward the shortened position allows the best observation of the stretch response. This reaction can usually be observed or palpated best at the tendon of insertion. When the muscle is quickly stretched and then slowly returned to the shortened position while the tendon is observed or palpated, a persistence of tension can occur during shortening only if there is active muscular contraction. Multiple quick short stretches may be more effective in initiating the response but the response is harder to observe. Elicitation of the stretch reflex demonstrates that the lower motor neuron pathway is intact. In a paralyzed muscle following lower motor neuron disease, elicitation of the stretch reflex in this manner often is the first evidence of return of innervation. Stimulation is carried on a number of times daily prior to the beginning of neuromuscular reeducation.

For upper motor neuron disease, stretch stimulation is an unreliable index of an effective pathway for control of muscular contraction. Various facilitation techniques may be necessary to demonstrate that there is an upper neuron pathway for volitional control. However, production of activity in a muscle by facilitation techniques does not necessarily indicate that there is a neural pathway which can be retrained so that volitional control of that muscle may be reestablished.

CUTANEOUS REINFORCEMENT OF STIMULATION. Stimulation of the skin over the belly of the muscle reflexly increases the sensitivity of the stretch reflex (gamma motoneuron reflex). Stroking, tapping, cold, histamine by iontophoresis or electrical stimulation of the skin over the muscle belly may be effective to increase the stretch reflex response.

MENTAL AWARENESS. Instruct the patient in the function of each muscle, indicating the origin and insertion of the muscle, the line of pull and the action produced by the muscle. Demonstrate the action while the patient remains passive. Instruct the patient to think of the pull as coming from the insertion and moving in the direction of the shortening muscle. Stroke the skin over the insertion in the direction of pull and tell the patient to concentrate on the sensation of motion occurring during this sensorially reinforced passive motion.

Control exercises must be initiated against minimal resistance if specific sensations of the contraction of the prime mover are to be perceived, because isolated contraction of an individual muscle can be performed only when the muscle is contracting against a resistance that is small in relation to the total strength of that muscle. Spread of excitation resulting in contraction of synergists, stabilizers or antagonists must not be allowed. If spread of excitation does occur, the stronger sensations produced by the contractions of the stronger synergists or antagonists or both are perceived more readily than sensations arising from the weaker prime mover. The patient then learns to monitor the wrong motor activity because he perceives these stronger sensations. He does not become aware of the sensations arising from the activity of the paretic prime mover so he does not relearn to control it. As a result, the paretic prime mover does not redevelop its potential strength and usefulness. If this type of incoordination is allowed during therapeutic exercise, a motor pattern is developed which does not include the paretic prime mover. The final result is an incoordinated contraction of less than the potential strength.

If the muscle is weak, the weight of the part may constitute a heavy resistance in relation to the maximal strength of the muscle and cause irradiation of impulses and incoordination. Therefore, reeducation exercises are begun with *maximal assistance* so that the muscle contracts against no resistance, and the resistance is increased only as ability is developed to contract the prime mover without activating the other muscles.

SEQUENCE OF TRAINING IN NEUROMUSCULAR REEDUCATION. (1) Instruct the patient to think about the motion while it is carried out passively by the therapist in order that the patient may feel the sensation of proper motion. Stroke the skin over the tendon of insertion in the direction of the motion to reinforce the sensation of the motion. (2) Have the patient assist only slightly by contracting the prime mover as the therapist carries out the motion, together with cutaneous stimulation. (3) Have the patient move the part through the range of motion with assistance and cutaneous stimulation from the therapist with emphasis on contraction of only the prime mover. (4) Have the patient carry out the activity alone using the individual prime mover.

Progression from one step to the next occurs only when the first step can be performed accurately without substitution. Each of the steps is carried out three to five times for each muscle at each training session depending upon the fatigability of the patient. Throughout control training avoidance of substitution must be emphasized. Control of the individual muscles should be achieved before more complex coordination is attempted.

Facilitation techniques which utilize overflow of nerve impulses from one motor pathway to another by mass activation of muscles in order to activate a weak muscle are incompatible with the training of precise control. Facilitation of this type can demonstrate a potential pathway to a muscle, but it interferes with, rather than aids in, the development of control.

Therapeutic Exercise to Develop Neuromuscular Coordination

Coordination is the combination of the activities of a number of muscles into the smooth patterns seen under normal conditions. The activities of the component parts of a well coordinated motion are automatic and not consciously perceived, although the accomplishment of the activity is perceived. Control of coordinated activity is monitored primarily through the feedback of sensory stimuli transmitted through proprioceptive pathways, although to a limited extent it may be monitored by visual or tactile stimuli. The patient must have intact proprioception and intact subcortical centers for integrating proprioceptive sensory impulses with motor responses in order to achieve a high degree of coordination. When there is damage to the proprioceptive pathways or centers, visual control must be substituted for proprioceptive control, but the degree of coordination achieved is never as great as when the proprioceptive pathways are intact.

The development of coordination depends upon the *repetition* of a precisely performed pattern of activity many times to produce an integration of sensory stimuli with the motor response. As training for coordination is carried out, the rate of movement must be slow enough so that the person is aware of the sensations related to the various components of the action.

As the activity is repeated precisely many times, a habit pathway is formed. The activity then can be performed with less effort. The speed of performance increases. The attention required for precise performance becomes less and there is less spread of excitation to other neurons outside of the activity pattern. Eventually, the activity can be carried on with little cerebral perception of its individual components and it is said to be automatic.

How the sensory feedback is improved and how the flow of stimuli is limited to the specific neural pathway by repetition is not understood. Nevertheless, all skilled muscular activities are developed in this way. Repetition of activity with sensory feedback to regulate performance is the basis for the development of motor skills in the infant and child. Likewise, it is the basis for relearning coordination for the patient who has suffered injury to the neuromuscular system.

High degrees of coordination and speed do not develop until the activity pattern becomes so well developed that it does not require constant awareness of all phases of the activity. For example, the pianist or typist does not need to think of the contraction of the muscles involved in the individual placement of each finger because a symbol on a page signifies a whole pattern of response and the cerebral cortex provides general direction without specific attention to the performance of all components of the activity. During motor activities, the brain is aware of the general performance rather than the precise motion of each muscle and joint. The more frequently an activity is repeated, the greater the speed and precision of its performance becomes. Development of coordination results in greater preciseness of motion and greater economy of muscular effort because of less involvement of extraneous muscular activity. This precision of motion depends upon active inhibition of impulse transmission to neurons other than those involved in the precise motion.

Training in coordination, therefore, increases the capacity of the central nervous system to inhibit irradiation. When the capacity for inhibition increases, cerebral effort to increase a specific motor activity can be increased while neuronal excitation remains restricted to the desired neuromuscular pathway. By developing increased ability to inhibit the irradiation of activity, training of coordination increases precision, speed and strength of contraction.

Coordination of movement is complex. There are multiple components, even for simple activities. All components must be integrated into a timed sequence of interrelated responses. To grasp with the hand, for example, *prime mover* responses involve the use of the fingers and thumb. *Synergistic* muscles contract with the prime movers to assist or modify the activity. *Stabilizer* cocontractions occur in the muscles of the wrist, elbow and shoulder. Before this apparently primary activity can begin, a stable base must be established in relation to gravity by the properly coordinated contraction of the muscles which establish a *stable posture* for the body. To change the location of the hand requires *translatory* motion produced by contraction of the muscles of the shoulder and elbow. As the arm moves there must be *postural adjustments* to maintain balance. Each of these muscular contractions must be monitored by sensory feedback from the joints, fascia and skin to the central nervous system.

The monitoring of position and motion for skilled motor patterns is largely automatic through the interaction between the cerebellum and the basal ganglia and premotor cortex. Awareness of the activities being performed and volitional monitoring of them are only superficial. Development of a habit pattern of activity, or motor engram, is dependent upon the establishment of a cerebellar-basal ganglionic internuncial network, which programs each motor pattern. Repetition of each pattern with precision and at the maximal speed and tension consistent with precision results in the development of a coordinated motor engram which requires minimal volitional effort to perform. Highly coordinated movement, therefore, is largely a subcortical neuromuscular response. The function of the cerebral cortex is to select those motor engrams to be used to accomplish a specific task.

The goal of coordination training is to reproduce precise activities enough times so that motor engrams are developed which do not need voluntary regulation to be performed rapidly and precisely. Volition is used to select or modify the sequence of engrams. Although information is scant, it appears that a coordinated activity must be performed with precision several million times before the peak of performance is reached.[15]

Time is also a significant factor in the training and maintenance of coordination. There is a progressive decline of ability to control motor responses during any period of inactivity; this decline in ability increases with the duration of the inactivity. Each component of sensorimotor performance must be tested frequently in order to perform at the highest level of precision. Integration of sensorimotor coordination begins to deteriorate with the onset of inactivity and this deterioration of coordination continues throughout prolonged inactivity. Rest, therefore, results in diminished coordination. If an activity is performed infrequently the degree of coordination developed is less than that resulting from frequent activity. One exercise period each day, or even less frequent exercise periods, with inactivity throughout the intervals, is not conducive to the development of a high level of coordination. As a matter of fact, skill may be lost progressively rather than gained on such a program.

Coordination training should be based on the following criteria:

The coordination exercise should be performed precisely and frequently each day in a program which is continued without interruption until the desired level of coordination has been gained.

Avoid extraneous muscular activity during the training exercise. Repetition of the same extraneous muscular contractions will make them a part of the motor engram. If random motor activity is allowed, inhibition is not developed and precision of motion remains poor.

Reinforce sensory perception of correct performance by every possible means: instruction, pictures or diagrams, cinegraphic recording, verbal monitoring.

Train the patient in a location where he is able to concentrate on the coordination training. Protect him from the diverting influence of external stimuli during training. Allow frequent short rest periods to avoid fatigue and reduce the tension associated with concentration and effort. Frequent yawning is evidence of fatigue from concentration rather than boredom.

Precise control of a prime mover requires that resistance to the muscle should be very low in relation to total strength of that muscle in order that the effort to initiate the activity may be slight and irradiation of impulses in the central nervous system will be low. For beginning training, resistance should be minimal. If a patient must use a large proportion of his strength during an activity, there will be poorer coordination than if the activity requires only a small portion of his strength. Even normal, well-coordinated muscles develop fatigue within a few minutes at a resistance as low as 10 per cent of maximal[16], and with fatigue, irradiation increases throughout the internuncial pool. Increasing the strength of a muscle may improve coordination during activity against moderate resistance because a smaller proportion of the strength of the muscle need be used.

Coordination Activities for the Hand and Upper Extremity. In the hand, the complex activities of pinch and grasp require flexion and extension of the fingers, and flexion, extension and opposition of the thumb. There is simultaneous movement of wrist, elbow and shoulder to carry the hand to the desired place of activity. The upper extremity is a derrick carrying the hand as a prehensile organ. Motions of the shoulder, elbow and wrist to carry the hand to the site of activity usually are automatic and not under specific attention. This automatic habit of positioning the upper extremity occurs through practice. During coordinated motion, the preliminary approach to a position is faster and requires less precision and less attention than the final positioning of the hand which usually is under visual and proprioceptive perception.

Prehension occurs mainly as a pinch between the thumb, index and middle fingers like a three-pronged chuck (Fig. 16-17). Seventy per cent of prehensile activity is carried out in this way. Power grasp performed by approximating the four fingers toward the thenar eminence occurs for about 20 per cent of activities. Apposition of the thumb to one fingertip or to the radial side of the index finger occurs much less frequently. Most of these activities are under direct perception unless they are performed repeatedly in which case they become semiautomatic.

The best way to develop precision and speed of coordination for a specific activity is to practice that activity for prolonged periods at maximal speed and with maximal precision. Performance is improved only when the activity is practiced at the peak of skill.

Variation of activities is necessary to prevent monotony and frustration, especially if the coordination of the patient is poor. Participation in multiple activities increases general skill and coordination and aids in maintaining attention.

Occupational therapy can be used to develop varying degrees of strength and endurance at the same time that coordination is stressed. Occupational therapy is especially suited to the development of dexterity of the fingers and

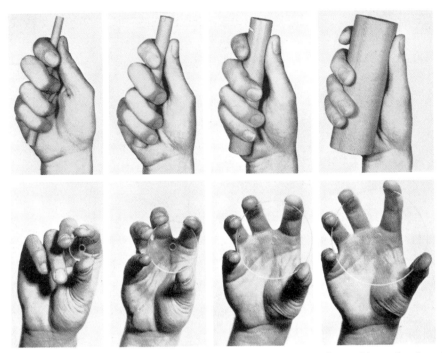

Figure 16–17   Prehension using the power grip or the precision grip on objects of various sizes. (From Napier, J. Bone Joint Surg., *38B:*902, 1956.)

hand. The constructive aspects of occupational therapy aid in maintaining attention (Fig. 16-18). Similar training may also be carried on in a prevocational shop. Such activities should be designed to encourage the patient to work at his maximal rate of speed and with maximal precision. Modification of craft activities by incorporating artificial maneuvers or excessive resistance not only discourage the patient from participation but also interfere with the improvement of coordination.

Coordination Activities for the Lower Extremities.   *Frenkel's exercises* are a series of exercises of increasing difficulty to improve proprioceptive control in the lower extremities. These exercises begin with simple movements with gravity eliminated and gradually progress to more complicated movement patterns utilizing simultaneous hip and knee motions carried on against gravity. They are especially useful when there is impairment of proprioception due to disorders in the central nervous system. Repeated practice helps to develop the usefulness of any proprioception which the patient has available to aid him. If the patient does not have adequate proprioception, he must be positioned so that he can monitor his activity by vision.

The initial exercise training is conducted under the supervision of a therapist and the emphasis is on slow precise motion and positioning. To avoid fatigue each exercise is performed not more than four times at each session. The first simple exercises should be accomplished adequately before progressing to the more difficult patterns. As the patient gains the ability to perform each exercise, he is instructed to perform it every three or four hours.

Exercises While Supine.   The patient lies on a bed or plinth with a

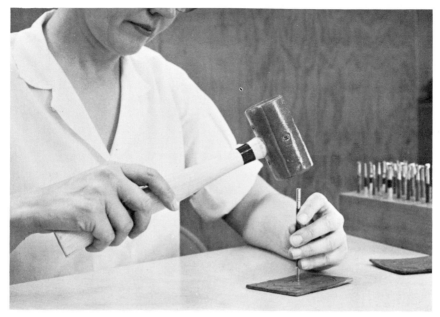

Figure 16–18 Leather stamping in occupational therapy requires the use of the power grip with the dominant hand and the precision grip with the nondominant hand.

smooth surface along which the heels may slide easily. The head should be supported so that the patient can see his legs and feet.

1. Flex the hip and knee of one extremity, sliding the heel along in contact with the bed. Return to the original position. Repeat with the opposite extremity.

2. Flex as in exercise 1. Then abduct the flexed leg. Return to the flexed position and then to the original position.

3. Flex the hip and knee only halfway and then return to the extended position. Add abduction and adduction.

4. Flex one leg at the hip and knee, stopping at any point in flexion or extension on command.

5. Flex both lower extremities simultaneously and equally; add abduction, adduction and extension.

6. Flex both lower extremities simultaneously to the halfway position; add abduction and adduction to half-flexed position. Extend. Stop in the pattern on command.

7. Flex one extremity at the hip and knee with the heel held 2 inches above the bed. Return to the original position.

8. Flex as in exercise 7. Bring the heel to rest on the opposite patella. Successively add patterns so that the heel is touched to the middle of the shin, to the ankle, to the toes of the opposite foot, to the bed on either side of the knee and to the bed on either side of the leg.

9. Flex as in exercise 7 and then touch the heel successively to the patella, shin, ankle and toes. Reverse the pattern.

10. Flex as in exercise 7 and then touch the heel on command to the point indicated by the therapist.

11. Flex the hip and knee with the heel 2 inches above the bed. Place the

heel on the opposite patella and slowly slide it down the crest of the tibia to the ankle. Reverse.

12. Use the pattern in exercise 11, but slide the heel down the crest of the opposite tibia, over the ankle and foot to the toes. If the heel is to reach the toes, the opposite knee must be flexed slightly during this exercise. Stop in the pattern on command.

13. With malleoli and knees in apposition, flex both lower extremities simultaneously with the heels 2 inches above the bed. Return to the original position. Stop in the pattern on command.

14. Reciprocal flexion and extension of the lower extremities with the heels touching the bed.

15. Reciprocal flexion and extension of the lower extremities with the heels 2 inches above the bed.

16. Bilateral simultaneous flexion, abduction, adduction and extension with the heels 2 inches above the bed.

17. Precise heel placement where the therapist indicates with the finger on the bed or the opposite extremity.

18. Follow with the toe the movement of the therapist's finger in any combination of lower extremity motion.

EXERCISES WHILE SITTING

1. Practice maintaining correct sitting posture for two minutes in an armchair with back support and the feet flat on the floor. Repeat in a chair without arms. Repeat without back support.

2. Mark time to the counting of the therapist by raising only the heel from the floor. Progress to alternately lifting the entire foot and replacing it precisely in a marked position on the floor.

3. Make two cross marks on the floor with chalk. Alternately glide the foot over the marked cross: forward, backward, left and right.

4. Practice rising from and sitting on a chair to the therapist's counted cadence: (1) Flex the knees and draw the feet under the front edge of the seat. (2) Bend the trunk forward over the thighs. (3) Rise by extending the knees and hips and then straightening the trunk. (4) Bend the trunk forward slightly. (5) Flex the hips and knees to sit. (6) Straighten the trunk and sit back in the chair.

EXERCISES WHILE STANDING

1. Walking sideways. Balance is easier during sideward walking because the patient does not have to rise on his toes, which decreases his base of support. The exercise is performed to a counted cadence: (1) Shift the weight to the left foot. (2) Place the right foot 12 inches to the right. (3) Shift the weight to the right foot. (4) Bring the left foot over to the right foot. The size of the step taken to the right or left may be varied.

2. Walk forward between two parallel lines 14 inches apart placing the right foot just inside the right line and the left foot just inside the left line. Emphasize correct placement. Rest after 10 steps.

3. Walk forward placing each foot on a footprint traced on the floor. Footprints should be parallel and 2 inches lateral to the midline. Practice with quarter steps, half steps, three-quarter steps and full steps.

4. Turning. (1) Raise the right toe and rotate the right foot outward, pivoting on the heel. (2) Raise the left heel and pivot the left leg inward on the toes. (3) Bring the left foot up beside the right.

Ambulation Training. Training of stance and balance must precede training in walking if optimal patterns are to be developed. Early training is best done in the parallel bars to allow security for stance, weight shifting and development of perception of balance. For severely involved patients, the initial upright posture may be attained on a tilt table to which the patient is securely strapped (Fig. 16-19). As the patient develops stability of his trunk he can be transferred to the parallel bars.

Drills which develop balance should precede attempts to walk. These drills include removing one hand at a time from the bar, balancing with one hand, shifting from one leg to the other, shifting forward and backward, unlocking one knee and locking it again, picking up one foot and replacing it, and forward and backward foot placement. If it is anticipated that the patient must walk with crutches, it is better to teach him to walk using crutches rather than using the parallel bars after he has developed his balancing techniques, to avoid substitution of improper pressure or pulling on the bars instead of the necessary maneuvers which he must perform when using crutches.

Factors Increasing Incoordination.   Irradiation of impulses in the central nervous system from the pathway of one coordinated activity to neurons activating other muscles results in incoordinated motion. Constant repetition of an activity in combination with the same extraneous motion will incorporate that extraneous motion into the activity pattern and produce a persistant incoordination.

When a patient is insecure or fearful, there is a greater spread of excitation within the central system with activation of more motor neurons than those essential for an activity pattern. This results in a greater expenditure of

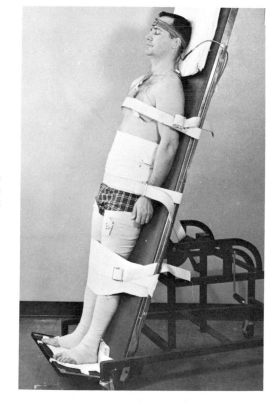

Figure 16–19 The tilt table may be used to provide security for a patient while he is developing tolerance to the upright position.

effort, less precision of motion and interference with the desired pattern of activity.

If a patient has to support himself against gravity, if he is weak or if he must overcome resistance which is great in relation to the strength of a muscle, incoordination will be increased.

Strong emotions increase incoordination.

Pain or increased sensory stimuli reaching the central nervous system increase irradiation from an activated pathway to other motor neurons.

Fatigue increase incoordination, probably because of the inability of the inhibitory centers to restrict impulses from irradiating beyond the desired activity pathway.

Just as coordination is produced by repetition, it is lost through periods of inactivity. It is necessary to reteach coordination to muscles that have been inactive or paretic. If the prime mover of a motion is weak, it is necessary to reteach coordination utilizing the prime mover in relation to the synergists; otherwise the prime mover may be dropped from the pattern of activity. The alienation of paretic muscles from an activity pattern in this manner occurs frequently. Only through specific training of control and coordination do these muscles again become incorporated as a part of the normal activity pattern.

EXERCISES TO DEVELOP MUSCULAR STRENGTH AND ENDURANCE

General Considerations

Strength may be defined as the maximal tension that can be exerted by a muscle during a contraction. Endurance is the ability of the muscle to contract and to exert tension for a prolonged period of time. Power is the rate of doing work or the work done per unit of time.

Although improvement in the tensile strength of a weak muscle is most frequently used as the index of improvement of muscular capability, it appears that for useful activity the development of power, i.e., work per unit time, might be a better index of muscular function. Instantaneous maximal strength is rarely required of a muscle for functional activities. All voluntary muscular contractions are sustained for a period of time. A maximal contraction of even a few seconds' duration will show the effect of fatigue[16] (Fig. 16-20). Repetitive muscular contractions at far less than maximal tensile strength, continued for a few minutes, will produce demonstrable fatigue (Fig. 16-21). Since activities are normally repetitive in this manner, assessment of muscular power might be more useful to predict performance than assessment of tensile strength.

Hypothetical Bases for Increase of Muscular Strength

Tension.   Tension during contraction of the muscle fiber is postulated to be the stimulus causing hypertrophy and an increase in the strength of the muscle fiber. Maximal or near maximal tension is most effective in causing an increase of strength.[17]

The time during which the maximal tension is exerted appears to be relatively insignificant. A muscle contracting at two-thirds of its maximal ten-

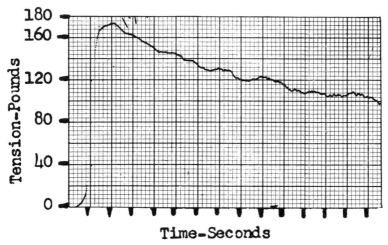

Figure 16–20 Decrease of tension from fatigue during maximally sustained isometric contraction of the muscles of hand grip of an athletic young man.

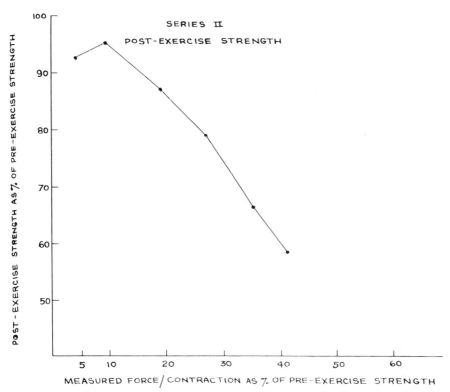

Figure 16–21 Decrease of strength of the muscles of hand grip after 10 minutes of intermittent isometric exercise at various proportions of maximal strength. The abscissa indicates the force exerted as per cent of maximal strength during 10 minutes of two second contractions alternating with one second rest periods. The ordinate indicates the maximal strength at the end of 10 minutes of exercise as per cent of preexercise maximal strength. (From Mundale.[18])

sion for six seconds once daily was reported to increase in strength as rapidly as when it was contracted for 45 seconds once daily. One contraction per day, maintained for six seconds, was reported to increase the strength of a muscle as rapidly as a similar exercise five times each day.[19] After further research, Müller and Rohmert reported that five daily maximal contractions of six seconds each at intervals of two minutes, which produced a total contraction time of 30 seconds, resulted in greater final or limiting strength than did maximal contractions for only six seconds daily.[17] Persons trained to limiting strength with one-second maximal isometric contractions each day and then continuing with six-second maximal isometric contractions each day responded with a further increase in strength of 10 to 40 per cent in about half of the subects. Müller suggests that training at 65 per cent of maximal strength, or at maximal strength for one, six or 30 seconds daily, results eventually in the same limiting strength but that the stronger contractions and longer contraction time each day accomplish this in a shorter time. Likewise, Liberson[20] reported that when isometric exercises of six seconds' duration were performed by the abductors of the fifth finger, exercising 20 times per day, they increased both tensile strength and endurance above the levels achieved when exercising only once daily.

In the hypothesis that tension is the stimulus causing an increase in the tensile strength of a muscle it is assumed that one maximal contraction of each muscle fiber is the adequate stimulus to cause the alterations of the metabolism leading to an increase in tensile strength of that muscle fiber. The contraction may be isometric or concentric (contraction with shortening) but it is easier to attain maximal tension during an isometric contraction than during a concentric contraction. It has been postulated that in a five- or six-second isometric contraction there is alternation of motor units which allows each muscle fiber of each unit to contract a number of times against nearly maximal tension. One maximal tension of each muscle fiber per day creates the adequate stimulus to increase strength.

When there was complete inactivity, strength was lost at the rate of 5 per cent per day.[17] Brief isometric exercise at longer than daily intervals caused strength to increase more slowly than during daily exercises because of this daily decrement due to inactivity.

Regularly recurring exercise in which tension exceeded 35 per cent of the strength of the muscle was reported to result in an increase of muscular strength. Exercise in which a muscle exerted 20 to 35 per cent of its maximal tension was reported to maintain muscular strength. A tension of less than 20 per cent was an inadequate stimulus to maintain muscular strength.

Brief isometric exercise in which tension exceeded 65 per cent of maximal was reported to increase strength at the rate of approximately 5 per cent per week over a 20 week period.[19] There was considerable variability of the response to this type of exercise. Numerous other reports have shown considerable variation, but the rate of increase of strength is of a similar magnitude. Strength usually reached a plateau in 12 to 20 weeks. Exercise programs of less than 12 weeks' duration were followed by a rapid loss of strength when the exercise was discontinued.[21] If the subject produced a brief isometric contraction once per week, strength was maintained near its peak level.

Müller[17] suggested that the relative increase in strength per week on maximal isometric exercise is a function of the state of training of the muscle. As strength approaches *limiting strength*, the maximal strength which can be attained by daily maximal isometric exercise, the increase of strength per week diminishes progressively (Fig. 16-22). Assuming that limiting strength repre-

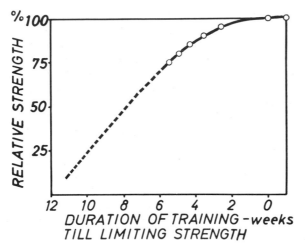

Figure 16–22 Increase of relative strength up to limiting strength by one daily maximal isometric contraction. (From Müller.[17])

sented the same state of training for all muscles, Müller and Rohmert[22] concluded that equal percentages of limiting strength represented similar states of training and termed strength in percentage of limiting strength the *relative strength*.

A system of brief maximal exercise described and studied by Rose et al.[23] consisted of a contraction of the quadriceps femoris muscle against maximal resistance through the range of knee extension from 90 to 180 degrees with sustained contraction in the fully shortened position for five seconds. Each day the resistance was increased by a constant small increment. There was a regular increase in strength on this regimen for 60 days or longer. Once a plateau was reached, strength could be maintained near that level by exercising only once each week. This increase in strength was not accompanied by a comparable hypertrophy of the muscle, although previously nonconditioned muscles became firmer to palpation.

Power. Work per unit time exceeding metabolic capacity (overload) has been proposed to be the stimulus causing muscular hypertrophy, increased strength, increased ability to recruit motor units and increased ability to withstand the discomfort of heavy exercise.[24]

DeLorme[25] in 1945 described a system of progressive resistive exercises consisting of a series of contractions of a functional muscle group beginning with 10 contractions against a light load and progressing through bouts of contractions against increasing resistance until the final bout of contractions each day was against maximal resistance. The progressively increasing submaximal contractions in this series were postulated to exert a "conditioning" effect on the neuromuscular system to prepare it for maximal effort. The final bout of 10 contractions against maximal resistance was considered to be the stimulus causing the increase in muscular strength and hypertrophy of the muscle. These exercises caused considerable fatigue in the exercised muscles by the end of the daily exercise period. On this program in which the maximal resistance against which the patient worked was increased each week, there was a progressive increase of the strength of the muscle. Modifications of this routine in which the number of contractions against submaximal resistance was decreased were reported to be equally effective to increase strength.[26-28] Decreasing the final maximal bout of exercise from 10 to 5 contractions was reported not to decrease the effectiveness of the exercise although the fatigue was less.

Hellebrandt[24] considered that hypertrophy and increased muscular strength occurred only when the muscular work per unit time exceeded the metabolic capacity (overload) and when such exercises were continued until marked fatigue had occurred. Hellebrandt emphasized that a person must exert maximal effort in order to achieve the maximal rate of increase of function. To reinforce maximal effort, a number of methods including verbal encouragement, competition and physiologic facilitation were utilized. Exercise against resistance was carried on through the fullest possible range of motion. When, because of fatigue, the muscle was unable to contract through the full range, the exercise was continued through the progressively restricted range until the muscle was unable to lift the load. Bouts of contractions were interspersed with short periods of rest to allow some recovery from fatigue so that more work could be done. This type of exercise resulted in postexercise fatigue, muscular swelling, redness and soreness. Recovery from these symptoms usually occurred in a day or two.

Conditioning of the central nervous system by increasing motivation, learning to recruit and utilize more motor units, and increasing tolerance to pain was considered to increase effort and contribute an increase in performance of at least 40 per cent of the initial maximal level. The more frequently the exercise was performed, the more rapidly performance increased. In these studies the increase in power was measured rather than the increase in tension produced by muscular contraction. Data do not show whether power per se is the stimulus to increase strength. Since, in these studies, increase of power rather than increase of tensile strength was measured, these data do not show whether prolonged power overload is a greater stimulus to increase strength than is briefly applied tension.

Liberson[20] has compared the effects of the modified progressive resistive exercise of DeLorme and Watkins[26] with single and multiple daily brief maximal isometric exercise. The descending order of value of these exercises to increase tensile strength and endurance is shown in Table 16-1.

TABLE 16-1   EFFECT OF ISOMETRIC AND CONCENTRIC ISOTONIC EXERCISE ON THE INCREASE OF TENSILE STRENGTH AND ENDURANCE OF MUSCLES OF NORMAL SUBJECTS*

TYPE OF EXERCISE	INCREASE IN STRENGTH IN PER CENT		ENDURANCE INDEX (50%)†
	Concentric Tension (1 R.M.)	*Isometric Tension*	*Sec.*
Multiple daily brief isometric maximal exercise	150	203	170
Single daily brief isometric maximal exercise	130	174	101
Progressive resistive concentric exercise	113	111	63

*From studies by Liberson of the hypothenar muscles abducting the fifth finger.[20]
†The endurance index is the elapsed time from the beginning of a sustained maximal isometric contraction until the tension falls to 50 per cent of maximum.

Techniques of Exercises to Increase Strength

Progressive Resistive Exercise.   This is the original long sequence exercise of DeLorme.[25]

Determine the 10 repetition maximal resistance (the maximal resistance which the muscle can lift through the range of motion 10 times), by contracting the muscle to the shortened position against a light load for 10 contractions and progressively increasing the load for bouts of 10 contractions each until the maximal load which can be lifted 10 times is reached. This is the 10 repetition maximum, i.e., 10 R.M.

For each exercise, five days weekly, have the patient perform bouts of 10 contractions each, beginning at 10 per cent of the 10 R.M. and increasing by deciles to the final 10 repetition maximum:

> Bout of 10 contractions at 10 per cent of 10 R.M.
> Bout of 10 contractions at 20 per cent of 10 R.M.
> ....
> ....
> Bout of 10 contractions at 100 per cent of 10 R.M.

Allow a rest period of two to four minutes between successive bouts.

Once weekly test the ability to exceed the 10 R.M., which shows the gain in strength and establishes the new 10 R.M. for the following week.

Shortened sequences of progressive resistive exercise have been reported to be equally effective to increase muscular strength.

The modification of DeLorme and Watkins[26] is:

> 10 repetition bout at 50 per cent of 10 R.M.
> 10 repetition bout at 75 per cent at 10 R.M.
> 10 repetition bout at 100 per cent of 10 R.M.

The modification of McMorris and Elkins,[27] done once daily, five days per week, increased strength by 5 per cent per week over a 12 week period:

> 10 repetition bout at 25 per cent of 10 R.M.
> 10 repetition bout at 50 per cent of 10 R.M.
> 10 repetition bout at 75 per cent of 10 R.M.
> 10 repetition bout at 100 per cent of 10 R.M.

McGovern and Luscombe[28] reported that their modification is equally as effective as the original progressive resistive exercise of DeLorme to increase strength but causes less fatigue:

> 5 repetition bout at 50 per cent of 10 R.M.
> 10 repetition bout at 100 per cent of 10 R.M.

Progressive Assistive Exercise.   If the muscle will not lift the part against gravity, progressive loading is utilized with gravity eliminated or counterbalanced. Horizontal exercises may be employed against progressive resistance by suspending the extremity or supporting it on a skate board or a powder board. Vertical exercises may be utilized by counterbalancing the weight of the part with a pulley system and then progressively increasing the resistance to muscular contraction by decreasing the counterbalancing weight. In progressive assistive exercise the principle of increasing the resistance against which the muscle must contract in successive bouts is the same as for progressive resistive exercises.

Regressive Resistive Exercise (Zinovieff[29]).   Determine the 10 R.M. as described for progressive resistive exercise. For each exercise, five days weekly, have the patient perform bouts of 10 contractions each, beginning at 100 per cent of the 10 R.M. and decreasing by deciles to a final bout at 10 per cent of the 10 R.M.:

> Loosen muscles with wand or calisthenic exercises.
> 10 repetition bout at 100 per cent of 10 R.M.
> 10 repetition bout at 90 per cent of 10 R.M.
> ....
> ....
> 10 repetition bout at 10 per cent of 10 R.M.

Each week test the increase in strength beyond the 10 R.M. to establish the maximal load for the subsequent week.

The rationale for this procedure is to decrease the resistance as the patient fatigues so that the muscles perform maximal work throughout the exercise period.

McGovern and Luscombe[28] reported that their modified sequence is slightly more effective to increase strength than either the regular or the short modification of progressive resistive exercise:

> 10 repetition bout at 100 per cent of 10 R.M.
> 10 repetition bout at 75 per cent of 10 R.M.
> 10 repetition bout at 50 per cent of 10 R.M.

Brief Maximal Exercise (Rose et al.[23]).   Establish, by progressive loading, the maximal load that can be lifted from the dependent position to the antigravity position and held for five seconds. On each succeeding day lift the weight of the previous day plus one standard increment and hold for five seconds.

One successful lift constitutes the exercise for that muscle group for that day.

If a patient fails to lift the weight as scheduled and to hold it for five seconds, after a four minute rest he is retested at the weight minus one increment. If the patient again fails, after a four minute rest he is retested with the weight minus two increments. Whether he succeeds or fails, this constitutes the complete exercise for that day. On the succeeding day increase the weight by one increment if he was successful on the previous day or decrease it by one increment if he failed on the previous day. Record the weight used in the final exercise and the success or failure each day.

Standard Weight Increments Per Day for Various Muscle Groups

Shoulder abductors	0.625 lb.
Elbow flexors	0.625 lb.
Elbow extensors	0.625 lb.
Wrist flexors	0.5 lb.
Wrist extensors	0.5 lb.
1st dorsal interosseus	0.125 lb.
Hip abductors	1.25 lbs.
Knee extensors	1.25 lbs.
Ankle plantar flexors	2.5 lbs.

Brief Maximal Isometric Exercise.   Contract the muscle against a fixed resistance and hold for five to six seconds. To monitor the force exerted, some type of isometric tension gauge must be used, such as a strain gauge or a cable tensiometer. A spring scale allows too much shortening of the muscle to provide true isometric contraction. All linkage mechanisms should be nondistensible. Hettinger and Müller[19] reported that the maximal rate of increase of strength occurred when the isometric tension exceeded 67 per cent of the maximal tension.

Studies by Liberson of the electrogenic response of a muscle to the degree of tension suggest that maximal effort is a better stimulus to increase strength than any submaximal effort and also that the angle of the joint that permits the highest mechanical output of the muscle is the most efficacious.[20]

If some type of recording device is not used, there is no way to be sure that optimal tension is being exerted. This becomes especially important if the patient is poorly motivated to exercise. Even for well motivated individuals when maximal effort is to be exerted periodically over a prolonged period of time, natural lethargy is likely to cause a submaximal effort. Proprioceptive evaluation of tension even by a well motivated individual is inaccurate. A reliable dynamometer provides both a stimulus to greater effort and a true record of the tension achieved.

Exercise to Increase Muscular Endurance

Endurance is the ability to carry on an exercise or activity for a prolonged period of time. Muscular endurance is related to the factors of muscular strength, circulation and muscular metabolism. It is also related to the less clearly definable factors of central nervous system fatigue and motivation to carry on the activity.

There is a direct relationship between the maximal tension that a muscle can exert and its ability to contract repeatedly against a constant load. As a muscle becomes stronger, work against a constant load requires proportionately less of the muscle to be contracting at any instant and leaves a greater recovery time for muscle fibers after contraction. During muscular activity, motor units contract intermittently. Tension is sustained because the irregular contractions and relaxations of many motor units fuse into a smoothly sustained contraction of the total muscle.

The activation of motor units during a contraction is not entirely random. Small motor units with a low threshold for excitation initiate contraction and are most active during weak contractions. As the contraction becomes stronger or the muscle begins to fatigue, larger motor units are activated. These larger motor units provide less precise responses than do the small motor units. Thus, during great effort or fatigue the precision of muscular contraction is diminished.

Voluntary muscle fibers do not remain contracted but undergo relaxation and metabolic recovery after each contraction. If the rest period between successive contractions of a muscle fiber is not long enough for full metabolic recovery, the muscle fiber becomes fatigued. It requires for full metabolic restoration of a muscle fiber, a rest period approximately 200 times as long as the contraction time (Fig. 16-23).[30] If there were completely random alternation of activity of motor units, fatigue should develop during any alternating muscular contraction in which the tension exceeded 1 per cent of maximal. The greater the tension relative to the maximal strength of the muscle, the more rapidly the fatigue occurs. Mundale[16] observed fatigue in hand grip (repetitive contractions for one second with one second intervals of rest) at the end of a 10 minute exercise period at a tension of 5 per cent of maximum (Fig. 16-24). As the exercise load was increased, the amount of fatigue also increased. The decrease in the maximal tension which could be produced at the

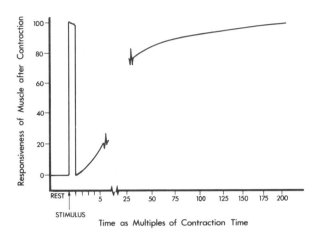

Figure 16–23 Relative rate of recovery of responsiveness of a muscle fiber after a maximal contraction.

end of such an exercise was roughly proportional to the isometric tension during the exercise (see Fig. 16-21).

The cardiovascular capacity to sustain work increases as the result of repeated prolonged effort. If a bout of work is very short, muscular needs can be provided by the development of an oxygen debt or depletion of the nutrient stores in the muscles and blood. For a longer period of activity, circulation and respiration must be increased by increased cardiac output, increased respiratory exchange and redistribution of peripheral circulation in relation to the demand. Metabolites produced in the muscle during work are effective stimuli to increase the local circulation, cardiac work and respiration. For the patient in poor condition, short periods of moderately heavy work followed by periods of rest appear to be most effective to increase circulatory and respiratory capacity. As the circulatory capacity improves in response to the exercise program, the duration of the activity can be increased.

The metabolites released as the result of muscular contraction provide stimuli locally to increase the circulation. A decrease in the pH of the blood due to muscular metabolites dilates arterioles, capillaries and veins and increases

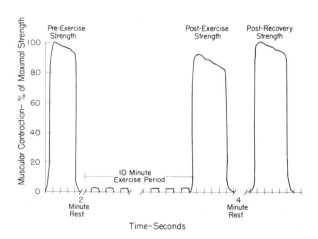

Figure 16–24 Record of fatigue produced by 10 minutes of isometric exercise of the muscles of hand grip at 5 per cent of maximal pre-exercise strength. One second contractions alternated with one second intervals of rest for the 10 minute exercise period. The post-exercise strength was reduced by fatigue to 92 per cent of the pre-exercise strength. (From Mundale.[16])

the dissociation of oxyhemoglobin. During exercise the number of open capillaries in the muscle is greatly increased. There is a profuse network of capillaries running through the endomysium in close proximity and parallel to each muscle fiber. When the muscle is at rest many of the capillaries are closed. During muscular activity there may be more than 4000 capillaries per square millimeter of cross-sectional area of muscle. Repeated prolonged exercise may increase the number of capillaries in muscles by 40 per cent.[31] The increased size of muscles resulting from frequent exercise is due, in part, to the number of open capillaries in the muscle.

The major stimulus for vasodilatation during muscular contraction appears to be directly on the blood vessels since the responses are similar in denervated and innervated muscles. Dilatation of the arteriolar supply to an active muscle may be due to an axon reflex. The cardiac output may increase as much as 10 times the basal value during maximal exercise, and because of regional redistribution of blood flow, the circulation of blood through the active muscles is even greater. As a consequence, in man the oxygen consumption of the muscles may be increased from 20 to 30 times and in well conditioned athletes to 50 times the resting value. This increase of oxygen consumption is due in part to the increased circulation and in part to a greater oxygen utilization.

Alternating kinetic contractions of antagonistic muscle groups mechanically aid venous and lymphatic flow. Compression of the vessels by the contracting muscle produces centripetal flow while the valves in the vessels prevent retrograde flow. Thus, alternating muscular contraction produces a "muscle pump" action aiding the circulation. On the other hand, a muscular contraction of 35 per cent or more of maximal tension will collapse the intramuscular blood vessels during the period of contraction. Therefore, muscles are ischemic during strong isometric contractions. The metabolites accumulating during this ischemic contraction act directly and reflexly to increase the circulation to the active muscle.

The metabolic changes associated with prolonged muscular activity result in an increase in the cellular stores and in the cellular metabolic capacity. Muscle conditioned to prolonged work has a higher myoglobin content and more intracellular lipids. Exposure of the muscle fibers to moderately fatiguing activity for progressively longer periods of time with intervals for rest allows these changes to occur without exposing the cell to the detrimental effects of exhaustion.

The development of tolerance for discomfort, of willingness to continue the activities for prolonged periods of time and probably of readjustments in neuronal metabolism are also built up by bouts of fatiguing activity for increasingly longer periods of time.

Techniques of Exercise to Increase Endurance

Endurance exercises have been described as low resistance-high repetition exercises. These exercises against low or moderate resistance should be repeated hundreds of times each day and should result in fatigue of the exercised muscles by the end of the exercise period. In order to be able to continue the exercise through many repetitions and to stimulate the cardiovascular system to respond before fatigue terminates the activity, the load on the muscle should be between 15 per cent and 40 per cent of maximal strength. The

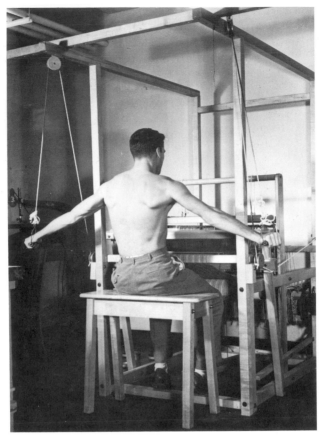

Figure 16–25   The floor loom may be adapted so that beating is performed by the shoulder depressor muscles. This is an excellent exercise to increase the strength and endurance of the upper extremities for crutch walking.

greater the proportionate load, the more rapidly fatigue will occur. Endurance does not develop unless the muscle exercises until some fatigue is produced. To develop great endurance an individual must work until he is markedly fatigued.

During this prolonged activity the factors of boredom or loss of interest in the activity, discomfort and lack of application to the exercise become important. For this reason, insofar as possible, exercises should be designed which provide an intrinsic interest in the activity. Construction crafts in occupational therapy attract or maintain the interest of most patients because of the constructive aspect of the activity. Group games or group activities also are usually of greater interest to patients than individual or isolated activities. Competition during exercise also stimulates greater effort.

In the therapeutic gymnasium any of the weight lifting or pulley exercises can be modified to become endurance exercises. Concentric muscular contractions through the range of motion of the joint rather than isometric contractions are preferred because of the aid to venous and lymphatic flow and the stimulation of cardiorespiratory function. The muscles are loaded so that fatigue begins to occur at the end of a bout of 20 to 30 contractions. Ten or more bouts are performed with short rest periods between bouts. Hellebrandt

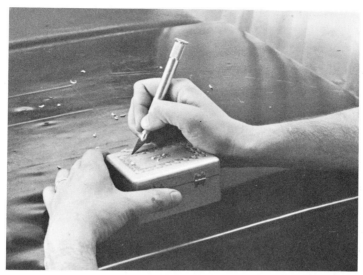

Figure 16–26 Chip carving requires strong contraction of the fingers and thumb and fixation of the wrist by co-contraction of the extensors and flexors.

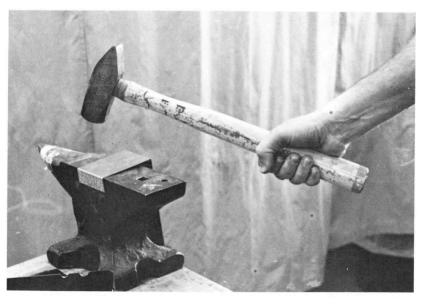

Figure 16–27 The use of a hammer or mallet in occupational therapy provides excellent exercise for muscles of the hand, wrist and arm. The resistance to muscular contraction varies with the weight of the hammer.

and Houtz found that such exercises three times weekly for eight weeks increased performance to 300 per cent of the initial value.[32] Such exercises for shoulder depressors, hip extensors or combined hip and knee extensors are useful for increasing the endurance of patients who ambulate with crutches.

Whenever possible, multiple muscles should be exercised in the same endurance activity. Rowing or bicycling provides such an opportunity. Stair climbing is excellent to increase the endurance of the lower extremities and also the cardiorespiratory system, but it must be used with caution for patients who have cardiac disease.

Occupational therapy provides a variety of activities useful to develop endurance, especially of the upper extremities. The adapted floor loom may be used to develop the endurance of the shoulders and arms[33] (Fig. 16-25). Woodworking, sawing, planing and sanding develop endurance of the hands, arms and trunk. Printing on a platen press may be adapted to develop endurance in the trunk and extremities. Patients who work while standing develop endurance of the muscles of the trunk and lower extremities. Patients who work while sitting on a bench without trunk support develop both balance and endurance of the muscles of the trunk.

Endurance of the fingers and wrists can be increased by leather or metal stamping, chip carving (Fig. 16-26) and clay wedging. Wielding a mallet or hammer provides good exercise for the muscles of the hand and wrist (Fig. 16-27). It is important in directing the patient in the selection of these activities to be certain that prolonged repetition of the desired activity is required so that endurance may be developed.

ISOKINETIC EXERCISE

The usual muscular contraction varies in length, force, and rate of shortening of the muscle. In order to analyze muscular contractions, it is necessary to stabilize the variables. Many studies have been reported of isometric or isotonic contractions. Recently an apparatus has been described which maintains the speed of motion constant, or isokinetic, independently from the force applied,[34] so that the effects of the speed of contraction may be studied on patients in a clinical setting.

A. V. Hill in 1922,[35] studying the speed and efficiency of contraction of the elbow flexors, showed that at maximal voluntary effort the speed of shortening decreased as the resistance increased. Fenn, Brody and Petrilli[36] calculated that when the rate of shortening of a muscle increased 10 per cent of the length of the muscle per second the maximal tension decreased 3.1 per cent. A logarithmic relationship between speed of shortening and maximal force exerted has been found, a relationship which indicates that chemical response time rather than viscous resistance is the factor limiting speed.[37]

Scudder[38] compared the maximal torques produced by flexion or extension of the knee during isometric contraction at four selected angles to the maximal torque curves throughout the range from 80 to 180 degrees during isokinetic contractions at five different speeds. Isometrically, maximal extensor torque occurred at 120 degrees while maximal flexor torque occurred at 150 degrees. The muscles exerted maximal force during isometric contraction and the force diminished as the speed increased (Fig. 16-28). The angle at which the maximal torque was exerted varied little with changes in the speed of isokinetic contraction.

During maximal effort through multiple cycles of isokinetic extension and flexion of the knee, uniform smooth torque curves were recorded, which varied in amplitude with the angle of the knee (Fig. 16-29). The maximal torque for flexion or for extension occurred at a constant angle of the joint. The maximal force that could be exerted diminished as the rate of motion increased.

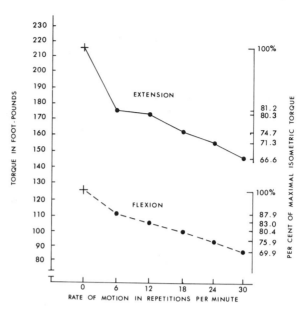

Figure 16–28 Maximal torques produced during isometric and isokinetic contractions of the knee extensors and flexors by normal young men, recorded as foot-pounds of torque and as per cent of maximal isometric torque. Maximal torque decreased as speed of motion increased.[38] (+ Isometric; • Isokinetic.)

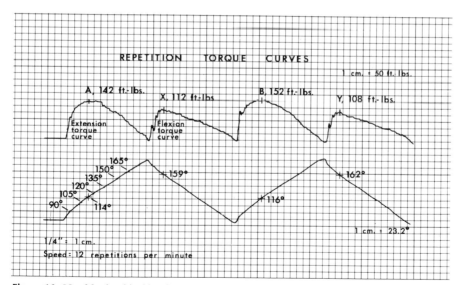

Figure 16–29 Maximal isokinetic torque curves of knee extensors and flexors during reciprocal motion of the knee through the range from 80° to 180° at a rate of 12 repetitions per minute. Maximal extensor torque was exerted at 115°. Maximal flexor torque was exerted at 160°.

Isokinetic motion allows concentric contractions to be performed at a controlled rate—a technique which helps to develop a smooth coordination pattern. If there are variations in muscular strength through the range of motion, these are recorded. Pain occurring in the range of motion is signaled by a sudden decrease of force at that point. However, if the force is decreased it may be possible to complete the motion without pain. Since the mechanism can start, stop or reverse at any point in the range, it is possible to use isokinetic exercise as an active, recorded exercise to increase range of motion as well as to increase coordination, strength or endurance.

EXERCISES TO TEACH RELAXATION

Anxiety produces a state of tension which causes increased activity in the central nervous system and affects many systems. The neuromuscular system responds by prolonged muscular contraction causing discomfort in muscles and joints, neckache and headache. As a result of the discomfort produced by prolonged muscular contraction, secondary reflex effects develop. The anxiety and tension of the patient are increased. Hyperventilation frequently occurs. Effective reversal of these secondary effects may be achieved by teaching the patient awareness of muscular tensions and how to control and inhibit them.

Technique of Relaxation Exercises

Relaxation is taught in a quiet semidarkened room with the patient comfortably positioned on a treatment table or bed. A small pillow should be placed under the head and another pillow should be placed under the knees to relax the hip and knee musculature. The feet should be supported so that the muscles in the legs can relax. Constricting garments should be loosened.

Breath control by prolonged slow breathing using proper diaphragmatic and abdominal coordination together with intercostal breathing is taught. The patient is taught to exhale slowly through the teeth to emphasize awareness of breathing rate and breath control. As the patient gains control of breathing in the fully relaxed position, he then begins to practice breathing while sitting or standing.

Awareness of muscular contraction in the extremities is taught by having the patient flex and extend each joint in the extremity, feeling the difference between tightness and relaxation of the contracting muscles.

Functional muscle groups at each joint are considered individually in the alternate tensing and relaxation so that the patient becomes fully aware of muscular activity in each region of the extremity. The patient should perceive the tenseness of the muscle, rather than any tension, position or motion of a joint. As the patient becomes aware of the sensations associated with a muscular contraction, he becomes able to initiate or inhibit that contraction.[39]

Electromyographic monitoring by cutaneous or intramuscular electrodes may be used to indicate whether complete relaxation has occurred. This monitoring provides auditory reinforcement of perception of tension or relaxation and hastens learning.

Following a strong voluntary contraction, the patient is asked to relax and feel the difference between contraction and relaxation. Then progressively weaker contractions are alternated with complete inhibition of muscular activity so that the extremity becomes fully relaxed. Dropping of the completely limp arm or leg is one method used to demonstrate the difference between partial contraction and relaxation.

The sequence of training is applied to all four extremities, to the shoulders by shrugging and relaxing, to the chest by tightening and relaxing the pectoral muscles, to the back by arching and relaxing and to the facial muscles by contracting and relaxing the muscles about the mouth and eyes and on the forehead.

The patient should be instructed that selective muscular relaxation is possible at the same time that a person is thinking or carrying on an activity. It is not necessary for the mind "to become a perfect blank" nor for the person to forego all activity in order to inhibit muscular tension. Even in the initial training the patient will soon observe that the muscles may be relaxed even though the mind remains active. However, disturbing stimuli or ideas make relaxation more difficult. In spite of this, the patient can learn to relax his muscles to avoid prolonged muscular tension even during periods of active cerebration.

When the patient is able to inhibit muscular contraction adequately in the various segments of the body while recumbent, he is taught to reproduce the same relaxation when sitting in a fully supporting arm chair, and later when sitting in a straight chair.

Through controlled relaxation the individual learns to relax the muscles which do not need to be used for a specific activity and thereby decreases the energy used during ordinary activity. As a result he is less fatigued by his work. Selective relaxation of the unneeded muscles during activity avoids the pain arising secondary to prolonged muscular tension.

For the tense patient, the sessions may have to be repeated a number of times before the patient learns to relax completely. Patients are instructed to practice this relaxation at home or at work when they become tense during the day or in the evening at bedtime if they have difficulty in relaxing before they go to sleep.

REFERENCES

1. Buck, R. C.: Regeneration of Tendon. J. Path. Bact., *66*:1–18, 1953.
2. Fernando, N. V. P., and Movat, H. Z.: Fibrillogenesis in Regenerating Tendon. Lab. Invest., *12*:214–229, 1963.
3. Lindstedt, S., and Prockop, D. J.: Isotopic Studies on Urinary Hydroxyproline as Evidence for Rapidly Catabolized Forms of Collagen in the Young Rat. J. Biol. Chem., *236*:1399–1403, 1961.
4. Viljanto, J.: Biochemical Basis of Tensile Strength in Wound Healing. An Experimental Study with Viscose Cellulose Sponges in Rats. Acta Chir. Scand. Suppl., *333*:1–101, 1964.
5. Watson-Jones, R.: Fractures and Joint Injuries. Vol. I, 4th Ed. Baltimore, Williams and Wilkins Co., 1952, p. 5.
6. Jackson, D. S., Flickinger, D. B., and Dunphy, J. E.: Biochemical Studies of Connective Tissue Repair. Ann. N. Y. Acad. Sci., *86*:943–947, 1960.
7. Perkins, G.: Rest and Movement. J. Bone Joint Surg., *35B*:521–539, 1953.
8. Kelton, I. W., and Wright, R. D.: The Mechanism of Easy Standing by Man. Aust. J. Exp. Biol. Med. Sci., *27*:505–515, 1949.
9. Kottke, F. J., and Kubicek, W. G.: Relationship of the Tilt of the Pelvis to Stable Posture. Arch. Phys. Med., *37*:81–90, 1956.
10. Mundale, M. O., Hislop, H. J., Rabideau, R. J., and Kottke, F. J.: Evaluation of Extension of the Hip. Arch. Phys. Med., *37*:75–80, 1956.
11. Lippmann, R. K.: Arthropathy Due to Adjacent Inflammation. J. Bone Joint Surg., *35A*:967–979, 1953.
12. Mennell, J.: The Science and Art of Joint Manipulation. Vol. I: The Extremities. 2nd Ed. Philadelphia, The Blakiston Co., 1949, pp. 51–69.

13. Simard, T. G., and Basmajian, J. V.: Methods in Training the Conscious Control of Motor Units. Arch. Phys. Med., *48*:12-19, 1967.
14. Herman, R.: Electromyographic Evidence of Some Control Factors Involved in the Acquisition of Skilled Performance. Amer. J. Phys. Med., *49*:177-191, 1970.
15. Crossman, E. R. F. W.: A Theory of the Acquisition of Speed-Skill. Ergonomics, *2*:153-166, 1959.
16. Mundale, M. O.: The Relationship of Intermittent Isometric Exercise to Fatigue of Hand Grip. Arch. Phys. Med., *51*:532-539, 1970.
17. Müller, E. A.: Influence of Training and of Inactivity on Muscle Strength. Arch. Phys. Med., *51*:449-462, 1970.
18. Mundale, M. O.: The Relationship of Isometric Grip Strength to Isometric Grip Endurance. M. S. Thesis, University of Minnesota, 1964.
19. Hettinger, T., and Müller, E. A.: Muskelleistung und Muskeltraining [Muscular Strength and Muscular Training]. Arbeitsphysiol., *15*:111-126, 1953.
20. Liberson, W. T.: Brief Isometric Exercises. In Licht, S.: Therapeutic Exercise. 2nd Ed. New Haven, Conn., Elizabeth Licht, 1961, pp. 307-326.
21. Müller, E. A.: Training Muscle Strength. Ergonomics, *2*:216-222, 1959.
22. Müller, E. A., and Rohmert, W.: Die Geschwindigkeit der Muskelkraft-Zunahme bei Isometrischen Training. Int. Z. Angew Physiol., *19*:403-419, 1963.
23. Rose, D. L., Radzyminski, S. F., and Beatty, R. R.: Effect of Brief Maximal Exercise on the Strength of the Quadriceps Femoris. Arch. Phys. Med., *38*:157-164, 1957.
24. Hellebrandt, F. A.: Application of the Overload Principle to Muscle Training in Man. Amer. J. Phys. Med., *37*:278-283, 1958.
25. DeLorme, T. L.: Restoration of Muscle Power by Heavy-Resistance Exercises. J. Bone Joint Surg., *27*:645-667, 1945.
26. DeLorme, T. L., and Watkins, A. L.: Technics of Progressive Resistance Exercise. Arch. Phys. Med., *29*:263-273, 1948.
27. McMorris, R. O., and Elkins, E. C.: A Study of Production and Evaluation of Muscular Hypertrophy. Arch. Phys. Med., *35*:420-426, 1954.
28. McGovern, R. E., and Luscombe, H. B.: Useful Modifications of Progressive Resistive Exercise Technique. Arch. Phys. Med., *34*:475-477, 1953.
29. Zinovieff, A. N.: Heavy-Resistance Exercises: The "Oxford Technique." Brit. J. Phys. Med., *14*:129-132, 1951.
30. Wright, D. L., and Sonnenscheins, R. R.: Relations among Activity, Blood Flow and Vascular State in Skeletal Muscle. Amer. J. Physiol., *298*:782-789, 1965.
31. Petrén, T., Sjöstrand, T., and Sylvén, B.: Der Einfluss des Trainings auf die Häufigkeit der Capillaren in Herz- und Skeletmuskulatur [The Influence of Exercise on the Frequency of Capillaries in Cardiac and Skeletal Musculature]. Arbeitsphysiol., *9*:376-386, 1936.
32. Hellebrandt, F. A., and Houtz, S. J.: Mechanisms of Muscle Training in Man: Experimental Demonstration of the Overload Principle. Phys. Ther. Rev., *36*:371-383, 1956.
33. Kooiman, C. A., and Kottke, F. J.: Adapted Floor Loom for Upper Extremity Involvement. Arch. Phys. Med., *37*:358-359, 1956.
34. Thistle, H. G., Hislop, H. J., Moffroid, M., and Lowman, E. W.: Isokinetic Contraction: A New Concept of Resistive Exercise. Arch. Phys. Med., *48*:279-281, 1967.
35. Hill, A. V.: The Maximum Work and Mechanical Efficiency of Human Muscles and Their Most Economical Speed. J. Physiol. (London), *56*:19-41, 1922.
36. Fenn, W. O., Brody, H., and Petrilli, A.: The Tension Development by Human Muscle at Different Velocities of Shortening. Amer. J. Physiol., *97*:1-14, 1931.
37. Fenn, W. O., and Marsh, B. S.: Muscular Force at Different Speeds of Shortening. J. Physiol., *85*:277-297, 1935.
38. Scudder, G. N.: A Study of Torque Produced at Controlled Speeds of Voluntary Motion. M. S. Thesis, University of Minnesota, 1969.
39. Jacobson, E.: You Must Relax. 4th Ed. New York, McGraw-Hill Book Co., Inc., 1957.

Chapter 17

TRANSFERS—METHOD, EQUIPMENT AND PREPARATION*

by Paul M. Ellwood, Jr.

A transfer is a pattern of movements by which the patient moves from one surface to another. This chapter is limited to a discussion of transfers to and from wheelchairs, since these are the earliest and most common types of transfer for the patient with neuromuscular disability. The ingredients of safe and efficient transfers are a combination of physical and perceptual capacities, proper equipment, and techniques that are suited to the patient's abilities. Firm, stable surfaces for the patient to move to and from are required for all transfers. It is also necessary that the patient have the ability to learn motor skills.

ASSISTED TRANSFERS

Techniques for assisted transfers are not demonstrated in this chapter. However, assistance by another person for physical support and reinforcement of learning may be required during early learning, or permanently for more severely disabled patients. In an assisted transfer, the same general techniques

---

*The author is indebted to the staff of Kenny Rehabilitation Institute for the preparation of photographs and drawings used in this chapter.

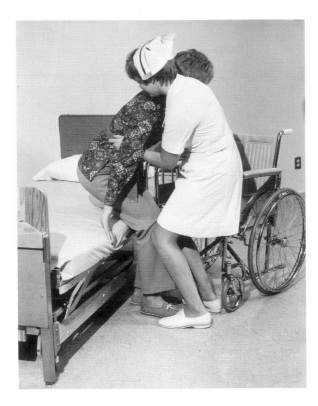

Figure 17–1 Using a belt around the patient's waist, the nurse assists her in a standing transfer.

are used, with the assistant compensating for the patient's inabilities. Providing support at the waist with a transfer belt assures a good grip on the patient without restricting him from using his arms (Fig. 17–1).

STANDING TRANSFERS

Physical Requirements. The unassisted standing transfer requires good sitting balance without postural hypotension; the ability to maintain the hip and knee in a position of extension by means of voluntary muscle contraction, long leg braces, or extensor spasticity; reasonably strong shoulder depressors and adductors, elbow flexors and extensors; and, preferably, hand and wrist function on one side.

Preparing the Patient for Standing Transfers. Activities helpful in preparation for standing transfers are sitting on the edge of the bed without making a transfer; daily use of the standing bed, followed by actual standing at the parallel bar and practice in locking the knee; exercises designed to strengthen hip and knee extensors, shoulder depressors and adductors and elbow and wrist extensors on the normal side; and mat work and bed activities to improve the ability to roll, balance and shift weight.

Teaching Transfers. The process of teaching the patient to make a transfer with assistance is begun as soon as he is able to balance in the sitting position. Patients should be taught in short sequences and they should master each step before proceeding to the next. Even patients with no verbal language can be taught to transfer by repetition and demonstration. Visual motor-perceptual defects may prevent motor learning.

Technique.   Most transfers are made toward the more normal or stronger side, regardless of the cause of the disability. This text uses as an example a hemiplegic patient, but the principles set forth apply to any patient who can attain a stable standing position during the course of his transfer.

BED TO WHEELCHAIR TRANSFER

Equipment.   The necessary equipment includes a stable bed approximately the same height as the wheelchair (a short side rail attached at the head end of the bed is optional) and a wheelchair with brakes and detachable footrests. For the hemiplegic patient, the footrest on the normal side should be removed.

Layout.   The wheelchair is on the patient's normal side; it is slightly angled toward the foot of the bed for the transfer out of bed (Fig. 17–2) and toward the head of the bed for the transfer into bed. The footrest adjacent to the bed is removed or swung aside.

Coming to a Sitting Position.   The patient begins the sequence lying in the center of the bed. With her normal hand, she picks up her involved arm at the wrist and places the forearm across her abdomen (Fig. 17–3).

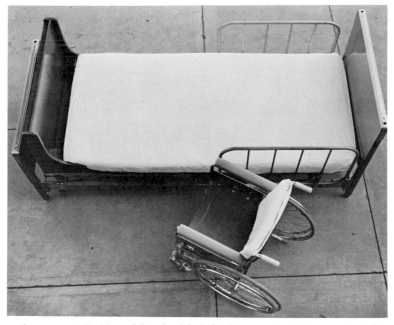

Figure 17–2   Position of the wheelchair for the standing transfer out of bed.

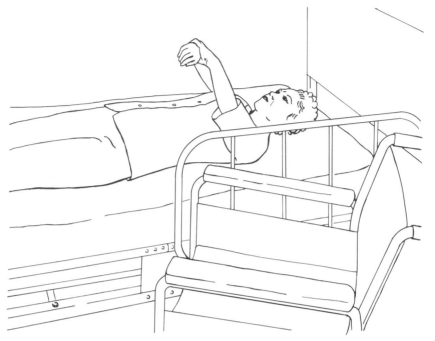

Figure 17–3   The patient moves her involved arm in preparation for coming to a sitting position.

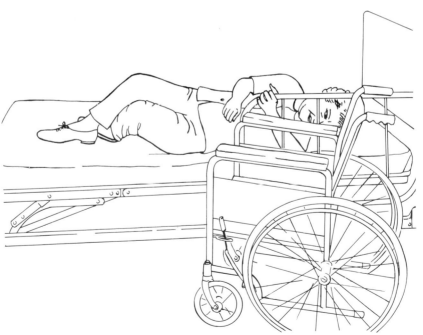

Figure 17–4   She moves her involved foot and leg, grasps the side rail and turns onto her normal side.

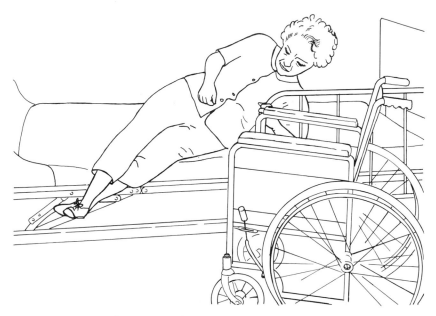

Figure 17–5   She swings into a sitting position.

The patient places her normal foot under the knee of her involved leg and slides her foot down the leg to her ankle. She then partly flexes and lifts her involved leg with her normal foot and leg. Keeping the same foot-support position, she grasps the side rail with her normal hand and, rolling her legs toward her normal side, turns onto her side (Fig. 17–4).

Then, as she moves her legs over the edge of the bed, she grasps and pulls on the side rail and swings herself to a sitting position (Fig. 17–5). She makes full use of gravity and momentum by performing these motions in one unit. She then uncrosses her feet and places them firmly on the floor to maintain balance.

Coming to a Standing Position and Completing the Transfer. From her sitting position at the edge of the bed, the patient locks the brakes on both sides of the wheelchair, locking the rear brake first. By leaning her trunk forward and pushing down at the same time with her normal hand and foot, she moves forward toward the edge of the bed. She then flexes her normal knee more than 90 degrees and moves her normal foot slightly behind the involved foot so that her feet will be free to pivot. Grasping the side rail (or the middle of the farther armrest of the wheelchair if balance is poor), the patient is now in a position for standing (Fig. 17–6).

She moves her trunk forward, pushes down with her normal arm, and, bearing most of her weight on the normal leg, comes to a standing position (Fig. 17–7).

She moves her hand to the middle of the far arm of the wheelchair and pivots on her feet, bringing herself into a position to sit down (Fig. 17–8). After sitting down in the chair, she adjusts her sitting position, unlocks the brakes, lifts her involved foot with her normal foot and backs the wheelchair away

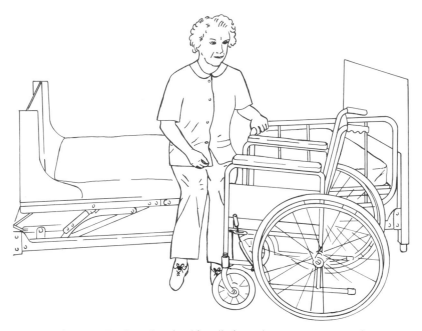

Figure 17–6   Grasping the side rail, the patient prepares to stand.

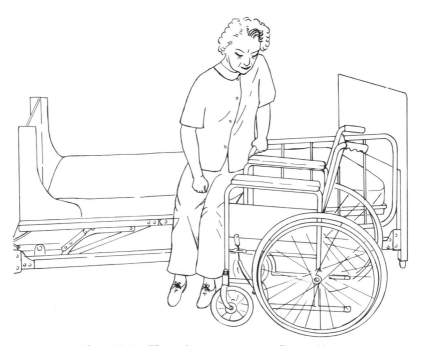

Figure 17–7   The patient comes to a standing position.

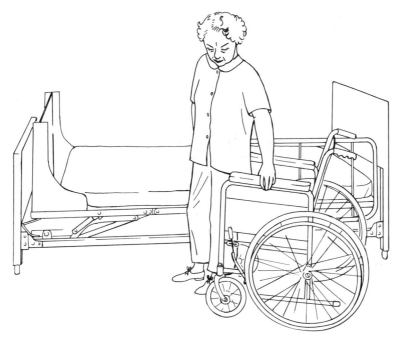

Figure 17–8 Grasping the far arm of the wheelchair, she pivots and prepares to sit down.

from the bed. Finally she swings the footrest into position and, lifting her involved leg with her normal hand, places her foot on the footrest.

The Standing Transfer from Wheelchair to Low Bed

Again, the transfer is made toward the normal side. The wheelchair faces the head of the bed (Fig. 17-9). After locking the brakes and taking her involved foot off the footrest, the patient swings the footrest out of the way. By leaning forward and pushing down, she moves forward toward the edge of the wheelchair until her feet are under her and her normal foot is slightly behind the involved foot. Holding onto the wheelchair armrest (or the side rail), the patient moves her trunk forward and, bearing her weight on her normal leg and arm, comes to a standing position. After standing erect, she moves her hand to the side rail and pivots on her feet, bringing herself into a position to sit on the bed. Seated on the edge of the bed, she moves the wheelchair away so that she can swing her legs onto the bed and lie down.

Standing Transfer from Wheelchair to Toilet

A special requirement for an unassisted toilet transfer is that the patient be able to manage his clothing.

Equipment. Preferably, the toilet seat is mounted 20 inches from the floor. Raised seats that can be fastened securely to the toilet bowl are available

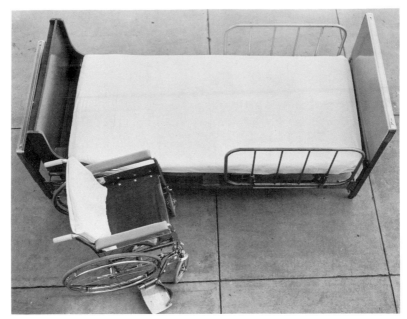

Figure 17–9 Position of the wheelchair for the standing transfer from chair to bed.

Fig. 17–10

Fig. 17–11

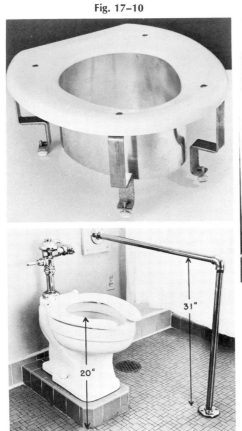

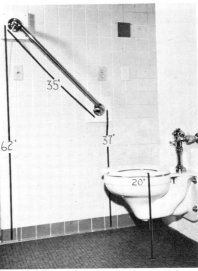

Figure 17–10 A raised toilet seat attached to the toilet bowl facilitates transfer.

Figure 17–11 Position of the 45-degree angle handrail at the toilet for transfers.

Figure 17–12 Position of the right-angle handrail at the toilet.

Fig. 17–12

from hospital supply companies (Fig. 17–10). The placement of a handrail generally depends on the position of the toilet in relationship to the side walls of the bathroom. The rail should be on the same side as the normal extremities when the patient is seated on the toilet. It is mounted on the wall at a 45 degree angle with the lower part of the bar placed 2 inches behind the leading edge of the toilet (Fig. 17–11). The length of the bar may vary from 15 to 35 inches. If for any reason the handrail cannot be attached to the wall beside the toilet, a right-angle rail may be bolted to the floor and wall (Fig. 17–12). The right-angle rail should extend 6 inches in front of the leading edge of the toilet.

Layout.   The chair is angled with the patient's normal side adjacent to the toilet.

Transfer Procedure.   After locking the brakes and removing her foot from the footrest, the patient swings the footrest out to the side (the clothing may be loosened at this time). Pushing down on the armrest with her normal hand, she moves forward in the chair, leans forward (Fig. 17–13), bearing most of her weight on her normal leg, and rises from the chair (Fig. 17–14). Most of her lifting power should come from her normal leg. When standing, she uses the handrail to keep her balance and pivots on her feet until she is standing in front of the toilet. Clothing is lowered and she sits down on the toilet.

To transfer from the toilet to the wheelchair, she reverses the procedure.

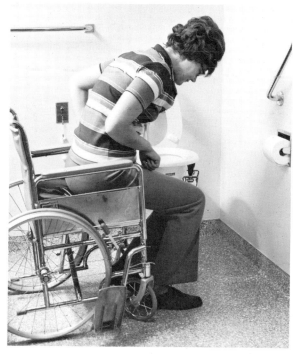

Figure 17–13   The patient has locked her wheelchair brakes, swung the footrest out of the way and moved to the edge of the chair.

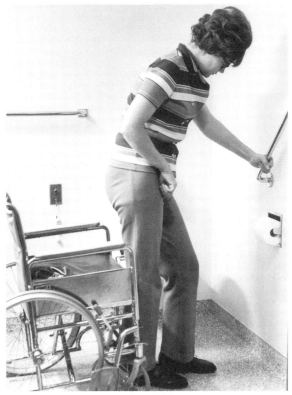

Figure 17–14 She pushes on the armrest to stand and reaches to the wall rail for support while turning and sitting down.

Bathtub Transfer

Getting in and out of the bathtub can be one of the most dangerous procedures for the patient and should always be supervised. Unlike most transfers, which should be made toward the patient's normal side, a tub transfer may be made toward either side, whichever is easiest for the patient.

Layout. A firm wooden chair should be placed beside the tub and another in the tub. These are used until the patient gains enough strength and confidence in his ability to transfer to a 9 inch or 5 inch stool or to the bottom of the tub. The legs of the chair placed in the tub should be shortened so that the seats of both chairs are the same height as the edge of the tub. Rubber tips attached to the bottom of the chair legs on the shorter chair protect the tub and prevent the chair from slipping. A shampoo hose is attached to the faucet. Safety tread tape is used in addition to a bath mat. The bath mat covers the rough surface of the tape and the tape keeps the mat from moving.

Transfer Technique. Pushing down on the chair seat with her normal hand, and on the floor with her normal leg, the patient moves to the edge of the chair and onto the edge of the tub. Then she picks up her involved leg with her normal hand and places it in the tub (Fig. 17–15).

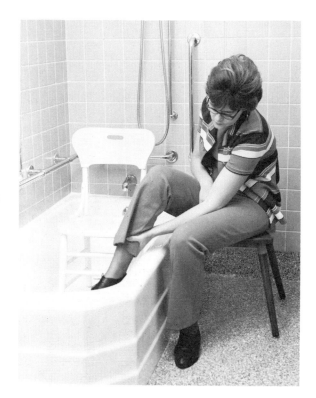

Figure 17–15 The patient places her involved leg in the tub.

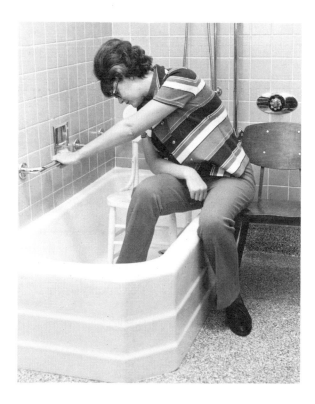

Figure 17–16 Using the wall rail for support, she slides onto the tub chair. She then moves her normal leg into the tub.

Again pushing down with her normal arm and leg, she slides onto the chair in the tub (Fig. 17-16). She then lifts her normal leg into the tub.

SITTING TRANSFERS

There are three basic types of sitting transfers: a lateral sliding transfer requiring the use of a sliding board to bridge the space between the two surfaces; an anterior-posterior sliding transfer; and a lateral transfer without a sliding board.

In the sitting transfers described in this section, paraplegic patients are used as examples. The transfer techniques apply unmodified to patients with other lower extremity disabilities (e.g., double amputees). If upper extremity weakness is present, the assistance of another person may be required for the transfer. The type of transfer used depends upon the patient's ability and the specific situation.

Preparing the Patient for Sitting Transfers. The following activities are valuable in preparation for sliding and swinging transfers: daily use of the standing bed, leading to the ability to stand at 80 degrees without postural hypotension; training in coming to a sitting position and sitting on the edge of the bed without making a transfer (transfer training is begun when the patient can balance in sitting position); progressive resistive exercises designed to strengthen shoulder depressors and adductors, elbow flexors and extensors and wrist extensors and flexors; intensive mat work in the long sitting position to improve the ability to roll and balance and to elevate the hips; and hamstring stretching. For quadriplegic patients with weak triceps, training in locking the elbow is also included.

Bed to Wheelchair Lateral Transfer Using a Sliding Board

Physical Requirements. Good sitting balance and arms powerful enough to lift the hips from the bed (strong shoulder depressors and adductors and elbow and wrist extensors) are necessary. This transfer is seldom accomplished unassisted by patients with lesions above the seventh cervical vertebra. Unusual quadriplegics with lesions at the fifth to sixth cervical segments who have weak triceps can use their biceps to lock their elbows in hyperextension sufficiently well to accomplish a sliding board transfer without assistance.

Equipment. A stable bed approximately the same height as the seat of the wheelchair; a wheelchair equipped with brakes, swinging detachable footrests and detachable armrests; and a sliding board are needed.

Layout. The wheelchair is placed next to the bed and facing the head or foot of the bed at a slight angle. The principle of transfer toward the stronger side applies here also. The armrest is removed from the side next to the bed and is hung on the back of the chair. After the patient is sitting, the sliding board is placed between the chair and the bed (Fig. 17-17).

Coming to a Sitting Position. Paraplegics in the early stages of training and some quadriplegics attain sitting positions in a manner similar to the hemiplegic; i.e., after the patient rolls onto his side, his legs are brought independently or

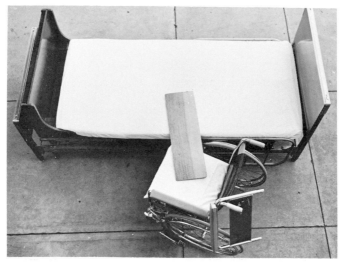

Figure 17–17 Position of the wheelchair and sliding board for a lateral sliding transfer.

Fig. 17–18

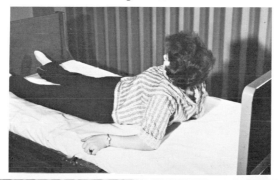

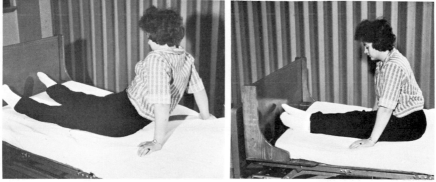

Fig. 17–19   Fig. 17–20

Figure 17–18 To come to a sitting position the patient raises her shoulders by pushing down on her forearms and gradually moving them backward.

Figure 17–19 She straightens her elbows, one at a time.

Figure 17–20 She "walks" her hands forward one at a time until her trunk is forward and she has reached an upright sitting position.

with assistance over the side of the bed. For more advanced patients, particularly those with good sitting balance and loose hamstrings, the following procedure can be used in coming to a sitting position.

The patient raises her head and bends it forward, then places her hands on the bed beside her hips, palms down, elbows flexed. She raises her shoulders by pushing down on her forearms and gradually "walking" her forearms backward (Fig. 17–18).

She transmits her weight to her right forearm and flexes her head to the right as she quickly straightens her left elbow. Keeping her left elbow in this locked position, she shifts her weight to her left arm and straightens her right elbow (Fig. 17–19).

To come to an upright sitting position, she must "walk" her hands forward one at a time until her trunk is forward. She must keep her head and shoulders slightly forward to maintain her balance and to keep from falling backward (Fig. 17–20). She performs lateral and anterior-posterior movements by using her upper extremities to push against the bed to raise her hips off the bed, moving in the desired direction while her hips are raised. She uses her fist rather than the palm of her hand for added height.

Transfer to the Chair. The patient reaches a sitting position on the side of the bed by moving her legs with her hands. She moves toward the edge of the bed, turning herself so that her knees are away from the wheelchair and her hips are toward the wheelchair (Fig. 17–21). As she turns, she must adjust her feet with her hands to bring them directly under her.

The patient leans over onto her right forearm, raising her left buttock off the bed enough to place one end of the sliding board under her (Fig. 17–22). Two corners of the board must rest securely on the bed and two corners must rest on the wheelchair seat or the board may slip or break.

Using her upper extremities for balance and movement, the patient carefully moves laterally across the sliding board into the wheelchair (Fig. 17–23). She then leans over onto her left forearm to raise her buttock off the board and removes the sliding board.

She replaces the armrest on the wheelchair and swings the left footrest into place. After placing her left foot on the footrest, she unlocks the brakes and moves away from the bed. Finally she swings the right footrest into place and places her right foot on the footrest. When the patient becomes adept at using the sliding board, she may be able to progress to transferring without it. The movement would then be performed by using her upper extremities to boost her hips short distances rather than by sliding.

Bed to Wheelchair: Anterior-Posterior Sliding Transfer

Physical Requirements. This transfer requires loose hamstrings and slightly more strength, particularly in the elbow extensors, and better balance than the lateral transfer.

Equipment. A bed that can be immobilized and set at approximately the same height as the wheelchair is needed.

Layout. The wheelchair is braked and placed with the front of the seat directly against the bed and the footrests are swung aside (Fig. 17–24).

Fig. 17–21   **Fig. 17–23**

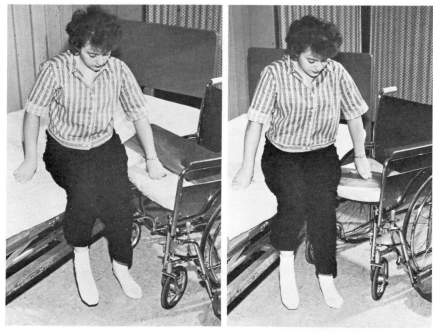

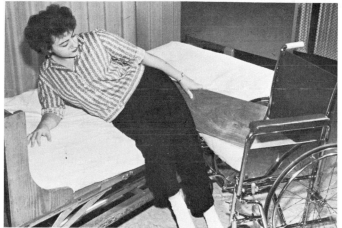

Fig. 17–22

Figure 17–21   She moves her legs over the side of the bed with her arms and slides to the edge of the bed in position for the sliding transfer to the wheelchair.

Figure 17–22   Leaning on her right forearm, the patient places one end of the sliding board under her.

Figure 17–23   She moves across the sliding board to the wheelchair.

Transfer Techniques.   During the entire transfer, the patient keeps her head and shoulders slightly forward to maintain her balance and prevent her from falling backward. She moves her legs to the side of the bed away from the wheelchair by moving one leg at a time with her hands.

By pushing with her fists, the patient moves sideways and backward,

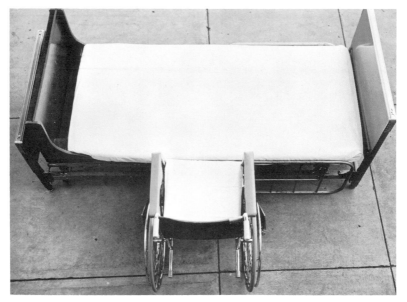

Figure 17–24   Position of the wheelchair for the anterior-posterior sliding transfer.

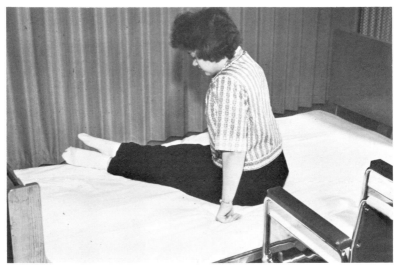

Figure 17–25   The patient pushes with her fists to move into position for the anterior-posterior transfer.

moving each leg and hip alternately to bring her hips close to the wheelchair (Fig. 17-25).

When the patient is near the edge of the bed, she reaches behind her, places her hands on the middle of the wheelchair armrests and lifts herself gently back into the wheelchair (Fig. 17-26). It is for this stage of the maneuver that strength in the elbow extensors is essential.

She moves the chair away from the bed until only her heels are resting on the edge of the bed. She locks her brakes; then using the armrests for support, the patient leans to each side to swing the footrests into place (Fig. 17-27) and

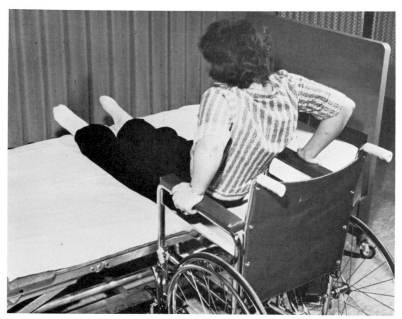

Figure 17–26   Grasping the middle of the wheelchair armrests, she lifts herself into the chair.

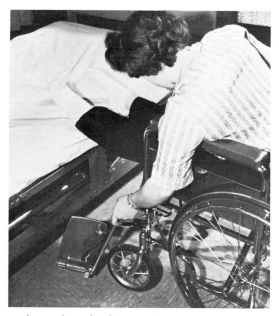

Figure 17–27   The patient swings the footrests into place and positions her feet on them.

carefully places her feet on the footrests, watching to see that they are properly positioned. To get back into bed, she reverses the procedure.

Sitting Toilet Transfers

Equipment. It is recommended that the toilet seat be approximately the same height as the wheelchair seat. In a rehabilitation center where many patients need a higher toilet, the fixture may be installed at a height of 20 inches. When a standard toilet seat 16 inches high is the only one available, a securely fastened raised toilet seat may be used (see Fig. 17-10).

Layout. Depending upon the space in the bathroom, the patient should position the wheelchair parallel or at an angle to the toilet. If space does not permit the use of the wheelchair in the bathroom, an ordinary sturdy wooden straight-back chair with small casters or gliders may be used instead of the wheelchair, provided the patient has sufficient balance to manage a chair without the support of armrests.

Transfer Technique. The patient lifts his feet off the footrests, places them on the floor one at a time, and swings the footrests out of the way. Next, he moves the chair until his knee is as close as possible to the toilet. He locks the wheelchair brakes (Fig. 17-28).

He shifts his hips so that he is sitting sideways on the chair and moves his legs so that his knees are away from the toilet (Fig. 17-29). He unlocks the brakes and moves the wheelchair as close as possible to the toilet. Then he relocks the brakes (Fig. 17-30). This final moving of the wheelchair is an important clue to a good transfer: it eliminates the space between the wheelchair seat and the toilet seat, thus reducing the distance the patient must cross. At this point, while he still has the support of the wheelchair armrests, the patient loosens his trousers and, by leaning from side to side, gradually works them under his buttocks to about midthigh.

Next he removes the armrest and places it on the back of the chair so that it will be within easy reach. He places one hand on the opposite side of the toilet seat and the other hand on the wheelchair seat. He uses his upper extremities to raise his hips and move toward the toilet (Fig. 17-31).

Several moves may be needed to complete the transfer. When the transfer procedure is completed, the patient must position his lower extremities.

Tub Transfers

Caution: When the patient has lost sensation to pain and temperature, the water temperature must be checked.

Equipment and Layout. See the bath tub transfer on page 438.

Transfer Technique. The patient transfers from a wheelchair to a straight chair next to the tub. Using his hands, he lifts each leg into the tub. He then straightens his knees and directs his feet toward the end of the tub so that his legs will move forward as he lowers himself into the tub. This is essential to a safe and efficient transfer. The patient positions his hands on the seat of the chair and on the handrail. Sometimes the edge of the tub may be used instead of a rail. Keeping his head and upper trunk forward, he gently lowers his body into the tub (Fig. 17-32). Gradual flexion of the elbows gives better control.

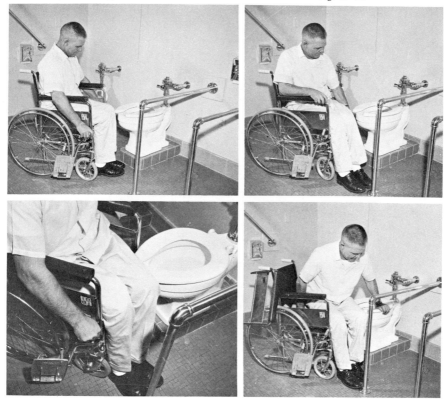

Fig. 17–28 ·   Fig. 17–29

Fig. 17–30   Fig. 17–31

Figure 17–28   For the lateral transfer to the toilet the patient swings the footrests to the side and moves the wheelchair so that his knee is close to the toilet.

Figure 17–29   The patient moves so that he is sitting sideways on the wheelchair.

Figure 17–30   He then moves the wheelchair as close as possible to the toilet.

Figure 17–31   Removing the armrest and placing one hand on the opposite side of the toilet seat, the patient lifts himself to the toilet seat.

The Lateral Sitting Transfer Without Sliding Board — Bed to Wheelchair

Physical Requirements.   This transfer method can be used only by paraplegics with exceptionally good shoulder depressors and abductors as well as good balance. The patient must have the ability to lift his buttocks off the bed and move himself from the bed to the wheelchair in one motion. Male paraplegics who develop very strong upper extremities may even be able to transfer to different levels with ease.

Layout.   The wheelchair is set at a 45 degree angle next to the bed. For close placement, the footrests are swung aside. Very strong patients find this maneuver unnecessary.

Transfer Techniques.   The patient comes to a sitting position on the side of the bed. She turns so that her knees are away from the wheelchair and her hips

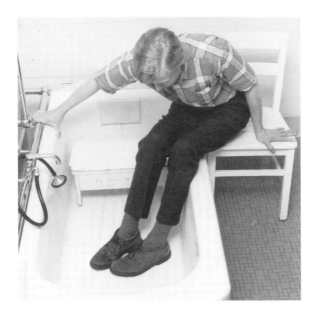

Figure 17–32 After placing his feet in the bathtub, the patient, using the handrail and the seat of the chair, lowers himself to a stool in the tub.

are directed toward the wheelchair. She adjusts her legs to bring her feet directly under her. She moves her hand to the middle of the farther armrest. By pushing down with her upper extremities, she raises herself off the bed and swings in one motion to the wheelchair (Fig. 17–33). She turns her trunk as she lowers herself into the chair.

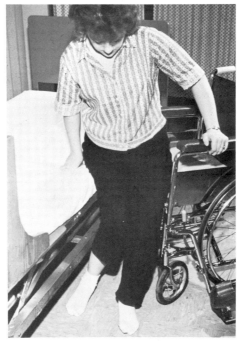

Figure 17–33   The patient pushes up on her arms to lift her buttocks from the bed to the wheelchair.

Car Transfers

Physical Requirements.   This is an advanced transfer and can be accomplished unassisted only by patients with strong upper extremities.

Transfer Techniques.   There are several methods by which patients can make a car transfer. If the patient wears long leg braces or has sufficient extensor spasticity or one strong leg, he may be able to perform a standing transfer in which he stands, pivots and sits on the edge of the car seat. If the windows are rolled down, he can grasp the window opening for support during the transfer.

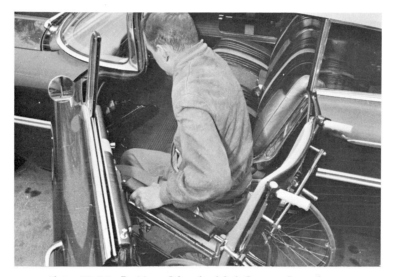

Figure 17–34   Position of the wheelchair for transfer to the car.

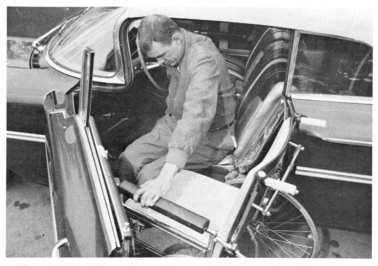

Figure 17–35   The patient performs a swinging transfer to the car seat.

If the car door opens wide enough, the wheelchair can be placed directly facing the seat of the car. The patient's legs can be placed on the seat of the car and the patient can then slide forward into the car. This method is exactly the same as the one described for the anterior-posterior transfer from the wheelchair to the bed. A wide sliding board facilitates this transfer, particularly for the bilateral lower extremity amputee with prostheses.

The wheelchair can be placed at an angle to the car and the patient may be able to perform a swinging transfer, moving to the side (Figs. 17–34 and 17–35). This again is the same procedure that is so frequently used for bed or chair transfers except that there is a wider space between the wheelchair seat and the car seat. If the patient does not have sufficient strength to bridge this gap, a sliding board 28 to 34 inches long may be used. A completely independent transfer includes the ability to bring the wheelchair into the car after the transfer has been made and to remove the wheelchair before transferring out of the car.

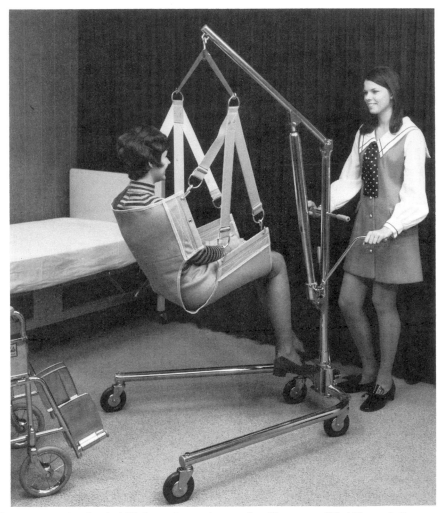

Figure 17–36   Mechanical lift for assistance in transfer. (Courtesy of Ted Hoyer & Company.)

LIFTS

For patients who cannot accomplish a transfer without extensive assistance, the various hydraulic or mechanical lifts have been found to be very effective (Fig. 17-36). A properly trained small woman, using these devices, can successfully lift and transfer a man more than twice her size. Family members or attendants should be trained to use such equipment if excessive lifting is required to assist a transfer. The rehabilitation center should have lifts available for training demonstrations.

REFERENCES

1. Audiovisual Aids Utilized in Teaching Rehabilitation Nursing. New York, Educational Services Division, American Journal of Nursing Company, 1970.
2. Flaherty, P., and Jurkovich, S.: Transfers for Patients with Acute and Chronic Conditions. Minneapolis, American Rehabilitation Foundation, 1970.
3. Fowles, B. H.: Syllabus of Rehabilitation Methods and Techniques. Cleveland, Stratford Press Co., 1963.
4. Lawton, E. B.: Activities of Daily Living for Physical Rehabilitation. New York, McGraw-Hill Book Company, Inc., 1963, Chapter 3.
5. Narrow, B. W.: A Hydraulic Patient Lifter. Amer. J. Nurs., *60:*1273–1275, 1960.
6. Rusk, H. A.: Rehabilitation Medicine. 2nd Ed. St. Louis, The C. V. Mosby Company, 1964, Chapter 6.

Chapter 18

PRESCRIPTION OF WHEELCHAIRS

by Paul M. Ellwood, Jr.

Whenever a person must spend much of his time in a wheelchair and whenever it is to be maneuvered by the patient rather than by other persons, a wheelchair prescription is a must. The prescription of wheelchairs by physicians is analogous to the prescription of drugs and requires attention to many of the same factors. The most important considerations include patient size, body weight, safety, diagnosis, prognosis, transfer technique, mode of propulsion, style of living and cost. Wheelchair features can be selected to assist the patient in these individual matters. A rehabilitation nurse or physical therapist may be able to prescribe a wheelchair capably, but the physician should make sure that such persons are knowledgable about both the patient and the types of basic chair variations available.

Since hundreds of possible combinations of wheelchair features are available, many extended care facilities and rehabilitation units have found it essential to use a special form to ensure complete, rapid and accurate wheelchair prescriptions (Fig. 18-1). Since a wheelchair is a costly item for the patient, it is imperative that his chair have only those features that are necessary to serve him optimally.

The major wheelchair manufacturers publish excellent catalogues which describe features and dimensions available on their chairs. Since wheelchairs are fitted to patients, not patients to wheelchairs, a rehabilitation facility should have available a group of sample chairs of different sizes with varied special features, such as detachable armrests and footrests and reclining backs. In this way, the patient and the staff can evaluate a wheelchair before actual purchase for an individual. If a variety of chairs are not available for trial, a wheelchair

```
                    WHEELCHAIR PRESCRIPTION

 Name _____ Date Ordered _____

 Address _____

 To Whom Billed _____ Dealer _____

 Brand Name _____ Model _____

 Size:  Adult _____           Wheels - 24":   36 spokes _____
        Junior _____
        Large child _____      Tires - 24":  Regular _____
        Small child _____                   Pneumatic _____
        Special _____

 Type:  Fixed back _____
          Added Height_____    Axle:  Regular _____ Heavy duty _____
        Semi-reclining _____
        Full reclining _____    Handrims:
        Amputee _____        Regular _____
                                     Vertical projections - No. _____
 Brakes:  Lever _____              Other _____
          Toggle _____
                                  Front Casters:  8" regular _____
 Detachable Footrests:                            8" semi-pneumatic _____
          Lift off _____
          Button _____        Cushion:   Seat: 2"____ 3"____ 4"____
          Swinging _____
          Elevating _____                 Horseshoe _____
                                           Measurement _____
 Footplates:  Regular _____              Protective Covering _____
             Large _____                 Other _____

 Heel Loops:  Right _____ Left _____
                                 Back:  1" _____  2" _____
 Armrests:  Padded _____
            Fixed _____       Measurement _____
            Removable _____      Protective Covering _____
                Regular _____
                Adjustable _____
                desk_____       Color of Upholstery: _____

 Additional instructions:




 Ordered By _____, M.D.
```

Figure 18–1   Wheelchair prescription form.

sales representative should be consulted about arranging to borrow or rent a chair for a brief period of time.

IMPORTANT FACTORS IN WHEELCHAIR SELECTION

Experience has shown that certain wheelchair features are virtually a requirement for a majority of handicapped persons. These include (1) a high degree of durability, (2) ease of folding, (3) easy propulsion, (4) brakes, (5) removable footrests and (6) 8 inch front casters. These are not luxury but essential features for persons who use a wheelchair regularly. The following discussion considers the factors that must be considered for each individual.

The Patient's Size.   Wheelchairs are available in three major sizes: a standard adult size, suitable for most adults; an intermediate or junior chair for

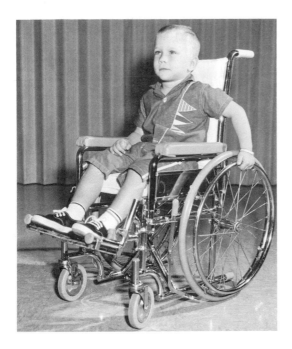

Figure 18–2 Child's wheelchair. (Courtesy of Kenny Rehabilitation Institute, Minneapolis.)

small adults and older children; and a children's size, which is ideal for children up to the age of six years (Fig. 18-2). "Growing chairs" are available for those undergoing the period of rapid growth between ages 6 and 12 years. In determining wheelchair size, the critical dimensions are seat width and depth, the height of the seat from the floor, armrests of a height that allows the patient to rest his forearms comfortably without slumping or excessive shoulder abduction, and adjustable footrests set to provide an ideal distance from the popliteal fossa to the heel. (Figure 18-3 shows typical variations in wheelchair dimensions.) The patient's weight should be distributed over as great an area of skin surface as possible. In rare instances, custom sizes may be necessary.

Safety.   For safety, particularly in making transfers, brakes are required on all chairs. It is essential that the bilateral lower extremity amputee with his higher center of gravity have a chair with more posteriorly placed rear wheels to prevent instability of the chair (see Fig. 18-12). The use of weights placed on the footrests of a regular chair will also compensate for this change in center of gravity. Another important safety measure is the seat belt, which can be attached at the hips, waist, or chest area.

Diagnosis and Prognosis.   The patient's prognosis should be carefully considered in making the proper wheelchair selection. For instance, in progressive muscular dystrophy, future trunk weakness can be anticipated by selecting a chair with a semireclining back. Trunk weakness may be compensated for by a semireclining or reclining back or perhaps by added back height. A head extension is attached to the back of the chair for patients with neck weakness (Fig. 18-4). Patients who have been bedridden for prolonged periods or those with postural hypotension may require a semireclining chair during the early stages of their rehabilitation program. Elevating foot and leg rests are available

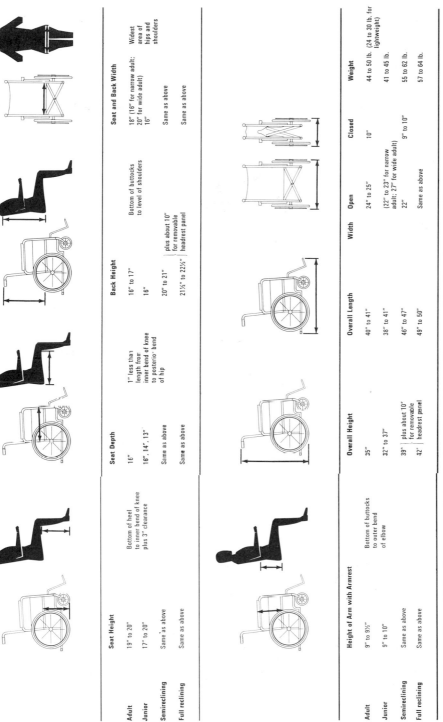

Seat Height

Adult	19" to 20"	Bottom of heel to inner bend of knee plus 3" clearance
Junior	17" to 20"	
Semireclining	Same as above	
Full reclining	Same as above	

Seat Depth

Adult	16"	1" less than length from inner bend of knee to posterior bend of hip
Junior	16", 14", 13"	
Semireclining	Same as above	
Full reclining	Same as above	

Back Height

Adult	16" to 17"	Bottom of buttocks to level of shoulders
Junior	16"	
Semireclining	20" to 21"	plus about 10" for removable headrest panel
Full reclining	21½" to 22½"	

Seat and Back Width

Adult	18" (16" for narrow adult; 20" for wide adult)	Widest area of hips and shoulders
Junior	16"	
Semireclining	Same as above	
Full reclining	Same as above	

Height of Arm with Armrest

Adult	9" to 9½"	Bottom of buttocks to outer bend of elbow
Junior	9" to 10"	
Semireclining	Same as above	
Full reclining	Same as above	

Overall Height

Adult	35"
Junior	32" to 37"
Semireclining	39" plus about 10" for removable headrest panel
Full reclining	42"

Overall Length

Adult	40" to 41"
Junior	38" to 41"
Semireclining	46" to 47"
Full reclining	49" to 50"

Width

	Open	Closed
Adult	24" to 25"	10"
Junior	(22" to 23" for narrow adult; 27" for wide adult)	9" to 10"
Semireclining	22"	
Full reclining	Same as above	

Weight

Adult	44 to 50 lb. (24 to 30 lb. for lightweight)
Junior	41 to 45 lb.
Semireclining	55 to 62 lb.
Full reclining	57 to 64 lb.

Figure 18–3 Common variations in sizes of wheelchairs. (Courtesy of the American Rehabilitation Foundation.)

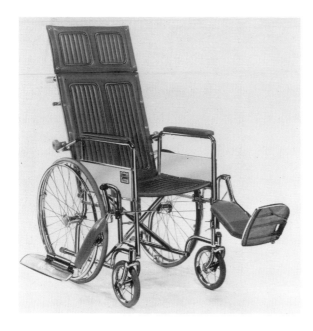

Figure 18–4 Wheelchair with semireclining back and headrest extension for trunk and neck weakness. (Courtesy of Everest & Jennings, Inc., Los Angeles, California.)

for situations in which incomplete knee flexion or dependent edema are problems (Fig. 18–5).

Most patients find that they are more comfortable using a cushion of some type. The presence of sensory loss from the fifth lumbar vertebra downward calls for the use of a foam rubber cushion, preferably 4 inches thick and horseshoe-shaped (Fig. 18–6). Cushions may also be filled with water, resin, gel or air. Seat boards used under cushions can improve lower extremity posture (Fig. 18–7).

Transfer Techniques.   Brakes are necessary for all transfers, and the transfer technique itself dictates the type of armrests and footrests chosen. For anterior sliding transfers, swinging detachable footrests permit placement of

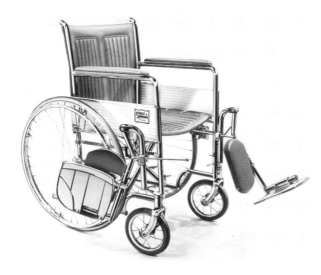

Figure 18–5 Elevating footrest and legrest. (Courtesy of Everest & Jennings, Inc., Los Angeles, California.)

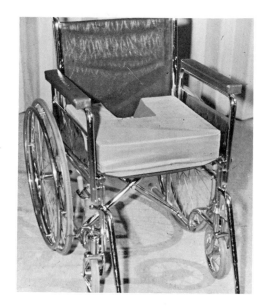

Figure 18–6 Horseshoe-shaped cushion used when there is sensory loss. (Courtesy of Kenny Rehabilitation Institute, Minneapolis.)

the chair closer to the surface to or from which the patient is moving. Lateral transfers (toward the arm of the wheelchair), with or without the use of a sliding board, require detachable arms plus a removable footrest (Fig. 18–8). For a standing transfer, footrests may not be a problem. If they are, a simple detachable footrest is adequate.

Propulsion Techniques. The mode of propulsion influences footrest and hand rim selection. Hemiplegic patients who propel the chair with their normal arm and leg require a detachable footrest on the uninvolved side. Chairs that are equipped with one-wheel drive are necessary only in triplegia, with weak-

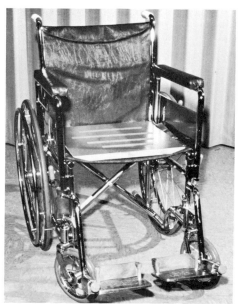

Figure 18–7 Seat board used under cushions. (Courtesy of Kenny Rehabilitation Institute, Minneapolis.)

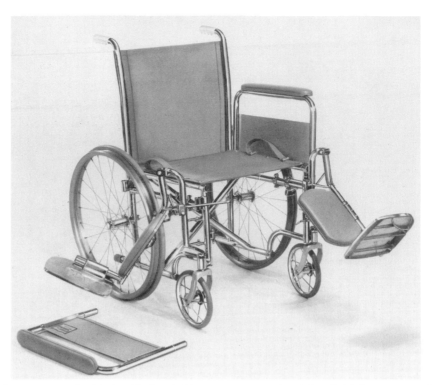

Figure 18–8   Wheelchair with detachable armrest removed and detachable leg rest swung back. (Courtesy of Everest & Jennings, Inc., Los Angeles, California.)

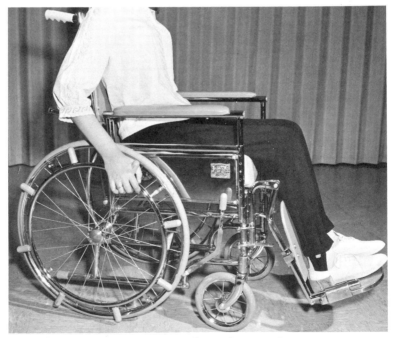

Figure 18–9   Vertical hand rim projections for weak grasp. (Courtesy of Kenny Rehabilitation Institute, Minneapolis.)

ness of both lower extremities and one upper, or in very unusual cases, such as a hemiplegic patient with a lower extremity amputation on the normal side.

For the patient with a poor grasp, as in quadriplegia or arthritis of the hands, vertical projections on the hand rim substantially assist propulsion (Fig. 18-9). Vertical projections (rather than horizontal) are preferred since they do not widen the dimensions of the chair. Battery-powered wheelchairs are available for individuals with minimal arm power or control, who by one means or another can operate a small control stick which activates the wheels. These chairs weigh from 70 to 80 pounds without the batteries and cost $900 and up.

Style of Living.   To circumvent certain architectural barriers of the household, the physician will need specific information from the family in order to prescribe chair modifications. Doorways should be measured to make sure they are wider than the overall open width of the open chair. Special narrowers can be attached to the chair to temporarily narrow its width by 2 to 4 inches (depending on the brand) to permit passage through slightly narrow doorways. Doorways can often be widened by 1 to 2 inches by simply removing inner moldings. In some instances an adult can be comfortably fitted with a junior chair, which is on the average 2 inches narrower than similar full size models. Some brands of junior size wheelchairs, when equipped with removable arms, will often accommodate adults.

Several other important architectural dimensions for wheelchair living are found in the *American Standard Specifications for Making Buildings and Facilities Accessible to, and Usable by, the Physically Handicapped.** This document states, "The average turning space required (180 and 360 degrees) is 60 by 60 inches. . . . The average horizontal working (table) reach is 30.8 inches, and ranges from 28½ inches to 33.2 inches. An individual reaching diagonally, as would be required in using a wall-mounted dial telephone or towel dispenser, would make the average reach (on the wall) 48 inches from the floor."

If ramps are installed for wheelchairs, a 5 degree incline may be lengthy but is most desirable. A recommended slope is not greater than a 1 foot rise in 12 feet. Guard rails are highly recommended on ramps to prevent the patient from slipping off the edge.

If the person's life takes him to areas where the ground is soft or uneven, pneumatic tires can be helpful in maneuvering such surfaces (Fig. 18-10).

Detachable desk arms are available for individuals who need to work closely at low desks and tables. The front 6 inches of the desk armrest are lowered to permit the wheelchair arms to pass under the table top (Fig. 18-11). These armrests can also be reversed. Another type of adjustable armrest is also available. These can be raised and lowered not only to clear under desks and tables but also to adjust for arm comfort and shoulder level of the individual.

It should be kept in mind that table legs or partitions also may inhibit the close approach to a work surface, unless the footrests can be swung aside or detached. A lap board can be placed over the arms of the chair when other adjustments are difficult.

Persons who will give a chair rugged daily use with frequent moves in and out of cars and over curbs and other forms of abuse require either a heavy-duty chair or a regular chair with a heavy-duty axle. When a chair must be

---

*American Standard Specifications for Making Buildings and Facilities Accessible to, and Usable by, the Physically Handicapped. New York, American Standards Association, published by National Society for Crippled Children and Adults, 2023 W. Ogden Avenue, Chicago, Ill. 60612. 1961.

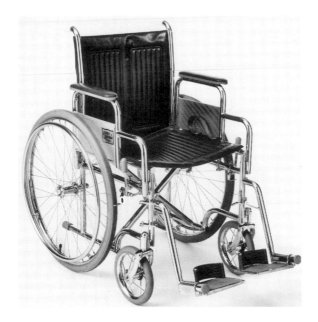

Figure 18–10 Wheelchair with pneumatic tires for use on soft or uneven surfaces. (Courtesy of Everest & Jennings, Inc., Los Angeles, California.)

lifted up and down stairs frequently, or handled by a woman, consideration might be given to a lightweight but slightly less durable steel and aluminum chair, which weighs approximately 20 pounds less than comparable models.

Cost.   Each special feature increases the cost of the chair. In most instances, quality is a function of price, but economy should never be sacrificed for essential individual needs.

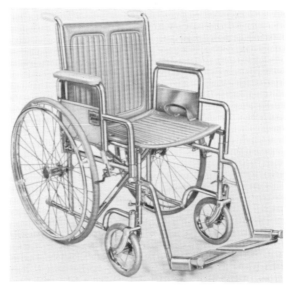

Figure 18–11   Wheelchair with desk arms positioned for close work at low tables. Arms can be reversed for comfort. (Courtesy of Everest & Jennings, Inc., Los Angeles, California.)

SOME TYPICAL WHEELCHAIR PRESCRIPTIONS

Hemiplegia

PATIENT. The chair is for a 170 pound, 5 foot 8 inch, right or left hemiplegic patient who is able to perform a standing transfer with assistance.

PRESCRIPTION. Adult chair, 8 inch front casters, 24 inch rear wheels, regular tires, button-detachable footrests with heel loops, padded armrests, fixed back, and 2 inch cushion for comfort.

Paraplegia

PATIENT. The chair is for a strong, 180 pound, 6 foot, paraplegic man who performs a sitting transfer. He expects to use his chair outside extensively on hard and soft surfaces.

PRESCRIPTION. Adult size wheelchair, 8 inch front casters with semipneumatic tires, 24 inch rear wheels, air cushion tires and heavy-duty axle (or a heavy-duty wheelchair), brakes, swinging detachable footrests with heel loops, padded removable armrests, fixed back, seat board and a special horseshoe cushion (filled with air, gel, water, resin or sponge rubber).

Quadriplegia

The chair is for a small quadriplegic female college student with a lesion at the sixth to seventh cervical segment who uses a sliding board to transfer.

PRESCRIPTION. Junior size, semireclining wheelchair, 8 inch front casters, 24 inch rear wheels, regular tires, hand rim with vertical projections, brakes, swinging detachable footrests with heel loops, adjustable detachable padded arms, seat board, and a special 4 inch horseshoe cushion (filled with air, gel, resin, water or sponge rubber), as shown in Figure 18–6.

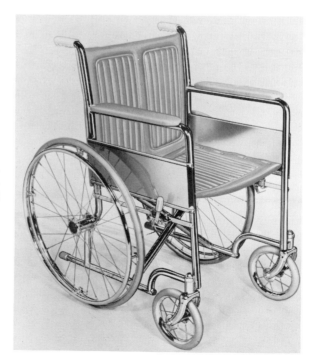

Figure 18–12 Amputee wheelchair. (Courtesy of Everest & Jennings, Inc., Los Angeles, California.)

Amputee

PATIENT.　The chair is for a 5 foot 10 inch, 145 pound, bilateral lower extremity amputee.

PRESCRIPTION.　Narrow adult size amputee chair. Until an amputee chair (Fig. 18-12) is available, place sandbags on the footrests on a regular chair to prevent tipping of the chair due to the patient's altered center of gravity.

SUGGESTIONS FOR PURCHASE OF WHEELCHAIRS FOR INSTITUTIONS

Many institutions use chairs principally to transport non-disabled patients to and from such departments as admitting, x-ray, laboratory, physical therapy and recreational therapy. A lightweight, folding, easy-to-push chair with brakes and a luggage rack and footrests is a good general purpose chair which can be used by a majority of patients.

Once chairs for this requirement have been satisfied, an institution must look further into its needs to serve the kinds of patient who come for care. For a rehabilitation center or extended care facility where patients with a variety of disabilities are served, it is essential to have one or more chairs with brakes, removable armrests and removable footrests. Such removable features permit exchange of parts and versatility within one chair. Certainly orthopedic areas and emergency areas require chairs with reclining back and elevating legrests. While a wheelchair must be individually prescribed for a handicapped person, careful thought must go also into the selection of chairs for an institution in order to prevent excessive expenditure on equipment which does not serve its particular patient population.

REFERENCES

1. Bergstrom, D. A.: Report on a Conference for Wheelchair Manufacturers. Bulletin of Prosthetics Research, Spring, 1965, pp. 60–89.
2. Cicenia, E. F. et al.: Maintenance and Minor Repairs of the Wheelchair. Amer. J. Phys. Med., 35:206, 1956.
3. Fahland, B. B.: Wheelchair Selection—More Than Choosing a Chair With Wheels. Minneapolis, Kenny Rehabilitation Institute, 1967.
4. Fowles, B. H.: Evaluation and Selection of Wheelchairs. Phys. Ther. Rev., 39:525–529, 1959.
5. Goldsmith, S.: Designing for the Disabled, 2nd ed. New York, McGraw-Hill Book Company, 1967.
6. Kamenetz, H. L.: The Wheelchair Book. Springfield, Illinois, Charles C Thomas, 1969.
7. Lawton, E. B.: Wheelchair Prescription, In Lowman, E. W.: Arthritis—General Principles, Physical Medicine, Rehabilitation. Boston, Little, Brown and Company, 1959.
8. Lee, M. H. M., et al.: Wheelchair Prescription. Public Health Service Publication No. 1666, undated. Superintendent of Documents, Washington, D.C. 20402.
9. Lowman, E. W., and Rusk, H. A.: Rehabilitation Monograph XXI: Self-Help Devices, Part 2. The Institute of Physical Medicine and Rehabilitation, New York University Medical Center, 1963.
10. Peizer, E., et al.: Bioengineering Methods of Wheelchair Evaluation. Bulletin of Prosthetics Research, Spring, 1964.

Chapter 19

BED POSITIONING

by Paul M. Ellwood, Jr.

The prevention and treatment of contractures and decubiti through an effective bed positioning program is contingent upon proper equipment, a well trained and well motivated nursing staff and appropriate physician's orders.

THE POSITIONING PRESCRIPTION

The positioning prescription should identify the equipment specifically needed for the positioning program, positions to be used, motions and positions to be avoided and frequency of turning. In addition, it is important to recognize that the patient should assume increasing responsibility for his positioning program. If he is able, the patient should remind the staff when he needs to be turned, know where positioning equipment is kept, actually assist in changing positions and ultimately assume full responsibility.

THE EQUIPMENT FOR EFFECTIVE BED POSITIONING

High-Low Bed. The use of beds that are adjustable to high (30 inches including the mattress) and low (20 inches including mattress) positions is recommended. With the bed in the high position, more comfortable and efficient nursing care and range of motion exercises can be carried out. In the low position, the bed can be set at the ideal height for wheelchair transfers or crutch walking.

Bed Boards. A ¾ inch plywood bed board equal in size to the spring frame is bolted between the spring and mattress (Fig. 19-1). Jointed (Gatch)

463

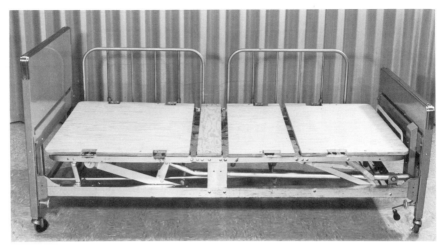

Figure 19-1   Three-quarter inch plywood bed board.

features can be retained by breaking the continuity of the board at the hinge points. Some hospital beds now have a metal panel which substitutes for springs and provides excellent mattress support. Also available are slatted bed boards which have the advantage of flexibility.

Mattresses.   Firmness and durability are sought in mattress selection. Uniform firm support is obtained through a foam rubber mattress. A 4 inch foam rubber mattress made of 34 pound compression ratio material is the firmest available. Urethane foam of the same compression ratio is still undergoing evaluation for rehabilitation uses. The firm support provided by bed board and mattress is especially valuable in preventing hip flexion contractures.

Footboards.   Heel cord contractures are prevented by the use of a footboard. It has been suggested, but not proved, that the footboard provides a valuable source of sensory input to the plantar surface of the feet so that the desirable extensor reflex dominance is maintained and the neuron networks normally involved in the standing position are activated. The board should be ½ inch thick and sufficiently high to keep the bed clothes from contact with the toes. To prevent decubiti over the posterior calcaneus and to facilitate prone positioning without knee flexion, the board is blocked 4 inches away from the end of the mattress (Fig. 19-2).

Short Side Rails.   Side rails are used for safety, moving about, coming to a sitting position and transferring in and out of bed (Fig. 19-3). Commercial short side rails are 33 inches long and should extend 11 inches above the level of the mattress. For most patients, the rails are attached only to the head end of the bed. If side rails are not required for protection, a single short rail is attached at the head end of the bed on the patient's stronger side to which he transfers.

Overhead Trapezes.   Trapezes are rarely necessary to facilitate moving about in bed or for upper extremity exercise. In making unassisted transfers,

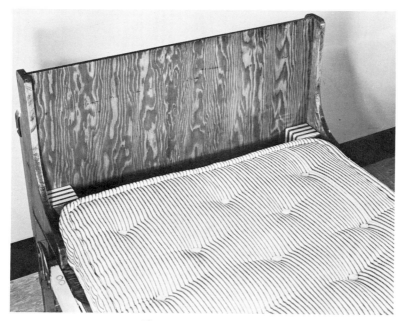

Figure 19–2 Foot board.

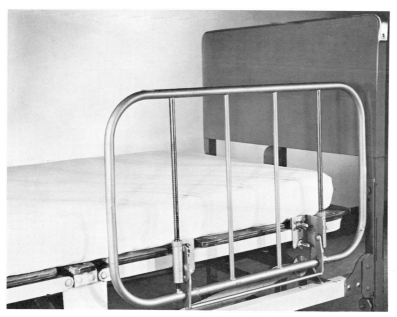

Figure 19–3 Short side rail.

they are not as useful as short side rails. They do simplify nursing care of very large patients or those in casts.

Positioning Frames (Foster, Stryker and Others).   When immobility of the spine is required, a bed consisting of canvas stretched on anterior and posterior frames that can be rotated along their long axes is used. Footboards for frames are often available and should be used. The narrow metal-rimmed canvas surface of the frame can be satisfactorily padded with 1 inch foam rubber covered with plastic. The foam rubber for the trunk section of the prone unit should be wider than the metal frame to protect the shoulders from pressure when the patient's arms are dropped downward for eating or reading. The foam rubber of the lower extremity section of the prone unit should be slightly longer than the canvas frame to protect the front of the patient's ankles. The foam rubber pieces of the supine section should cover the canvas to protect the patient's sacral area when using the bed pan. Arm boards are available for positioning the upper extremities of the quadriplegic patient.

Powered Rotating Frames.   Electrically powered frames which rotate along their short axes can be used to substitute for both canvas frames and standing beds. They permit more comfortable positioning and changes in position by the patient or a single staff member by the operation of remote control switches. They are costly, however, and because of their complexity are more subject to mechanical failure.

Standing Beds.   Electrically or manually controlled beds to elevate patients to the upright position are thought to aid in the reduction of osteoporosis and renal calculi, the maintenance of vascular tone (thus preventing postural hypotension), preservation of morale, and the shifting of weight bearing to relieve pressure in other areas. Postural hypotension owing to pooling in splanchnic and lower extremity veins is prevented in part by the use of scultetus binders and by wrapping the legs with 6 inch elastic bandages. Blood pressure should be taken at frequent intervals by the attendant. No patient on a standing bed should be left unattended. Many patients cannot attain the upright position on the first occasion on the standing bed. A useful routine is to begin at 30 degrees for 30 minutes. When this is readily tolerated, increase by 5 to 10 degree increments. Binders and bandages are progressively eliminated after the patient attains 80 degrees.

Small Positioning Devices.   Most quadriplegic patients will require two trochanter rolls, two shoulder rolls, three hand rolls, two small pillows, six large pillows, 6 inch wide canvas straps and, in the presence of lower extremity abduction spasticity, a 6 inch wide canvas strap lined with soft leather. The application of these devices is described later in this chapter.

THE POSITIONING PROGRAM

Positioning instructions and turning schedules are based on individual patient needs, but certain generalizations can be made about most disabilities that are associated with muscle weakness or joint deformity. In some institutions that serve large numbers of the chronically disabled, it has been found desirable to establish a set of positioning procedures for hemiplegia, quadriplegia and paraplegia. The physician's order then may specify variations from the

TABLE 19–1 SOME COMMON DEFORMING FORCES

Force	Resultant Deformity	Method of Prevention
Gravity	Sagging mattress and springs + gravity = hip flexion contractures	Firm mattress plus bed board, prone position, prone cart
Shape of the extremity surface	Configuration of the ankle and foot + gravity = external rotation of the lower extremity and a tight gastrocnemius	A trochanter roll and footboard
Muscular imbalance	High, above-knee, amputation + strong hip abductors = hip abduction contracture	Prone positioning with leg adducted and internally rotated
Spasticity	Paraplegia + flexor spasticity = hip and knee flexion contractures	Prone position, buttocks plus knees strapped in extension, prone cart, knee lockers during gait training

routine positioning procedure, positions to be avoided and areas to be kept immobilized. Positions are prescribed to overcome certain natural and pathologic forces, to provide a variety of joint positions for maintaining joint range and to place the extremity in a more functional position.

The Supine Position

Lower Extremities. The feet are positioned with the entire plantar surface firmly against the footboard. Contact with the posterior heel is avoided by placing it in the space between the mattress and the footboard which has been created by 4 inch thick blocks. The legs are placed in a neutral position with the toes pointed toward the ceiling (Fig. 19–4). This position is maintained by friction of the feet against the footboard and a cloth roll placed under the greater trochanter (trochanter roll).

The knee and hips are positioned in extension (Fig. 19–5). Perhaps the most critical element of the lower extremity positioning program is the prevention of

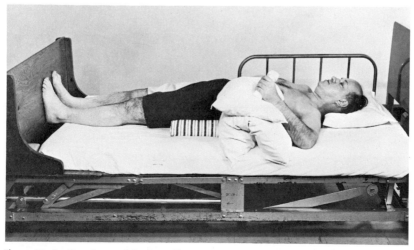

Figure 19–4   Routine positioning of lower extremities, plus one possible arm position.

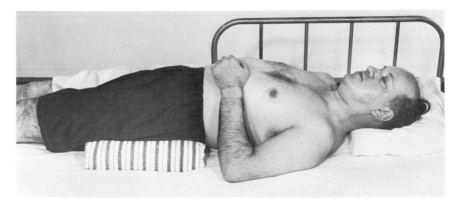

Figure 19–5   Use of trochanter roll in positioning of lower extremities.

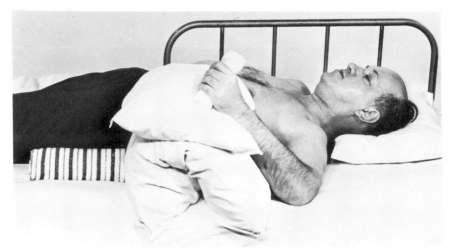

Figure 19–6   Positioning of the upper extremities, position 1.

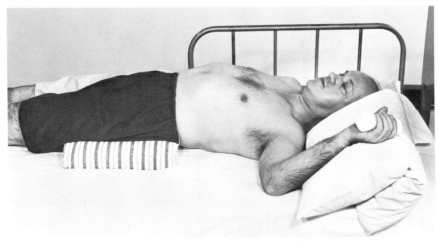

Figure 19–7   Positioning of the upper extremities, position 2.

hip and knee flexion contractures. Hip flexion contractures in the presence of lower extremity weakness are the principal deterrents to ambulation for patients with hemiplegia, paraplegia and above-knee amputations. Stance phase stability of the knee and hip joints requires full extension so that gravitational forces are applied against ligaments and the normal configuration of the joint rather than requiring muscle power.

Upper Extremities.   Nurses should be cautioned to position only within the painless or nonresistive range of motion. Spasticity must, however, be differentiated from other forms of resistance to joint motion.

POSITION 1.   The shoulder is abducted to 90 degrees and slightly internally rotated, the elbow is at 90 degrees and the forearm is partially pronated (Fig. 19-6).

POSITION 2.   The shoulder is abducted to 90 degrees or more and externally rotated to the greatest degree compatible with comfort. The elbow is flexed at 90 degrees and the forearm is pronated (Fig. 19-7).

POSITION 3.   The shoulder is in slight abduction, the elbow extended and the forearm supinated (Fig. 19-8).

Wrist and Hand

POSITION 1.   The wrist is extended, the fingers are partially flexed at the interphalangeal and metacarpal phalangeal joints and the thumb is abducted, opposed and slightly flexed at the interphalangeal joint (Fig. 19-9). Maintenance of these positions is facilitated by the use of a hand roll (Fig. 19-10).

POSITION 2.   This position is similar to position 1 except that the fingers are extended at the interphalangeal and metacarpal phalangeal joints. A palmar positioning splint can be used to maintain this position (Fig. 19-11). The positioning program for the wrist and fingers should be particularly directed to *maintenance of joint motion of the wrist* from neutral to a fully extended position, *a full range of motion in the metacarpal phalangeal joints,* flexion of the interphalangeal joints and opposition of the thumb. To obtain tenodesis grasp in the quadriplegic patient who retains wrist extensor function, arthrodesis of thumb joints and interphalangeal joints to form a three-jawed chuck may be sought.

Side-Lying Position

Hemiplegic patients are most comfortable lying on their uninvolved side. Paraplegics and quadriplegics should be positioned on either side when they can tolerate it. The top leg is placed in a position of flexion at the hip and knee. Through use of pillows, contact with the under leg is avoided. The inner (bottom) arm is externally rotated and partially extended. The outer (top) arm is kept away from the patient's chest (Fig. 19-12).

The Prone Position

The prone position is ordered when pulmonary, cardiac and skeletal status permit. Many patients do not tolerate it well at first. It is highly advantageous in maintaining full extension of the hips and relieving pressure over vulnerable posterior bony prominences that so commonly are sites of decubiti. The prone position also has its vulnerable points such as the skin over the sternum, the iliac spines, the patella and the dorsum of the foot. These areas should be

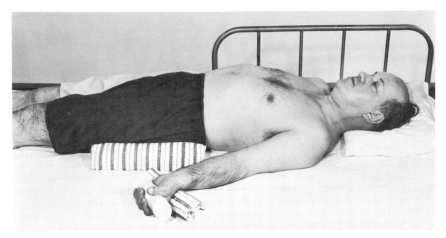

Figure 19–8   Positioning of the upper extremities, position 3.

Fig. 19–9   **Fig. 19–10**

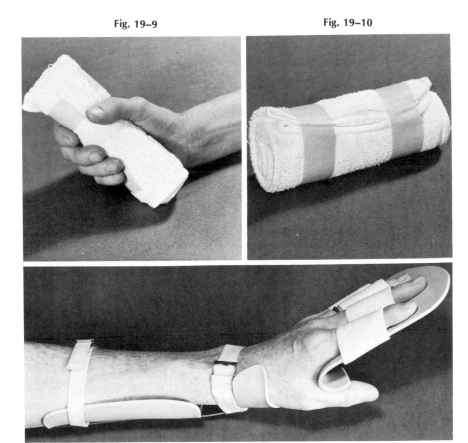

Fig. 19–11

Figure 19–9   Positioning of the wrist and hand, position 1.

Figure 19–10   Hand roll for use in wrist and hand positioning.

Figure 19–11   Palmar positioning splint for use in wrist and hand positioning.

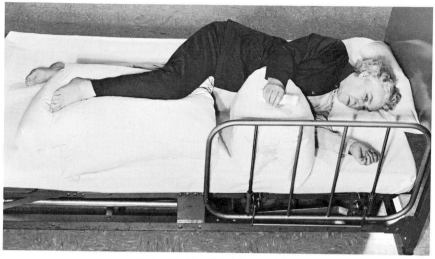

Figure 19–12   Side-lying position.

inspected frequently. Foam rubber can be used above and below the contact points when pressure is producing focal ischemia. Synthetic fibers or sheepskin are also useful to protect the bony prominences. Narrow doughnut-shaped devices should *not* be used. They actually inhibit circulation to ischemic areas.

The prone position (Fig. 19-13) is simply one of good alignment with hips and knees extended. Toes should not be allowed to touch the footboard. The feet can be elevated slightly using a trochanter roll under the anterior ankle.

The arm is abducted slightly, extended at the elbow, extended and supinated at the wrist. Finger flexion and wrist extension is achieved through the use of a hand roll. Shoulder rolls are placed lengthwise under each shoulder.

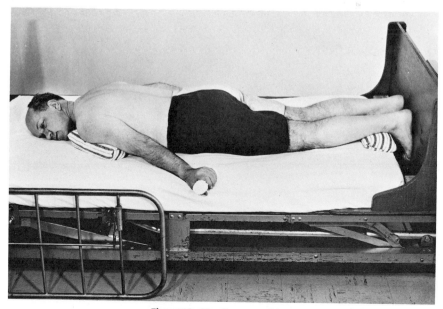

Figure 19–13   Prone position.

FREQUENCY OF TURNING

Turning the patient every two hours is usually a safe routine to follow until the patient's skin sensitivity and tolerance of the positions have been determined. It may be necessary to decrease the amount of time spent in certain positions or it may be found that time in other positions can be increased to two and a half or three hours. Generally it is best to order the more prolonged positioning periods for the night hours, thus lessening the amount of turning at night and enabling the patient to sleep more satisfactorily. More frequent turning will automatically be needed during the day to allow for the desired positions for the patient's daily activities. Nursing staff should be encouraged to set up a definite schedule so that the patient will be in a proper position for activities (such as supine for physical therapy).

The physician should frequently check the skin in vulnerable areas to make certain that no decubiti are developing and to emphasize to the attending staff the importance of a proper turning schedule. Increased activities in the use of various appliances should call attention to new possible areas of ischemic ulceration. The patient who is spending a great deal of time in a wheelchair should have particular close observation for the possible ischemia in the region of the ischial tuberosities.

REFERENCES

1. Coles, C. H., and Bergstrom, D. A.: Bed Positioning Procedures. Minneapolis, American Rehabilitation Foundation, 1969.
2. Elson, R.: Practical Management of Spinal Injuries for Nurses. Baltimore, Williams & Wilkins Company, 1965.
3. Hicks, D., Scarlisi, S., Woody, F., and Skinner, B.: Increasing Upper Extremity Function. Amer. J. Nurs., *64:*8:69-73, 1964.
4. Hirshberg, G., Lewis, L., and Thomas, D.: Rehabilitation: A Manual for the Care of the Disabled and Elderly. Philadelphia, J. B. Lippincott Co., 1964.
5. Kosiak, M.: Etiology and Pathology of Ischemic Ulcers. Arch. Phys. Med., *40:*1:62-69, 1959.
6. Kosiak, M.: Etiology of Decubitus Ulcers. Arch. Phys. Med., *42:*1:19-29, 1961.
7. Larson, C., and Gould, M.: Orthopedic Nursing. St. Louis, C. V. Mosby Company, 1970.
8. Strike Back at Stroke. U.S. Department of Health, Education and Welfare, Public Health Service Publication No. 596. U.S. Government Printing Office, Washington, D.C. 20201, 1960.
9. Sverdlik, S. S., and Chantraine, A.: A Spongy Cushion Over Hypersensitive Areas of the Skin to Increase Threshold to Pain. Arch. Phys. Med., *45:*1:430-432, 1964.

Chapter 20

TRAINING FOR FUNCTIONAL INDEPENDENCE

by Frederic J. Kottke

The achievement of functional independence in the performance of those activities which must be accomplished each day in order for a person to live at home and participate in modern society is one of the goals of rehabilitation. These activities are frequently referred to as activities of self-care or activities of daily living, i.e., A.D.L.

In the course of each day each person must perform or be assisted in performing such activities as arising from bed, caring for hygiene, eating, dressing, using the wheelchair, ambulating and performing a wide variety of manual tasks. Any person who cannot accomplish all of these activities will be dependent on others for help each day.

Although such a person may have a great deal of useful physical ability, the inability to perform one or more of the essential activities of daily living leaves him dependent on others. This dependence for help in self-care often prevents the handicapped person from returning to his home or holding a job. In many cases, because no member of the family is able to provide the necessary assistance, handicapped persons must live as patients in nursing homes. The cost of providing this daily assistance for persons who are not completely independent is extremely high. If a handicapped individual is to resume a normal social status he must be able to care for himself without daily dependency on others.

To ascertain the level of independence, the ability of each patient to perform these necessary daily activities must be checked. If a patient lacks the ability to carry out any of these tasks which are within his capacity he should receive special training to develop that ability. Programs for training physically

TRAINING FOR FUNCTIONAL INDEPENDENCE

SCORING KEY

INDICATE SPECIAL CONDITION OR EQUIPMENT

SCORE   DATE

B—Bed

Black—Independent

W—Wheelchair

Red—Partially Independent

C—Crutches

Activity Attempted, Failed

Ca—Cane

Possible But Not Practical

O—Doesn't Apply

Bed Activities	*Eating*
Move place to place	With fingers
Turn, lie on abdomen	With spoon
Sit erect from lying position, return	With fork
	From glass
Lift object from bed-side table	From cup
	Use knife
Hygiene	*Dress, Undress*
Wash face, hands	Pajamas
Sponge bath	Shorts
Brush teeth	Bra
Shave, make-up	Girdle
Comb, brush hair	Slip-over garment
Clean, trim nails	Buttoned shirt or blouse
Use handkerchief	Slacks
Shampoo hair	Hose, Socks
On, off bedpan	Slipper shoes or Tie shoes
On, off toilet	Braces, prosthesis
In, out bath	Tie a bow, necktie
Feminine hygiene	Outdoor clothing

Figure 20–1   Form for recording performance of activities of daily living.

Wheelchair Activities		*Manual Utilities*	
Sitting tolerance, hours		Write	
Bed to chair, return		Type	
Manipulate wheelchair		Use dial phone	
Pass through doors with wheelchair		Fold, place letter in envelope, remove	
Chair to wheelchair, return		Hold book, turn pages	
Chair to floor, return		Handle newspaper	
Control chair on incline		Use scissors	
Wheelchair to car, return		Wind wrist watch	
Ambulation		Open, close drawers	
Chair to standing, and return		Open, close windows	
Walk forward 30 ft.		Open, close door locks	
Walk sideways 10 ft.		Operate light switch	
Walk backward 5 ft.		Turn faucets	
Pass through doors		Pick objects from floor	
Up, down ramp		Handle money	
Up stairs with rail		Light cigarette	
Down stairs with rail		Plug in cords	
Up stairs without rail		Open, close containers	
Down stairs without rail		Others	
Crutches to car, and return			
Up, down 8 in. curb			
Up, down bus steps			
Cross street on light			

Comments:_____

_____

_____

_____

Figure 20–1 *Continued.*

handicapped patients to become independent in the activities of daily living are adapted from the original work of George G. Deaver and Mary Eleanor Brown at the Institute for the Crippled and Disabled, New York City.[1]

There are many variations in the techniques for training, the use of assistive devices and the means of recording the performance of the activities of daily living. This chapter presents a short review of the basic principles involved in making a physically handicapped patient independent in the performance of those activities that are essential in order that he may return to a normal social environment. Details of techniques and the special problems of specific diseases are presented in articles referred to in this chapter.

Tests of the ability to perform the activities of daily living provide one type of functional assessment of the effectiveness of procedures used in rehabilitation. Other quantitative tests of physical function are also used to define the factors limiting current or potential performance. These factors include joint mobility, muscular strength and endurance, coordination and sensory perception of the segments of the body. The movements necessary for each activity may be broken down into component parts for analysis. However, the ability to perform the component activities is not a sure criterion of ability to perform a total activity. Likewise, unless the performance of each of these essential activities is evaluated, the patient may go through a rehabilitative program and be discharged from the hospital still unable to perform certain activities which leave him dependent on others for care each day. Moreover, handicapped patients frequently must be taught modifications of activities or how to use special equipment in order to make themselves independent in self-care. Therefore, testing of the ability to perform the activities of daily living provides a necessary objective test of the independence of the patient. In addition, the tests direct attention to the areas of significant residual disability and indicate the types of training that should be prescribed in order to develop the greatest possible independence.

The activities that must be performed to achieve functional independence may be classified as bed activities, hygiene, eating, dressing, wheelchair activities, ambulation and manual utilities (Fig. 20–1). A systematic method of assessing and recording all these activities is essential in order that none be overlooked in the rehabilitation program.[2, 3] A more extensive and detailed list can be made but if the tabulation becomes too involved it is difficult to induce all members of the rehabilitation team to use the list as a daily working instrument.[4]

The ability of the patient to perform each activity is tested and the result recorded, indicating whether or not special equipment must be used. Activities that can be performed become the daily activities required of the patient on the ward. Any activity that cannot be performed is analyzed by breaking it down into the simplest components and exercises are selected that will increase the ability of the patient to perform each component motion until he can perform the total activity.[2, 4, 5] These exercises become a part of the daily program of rehabilitation.

Many of the activities of daily living can be performed in a number of ways with a variety of mechanical aids.[6-9] It is often necessary for the patient to use more apparatus early in his program than later, when he has developed more flexibility, strength and coordination. Whenever practical, the patient is taught to perform these activities without the use of special apparatus. However, successful performance of self-care by the disabled patient is a strong motivating force to encourage him to seek further independence so that means should be devised to achieve success as quickly as possible with the necessary equipment and then to develop abilities further, using methods that require less equipment.

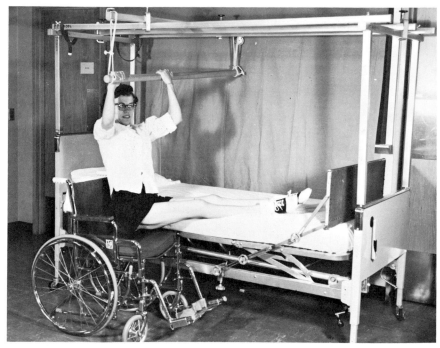

Figure 20–2 Transfer from bed to wheelchair by a paraplegic patient using a 4-foot trapeze bar. The long bar makes lateral transfers less difficult for any patient who has good strength in the upper extremities.

BED ACTIVITIES

The handicapped patient should be provided with a physiatric bed[10] both to prevent the development of further disabilities and to make it easier for him to become independent. Such a bed should have a ¾ inch plywood board under a firm flat mattress, a footboard fixed at a right angle to the bedboard at a distance of 4 inches from the lower end of the mattress and a half-length side rail which provides both protection against falls and a handgrip when sitting up or turning (see Figs. 19–1, 19–2, and 19–3 on pages 464 and 465).

A 4 foot trapeze bar suspended from a Balkan frame enables the patient to pull up to a sitting position or to lift the trunk to transfer to a wheelchair beside the bed (Fig. 20-2). Patients with good arms can push to the erect sitting position (see Figs. 17–18 to 17–20 on page 441), or grasp the side rail to pull themselves erect (see Figs. 17–3 to 17–6 on pages 432, 433 and 434).[10]

The patient should be trained to shift about in bed, turn in both directions, sit erect and reach objects on the bedside table.

HYGIENE

The usual hygienic activities of washing, brushing teeth, shaving or applying makeup, combing hair and using a handkerchief may require adapted equipment so that the patient can hold, control or reach. Limitations of arm mobility or of grasp interfere with the performance of these activities. If the grasp is inadequate but the arm can be controlled, a holding device for such

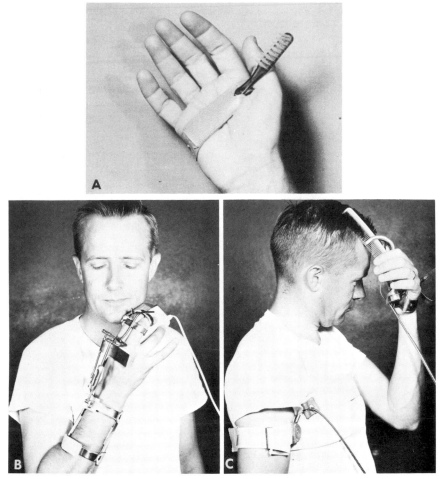

Figure 20–3 *A.* Cuff with pocket to hold the handle of a toothbrush. *B.* Finger flexion splint activated by wrist extension to hold a razor or other equipment for daily self-care. *C.* Robin-Aid splint hook attached to the hand for prehensile activities. The hook is closed by elastic bands and opened by abduction of the opposite arm.

articles as a toothbrush, comb or razor allows independence. Such a device may vary from a simple cuff to an elaborate splint or a motorized orthesis (Fig. 20-3). If the muscles of the shoulder or elbow are weak or incoordinated, a counterbalanced deltoid aid greatly increases the sphere of useful motion of the upper extremity (Fig. 20-4). Motorized equipment such as electric razors or toothbrushes also makes self-care easier for the patient with a severe physical impairment.

Bladder Control. The establishment of bowel and bladder continence is an urgent need in the rehabilitation program to prevent perineal and sacral irritation and ulceration and to decrease the requirements for personnel and linen. For the patient with urinary incontinence, control may be achieved by an indwelling catheter. Because of the multiple hazards of prolonged catheterization it is desirable to achieve a catheter-free status whenever practical.[11-13]

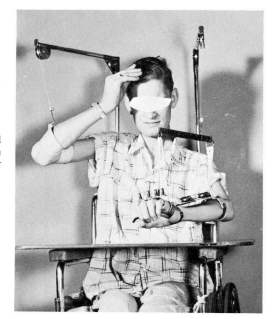

Figure 20–4   A counterbalanced deltoid aid allows flexion, abduction and adduction of the shoulder with minimal muscular strength.

EXTERNAL CONDOM TYPE DRAIN

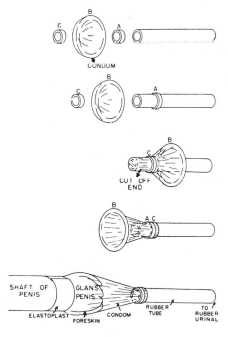

Figure 20–5 Assembly of a condom-catheter drainage system for the male patient with urinary incontinence. (From Comarr, A. E., Brit. J. Urol. *31*:1, 1959.)

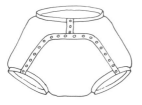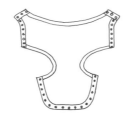

Figure 20–6 Waterproof snap-fastened pants for incontinent patients are worn over absorbent pads. Patients who require long leg braces can take off and put on these pants when toileting without removing their braces.

Bladder training is described in greater detail in Chapter 31. For the male patient who can void but is incontinent, condom-catheter drainage to a bottle or a plastic reservoir attached to the leg is the most satisfactory procedure, whether he is in bed or ambulatory (Fig. 20-5). The patient who requires such equipment must learn how to apply, change and maintain it as part of his self-care.

Methods of maintaining incontinent female patients without soiling are much less satisfactory. An indwelling catheter is the only mechanism by which a woman with urinary incontinence may be kept dry. Rubber or plastic urinals are unsatisfactory because they cannot be attached in a manner that prevents leaking. During the day special waterproof snap-fastened pants may be worn over absorbent pads that are held in place by an elastic belt (Fig. 20-6). This will keep outer clothing dry, although the perineal skin is exposed to irritation and maceration. In order to keep the bed dry at night absorbent cotton or paper pads are placed under the patient. These pads must be changed as frequently as they become wet to decrease the problems of maceration and irritation which increase the susceptibility to ischemic ulcers over the ischial tuberosities, sacrum and trochanters. The use of incontinence pads prevents the automatic shifting of pressure by an alternating air pressure pad and makes hourly turning of the patient necessary if ischemic ulcers are to be avoided.[14]

Bowel Control. Bowel control is somewhat easier to manage than bladder control. If normal bowel function cannot be restored, management of the bowel should prevent fecal incontinence, diarrhea, impaction and irregularity.[15] Patients with neuromuscular diseases must develop regular bowel habits if they are to obtain optimal function. Each day at the same time, 20 to 40 minutes after a meal (to utilize the gastrocolic reflex), the patient should attempt a bowel movement on a toilet or commode. The postprandial period selected depends to some extent on the patient's schedule of activities. Adequate time without emotional stress must be allowed so that the patient can relax, adequate peristalsis can occur and the bowel can be emptied. The gastrocolic reflex is greater after a large hot meal than following a small or cold one.

Other stimuli of colonic peristalsis may also be used. Since nicotine has an immediate ganglionic stimulating action as well as a central sedative action, smoking a cigarette may help to initiate defecation. Hot tea or hot coffee may also be effective. Stimulation of the anorectal reflex by tickling or dilating the anal sphincter with the gloved finger or by the use of a glycerine suppository is a highly effective means of initiating defecation.

Irritation of the rectum by irritant suppositories, cathartics or enema should be avoided except for thorough pre-examination cleansing. However, at times, an atonic bowel may require such a stimulus as a glycerine or Dulcolax suppository, milk of magnesia, cascara sagrada or a tap water or Phospho-soda enema in order to initiate peristalsis. Since the regimen for evacuation of the bowel must be maintained for years, the least irritating procedure that is effective should be used. Mineral oil is unsatisfactory as a laxative for patients with neuromuscular disease since leaking of oil from the rectum may occur. Likewise, saline cathartics may cause fecal incontinence.

The optimal physiologic position for defecation and urination is the squat. The posture on a toilet of standard height approaches this position. Toilet seats that have been built up to allow easy transfer from a wheelchair should have a footrest so that the hips are flexed to the "squat" position. The patient should lean forward, if possible, to increase abdominal pressure by compression against the thighs.

Fecal incontinence due to soft or loose stools is controlled best by dietary management. Decreasing condiments or roughage in food or adding such foods as cheese, apple sauce or tea may be adequate to solve the problem. Pectin, kaolin and tannic acid decrease bowel motility. On occasion anticholinergic drugs or smooth muscle depressants such as adiphenine may be necessary to decrease intestinal motility. The use of opium preparations to control fecal incontinence is unsatisfactory since the patient may fluctuate between incontinence and constipation.

The use of the bedpan or bedside commode requires that the patient learn to lift the body or to transfer out of bed.[2, 10] The commode is far more satisfactory than the bedpan from the standpoints of comfort, energy requirement[16] and successful bowel evacuation. Except for the completely helpless patient, it is best to begin to train each patient to transfer to the commode or toilet as quickly as possible. In addition to the need to develop the strength of the upper extremities in order to transfer to a toilet (see Figs. 17–11 to 17–14 on pages 436, 437 and 438), consideration must be given to the procedure for adjusting the clothing before transferring onto the toilet and after transferring off.

Likewise, bathing in a tub or shower requires the ability to transfer. Suitable handrails are essential to minimize the danger of a fall.[2, 10] The bathtub or shower should have a nonskid rubber mat or adhesive on the bottom for safety. A stool in the tub or shower makes independent transfer easier.

The patient should perform all of the activity of which he is capable and assistance should be limited to those activities that he is unable to perform. It must be emphasized that although having the patient perform these activities for himself may require more of the attendant's time than having the attendant do the activity for him, the patient will achieve independence only if he is able to practice repeatedly until he becomes completely independent.

EATING

The patient may be unable to feed himself adequately because of loss of grasp, range of motion or coordination. A holding device may be necessary for the knife, fork, spoon or cup (Figs. 20–3 and 20–7). Adapted utensils may be needed to make use easier (Fig. 20–8). If the mobility or coordination of the upper extremity is limited, devices such as a Warm Springs feeder, a rocker feeder or a balanced deltoid aid may be required (Figs. 20–4 and 20–9).

Again it should be emphasized that rehabilitation training for self-care becomes only an academic exercise unless the methods developed in A.D.L. testing and training are made a part of the daily eating pattern. Methods or

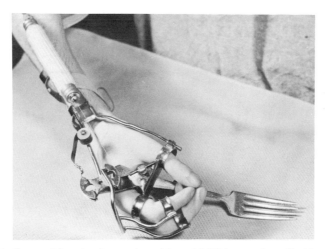

Figure 20–7   Powered hand splint, activated by a McKibben carbon dioxide artificial muscle, to provide grasp for a flail hand.

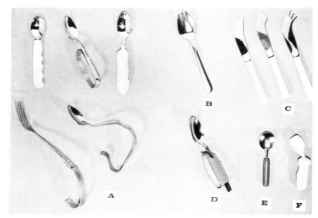

Figure 20–8   Adapted eating utensils for patients with impairment of grasp or reach.

equipment that are not practical for daily use are of no value. Unless the patient learns and adopts his A.D.L. routines while he is in the rehabilitation program, he will not continue them after he goes home.

DRESSING

Patients should be tested for the ability to put on and take off the usual types of clothing. Limitations of mobility may make it difficult or impossible to put the arms through sleeves or to slip clothing of usual design over the feet. Impairment of finger coordination may interfere with such activities as buttoning, lacing, tying and other small motions. Frequently minor adaptations in clothing such as putting buttons, hooks and zippers on the front rather than the side or back of the clothing increases the ability to dress. Elastic or Velcro may be substituted for buttons, belts or laces to make dressing easier.

Research has resulted in the development of specially designed clothing which the severely handicapped person can put on and remove more eas-

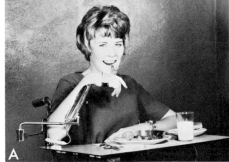

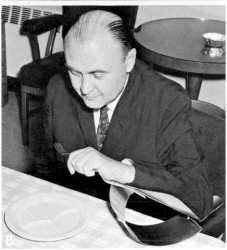

Figure 20–9 *A*. A Warm Springs feeder allows the patient to substitute shoulder depression to elevate the hand during eating. This device also assists the function of weak shoulder flexors, adductors and abductors, and weak elbow flexors. *B*. A forearm rocker feeder aids in the elevation of the hand during eating.

ily.[7, 17, 18] Special utility rods, extension hooks and reachers have been described to enable patients with limited mobility or paralysis of the upper extremities to put on or remove various articles of clothing.[5, 6, 9, 19] Special adaptations of techniques for dressing for various types of disability have also been described.[2, 10, 20] In dressing, as in eating, adaptations must be made according to the abilities and limitations of each patient. Enough time must be allowed in the patient's daily schedule for dressing or training in dressing. Patients in rehabilitation should dress each morning as they will when they return home. Orthotic devices should be worn daily as a part of the regular wearing apparel.

WHEELCHAIR ACTIVITIES

Wheelchair activities include transfers to and from the wheelchair, management of the wheelchair and sitting tolerance. Ability to transfer requires strength to lift or shift the weight of the body, balance and coordination. There are numerous types of chair transfers that use a wide variety of equipment.[1, 2, 10] Chapter 17 describes transfer techniques. The method that should be selected for any patient should be the most convenient one in relation to his residual abilities. Patients should be trained to transfer from bed to chair, from one chair to another, onto and off the toilet and from the wheelchair to and from a car seat. *Patients should also be taught to transfer to the floor from a wheelchair and to return.* This transfer requires both flexibility and strength and requires considerable practice.[2] To improve ability to transfer, exercises are directed particularly at the muscles for shoulder depression, elbow extension, hand grip, hip extension and knee extension.

For the patient with hemiplegia or general paresis who has head and trunk balance, the pivot transfer with the assistance of one person can be performed with little effort (see Fig. 17–1 on page 430). This is probably the most frequently used transfer when assistance is available. The nurse or therapist prevents buckling of the patient's knees with her knee and by supporting him at the hips she assists the patient to stand and balance on the lower extremities without lifting his full body weight. The patient may then be pivoted on his feet to change direction for seating. This transfer is stable and safe for institutional use. Its relatively low energy requirement permits a small attendant to assist a large patient and decreases the likelihood of a back injury.

For the patient who has lower extremity paralysis, transfer to and from the bed by use of the 4-foot trapeze bar is convenient (Fig. 20–2). As the patient becomes more adept at self-care he will learn to transfer without this equipment. The bed should be at the same height as the seat of the wheelchair so that the patient transfers horizontally without having to lift the body vertically.

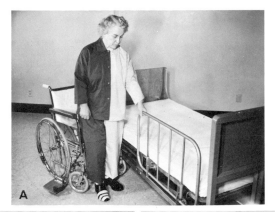

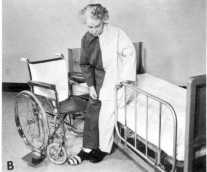
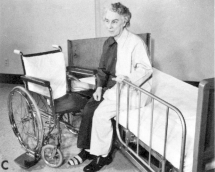

Figure 20–10   Sequence for independent transfer by a hemiplegic patient from a wheelchair to bed. The patient approaches the bed, locks the chair and swings the footrest out of the way. She moves forward toward the edge of the chair seat and, grasping the arm rest, leans forward and pushes herself erect. After she is standing erect she grasps the side rail of the bed, pivots on her feet and lowers herself to sit on the bed. (From A Handbook of Rehabilitative Nursing Techniques in Hemiplegia. Minneapolis, Kenny Rehabilitation Institute, 1964.)

If the arm of the wheelchair is removable, the patient can slide sideways onto the bed or toilet rather than having to lift himself over the arm of the chair (see Fig. 17–31 on page 447). The patient with severe paresis may find it easier to slide straight forward onto the toilet, straddling the bowl, rather than trying to slide onto it from the side. Chairs with swinging detachable footrests can be wheeled close to the bed, toilet or chair so that the distance for transfer is minimal (Fig. 20-10).

The method of independent transfer that requires the least strength utilizes a transfer board along which the patient slides (see Figs. 17-21 to 17-23 on page 443).

Manipulation of the wheelchair by the patient should also be checked. The patient should be able to lock both wheels and adjust the footrests. He should be able to remove and replace the removable arm if one is used. He should be able to wheel his chair on level surfaces or on an incline and to turn in either direction. The hemiplegic patient should be taught to use his uninvolved leg as well as his arm to propel his wheelchair; this allows him to travel in a straight line.

The length of time that a wheelchair patient is allowed to sit is very important. When a person sits on any surface, whether it is flat, contoured or cushioned, the weight of the body is so great in relation to the contacted surface area that the pressure exceeds capillary blood pressure over parts of the sitting surface at all times.[14] Usually this pressure is greatest beneath the ischial tuberosities and the greater trochanters. Therefore, during sitting a pressure ischemia occurs in the soft tissues that are compressed. If that pressure is maintained for more than 30 minutes, ischemic damage begins to occur to the tissues in that area. Normal persons shift position frequently enough so that this does not become a problem. The disabled person who has sensation in the sacral area and who can shift his weight experiences no problem because discomfort warns him of developing ischemia and he has the ability to shift his weight to allow the circulation to be restored.

On the other hand, the disabled person who has no sensation or lacks the ability to shift his weight is in danger of tissue damage at all times when he sits. Because he has no sensory warning he is likely to neglect to shift his position and ischemic necrosis may develop. All persons with sensory loss in the saddle area should be taught to relieve the ischemia by lifting themselves on the arms of their chairs for a few seconds every ten minutes. They should be encouraged to shift positions frequently. In addition, they should have a 3-inch foam rubber cushion on the seat of the wheelchair to distribute the sitting pressure more evenly. Each morning and evening each wheelchair patient should use a hand mirror to inspect the skin over the ischial tuberosities for evidence of injury. Sitting time must be limited to that time during which the patient can sit without evidence of injury to the skin. In general the less freely mobile the patient, the shorter his sitting tolerance.

AMBULATION AND TRANSFERS

Ambulation training is dealt with elsewhere in this text (see Chapters 4, 16, 23 and 33). Successful ambulation requires that the patient be able to transfer from sitting to standing independently and with ease in order to make walking practical. He must be able to handle his crutches, canes or other appliances without aid. He should be able to get to and from a variety of seating: chair, bed, toilet, car. He should be able to climb stairs and curbs. If he will be using public transportation he should be able to enter and leave a taxi or bus. All of these phases of ambulation should be checked and recorded in order to be sure that the patient will be independent in ambulation when he is discharged.

MANUAL DEXTERITY

There are a number of activities encountered in daily life that require varied types of manual dexterity. These have been listed in Figure 20-1. Performance of these activities is necessary for normal independent living. Any patient who has impairment of manual function may have to use special techniques, special equipment or special procedures to be independent in these activities. Patients with a manual prosthesis or orthesis may need training in order to become adept at these activities. Development of speed as well as precision of performance may be important in order to make the patient independent and vocationally productive.

THERAPY TO IMPROVE FUNCTIONAL INDEPENDENCE

Based on the performance recorded during the testing of the activities of daily living, therapeutic exercises are prescribed to improve the abilities necessary to carry out these daily tasks. The activities of daily living may be analyzed in terms of the component musculoskeletal actions which must be combined to make performance of the full activity possible. These components include flexibility of the joints, range and strength of contraction of the muscles, muscular endurance and coordination.

Coordination in turn has a number of aspects such as balance of the head, balance of the trunk for sitting and balance of the pelvis and lower extremities for standing and walking. Coordination of the fingers and thumb for grasp and of the hand with the joints of the upper extremities for reaching may require special training. Lifting or transferring the weight of the body from place to place is heavy exercise and requires considerable strength and endurance.

To develop mobility, strength or endurance, exercise for the muscles concerned should be carried out according to the principles in Chapter 16, Therapeutic Exercise. For the development of coordination and skill in the specific activity of daily living, practice of that activity is the most effective procedure. These activities are practiced in their component parts on a regular daily schedule until they can be achieved. Specific techniques of training of the component aspects of rehabilitation have been described in detail.[2, 5]

Evaluation of improvement in self-care becomes meaningful only when effective comparison can be made of the patient's abilities before and after rehabilitation. A number of methods of evaluating and scoring the patient's functional performance in self-care have been reported.[1–4] Of these the Kenny Self-Care Index on six categories of activities has been studied most extensively.[4, 21] Standardized methods were developed for evaluating self-care abilities of patients in bed activities, transfers, locomotion, dressing, personal hygiene and feeding. Items in each category were rated on a 5-point scale. Inter-rate reliability has been shown to be good. An increased rating is reliably related to increased independence during the course of rehabilitation. This quantitative measure of functional improvement can be used to provide an index of the improvement of the patient, the effectiveness of therapy, or the accuracy of the estimation of the degree of recovery.

Patients frequently need equipment in order to perform activities of daily living. Some patients can perform satisfactorily using standard equipment. For others equipment must be modified or special equipment made in order to make self-care possible. Some patients can be completely or partially independent only with orthotic or prosthetic devices. The determination of the use of such equipment or assistive devices is a necessary part of the prescription for a rehabilitation program.

Since activities of daily living are practical and of value only when applied and used regularly, the testing should be followed by the assignment of all items successfully passed as a part of the patient's independent self-care. Each day, the patient should do those activities. As he accomplishes each new activity he should be required to add it to his daily performance. In that way he is moving at optimal speed toward self-sufficiency at home.

REFERENCES

1. Deaver, G. G., and Brown, M. E.: Physical Demands of Daily Life. New York, Institute for the Crippled and Disabled, 1945.
2. Lawton, E. B.: Activities of Daily Living for Physical Rehabilitation. New York, McGraw-Hill Book Co., 1963.
3. Dinnerstein, A. J., Lowenthal, M., and Dexter, M.: Evaluation of a Rating Scale of Ability in Activities of Daily Living. Arch. Phys. Med., 46:579-584, 1965.
4. Schoening, H. A., Anderegg, L., Bergstrom, D., Fonda, M., Steinke, N., and Ulrich, P.: Numerical Scoring of Self-Care Status of Patients. Arch. Phys. Med., 46:689-697, 1965.
5. Rusk, H. A., and Taylor, E. J.: Living With a Disability. Garden City, New York, The Blakiston Co., 1953.
6. Self-Help Devices for Rehabilitation: Part I. New York University–Bellevue Medical Center Institute of Physical Medicine and Rehabilitation. Dubuque, Iowa, Wm. C. Brown Company, Publishers, 1958.
7. Self-Help Devices for Rehabilitation: Part II. New York University–Bellevue Medical Center Institute of Physical Medicine and Rehabilitation. Dubuque, Iowa, Wm. C. Brown Company, Publishers, 1965.
8. Goldsmith, S.: Designing for the Disabled, Second ed., New York, McGraw-Hill Book Co., 1967.
9. Rosenberg, C.: Assistive Devices for the Handicapped. Minneapolis, American Rehabilitation Foundation, 1968.
10. A Handbook of Rehabilitative Nursing Techniques in Hemiplegia. Minneapolis, Kenny Rehabilitation Institute, 1964.
11. Stolov, W.: Rehabilitation of the Bladder in Injuries of the Spinal Cord. Arch. Phys. Med., 40:467-474, 1959.
12. Morales, P., and Tsov, A. Y.: Quantitative Bacteriologic Study of Urinary Infection Among Paraplegics. J. Urol., 87:191-198, 1962.
13. Price, M., Tobin, J. A., Reiser, M., Olson, M. E., Kubicek, W. G., Kottke, F. J., and Boen, J.: Renal Function in Patients with Spinal Cord Injuries. Arch. Phys. Med., 47:406-411, 1966.
14. Kosiak, M.: Etiology of Decubitus Ulcers. Arch. Phys. Med., 42:19-29, 1961.
15. Mead, S.: A Bowel Training Program in a Rehabilitation Center. Arch. Phys. Med., 37:210-213, 1956.
16. Benton, J. G., Brown, H., and Rusk, H. A.: Energy Expended by Patients on the Bedpan and Bedside Commode. J.A.M.A., 144:1443-1447, 1950.
17. Rusk, H. A., and Taylor, E. J.: Functional Fashions for the Physically Handicapped. J.A.M.A., 169:1598-1600, 1959.
18. Cookman, H., and Zimmerman, M.: Functional Fashions for the Physically Handicapped. New York University–Bellevue Medical Center, Institute of Physical Medicine and Rehabilitation, New York, 1961.
19. Cicenia, E. F., Rosenthal, J., and Springer, C. F.: Solving the Problem of Self Care with Self-help Devices. Phys. Ther. Rev., 37:726–735, 1957.
20. Rikert, G. C., Sloane, N., Sosnowski, G., and Wiencrot, B.: Dressing Techniques for the Cerebral Palsied Child. Amer. J. Occup. Ther., 8:8-10, 37-38, 1954.
21. Anderson, T. P., Bourestom, N., and Greenberg, F. R.: Rehabilitation Predictors in Completed Stroke. Minneapolis, American Rehabilitation Foundation, 1970.

Chapter 21

TRAINING IN HOMEMAKING ACTIVITIES

by Bernard Sandler

Homemaking is probably the oldest vocation in history. It is also one of the most neglected areas in the field of rehabilitation. As early as 1954 the Federal Rehabilitation Law was interpreted to include homemakers, yet only a few states have used this opportunity to advantage.[1] Even earlier, in 1943, federal rehabilitation programs were included in the Social Security Law, and in 1946 homemaking was declared a vocation by the Vocational Rehabilitation Administration.[1]

Homemakers constitute the largest group among the disabled. A recent survey[3] pointed out that there were 1,875,000 women with arthritis, 4,000,000 women with cardiovascular disease, 175,000 women with active or arrested tuberculosis, 650,000 women with hemiplegia and 800,000 women with orthopedic disabilities. The last group runs the gamut from tetraplegia to osteoarthritis of the hip. The total number of physically handicapped homemakers is now well over 10,000,000.

The disabled housewife is not the only one who can benefit from training in homemaking.[1, 4] Men with physical impairment often must assume homemaking roles in order to allow other members of the family to work outside the home (Fig. 21-1). The enormous number of aged of both sexes could benefit greatly from training in homemaking skills. Men and women with a chronic illness are often relegated unwittingly to a condition of complete dependency. Their potential for at least partial independence through training has never been realized. Children and young people with handicaps are certainly candidates for training. Development of homemaking skills may contribute to development of self-confidence and initiative.

488

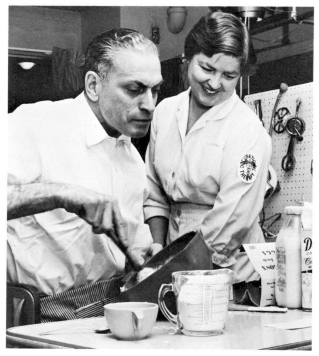

Figure 21–1 Men sometimes need homemaker training. (Connecticut Society For Crippled Children and Adults.) (From U.S. Department of Health, Education and Welfare, Vocational Rehabilitation Administration: Rehabilitation of the Physically Handicapped in Homemaking Activities, 1963.)

The disruption of family life that may follow disability is incalculable. If the disabled member happens to be the wife and mother—the very hub of the family—the disruption may be irreversible. At what cost can the handicapped housewife be replaced by a cook, seamstress, governess, companion, chauffeur, laundress, nurse and cleaning woman?

Training in homemaking, as in every other phase of rehabilitation, is expensive in terms of time, money and effort. Lack of such training, however, leads to economic and human waste. We must make available to every handicapped person facilities for training, but we must also be realistic. Not all disabled homemakers will achieve complete independence. For those who do not, we must consider these possibilities in our training program:[1]

(1) Some homemaking jobs are better left undone.

(2) Some other member of the family must do them.

(3) Someone must be employed to do them either inside or outside the home.

DEFINITION AND SCOPE OF HOMEMAKING ACTIVITIES

"Homemaking activities—whether carried out by men, by women, or by children—contribute to the welfare of the family and to its economic productiveness and well-being. Homemaking itself is a composite of physical tasks, managerial functions, spirit, and emotional climate that holds the family or personality together and fosters development. Damage to this complex at any point weakens its total capacity to function. Where possible, the damage must be repaired; where this is not possible, other measures must be taken: Perhaps the environment can be changed so that the function can continue. Perhaps other areas of the complex must be brought into greater prominence and use; perhaps the very depths of personality must be touched and a new role learned."[2] This definition implies that homemaking is much more than the development of work skills alone. Rehabilitation of the homemaker may be further defined as concern with the following areas:[5, 6]

(1) Work simplification and selection and adaptation of household equipment.

(2) Remodeling or rearranging of home facilities.

(3) Clothing selection and care.

(4) Psychologic needs and family relations.

(5) Child care.

(6) Nutrition exercise and energy expenditure.

ORGANIZATION OF A TRAINING PROGRAM

Training may be arranged as a community service, as part of a hospital service or, when possible, as a combination of the two.[7]

There are many agencies and facilities in most communities with an interest in homemaking. If there is a physiatrist and a rehabilitation center in the community, so much the better. In planning the program, one should consider the local medical society, physical and occupational therapists, visiting or public health nurses, social workers, voluntary agencies, such as the National Society for Crippled Children and Adults, homemaker services in welfare departments or family service groups, home economists, dietitians, architects, designers, builders and industrial engineers. Other physicians in addition to physiatrists, such as orthopedic surgeons, neurologists and cardiologists, should be encouraged to help in the planning.

The ideal training program, however, should be based in a rehabilitation center or in a hospital with a department of physical medicine and rehabilitation and should begin when the homemaker is in the hospital.[8] Here the team concerned with the patient's rehabilitation is ready at hand and can plan homemaking as an integral part of the general rehabilitation program. In addition, after discharge, liaison for continued training and follow-up can be arranged. If this is not practicable because the patient lives too far away from the rehabilitation facility, then agencies in the patient's community can be alerted to his or her needs after return to the home.

The team may include all medical and nonmedical personnel in a department of physical medicine and rehabilitation. People most concerned are the physician (preferably a physiatrist), who directs training; the social worker, who acquaints the patient's family with the patient's particular needs and maintains the link with the physician, evaluates the possibilities for adaptations in the home and helps in the purchase or procurement of special aids or devices; the physical therapist, who helps evaluate the patient's proficiency in activities of daily living and plans a conditioning program to maintain physical fitness; and the occupational therapist, who instructs in household management and the use of adaptive devices.[9] Most often the actual home evaluation is carried out by a physical or occupational therapist who collaborates with the social worker. When the patient is a client of an outside agency, coordination of the rehabilitative program may be directed by a rehabilitation counselor. A very useful addition to the team is the home consultant or home economist who is trained in many areas of homemaking and whose skills are too often overlooked by the other members of the rehabilitation team.[1] Duties of team members will vary and overlap and complement each other.

TRAINING CONTENT

The goal of homemaker training is efficient resettlement of the patient in her place of work—the home. Considered in this light, training should anticipate problems or difficulties which the patient will encounter in the home. Domestic activities involve consideration of the following:[10]

(1) Range of reach. One should consider the maximal reach required, both in a vertical and a horizontal direction. Prescription of tools for reaching, allocation of equipment and arrangement of working surfaces depend on these measurements (Figs. 21-2 to 21-4). Conditions that limit range of reach are those requiring working sitting down, such as paraplegia, and those severely limiting motion, such as crippling rheumatoid arthritis.

(2) Movement from one place to another. A housewife may walk as much as 25 kilometers during her day's work. Cardiac patients, those limited to wheelchairs and those requiring the use of canes, crutches or leg braces are obviously limited.

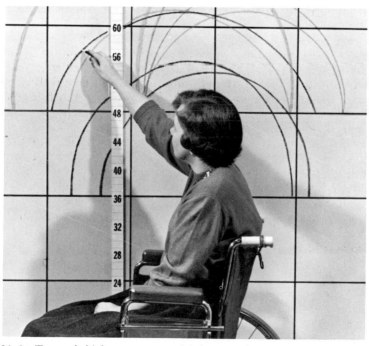

Figure 21–2 To reach high a woman confined to a wheelchair works from the side to get maximum reach. This wheelchair woman adds her maximum reach on the chart with marking of the normal homemaker and the one-handed woman. (From May, E. E., and Waggoner, N. R.: Work Simplification in Child Care, 1962.)

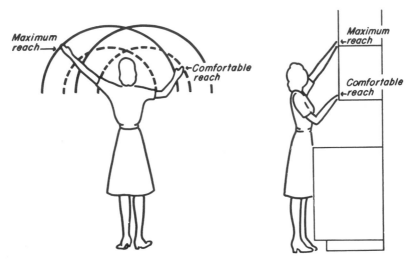

Figure 21–3 Determining vertical reaching areas. (From Rusk, H. A., et al.: A Manual for Training the Disabled Homemaker, 2nd Ed., 1961.)

(3) Manual activities. Patients with impaired use of hand or arm because of weakness, incoordination or amputation may suffer severe limitation. It is this group that will call upon all the ingenuity the occupational therapist can muster (Fig. 21-5).

(4) Energy consumption. Patients with cardiorespiratory diseases will usually find this the chief limiting factor. Bed making, ironing or washing up requires the same rate of energy expenditure as house painting, cabinetmaking or plastering—3 to 4.5 calories per minute. Passmore and Durnin[11] in an excellent review describe the energy costs of many common household activities. Steidl and Bratton[83] in their book "Work in the Home" compare various energy cost studies.

(5) Safety. Lack of coordination, of sensation and of spatial orientation may prove dangerous when one handles hot or sharp objects. The danger of falling because of vertigo, loss of consciousness, syncopal attacks or epilepsy must be guarded against. It is in this group that one should consider elimination of certain household tasks altogether.

(6) Communication. Contact with the outside world through the telephone or directly in such activities as shopping is difficult for patients with language difficulty. The aphasic patient is an example of this problem.

THE HOMEMAKER TRAINEE

It can be inferred from the previous discussion that trainees will fall into three broad categories: (1) Those with conditions involving hand or arm or calling for one-handedness, e.g., arthritis, poliomyelitis, amputation, hemiplegia. (2) Those with disabilities requiring sedentary work or a wheelchair, e.g., paraplegia, severe athetosis, crippling arthritis. (3) Those with conditions calling for maximal energy saving, e.g., congestive failure, severe emphysema, tuberculosis.[10]

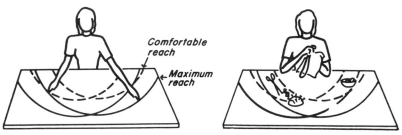

Figure 21–4   Determining horizontal reach areas. (From Rusk, H. A., et al.: A Manual for Training the Disabled Homemaker, 2nd Ed., 1961.)

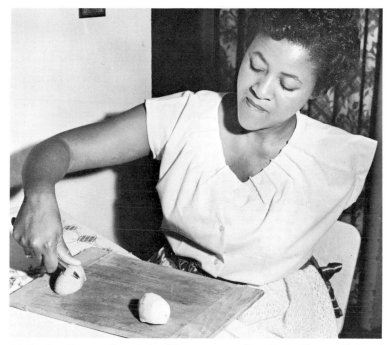

Figure 21–5   A spike on a board simplifies potato peeling. (J. A. Manter, University of Connecticut.) (From U. S. Department of Health, Education and Welfare, Vocational Rehabilitation Administration: Rehabilitation of the Physically Handicapped in Homemaking Activities, 1963.)

Gordon[12] discusses disability under two broad headings—motor impairment and impairment of endurance. The first includes disability due to neural, muscular or articular involvement, and the second, the cardiorespiratory diseases. The first category may logically be further refined as disability involving loss of strength, e.g., amyotrophic lateral sclerosis; loss of a part of the body, e.g., amputation of a limb; loss of coordination, e.g., cerebral palsy with severe athetosis; loss of speed, e.g., the aged patient without any crippling disease; loss of range, e.g., the arthritic patient with severe contractures or ankylosis.

We are not concerned here with the problems of the deaf, blind or mentally deficient because they require special training facilities. Nor is it necessary to outline disabilities resulting from various diseases.

Evaluation of the Trainee

Almost all rehabilitation centers and physical medicine and rehabilitation services in general hospitals have a training kitchen facility.[14] In addition, bathroom and bed and sitting room training areas are often standard equipment.[15] The Rehabilitation Center of the City of Stockholm houses a training apartment consisting of two kitchens (a functional kitchen for experimenting with new techniques and a standard kitchen that conforms to Swedish housing standards), a living room, a bedroom and a bathroom—an area of approximately 106 square meters.[16] In such facilities, patients' skills in cleaning activities, meal preparation, meal service, laundry tasks, sewing, heavy household duties, marketing, child care and special tasks may be thoroughly evaluated and plans made for adaptations in the home.[17] Forms on which careful records are kept are an essential part of the training program. Accurate assessment of progress or changes in technique cannot be made any other way. Evaluation of skills in activities of daily living, such as bed, wheelchair, transfer, walking, climbing, traveling, hand dressing, eating, and toilet activities, cannot be excluded from the program.[18] Training in these areas must go on concomitantly with training in homemaking.

All members of the rehabilitation team try to help the homemaker to help herself. The therapeutic keys are: work simplification—a scientific process of improving job method—and human engineering—adapting mechanical facilities to fit the physiologic capacity of the worker.[13] We may add two more: improved physical fitness—increased capacity for work—and improvement in psychosocial milieu so that the patient is encouraged to become proficient in her duties.

PRINCIPLES OF WORK SIMPLIFICATION OR ECONOMY OF MOTION

This is of primary concern in homemaking training. The following outline is an excellent working guide:[19]

(1) Whenever the condition allows, use both hands in opposite and symmetric motions while working.

(2) Lay out work areas within normal reach. Arrange supplies in a semicircle.

(3) Slide—do not lift and carry. Use a table with wheels when moving from one work surface to another (Fig. 21–6).

(4) Use fixed work stations. Have a special place to do each job so that supplies and equipment may be kept ready for immediate use.

(5) Use the smallest number of work elements. Select equipment that may be used for more than one job; eliminate unnecessary motions.

(6) Avoid the work of holding. Use utensils that rest firmly and are secured by suction cups or clamps. This will free hands for work (Fig. 21-7).

(7) Let gravity work. Examples are a laundry chute, refuse chute, gravity-feed flour bin.

(8) Position tools in advance. Store them so they are placed in position for immediate grasping and use. Hang measuring cups and spoons separately within sight (Fig. 21–8).

(9) Position machine controls and switches within easy reach. Household appliances should be chosen on the basis of ease of operation.

(10) Sit to work whenever possible. Use a comfortable chair and adjust

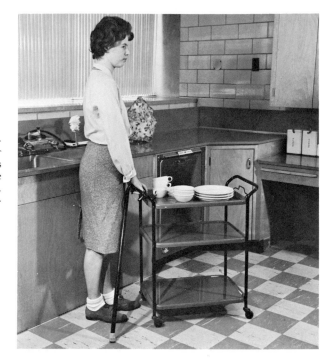

Figure 21–6 Wheeled utility table. The patient hangs her cane on the table rail and uses the table for support as she wheels it from place to place. (Courtesy of Kenny Rehabilitation Institute.)

Figure 21–7 Suction bowl holder. (From Steinke, N., and Ericksson, P.: Homemaking Aids for the Disabled, 1963.)

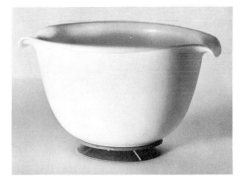

Figure 21–8 Perforated masonite gives flexibility in arranging storage. (From Rusk, H. A., et al.: A Manual for Training the Disabled Homemaker, 2nd Ed., 1961.)

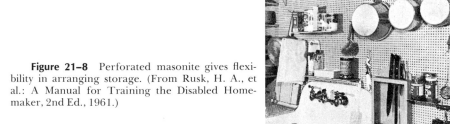

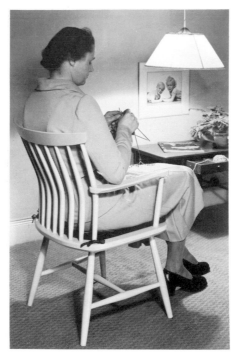

Figure 21–9   On the new type of chair the back is comfortably supported. (Courtesy of Bengt Åkerblom.)

work place height to the chair. Or use an adjustable stool or chair. Akerblom[20] describes a chair designed to fulfill anatomic and physiologic needs (Fig. 21-9).

(11) Use a correct work place height. The height should be right for the homemaker and the job. There are no standard heights. Morant[21] points out that the dimensions of a work space suitable for persons of normal size may differ appreciably from the best that can be found to accommodate workers of all sizes and that in a work space, a change of even ½ inch may make an appreciable difference in the ease of operation and comfort of a considerable proportion of workers. For example, the Cornell study on ironing demonstrates that a 34 inch height for the ironing board is far more suitable in general than a 31 inch height.[22]

(12) Good working conditions are important—good light and ventilation, comfortable clothing and ambient temperature.

Rules of work simplification are not enough. The patient must learn to manage herself and her needs before she can manage homemaking activities and her family. She must become proficient in her activities of daily living.[23–26] She must begin to think like an industrial engineer. Is her strength adequate for certain jobs? What is her need for rest periods; what is the best time of day for the performance of certain duties; ought she to plan some jobs as a daily chore, a weekly chore or even monthly; in what quantities ought food to be prepared? It is these and countless other questions that the homemaker tries to answer as she becomes more skillful in her job. In short, the efficient disabled homemaker ought to become a time-and-motion expert. Two excellent bibliographies on home management and food preparation have been published by the University of Connecticut.[27, 28]

SELF-HELP DEVICES OR AIDS, AND SELECTION AND ADAPTATION OF HOUSEHOLD EQUIPMENT

Much has been written about self-help devices or aids for the homemaker. In general, it is fair to say that, whenever possible, jobs should be attempted

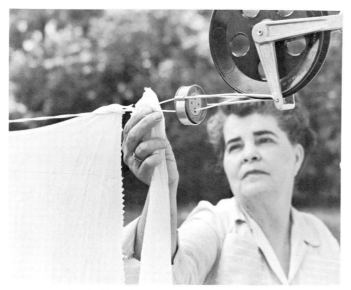

Figure 21–10 A twist line holds without pins. Just insert the edge of the garment between the lines and push the line ahead. It will twist and hold the garment. (From Zmola, G. M.: You Can Do Family Laundry With Hand Limitations.)

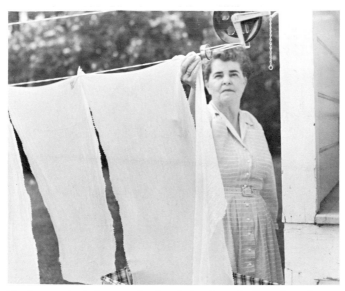

Figure 21–11 Let gravity help you take the clothes from the line. Place the cart under the line in order that the clothes may drop directly into it as you pull them toward you. (From Zmola, G. M.: You Can Do Family Laundry — With Hand Limitations.)

without special aids. If it is decided that the homemaker will continue certain activities that require them, then plans can be made for the adaptation of a special aid or device. It would be foolish to plan for aids if the homemaker is not going to carry out activities for which the aids are designed. Lowman and Klinger[74] have compiled a very detailed source-book on aids and devices. Agerholm[75] has edited a four-volume compendium on equipment for the disabled.

Before planning to make a device, it is wise to see whether it is already available. Very often aids can be purchased more cheaply than they could be made. If a device has to be made, it is wise to consider in detail its weight, ease of handling, washability and durability. It should be as inconspicuous and as simple as possible.

After the device is made the homemaker must still take a great deal of time to learn its use and to practice until maximal efficiency is achieved.[29] A very useful bulletin entitled "Homemaking Aids for the Disabled" has recently become available.[30] Another excellent source of instruction is "Do It Yourself Again."[72]

Zmola[31] shows how a one-armed homemaker develops efficiency in laundry tasks because of proper equipment, tools and procedures rather than dependence on special devices (Figs. 21-10 and 21-11). Again, one must emphasize that a device is important only when one cannot get along as well without it. Figure 21-12 illustrates a very simple kitchen aid.

Selection of proper appliances also can be of immense help to the homemaker. Care should be taken to see that all machines and appliances have

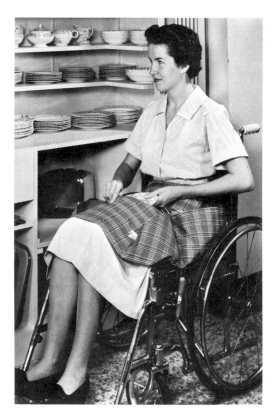

Figure 21–12 A wheelchair apron simplifies housework. (U. S. Department of Agriculture.) (From U. S. Department of Health, Education and Welfare, Vocational Rehabilitation Administration: Rehabilitation of the Physically Handicapped in Homemaking Activities, 1963.)

openings and controls that can be reached and operated easily. It is also important that such appliances are placed in a convenient location. In general, it can be said that for the limited homemaker, front-opening equipment is better than top-opening equipment and that doors hinged on the side are best. A piece of equipment, such as a refrigerator, should not be purchased until the needs of the homemaker are clearly understood. Gas and electric utility companies can give very helpful advice. The Scottish Gas Board, for example, visits its disabled customers every year.[73]

REMODELING AND REARRANGEMENT OF HOME FACILITIES

In recent years there has been a great deal of emphasis on remodeling and rearrangement of home facilities, particularly kitchens.[32-34] This work has emphasized space requirements for maneuvering a wheelchair, for vertical and horizontal reaches of the homemaker, for comfortable working heights, for necessary clearances of work areas, and for arrangement of the various centers such as the sink center, the range center and the mix center. Three basic kitchen arrangements, the U, the L and the corridor, have been thoroughly worked out. There are advantages and disadvantages to each. Which one is best for a particular homemaker depends on her disability. Wheeler's monograph[76] can be particularly recommended as a guide for the vocational rehabilitation of disabled homemakers. A new British source[77] stresses that success in the kitchen is indispensable for success in homemaking or maintenance of independence. Very recently a practical manual on cooking and serving[78] has become available. It will be particularly helpful to the aged and disabled because of emphasis on nutrition and labor-saving techniques.

A logical extension of kitchen planning is the design of complete dwellings for the disabled. Obviously the limitations here are chiefly economic. In addition to the financial problem, however, there is lack of interest among architects. In spite of these drawbacks, several approaches to housing for the disabled have been made. In Sweden,[35] a special housing committee is in charge of housing for the disabled. Apartments are purchased with funds granted by a state subsidy. The apartments are remodeled under an architect's direction. Plans have been carefully worked out in relation to the location of the apartments, location of streets and other approaches, kitchen layout, bathroom layout, and design of fittings, sanitary equipment and electric installation. Design of dwellings for the disabled who require wheelchairs has been extensively discussed in two communications from the Testing and Observation Institute at Hellerup, Denmark.[36, 37]

At a recent conference of the International Society for Rehabilitation of the Disabled the following criteria were stressed.[38]

(1) The dwelling must allow the individual, whatever his handicap, to move about with maximal convenience and minimal effort.

(2) The disabled person must be able to use all the facilities, not just the kitchen.

(3) The dwelling must have maximal ease of communication with the outside world.

(4) The house must have an adequate heating system.

(5) Everything in the house must be planned for maximal serviceability and ease of maintenance.

(6) The house must be usable regardless of the type of disability. It must never be planned for one disability only.

(7) The price of every single component must be reduced to the absolute minimum.

The Dutch approach to housing for the disabled is directed toward two general groups of disabled — those restricted to wheelchairs and those who can move about with the aid of crutches or sticks.[39] This in no way is contradictory to one of the criteria previously laid down — that housing for the disabled should be multipurpose in character.

An American plan for single family dwellings[40] alters standard building plans in a way which makes an immensely more livable home. A built-in vacuum cleaning system is an outstanding feature. In the kitchen, equipment needed in each work area is easily accessible from either a sitting or a standing position. Many other useful features are described. However, in this case too, cost would be a compelling deterrent. Smith[79] points out that planning the home for a disabled person requires accurate information concerning the physical limitations imposed by the disability or illness and the actual space available in the house. A planning consultant can save time and money. An apartment building designed especially for the handicapped and taking into account kitchen, bathroom, door, parking and safety requirements has been erected in Seattle.[80] It is the first of its kind in this country.

CLOTHING SELECTION AND CARE

The disabled have many problems related to clothing. They have trouble putting on and taking off their clothes. They have difficulty with fastenings on clothes as well as on shoes. Most clothes do not give adequate freedom of movement during various activities, especially when crutches and wheelchairs are used. The wheelchair, crutches and braces also cause wear and tear of fabric. Transfer activities that involve sliding require, in addition to freedom of movement, fabrics that do not stick. Incontinence is an added problem. Another problem is that of the handicapped mother who must dress not only herself but her young children. Zimmerman[41] summarizes some solutions:

(1) Large flat buttons for easy handling; extra-long, side-front opening zippers on skirts; Velcro closures for ease in putting on and taking off clothes. Velcro consists of two surfaces of nylon which adhere to each other securely with minimal pressure and which can be pulled apart easily.

(2) Skirts with center-front openings and elasticized webbing waist band. There are side vents for hip adjustments.

(3) Flared skirts with slight fullness in order to cover braces; wrap-around dresses with extra width across the bodice.

(4) Slacks for men and women with full-length side-seam zipper with two-way slide action. Opening from bottom allows easier putting on and taking off over braces.

(5) Undershirts with no underarm seam.

(6) Aprons with waist hoops to eliminate tying.

(7) Blouses that open completely flat and need only to be placed around a person.

For children, Zimmerman suggests the following:

(1) Overalls, dresses, skirts and snowsuits with full-length center-front openings.

(2) Over-the-head type openings or expandable necklines.

(3) Easy fasteners, such as large buttons with long thread shanks, large grippers, large trouser-type hook-and-eye fasteners, zippers with pull tabs.

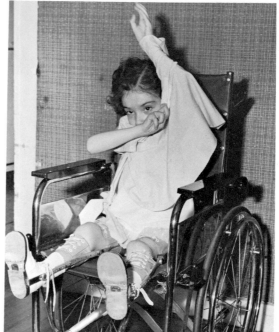

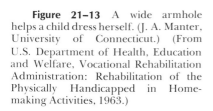

Figure 21–13 A wide armhole helps a child dress herself. (J. A. Manter, University of Connecticut.) (From U.S. Department of Health, Education and Welfare, Vocational Rehabilitation Administration: Rehabilitation of the Physically Handicapped in Homemaking Activities, 1963.)

(4) Raglan or kimono sleeves for ease of getting in and out (Fig. 21-13).

(5) Wide hems and adjustable shoulder straps.

(6) Magnetic buttons.

We have listed only a few possibilities. Suffice it to say that much more work has to be done on clothing for the disabled. Lowman and Rusk[42] give valuable information on aids to dressing and functional fashions designed for the disabled person. The "Fashion-Able" line of undergarments emphasizes replacement of hooks and eyes with Velcro, and the use of zippers.[81]

CHILD CARE

Child care may be a particularly vexing problem for the disabled homemaker. It is important for her to develop a sense of discipline and responsibility in her children. May and Waggoner[43] and Waggoner and Reedy[44] have written very helpful bulletins on work simplification in child care and child care equipment (Fig. 21-14). Dressing the young child may be especially difficult for the handicapped mother. Boettke[45] has made some very practical suggestions concerning clothes for preschool children which make dressing much easier.

It may happen on occasion that a handicapped homemaker has handicapped children. In such cases the inculcation of good work habits and a sense of pride in accomplishment is invaluable. Bare, Boettke and Waggoner[46] describe self-help clothing for handicapped children. This is an excellent way to encourage independence.

All children, whether handicapped or not, work better under established rules and regulations. Disciplinary problems arise more often when there are no standards and when the child is not made responsible. A model program in homemaking for handicapped children is taught at the Orthopedic Hospital

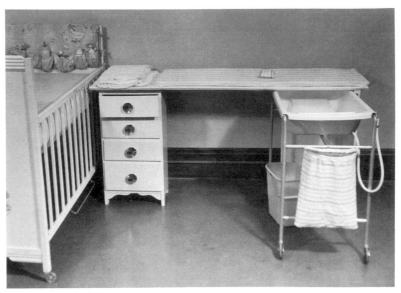

Figure 21–14　This bathing and dressing area designed for a wheelchair mother provides for: a comfortable working height, plenty of knee room to work in a forward position, "easy flow of work" from crib to dressing counter and chest with baby's clothes within easy reach; hose allows for "use of gravity" in emptying the tub. (From May, E. E., and Waggoner, N. R.: Work Simplification in Child Care, 1962.)

School in Helsinki. Here parents, too, are educated to appreciate their child's potential and limitations and to encourage independence. Wall[48] points out that the desire to be helpful and independent is often at its height when the child is four years old. Instead of making the child more dependent, the mother should give him the opportunity he needs to develop into a cooperative member of the family.

A mother who teaches her children to be independent early, whether they are handicapped or not, will make time available for her own needs—needs for rest, for cultural enrichment and for other tasks not related to child care.

NUTRITION, ENERGY EXPENDITURE AND EXERCISE

During her training in the hospital or rehabilitation center the disabled homemaker should learn the principles of sound nutrition. This is of importance not only for herself but also for her family. Since mixes and canned and dehydrated foods may be sources of work simplification, it is imperative that the homemaker learn to incorporate them in a balanced diet. The hospital dietitian has a very helpful role to play here.

It is probably true, however, that the homemaker will suffer far more often from overnutrition than from malnutrition. Because disability may limit markedly the homemaker's opportunity to perform tasks that require intense, prolonged physical effort, she will tend to eat more than she needs. The result is obesity, which in turn will increase the cost of work[12] (Fig. 21-15). An occasional patient, however, who is taking large doses of medication, or of several medications, may have little or no appetite. The goal in this instance is to control medication and encourage sound nutritional habits rather than give

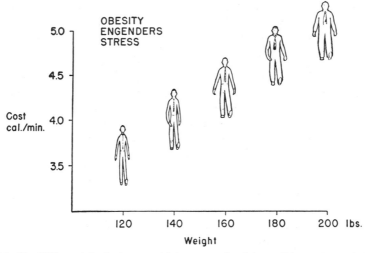

Figure 21–15 Differential calorie cost with increase of weight, walking at 2.5 mph. (From Gordon, E. E.: The Expenditure of Energy in Health and in Disease. Med. Sci. 3:19, 1958.)

the patient more pills to stimulate appetite and to substitute for impending nutritional deficiencies.

Gordon[12] defines ergonomics as the relationship between external work and internal energy expenditure. As applied to disability, it connotes maximal work performance for the least energy expenditure. This is precisely our goal for the disabled homemaker. Isherwood[82] defines ergonomics as "the study of man with regard to his total environment and the arranging of that environment to achieve his utmost comfort and efficiency." In this definition one senses the importance of the discipline of engineering in relation to medicine.

TABLE 21–1 RELATIVE EFFICIENCY OF LOCOMOTION IN DISABILITY*

Disability	Mechanical Aid	Efficiency Per Cent
Normal		20
A-K Amputee	Suction Socket	18
A-K Amputee	Standard Socket	16
A-K Amputee	Pylon	14
A-K Amputee	Forearm Crutches Only	11
Hemiplegia†		
Good Recovery		25
Hemiplegia		
Fair Recovery	With Cane	17
	Without Cane	17
Hemiplegia		
Poor Recovery	With Cane and Short-Leg Brace	11
	Brace Only	8
Paraplegia‡	Crutches and Long-Leg Brace, Pelvic Band	5

*From Gordon, E. E.: Development of the Applied Sciences to the Handicapped Homemaker. *In* Rehabilitation of the Physically Handicapped in Homemaking Activities. U. S. Department of Health, Education and Welfare, Vocational Rehabilitation Administration, 1963.
†Pace slower than normal.
‡Swing-thru gait.

In recent years standard tests have been developed that give better guidelines as to a patient's work tolerance than clinical observation alone. Changes in cardiac and pulmonary parameters, such as pulse rate and oxygen consumption, have been measured with a view to evaluating the patient's working capacity or readiness to return to remunerative employment.[49–51] Moreover, we have become much more aware of the tremendous energy requirements of ambulation in the severely disabled, particularly paraplegics.[52–54] The paraplegic walking with long leg braces, crutches and a pelvic band is only one-fourth as efficient as the individual without handicap (Table 21-1). It should be noted also that emotional stress itself causes increased cardiac work which is essentially wasted.[12, 51]

The recommendation for daily periods of cardiorespiratory and muscular exercise may appear contradictory after we have stressed work simplification and efficiency. On the contrary, short periods of graded exercise which are relatively intense are the basis of physical fitness and will increase the homemaker's ability to perform useful work. Rodahl and Issekutz[55] give a useful review of physical performance and training. Some activity aside from the fixed duties of homemaking is also necessary to maintain flexibility and optimal range of motion of joints. An exercise program may be contraindicated in the case of a patient with severe cardiopulmonary disease.

PSYCHOLOGY OF DISABILITY AND FAMILY RELATIONSHIPS

The handicapped homemaker has fears and anxieties which we, who are well, can only dimly perceive. She must learn to accept the difference in her appearance and she must finally adjust her life to a central fact—disability is permanent and the most fervent wishing will not make it disappear. She is perturbed by doubts concerning her abilities, her role as a wife and sexual partner and the way her children may respond to her altered appearance. It is all too true that a husband's sexual gratification and his companionship satisfaction are low when his wife is severely disabled.[84] Henrich and Kriegel[56] have described very well, through the words of disabled individuals, the turmoil caused by irreversible physical impairment. Wright[57] has written of disability as a psychosocial problem and defines difficulties in rehabilitation only indirectly related to the physical disability. Litman,[58] in a study of one hundred patients undergoing treatment in rehabilitation centers, has emphasized the importance of family support in the rehabilitation process.

If we are to help the homemaker achieve successful resettlement in her home, the family must be encouraged to take an active part in the training. Frequent visits to the hospital by family members help the patient, but also allow them to see the patient at work, to discover what she can do and to learn techniques of treatment which will be carried out at home.[59] Members of the rehabilitation team must learn to wait, to be patient and to understand that the patient's adjustment is a dynamic, constantly changing process.[60] Above all, society must learn tolerance and acceptance of "the differences among men"— especially those caused by disability.[61]

Two accounts of the trials and tribulations of disabled homemakers demonstrate that there are certain common factors in successful rehabilitation.[62, 63] They are courage, determination to succeed, family support, ability to change work habits and techniques and intelligent use of available facilities.

The question of marital counseling in families with a disabled member deserves more consideration. Certainly divorce is very common in situations where the wife or the husband becomes disabled.

HOME CARE AND HOMEMAKER SERVICES

These subjects have some relation to training in homemaking and deserve definition. Home care is the provision of health care and supportive services to the sick or disabled person in his place of residence. It may be provided in a diversity of patterns of organization and service running the gamut from nursing service under a physician's direction, to a program which is centrally administered and which through coordinated planning, evaluation and follow-up procedures provides for physician-directed medical, nursing, social and related services to selected patients at home.[64] Certainly the logical link between the homemaker and the hospital would be a hospital extension service.[65] Such a service would allow follow-up of patients' progress by team members such as the physician, rehabilitation nurse, social worker, dietitian, occupational therapist and physical therapist. There are administrative problems but the idea appears to be making headway in some hospitals.[66]

Homemaker services are services offered to families disrupted by death, illness or accident. A homemaker in this frame of reference is a trained housekeeper and cook who has skill in handling children. Such services are provided by many welfare and family agencies.[67, 68] There are even training programs available for persons who wish to qualify as visiting homemakers.[69] Home health aides have been added to homemaker services. Their function is to help the patient improve her level of independence by helping in the carrying out of instructions left by the occupational therapist, physical therapist, physician or other supervisor. The nutritionist or dietitian may offer useful services through consultation to staffs of home health agencies, membership on a professional advisory committee, and teaching programs for home health aides.[85] It is obvious that such services may be extremely helpful to individuals whose disability is so severe that independent function will never be possible.

CONCLUSION

There are many unsolved problems in the field of rehabilitation in general and homemaking training in particular. Physician and layman alike do not yet fully appreciate the problems of the disabled. "Although the able-bodied benefit from the best available brains and material, only crumbs from the table of science are devoted to the needs of the disabled. Because the applied sciences of metallurgy, plastics, electronics, biophysics, and biochemistry can fill these needs but fail to do so, handicap is today less an accident of nature than a condemnation by man."[70]

Krusen, appealing for new horizons for the handicapped, has written,[71] "Society continues to feel that the outlook for the handicapped patient is the ceiling or four walls at which he stares from his bed or wheelchair. It is up to us to widen this horizon to take in the new world of rehabilitation. . . . The needs of the physically handicapped represent one of our nation's most serious health problems. In fact, many of us could make a good case that it is now, or soon will be, our greatest health problem. But we must concede that we are a long way from convincing the general public and our legislative bodies of this fact. . . . The effort to arouse physicians to the need for rehabilitation must be part of a broader effort aimed at arousing all segments of our population to the compelling humanitarian needs of the disabled."

REFERENCES

1. May, E. E.: Vocational Rehabilitation for Handicapped Homemakers. Reprinted from American Vocational Journal, May, 1962.
2. Switzer, M. E.: Foreword. In Rehabilitation of the Physically Handicapped in Homemaking Activities. Proceedings of a Workshop. Highland Park, Ill., Jan. 27-30, 1963, U.S. Department of Health, Education and Welfare, Vocational Rehabilitation Administration.
3. Rusk, H. A., Kristeller, E. L., Judson, J. S., Hunt, G. M., and Zimmerman, M. E.: Introduction. In A Manual for Training the Disabled Homemaker. Rehabilitation Monograph VIII. 2nd Ed. New York, The Institute of Physical Medicine and Rehabilitation, New York University Medical Center, 1961.
4. Koch, A. R.: Significance and Scope of Rehabilitation in Homemaking Activities. In Rehabilitation of the Physically Handicapped in Homemaking Activities. Proceedings of a Workshop. Highland Park, Ill., Jan. 27-30, 1963, U.S. Department of Health, Education and Welfare, Vocational Rehabilitation Administration, p. 13.
5. Trotter, V. Y.: Home Economics. In Rehabilitation of the Physically Handicapped in Homemaking Activities. Proceedings of a Workshop. Highland Park, Ill., Jan. 27-30, 1963, U.S. Department of Health, Education and Welfare, Vocational Rehabilitation Administration, p. 103.
6. Jenson, I.: Representative Programs in Patients' Homes. In Rehabilitation of the Physically Handicapped in Homemaking Activities. Proceedings of a Workshop. Highland Park, Ill., Jan. 27-30, 1963, U.S. Department of Health, Education and Welfare, Vocational Rehabilitation Administration, p. 27.
7. Rusk, H. A., Kristeller, E. L., Judson, J. S., Hunt, G. M., and Zimmerman, M. E.: A Manual for Training the Disabled Homemaker. Rehabilitation Monograph VIII. 2nd Ed. New York, The Institute of Physical Medicine and Rehabilitation, New York University Medical Center, 1961, p. 2.
8. May, E. E.: Suggestions for the Rehabilitation of the Physically Handicapped Homemaker. Amer. J. Occup. Ther. 8:Part I, 1962, 1959.
9. The Physically Handicapped Housewife. SVCK's Publication Series No. 6. New York, The International Society for the Rehabilitation of the Disabled, 1959, p. 29.
10. Petrie, A.: Rehabilitation of the Housewife. Occup. Therapy, 27:19, 1964.
11. Passmore, R., and Durnin, J. V. G. A.: Human Energy Expenditure. Physiol. Rev., 35:801, 1955.
12. Gordon, E. E.: Development of the Applied Sciences to the Handicapped Homemaker. In Rehabilitation of the Physically Handicapped in Homemaking Activities. Proceedings of a Workshop. Highland Park, Ill., Jan. 27-30, 1963, U.S. Department of Health, Education and Welfare, Vocational Rehabilitation Administration, p. 159.
13. Zimmerman, M. E.: The Disabled Homemakers and Their Problems. In ISRD Conferences, The Physically Disabled and Their Environment. Stockholm, Oct. 12-18, 1961. New York, International Society for the Rehabilitation of the Disabled, 1962, p. 9.
14. Rusk, H. A., Kristeller, E. L., Judson, J. S., Hunt, G. M., and Zimmerman, M. E.: A Manual for Training the Disabled Homemaker. Rehabilitation Monograph VIII. 2nd Ed. New York, The Institute of Physical Medicine and Rehabilitation, New York University Medical Center, 1961, p. 144.
15. Cooksey, F. S.: Rehabilitation of the Disabled Housewife. Ann. Phys. Med., 1:120, 1952.
16. The Physically Handicapped Housewife. SVCK's Publication Series No. 6. New York, The International Society for the Rehabilitation of the Disabled, 1959, p. 25.
17. Rusk, H. A., Kristeller, E. L., Judson, J. S., Hunt, G. M., and Zimmerman, M. E.: A Manual for Training the Disabled Homemaker. Rehabilitation Monograph VIII. 2nd Ed. New York, The Institute of Physical Medicine and Rehabilitation, New York University Medical Center, 1961, p. 14.
18. Rusk, H. A., and Taylor, E. J.: Living with a Disability. New York, The Blakiston Company, Inc., 1953, p. 13.
19. Rusk, H. A., Kristeller, E. L., Judson, J. S., Hunt, G. M., and Zimmerman, M. E.: A Manual for Training the Disabled Homemaker. Rehabilitation Monograph VIII. 2nd Ed. New York, The Institute of Physical Medicine and Rehabilitation, New York University Medical Center, 1961, p. 49.
20. Åkerblom, B.: Chairs and Sitting. In Symposium on Human Factors in Equipment Design. The Ergonomics Research Society, Proceedings, Vol 2, edited by W. F. Floyd and A. T. Welford. London, H. K. Lewis & Co., Ltd., 1954, p. 29.
21. Morant, G. M.: Body Sizes and Work Spaces. In Symposium on Human Factors in Equipment Design. The Ergonomics Research Society. Proceedings, Vol. 2, edited by W. F. Floyd and A. T. Welford. London, H. K. Lewis & Co., Ltd., 1954, p. 17.

22. Knowles, W. E.: Some Effects of Height of Ironing Surface on the Worker. Bull. 833, Cornell University Agricultural Experimental Station, 1946.
23. Bed Positioning and Transfer Procedures for the Hemiplegic. Rehabilitative Nursing Techniques. 1. Minneapolis, Kenny Rehabilitation Institute, 1962.
24. Coles, C. H., Grendahl, B. C., Hannan, V. C., Plass, J. R., and Ulrich, P. G.: A Procedure for Passive Range of Motion and Self-Assistive Exercises. Rehabilitative Nursing Techniques. 3. Minneapolis, Kenny Rehabilitation Institute, 1964.
25. Up and Around. A Booklet to Aid the Stroke Patient in Activities of Daily Living. Public Health Publication No. 1120. U.S. Department of Health, Education and Welfare, Public Health Service, 1964.
26. Selected Equipment Useful in the Hospital, Home or Nursing Home. Rehabilitative Nursing Techniques. 2. Minneapolis, Kenny Rehabilitation Institute, 1962.
27. Callender, M. C., and Corcoran, S. P.: Bibliography on Home Management with Emphasis on Work Simplification for Handicapped Homemakers. Storrs, Conn., University of Connecticut, School of Home Economics, 1960.
28. Aho, S. M.: Bibliography on Work Simplification in Food Preparation for Handicapped Homemakers. Storrs, Conn., University of Connecticut, School of Home Economics, 1961.
29. Rusk, H. A., and Taylor, E. J.: Living with a Disability. New York. The Blakiston Company, Inc., 1953, p. 21.
30. Steinke, N., and Erickson, P.: Homemaking Aids for the Disabled. Minneapolis, Kenny Rehabilitation Institute, 1963.
31. Zmola, G. M.: You Can Do Laundry With Hand Limitations. Storrs, Conn., University of Connecticut, School of Home Economics, 1959.
32. McCullough, H. E., and Farnham, M. B.: Space and Design Requirements for Wheelchair Kitchens. Bull. 661, University of Illinois Agricultural Experimental Station, 1960.
33. Howard, M. S., Thye, L. S., and Tayloe, G. K.: The Beltsville Kitchen—Workroom with Energy Saving Features. Home and Garden Bulletin No. 60, U.S. Department of Agriculture, 1958.
34. McCullough, H. E., and Farnham, M. B.: Kitchens for Women in Wheelchairs. Circular 841, University of Illinois, College of Agriculture, Extension in Agriculture and Home Economics, 1961.
35. The Physically Handicapped Housewife. SVCK's Publication Series No. 6. New York, The International Society for the Rehabilitation of the Disabled, 1959, p. 17.
36. Leschly, V., Exner, I., and Exner, J.: General Lines in Designs of Dwellings for Handicapped Confined to Wheelchairs. Part I. Communications from The Testing and Observation Institute of the Danish National Association for Infantile Paralysis, No. 3. Hellerup, Denmark, 1959.
37. Leschly, V., Kjaer, A., and Kjaer, B.: General Lines in Designs of Dwellings for Handicapped Confined to Wheelchairs. Part 2. Communications from The Testing and Observation Institute of the Danish National Association for Infantile Paralysis, No. 6 Hellerup, Denmark, 1960.
38. Planning of Dwellings. In ISRD Conferences, The Physically Disabled and Their Environment, Stockholm. Oct. 12-18, 1961. New York, International Society for the Rehabilitation of the Disabled, 1962, p. 28.
39. Housing for the Disabled. Dwellings for Invalids Moving about in Wheelchairs. Dwellings for Invalids Moving about with the Aid of Crutches or Sticks. The Netherlands, Netherlands Central Society for the Care of Disabled, 1960.
40. Lowman, E. W., and Rusk, H. A.: Self-Help Devices. Rehabilitation Monograph XXI. New York, The Institute of Physical Medicine and Rehabilitation, New York University Medical Center, 1962, p. 59.
41. Zimmerman, M. E.: Clothing for the Disabled. In Rehabilitation of the Physically Handicapped in Homemaking Activities. Proceedings of a Workshop. Highland Park, Ill., Jan. 27-30, 1963, U.S. Department of Health, Education and Welfare, Vocational Rehabilitation Administration, p. 69.
42. Lowman, E. W., and Rusk, H. A.: Self-Help Devices. Rehabilitation Monograph XXI. New York, The Institute of Physical Medicine and Rehabilitation, New York University Medical Center, 1962, pp. 12-19.
43. May, E. E., and Waggoner, N. R.: Work Simplification in Child Care. Teaching Materials for the Rehabilitation of Physically Handicapped Homemakers. Storrs, Conn., University of Connecticut, School of Home Economics, 1962.
44. Waggoner, N. R., and Reedy, G. N.: Child Care Equipment for Physically Handicapped Mothers. Suggestions for Selection and Adaptation. Storrs, Conn., University of Connecticut, School of Home Economics, 1961.
45. Boettke, E. M.: Suggestions for Physically Handicapped Mothers on Clothing for Preschool Children. Storrs, Conn., University of Connecticut, School of Home Economics, 1957.

46. Bare, C., Boettke, E., and Waggoner, N.: Self-Help Clothing for Handicapped Children. Storrs, Conn., University of Connecticut, School of Home Economics, 1962.
47. May, E. E.: Homemaking Instruction for Handicapped Children. Children, *11:*32, 1964.
48. Wall, J. S.: Play Experiences Handicapped Mothers May Share with Young Children. Storrs, Conn., University of Connecticut, School of Home Economics, 1961.
49. Asmussen, E., and Molbech, S. V.: Methods and Standards for Evaluation of the Physiological Working Capacity of Patients. Communications from the Testing and Observation Institute of the Danish National Association for Infantile Paralysis, No. 4. Hellerup, Denmark, 1959.
50. Asmussen, E., Brandt, M., Molbech, S. V., and Mortensen, K.: A New Test for Estimating Fitness for Housework. Communications from the Testing and Observation Institute of the Danish National Foundation for Infantile Paralysis, No. 10. Hellerup, Denmark, 1961.
51. Kottke, F. J., Kubicek, W. G., Olson, M. E., Hasting, R. H., and Quast, K.: Five Stage Test of Cardiac Performance during Occupational Activity. Arch. Phys. Med., *43:*228, 1962.
52. Clinkingbeard, J. R., Gersten, J. W., and Hoehn, D.: Energy Cost of Ambulation in the Traumatic Paraplegic. Am. J. Phys. Med., *43:*157, 1964.
53. Gordon, E. E., and Vanderwalde, H.: Energy Requirements in Paraplegic Ambulation. Arch. Phys. Med., *37:*276, 1956.
54. Bard, G., and Ralston, H. J.: Measurement of Energy Expenditure during Ambulation, with Special Reference to Assistive Devices. Arch. Phys. Med., *40:*415, 1959.
55. Rodahl, K., and Issekutz, B.: Physical Performance Capacity of the Older Individual. In Muscle as a Tissue. Edited by K. Rodahl and S. M. Horvath. New York, McGraw-Hill Book Company, Inc., 1962, p. 272.
56. Henrich, E., and Kriegel, L.: Experiments in Survival. New York, Association for the Aid of Crippled Children, 1961.
57. Wright, B. A.: Physical Disability—A Psychological Approach. New York, Harper and Brothers, 1960.
58. Litman, T. J.: An Analysis of the Sociologic Factors Affecting the Rehabilitation of the Physically Handicapped. Arch. Phys. Med., *45:*9, 1964.
59. Peszczynski, M., Fowles, B. H., and Mahan, S. P.: Function of Home Evaluations in Discharging Rehabilitated Severely Disabled from the Hospital. Arch. Phys. Med., *42:*109, 1961.
60. Christopherson, V. A.: The Patient and the Family. Rehab. Lit., *23:*34, 1962.
61. Harlem, G.: The Place of Persons with Disabilities in Society. In Rehabilitation and World Peace. Proceedings of the Eighth World Congress of the International Society for the Welfare of Cripples. Edited by E. J. Taylor, New York, Aug. 28–Sept. 2, 1960.
62. Where There's A Will. Storrs, Conn., University of Connecticut, School of Home Economics, 1958.
63. One-Armed Mother. Reprinted from the Ladies' Home Journal, July, 1959.
64. Statement on the Role and Responsibilities of Hospitals in Home Care. Reprinted from Hospitals, July 1, 1964.
65. Kovell, J.: A Home Care Program for King County. Am. J. Occup. Ther., *18:*255, 1964.
66. Kissick, W., Rudnick, B., and Rossman, I.: Procedure Manual for Home Care—Montefiore Hospital. New York, 1962.
67. Homemaker Services in Public Welfare. U.S. Department of Health, Education and Welfare, Welfare Administration, April, 1964.
68. Morlock, M.: Homemaker Services: History and Bibibliography. Children's Bureau Publication No. 410, U.S. Department of Health, Education and Welfare, Welfare Administration, 1964.
69. The Visiting Homemaker, A Suggested Training Program. U.S. Department of Health, Education and Welfare, Office of Education, Division of Vocational and Technical Education, 1964.
70. Gordon, E. E.: Development of Community Responsibility in Handicapped Youth. Med. Times, *90:*60, 1962.
71. Krusen, F. H.: Concepts in Rehabilitation of the Handicapped. Philadelphia, W. B. Saunders Company, 1964, p. 63.
72. Gordon, E. E.: Do It Yourself Again. Self-Help Devices for the Stroke Patient. New York, American Heart Association, 1969.
73. Helping the disabled housewife. Brit. Med. J. *3:*598–599, 1970.
74. Lowman, E. W., and Klinger, J. L.: Aids to Independent Living. Self-Help for the Handicapped. New York, McGraw-Hill, Inc., 1969.
75. Agerholm, M. (Ed.): Equipment for the Disabled. An Index of Equipment, Aids and Ideas for the Disabled. London, National Fund for Research into Poliomyelitis and other Crippling Diseases. Vincent House, Vincent Square, ed. 2, 1966.
76. Wheeler, V. H.: Planning Kitchens for Handicapped Homemakers. Rehabilitation Monograph XXVII. New York, Institute of Rehabilitation Medicine, 1965.
77. Disabled Housewives in Their Kitchens. London, Disabled Living Foundation, Vincent House, Vincent Square, 1970.

78. Klinger, J. L., Frieden, F. H., and Sullivan, R. A.: Mealtime Manual for the Aged and Handicapped. New York, Essandess, 1970.
79. Smith, C. R.: Home Planning for the Severely Disabled. Med. Clin. N. Amer., *53:*703, 1969.
80. Center Park for the Handicapped. Seattle Housing Authority, 1969.
81. May, E. E., Waggoner, N. R., and Boettke, E. M.: Homemaking for the Handicapped. New York, Dodd, Mead and Company, 1966, p. 85.
82. Isherwood, P. A.: Ergonomics and the Disabled. International Rehab. Rev., *21:*9, 1970.
83. Steidl, R. E., and Bratton, E. C.: Work in the Home. New York, John Wiley and Sons. 1968, Chapters 7 and 8.
84. Skipper, J. K., Fink, S. L., and Hallenbeck, P. N.: Physical Disability among Married Women: Problems in the Husband-Wife Relationship. J. Rehab., *34:*16, 1968.
85. Youland, D. M., Barry, M. B., Ames, J. L., Gemple, N., and Whitten, M. M.: Nutrition Services in Home Health Agencies. J. Amer. Diet. Ass., *56:*111, 1970.

Chapter 22

PRESCRIBING PHYSICAL AND OCCUPATIONAL THERAPY

by Gordon M. Martin

A well-written prescription for physical and occupational therapy containing sufficient specific detail is essential to the effective use of these methods of treatment. Such written prescriptions provide the physician an opportunity to plan, specify and correlate various techniques and procedures into a suitable program designed to improve or develop physical function to a realistic maximal goal. The prescription may be a simple one for short-term treatment or it may provide a complex and changing program over a prolonged period for the severely and chronically handicapped patient. In any case, the prescription must be concise, clear, specific and individualized. The suitability of the prescription and the effectiveness of the therapy are in large measure dependent on the physician's interest and knowledge of this field and his ability to work well with the therapists, at the same time keeping the patient interested, motivated and cooperative.

Purposes.   There are several important purposes of the detailed, specific written prescription. It provides the therapist with basic aims and specific directions for treating patients. It is designed to ensure the physician that his orders will be followed and that misunderstandings between physician and therapist will not arise. It will provide a permanent record of the treatment prescribed and administered. Such records are valuable for use in the future care of a patient and in insurance or compensation cases. It will serve to protect both physician and therapist in case of medicolegal complications.

510

The Physician as Prescriber. Certain qualifications are expected of the person prescribing physical therapy, occupational therapy or other rehabilitative procedures. Only a physician is licensed to prescribe. He need not be a physiatrist. He should, however, refer certain patients to, or consult with, a physiatrist when this would provide better service to the patient. The physician should have basic knowledge of the biophysical and physiologic effects of the various procedures used in physical and occupational therapy. He should know the indications for their use as well as the contraindications and limitations. He should have knowledge of the training, special abilities and possible limitations of the therapists. He should be aware of equipment, facilities and time available for physical treatment. He should be cognizant of the principle that an ethical, licensed therapist treats patients only with an adequate prescription or written instructions.

Preliminary Considerations.   Before the physician turns the patient and the prescription over to the therapist, an adequate working diagnosis should be established based on history, physical findings and laboratory tests as indicated. Only treatment and procedures that have been proven clinically to be beneficial should be prescribed. It should be ascertained that the prescription contains sufficient detail so that the therapist can proceed efficiently and with assurance and not have to question the patient or call the physician relative to proper position, removal of supports or mobility and strength of involved parts. A short summary of essential physical findings and diagnosis should accompany the prescription.

The type of treatment, the aims of treatment and the result expected in the immediate future or in the long run should be explained to the patient. The costs of treatment should be evaluated and discussed with the patient; the need or availability of insurance or other aid may have to be determined if prolonged treatment is expected. The patient should be informed about, and the prescription should indicate specific instructions for, any treatment measures or procedures to be used at home.

Common Errors

An awareness of common errors that are made in prescribing physical treatment can lead to more efficient or effective therapy.

Delay in starting treatments may unnecessarily prolong a period of disability and suffering. Often physicians err in assuming that stiffness or weakness following fractures or soft tissue trauma "will work itself out" with ordinary use or with some simple exercises that may merely be described superficially to the patient in an office visit. The patient, too, may be reluctant to undertake treatments that tend to be time-consuming and expensive, and he may want to gamble on nature's tendency to bring about spontaneous improvement.

A "shotgun" type of prescription can be disadvantageous, as, for instance, in prescriptions for several types of heat in one therapy session, or for heat, massage and exercise when only a concise prescription for therapeutic exercise is indicated. The type of treatment prescribed in the "shotgun" manner may detract from or miss the primary aim of the treatment. Such haphazard treatment is unnecessarily time-consuming for therapist and patient alike and hence is inefficient. These procedures tend to be seen when a checklist order sheet is used. Although a checklist order sheet may be satisfactory for ordering laboratory tests, it does not permit an adequately detailed, individualized prescription for physical treatment.

Selection of Patients. If patients are not selected with some discrimination, the results are poor and the therapist's time and effort are exploited or wasted; under such circumstances patients may understandably become disillusioned or discouraged.

The severe psychoneurotic patient with multiple somatic complaints and lack of insight either will not benefit from therapy or will become overly dependent on both treatment and physical therapist. However, many patients with functional neuromuscular complaints who have tension anxiety states but possess some insight into their problems may be benefited greatly by physical and occupational therapy and by instructions in a program of home treatment and diversional activities.

Patients having complaints of peripheral pains that are of thalamic or central nervous system origin do not benefit from physical therapy. Patients with progressive metastatic lesions are generally poor candidates for prolonged treatment. Patients with stroke or those with residual effects of cerebral trauma who remain semicomatose, confused and stuporous, or who are unable or unwilling to cooperate, usually do not benefit from unduly prolonged physical therapy and rehabilitation.

The severely involved arthritic cripple can rarely be helped significantly by physical treatment alone. Occasionally an intensive program utilizing the combined efforts of a rheumatologist, orthopedic surgeon and physiatrist will result in good progress.

Most patients who are antagonistic or uncooperative relative to treatment are poor candidates.

Other Errors. Vague, muddled or inadequate prescriptions are of little use to a therapist. These may lack sufficient detail or specify treatment that cannot be carried out or tolerated by the patient.

The therapist is sometimes expected or encouraged to select or prescribe the treatment. This is both illegal and unethical and it encourages the therapist to practice medicine without qualifications or license.

The patient should not be permitted to prescribe his own treatment nor should the therapist be permitted to "give him whatever he asks for."

Treatments that are given too infrequently may be a source of disappointing results. Generally, at first, daily or even twice-daily treatments are indicated. Later, the frequency may be decreased to two or three times weekly as progress is made and as the patient learns to carry on with treatment procedures at home. Treatment once weekly is worthless.

The use of so-called "routine" orders results in a gross misuse of physical therapy and permits, essentially, prescription by the therapist. There is no such thing as the "arthritis routine," "hemiplegia routine" or "low-back routine." The prescription should be individualized and specific for each patient.

Telephoned or verbal orders should be considered only a temporary expedient and should be followed up by a properly written prescription.

Inadequate or delayed follow-up and recheck by the physician is a common pitfall that may unnecessarily prolong treatment. Generally, orders must be changed as response to treatment is observed and progress is made.

ESSENTIALS OF THE PRESCRIPTION

The essentials of the physical therapy or occupational therapy prescription should be recorded on a departmental record or order sheet, which should become a permanent part of the patient's office or hospital history and record file.

The diagnosis should be given, whether it is a final diagnosis or a tentative one. A brief summary of history and physical findings will provide pertinent information for the physical or occupational therapist and for the consulting physicians, residents or interns who will be following the course of the patient. The patient's hospital, clinic or office record is generally not available with the patient at the time of each treatment. Thus, the statement "see record" or "see history" is useless to physicians and therapists who are treating or following the course of the patient in the department of physical medicine. Measurements of range of motion and muscle strength that are recorded with the original prescription provide base lines for evaluation of progress.

The part or parts to be treated are to be determined by the physician and indicated by him on the order sheet. Procedures to be used with specifications as to apparatus, techniques and time should have the most prominence on the prescription sheet.

Special instructions or cautions should be clearly indicated. If a splint or bandage is to be removed during treatment, this should be recorded. The presence of diabetes, convulsive disorder, angina or mental confusion should be clearly indicated so that the therapist can observe necessary precautions.

Home treatment instructions for the patient should be specifically ordered by the physician and the technical details of the instructions supplied by the therapists. Generally, instructions can best be given during the course of several treatment sessions. Printed or written instructions given to the patient serve as reminders of what to do, but "how to do it" can be learned properly only by actual *doing* it under close supervision of a competent instructor.

The number and frequency of treatments must be indicated and the date for the physician's recheck of the patient should appear on the prescription. In addition, the order sheet should include dates of treatment, names of therapists treating the patient, progress notes by physicians and therapists and the patient's condition at time of dismissal as well as the final recommendations. See the sample prescriptions at the end of this chapter.

Physical Therapy

Thermotherapy. The essential elements of a prescription for thermotherapy are the following: the source of heat to be used—heat lamp, shortwave diathermy, warm tub bath, contrast bath or others; the part to be treated, specifying local areas and the position of patient; the time or duration of application and number of daily applications; specifications regarding technique, listing of the type of applicator, such as coil, hinged drum or vaginal electrode for shortwave diathermy, with electrode temperature specified for the last-named technique; and the intensity in terms of output or temperature measurement when possible. *Low intensity* must be indicated for anesthetic areas and in debilitated individuals or for those with a possible intolerance or sensitivity to heat. The temperature of the water should be indicated when hydrotherapy is prescribed.

Massage. In the prescription for therapeutic massage, the type or types must be specified. This may be the *stroking* or *kneading* types, which are usually combined, or *friction* massage, which may be specified for certain limited areas. Other types of manual massage or the use of mechanical massage devices are infrequently prescribed.

Specifications include indication of quality, that is, *deep* or *light* and *sedative* (most common) or *stimulating* massage. Avoidance of recent surgical incisions and varicosities may have to be noted.

The parts to be massaged should be specifically listed. Patients frequently attempt to have the therapist massage more extensive areas, which would prolong treatment unreasonably. Therapeutic manual massage is time-consuming and should not be prescribed indiscriminately.

Electrical Stimulation. Prescription for electrical stimulation should be preceded by a manual muscle test, sensory test and electrodiagnostic tests when indicated.

The types of current and apparatus used are interrupted galvanic or slow sinusoidal (6 to 40 cycles per second) for denervated muscle and faradic-like current or sine wave current of 30 to 1000 cycles per second for muscles when the lower motor neuron is intact.

Specifications should include the number of contractions or surges per minute, the approximate number of contractions at each session (generally 60 to 150) and the intensity of the current or the strength of contractions. Individual muscles, muscle groups or nerves to be stimulated should be listed.

Therapeutic Exercise. The prescription for therapeutic exercise is generally the most complex and difficult part of the prescription for physical therapy. It must be preceded by a complete evaluation of malfunction, including manual muscle tests, evaluation of range of motion, status of bones and joints and noting of coordination problems. Frequently, several types of exercises should be prescribed for one or several different parts of the extremities or trunk. The prescription should indicate clearly just what exercise procedures the therapist is to employ. The type of therapeutic exercise is listed first.

PASSIVE. These are relaxed exercises without forcing or stretching. If stretching, forcing or manipulation is desired, it must be clearly specified since these are not true passive exercises.

ACTIVE ASSISTIVE. Exercises with assistance by the therapist or by an assistive apparatus are prescribed for parts with which the patient cannot carry out active exercise satisfactorily.

ACTIVE. These exercises are most frequently prescribed to maintain range of motion and increase strength and endurance.

RESISTIVE. Exercises against resistance are prescribed for strengthening muscles. Several satisfactory techniques and programs have been described for progressive resistive exercises. Indications are made regarding apparatus such as wall weights, sandbags, weighted boots and manual resistance.

REEDUCATION. Reeducation exercises are prescribed for retraining in individual function and coordination of recovering paralyzed or paretic muscles or tendon transplants. They may be prescribed in any condition in which there are poor coordination and muscle imbalances.

COORDINATION. Exercises for coordination are of several types. Originally they were designed to utilize visual reflexes in replacing poor proprioceptive reflexes. Now they may be combined with reeducation exercises and with occupational therapy for any condition involving poor coordination and muscle imbalances.

RELAXATION. The principles of relaxation and the appropriate exercises are prescribed for patients with persistent muscle guarding and spasm and persistently hypertonic muscles as observed in patients with tension states.

Other specifications essential to the prescription for exercise include the specific parts to be exercised (joints, muscles or an extremity), the number of exercise periods daily, the duration of each exercise period, indications as to grading or progression of the program, apparatus to be used and exercises to be done by patient at home or on his own.

There are several reasons for failure of a prescribed exercise program. The prescribed program may be overwhelming to the patient. It may exceed his capabilities and be overfatiguing or may aggravate pain or other symptoms; if so, it should be modified but not necessarily discontinued. There may be lack of cooperation, enthusiasm or understanding on the part of the patient. Lack of care and attention to detail by the therapist administering the exercises may occur when the therapist has too many patients to treat and thus leaves the patient to exercise without adequate supervision.

Ambulation.   Training and assistance with ambulation is often an important part of physical therapy. The decision as to the need for cane, crutches, walker, braces or other special assistive devices is the physician's prerogative.

Preliminary strengthening exercises may be needed and should be included in the prescription. Preparatory to crutch walking, progressive resistive exercises for latissimus dorsi, triceps and biceps may be indicated along with those for quadriceps and hip extensors and abductors. Mat exercises, crawling, rolling, sitting, balance or tilt-table procedures may precede ambulation for some patients (for example, paraplegics). Parallel bars may be prescribed for assistance and balance for patients learning correct patterns of gait.

The type of crutch gait—four-point or three-point, with or without weight bearing and the amount of weight bearing permitted; swing-to or swing-through; or walk-to or walk-through—should be specified.

Practice on curbs and steps is prescribed when the patient is competent in walking on level surfaces with cane or crutches. Getting in and out of chairs and bed correctly should be prescribed with the ambulation training. Crossing streets and getting in and out of cars are final steps in the ambulation prescription.

Occupational Therapy

The prescription for occupational therapy requires the same preliminary considerations and essentially the same evaluation and summary of history and physical status as are described for the physical therapy record. In some departments of physical medicine the prescription for occupational therapy is included on the same order sheet as that for physical therapy.

Certain factors are particularly important in the guidance of the occupational therapist. The diagnosis is again included. Present physical status and general condition of the patient should be given as well as the mental and emotional status and any significant psychologic factors. Indication should be made as to whether occupational therapy is to be done in bed or in the occupational therapy department and the time to be devoted to these activities should be specified.

Specific aims and desired results should be indicated on the prescription. Functional or kinetic activities are prescribed for mobilizing, coordinating or strengthening specific parts. Functional occupational therapy generally supplements physical therapy.

Training in certain phases of the activities of daily living is carried out by the occupational therapist on prescription. The physician should indicate whether the activities are to be done in bed or in a wheelchair, and what specific limitations will be encountered. Generally this work by the occupational therapist is correlated with certain phases of training in self-help, transfer and daily living activities that are taught by the nursing staff and physical therapists. Special assistive devices may be designed and fashioned by the occupational therapist for the severely handicapped patient at the request of the physician. The prescription for functional occupational therapy can specify areas for special attention, i.e., dressing, grooming, eating, homemaking activities, fine coordination, increasing speed or mobility.

Some occupational therapy departments can construct splints for preventing or controlling potential deformities of the hand of patients with rheumatoid arthritis or hemiplegia. Functional splints, such as a tenodesis splint for a tetraplegic, can be fitted in occupational therapy, and training and practice in their use may be prescribed.

Diversional, "tonic," recreational and avocational activities may be prescribed for the physically handicapped as well as for those with mental illness. Prevocational exploratory services are available on request or prescription in some occupational therapy departments.

The attitude the therapist is to take—whether he should insist on productive work or merely invite or encourage the patient—should be indicated on the prescription. Suggestions or information as to the patient's likes, dislikes, attitudes, previous occupations and hobbies may be of real value to the therapist in establishing good rapport and achieving an effective program of occupational therapy.

SAMPLE PRESCRIPTIONS

These sample prescriptions illustrate some of the principles that have been discussed. They are not to be considered as standard or routine prescriptions or necessarily ideal prescriptions for patients with the condition listed. Each prescription must be individualized and then modified as changing status indicates need for variations and progression.

DEGENERATIVE LUMBOSACRAL DISK WITH RADICULITIS, LEFT SIDE

Treatment	Time, Minutes	Specifications
Radiant heat	30	Lamp to low back and left hip (lying on right side)
Massage	10–15	Deep stroking and kneading, low back and left hip
Exercises		Abdominal strengthening exercises
		Non-weight bearing pelvic flexion
		Trunk flexion from sitting position
		Posture principles for low back and pelvis

Treat: Daily 3 times for instruction
Instruct: Heat lamp
       Exercises as listed above

ADHESIVE CAPSULITIS, RIGHT SHOULDER

Treatment	Time, Minutes	Specifications
Ultrasound	10	1.5 watts per sq. cm.
		Stroking technique, right shoulder
Massage	5–10	Deep stroking and kneading to right shoulder
Exercise	10–15	Active and assistive right shoulder
		Moderate stretch
		Wall ladder
		Overhead pulley
		Shoulder wheel
		Codman's exercise with 5 lb. sandbag

Treat daily. Physician's recheck after 5 treatments
Instruct: Infrared lamp 30 min. daily
  Active exercises and pulley and ladder assistive exercises, two times daily at home

LEFT HEMIPLEGIA (ONSET ON JANUARY 26)

Date	Treatment	Time, Minutes	Specifications
2–1	*Exercise* Passive	10	Left upper and lower extremities through normal range, 3–4 times each joint (remove footdrop splint for treatment)
2–7	Reeducation and coordination Active	20	Left upper and lower extremities
			Normal range, right upper and lower extremities (avoid fatigue; encourage use of normal extremities for activities of daily living)
2–16	Active and assistive		Left shoulder and elbow
			Left hip and knee
			Powder board with assistance for hip and knee flexion and extension, and hip abduction and adduction
	Resistive		Right quadriceps
			30 contractions daily—10 each of ½, ¾, and full 10 rep. max.*
2–18	*Gait training*	B.i.d.	Parallel bars with knee splint and foot support
			Sling left arm
			1. Standing balance
			2. Walking
2–22	Gait	B.i.d.	Start on glider cane with assistance (cane in right hand)
3–2	Gait	B.i.d.	Walk with regular cane and footdrop brace
3–6	Gait	B.i.d.	Climb stairs, ramp
			In and out of chairs
			In and out of car

2–1 Treat once daily in patient's room
  Physician check q. 3 days
2–7 Treat in physical medicine and rehabilitation department twice daily
2–8 Occupational therapy for left hand and arm. Help with activities of daily living
3–4 Instruct in normal range of motion exercises for home use

  *By "10 rep. max." (10 repetition maximum) is meant the number of pounds that can be moved through the full range 10 times.

RHEUMATOID ARTHRITIS (HANDS, ELBOWS, SHOULDERS, KNEES AND FEET)

Treatment	Time, Minutes	Specifications
Radiant heat	30	Two bakers—patient supine (alternate with hydrotherapy)
Hydrotherapy	30, 3 times weekly 30	Hubbard tank—water temperature 102° F., with active assistive underwater exercise of shoulders, elbows, knees Contrast baths, hands and feet; once for instruction
Massage	20	Deep stroking and kneading to hands, shoulders, knees
Exercise	10	Active and assistive, work toward normal range in above joints Resistive isometric with 5 lb. sandbag, 10 contractions for each quadriceps. Later progressive resistive exercise program Posture correction and principles, stand, sit, lie
Gait	5	Supervise walking short distances In and out of chair Stair climbing

Treat daily for 2 weeks
Instruct: Daily contrast baths at home, water temperature 110° F. and 65° F. for hands and feet
　　　　Warm tub bath twice a week, water temperature 102° F., 20 minutes

REFERENCES

1. Martin, G. M.: Physical Therapy in the General Practitioner's Office. Minnesota Med., *42*:235–239, 1959.
2. Martin, G. M.: The Physical Therapy Equipment for a Physician's Office. New Physician, *9*: 25–29, 1960.
3. Martin, G. M.: Prescription Writing in Physical Medicine and Rehavilitation. Mayo Graduate School Teaching Outline, 1960.
4. Martin, G. M.: Clinical Applications of Physical Medicine and Rehabilitation to General Medical Problems. Proc. Mayo Clin., *36*:75–87, 1961.
5. Martin, G. M.: Physical Medicine in Rheumatoid Arthritis. Arthritis Rheum., *6*:177–182, 1963.
6. Stillwell, G. K.: The Use of Physical Medicine in Office Practice With Particular Emphasis on the Aftercare of Fractures. J. Iowa Med. Soc., *53*:12–18, 1963.

Part III

EVALUATION AND MANAGEMENT OF SPECIFIC DISORDERS

Chapter 23

REHABILITATION OF THE STROKE HEMIPLEGIA PATIENT

by Carl Levenson

INTRODUCTION

Hemiplegia is one of the disorders most frequently referred for rehabilitation. The characteristic paralysis of the arm and leg is a neuromuscular functional residue caused usually by occlusion or rupture of an artery that supplies the contralateral hemisphere of the brain. This is the common stroke or cerebrovascular accident. It is a focal, neurologic disorder with an abrupt onset and rapid development due to pathologic changes in the blood vessel.

The need for a rehabilitation program arises from the functional deficits that follow the stroke. Many who suffer a cerebrovascular accident do not survive the first attack. Others recover completely with no apparent impairment. In still others varying degrees of functional impairment remain, producing disability that ranges from total, bedridden, incontinent dependency to almost complete self-sufficiency, with residual difficulties in the use of the involved upper extremity or in standing and ambulation. Rehabilitation is concerned with those survivors of cerebrovascular accidents who have some functional impairment and disability.

The aim in rehabilitation of the hemiplegic stroke victim is to afford the patient an opportunity to lead as fulfilling and self-sufficient a life as his physical, emotional and socioeconomic resources permit. The rehabilitation process seeks to accomplish this goal by narrowing any disparity that may exist between the patient's disability in performance and the potential capabilities present despite the neuromuscular physiologic impairment produced by the stroke. The sensory and motor deficits in the upper motor neuron involvements should not prevent most patients from relearning how to transfer, stand and ambulate but many are unable to accomplish these activities independently. The disparity between impairment and disability is narrowed not only by techniques and devices to improve performance, but also by helping the patient overcome the fears, depressions and anger that prevent him from accepting and using help.

The physiatrist, in guiding the rehabilitation of the stroke patient after he has made his evaluation, not only must prescribe various treatments and devices but also must assist the professional staff in their orientation to the psychologic and socioeconomic needs of patients.

Magnitude of the Problem

It is estimated that 1.8 million persons who have suffered a cerebrovascular accident are alive in this country. About one third, or 600,000 of them, are former wage earners who were made unemployable by the residuals of a stroke.[50] Today cerebrovascular diseases rank third as a cause of death in this country and are exceeded only by heart disease and cancer. The problem, although its magnitude is already appalling, is expected to become more prevalent because of the increase in longevity of the population in this country. It is the increase in numbers of older persons that will provide the anticipated increased numbers of stroke patients. There were about 17 million people 65 years of age and older in this country in 1964. This number is estimated to be 20 million in 1970. Preliminary studies by the United States Public Health Service indicate that a member of one in 10 households will fall victim to a stroke during a 10 year period.

Physical medicine and rehabilitation has made a notable contribution to the rapidly growing international interest in strokes. The immensity of the problem has created concern. The literature is growing rapidly and many research projects are devoted to this area. Numerous methods for investigating the causes, attempts to find means for prevention and tools for diagnosis are being developed. Anticoagulation has been used for some time to prevent repetition of arterial occlusion by emboli. Research attempts have been made to dissolve the already existing clot by the use of thrombolysins. Arteriography, ophthalmodynamometry, and isotope brain scanning are being used diagnostically at the clinical level (Fig. 23–1).

The most effective impetus to medical interest in strokes has come from the positive, hopeful approach of the proponents of physical medicine and rehabilitation toward management of patients who have had strokes. Before World War II, except for the efforts of a few doggedly persistent physicians, the long-term medical approach to survivors of strokes was enshrouded in a fog of indifference. During and after the war, physiatrists demonstrated the validity of a hopeful attitude toward rehabilitating patients with quadriplegia, paraplegia and hemiplegia.

Dr. Trevor H. Howell, physician to the Geriatric Research Unit, St. John's Hospital, London, told his confreres attending the London Rehabilitation Stroke Conference in 1961:

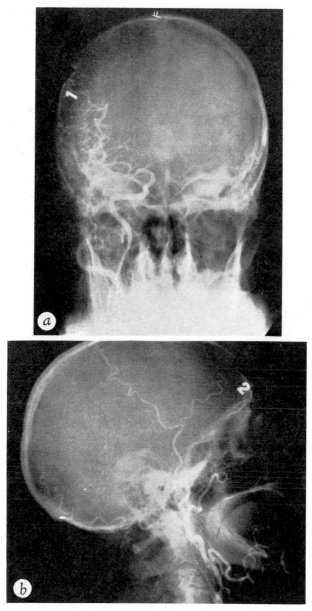

Figure 23-1   Right carotid arteriogram. *a.* Anteroposterior view reveals filling of intracranial vessels. *b.* Lateral view three minutes later. The internal carotid artery is occluded at its origin. The needle tip can be seen at the point of occlusion. This is an example of diagnostic value of arteriograms in cerebrovascular disease. (From Baker, H. L., Jr.: Angiographic Investigation of Cerebrovascular Insufficiency. Radiology, 77:399–405, 1961.

The approach to stroke rehabilitation nowadays is a positive one. New methods of treatment help to bring about a quicker and better recovery. Among one series of 200 elderly patients sent to a hospital for the chronic sick, more than one-half recovered while over one-quarter were able to resume a normal life at home. All of these were serious cases, some having failed to benefit from treatment in a general hospital. We must still fight hard against incontinence, contractures, and bed sores, but the outlook for the future is promising. The day is now past when a stroke meant inevitable paralysis and a hopeless future.[51]

Effectiveness of Rehabilitation

At a national stroke conference held in 1964 in Chicago under the chairmanship of Dr. Frank H. Krusen, it was estimated that with the help of rehabilitation programs 90 per cent of patients with hemiplegia can be taught to get out of bed, 70 per cent can become self-sufficient and 30 per cent of those in the employable age group can return to work.*

The effectiveness of an organized rehabilitation program for severely involved patients with hemiplegia was demonstrated in 1957 by Lowenthal, Tobis and Howard of New York City, who followed 232 cerebrovascular accident patients admitted that year to Metropolitan Hospital, a 1000 bed institution.[34] This group of patients represented 4 per cent of all medical admissions. A comprehensive rehabilitation program was available to those who survived. The investigators found that only 3 per cent of the stroke patients remained dependent at the end of their hospital stay. This small percentage of dependency contrasted with results of a similar study among 206 patients in a Glasgow, Scotland, hospital by Rankin.[45a] Among a similar group of stroke patients to whom no organized rehabilitation program was available, Rankin found that dependency on discharge was 18 per cent. Lowenthal et al., in assessing the two sets of figures, believed that the difference was the result of the effectiveness of an organized rehabilitation effort.

Importance of Attitudes

A rehabilitation program for severely involved stroke survivors is most effective when it represents a comprehensive approach under trained medical guidance that is supported by trained paramedical personnel. The staff involved in management of the patient must be aware of the neuromuscular dysfunction and concomitant medical disorders. The staff must also evaluate the influence of emotional, intellectual, social and vocational problems.

The attitude of the staff members toward the hemiplegic patient has a far-reaching, if not determinative, influence. The entire staff must recognize and support the patient in his emotional struggle to overcome the profound shock, frustration and fear that he experiences when he finds himself reduced to complete dependence due to his inability to make his own body respond to his commands. It is not enough to "urge" the patient to become independent and useful again. Those about him must help him feel his worthiness as a human being. To overcome depression the hemiplegic patient must realize that his life still has meaning and purpose. The attitude of the staff should communicate acceptance of a patient's worthiness. The physiatrist, as the guiding influence, should diffuse this attitude throughout the staff. It helps the fearful hemiplegic patient to struggle free of frustrations and resentments that bind him to his disability even more than does his neuromuscular impairment. If the patient believes in his own worth, in his own emotional and physical strength, in his

---

*Proceedings of the National Stroke Congress, 1964.

own integrity, he then may accept a revised physical image of himself and accept his physical limitations. He becomes free to accept help and to develop independence. He can then reap the splendid reward of his own sense of achievement without which his life would have little meaning.

ETIOLOGY

Three basic processes account for most strokes: thrombosis, embolism and hemorrhage.

Thrombosis. Most stroke patients referred for rehabilitation have suffered strokes caused by thrombosis. Seventy-nine per cent of victims of stroke due to thrombosis survive the initial stroke, but a large percentage succumb to subsequent thrombi. Thrombosis commonly occurs during sleep, during vascular collapse in myocardial infarctions and following surgery (Fig. 23–2).

Embolism. Victims of strokes caused by embolism are least frequently encountered in rehabilitation programs because they usually recover more quickly with less residue than victims of other kinds of strokes. Embolism usually originates in the heart. It occurs in all age groups and is seen in the young although it is more common in the fifth and sixth decades. It is often associated with mitral stenosis and rheumatic fever, with coronary thrombosis and with auricular fibrillation. Subacute bacterial endocarditis can produce it and sometimes must be excluded.

Hemorrhage. Other stroke patients in rehabilitation are victims of a process that is caused by bleeding from the rupture of a vessel into the substance of the brain. Large hemorrhages usually stem from an artery. Small extravasations may arise from capillaries and veins. Causes for leakage from vessels include hypertension, aneurysm, hemorrhagic blood disease, trauma and erod-

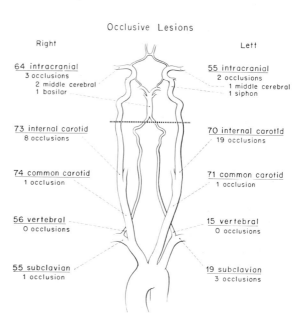

Occlusive Lesions

Right   Left

64 intracranial   55 intracranial
  3 occlusions   2 occlusions
  2 middle cerebral   1 middle cerebral
  1 basilar   1 siphon

73 internal carotid   70 internal carotid
  8 occlusions   19 occlusions

74 common carotid   71 common carotid
  1 occlusion   1 occlusion

56 vertebral   15 vertebral
  0 occlusions   0 occlusions

55 subclavian   19 subclavian
  1 occlusion   3 occlusions

Figure 23–2 The incidence and distribution of vascular occlusions observed in 154 angiograms. (From Baker, H. L., Jr.: Angiographic Investigation of Cerebrovascular Insufficiency. Radiology, 77:399–405, 1961.)

ing tumors. Hemorrhages cause the most profound residual functional deficits and the slowest recoveries.

An official classification and clarification of cerebrovascular diseases was evolved and published by an Ad Hoc Committee established by the Advisory Council of the National Institute of Neurological Diseases and Blindness, U.S. Public Health Service.[7] This classification, developed to clarify and standardize nomenclature in cerebrovascular disease, is now undergoing revision because of progress in knowledge and concepts of cerebrovascular diseases and continued need for greater clarification. The revision, not yet completed, will include guidelines for evaluation of patient performance and placement status. The addition of performance and placement status evaluations constitutes recognition of the significant role rehabilitation has in management of stroke patients.

Associated conditions that account for strokes have a significant influence upon physiatric planning and management during rehabilitation. The principal conditions that account for the majority of cerebrovascular lesions are: cerebral infarction due to atherosclerotic thrombosis, 40 per cent; cerebral infarction due to embolism, 25 per cent; hypertensive intracerebral hemorrhages, 20 per cent; ruptured saccular aneurysm or angioma, 6 per cent; and, occasionally, brain tumors and trauma.

Atherosclerosis produces changes in the arteries of the heart, kidney and other organs and in the extremities and the brain. The associated pathologic changes produced create disorders that often determine when the rehabilitation program can be started, how it should be paced and what goals may be set. Diffuse cerebral atherosclerosis with organic brain syndrome interferes with the ability to learn and can seriously impede progress in rehabilitation. Organic brain syndrome permits the patient to learn to ambulate, with assistance or independently, but it limits such goals of self-sufficiency as living alone.

A myocardial infarction may be related to the onset of a stroke, and its existence obviously will limit rehabilitation activities. Atherosclerotic cardiovascular disease with an enlarged heart and limited cardiac reserve may prevent the hemiplegic patient from learning to negotiate stairs because of the amount of physical effort required. Intermittent claudication due to arterial occlusive vascular disease sometimes seriously interferes with attempts to ambulate.

Associated pathologic and clinical disorders must be evaluated and should be considered in determining when to start, how to pace and what goals are feasible for rehabilitation. Cardiac and peripheral vascular disease, hypertension, diabetes and other clinical problems must be adequately managed during rehabilitation. Cerebroatheromatosis is chiefly a disease of late middle life and old age, but it sometimes occurs in patients as young as 40 years of age.

The atherosclerotic patch protrudes into the lumen and forms a nidus upon which a clot may form. Anticoagulant therapy is currently advocated to prevent this clot formation. There is considerable debate about the use of anticoagulants. Its proponents recommend anticoagulation to prevent repetition of embolization and to prevent transient ischemic attacks or thrombosis in evolution from becoming completed strokes. Anticoagulants currently are considered most clearly indicated in recurrent transient ischemic attacks but are definitely contraindicated in cerebral infarction, in the completed stroke or in the patient with prolonged neurologic deficit. Close clinical control and laboratory observations of the clotting mechanism are necessary.

If bleeding occurs anticoagulation therapy should be stopped immediately but otherwise it is most safely stopped gradually, instead of suddenly, because of the danger of oozing and hemorrhage in an area of brain softening. A history of hemorrhage or hypertension contraindicates the use of an anticoagulant. It is imperative that the physiatrist and his professional staff know when a patient in physical therapy is being treated with an anticoagulant, particularly when the patient is a hemiplegic who is learning to walk.

Three classes of focal cerebral dysfunction have been designated: transient ischemic attacks, actively changing neurologic deficit and prolonged neurologic deficit. In *transient attacks* the loss is temporary, with recovery occurring in minutes or hours. Some patients who have numerous brief attacks incur one final irreversible stroke; others do not. A *thrombosis in evolution* (actively changing neurologic deficit) is one in which the neurologic deficits develop in a steplike fashion. Neurologic impairment increases during the hours or days after onset. Anticoagulation is advocated by some to prevent transient ischemic attacks and thrombosis in evolution from becoming completed strokes. A *completed stroke* (prolonged neurologic deficit) is a stabilized neurologic deficit that is no longer progressive.

MANAGEMENT

The Evaluation Process

The initial step in the rehabilitation program is to determine goals for the patient and means to help him achieve them. The objectives may range from complete functional restoration and return to former work to healing decubitus ulcers, overcoming contractures and partial independent self-care in a wheelchair. The staff must decide whether the patient can and desires to return to full-time or part-time, modified employment, or whether he is willing to settle for partial independence at the wheelchair level. The goals must be feasible and attainable, lest rehabilitation hold within it the seeds of frustration and defeat. The aims of rehabilitation must not be merely projections of someone else's wishes but they should meet the patient's needs as fully as possible in terms of his emotional and functional potentials.

The objectives of rehabilitation are influenced by the patient's prestroke vocation and skills, his age, his education and his social environment. Some factors have an even more critical effect upon the feasibility of his goals, for instance, the possible level of function as determined by his physical and intellectual resources and his emotional and psychologic reactions. The goals actually are determined by the patient. The rehabilitation staff members, under the leadership of the physiatrist, collaborate to help the patient establish and work toward his objectives. Modifications in goals and methods are made as the patient's needs and his performance in rehabilitation activities indicate. The rehabilitation nurse, the therapists, the psychologist and the social worker join forces with the physicians in this program. Evaluation and rehabilitation really are phases of one dynamic process that, at times, merge imperceptibly with each other. Evaluation often requires a prolonged trial of rehabilitation, for a month or even longer, before objectives begin to take definitive shape.

The traditional neurologic examination of the stroke patient for diagnostic purposes is not sufficient for purposes of rehabilitation. The evaluation for rehabilitation has four areas of study: neurologic aspects, general medical status, functional performance and emotional and social aspects.

The hemiplegic patient in bed may demonstrate the positive Babinski sign, hyperactive deep tendon reflexes, ankle clonus and all the neurologic hallmarks of upper motor neuron paralysis. Yet when he is placed between parallel bars, he may move the involved extremities in the associated reciprocal movements required for walking. Only actual clinical tests determine the ability to perform. Often performance tests also reveal the reasons for failure. Performance emphasizes to the patient what he can do and reveals to him what he has to learn in order to achieve the goals that have been set.

Neurologic Aspects

The physiatrist, to write his prescriptions for various therapies, must have specific information about the patient's neurologic deficits. He must know whether the middle, anterior or posterior cerebral artery is involved because each involvement requires different management. The physiatrist must notify the other members of the rehabilitation team that homonymous hemianopia, astereognosis or global aphasia are present or that the patient has cerebellar ataxia, pseudobulbar palsy, organic brain syndrome or a brain tumor. These conditions influence rehabilitation goals and management.

A wide variety of neurologic abnormalities are found in stroke patients. The specific neurologic findings depend upon the location and size of the brain area involved in the ischemia or infarction.

The artery involved in the stroke process determines the neuromuscular and sensory dysfunctions that result. In 25 per cent of the patients the ischemic brain involvement originates in one of the four principal brain arteries as they course through the neck. The extracranial location of these four major arteries on the way to the brain makes them accessible to surgeons. When there is occlusion of an extracranial artery that supplies the brain, some surgeons recommend vascular surgery to alleviate the threat or presence of a stroke. Without arteriography, it is often impossible to determine whether circulation is impeded below or beyond the Circle of Willis (Fig. 23–3). It can be critically important to find indisputable evidence of occlusion in the neck early. At present only those strokes caused by occlusion of vessels in the neck are amenable to vascular surgery.

The two major arterial blood supply routes to the brain, the internal carotid system and the vertebral-basilar system (Fig. 23–4), furnish the basis for classifying the neurologic disorders of cerebrovascular lesions into two categories.

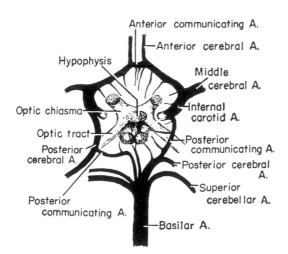

Figure 23–3 Circle of Willis. The frequency of abnormalities of the circle of Willis is stressed. This drawing from a human brain shows derivation of posterior cerebral artery from left internal carotid. The typical pattern is shown on the right. Only a few basal penetrating arteries arising from the arterial circle are shown. (From Peele, T. L.: The Neuroanatomic Basis for Clinical Neurology. 2nd Ed. New York, McGraw-Hill Book Co., Inc., 1961.)

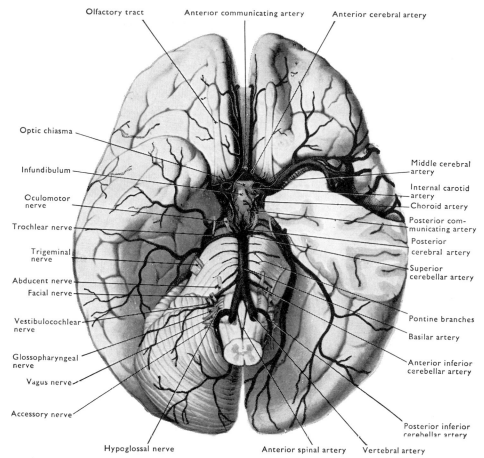

Figure 23–4   Arteries of the base of the brain. (From Brain: Diseases of the Nervous System. 6th Ed. New York, Oxford University Press, 1962.)

Internal Carotid System.   This artery, a branch of the common carotid, gives off the middle and anterior cerebral arteries (Fig. 23-5) and the ophthalmic arteries.

Disease of this system produces a contralateral spastic hemiplegia of varying degree and extent. Occlusion of the main trunk of the middle cerebral arteries produces paralysis of the opposite side of the body with preponderant effects in the face and upper extremity, hypesthesia in the same areas and homonymous hemianopia (Fig. 23-6). In a right-handed person, when the left hemisphere is involved, there is aphasia, sometimes both motor and sensory. When individual cortical branches are occluded, symptoms are limited to loss of function of the particular region supplied by the branch. If the inferior frontal branch on the left is occluded, weakness of the right side of the face and tongue and motor aphasia result. Thrombosis of the anterior cerebral artery produces paresis and hypesthesia of the opposite leg (Fig. 23-7). Occlusion of the ophthalmic artery produces homolateral amaurosis.

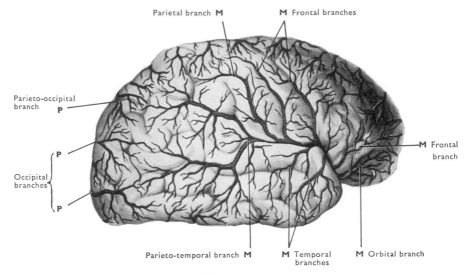

M   Middle cerebral artery
P   Posterior cerebral artery

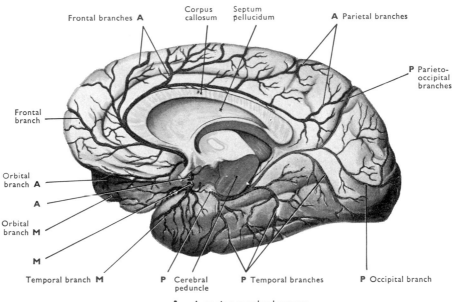

A   Anterior cerebral artery
M   Middle cerebral artery
P   Posterior cerebral artery

Figure 23–5   *Top:* Demonstration of the internal carotid system with the anterior and middle arterial branches, and the vertebral basilar system with the posterior cerebral arterial branch. This figure demonstrates distribution of cerebral arteries on superolateral surface of the right cerebral hemisphere. *Bottom:* Distribution of cerebral arteries on the medial and tentorial surfaces of the right cerebral hemisphere. (From Brain: Diseases of the Nervous System. 6th Ed. New York, Oxford University Press, 1962.)

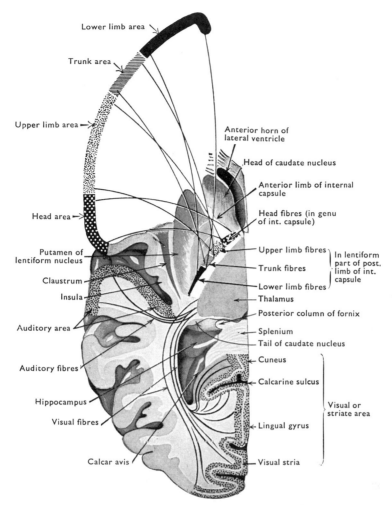

Lower limb area

Trunk area

Upper limb area

Head area

Putamen of lentiform nucleus

Claustrum

Insula

Auditory area

Auditory fibres

Hippocampus

Visual fibres

Calcar avis

Anterior horn of lateral ventricle

Head of caudate nucleus

Anterior limb of internal capsule

Head fibres (in genu of int. capsule)

Upper limb fibres ⎫
                  ⎬ In lentiform
Trunk fibres   ⎪ part of post.
                  ⎬ limb of int.
Lower limb fibres ⎭ capsule

Thalamus

Posterior column of fornix

Splenium

Tail of caudate nucleus

Cuneus

Calcarine sulcus ⎫
                 ⎬ Visual or
                 ⎪ striate area
Lingual gyrus   ⎭

Visual stria

Figure 23–6   The structural relationships of the internal capsule of the left hemisphere, particularly the posterior limb and knee, or angle, are shown. The internal capsule frequently is the site of infarction. It is supplied by the middle cerebral artery. This diagram of motor, auditory and visual areas of the left hemisphere and their relations to the internal capsule explain why involvement of the middle cerebral artery produces its clinical manifestations. (From Brain, Sir Russell: Clinical Neurology. London, Oxford University Press, 1960.)

Vertebral-Basilar System.   This system supplies the brain stem, the cerebellar, medial and inferior aspects of temporal lobe and the occipital lobe. It supplies the visual cortex and the posterior and lateral parts of the thalamus and subthalamus. The vertebral arteries fuse at the lower border of the pons to form the basilar artery. At the upper rostral border of the pons, the basilar artery bifurcates into two posterior cerebral arteries.

Occlusion within this system produces a wide variety of clinical neurologic disorders—hemiplegia, quadriplegia and ipsilateral ataxia. Occlusion of the thalamic branches produces the thalamic syndrome. Sensations of touch, pain and temperature on the opposite side of the body are distorted; agonizing, burning pain may occur spontaneously. Cerebellar asynergia and tremor of the opposite limbs may be present. Clinical manifestations of vertebral artery dis-

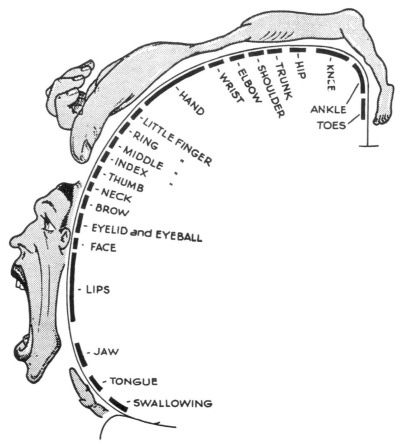

Figure 23–7   Localization in the cortex of motor functions. The premotor areas of frontal lobes are said to be association areas. They control the motor areas and are involved in planning movements. They are important in learning processes. (In McNaught, A. B., and Callander, R.: Illustrated Physiology. Baltimore, The Williams and Wilkins Co., 1963, adapted from Penfield, W., and Rasmussen, T.: The Cerebral Cortex of Man. New York, Macmillan Co., 1955.)

ease are chiefly those of the posterior cerebellar artery—homolateral cerebellar ataxia, dysphagia, dysphonia, Horner's syndrome, facial paralysis and contralateral loss of pain and temperature sensation from spinothalamic involvement. Complete basilar artery occlusion usually is fatal. It leads to small fixed pupils, pseudobulbar palsy and quadriplegia. Incomplete occlusion of the basilar artery is more common; it causes disorders of the brain stem and of the corticospinal tracts.

In the sensory area the neurologic deficits involve three major groupings (Fig. 23–8): visual problems; position, motion and vibration sense in the subcutaneous tissues; and pain, touch and temperature sensations, essentially in the skin.

Visual deficiency problems are common in hemiplegia. They prevent the patient from seeing recognizable cues and interfere with his ability to relearn motor skills. The field of vision lost in homonymous hemianopia forces the patient to turn his head in order to see where he is walking (Fig. 23–9). This

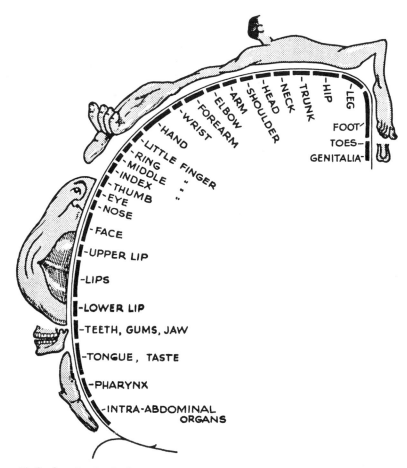

Figure 23–8 Localization in the cortex of sensory function. (In McNaught, A. B., and Callander, R.: Illustrated Physiology. Baltimore, The Williams and Wilkins Co., 1963, adapted from Penfield, W., and Rasmussen, T.: The Cerebral Cortex of Man. New York, Macmillan Co., 1955.)

requires special attention from the therapist in the patient's training. Patients with this visual deficit are exposed to accidents and physical hazards. Depth perception and perception in the horizontal and vertical planes may also be impaired in the hemiplegic and create problems in gait and posture (Fig. 23-10).

The loss of touch and position in half of the body sometimes poses considerable motor difficulties even when no motor paralysis is present. When there is motor paralysis in combination with a sensory deficit, plus the visual problems of a hemianopia—a combination that is not unusual in hemiplegic patients in rehabilitation—the patient requires a great deal of attention and time with short periods of repetitive teaching to reacquire new points of reference and cues in order to relearn how to walk.

Pain may be a prominent feature in cerebrovascular disease and it sometimes seriously interferes with rehabilitation activities. Fortunately the diffuse burning pain of the thalamic syndrome is not very common, but when it is

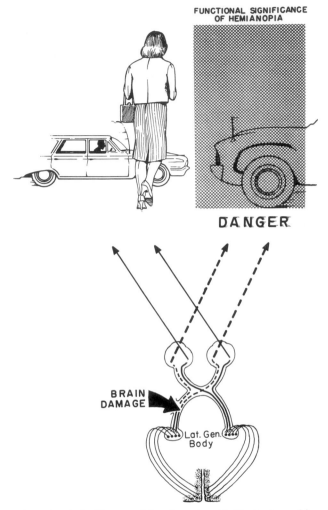

Figure 23–9 Functional significance of hemianopia with illustration of how hemianopia may lead to accident. Diagram of a visual deficiency common in hemiplegia. (From Tobis and Lowenthal: Evaluation and Management of the Brain-Damaged Patient. Springfield, Ill., Charles C Thomas, 1960.)

present, it can be extremely disabling. Thalamic pain is difficult to manage under the best of circumstances.

General Medical Status

Serious concomitant disorders are common among hemiplegic patients. These disorders may restrict, postpone or preclude full-scale rehabilitation. The evaluation of the cardiovascular status is of paramount importance. The presence of myocardial infarction or congestive heart failure requires management. Every patient who has an acute stroke requires a general medical examination. Glathe and Achor[25] reported that 12 per cent of the acute stroke

DEGREE OF VERTICALITY

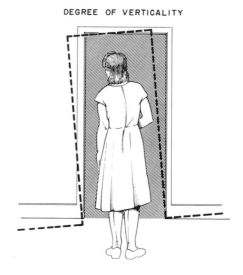

Figure 23–10 Perceptual disturbances: displacement of verticality in hemiplegia contributes to disturbances of motor performance, both in posture and gait. (From Tobis and Lowenthal: Evaluation and Management of the Brain-Damaged Patient. Springfield, Ill., Charles C Thomas, 1960.)

patients in their study had a simultaneous myocardial infarction, and that 23 per cent had associated heart disease. Early recognition and appropriate management of heart disease influence the prognosis of the stroke because adequate treatment of the heart makes more circulating oxygen available to the brain. Electrocardiograms and chest x-rays are routine in the evaluation of a new patient. Diagnostic enzyme studies are sometimes indicated. A complete blood count is done routinely. If anemia is present, it is corrected. An already damaged brain can be impaired further if anemia diminishes its supply of oxygen. The nutritional status of the patient should be assessed, particularly in elderly patients because they often eat little. Vitamins and a full protein and carbohydrate intake sometimes must be prescribed. Obesity is reduced when possible. Electrolyte balance must be maintained.

Hypertension and diabetes are very common among hemiplegic patients and must be carefully watched. They require treatment and they occasionally interfere with ability of patient to continue his rehabilitation program. The vascular status of the lower limbs should receive attention. Arteriosclerotic and diabetic peripheral vascular disorders can lead to gangrene and amputation if early and persistent foot care and preventive measures are ignored. Preventive attention sometimes allows hemiplegic patients to become independently ambulatory despite arterial circulatory problems of the lower extremities. These patients must be kept under continual medical observation. It is dangerous to lower hypertensive blood pressure profoundly and precipitously in a hemiplegic with arteriosclerotic cerebrovascular disease.

Genitourinary problems, including incontinence, are common both during the acute and later phases of stroke management and they require care and evaluation. The bladder is often flaccid at the onset of a stroke. It is common practice to use the indwelling catheter freely to avoid the aftermath of incontinence. While the patient is in a coma, there may be bladder flaccidity with retention. If the bladder is distended with more than 500 cc. of urine, it may be necessary to decompress it slowly by catheter. To avoid using an indwelling catheter during the first two or three days after the onset of a stroke, repeated catheterizations are done and the bladder is emptied each time with a new catheter. Repeated catheterization for two or three days determines whether it is necessary to install an indwelling catheter.

A few days after stroke onset, the flaccid bladder becomes spastic. An indwelling catheter enhances spasticity and lowers the capacity of the incontinent bladder. When an indwelling catheter proves necessary, it should be removed as early as possible. Bladder training using time voiding and methods similar to those used with the paraplegic is started. When a patient has attained bowel continence but remains incontinent of bladder despite efforts at training, urologic investigation is necessary. Urinary incontinence in hemiplegia often is not due to brain damage but is the result of urologic disease, such as prostatism, cystitis, urethral caruncles or bladder tumors.

Bowel incontinence must be investigated. Rectal impaction with a diarrhealike incontinence must be excluded by rectal examination. Elderly patients with hemiplegia and gastrointestinal disease may appear to have bowel incontinence. It is important also to rule out local causes. Polyps, diverticulosis and even intestinal malignancy may be present. The elderly hemiplegic who has had a recent cerebrovascular accident and remains incontinent after a month of bowel training is usually a poor candidate for self-care status.

Functional Performance

The most effective way to test the hemiplegic patient's ability to perform a purposeful act is to have him attempt to do so. When a patient fails in attempts to rise from a sitting position in a chair, it is therapeutically important to find out why he did not succeed in standing. Whenever possible, corrective measures are used. The causes of failure to perform this act independently may include bilaterally weak quadriceps, poor truncal balance, the use of a chair that is too low, improper placement of feet in preparation for standing and others.

The motor usefulness of hemiplegic extremities may be impaired by many factors. These factors include sensory disturbances as well as disorders of cortical motor control and also may involve cerebellar function. Muscular weakness and spasticity, soft tissue contractures, pain and intellectual and emotional difficulties may interfere with patient's ability to perform adequately. Yet patients with these problems do learn to stand and to walk. Skillful examination by the physiatrist at the beginning of the rehabilitation program reveals which factors — weakness, contractures, pain — are reversible by treatment and steps to overcome them are prescribed. Other factors may be managed by the use of substitutes or supports or by prolonged training in a favorable environment. Braces and assistive devices sometimes make the difference between functional success or failure.

The hemiplegic often holds his involved limbs in adduction. The upper extremity is held in the withdrawal flexed position with the shoulder internally rotated. The joints are in various degrees of flexion and the forearm is pronated at the elbow. The involved lower extremity is most often held in extension with the foot supinated.

Functional examination of the patient by the physiatrist before standing and ambulation includes having the patient attempt to voluntarily flex the hip, extend the knee and dorsiflex the foot. While the patient lies supine in bed, he is requested to lift his hemiplegic leg so that the heel is brought off the bed. Extension of the knee is followed by tests of knee flexion. A hemiplegic patient who demonstrates voluntary control and can move the joints under these conditions has a good chance for success in standing and ambulation. After the patient can stand and begin to ambulate, evaluation determinations are done in the parallel bars to establish whether he requires someone to help him walk in the bars, whether he requires someone nearby for psychologic support or whether he is able to walk independently. The distance the patient can walk in the parallel bars is an indication of his endurance level. After he has learned to walk in the parallel bars, the patient is tested to determine whether independent walking is possible. The need for a brace or cane or the support of a walker is determined.

Most hemiplegic patients can be taught to walk because standing and walking are gross motor functions; the greatest demands of weight bearing are placed upon the larger proximal hip and knee joints. Many patients who remain aphasic and have no functional use of the involved upper extremity learn to ambulate over rough ground and negotiate stairs and ramps.

Most hemiplegic patients have more intact voluntary control in proximal muscles than in distal muscles. The patient may be able to shrug his shoulders or abduct his hemiplegic shoulder and bend his elbow, but be completely unable to move his wrist or fingers. In his evaluation the physician describes the most distal motor function the patient can accomplish with his involved extremity. While the patient is lying in bed, the physiatrist notes whether the patient can voluntarily flex the elbow, extend the forearm, move the joints, including the thumb and fingers, and move the hand in extension, flexion and grasping. The ability of the patient to use the so-called "good" arm to feed, dress or write is important.

The rehabilitation nurse tests the patient's performance in the activities of daily living—feeding, dressing, undressing, washing and shaving. Members of the rehabilitation staff report whether the patient requires help in transfer, standing or walking and the type of help that is required.

The functional approach is ecologic. By actual performance, it determines what gaps exist in the patient's ability to adapt to independent living in modern society. It also establishes which steps must be taken to overcome adaptive problems.

The scope of rehabilitation of the hemiplegic includes good nursing care as well as the active processes required in meeting the demands of daily living, such as self-care, transfer and ambulation. Such an extensive scope precludes any absolute contraindications. Even the most seriously ill patient is to be afforded protection from decubitus ulcers, deformities due to poor positioning and the adverse effects of bed rest. Malnutrition and secondary anemias produce weakness, which in turn causes dependency. Adverse effects of inactivity in bed rest should be prevented. Rehabilitation of the hemiplegic should not be excluded without a thorough trial of evaluation.

Emotional and Psychologic Aspects

Cerebrovascular disease produces profound emotional and psychologic changes in addition to the physical changes of hemiplegia. Rehabilitation is essentially an educational process. The hemiplegic patient must be able to participate in the rehabilitation program and desire the long learning experience. He must be aware of the goals and accept them as his own. His emotional reactions to the stroke can present major obstacles to learning; for example, he may not wish to become self-sufficient, because independence may be unacceptable or undesirable emotionally. His ability to learn also may be impaired because of loss of integrative mechanisms and sensory contact with the environment. The emotional reactions of the hemiplegic patient to the loss of control of the body may be overwhelming. The ensuing depression, anxiety, fear, frustration, anger and hostility, or a denial pattern, prevent the hemiplegic from having a cooperative, receptive learning attitude in rehabilitation.

The patient's ability to learn and desire to become rehabilitated must be evaluated. The material obtained during the evaluation by the physiatrist, psychiatrist, psychologist and social worker must be correlated and presented to the other members of the rehabilitation staff to aid them in their efforts.

The physiatrist often must evaluate grossly the patient's potential for rehabilitation at his initial examination. Several tests for orientation as to time, place and person, concentration and memory, perceptivity and emotional lability are carried out. The patient is asked to name the year, month, date and day of the week. He is asked whether he knows where he is and why he came. He is asked to name and locate the place of his examination. His replies are noted exactly. The manner of answering—whether he rambles or gropes for answers—is described. His emotional state is observed.

If the patient is not upset by the questioning, he can be asked whether he has any problems with his memory. Patients frequently will describe their difficulties in remembering but they often are unreliable observers, particularly concerning memory. Very often elderly people will recall memories of their earlier days in an attempt to conceal loss of recent memory and inability to be attentive. Old memory frequently is retained by a patient with extreme deficits in recent memory. An engineer who becomes a hemiplegic may be able to retain some highly technical material although he cannot remember instructions in how to stand. A rapid screening test for concentration and memory is to have the patient subtract sevens beginning with one hundred.

Elderly people often have a very narrow reserve of ability to adapt to a new environment and to a new experience. Sometimes when he is brought to the hospital from old familiar surroundings, the elderly patient's adaptive mechanisms decompensate. He becomes completely disoriented and even agitated. It is often not possible in such circumstances to undertake a rehabilitation program. Slow treatment at home is better for these patients. A member of the family can be taught to supervise patient's daily exercise and his activities in learning self-sufficiency. A visiting rehabilitation nurse and physical therapist who come two or three times a week can vary and pace these activities as necessary. Some patients require the warm support of a devoted family and the familiar surroundings of the home.

If intellectual and perceptive deficiencies or severe personality disorders are present, detailed studies by a psychiatrist and psychologist are necessary. Appropriate tests are administered to the patient and the results and implications are reported to the medical and paramedical personnel involved with the patient's rehabilitation.

It is important to have a picture of the patient's premorbid personality, occupations and skills, as well as a picture of his family and social relationships. This information, which is obtained by the social worker, is integrated with the data from the psychologist and the psychiatrist, and a picture of the patient's problems in the nonorganic, functional psychosocial sphere is brought into focus. The patient's reactions to his stroke and his current situation must be understood so that steps can be taken to resolve the obstacles they present to rehabilitation.

The Early Phase of Treatment

Most cerebrovascular accident patients are admitted initially to a general hospital. It is more and more common for the physiatrist to participate early in the care of stroke patients. At admission or shortly thereafter, stroke patients often are helpless, comatose and in severe shock. General medical management in the acute phase is that used for any comatose patient. Treatment during the acute phase is directed toward maintaining life and preventing complications. As soon as the patient's condition allows, rehabilitation efforts are started. Early rehabilitation treatment is directed toward prevention of complications.

The early management of hemiplegic patients is equated with good nursing care. The strongest ally of the physician and his patient at this time is a devoted skillful rehabilitation nurse. The essential aim is to prevent complications. The ultimate success or failure in achieving rehabilitation goals often is determined not by the paralysis of the stroke but by the presence or absence of preventable complications. Contractures and stiffness with deformities are prevented by full range of motion exercises of the joints at the time nursing care is given. Proper positioning of the body and of the involved arm and leg helps prevent crippling deformities. Bed sores are prevented by frequently changing patient's bed position. When intravenous feeding is not used, the nurse must be sure that the patient's fluid intake is adequate, because fluid intake is an important factor in the prevention and management of urinary tract infections.

In addition to prevention of decubitus ulcers, contractures, urinary tract infections and other complications from prolonged bed rest, management of emotional factors is another important aspect of early rehabilitation management. As soon as the patient regains consciousness, he begins to react to a growing awareness of restrictions to his muscle control imposed by the brain injury. At this time, the physician and nurse make a major contribution by understanding and skillfully handling the patient's emotional reactions. Emotional lability, intense fears, sometimes even panic, and frustrations are present. The patient must have reassurance and support from the persons caring for him. Warm understanding and persistent nursing attention to the patient's practical needs should be provided. The problems of aphasia and dysphagia also are often present in the same patient. The nurse and others who care for him must learn how to interpret and anticipate his needs when he cannot speak. Bowel and bladder routines become important. Often so-called incontinent patients really need only the opportunity to void into a receptacle.

The reassurance and support that stroke patients receive in the early phase and the measures to prevent complications are essential for long-term progress. Early care determines whether or not the patient later stands, walks and is self-sufficient. The sooner rehabilitation measures are instituted the greater the potential for independence.

Positioning in Bed. Rehabilitation of the hemiplegic patient begins with proper positioning in bed. The nurse traditionally concerns herself with posturing and turning the patient in bed. Bed posturing in the early phase of hemiplegia is extremely important, particularly for prevention of aspiration pneumonia. A good bed that can be raised and lowered automatically and a firm mattress are essential. A board under the mattress prevents low back stress from faulty sags. The nurse arranges for the patient who recovers consciousness to have a level body position by placing a small pillow under his head. The patient should be placed in bed lying straight. The head and neck should not be flexed. The shoulders and hips are placed level with each other. The feet should be placed against a footboard with the toes up straight, the feet at right angles to the legs. There should be about 4 inches of space between the mattress edge and footboard where the heels rest to prevent decubitus ulcers of the heels, which may delay wearing of shoes and walking exercises for as long as three months.

The patient's position should be changed frequently, not only for his comfort, but also to prevent decubitus ulcers about bony prominences. Bed sores develop at pressure points when the pressure upon the capillaries over bony prominences produces tissue necrosis. The best way to prevent tissue necrosis is to turn the patient every two hours. Adequate nutrition and good skin care also are factors in preventing extensive decubitus ulcers.

The hemiplegic often prefers to lie on the involved side and he may resent attempts to turn him over to lie on his good side. He develops pressure sores and skin breakdown over the external malleoli and the greater trochanters if he lies on one side too long. When he lies on his back too long, he may develop decubitus ulcers over the sacral and heel areas.

To help him lie on his good side, a pillow is placed under the weak side of the body. In the side-lying position, a pillow helps support the involved arm and leg. The classic position of the lower extremity in hemiplegia is extension with the hip held in external rotation and the foot in extension. This positioning, if uncorrected, produces talipes equinus.

The classic deformity of the hemiplegic upper extremity is one of flexion, with the shoulder held in adduction and internal rotation so that it frequently becomes painful. The upper extremity is held against the body and subluxation of the shoulder frequently occurs. Pain and contractures from advanced deformities of this type prevent any use of the entire upper extremity. The shoulder pain sometimes also involves the hand. A shoulder-hand dystrophy can become painful enough to limit or halt the rehabilitation program. The hemiplegic patient should not be permitted to lie with his arm adducted across the abdomen because this position encourages contractures of the adductors and internal rotators of the hemiplegic shoulder and fosters the development of painful shoulder deformities.

To prevent external rotation of the hip, the nurse tucks a rolled bath towel or a light cotton blanket about 2 inches under the lateral aspect of the involved thigh and leg to prevent the leg from rolling over. Sometimes a long sandbag may be used instead of a towel or blanket. The foot should rest against the footboard. Sometimes when the head of the bed is raised, there is a tendency for the patient to slip down in bed and flex the knee and this should be prevented. Protracted knee flexion can lead to flexion contractures of the knee which may be disabling.

To prevent the adduction and internal rotation deformity of the hemiplegic shoulder, the arm is kept in abduction at an angle of about 60 degrees while the patient is on his back in bed. This is done by placing a pillow between the chest wall and arm. The forearm should be placed on a pillow with the elbow above the shoulder and the wrist above the elbow. The effect of this modified "Statue of Liberty" position is to stretch tight internal rotators of the shoulder. The wrist and fingers are kept in a neutral functional position. A rolled towel or bandage is placed in the hand to keep the fingers from tight flexion. The characteristic spastic flexion deformity of the hemiplegic elbow, wrist and fingers can be kept to a minimum to avoid contractures and deformities that would prevent the use of any muscles that might become usable.

Passive Exercises.   Passive exercises to the joints of the hemiplegic extremities are even more important than positioning for prevention of stiffness and contractural joint deformities. Exercises are begun as soon as the patient recovers consciousness, usually two or three days after onset of the stroke. The physical therapist administers the initial passive range of motion exercises to all joints of the paralyzed side and shows the bedside nurse the exact techniques to be used. The nurse performs the passive exercises at least three times a day. The passive exercises include full range of movement of the involved elbow, wrist, fingers, hip, knee, ankle and foot. As soon as the patient becomes strong enough, he is taught to exercise the muscles of the uninvolved side and the trunk. These activities also are started as early as possible.

Devices such as a single knotted sheet tied to the foot of the bed or an overhead trapeze at the head of the bed are used to help the patient learn to sit up independently by pulling with his uninvolved upper extremity. Many hemiplegics lean toward the paralyzed side and lose their balance when they attempt to sit up and must be taught to lean toward the uninvolved side. Head balance activities also are taught. At first the patient's back is assisted while he is in sitting position and his head is supported but he gradually progresses to independent sitting and then he is taught to sit at the edge of the bed and dangle his feet. If these early activities are done properly and often, they will shorten a patient's stay in bed, and thus permit the more intensive program out of bed to begin.

While he is in bed, the patient is taught to use the uninvolved upper extremity in feeding, grooming, rolling over and sitting up. The length of time he remains in bed depends upon the severity of the stroke. Patients with very mild attacks and no complications get out of bed in 24 hours and walk with little difficulty. Most patients with severe involvement remain in bed for about 14 days. Occasionally, especially when there is a serious concomitant disorder, the patient remains in bed for a longer period. To prevent weakness and atrophy of the uninvolved side, key muscles like the quadriceps require active exercises. Mild progressive resistive exercises to muscles of the uninvolved side are administered as early as possible. As the patient becomes stronger, he is taught to use his uninvolved arm to give assistive exercises to the hemiplegic upper extremity.*

If the patient's shoulder becomes painful while he is still in bed, the application of heat, with hot packs for example, and massage are started in conjunction with early active mobilization of the shoulder joint.

Getting the patient out of bed into the upright position moderates the dangers of prolonged bed rest. These dangers include: atrophy of the muscles, "atrophy of the spirit" and development of a need to remain dependent, the threat of thrombophlebitis and pulmonary embolism. The great fear of falling that so many hemiplegics develop is mitigated when a patient stands as soon as possible, on a tilt table if necessary. When severe problems prolong bed rest, the transition from bed to the upright position may be difficult and the use of a tilt table may be necessary for the patient to achieve the upright position.

Most hemiplegic patients are able to get out of bed and stand between parallel bars without great difficulty. Usually the patient is out of bed, in a wheelchair and started on training in transfer and standing not later than two weeks after the onset of the stroke.

---

*Strike Back at Stroke, a well-illustrated brochure by the Public Health Service, Publication No. 596, may be obtained from the Superintendent of Documents, U.S. Government Printing Office, Washington, D.C.

The Later Phase of Treatment

Training in Standing and Ambulation.   Usually about two days of training in standing up with assistance from the physical therapist are needed to teach the hemiplegic how to pull himself up to the parallel bars. Severely handicapped hemiplegics, including those with chronic brain syndromes, those who are debilitated and those who have had multiple strokes involving both sides, may require a training program of progressive standing exercises to learn to transfer from the bed to a chair and from sitting to the standing position.[27] With aid of the physical therapist the patient must develop balance and power in the antigravity muscles of both sides and he must be reminded to keep the weight of his body forward over his feet.

As soon as the patient learns to stand up and transfer from the chair to the parallel bars, training in ambulation is begun with balancing exercises at the rails. At first the therapist assists and gradually the patient learns to walk in parallel bars unassisted. He then is taught to walk outside the parallel bars. At first he may require some assistance from the therapist and possibly a walker or a cane. Then he learns to walk with the aid of a cane. Gradually, as the fears subside and ability increases, he walks independently and is taught to negotiate stairs, inclines, curbs and rough ground.

If the hemiplegic is to achieve these objectives in transfer, standing and ambulation, his muscle strength, muscle coordination, balance and endurance must be improved by means of the physical therapy exercise program. While the patient is bedridden, passive exercises are used on his upper and lower extremities. Active exercises to the uninvolved side next are added, followed by assistive exercises in which the patient uses his good arm to move the hemiplegic arm.

Later, when the patient goes to the therapeutic gymnasium, assistive exercises that require overhead pulleys are added. A shoulder wheel is used in conjunction with overhead pulleys for passive exercise of the hemiplegic shoulder. Stall bars help him practice coming to a standing position and balance. Exercises on the floor mat, where there is no fear of falling, are used to improve mobility and balance in preparation for ambulation. Exercises on a powder board improve mobility of the hip and shoulder joints of the hemiplegic upper and lower extremities.

The exercise program is progressive. The early use of associated movements is extremely helpful. Patients are capable of reflex movement in ambulation with muscles that they cannot control voluntarily. Reciprocal movements improve associated movements; the stationary bicycle helps develop these movements. Initially, the exercise program is designed to promote joint motion. Later it represents a systematic attempt to improve power and coordination. Power building exercises are amplified by the addition of resistance, weights and sandbags. The use of heavy resistive exercises is the most rapid method of building power. Muscle reeducation in the associated and reciprocal movements improves function that is based upon coordination. More difficult obstacles including stairs, ramps and rough ground are gradually added to the ambulation program.

Training in Use of the Upper Extremity.   The majority of patients with hemiplegia can be taught once again to transfer, stand and walk independently. Unfortunately success in functional use of the involved upper extremity is not so universal. If, after five to six months of persistent effort, there is no evidence of return of function to the upper extremity, there is little likelihood that useful function will be restored. Most often the objective for the upper extremity is to develop the involved hand as an assistive member. If the involved hand is not the dominant one, the aim in occupational therapy is to train the patient in self-care and writing as one-handed activities using the good hand.

The occupational therapist, guided by the physiatrist's prescription, provides a graded and controlled program of activities for the hemiplegic. The patient regains proximal muscle control of the upper extremity first. The initial activities are directed toward developing gross coordination of shoulder and elbow motion and reciprocal exercises for the lower extremities, using a treadle sander or bicycle jig saw. Standing and transfer activities also are begun early in occupational therapy to help develop tolerance and balance.

While he is in a wheelchair, the patient can use a suspension sling to provide fuller range of motion, to support the hemiplegic upper extremity and to prevent subluxation of the humerus. This type of sling is useful when shoulder deformities and pain threaten or are present.

At the first evidence of wrist and hand motion, the patient begins to work for grasp, placement and release. If the flexors of the fingers and wrist are spastic, the patient's occupational therapy is directed toward achievement of simple placement and release. If he is able, he proceeds to skills that require fine coordination. The physical therapist, occupational therapist and rehabilitation nurse work closely to integrate their efforts toward these goals.

In choosing the treatment media for the patient, the occupational therapist considers any special requirements of the patient's occupation, depending, of course, upon whether there is any possibility of return of function. Memories and reflex patterns of coordinated activities of the past help develop function.

When prevocational exploration is required it is provided by the psychologist and vocational guidance counselor. Adequate management of sensory and perceptive impairment is necessary before prevocational exploration can be begun. The patient with hemianopia must learn to position his head to increase his visual field and to help reestablish the body image. The aphasic requires simple repetitive instruction with visual directions.

The emphasis in occupational therapy, as in rehabilitation nursing and physical therapy, is on helping the patient attain independence whether the upper extremity is functional or not. If necessary, special procedures in dressing, transferring, feeding and personal hygiene are taught. Assistive devices are helpful for some patients, particularly homemakers.

The occupational therapy program contributes in a planned and progressive manner in guiding the hemiplegic patient gradually toward social adjustment. The patient's relation with the occupational therapist and the sense of achievement he derives from performance of functional activities contribute to the process of return of self-esteem and independence.

Shoulder Pain

Subluxation of the flail shoulder joint may cause pain that is severe enough to interfere with the hemiplegic's rehabilitation program. This pain results from subluxation of the humeral head out of the glenoid cavity and pull on the soft tissues of the joint (Figs. 23-11 and 23-12). The upper extremity requires the support of a fitted sling. In extreme cases, orthopedic fusion of the shoulder joint in a functionally advantageous position is advocated.

The so-called shoulder-hand dystrophy is another common cause of pain

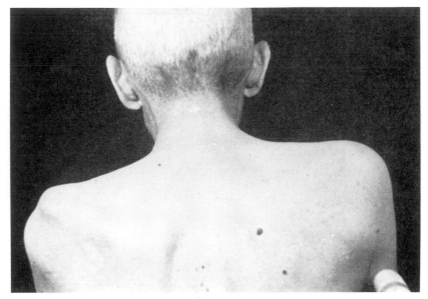

Fig. 23–11

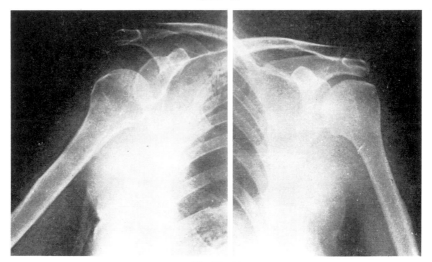

Fig. 23–12

Figures 23–11 and 23–12   Subluxation of left shoulder of hemiplegia. Fig. 23–11 is a photograph of a patient showing the subluxation when viewed from the back. Fig. 23–12 shows x-rays of the subluxed left shoulder of the patient. (From Tobis and Lowenthal: Evaluation and Management of the Brain-Damaged Patient. Springfield, Ill., Charles C Thomas, 1960.)

in hemiplegia. There is contracture and often fixation and spasm of the muscles around the shoulder joint. The hand swells and sometimes is cold and there are color changes associated with autonomic nervous system involvement. There is pain in the shoulder and sometimes also in the hand and it is intensified when the patient attempts to move the joints of the affected areas. Oral steroid therapy for 10 to 14 days and mobilization of the shoulder joint are usually sufficient. The problem can and should be prevented by early

Figure 23–13 The abduction outrigger consists of a spring steel wire hoop attached to the upper portion of either a straight or an axillary type shoulder suspension hoop. The outrigger projects laterally like a wing, as shown in the illustration. A forearm cuff is used with rubber bands running from it to a steel trolley ring that is free to slide on the outrigger. By varying the number and arrangement of rubber bands the patient's forearm can be supported to any extent desired, and he can be encouraged to exercise his weakened muscles by reaching to one side as shown in the illustration, then bringing his arm back to his body. In some cases this is reversed when the abductors are weak and the adductors retain some strength. (From Anderson, M. H.: Functional Bracing of the Upper Extremities. Springfield, Ill., Charles C Thomas, 1958.)

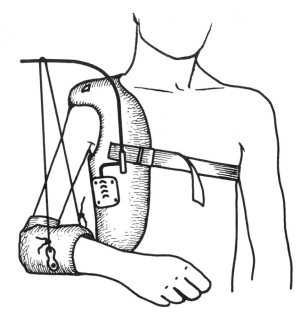

mobilization of the shoulder joint through passive, assistive and, when possible, active exercises. Suprascapular and stellate ganglion blocks also are used to relieve the symptoms in the shoulder area. A special shoulder suspension bracing device is available that permits the involved upper extremity to be held in abduction and utilized in a functional level (Fig. 23-13). This abduction outrigger was designed by Rancho Los Amigos, Downey, California. The parts are supplied by Hosmer Company, P.O.B. 152, Santa Clara, Calif.

Spasticity

Spasticity is one of the factors that determines the functional status of a hemiplegic patient. It results from partial or complete interruption of the upper motor neurons and is most commonly seen after lesions in the motor cortex and the internal capsule. When central structures that inhibit the stretch reflex are removed, the muscles are hypertonic. In spasticity the hypertonia is confined to the antigravity muscles; for example, in the spastic lower extremity, flexion of the hip, knee or ankle meets resistance. Resistance in the arm is most prominently displayed in the flexors, for these are the muscles which counteract the forces of gravity. Spasticity is a release phenomenon.

Any lesion that separates the efferent neurons from central control may produce spasticity. Anger, excitement, cold air and pain can intensify it and walking may be more difficult for spastic hemiplegics during cold weather.

Spasticity may seriously mask voluntary motor power; if this is the case, a block of the obturator nerve may make ambulation possible by eliminating adductor spasm and permitting more effective use of motor power in the leg. A short leg brace may be helpful and sometimes a long leg brace is necessary to assist in standing and walking by maintaining both knee joints and ankles in a stabilized functional position. Dilute procaine solutions have been used by Rushworth[46] to relax spastic hemiplegic muscles with selective blocking of gamma motor fibers.

Spasticity in the upper extremity causes the patient to hold the shoulder adducted and internally rotated and the fingers, wrist and elbow in flexion. If the patient is in a wheelchair, there is danger of flexion at the hip and knee. Spasticity contributes to the abnormal gait and posture of the hemiplegic and it is a significant factor in the development of the contractures. Early treatment is important to prevent contractures and deformities while the patient is bed-ridden.

Bracing

The decision regarding the need for leg bracing is usually deferred until after training for standing and ambulation has begun because often the hemiplegic does not require any leg bracing for ambulation. However, a severe inversion of the foot or instability of the ankle require protection against possible injury during early ambulation and a short leg brace with T-strap may be necessary.

Spasticity of the gastrocnemius overwhelms the dorsiflexors of the foot, causing the foot to be held in the equinus position. A toe drag results; i.e., the patient cannot clear the floor with his toes when he picks up the hemiplegic foot and he cannot get his foot over the top of a step when he climbs stairs. The purpose of bracing the lower extremity is to help the foot clear the floor and to support the ankle in a functional position.

The most commonly used short leg brace for hemiplegics is the double bar 90 degree ankle stop with a posterior metal calf band (Fig. 23–14). The single bar short leg brace usually is inadequate. For inversion of the foot a T-strap is used to support the foot in a better functional position. When T-straps are prescribed, the part to which the buckle is attached should be long enough so

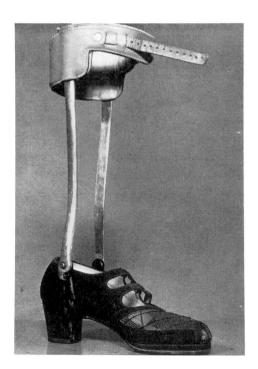

Figure 23–14 The most common short leg brace used for hemiplegias is this short double bar brace with stirrup attachment and 90° stop. (From Rusk: Rehabilitation Medicine. St. Louis, C. V. Mosby Co., 1958.)

that the hemiplegic patient can bend over and fasten the strap. The Klenzak adjustable spring type brace is not used for spastic hemiplegics when ankle clonus is present.

The patient must be taught to put on the brace independently. Long leg braces are usually avoided because hemiplegic patients find it difficult to walk with them. However severe spasticity with contractures at the knee and severely painful or unstable knees with extreme quadriceps weakness or ligamentous destruction may require the support of a long leg brace with a knee lock on the medial aspect to keep the knee in weight bearing position and stabilized for walking.

A good orthopedic type oxford shoe that is fitted properly to the patient is used as a basis and support for the brace. A rigid shank with a steel bar helps maintain the 90 degree angle in which the foot is held by the brace and the shoe. The heel counter should support the heel snugly without rubbing the skin. The inner part of the counter should be long enough to support the foot. A shoe that fits correctly is an asset of great value in helping hemiplegics stand and walk.

CONCOMITANT MEDICAL CONDITIONS

Severe chronic obstructive pulmonary disease interferes with the patient's ability to develop strength and endurance. Breathing exercises, apparatus for forced respiration, administration of oxygen and aerosol and a carefully "custom-tailored" slow, persistent program of rehabilitation enable the hemiplegic patient with chronic pulmonary disease to become self-sufficient in transfer, walking and activities of daily living.

Since the destructive pallidectomy approach has come into use, postoperative Parkinsonism patients with hemiplegia are more common. The surgical procedure causes athetosis to subside, but the rigidity, the festinating gait and the flexed truncal posture frequently persist and present difficult problems for training in ambulation. However, these patients can be taught to walk, stand straighter and become self-sufficient.

In elderly hemiplegics painful osteoarthritis of the hip and knee can be severe enough to prevent weight bearing and ambulation. Sometimes training in standing, ambulation and transfer must be delayed until pain in the hip and knee subsides. Exercises to strengthen the supporting musculature of the involved joints, such as the quadriceps and hip muscles, and the use of such supporting devices as braces, canes or walkers, can prove very helpful in getting these patients slowly to stand upright again and walk. In the case of fracture of the involved hemiplegic hip the patient does standing exercises but does not bear weight on the involved leg until the fracture is healed.

Severe flexion knee contractures of the hemiplegic leg combined with a nonfunctional upper extremity prevent the patient from transferring unassisted to and from the bed and wheelchair. Sometimes surgical procedures are used to overcome irreversible contractures when progressive casting and passive and active exercises fail.

SPEECH AND LANGUAGE DISORDERS

A large proportion of hemiplegic stroke patients have some impairment in the ability to speak or understand language. Language disorders, it is estimated, are present initially in about 40 per cent of hemiplegics. They are especially common in right hemiplegia (Fig. 23-15). About 80 per cent of those

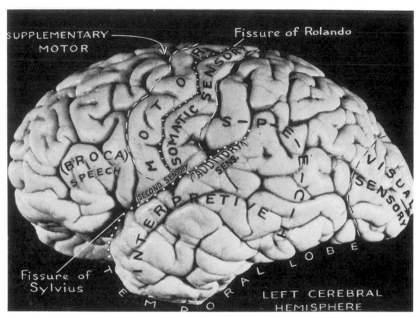

Figure 23–15 Left hemisphere of the human brain. (From Penfield, W., and Roberts, L.: Speech and Brain Mechanisms. Princeton, N. J., Princeton University Press, 1959.)

who have a language disorder with hemiplegia make some improvement. In some patients the loss of speech is evanescent, but in others, disorders in language communication or speech may be prolonged. Sometimes, the inability to speak persists after the patient has become ambulatory and self-sufficient in other areas.

Speech disorders, even mild ones, are distressing to the patient. The inability to communicate produces profound frustration and irritability. The patient fears that he may make an error, that he may be misunderstood and even that he may be insane.

Dysarthria. Two main types of speech disorders are common in stroke patients, *dysarthria* and *aphasia*. In dysarthria, the patient cannot form words clearly and cannot articulate sounds because the muscles of the lips, tongue and larynx do not function properly. Any mechanical defect in speech production caused by muscle dysfunction that results from brain injury is a dysarthria. The difficulty may be due to a weakness or paralysis of the muscles or a loss of sensation. The patient has no difficulty in reading to himself and in understanding what is said and he can write if his hand and fingers are not paralyzed. Dysarthria is a defect in articulation. The evaluation of dysarthria usually includes an examination of the peripheral speech mechanism, otolaryngological consultation, tests for specific speech skills and an assessment of functional ability based on patient's clarity of speech in conversation.

Aphasia

Aphasia is a language disorder. It is most common when the hemiplegia involves the dominant side and the brain lesion implicates the posterior aspect of the inferior frontal gyrus. Aphasias actually are a symptom complex concerned with all aspects of language: understanding spoken language, speaking, reading and writing. The severity may range from complete inability to communicate to minor deficiencies with relatively normal language command. The aphasia may involve all avenues of communication, including the ability to make an appropriate movement, to imitate and to gesture.

The types of aphasias are those based on sensory deficiency, *receptive aphasia;* those based on motor deficiency, *expressive aphasia;* and the *mixed type* in which both expressive and receptive elements are affected. In *global aphasia* there is neither receptive nor expressive language ability.

Total expressive aphasia poses troublesome problems in making a differential diagnosis. It is most difficult to differentiate between apraxia and expressive aphasia. Agnosia and receptive aphasia also present problems in diagnosis. Wepman[58] differentiates between the integrative functions and the dynamics of modality-bound functions in language to distinguish aphasia, which is an integrative disturbance, from agnosia and apraxia.

Agnosia. Agnosia, a modality-bound disturbance of input, signifies the loss of the ability to recognize objects. In any type of agnosia, whether it is visual, auditory or tactile, the patient exhibits impairment in transmission of sensory signals. It should not be mistaken for deafness, blindness or loss of touch. Rather, agnosia is a loss of transmission of the signal to the conceptual level.

Apraxia. Apraxia is a transmission disturbance on the output side. Although he is able to conceive or conceptualize the content of the message to be conveyed to the muscles, the apraxic patient cannot reconstruct the schema or motor pattern necessary to convey the message. Apraxia presumes loss of memory associations needed to carry out certain purposive movements that are not related to speech itself. Apraxia may be apparent in any or all modalities, and may vary from one modality to another. A patient may have less difficulty with writing than with speaking or vice versa. A patient with verbal apraxia may be unable to imitate the words of the examiner, although at other times he can produce the same words spontaneously. The patient with apraxia usually has difficulty in imitating oral movements. Tests that require imitation may be used to differentiate between expressive aphasia and apraxia. Apraxia interferes with skilled motor acts. Agnosia does not lead to clumsy movements, but to inappropriate ones. These disorders in language and communication lead to disturbances of motor behavior.

In contrast to agnosia and apraxia, true aphasia is not modality-bound. Aphasia is the result of loss of integrative ability and of use of any or all types of symbols. The patient appears to hear, see or feel, but he demonstrates difficulty in making use of the symbols he has received. The aphasic demonstrates deficiencies in creating or constructing the "schema" of language to bring it into a meaningful state, either on the side of comprehending messages or on the side of conveying messages to his audience. Sir Russell Brain[14] has referred to aphasia as "disturbance in schema."

The modality-bound disorders—agnosia and apraxia—are more responsive than aphasia to direct therapy. The patient can learn to handle symbols receptively and expressively with repeated drills and support from the speech therapist when a partial disability exists.

The patient with true aphasia must be stimulated to concentrate or focus on language symbols in order to learn to reconstruct the schema, or integration of the sensory stimuli. The tools for evaluation of aphasics are not sensitive enough to prognosticate accurately what the patient will accomplish. At best, aphasic rehabilitation is a slow process. It is requires short, frequent training sessions which are individual and "custom-tailored" to the patient's needs. The psychologic problems, premorbid personality and psychologic states of the aphasic patient have a profound effect on the rehabilitation process.

The speech therapist should see the patient early to assess the speech and language problem. Speech sessions should be daily. It may be necessary to continue treatments for weeks, months and even years. It is never too late to seek speech therapy help. Some benefit may be derived even two and more years after the initial illness. Patients with persistent language problems should be treated by a specialist in language disorders. It is important to talk to the patient without exerting any pressure upon him to respond verbally.

Motor experience is essential for language experience. Aphasics who learn to get out of bed alone and are taught to stand and walk improve in their ability to speak and communicate. There appears to be a close relationship between learning to use the upper extremity of the involved side and learning to speak. The tools of language are said to develop out of manual function. J. B. S. Haldane said, "The human brain has two superanimal activities: Manual skill and logical thought. Manual skill appears to be the earlier acquisition of the two and the capacity for language and thought has grown up around it."[26] Improvement in speech function often empirically appears to bear a definite time relationship to improvement of neuromyoskeletal function. The greater the level of motor skill the patient achieves, the more likely he is to find means for communicating.

Rehabilitation activities other than speech therapy become language experiences. Thus, when the patient is learning to brush his teeth and groom himself, he may also be developing his language ability. The aphasic has a disorder in a motor area which causes difficulties in lip and tongue movements. The speech therapist should work closely with the other members of the rehabilitation team—the physician, physical therapist, occupational therapist, rehabilitation nurse, psychologist and social worker. All those who help the patient redevelop patterns of work skill are aiding the speech therapist in his efforts to help the hemiplegic reestablish communication with the world around him.

Dr. Leonard Pearson, discussing the aphasia problem among hemiplegics at 1963 Stroke Conference in Chicago, said, "There is no justification for the prevailing pessimism about the treatment of this condition today."* He believes that the present rate of improvement of 75 per cent of aphasics may be extended in the future as we develop more knowledge about special neurologic and psychologic mechanisms. He advocated such simple procedures as tactile stimulation in unaffected areas, orientation of the patient to the reality of his environment and utilization of group therapy to reinforce the measures of speech therapy programs. He suggested the use of so-called facilitation techniques of various controlled external stimuli to enhance the patient's capacity to reach his potential for verbal communication.

TRANSITION PERIOD AND FOLLOW-UP

The hemiplegic patient who achieves his goals of self-sufficiency and independent ambulation in the hospital has not necessarily completed the

---

Proceedings of the National Stroke Congress, 1964.

rehabilitation process. He must learn to use these skills at home and in his cultural environment. The transition from the hospital to the home environment can be difficult. The social worker is of great help in this transition period, and with the cooperation of the psychologist and the vocational guidance counselor, he may help those patients who are able to return to employment.

Hemiplegic patients often require continued training and supervision in their exercise and kinetic activities as outpatients in physical therapy and occupational therapy programs. The aphasic patient may have to return for a year or more as an outpatient for speech therapy. The rehabilitation program continues until the patient reaches the goal of maximal use of his remaining resources. Long-term follow-ups enable the physician to study the long-range effects of the rehabilitation program on the patient. The rehabilitation process is a continuous long-term one, and is completed only when the patient has demonstrated that he is able to adapt successfully to life among his family and in the society in which he lives, limited only by the physical impairments that have proved to be irreversible.

REFERENCES

1. American Medical Association: Handbook of Physical Medicine and Rehabilitation. Philadelphia, The Blakiston Co., 1950.
2. American Physical Therapy Association Symposium: Rehabilitation of the Brain-injured. Phys. Therapy Rev., *34:*605–625, 1954.
3. Anticoagulant Therapy in Cerebrovascular Disease. Editorial by Roland P. Mackay. J.A.M.A., *187:*450–451, 1964.
4. Archibald, K. C.: Leg Bracing in Hemiplegia. J.A.M.A., *171:*1061–1065, 1959.
5. Aring, C. D.: Flaccid Hemiplegia in Man. Arch. Neurol. and Psychiat., *43:*302–317, 1940.
6. Aring, C. D.: Differential Diagnosis of Cerebrovascular Stroke. Arch. Intern. Med., *113:*195–199, 1964.
7. Advisory Council, National Institute of Neurological Diseases and Blindness, U.S. Public Health Service: A Classification and Outline of Cerebral Vascular Disease—A Report by an Ad Hoc Committee. Neurology, *8:*397–434, 1958.
8. Bard, G.: Energy Expenditure of Hemiplegic Subjects During Walking. Arch. Phys. Med., *44:*368–370, 1963.
9. Bean, W. B.: Cerebrovascular Accidents and Myocardial Infarctions. Heart Bull., *7:*73–75, 1958.
10. Bierman, W., and Licht, S.: Physical Medicine in General Practice. 3rd Ed. New York, Paul B. Hoeber, 1960.
11. Birch, H. G., Proctor, F., and Bortner, M.: Perception in Hemiplegia: III. The Judgment of Relative Distance in the Visual Field. Arch. Phys. Med., *42:*639–644, 1961.
12. Birch, H. G., Proctor, F., Bortner, M., and Lowenthal, M.: Perception in Hemiplegia: I. Judgment of Vertical and Horizontal by Hemiplegic Patients. Arch. Phys. Med., *41:*19–27, 1960.
13. Birch, H. G., Proctor, F., Bortner, M., and Lowenthal, M.: Perception in Hemiplegia: II. Judgment of the Median Plane. Arch. Phys. Med., *41:*71–75, 1960.
14. Brain, R.: Speech Disorders: Aphasia, Apraxia, and Agnosia. Washington, D.C., Butterworth Inc., 1961.
15. Brain, R.: Diseases of the Nervous System. 6th Ed. New York, Oxford University Press, 1962.
16. Brown, J. R.: Management of Patients with Brain Damage. Neurology, *2:*273–283, 1952.
17. Bruell, J. H., Peszcynski, M., and Volk, D.: Disturbance of Perception of Verticality in Patients with Hemiplegia. Arch. Phys. Med., *38:*677–679, 1957.
18. Bruell, J. H., and Simon, J. I.: Development of Objective Predictors of Recovery in Hemiplegic Patients. Arch. Phys. Med., *41:*564–569, 1960.
19. Casella, C.: A Behavioral Test of Activation Theory for Hemiplegic Patients. Arch. Phys. Med., *43:*321–323, 1962.
20. Covalt, N. K.: Preventive Techniques of Rehabilitation for Hemiplegic Patients. GP, *17:*131–142, 1958.
21. Deaver, G. G., and Brittis, A. L.: Braces, Crutches, Wheelchairs. Rehabilitation Monograph V,

Institute of Physical Medicine and Rehabilitation, New York University–Bellevue Center, 1953.

22. Dooley, D. M., and Perlmutter, I: Spontaneous Intracranial Hematomas in Patients Receiving Anticoagulation Therapy. J.A.M.A., *187*:396–398, 1964.

23. Fink, S. L., and Hallenbeck, C. E.: Assessment of Intellectual Potential of Persons with Hemiplegia. Arch. Phys. Med., *43*:324–331, 1962.

24. Gillette, H. E.: Recovery of Motion Following Cerebral Insult: An Appraisal of Current Methods of Management. Arch. Phys. Med., *45*:167–176, 1964.

25. Glathe, J. P., and Achor, R. P.: Frequency of Cardiac Disease in Patients With Strokes. Proc. Mayo Clin., *33*:417–422, 1958.

26. Haldane, J. B. S.: Human Evaluation Past and Future. In Burnett, W.: This Is My Philosophy. New York, Harper and Brothers, 1957, p. 39.

27. Hirschberg, G. G.: The Use of Stand-up and Step-up Exercises in Rehabilitation. In DePalma, A. F.: Clinical Orthopaedics. Vol. 12, Rehabilitation. Philadelphia, J. B. Lippincott, 1958, pp. 30–46.

28. Hoerner, E. F.: Rehabilitation of the Hemiplegic. In DePalma, A. F.: Clinical Orthopaedics. Vol. 12, Rehabilitation. Philadelphia, J. B. Lippincott, 1958.

29. Knapp, M. E.: Problems in Rehabilitation of the Hemiplegic Patient. J.A.M.A., *169*:224–229, 1959.

30. Knapp, M. E.: Results of Language Tests of Patients with Hemiplegia. Arch. Phys. Med., *43*:317–320, 1962.

31. Krusen, F. H.: Physical Medicine. Philadelphia, W. B. Saunders Co., 1941.

32. Liberson, W. T., Holmquest, H. J., Scot, D., and Dow, M.: Functional Electrotherapy: Stimulation of the Peroneal Nerve Synchronized with the Swing Phase of the Gait of Hemiplegic Patients. Third International Congress of Physical Medicine, Washington, D.C., 1960.

33. Lorenze, E. J., Simon, H. B., and Linden, J. L.: Urologic Problems in Rehabilitation of Hemiplegic Patients. J.A.M.A., *169*:1042–1046, 1959.

34. Lowenthal, M., Tobis, J. S., and Howard, I. R.: An Analysis of the Rehabilitation Needs and Prognoses of 232 Cases of Cerebral Vascular Accidents. Arch. Phys. Med., *40*:183–186, 1959.

35. McDevitt, A., Carter, S. A., Gatje, B. S., Foley, W. T., and Wright, I. S.: Use of Anticoagulants in Treatment of Cerebral Vascular Disease. J.A.M.A., *166*:592–597, 1958.

36. Miglietta, O., Lewitan, A., and Rogoff, J. B.: Subluxation of the Shoulder in Hemiplegic Patients. New York J. Med., *59*:457–460, 1959.

37. Millikan, C. H., Siekert, R. D., and Whisnant, J. P.: Anticoagulant Therapy in Cerebral Vascular Disease – Current Status. J.A.M.A., *166*:587–592, 1958.

38. Millikan, C. H., Siekert, R. G., and Whisnant, J. P.: Cerebral Vascular Diseases – Third Conference Held Under the Auspices of the American Neurological Association and the American Heart Association, 1961. New York, Grune and Stratton, Inc., 1961.

39. Mosley, D. H., Schatz, I. J., Breneman, G. M., and Keyes, J. W.: Long-Term Anticoagulant Therapy. J.A.M.A., *186*:914–916, 1963.

40. Nathanson, M., Bergman, P. S., and Gordon, G. G.: Denial of Illness, Its Occurrence in 100 Consecutive Cases of Hemiplegia. Arch. Neurol. and Psychiat., *68*:380–387, 1952.

40a. Penfield, W., and Rasmussen, T.: The Cerebral Cortex of Man. New York, The Macmillan Co., 1955.

41. Peszczynski, M.: Ambulation of the Severely Handicapped Hemiplegic Adult. Arch. Phys. Med., *36*:634–639, 1955.

42. Peszczynski, M.: Exercises for Hemiplegia. In Licht, S.: Therapeutic Exercise. 2nd Ed. New Haven, Conn., Elizabeth Licht, 1961, pp. 721–745.

43. Posniak, A. O., et al.: Rehabilitation of the Hemiplegic Amputee. J.A.M.A., *155*:1463–1465, 1954.

43a. Rankin, J.: Cerebral Vascular Accidents in Patients Over the Age of 60. Prognosis. Scot. Med. J., *2*:200–215, 1957.

44. Reivich, M., Holling, E. H., Roberts, B., and Toole, J. F.: Reversal of Blood Flow Through the Vertebral Artery and Its Effects on Cerebral Circulation. New Eng. J. Med., *265*:878–885, 1961.

45. Roth, M.: Disorders of the Body Image Caused by Lesions of the Right Parietal Lobe. Brain, *72*:89–111, 1949.

46. Rushworth, G.: Spasticity and rigidity: An Experimental Study and Review. J. Neurol. Neurosurg. Psychiat., *23*:99–118, 1960.

47. Rusk, H. A.: Rehabilitation Medicine. St. Louis, C. V. Mosby Co., 1958.

48. Russell, W. R.: Brain, Memory, Learning. London, Oxford University Press, 1959.

49. Schuell, H.: A Short Examination for Aphasia. Neurology, *7*:625–634, 1957.

50. Survey Report. Cerebral Vascular Study Group, Institute of Neurological Diseases and Blindness, National Institutes of Health, 1961.
51. "Stroke" Rehabilitation. Trans. of Conference, London, June 1961. London, The Chest and Heart Association, 1961.
52. Tobis, J. S.: Posthemiplegic Shoulder Pain. New York J. Med., *57*:1377–1380, 1957.
53. Tobis, J. S.: Physical Medicine and Rehabilitation Management in Aphasia. J.A.M.A., *171*:393–396, 1959.
54. Tobis, J. S.: Pathophysiologic Considerations in the Evaluation of the Stroke Patient. Bull. N.Y. Acad. Med., *39*:569–589, 1963.
55. Tobis, J. S., and Lowenthal, M.: Evaluation and Management of the Brain-Damaged Patient. Springfield, Ill., Charles C Thomas, 1960.
56. Ullman, M.: Behavioral Changes in Patients Following Strokes. Springfield, Ill., Charles C Thomas, 1962.
57. Walshe, F.: Diseases of the Nervous System. Baltimore, The Williams & Wilkins Co., 1963.
58. Wepman, J. M.: The Language Disorders. In Garrett, J. F., and Levine, E. S.: Psychological Practices with the Physically Disabled. New York, Columbia University Press, 1962.
59. Wylie, C. M.: Late Survival Following Cerebrovascular Accidents. Arch. Phys. Med., *43*:297–300, 1962.
60. Zane, M. B.: Role of Personality Traits in Rehabilitation Problems. Arch. Phys. Med., *40*:197–202, 1959.

Chapter 24

CONNECTIVE TISSUE DISEASES*

by Edward W. Lowman

NONARTICULAR CONDITIONS

SHOULDER

Subdeltoid Bursitis

Subdeltoid bursitis with or without associated calcific deposit probably occurs far less frequently than it is diagnosed. The entity is, however, a real one and its etiology is usually indeterminate.

Treatment. The objectives of treatment are to maintain normal mobility of the shoulder joint and thus prevent the complicating sequela of a "frozen shoulder" after the acute pain has subsided, to provide analgesia for relief of pain so that the exercises necessary to maintain normal ranges of motion of joints may be accomplished and to assist the healing process of the bursitis through the use of heating agents which promote resolution by vasodilatation.

---

*This chapter includes only those more common conditions for which physical medicine and rehabilitation may be helpful.

Heating by infrared, hot packs, diathermy or other forms should be applied locally for 20 to 30 minutes, followed by passive range of motion exercises carried out at least once daily, even though the acuteness of the condition may require immobilization between treatments.

Rotator Cuff Syndrome

This is the most common cause of shoulder pain after the age of 40 years. It may be a chronic discomfort related to use or it may have acute exacerbations. Its development is usually insidious, resulting from degenerative and attritional changes within the rotator cuff of the shoulder which impair the normal elasticity of these tissues.

Treatment. The objectives of treatment are the same as those for subdeltoid bursitis, plus protection of the shoulder against further damage to the cuff.

The treatment for subdeltoid bursitis is used. In addition, the patient must be made aware of the basic pathologic defect causing the problem and of the need to spare the cuff of work stresses for the prevention of future exacerbations.

Scapulocostal Syndrome

Scapulocostal syndrome is a chronic traction fatigue syndrome resulting from long-standing forward riding of the scapulae on the thorax caused by postural or occupational factors.

Treatment. Relief of pain and correction of the abnormal anatomic scapulocostal alignment that produces the symptoms are the aims of treatment.

Immediate relief of pain is best accomplished by local infiltration of trigger points with local anesthetics or steroids or both. To prevent recurrences the patient must be taught postural exercises to restore the normal scapulocostal relationship. If occupational factors are contributory, they must be identified and corrected.

Shoulder-hand Syndrome

In its classic form, it is reflexly induced, but it may also result from chronic traction, as commonly occurs in the flail hemiplegic upper extremity.

Treatment. The goals of treatment are maintenance of ranges of motion in the fingers, wrist and shoulder, analgesia, and support of the shoulder to counterbalance downward traction if this is a factor.

Local application of heat (packs are usually the easiest) to the shoulder and hand for 20 to 30 minutes is followed by passive range of motion exercises to all joints of the hand, wrist and shoulder at least once daily. Active exercises and the use of the extremity are encouraged. If the extremity is paretic, support on a pillow or in a sling relieves traction at the glenohumeral joint and elevates the hand above elbow level.

ELBOW

Tennis Elbow

Tennis elbow results from microscopic rupture of fibers of origin of the main wrist extensors. Though most commonly associated with tennis, it may originate from occupational or other sources of trauma to wrist extensors.

Treatment.   Healing of the immediate damage, analgesia and protection against subsequent recurrences are the objectives.

The treatment consists of application of heat, radiant (lamp, baker) or conversive (diathermy, ultrasound), to the local area of elbow tenderness at least once daily; rest for the wrist; and, if need be, splint immobilization to prevent use of the extensors until repair at the elbow is complete. The patient should be instructed to avoid physical activities that cause excessive stress to the wrist extensors and may predispose to recurrences.

HAND AND WRIST

Carpal Tunnel Syndrome

Carpal tunnel syndrome results from carpal tunnel entrapment of the median nerve and is a problem for surgical treatment. When diagnosis is uncertain or obscure, electrical conduction times of the median nerve are helpful in positively identifying the problem. (See p. 245 in Chapter 9.)

Dupuytren's Contracture

This contracture may occur idiopathically or it may be identified with chronic trauma, occupational or otherwise, to the palmar fascia of the hand.

Treatment.   The aims of treatment are to prevent flexion contracture deformities of the fingers or to restore mobility where tightness has already developed and to promote pliability in the fibrotic scarring of the palmar fascia to deter fixation.

Local heating of the hands in a paraffin or whirlpool bath (ultrasound may also be of value) for 20 to 30 minutes daily is followed by carefully graded deep friction massage for palmar stretching and range of motion stretching exercises of the finger flexors to maintain or restore full extensor range. The patient should be taught extension exercises that will assist in maintaining mobility of the hand and he should be told to avoid hand activities that may be potentially traumatic and aggravating to the basic pathologic process. Severe contracture may necessitate surgical excision of the involved palmar fascia.

BACK

Hypokinetic Low Back Pain

This is a frequently encountered and frequently overlooked syndrome in which muscle imbalances due to disuse weakness and tightness of truncal and axial musculature result in abnormal postural stress, fatigue and skeletal discomfort. The usual findings are decrease in flexion mobility of the hips and the spine, decrease in strength in the abdominal musculature and to a lesser degree in the upper and low back and lordotic and kyphotic postural changes compensatory to the resultant imbalances.

Treatment.   Regaining full normal skeletal mobility, strengthening truncal muscles and restoring a normal balance to posture are the objects of therapy.

Hypokinetic low back pain is treated by an exercise program, including active and assistive exercises for stretching out tightness in the legs and trunk, especially for improvement of spine and hip flexion, active exercises for strengthening back and abdominal muscle groups and postural exercises.

Fasciae Latae Syndrome

This syndrome is a source of low backache usually hypokinetically induced. The tightened, shortened fasciae latae bands exert abnormal stresses on the low back with resultant symptoms.

Treatment.   Treatment is directed toward restoration of normal length to the shortened fasciae latae.

Although surgical clipping is resorted to at times, most cases respond to a more conservative approach. Local heating (in a sitting whirlpool bath or with hot packs) precedes active stretching of the tight bands by the physical therapist. This is carried out daily in a graduated fashion while at the same time the patient is taught an active exercise program of self-stretching to supplement the therapist's stretching and for future maintenance of mobility.

Psychogenic Rheumatism.   Psychosomatic tension fatigue of musculoskeletal structures produces upper as well as low backache. Since its etiology is psychogenic, the basic approach to its correction is psychiatric. Symptomatic physical therapy, however, is of help in support of the psychiatric treatment.

Treatment.   The patient must be reassured that the syndrome is not arthritis and that no organic crippling will ensue and he should be encouraged to accept the tension-fatigue relationship of the symptoms. Psychologic or psychiatric assistance in resolving the problems that cause the somatic condition and analgesia for pain relief are the objectives of treatment.

Treatment consists of psychotherapy and instruction in home measures of physical therapy for relaxation and for relief of the tension-induced musculoskeletal discomfort, for example, hot tubs, contrast showers, tub whirlpools, general stretching and conditioning exercises and relaxation exercises.

ARTICULAR CONDITIONS

Infectious Arthritis

Specific bacterial infections of joints are rare and usually respond promptly to chemotherapies. In the process of eradication, however, there may be the sequelae of articular damage, disuse weakness in the muscles about the joint and restricted joint mobility that must be dealt with *after* the infection is eradicated.

Treatment.   The goals of treatment are to restore joint mobility, to restore muscle strength about the joint and, if articular damage has resulted, to protect the joint against further deterioration from excessive use.

After the infection is quiescent, heat of a type appropriate to the involved joint should be applied locally as a preliminary to stretching exercises to restore normal joint ranges of motion. This is done on a daily basis. The exercises prescribed depend on the particular patient and include assistive, manual resistive or progressive resistive graduated exercises. Occupational therapy often provides the needed exercise.

If there is significant residual articular damage, crutches, canes, bracing, self-help devices or other protective measures may be necessary to impede further structural and functional deterioration.

Rheumatic Fever

Rheumatic fever never leaves residual joint damage. However, prolonged bed rest and immobilization of specific joints because of pain may result in local and general muscle weakness that requires attention in the convalescent stage.

Treatment.   Treatment seeks to provide general reconditioning and to identify and strengthen local muscle weaknesses.

A graduated program of general conditioning exercises is prescribed. Manual resistive or progressive exercises may be necessary for more pronounced, isolated, disuse muscle weaknesses.

Rheumatoid Arthritis (and Variants*)

Rheumatoid arthritis remains a disease of unknown etiology and treatment is nonspecific or empirical. The effective though nonspecific anti-inflammatory action of steroids is so heavily counterbalanced by serious and catastrophic side effects that their usefulness is limited to a small group of more fulminating rheumatoid arthritics. Conservative management is still the bulwark of treatment for the great majority.

Of major import in this regimen is the intelligent prescription of a good program of physical medicine. Since the pathologic process of rheumatoid arthritis takes place primarily within the peripheral joints, the greatest danger

---

*Still's disease, psoriatic arthritis, intermittent hydrarthrosis, palindromic rheumatism, Reiter's disease and arthritis accompanying ulcerative colitis.

is to these structures. Physiatric measures have no curative or deterrent effect on the basic rheumatoid disease process but, rather, are useful in preventing and protecting the involved joints against deformity and other residual stigmata.

The inflammatory synovitis of the disease produces synovial effusion, joint capsular distention and pain. Movement of the joint in any arc of motion may be painful but the extremes of ranges of motion are especially painful because of the maximal intra-articular pressure induced. The patient functionally tends to favor the joint to avoid discomfort associated with use and he especially guards against those extremes of motion which result in the greatest degree of pain. As a result of this constant factor of disuse, the danger of structural complications to the mechanics of the joint is fostered and the threat persists as long as the synovitis persists and in direct ratio to the acuteness of the synovitis.

The results may be threefold: (1) loss of mobility of the joint due to shortening of para-articular supporting tissues (the extremes of joint motion are lost first; in the extreme, the joint may lose all mobility and become fixed from intra-articular fibrous or bony ankylosis); (2) muscular weakness about the joint resulting from functional disuse; and (3) distortion of joint alignment with resultant deformity as the consequence of inadequate protection with splints or assistive devices or from permitting the patient to perform physical activities that cause trauma to the articular structure. To a large extent all these complications are preventable.

Treatment. The goals in treating rheumatoid arthritis are to maintain normal ranges of motion of involved joints, to maintain strength in the supporting musculature about involved joints and to relieve joint pain so that the other objectives may be successfully attained. It is also important to anticipate and protect joints against avoidable trauma that may damage articular structure further.

To accomplish the objectives treatment must be carried out daily. The more acute the inflammatory synovitis, the more imperative is the demand and the greater the need that it be performed by a professionally trained technician. Conversely, as the inflammation subsides, so also does the threat of the complicating sequelae, and the urgency for need of a daily treatment program similarly and in measure lessens.

Heat is usually applied locally to the joint or joints involved. Moist heat generally is tolerated better than dry. Selection of the type and source of heat depends upon ease of application and the breadth of body coverage needed; no one type of heat source possesses any significant specificity over another. The purpose of the heating is to relax muscular spasm and to effect as much local relief of pain as possible in order to achieve the objectives of mobility and strengthening. Since the treatment program must be carried out indefinitely as long as the disease is active and threatens the joints, it is important to select a means of applying heat that can be used in the home. After instruction (and after discharge from the hospital) the patient can carry on the program within the home without continuous professional help. Hot packs, body bakers, tub immersion baths, paraffin, contrast baths, home whirlpools and the like are most likely to fulfill these criteria.

Following the preliminary application of heat, the joints are each passively carried through all of their normal ranges of motion to preserve full mobility. Since restriction of motion begins at the extremes, it is important to emphasize forcing these areas of range. The patient must be taught the various ranges of motion that are normal for each joint and the various maneuvers to be carried out if he is to preserve them effectively.

Repetitive non-weight bearing exercises then are carried out to maintain power in the supporting muscles about the involved joints. The exercises must be specified in detail and preferably in writing for the patient. These exercises are less important than passive mobilization since muscular power can always be restored *if* joint mobility has been preserved to provide the arc of excursion through which the muscle can be worked with exercise. Further, in the more acute phase of rheumatoid arthritis the patient may be systemically too ill or the pain may be too severe to carry out repetitive exercises effectively. The exercises may have to be delayed or initiated gradually with increasing increments adapted to the patient's general clinical condition.

The joints must be protected. Articular damage that compromises the functional integrity of the joint, weakness in the supporting muscles about a joint and contractures that impair the normal mechanics of the joint will deleteriously predispose to abnormal trauma and to further structural deterioration. Protective, preventive measures should be initiated in anticipation of complications, rather than waiting until they arise. Crutches, canes, wheelchairs, splints and energy-saving self-help devices too frequently are resorted to in need rather than with judicious forethought for conservation of function and preservation of structure. Appliances often can be used temporarily as protective measures until the skeletal deficit is corrected; for example, crutches may be prescribed for knee support until quadriceps support is strengthened by exercise to provide adequate knee stabilization without need for crutches or the patient with knee flexion contractures may use a wheelchair until the contractures can be corrected by physiatric or surgical means.

Rheumatoid Spondylitis

Like rheumatoid arthritis, this is a disease of unknown etiology for which treatment is nonspecific or empirical. At present the most widely practiced conservative regimen of medical management places heavy emphasis on measures of physical medicine.

When, as often is the case, there is peripheral joint involvement in conjunction with the spinal involvement, the objectives and treatment measures for this peripheral disease component are the same as those for rheumatoid arthritis.

The spinal problem and its method of management with physiatric means are unique. The characteristic deformity that threatens the rheumatoid spondylitic is a progressive spinal kyphosis with ankylotic fixation. Once fixation occurs there is no further progression, nor is there any possibility of regression of the deformity.

Treatment.   The objective of the therapeutic exercise program is to maintain the spine in an erect position that is as near normal as possible so that if and when fixation occurs it will impose the least degree of deformity.

Attempts are made to preserve as much cervical range of motion as possible in the hope that the progression of the disease process upward in the spine will abate short of total vertebral involvement and to stretch hip flexion to a maximum so that functionally this hypermobility may be used in compensation for the decrease in spinal mobility.

The treatment procedures are the same as those for rheumatoid arthritis. The program is preventive in objective, and must be carried out daily. Its urgency is in direct ratio to the acuteness of the disease process.

Preliminary heating is best carried out in a contrast shower, in an immersion tub or under a body baker for 15 to 30 minutes to obtain muscle relaxation and analgesia.

Three types of exercise are used after heating: upper back hyperextension and deep breathing exercises to counteract the tendency toward kyphotic deformity (measurements of height and chest expansion are good indices as to the effectiveness of the patient's efforts and should be regularly checked); range of motion exercises for the cervical spine to maintain mobility (note that no attempt is made in rheumatoid spondylitis to maintain general mobility in the dorsal and lumbar spine); and flexion stretching exercises for the hips, including stretching of the hamstrings and fasciae latae, to retain hypermobility of flexion in these joints.

Factors that may environmentally, occupationally or otherwise contribute to kyphosis should be eliminated. This may include discarding of bed pillows, use of a firm solid bed, avoidance of soft, overstuffed chairs and so forth.

Degenerative Arthritis

Degenerative arthritis may occur as a deterioration process concomitant with aging, i.e., a wear and tear process. With the exception of the Heberden node involvement of the terminal interphalangeal joints, the joints most prone to deterioration are, as might be anticipated, those weight bearing joints most subject to trauma—the knees, hips, lumbosacral spine and cervical spine. Specific factors, however, may acutely or chronically focus trauma on certain joints and predispose them to a local traumatic arthritis, the pathology of which is the same as the more generalized senescent variety. Acute damage such as a fracture extending intra-articularly may heal leaving permanent disruption to the architecture of the joint. Chronic local traumata such as in an unstable knee joint similarly may produce a prolonged process of articular damage. This type of arthritis, regardless of cause, is thus basically one of attrition.

Treatment.   Treatment measures seek to maintain mobility of the involved joints, to maintain power in those muscle groups upon which the joints depend for stability and mechanization and to protect the joints against progression of the arthritis.

Since the joint defects are permanent and progressive, the physiatric measures to be prescribed must be carried on indefinitely. It is important, therefore, that an independent home program be devised which the patient can perform daily with only periodic professional reevaluations to assure its effectiveness. Indoctrination of the patient in an appropriate program must be done by a therapist in a series of instruction-treatment sessions in a physical therapy department.

The basic ingredient of such a program is heat for its muscle relaxant and analgesic effect preliminary to the more definitive objectives of range of motion and muscle exercise. As in rheumatoid arthritis, selection of the type and source of heat depends upon availability and simplicity of application to the joints to be treated. Such methods as hot packs, heat lamps, bakers and hot tubs may be employed. It should be emphasized that there is no specificity in any one source of heat and this is, therefore, not a selection factor.

Stretching exercises to maintain normal ranges of motion and full mobility of the joints involved must be taught to the patient and in addition he should be given a written description of them for reference.

Exercises to maintain power in the para-articular musculature are repetitive antigravity exercises aimed at keeping the supporting musculature as strong as possible so that there is maximal stabilization and external support for the internally impaired joint mechanism. These procedures are all to be done daily indefinitely.

The joint should be protected against progression of the deterioration by relieving it of as much work as possible. Crutches, canes, energy-saving self-help devices, wheelchairs, restriction of weight bearing activities, reduction of body weight, correction of postural faults, elimination of occupational or other specific and avoidable sources of trauma—all should be taken under consideration and utilized as anticipatory measures for conservation rather than waiting until further deterioration demands them.

Rehabilitation of the Arthritic Cripple

For the patient in whom chronic progression of the arthritis has already resulted in severe musculoskeletal disability, the problem of reversal or of rehabilitation is of considerable complexity. This is true regardless of basic etiology, whether it is gout, rheumatoid arthritis, rheumatoid spondylitis, degenerative joint disease or some other condition. Not only does the disability require a more active physical medicine program, but since some residual derangement of function is to be expected, adjustments must be made in vocational, social, psychologic and, indeed, all areas of living. Coordinated attention to all of these peripheral ramifications of the problem may thus be needed if the patient is to be rehabilitated to his maximal capability. A team approach of many disciplines, medical and paramedical, for the resolution of a total problem created by disability usually can be effectively provided only in a rehabilitation hospital facility appropriately staffed and oriented for such service.

Methods. The objective in rehabilitation of the arthritic cripple is maximal restoration of function physically, vocationally, socially and psychologically so that despite residual limitations the patient may make the greatest use of his capability within the limits of his disability.

Evaluation of the patient's total problem medically, physically, psychologically, vocationally and socially by an appropriate team of professionally qualified persons is the first step.

A coordinated program is instituted with measures designed to reduce to a minimum the disability effects in each of the five areas mentioned. The program includes medical measures for the stabilization of the arthritis, physical and occupational therapy for reducing restrictions in joint mobility and for increasing power in weakened muscles, training in independent performance of physical activities of daily living, provision of protective appliances or self-help devices, social service for the resolution of living and other environmental problems, psychologic support and assistance in personal adaptation to disability and vocational exploration, guidance and, when necessary, job retraining for ultimate return to productive employment.

Hemophilia

Because of the amount of physical trauma to which they are subjected, joints are frequently the sites of hemorrhage in hemophilia. The hemarthrosis may involved not only the synovia but also cartilage and subchondral bone. Repeated insult to the latter two tissues may result in severe structural damage within the joint.

Treatment. The objectives of treatment are prevention of deformity during the acute phase of hemarthrosis, promotion of resolution of the acute hemorrhage and protection against joint trauma and subsequent episodes of hemorrhage.

In the *acute phase* daily passive range of motion exercise to prevent formation of contractures and traction, posterior splints or other methods for immobilization between exercise sessions are prescribed. Ultrasound may be helpful in speeding resolution of the hematoma.

Interim treatment consists of range of motion exercises to restore full normal joint mobility if contractures have developed, repetitive and resistive exercises to maintain or restore maximal power to the muscles about the joint to assure the greatest degree of stability and protection of joints against avoidable trauma by restriction of physical activity, external support with bracing, energy-saving devices and so forth.

Gouty Arthritis

The basic approach to management of gouty arthritis is early diagnosis and medical treatment of the metabolic defect for the prevention of complications. It should be stressed that the unrecognized and untreated case has the potential for severe and diffuse articular damage and crippling. Patients with neglected gouty arthritis may present as profound a problem to the rehabilitation team as the rheumatoid cripple. With the adequacy of modern medical measures for management, the need for physical medicine is infrequent except in the obstinate or protracted joint problem in which disuse atrophy or loss of range of motion may develop. In these instances an exercise program may be prescribed.

Osteoporosis

Osteoporosis of the spine is a common cause of back pain especially in the postmenopausal female. Although several medical approaches to treatment are recommended, the most unanimously endorsed, as well as the most definitive, is the use of anabolic steroids. Their effectiveness is cumulative over months.

Treatment. Conjunctive treatment, used until the anabolic steroids become effective, has as its objectives protection of the spine against stresses that may produce vertebral compression fracture and analgesia.

External back support in the form of a back brace or a custom-tailored full body garment with paravertebral reinforcement is usually necessary to supplement muscle support of the spine.

At the same time, a repetitive exercise program should be instituted to maintain and improve to a maximum the strength in the back and abdominal musculature which supports the spine.

Wet or dry heat, diathermy or ultrasound therapy locally to the back preceding exercise has analgesic value and promotes successful performance of the exercises. There is no convincing evidence that any of these techniques exerts any specificity in assisting directly in reversal of the basic bone metabolic problem.

Disseminated Lupus Erythematosus

The peripheral joint involvement by this multisystem disease is the same as that seen in rheumatoid arthritis; the degree of crippling is usually less, but this is not categorically true. The objectives and methods of management from a physical medicine standpoint are identical to those listed under rheumatoid arthritis.

Dermatomyositis

Dermatomyositis is not a true arthritis, but an inflammatory disease of muscle which may result in fibrotic replacement of muscle. More important, the reluctance of the patient to use painfully involved muscles predisposes to shortening and contractures of soft tissues with resultant compromise of joint mobility.

Treatment.   During the active inflammatory phase of the disease, range of motion exercises are used to maintain normal joint mobility (and thus normal muscle length). In the more acute phase this may have to be a passive procedure carried out by the therapist at least once daily. As the acute phase subsides, the patient more actively becomes a participant in this prophylactic procedure.

In remission, treatment emphasis shifts to an active repetitive exercise program for restoration of strength to muscles that are residually weak either because of damage from the basic pathologic condition or as the result of disuse.

Heat is often employed as a preliminary to exercise for its relaxant and analgesic effects.

Scleroderma

Like dermatomyositis, scleroderma inflicts its damage primarily extra-articularly. In contrast to the muscle focus of the latter, scleroderma is pathologically insulting to the soft subcutaneous tissues. The initial inflammation and edema may lead to fibrosis, soft tissue fixation and deformity. The objectives and methods of physiatric management are the same as those for dermatomyositis.

Polyarteritis Nodosa

Polyarteritis nodosa may involve joints with synovitis and effusion when there is necrosis of a nutrient vessel to such an area. Because of the random nature of this process, polyarticular involvement is unusual. In addition, since the pattern of the pathologic process is more a focal one than panarterial, the degree of joint reaction is usually not so profound as that of rheumatoid arthritis. In the patient who survives the disease, a more disabling sequela is peripheral neuropathy, the result of necrosis of the nutrient vessel in the nerve trunk.

Treatment. In cases of peripheral neuropathy physical medicine has as its objectives evaluation of the location and extent of nerve involvement, protection of the involved muscles and of the part against structural change complicating the paresis and restoration of muscle function and of muscle power.

Therapy includes electrodiagnostic procedures for assessing the degree and extent of denervation with serial examinations for continuing determination of the prognosis for resolution; static or functional splinting to protect against attritional derangement of structure; passive range of motion exercises to prevent contractures from occurring during the paretic stage; and assistive and graduated strengthening exercises during reinnervation within the involved muscles, if it takes place.

REFERENCES

1. Austin, E., Rolland, W., and Clausen, D.: Use of Physical Therapy Modalities in the Treatment of Orthopedic and Neurologic Residuals in Hemophilia. Arch. Phys. Med., *42:*393-397, 1961.
2. Hollander, J. L.: Arthritis and Allied Conditions. 7th Ed. Philadelphia, Lea & Febiger, 1966.
3. Home Care Programs in Arthritis, A Manual for Patients New York, The Arthritis Foundation.
4. Johnson, E. W., Wells, R. M., and Duran, R. J.: Diagnosis of Carpal Tunnel Syndrome. Arch. Phys. Med., *43:*414-419, 1962.
5. Kraus, H., and Raab, W.: Hypokinetic Disease. Springfield, Ill., Charles C Thomas, 1961.
6. Lowman, E. W.: Arthritis. General Principles, Physical Medicine, Rehabilitation. Boston, Little, Brown and Co., 1959.
7. Lowman, E. W., Klinger, J. L.: Aids to Independent Living. New York, McGraw-Hill Book Co., 1969.
8. Michele, A. A., Davies, J. J., Krueger, F. J., and Lichtor, J. M.: Scapulocostal Syndrome. New York J. Med., *50:*1353-1356, 1950.
9. Moseley, H. F.: Shoulder Lesions. 2nd Ed. New York, Paul B. Hoeber, Inc., 1953.
10. Osteoarthritis, A Handbook for Patients. New York, The Arthritis Foundation, 1958.
11. Russek, A. S.: Diagnosis and Treatment of Scapulocostal Syndrome. J.A.M.A., *150:*25-27, 1952.
12. Zohn, D. A., Hughes, A. C., and Haase, K. H.: Carpal Tunnel Syndrome—A Review. Arch. Phys. Med., *43:*420-425, 1962.

Chapter 25

CONGENITAL AND TRAUMATIC LESIONS OF THE SPINAL CORD

by Charles Long, II

This chapter presents a means of dealing with patients with spinal cord injuries, a method of evaluating and treating them and the complications which occur during recovery.

The cause of the lesion, whether it is congenital, traumatic or infectious, is not as important as the level at which it strikes the spinal cord. Lesion level is the primary factor in determining the patient's ultimate rehabilitation goal, and hence the course he must follow to reach it. Management of the spinal cord injured patient requires specialized knowledge beyond the scope of any single physician, so that a team effort is required, regardless of the specialty of the primary managing physician. Further help is needed from paramedical personnel—physical and occupational therapists, social workers, psychologists, vocational counselors and trainers—who should work under the direction of the physician or rehabilitation team throughout the patient's rehabilitation, including outpatient follow-up. An excellent environment for such management is the spinal cord injury center, where patients can be treated from the day of injury to the ultimate vocational rehabilitation.

GENERAL MANAGEMENT

As in any rehabilitation program, management is directed toward encouraging the patient to achieve the best level of function consistent with his safety.

The patient is helped through a regimen of self-mobilization consisting of exercises, measures to assist circulatory homeostasis, wheelchair activities and, when applicable, ambulation training. These factors are listed in the following outline; their applicability will be apparent from the detailed descriptions of functional levels later in this chapter. Details of the specific methods are available in the chapters in Part II, Techniques of Management.

Mobilization of the Patient with Spinal Cord Injury
1. *Early exercise,* on frame or bed
   a. Passive Range of Motion (R.O.M.)
   b. Active R.O.M. (graded exercise to all functioning muscles)
   c. Resistance (weights) added gradually
2. *Tiltboard* to help adapt to erect position
   After vertebral healing is "safe," (30 to 60 minutes daily, graded tilt)
3. *Wheelchair training*
   a. Transfers (A.D.L.)
   b. Push-ups (prevention of decubiti), one every 10 minutes
   c. Occupational therapy in A.D.L. (feeding, grooming, dressing)
4. *Ambulation training* (injury below midthoracic level)
   a. Brace (long leg, with or without pelvic band and spinal attachment)
   b. Training from parallel bars to crutches
   c. Continued need for wheelchair in most cases
   d. Slow progress (takes 4 to 8 months)
5. *Vocational rehabilitation*
   a. Psychologic testing (aptitude and preference)
   b. Vocational testing (skills tests)
   c. Vocational training

Natural History of Spinal Cord Injury

Application of mobilization procedures depends on the physician's knowledge of the natural history of paraplegia. This natural history reflects changes occurring in the central nervous system and in the healing lesions of the skeletal system. During the period immediately after the injury there is flaccidity below the level of the lesion. This period of spinal shock lasts from weeks to months and is succeeded by the development of spasticity, favoring usually extensor but sometimes flexor groups. This return of tone to the muscles is accompanied by a similar increase in tone of the bladder and sometimes spasticity. As the change from flaccidity to spasticity is taking place, healing is occurring in fractured and dislocated areas of the spine. *Healing of ligaments, as after simple dislocation, takes 6 to 12 weeks; healing after fracture usually takes a full six months.*

Protective Bracing. Bracing of the spine depends on a judgment of its true value. In the patient with a *complete transection*, it is no longer necessary to protect the cord. The removal of bracing then depends only on assurance that a painful pseudarthrosis or recurring dislocation will not impede rehabilitation. *In the presence of a partial or healing lesion*, it is advisable to brace throughout the healing period to protect the cord from injury by excessive motion. In the quadriplegic with a spinal cord lesion at the level of the fifth cervical cord segment, increased protection is advisable, even in complete lesions, for the accidental damage of one more segment would be fatal.

Psychic Recovery. As the patient proceeds through his rehabilitation program, he goes through a natural course of recovery that is psychologic as well as physical. The severe, catastrophic and castrative (literally and psychodynamically) trauma early produces either profound depression or a denial of the disability or both. The process of recovery implies the acceptance of the fact of the disability and the growth of psychic ability to cope with the fact. Psychic recovery is essentially an ability to deal with reality. The patient's family is often involved in the dynamic mechanism with him. It is necessary for the physician to work with the family, pointing out reality and encouraging the family to support the patient along realistic paths. One of the major crises of rehabilitation arises when it is ascertained that a patient who wishes to walk will not be physically able to do so. The physician must use his judgment in determining whether to confront the patient directly with the fact that he will not walk, or to let him find out by implication.

Homeostasis.   The natural course of recovery includes an attempt by the body to recover some homeostasis in the circulatory response to the erect posture. When the patient first sits or stands he will be lightheaded and may even faint. This can be prevented by moving the patient gradually toward the erect posture. Tilting on a table or board is commonly used for this purpose. The tiltboard is also said to assist in preventing osteoporosis and the resultant "dumping" of calcium into the circulation; this in turn is supposed to prevent kidney stones. In spite of the lack of evidence to support these claims, the tiltboard is used by many clinicians, including the author.

Prevention of Complications

Complications common in patients with spinal cord injuries include urinary infection and stones, decubitus ulcers, autonomic hyperreflexia, contractures and heterotopic ossification.

Urinary Complications.   (See also Chapter 31.)   Urinary infection and stones, with eventual kidney failure, are inevitably fatal if unattended. Urinary stone formation in chronic disease patients is related to recumbency, infection and indwelling catheters. Each of these predisposing factors is present to some degree in patients with spinal cord injuries. Recumbency is to be avoided as much as possible, catheters are to be removed as soon as they safely can be and infection should be religiously controlled or prevented. The development of automatic voiding ability can probably be hastened through early "intermittent catheterization." In this technique a catheter is inserted to empty the bladder every six hours, and immediately withdrawn. After 24 to 48 hours of this treatment, automatic, low residual bladder emptying is often accomplished. Cystometrographic evidence of bladder tone is not essential for successful application of this technique. When automaticity has been developed the patient can wear a condom-type external catheter, or may go without any device if he has adequate local or reflex warnings of impending voiding.

Antibiotics are not used unless clinical urinary infection appears. lest the urinary flora develop resistance to each successive antibiotic, making it useless in major crises.

Prevention of Urinary Tract Complications
in the Catheterized Patient

1. Prevention of infection
   a. Fluid intake of more than 4000 cc. every day
   b. Frequent catheter change (every 2 weeks or 1 month)

    c. Twice daily irrigations with "solution G"* until returns are clear
    d. Mandelamine, 1 Gm. 4 times a day; ascorbic acid, 1 Gm. 4 times a day to acidify urine if needed
    e. Insertion of catheter if residual is more than 100 cc. after voiding
    f. Removal of catheter when automatic voiding is possible
2. Maintenance of bladder size without overstretching by clamping catheter for 1 to 2 hours twice a day
3. Prevention of stones (?)
    a. Restriction of milk intake to less than one glass per day
    b. Avoidance of citrus fruits and juices (to avoid alkaline urine)
4. Continuous monitoring of GU status
    a. Weekly urinalyses in hospital; monthly as outpatient
    b. Intravenous pyelogram every 6 to 12 months

---

*"Solution G" (Suby's Solution) is composed of citric acid monohydrate (U.S.P.), 32.4 Gm.; sodium carbonate monohydrate (U.S.P.), 5 Gm.; magnesium oxide (heavy) (U.S.P.), 3.8 Gm.; benzalkonium (17%), 0.4 cc.; and distilled water to make 1000 cc. The pH range of this solution is 3.5 to 4.5.

Decubitus Ulcers. (See Chapter 32.) Decubitus ulcers are more annoying than deadly, but may be a source of continuous frustration to the aims of the paraplegic and his physician. The major causative factor is pressure; the obvious preventive measure is the removal of pressure. The weight bearing points are rotated by turning the patient in bed once every two hours. This strict regimen is followed at the beginning of the rehabilitation course. Later it becomes practical to determine, by balancing the patient's comfort against his safety, a more workable schedule.

If a decubitus ulcer has already developed, the most important method of treatment is removal of offending pressures. It is sometimes necessary to allow short periods of pressure on the decubital side in order to rest the nondecubital surfaces. The use of doughnuts for sitting or lying positions does not solve the problem; most commonly the doughnut shifts position so that its edge is right over the ulcer.

Turning frames may be used until the patient is spending several hours daily in a wheelchair. The patient should then be weaned to a hospital bed because when he goes home a hospital bed is part of his discharge equipment. His turning schedule and detailed descriptions of the length of time he is allowed to be up are essential components of discharge orders.

Autonomic Hyperreflexia. Certain complications are more frequently seen in quadriplegics than in paraplegics. Such complications are therefore becoming more common as increasing numbers of quadriplegics are being produced by automobile trauma and increasing numbers are surviving the initial episode through early, effective treatment. Among these complications is autonomic hyperreflexia. This state may occur in many degrees, ranging from the most simple circumoral blanching and mild sweating to severe hypertension with excruciating headache, massive diaphoresis and a subjective feeling of impending doom. In its most malignant form the hypertension can produce intracerebral hemorrhage and death. The condition is apparently related to release of norepinephrine at ganglia of the sympathetic nervous system no longer under effective spinal cord control. This release may be triggered by a variety of stimuli, including skin pressure or stroking, change of position or the presence of systemic infection; the most common cause is stimulation of the bladder through overstretching or during the process of irrigation. The most common cause of severe headache in quadriplegics is probably bladder distension due to a plugged catheter, with resultant autonomic hyperreflexia and hypertension. Relief of the catheter obstruction usually produces an immediate drop in blood pressure and relief of symptoms.

Once a patient has developed the tendency to sympathomimetic response, certain preventive measures can be taken. Irrigations of the bladder in such patients should be performed with the patient in the sitting position; intracranial hypertension is minimized by this position. Probanthine (15 mg. three or four times daily) can be used over the long term to reduce bladder reflex sensitivity to distension, thus subduing the reflex arc at its source. Bladder sensitivity is also reduced by keeping incumbent infection at a minimum by using the measures just described.

Treatment of a major hypertensive response is an emergency. The patient should be made to sit up, and his blood pressure constantly monitored. Specific precipitating causes, especially catheter obstruction, should be sought and relieved. If relief of the cause does not produce immediate lowering of the blood pressure, alpha-adrenergic blocking agents should be used. Tetraethylammonium chloride may be effective in the midst of hypertensive crisis. Phentolamine or phenoxybenzamine may be useful to reduce the effect of further stimuli in producing hypertension. After a few days on such therapy, it may be possible to discontinue the use of the protective drug and to institute the general measures described previously.

Contracture.   Contractures, which result primarily from allowing joints to remain in one position for a long enough period to permit shortening of supporting structures, are prevented by motion. Passive motion is started early (the day after the accident is not too soon) and continued until functional movement takes over the process of daily exercise. Range can be maintained by three to five repetitions of gentle passive stretching in one daily bout. Any joint that is moved by the patient through a reasonable range in the course of daily activities can be dropped from the passive stretching routine. The back should not be stretched because of the danger of increasing its flexibility and instability.

Heterotopic Bone Formation.   A further complication is the laying down of new bone in soft tissues, often around joints or along the femoral shaft. Although the joint itself is not attacked, limitation of motion often occurs as a result of encroachment by the extra-articular formations, especially at the hip. During development of these processes, active inflammation and swelling may surround the area, mimicking an acute arthritic process. The condition most often occurs within months after injury but may occur years later, always below the level of the spinal lesion. It is self-limited, usually progressing over several months to its ultimate anatomic limit; at that point it is usually limited to a specific muscle group. It occurs most frequently at a level between the upper pelvis and the knee; however we have seen it also in paraspinal muscles. There is no known method of treatment of this complication. There have been suggestions that it is related to the trauma of passive motion and of turning frames, but these methods of treatment are so important that they cannot be omitted because of an unproved relationship to heterotopic bone formation. Surgical removal, when indicated, must be carefully timed to allow resection while the bone is still soft enough to be removed relatively easily, but must be done late enough for the process to have reached maturity. Surgery is performed only when restriction of motion causes severe limitation of activity, generally at the hip joint.

FUNCTIONAL SIGNIFICANCE OF SPINAL CORD LESION LEVEL

Although general principles can be mentioned for the management of patients with spinal cord injuries, the specific program for an individual patient must be modified according to the level of the lesion. The lower the level of the injury, the greater the amounts of muscle power available to the patient for his rehabilitation. Because certain functional groups of muscles are activated at particular levels of the spinal cord it is possible to categorize the performance to be expected of patients injured at and between these levels (Table 25-1).

Fourth Cervical Level

The quadriplegic in whom the fourth cervical segment is spared has good use of the sternomastoids and the trapezius and upper cervical paraspinal muscles. He is incapable of voluntary function in the arms, trunk or lower extremities. Upper extremity function is possible only with the use of externally powered devices. Electric motors, when attached to a terminal device such as the Rancho Los Amigos flexor hinge splint, can be used to drive the hand. Springs are used to open the hand and the motor provides "voluntary" closure. The completely paralyzed arms are supported on balanced forearm orthoses (mobile arm supports; feeders). The patient then uses "body English" and changes in head position to raise and lower the hand. External power devices can be used to assist elbow flexion in the feeder. Patients at this level often do not accept these devices because they are so cumbersome and do not add enough to the patient's abilities. A mouthstick may be useful in typing, writing, dialing, and turning pages. Another approach can be taken through application of the Rancho Electric Arm, a multi-axis device which drives the entire arm through geared electric motors. The device is controlled usually by a bank of tongue switches mounted before the patient's face. Some patients have apparently accepted this device and use it in a clinical setting; evaluation of the device in the field is still in progress. All quadriplegics with functioning fourth cervical segments should have electric wheelchairs if they have adequate space

TABLE 25-1   CRITICAL LEVELS OF CORD FUNCTION

LEVEL	MAJOR MUSCLES ADDED
C 4	Diaphragm, midcervical extensors and flexors
C 5	Deltoid, biceps
C 6	Radial wrist extensors, serratus, latissimus, pectorals
C 7	Triceps, long finger flexors and extensors, wrist flexors and extensors
T 1	Hand intrinsics, ulnar wrist
T 12	Full abdominal innervation, full intercostal innervation
L 4	Hip flexors, knee extensors

in which to maneuver them. Special control systems (tongue switches or touch-plate microswitches) are necessary. With this combination of aids the patient should be able to control his own electric wheelchair, turn pages, operate an electric typewriter, dial a telephone and sometimes feed himself.

Fifth Cervical Level

The patient with a functioning fifth cervical segment can use the deltoid and biceps muscles to accomplish activities of daily living. Partial continued weakness of the deltoid and biceps may make it necessary to use "feeders" for support of the elbow and shoulder, especially in the early stages of the rehabilitation program. Overhead sling suspension may be used as an interim measure if it appears that permanent feeders will not be necessary. The patient needs some sort of substitute for nonfunctioning hand and wrist musculature. The use of electric motor splints has already been described. For patients who do not tolerate external power (and these are becoming increasingly rare), fixed support of the wrist and fingers may be used. Adapted devices are then applied to the patient's hand by another individual and kept in place until a new activity is started. Skillful use of these devices requires much training and practice.

The quadriplegic whose lesion is below the fifth cervical segment can be expected to feed himself, perform some grooming activities, help a little with upper extremity dressing, help apply bracing, push his wheelchair for short distances (with special projections on the wheelchair rims), turn pages, use the electric typewriter and play board games requiring grasp and release.

Patients with lesions at the fourth and fifth cervical levels require full-time help for lifting and assisting. A hydraulic lift is necessary to help the family move the patient from bed to wheelchair. Beds for all patients with spinal cord injuries should be adjusted to wheelchair height. The patient's wheelchair should be reclinable to permit non-weight bearing rest periods during the day. Removable armrests are essential components of all wheelchairs for the spinal cord injured.

Sixth Cervical Level

At the sixth cervical level of involvement, the quadriplegic has the added use of the radial wrist extensors. This addition permits graded control of the wrist, with gravity performing the flexion movements. Wrist extension can be harnessed through special "tenodesis' splints to drive the fingers into flexion; sometimes a surgical finger flexor tenodesis can be performed for the same purpose. Many patients prefer simply to use leather cuffs strapped to their hands, into which such implements as tooth brushes, forks and spoons can be inserted.

The patient injured below the sixth cervical segment can perform all the activities of patients with higher level lesions and in addition can be more helpful in dressing himself, often doing it completely, can propel his wheelchair long distances and usually can transfer himself from bed to chair using the overhead trapeze or a modified push-up with elbow stabilization by shoulder adduction. Automobile transfers are often possible; driving with hand controls is often possible for young patients.

Seventh Cervical Level

The major functional additions at the seventh cervical segment are associated with the use of the triceps and the finger flexors and extensors. This patient is able to do push-ups in the sitting position and therefore can transfer himself from bed to chair. He can grasp and release and is usually able to operate his hands without splints. Sometimes the vagaries of innervation of either the flexors or extensors make it necessary to apply a hand splint with a spring to assist the uninnervated group.

This patient is independent at the wheelchair level.

As the patient grows older, less functional independence should be expected from him. Reductions in capability vary with the individual, his physiologic age and his physical abilities.

Upper Thoracic Level (First to Tenth Thoracic Segments)

The paraplegic whose lesion is at the upper thoracic level has full innervation of upper extremity muscles and varying degrees of upper back, abdominal and intercostal innervation. He may be braced for standing, but should not be expected to walk functionally. Long leg braces, sometimes with pelvic band and spinal attachment, are necessary for daily standing and if ambulation is to be attempted.

This patient is a completely independent individual in the wheelchair; he can dress and feed himself, tend to his toilet, transfer to and from his wheelchair and in and out of a car, drive a car* and hold a job away from home requiring self-transportation.

Lower Thoracic-Upper Lumbar Level (Tenth Thoracic to Second Lumbar Segments)

The paraplegic with a lesion at this level has full abdominal control, full upper back control and respiratory reserve. Full innervation of the abdominal muscles may permit ambulation in long leg braces. The patient is completely independent in all activities of daily living; he can drive, perform transfers and attend an outside job. He stands fair chance of being ambulatory and free of the wheelchair.

Low Lumbar Level (Fourth Lumbar Segment)

The patient injured at or below the fourth lumbar segment has the use of at least the hip flexors and quadriceps and he can stand without braces and walk without external support. However, because of severe weakness of the gluteus maximus and medius, coupled with paralyzed ankles, the patient has a laborious, waddling gait. Ambulation can be greatly assisted by the application

---

*Hand controls can be obtained commercially for all automobiles with automatic transmission. The brake and gas pedal operate reciprocally with one hand; as the brake is applied, the accelerator releases.

of short leg (ankle) braces and by the bilateral use of crutches. If these supports are not used, the patient's unusual method of ambulation will cause recurvatum at the knees and abnormal strain in the lumbar spine.

Since most injuries at this level occur in the cauda equina, the bladder denervation is of the lower motor neuron type. Recovery of reflex function does not occur and the bladder becomes large and atonic. Bladder care is as important in these patients as in those with higher lesions and should not be forgotten just because the patient is ambulatory.

CONGENITAL SPINAL CORD LESIONS

The most common group of congenital spinal cord lesions are those associated with spina bifida. Spina bifida implies the presence of an external sac of meninges, such as a meningocele or myelomeningocele. Spina bifida occulta implies a bifid malformation of the spinal column without external "cele" formation. Either type may result in spinal cord destruction ranging from partial involvement to complete transection. The most common levels of involvement are thoracic and lumbar. The level of the neural arch defect is not necessarily related to the level of spinal cord or cauda equina involvement.

Many physicians hesitate to assume the task of treating these children because, as will be seen from the accompanying guides to management, the care of the spina bifida child is a complex life-long process. Treatment must encompass all the factors involved in the care of the adult paraplegic, plus the emotional and educational problems inherent in pediatric management.

Management of Spina Bifida Paraplegics

General Mobilization.   The spina bifida child can usually become ambulatory. He requires bracing consistent with his spinal cord level of involvement. Training is best accomplished on wooden axillary crutches, with a drag-to gait advancing to a swing-through or four-point gait if possible.

Regular range of motion exercise should be prescribed and administered by the family daily to maintain range in the lower extremities. Commonly occurring contractures, such as equinovarus feet, may respond to stretching but sometimes require plaster wedging or orthopedic surgical correction.

Genitourinary Complications.   Genitourinary complications are common in children with spina bifida paraplegia and may be lethal. Urethal reflux and hydronephrosis eventually lead to renal failure and the premature death of the patient. Although antibiotics have effectively lengthened the life span of these patients, control of genitourinary problems still leaves much to be desired.

Control measures are aimed particularly at the relief of urinary obstruction and the prevention of infection. Measures for prevention of infection are similar to those for adults listed on page 568. Doses of Mandelamine and ascorbic acid must be appropriately reduced depending on the age of the child.

Obstruction of ureteral outflow into the bladder must be corrected by reconstructive surgery of the ureterovesical junction. Although obstruction at the urethral level is sometimes treated by transurethral bladder neck resection, it is usually possible to relieve the obstruction and its consequent ureteral and renal hydrops by inserting an indwelling catheter. The use of a catheter must not be considered an admission of defeat, for it may be life-saving. The surgical, ileal-pouch bladder is presently being evaluated; it is useful in selected cases with obstruction and reflux.

Every possible attempt should be made to train the child's bladder to void voluntarily or on a schedule. Stimulating areas of the skin of the groin or thigh helps initiate reflex bladder emptying and the child should be encouraged to push with his hands on the lower abdomen (Credé method). Residual urine must be kept low to prevent infection and reflux.

In spite of all attempts at bladder training, the majority of patients will not be satisfactorily trained. Absorbent pads may be used to collect the incontinent urine, or condom-type prophylactic kits may be used in the older male child.

SPASTICITY

Almost every spinal cord patient becomes spastic to some degree during his rehabilitation. In the natural history of the lesion, flaccidity occurs first (spinal shock) and spasticity begins to appear some time during the first few months. The spasticity increases to some maximum for the individual, this maximum either being maintained indefinitely or waning gradually over the course of years.

Patients with cauda equina lesions do not develop spasticity because the abnormality is located in peripheral nerves instead of in the cord.

The spastic patient may have many problems. The most important is a general inability to perform at a top level in activities of daily living because of the encumbering effect of relatively rigid extremities. Spasticity may involve specific groups of muscles, especially the extensors in the lower extremities. This spasticity may actually be useful at times, responding reflexly to attempts at standing by assisting the patient in keeping his knees straight. The presence of spasticity in the bladder may be either an aid or a detriment. It may be the basis for automatic bladder function or the bladder may become so spastic that it is useless as a reservoir of urine. Spasticity may appear as "spasms" superimposed on a background of increased stiffness of the limbs; these spasms may occur in response to minimal stimuli directed against the body at any level below the lesion. Such spasms can keep the patient awake at night, or throw him from his wheelchair. Local examples of rehabilitation obstacles imposed by spasticity include: secondary tightening of heel cords with limited ambulation; extension or flexion contractures of the knees preventing sitting or standing, respectively; extension contractures of the hips preventing sitting; and adductor spasm preventing ambulation.

In judging the need for surgical correction of spasticity to overcome any of these obstacles, the possible detriment to other phases of the patient's existence must be carefully weighed. For instance, surgery that involves the upper sacral roots or cord area precludes any return of bladder control. The decision for surgery must also be weighed against the time allowed for spontaneous recovery; if any return is occurring at the level of injury, the decision should be put off until at least a year after onset to give the cord a chance to do its own recovering.

Mechanism of Spasticity. The exact mechanism of spasticity is not known. Spasticity may be defined as an increased resistance to passive stretch, accompanied by increased tendon reflexes. Pragmatically it is represented at the spinal cord level by a hypersensitive stretch reflex and a tendency for incoming impulses to spread within the cord beyond their normal boundaries. Thus there is a summation of many impulses entering the cord from skin, ligaments and muscle and other receptors, directed toward the oversensitive alpha and gamma systems.

Conservative Management of Spasticity.   Conservative therapy begins with the reduction of sensory bombardment of the cord. This implies careful treatment of decubitus ulcers, bladder infections and other intercurrent infections, and the early removal of bladder stones.

In addition, if spasticity is present to a significant degree, the patient must receive daily stretching to maintain full range of motion of all involved segments and to prevent contracture. If the muscle is not threatened by spasticity, has been declared unresponsive to conservative therapy or is of so little importance to the patient that it is not worth the trouble to stretch it, stretching is not necessary. Stretching should be applied slowly and fairly forcefully and the muscle should be held at full range for the count of three.

Surgical Correction of Spasticity.   Spasticity can be corrected surgically only by destructive procedures that interrupt the reflex loop. These procedures may be used peripherally or centrally, locally or generally. The following outline describes the surgical measures that are used.

Surgical Management of Spasticity

A. Central. General control by sectioning many roots; local control by specific sections of one or two roots. Test by spinal anesthesia for effectiveness before surgery.
   1. Dorsal rhizotomy for lower extremity general spasticity if increased by external stimuli; in presence of voluntary motion. May avoid bladder segments.
   2. Ventral rhizotomy for lower extremity general spasticity in absence of voluntary control, or if voluntary control is to be sacrificed. Can avoid bladder segments. More certain spasticity control than dorsal rhizotomy.
   3. Alcohol block (intrathecal injection of alcohol). If done carefully the level of the block can be controlled; effect is often permanent, but can wear off; destroys ventral and dorsal roots; precludes bladder training.
B. Peripheral. Avoids necessity of laminectomy; can be directed more easily toward specific muscle groups rather than root outflows. Test by local block for effectiveness before surgery.
   1. Obturator neurectomy. Used in ambulation or nursing problems due to spastic adductors of hips; sometimes relieves lower extremity spasticity beyond obturator sphere due to reduction of cord input.
   2. Sciatic neurectomy. Still somewhat experimental, but logical for spastic hamstrings and heel cords.
   3. Gastrocnemius-soleus neurectomy. Logical and may work well when done by an experienced surgeon.
C. Adjunctive Surgery. Tight tendons often must be sectioned or lengthened, e.g., heel cords or hamstrings, in addition to the nervous system surgery.

When spasticity occurs in the upper extremities, as it may when the lesion is at the cervical level, the few activities possible to the quadriplegic patient may be lost. Unfortunately there are few effective approaches to upper extremity spasticity. If a significant imbalance exists, for instance between an active biceps and a spastic triceps, surgical lengthening, denervation, or section of the tendon of the spastic muscle is indicated.

"Antispastic" Drugs.   Diazepam has proved effective against general spasticity or recurrent spasms in the spinal cord patient. Individual tolerance to this drug varies widely, especially in susceptibility to somnolence. Within the patient's tolerance, spasticity or spasms may respond to 2.5 to 10 mg. of Diazepam taken orally three or four times daily.

SEXUAL PROBLEMS OF PATIENTS WITH SPINAL CORD INJURIES

Under the best of circumstances, the patient with complete spinal cord section cannot expect normal intercourse. The man, by virtue of paralysis, cannot assume a dominant physical role. The paraplegic woman becomes a passive partner without local genital sensation. In spite of these ultimate limitations, coitus is practiced with gratification by about a third of paraplegic men, and probably a higher percentage of paraplegic women. This is possible since a significant percentage of paraplegic men can have erections. These may be psychically induced in patients with lesion levels below T-9, leaving the upper splanchnic outflow intact. In patients with upper motor neurone lesions at any spinal level, reflex erections can be produced by local stimulation; in patients with lesions at higher levels, the probability of success is greater. The ability to have erections, psychic or reflex or both, usually appears within six months after injury. Eventually two-thirds to three-quarters of all men with complete spinal cord injury experience this ability.

Libido, in the sense of psychic desire, fantasy, and dreaming, apparently remains. The psychic accompaniments of intercourse in the paraplegic may be intense. Less than 20 per cent of patients achieve the "voluptuous sensation" of suffusive orgasm, but there may be a distinct sense of gratification of partner and fulfillment of the patient's libidinous need. For this type of intercourse to be successful, that is, gratifying, it often requires that the normal female be vigorously active to maintain her partner's erection. Both partners, therefore, face direct reversal of their customary roles, and all the adjustments and concessions demanded by that reversal. In the event that intercourse cannot be accomplished, other methods of sexual satisfaction are substituted which may be gratifying to the partners. The discussion of the adjustments necessary to the paraplegic are an integral part of the care of the paraplegic. Each physician develops his own style in bringing these problems into focus, or allowing the patient to bring them into focus. In any case, such problems can rarely be productively bypassed. The patient's silence on this topic, as on others, does not usually indicate lack of interest but more likely embarrassment, or fear of what he may find out.

Fertility of the completely paraplegic man is low. The contributory factors include decreased spermatogenesis, recurrent infection contributing to a decrease in semen and spermatogenesis, and failure to ejaculate. Only about 10 per cent of patients have ejaculation, and this may not be consistent. Some experimental methods of obtaining sperm for artificial insemination are under investigation. The total fertility rate for paraplegic men is probably about 5 per cent. In paraplegic women the situation is different. Ovarian function is not significantly affected by paraplegia, so oogenesis and ovulation occur as in normal women. Since intercourse is feasible for her, the paraplegic woman can conceive normally. She is also able to bear children. Uterine contractions and cervical dilatation occur in spite of the spinal cord lesion. There have been numerous deliveries of normal children to paraplegic mothers. Recognition of the onset of labor is difficult, so hospital admission is usually planned for about the thirty-second week of pregnancy. The actual diagnosis of labor and its progress depend mostly on observation of cervical dilatation.

REFERENCES

1. Berns, S. H., Lowman, E. W., Rusk, H. A., and Covalt, D. A.: Spinal Cord Injury—Rehabilitation Costs and Results and Follow-up in Thirty-One Cases. J.A.M.A., *164:*1551–1558, 1957.
2. Bluestone, S. S., and Deaver, G. G.: Habilitation of the Child with Spina Bifida and Myelomeningocele. J.A.M.A., *161:*1248–1251, 1956.
3. Bors, E.: Urological Aspects of Rehabilitation in Spinal Cord Injuries. J.A.M.A., *146:*225–229, 1951.
4. Bors, E., and Comarr, A. E.: Neurological Disturbances of Sexual Function with Special Reference to 529 Patients with Spinal Cord Injury. Urol. Survey, *10:*191–222, 1960.
5. Carr, T. L.: Orthopedic Aspects of One Hundred Cases of Spina Bifida. Postgrad. Med. J., *32:*201–210, 1956.
6. Guttmann, Sir Ludwig, and Frankel, H.: The Value of Intermittent Catheterization in the Early Management of Traumatic Paraplegia and Tetraplegia. Paraplegia, *4:*63–83, 1966.
7. Hardy, A. G., and Dickson, J. W.: Pathological Ossification in Traumatic Paraplegia. J. Bone Joint Surg., *45B:*76–87, 1963.
8. Kaplan, L. I., Grynbaum, B. B., Lloyd, K. E., and Rusk, H. A.: Pain and Spasticity in Patients with Spinal Cord Dysfunction. J.A.M.A., *182:*918–925, 1962.
9. Kennedy, H. C., and Hodges, C. V.: Urologic Problems in Spina Bifida. Trans. West. Sect. Amer. Urol. Ass., *23:*72–77; discussion, 78–80, 1956.
10. Long, C., II: Normal and Abnormal Motor Control in the Upper Extremities (Final Report SRS Grant RD 2377). Cleveland, Case Western Reserve University, 1970.
11. Long, C., II: Upper Limb Bracing. From Orthotics, Etc., edited by S. Licht. New Haven, Elizabeth Licht, Publisher, 1966.
12. Norton, P. L., and Foley, J. J.: Paraplegia in Children. J. Bone Joint Surg., *41A:*1291–1309, 1959.
13. Robertson, D. N. S., and Guttmann, L.: The Paraplegic Patient in Pregnancy and Labour. Proc. Roy. Soc. Med., *46:*381–387, 1963.
14. Sizemore, G. W., and Winternitz, W. W.: Autonomic Hyperreflexia—Suppression with Alpha-Adrenergic Blocking Agents. New Eng. J. Med., *282:*795, 1970.
15. Symington, D. C., and Mackay, D. E.: A Study of Functional Independence in the Quadriplegic Patients. Arch. Phys. Med., *47:*378–392, 1966.

Chapter 26

AFTERCARE OF
FRACTURES

by Miland E. Knapp

Problems in the aftercare of fractures may arise from bony causes, soft tissue injuries and edema. Bony causes, such as malunion, delayed union or nonunion, will not be discussed in this chapter since they do not properly come under the heading of physical medicine. Soft tissue injuries, including lacerations of nerves, tears of ligaments and joint capsules and injuries to tendons and muscles, also will not be discussed in this chapter since they require definitive treatment, often surgical in nature, and although physical measures are commonly useful in their treatment, most of these measures will be discussed under other headings. Persistent edema, in my opinion, is the most common cause of disability following fractures. This problem will be discussed in detail.

Traumatic edema fluid is produced either by the original injury or by mechanical factors following the injury. Extravasation of blood into the soft tissues is a constant accompaniment of fracture. In addition to this, extravasation of edema fluid into the soft tissues may result in so much swelling and interference with normal blood supply that extensive blisters may form, covering sometimes the entire extremity. The extravasated blood and edema fluid must be removed by one of two methods. If return flow circulation is restored adequately and early, both the blood and edema fluid may be removed by absorption into the general body circulation with no undesirable residual effects.

If, on the other hand, the swelling persists longer than a week or two, the swelling may be removed by organization instead of absorption, with the eventual production of fibrous scar tissue. This process is similar to and

579

proceeds at the same time as the organization which results in the production of fibrous callus in the process of normal bone healing. It is desirable that fibrous tissue develop between the bone ends since this is the first stage of fixation of the fracture. However, it is not desirable for fibrosis to occur in muscles or between such solid structures as tendon, joint capsule, bone and strong fascial layers since these parts are normally movable and the fibrosis limits movement.

"Oedema is glue," says Watson-Jones. Since the fibrous tissue produced between the bone ends and within the soft tissues is developed at exactly the same time, it is obvious one cannot wait for the bone to heal before treating the soft tissue damage. There are two apparently antagonistic objectives to be obtained simultaneously. First, the bone ends must be held immobile and in constant apposition until healing occurs. Second, the soft tissues must be kept moving to prevent fibrosis and subsequent limited painful motion. However, the objectives are really not as antagonistic as it might appear since pressure tends to promote bone healing and activity increases circulation to the part and this, too, aids in bone healing. It is necessary at the time of reduction to ascertain that the apparatus that maintains immobility of the bone ends is so arranged that maximal activity of soft tissues can be obtained starting immediately after the reduction of the fracture.

The aftercare of fractures may be divided into early and late stages.

TREATMENT IN THE EARLY STAGE

Active Motion.   The most effective, as well as the most available and the least expensive, method of removing edema fluid is active motion. However, in order that this may be accomplished the surgeon must trim the cast to allow function or apply the retaining apparatus in such a manner that maximal function is possible. For instance, if function of the metacarpophalangeal joints of the hand is to be retained, it is necessary that the immobilizing apparatus not extend distal to the flexion crease of the palm.

Active motion is effective in removing edema fluid because it assists return flow circulation. Normal return flow circulation is carried on to a large degree by muscle activity. The veins are provided with valves which will not allow the blood to flow distally so that when the muscle squeezes down on the vein, blood is forced proximally. The blood cannot return through the valve so the area fills up from below and blood is again ready to be forced back toward the heart. This same mechanism is present in the lymphatics.

Elevation.   If it is not feasible to remove the edema fluid by active motion, the next best method is elevation. However, it must be remembered that for elevation to be effective the distal part of the extremity must be above the proximal and the proximal part above the heart. This is a practical method in fractures of the lower extremity when the patient is in bed. Under these circumstances, elevation can be accomplished fairly easily. In the upper extremity, however, elevation is not usually practical because the hand would have to be up in a position above the elbow and the elbow above the shoulder. In fractures of the upper extremity the patient is not ordinarily put to bed so this method is not available. The use of a sling is not elevation because the hand and forearm in a sling are below the shoulder by the length of the arm.

Physical Therapy.   If neither of these methods is feasible or effective, treatment must be given by what is ordinarily designated as physical therapy. The usual procedures are heat, massage and motion.

HEAT. The physiologic effects of heat may be summarized briefly as relief of pain, increase in the arterial blood supply, increased edema because of the increased capillary pressure produced and softening of fibrous tissue.

The type of heat used is not usually important. Hot packs or hot soaks are quite convenient, as is infrared radiation. In a department of physical medicine whirlpool baths or similar methods of heat application are usually used. Diathermy is not advisable in the early stages following fractures because, as a result of its greater effectiveness, it often causes increased pain by increasing edema. Heat should always be followed by massage or exercise.

MASSAGE. The physiologic effects of massage are relief of pain if the massage is given efficiently and expertly, increase of venous circulation because the stroke of the massage is toward the heart, reduction of swelling as a result of the enhanced return flow circulation and stretching of fibrous tissue (see Chapter 15).

The massage should be mild so that pain is relieved instead of increased but it should be firm enough to give good edema reduction. Violent manipulation or painful types of massage should be avoided because of the possibility of displacing fragments before healing has occurred.

EXERCISE. If possible, massage should be followed by active exercise. If it is necessary to remove the supporting apparatus for exercise, the therapist should assist the patient in carrying out the exercise motion, either by overcoming gravity for him or by supporting a part of his body while the exercise is being performed. Passive motion should never be used in the early stage after fracture because fear of pain may cause the patient to resist any passive motion and the so-called passive motion is transformed into resistive motion with the patient doing the resisting. Assisted active exercise is the exercise of choice in early fractures.

To summarize, during the period of immobilization of the fracture, physical treatment is used to reduce swelling as soon as possible and to maintain range of joint motion, muscular strength and dexterity.

TREATMENT IN THE LATE STAGE

If the removal of edema fluid is delayed until the bone is healed, soft tissue adhesions will have become firmly established and may be solid enough to limit motion as well as cause pain. Unfortunately it is common practice to refer patients for physical therapy two months or more after the original injury, when fibrosis and contractures, painful motion, muscle atrophy and weakness, and persistent brawny edema make the danger of permanent impairment of function obvious. Treatment at this time is entirely different from treatment in the early stage. Now the objectives of treatment are: to remove whatever edema is still present, to soften and stretch fibrous tissue, to increase the range of joint motion, to restore circulatory efficiency, to increase muscular strength and to retrain muscular dexterity.

HEAT. Heat may be used for sedation, to increase circulation and to soften fibrous adhesions. The type of heat used is not extremely important and depends more upon the availability of the modality and the pathologic conditions present in the patient than on any specific properties of the various methods of heat application. In my experience, relaxation is best obtained by the use of moist heat. The whirlpool bath is valuable because heat, massage and active motion are possible simultaneously in it. Hot packs are often useful, particularly for areas that cannot be treated easily in the whirlpool. Diathermy and shortwave diathermy may be used. Infrared radiation is not as effective in the late stage as it is during the early stages.

MASSAGE.   Again, the heat is followed by massage with emphasis upon deep stroking and compression movements in order to stretch the fibrous adhesions as well as to get rid of any edema that may still be present. This treatment may be considerably more vigorous than that used during the early stage. Tender areas are made less tender by massage. The intramuscular movement produced by the kneading and friction motions helps to stretch adhesions so that a greater range of motion is possible.

EXERCISE.   Heat and massage should always be followed by exercise. The most effective regimen begins with assisted active exercise followed by free motion and then resistive exercise as the patient improves. Forced stretching of fibrous bands may be necessary in order to obtain maximal range of motion. It may be done manually or by prolonged stretch using a weight over a period of a half hour or more (see Chapter 16).

Manipulation under anesthesia should be used only if no other method is effective and then should be considered very carefully because of the danger of increasing the disability. If this method is used, it must be followed immediately by physical measures designed to overcome the pain and maintain the range of motion obtained by the manipulation. As the patient gains in range of motion and strength and as pain is decreased, occupational therapy becomes particularly useful because the patient's interest in the object he is making encourages prolonged effort (see Chapter 22). Projects may be chosen to increase range of motion, strength or coordination and manual dexterity. When the exercise is to be continued for months, the projects should be suitable for home use after discharge from the hospital.

SPECIAL PROBLEMS

A few special problems seem worth discussing in some detail because physical treatment may prevent serious complications if the condition is recognized before irreversible changes have occurred.

Myositis Ossificans

During the healing process, calcification may occur in the soft tissues as well as around the bone. Frequently it follows hemorrhage into the muscle or a hematoma in the tissue spaces. The patient usually complains of pain and limited motion. Examination shows palpable localized induration, which may be deep in the tissues. X-ray examination reveals calcification diffusely in the muscle or localized to fascial planes. Continuous hyperemia will assist absorption into the circulation, and the calcification will often disappear without surgical removal.

I have used the following technique: The involved part is wrapped in a bath blanket or other insulating material to prevent heat loss. Gauze bandage holds it in place. Short-wave diathermy is then applied to the part as frequently as is convenient. The insulating padding remains in place between treatments to maintain the hyperemia. The diathermy may be applied for a half hour every two hours, all day, if the patient is hospitalized. If he is an out-patient, it should be repeated at least twice daily for an hour at a time. This treatment must be continued consistently for at least a month. A follow-up x-ray may show beginning absorption at that time, but two or more months of treatment is usually needed. During the treatment period, unusual exercise and stretching of the contracted muscle is prohibited because trauma may further injure the muscle and increase the calcification. When the calcium has nearly disappeared from the muscle itself and the range of motion is approaching normal, treatment may be discontinued. Calcification remaining in the fascial planes is of no clinical significance.

Atrophy

Atrophy of Disuse. This form of atrophy follows any prolonged immobilization and involves not only the bone but the muscle as well. X-ray examination may show marked loss of bone density. Heat is often useful in relieving pain and in softening tissues to overcome contractures, but active exercise is the essential treatment. Roentgenograms should not be used to gauge improvement because recalcification is extremely slow and the patient will be clinically normal long before the x-ray becomes normal.

Reflex Sympathetic Dystrophy. This may follow minor fractures. Sudeck's acute post-traumatic bone atrophy, the shoulder-hand syndrome and causalgia are common examples of reflex sympathetic dystrophy. X-rays often show marked bone atrophy with a patchy distribution. It is important to recognize these causes of pain and disability because relief may be greatly accelerated by blocking, with local anesthetics, the sympathetic ganglia supplying the area. Such blocking should be done in addition to the usual physical treatment, as early as the diagnosis can be made, because results improve with early treatment. In these dystrophies hyperemia is present, as evidenced by swelling, redness of the skin and bone atrophy. Therefore, heat is not usually beneficial. If heat is desired to relieve pain, it should be used cautiously and if the pain is not relieved or is increased, as is common, the heat should be discontinued. The essential part of the physical treatment is active exercise. Increase in strength and decrease in atrophy results, even though active motion may be painful at first.

Volkmann's Contracture

Volkmann's ischemic contracture requires immediate recognition and treatment to prevent severe disability. It usually follows a supracondylar fracture of the humerus but may also follow fracture of both bones of the forearm. Arteriospasm or rupture of blood vessels causes swelling, which compresses the muscles and nerves within the fascial sheath. Necrosis of muscles, of nerves or even of bone and cartilage may result. The fibrosis produced during healing shortens the muscles on the flexor surface of the forearm, so the fingers contract down into the palm and become nonfunctional. Immediate emergency treatment to relieve pressure or repair arterial injury is imperative. This is a real emergency because even a few hours of delay may result in irreparable damage. When a patient with a forearm or elbow injury complains of pain, sedatives should not be given until the physician has examined the extremity to be sure that this condition is not developing.

If adequate treatment is delayed too long, developing contractures may be prevented or reduced by physical treatment started as early as possible and continued intensively until maximal improvement is obtained. Whirlpool bath followed by massage plus interrupted direct current stimulation to the paralyzed muscles should be started at once. A pancake splint with a malleable wrist section may be adjusted to maintain the length of the flexor muscles as it increases with intensive treatment. The treatment should continue for at least six months to a year. In some cases where severe damage has occurred, reparative or cosmetic surgery may be needed.

Shoulder Dislocation

Following shoulder dislocation, even though the dislocation is satisfactorily reduced, disability may result.

1. Scapulo-humeral contracture may limit motion. Treatment consists of heat, massage and scapulo-humeral motion.

2. The axillary nerve may be injured by pressure of the humeral head as it slips into the axilla. Its motor fibers supply the deltoid and teres minor muscles only, while its sensory distribution is to a variable but small area near and slightly posterior to the deltoid insertion. Nerve damage is often unrecognized because the symptoms are masked by a Velpeau bandage or similar retaining apparatus. Removal of the bandage a month or so later reveals that the patient cannot abduct his arm. Then physical therapy is prescribed. The true nature of the injury can be identified by merely stimulating the deltoid muscle with a tetanizing current. If the tetanizing current produces muscle contraction the nerve is intact. If the muscle does not respond to the tetanizing current, even though some voluntary motion may be present, nerve damage has occurred and the muscle should be treated to prevent fibrosis and limitation of motion.

Treatment consists of interrupted negative direct current stimulation in addition to heat, massage and scapulo-humeral motion. When good voluntary function has returned, the electric stimulation can be discontinued and active exercise prescribed to develop maximal strength.

3. Loss of function at the shoulder joint may also result from rupture of the short rotator tendons. In this case, the head of the humerus, which is normally held in place by the short rotator cuff during abduction, rides upward and strikes the acromion, which limits abduction. In complete rupture, the only effective treatment is surgical suture. In partial rupture, immobilization in an abducted position and cautious maintenance of range of motion may be adequate to maintain function while the tendon heals.

Hip Fracture

Hip fractures present special problems requiring careful treatment. Intertrochanteric fractures usually heal satisfactorily in about four months because the blood supply is adequate. Open operation with internal fixation secures accurate reduction and maintains contact. However, one must realize that the internal fixation is not intended to support weight bearing. Many older persons will not walk between parallel bars or on crutches without putting the injured foot to the ground. The plate may break or screws may loosen with weight bearing. Therefore, if the patient cannot be taught to walk without bearing weight on the fractured extremity, he should not be allowed to try independent ambulation until the bone has healed sufficiently to support his weight.

In intracapsular fractures, non-union is frequent because the major portion of the blood supply comes through the neck of the femur. Since this is broken, the femoral neck and head may not receive an adequate blood supply. Non-union is common and aseptic necrosis may supervene even when union is solid. Again, weight bearing should not be allowed until healing has occurred, and this may take six months. Therefore, the patient must be taught to walk with crutches or a walkerette with a three point type of gait. It is important to maintain range of motion and strength in both types of fracture. Treatment by whirlpool bath or Hubbard tank, followed by range of motion exercise is helpful and active exercise should be started as early as possible. Gait training in the parallel bars and graduating to underarm crutches should start as soon as the patient can be trusted to keep his weight off the injured extremity.

REFERENCES

1. Knapp, M. E.: Treatment of Fracture Sequelae. J. Lancet, 79:106-112, 1959.
2. Knapp, M. E.: Physical Medicine in the Treatment of Fractures. (Panel Discussion, American Medical Association, Atlantic City, N.J., June 12, 1947.) J.A.M.A., 137:136-139, 1948.
3. Knapp, M. E.: Physical Therapy in Fractures About Elbow Joint. (Read at Annual Session at Cleveland, Ohio, Sept. 3, 1940.) Arch. Phys. Therapy, 21:709-715, 1940.
4. Knapp, M. E.: Role of Physical Therapy in Fractures. (Read at American Congress of Physical Therapy, New York, Sept. 8, 1939.) Arch. Phys. Therapy, 21:401-407, 1940.
5. Watson-Jones, R.: Fractures and Other Bone and Joint Injuries. 2nd Ed. Baltimore, The Williams and Wilkins Co., 1941, p. 48.

Chapter 27

MANAGEMENT OF MOTOR UNIT DISEASES

by Ernest W. Johnson

Definitions

Motor unit diseases include those conditions affecting the anterior horn cell, its axon, the myoneural junction and muscle fibers.

Anterior Horn Cell. Examples of diseases that affect the anterior horn cell include acute anterior poliomyelitis, amyotrophic lateral sclerosis (progressive spinomuscular atrophy), Werdnig-Hoffmann disease and myelitis.

Axon. Conditions that affect the axon are peripheral nerve injuries, Guillain-Barré syndrome (idiopathic polyneuritis), toxic neuropathies, diabetic neuropathy, Charcot-Marie-Tooth disease and other heredofamilial peripheral neuropathies.

Myoneural Junction. Myasthenia gravis and myasthenic syndrome in small cell carcinoma of the lungs affect the myoneural junction.

Muscle Fiber (and Cell Membrane). Diseases that affect muscle fibers include progressive muscular dystrophy (Duchenne type), restrictive muscular dystrophy (fascio-scapulohumeral), myotonic dystrophy, polymyositis (dermatomyositis), metabolic myopathy (e.g., thyrotoxic) and hypokalemic and hyperkalemic myopathies.

586

Management

In a majority of motor unit diseases there is no specific treatment to effect a cure. The ideal approach would be prevention—vaccination for virus diseases, education to prevent toxic polyneuropathies, genetic counseling for hereditary diseases and such measures as desensitization for allergic diseases. Therefore, the treatment is directed largely toward symptoms that appear during the course of the disease.

Pain.   In acute poliomyelitis, polyneuritis or polymositis, pain may be a significant symptom. Physical treatment includes the application of various types of heat and massage.

Tightness.   Soft tissue shortening may be present at all stages in motor unit disease. Figure 27-1 shows the most common areas of soft tissue tightness. Physical treatment includes passive, active and active assistive stretching, usually after the application of heat. Positioning and bracing also are physical procedures used to prevent or alleviate tightness.

Weakness.   Weakness is present in all motor unit disease. It may be localized, asymmetric or generalized. Physical treatment includes reeducation, exercises (progressing to strengthening exercises) and, if needed, assistive bracing to compensate for weakness later in the course of the disease.

Deformity.   Malalignment of body segments represents a negative aspect of general management. Efforts to prevent malalignments are primary and correction if they occur is secondary. Malalignments are prevented by positioning, selective stretching and bracing. They are corrected by surgical procedures and occasionally by mechanical stretching with wedging casts and special bracing. Careful repeated observation is necessary to identify early deformities.

Functional Ability.   Translation of specific motor and sensory function into complicated and practical results is the essence of functional ability. Examples include walking, dressing and eating. Assistive devices, substitutive training and such surgical procedures as transplant and arthrodesis represent symptomatic management.

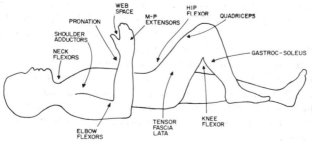

Figure 27–1   Diagram showing the most frequent areas of soft tissue tightness in prolonged immobilization or neuromuscular conditions.

Prognostic Categories

Symptomatic management is modified to relate to the expected prognosis. Motor unit diseases may be divided into four categories with respect to prognosis.

Progressive Conditions.   In progressive conditions the primary pathologic lesions worsen at various rates. Amyotrophic lateral sclerosis, which is fatal in three to five years, is rapidly progressive; progressive muscular dystrophy (Duchenne), which is fatal in 15 to 20 years, shows intermediate progression; and Charcot-Marie-Tooth disease (not fatal but causes progressive disability) progresses slowly.

Static Conditions.   Static conditions are those whose specific pathologic lesion occurs usually as a single insult leaving permanent deficit. Acute anterior paralytic poliomyelitis and severe peripheral nerve injury are examples.

Transient Conditions.   Conditions whose effects regress with complete, or nearly complete, recovery after specific tissue injury or disease or for which specific treatment is available for control or alleviation are called transient. Examples are Guillain-Barré syndrome (acute idiopathic polyneuritis), thyrotoxic myopathy and often, myasthenia gravis.

Miscellaneous Conditions.   There are some motor unit diseases, e.g., polymyositis, whose course is highly variable. Polymyositis (dermatomyositis) may regress with almost complete disappearance, it may become arrested at any stage, leaving residuals or it may be progressively fatal.

A distinction must be made between truly progressive diseases and those which apparently progress, by onset or worsening of secondary deformities. Individuals may lose functional abilities by becoming obese or children may seem to regress as they grow larger or reach a plateau in motor development. Motor unit disease in growing children is more likely to produce deformities whether the condition is progressive or static.

Deformities resulting from asymmetric tightness of an iliotibial band (tensor fasciae latae) are scoliosis (type I according to Bennett's classification[2]); pelvic tilt; subluxation of the opposite hip; flexion contracture, internal rotation deformity, abduction contracture and internal rotation of the hip; abduction and external torsion of the tibia; and supination deformity of the foot.

Adverse reactions to physical treatment in motor unit diseases may include burns from hot packs or other heating agents, soft tissue tearing with calcification, fractures of osteoporotic bones or weakness from overwork. Early unsupervised activities and substitutive movement may result in incoordination and asymmetric strengthening or ill advised ambulation may aggravate deformities. Overbracing may cause retardation or limitation of functional ability. Adverse psychologic reactions may occur; for example, depression when unobtainable goals are presented.

PROGRESSIVE MOTOR UNIT DISEASES

Amyotrophic Lateral Sclerosis

Physical Treatment. Treatment measures should anticipate progression. Minimal bracing and ambulation aids are helpful for prolonged and safe ambulation. To prolong ambulation efforts, the patient should be taught how to fall safely. Positioning and therapeutic exercise are prescribed to prevent deformities. Early in the course of the disease this will maintain ambulation and functional ability and later it will facilitate nursing care.

Medical Treatment. When there are bulbar symptoms and a prognosis of continuation for more than several months, a gastrostomy and tracheostomy are helpful. If there is a short-term prognosis, intramuscular injection of Prostigmin (1 cc. of a 1:1000 dilution) 30 minutes before eating may temporarily facilitate swallowing. Fasciculations will be intensified, however.

A home suctioning device is often necessary. Mechanical respiratory aid may be needed terminally. Home management is very possible even in the terminal stages with an understanding family. It is important to keep an enthusiastic attitude in dealing with the patient.

Progressive Muscular Dystrophy

This disease is characterized by an insidious onset of weakness and tightness.

Physical Treatment. Vigorous flexibility exercises should be begun early. Contractures occur early and are severe probably because the muscle itself is the site of the pathologic lesion. Tightness occurs early in the gastrocnemius-soleus groups, iliotibial band, hip flexors and hamstrings in the lower extremities. Weakness occurs first in the gluteus maximus, then in the abdominal muscles, foot dorsiflexors, neck flexors, lower pectorals; then in the quadriceps and deltoids.

Each patient should be examined for tightness and an individual home program should be prescribed. It is desirable to have a rather intensive and repeated home instruction period with the parents doing the exercises under the supervision of the therapist. In the upper extremity and the forearm pronators, wrist and finger flexors often are tight areas (Figs. 27–2 and 27–3).

Strengthening exercises are of unproven value and may even accelerate the degenerative process.[10] Functional training is often helpful, particularly as the patient moves from independent ambulation to assisted ambulation and then wheelchair ambulation.

Bracing and ambulation aids should be minimal since this is a generalized disease with the individual performing at his maximal energy expenditure. Gowers[6] in 1902 pointed out that deformities are the principal reason for early loss of ambulation in muscular dystrophy. If the patient is falling several times each day, long leg braces to stabilize the knees may prolong limited but functional ambulation for several years.

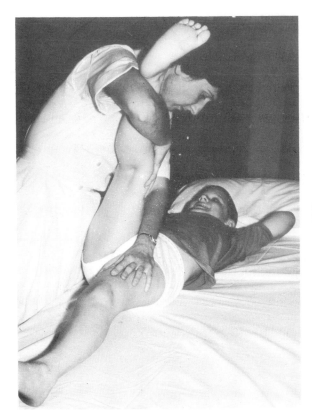

Figure 27–2 Stretching the hamstring muscles in a patient with Duchenne muscular dystrophy.

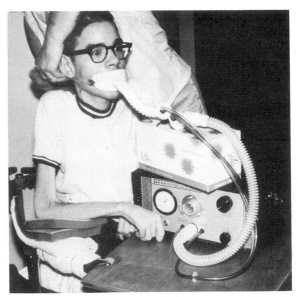

Figure 27–3 Parent applying intermittent positive pressure breathing device to her son with advanced Duchenne muscular dystrophy.

Medical Management.   Special attention should be given to respiratory infections. Patients with progressive muscular dystrophy usually die of pneumonia or cardiac failure. Patients should be vaccinated against all diseases possible. They should *not* be put to bed for minor illness but kept ambulatory. Home management in the late stages should include the use of a hand resuscitator for assistance in coughing and periodic pulmonary thoracic stretch. Dietary management includes gradual restriction of caloric intake, since the gradual loss of muscle bulk, and thus activity, predisposes to obesity.

Surgical Management.   Selective surgical release of tightness that resists conservative management may prolong and facilitate functional abilities, but rapid convalescence is imperative.

For early inversion instability of the foot, transplantation of the posterior tibial tendon to the lateral dorsum of the foot is indicated. A walking cast must be provided.

Lengthening of the Achilles tendon may be a disastrous procedure unless bracing is provided, since the tight soleus can provide knee stability during the stance phase of gait.

Surgical release of the iliotibial tract is often quite helpful in prolonging ambulation, since the tight tensor fosters knee instability as the patient increases his lumbar lordosis to stabilize the hip.

Surgical correction of severe scoliosis and the equinovarus foot deformities in the nonambulatory patient is of questionable value and the author prefers to use it sparingly at this stage. Surgical relief is primarily for cosmetic reasons.

General Management.   In this type of muscular dystrophy, which follows an x-linked recessive genetic pattern, counseling the parents is a necessity. Fewer than one half of the patients will have a family history of progressive muscular dystrophy, since this gene has an extremely high rate of mutation. Estimates suggest one mutation per 10,000 genes. When the mother has been identified as a carrier by the appearance of an affected son, her daughters are suspected of being carriers (one half will be). All parents of patients are urged to have their names put on the mailing list of the Muscular Dystrophy Association of America so that the newsletter will provide a means for keeping up with the latest facts. This contact with a reliable source of information is often a deterrent to "doctor shopping" and frustrating trips for "miracle cures" at the urging of well-meaning friends and relatives.

Empathetic attitudes and forthright advice may lessen the fears and frustrations that are inevitable. Periodic checks by a physician conversant with physical management should be done as needed, usually every three to four months. Attendance at regular school as long as possible is recommended.

STATIC MOTOR UNIT DISEASES

Acute Anterior Paralytic Poliomyelitis

Recent literature is replete with excellent descriptions of the proper management of this entity. Prevention by the Salk vaccine (formalin-killed virus) and more recently the Sabin vaccine (attenuated live virus) is now widely accepted.

Physical Management

EARLY STAGE.   Management is based on the three clinical manifestations in the early phase (the first six weeks) of the disease. For *muscle pain* hot moist packs (Kenny) are applied three or four times daily in mild to moderate cases or continuously in severely involved patients.

Muscle tightness in the early stage may represent altered physiology at the internuncial pool; later soft tissue tightness probably involves fascial tightness. Early proper positioning and passive exercises following applications of hot packs are indicated.

Asymmetric *muscle weakness* is the cardinal sign of poliomyelitis. In the early stage, weakened segments are protected by positioning; later, selective reeducation and strengthening exercises are begun while protection is continued with bracing and limited activity.

INTERMEDIATE STAGE.   Various authorities support different views about management in the intermediate stage (six weeks to six months). The author prefers to separate the growing child from the adult at this stage.

In the growing child the muscles are selectively reeducated in stretching to insure maximal function of weakened body segments to minimize deformity. Limited activities, especially in the upright position, and limited ambulation are necessary. Precise support with bracing and careful observation are essential. Substitutive patterns are allowed in the child after six months if they do not appear to contribute to deformity.

In adults substitutive patterns are permitted early as a compromise for increasing functional ability.

LATE STAGE.   Beyond six months of ideal management a clear estimation of the probable functional ability and potential sources of deformity is usually possible. The spine of the growing child should be checked radiographically at least yearly and more often during periods of rapid growth. Adults need periodic observation for orthetic adjustment and for detection of possible loss of function due to overwork.

There are several general rules of physical treatment. Active exercise should be deferred until the pain is relieved and selective strengthening should be deferred if there is a signficant tightness of the muscle group. Progressive resistive exercises and functional training unavoidably encourage substitutive patterns. Development of substitutive patterns usually inhibits activation of the prime movers; for example, the anterior tibial may drop out of the pattern of dorsiflexion if walking is initiated before this muscle is able to carry out its action. Asymmetric strengthening should be avoided because it may aggravate or initiate scoliosis. Overwork can cause further weakness in specific muscle groups. Tightness should be retained if it is symmetric and if weakness is present; for example, back extension tightness in the presence of severe weakness of back extensors.

Orthetic devices are used to prevent deformity (e.g., Hoke corset), to provide support (e.g., long leg brace), to protect a weakened muscle group (e.g., opponens splint) or to increase function (e.g., reacher-feeder).

Medical Management.   In the respiratory system it is important to recognize and treat reduced ventilation *early.* Having the patient count slowly and loudly will permit an adequate clinical estimation of the ventilation reserved. The number of counts is multiplied by 100 cc. to estimate the vital capacity. The patient should have mechanical respiratory aid if the vital capacity drops below 50 per cent or if it is dropping rapidly even if above 50 per cent. While the patient is in the respirator, coughing and periodic deep breathing will reduce the episodes of atelectasis and pneumonitis.

Swallowing difficulties require meticulous nursing care especially in the acute stage. If the patient is in a respirator a tracheostomy is usually indicated if there is pharyngeal muscle weakness. Tracheostomy is also indicated in vocal cord abductor muscle paralysis since the airway is compromised.

Early urinary retention is common; catheterization should be avoided if at all possible. Adequate urinary output is 1.5 liters per square meter of body surface per 24 hours. This will minimize urinary calculi and infection.

In the acute stage with encephalitis it is important to observe carefully for possible Cushing ulcer with gastrointestinal bleeding. In the convalescent stage constipation is often a problem. Severe muscle weakness and atrophy results in a loss of potassium stores which predisposes to episodes of paralytic ileus. This is a most common reason for an "acute" distention of the abdomen in severely involved polio patients.

Hypertension in the acute phase is usually secondary to hypoxia but it may be due to bulbar involvement. Bulbar involvement may also result in hypotension.

Surgical Management. In the acute stage tracheostomy may be necessary. In the intermediate stage surgical procedures are used for the release of soft tissue or urinary calculi removal. Tendon transfers and arthrodesis to improve function or correct deformity are done in the late stage.

General Management. Attendance at regular school is recommended whenever possible for children. A conference with the teacher to discuss positioning and modification of activities is usually necessary. A forthright but encouraging attitude on the part of the attending physician is essential for both the parents' and the child's well-being. Adult patients' questions regarding prognosis should be answered honestly with encouragement. Early vocational planning is imperative and the patient's emotional need should be identified and met at appropriate stages of his rehabilitation.

TRANSIENT MOTOR UNIT DISEASES

Guillain-Barré Syndrome (Acute Idiopathic Polyneuritis)

Full recovery is expected although some patients die because of respiratory failure and a few have residual weakness. In the author's experience this permanent weakness has usually resulted from prolonged periods of hypoxia during the acute phase.

Pain is treated as in poliomyelitis. Tightness is prevented and corrected by positioning and early stretching. Weakness is usually reversible over a period of two months to as long as two years. If the onset is acute, ordinarily the recovery is more rapid. An insidious onset may foretell improvement over a period of a year or two, and some patients may never regain full strength. Strengthening exercises and exhaustive activities may aggravate the weakness or result in a relapse.

Temporay ambulation aids include wrapping the foot early with an Ace bandage for dorsiflexion support, temporary splints at the knee and a light spring wire brace later for footdrop if needed. Ambulation is begun in the parallel bars, proceeding to underarm crutches, forearm crutches, canes and then no aid as progress continues. Temporary upper extremity aids include the reacher-feeder and other shoulder abductor supports and hand splints.

Pressure ulcerations are frequent complications in this condition, especially if the patient is in the respirator. Ventilation insufficiency should receive early mechanical aid as in acute poliomyelitis.

Myasthenia gravis, metabolic myopathy and similar reversible conditions ordinarily do not need physical treatment except for ambulation aids during the period of weakness and functional training in safe ambulation.

MISCELLANEOUS MOTOR UNIT DISEASES

Included in this category are motor unit diseases that may progress, become arrested or improve. Polymyositis (dermatomyositis) is a classic example. It appears to be a primary inflammatory disease of the muscle fiber.

Physical treatment is based on the following three principles: Maintaining flexibility, minimizing pain by application of heat (hot tub baths or home baker) and use of minimal bracing or ambulation aids if needed.

In medical management, some authorities feel that high doses of steroids are helpful during an exacerbation or an acute onset.

SUMMARY

The aim in management of progressive motor unit diseases is to prolong functional abilities; in static diseases, to protect from deformity and increase functional ability (Fig. 27-4 *A* and *B*); and in transient diseases, to maintain flexibility and anticipate return of function.

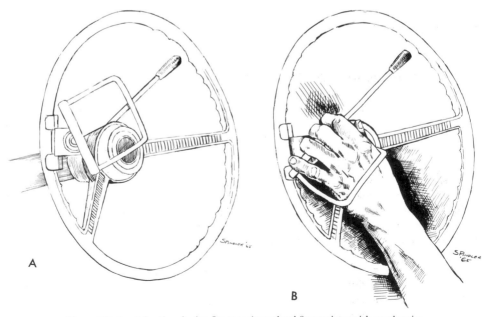

A

B

Figure 27-4   Adaptive device for steering wheel for patient with weak grip.

The key to management of motor unit diseases is *the maintenance of the patient's flexibility.*

REFERENCES

1. Archibald, K. C., and Vignos, P. J.: A Study of Contractures in Muscular Dystrophy. Arch. Phys. Med., *40*:150–157, 1959.
2. Bennett, R. L.: Evaluation of End Results of Acute Anterior Poliomyelitis. J.A.M.A., *162*:851-854, 1956.
3. Bennett, R. L.: Evaluation and Treatment of Lower Motor Unit Lesions Involving the Shoulder, Arm, Forearm and Hand. Arch. Phys. Med., *41*:54-61, 1960.
4. Bennett, R. L.: Use and Abuse of Certain Tools of Physical Medicine. Arch. Phys. Med., *41*:485-496, 1960.
5. Bosma, J. F.: Significance of the Pharynx in Rehabilitation of Poliomyelitis Disabilities in Cervical Area. Arch. Phys. Med., *38*:363-368, 1957.
6. Gowers, W. R.: Myopathy and a Distal Form. J.A.M.A., *2*:89-92, 1902.
7. Hoberman, M.: Physical Medicine and Rehabilitation: Its Value and Limitations in Progressive Muscular Dystrophy. *34*:109-117, 1955.
8. Jebsen, R. H., Johnson, E. W., Knobloch, H., and Grant, D. K.: Differential Diagnosis of Infantile Hypotonia. A.M.A. J. Dis. Child., *101*:8-17, 1961.
9. Johnson, E. W.: Examination for Muscle Weakness in Infants and Small Children. J.A.M.A., *168*:1306-1313, 1958.
10. Johnson, E., and Braddom, R.: Overwork weakness in fascio-scapulohumeral muscular dystrophy. Arch. Phys. Med., In Press.
11. Knapp, M. E.: The Contribution of Sister Elizabeth Kenny to Treatment of Poliomyelitis. Arch. Phys. Med., *36*:510-517, 1955.
12. Knowlton, G. C.: Physiologic Background for Neuromuscular Re-education and Coordination. Arch. Phys. Med., *35*:635-638, 1954.
13. Lowenthal, M., and Tobis, J. S.: Contractures in Chronic Neurologic Disease. Arch. Phys. Med., *38*:640-645, 1957.
14. Pearson, C. M.: Serum Enzymes in Muscular Dystrophy and Certain Other Muscular and Neuromuscular Diseases. New Eng. J. Med., *256*:1069-1075, 1957.
15. Plum, F.: Prevention of Urinary Calculi after Paralytic Poliomyelitis. J.A.M.A. *168*:1302-1306, 1958.
16. Stevenson, A. C.: Muscular Dystrophy in Northern Ireland. Ann. Eugenics, *18*:50-93, 1953.
17. Swinyard, C. A., et al.: Gradients of Functional Ability of Importance in Rehabilitation of Patients with Progressive Muscular and Neuromuscular Diseases. Arch. Phys. Med., *38*:574-579, 1957.
18. Vallbona, C., and Spencer, W. A.: Systematic Classification of the Chronic Sequelae of Poliomyelitis. Arch. Phys. Med., *42*:114-121, 1961
19. Walton, J. N., and Nattrass, F. J.: On the Classification, Natural History and Treatment of Myopathies. Brain, *77*:169-231, 1954.

Chapter 28

CRANIAL NERVE PALSIES AND BRAIN STEM SYNDROMES

by Bernard Sandler

This discussion will include only those affections which commonly fall within the purview of the physiatrist. For a more complete picture the reader is referred to neurologic texts.[1-4] We shall also include those conditions which do not properly involve *only* the cranial nerves or brain stem. For example, amyotrophic lateral sclerosis involves cortical neurons, the corticobulbar tracts, cranial nerve nuclei, the corticospinal tracts and anterior horn cells. In these cases we shall emphasize diagnosis and treatment as they relate to the cranial nerves and brain stem.

DEFINITIONS

The term brain stem refers to the medulla oblongata, pons and midbrain; their cranial nerve nuclei; and the ascending and descending tracts passing through them.

Lesions affecting pathways between the cerebral cortex and brain stem are called *supranuclear;* lesions in the brain stem nuclei are *nuclear;* and lesions of the cranial nerves are *infranuclear.* A fourth category involves lesions of the ascending and descending tracts connecting the spinal cord and supranuclear structures.

596

THE CRANIAL NERVES

Cranial nerves I and II, the olfactory and the optic, respectively, are from an embryologic point of view not nerves at all but extensions of the brain. Occasionally the physiatrist will see a case of anosmia produced by an olfactory groove meningioma. Multiple sclerosis is the chief cause of optic nerve involvement. At times the physiatrist may see patients with optic nerve involvement caused by leukemia, syphilis, arteriosclerosis of the brain, gliomas, meningiomas, pituitary tumors, metastatic carcinoma, aneurysms or trauma.

The oculomotor, trochlear and abducens nerves and their nuclei may be involved as a result of trauma, multiple sclerosis, encephalitides, tumors, aneurysms, alcohol poisoning, syringobulbia, diphtheria, diabetes, meningitides, venous sinus thrombosis, poliomyelitis, vascular accidents in the brain stem and heavy metal poisoning. Because of its long course the abducens is especially subject to damage from increased intracranial pressure.

The trigeminal nerve may be affected by neoplasms, trauma, aneurysms, meningitides and polyneuritides. The sensory and motor nuclei are damaged by tumors, vascular lesions, syringobulbia, multiple sclerosis, encephalitides and amyotrophic lateral sclerosis.

The facial nerve may be injured by neoplasms, meningitides, Paget's disease, osteomyelitis, herpes zoster, ear infections, leukemia, polyneuritides, diphtheria, tetanus and leprosy. Trauma from gunshot or knife wounds and forceps delivery is not uncommon. Neuromas growing from the acoustic nerve may frequently involve the facial nerve. Bilateral facial palsies are most frequently seen in the Guillain-Barré syndrome, leprosy, leukemia, syphilis and meningococcal meningitis. The facial nucleus is involved in poliomyelitis, amyotrophic lateral sclerosis, vascular accidents and multiple sclerosis.

Bell's palsy is an infranuclear affection of the seventh nerve which is frequently seen by the physiatrist. It commonly follows exposure to cold. Presumably the paralysis is caused by edema of the nerve, which results in compression against the hard walls of the facial canal and ischemia. The eye cannot be made to close, nor the forehead to wrinkle. This paralysis of the upper facial musculature distinguishes the condition from central facial palsy seen in hemiplegic patients (Fig. 28–1). Alter[5] believes there is a tendency for

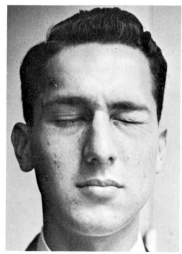

Figure 28–1   Right peripheral facial palsy (incomplete). (Courtesy of Dr. A. Ornsteen, Philadelphia.)

Bell's palsy to occur in family members because of inherited traits such as a narrow facial canal or a small stylomastoid foramen.

A conservative regimen of treatment consists of superficial heat and sympatholytic agents to increase blood supply, reduction of edema by use of steroids, maintenance of muscle tone by massage and electrical stimulation and muscle reeducation through exercise when voluntary function returns.[6] Taverner et al.[17] claim a marked decrease in severe denervation of the facial nerve in patients treated with ACTH gel intramuscularly when oral corticosteroids fail.

Surgical intervention is a subject of controversy. Kettel[7] has suggested the following as criteria for intervention: (1) Palsy accompanied by severe pain from the onset behind the homolateral ear. (2) No sign of return of function in two months. (3) Cases of incomplete spontaneous recovery. (4) Relapsing palsies. The value of surgery is predicated on the hope that some nerve fibers not yet undergoing degeneration may be preserved.[18] If this is true, then prompt decompression on evidence of beginning degeneration seems indicated.

Anastomosis of the facial nerve with the phrenic, spinal accessory or hypoglossal nerves has been proposed in those cases in which there is little or no return of function in one year. Cosmetic procedures for support of sagging facial musculature by means of muscle slings or fascial strips have been helpful. Lagophthalmos has been improved by tarsorrhaphy.[6] Edgerton[19] believes that dynamic muscle transfers have great advantages over nerve anastomoses or static support with fascia lata, tendons, or synthetic material.

Prognosis can be made more accurate through the use of electromyographic techniques. If fibrillation potentials are discovered two to three weeks after onset, one may infer that axonal degeneration has taken place and that recovery will be delayed. On the other hand, absence of such potentials points to a simple neurapraxia with a good prognosis. Langworth and Taverner[8] point out that a loss of response to electrical stimulation of the nerve is a grave sign and that conduction latency above 4 milliseconds signifies partial denervation. More recent electrodiagnostic tests such as electrogustometry[20] and the facial nerve excitability measurement[21] give information concerning impending degeneration of nerve fibers earlier than is possible with electromyography, and may help decide whether surgical intervention is warranted.

Annoying complications and sequelae of Bell's palsy are: associated movements, contractures, lacrimation during eating (crocodile tears), gustatory sweating, parageusia and hemispasm.

Herpetic palsy (Hunt's syndrome) is characterized by severe pain in and behind the ear and a herpetic eruption on the tympanum and in the external auditory canal.

The acoustic nerve may be injured by salicylates, streptomycin, quinine and many other drugs. It is also involved by meningitides, cerebellopontine angle tumors and degenerative processes in the middle and inner ear. The nuclei are damaged by tumors, demyelinating disease, vascular lesions and inflammatory processes.

The glossopharyngeal nerve and its nucleus are rarely damaged by isolated lesions. Neoplasms and vascular lesions will usually involve neighboring nerves as well.

The vagus nerve is damaged by various neuritides, particularly the diphtheritic and "infectious" types. It may also be compressed by tumors or aneurysms. Lesions of the pharyngeal branch result in swallowing difficulty. Involvement of the recurrent laryngeal branch produces hoarseness and dysphonia. Superior laryngeal involvement is reflected in a weak voice. The nuclei of the

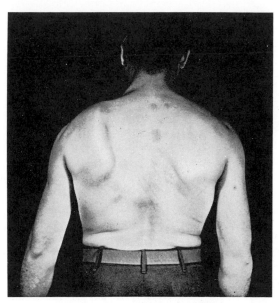

Figure 28–2 Trapezius palsy, left. The posterior triangle of the neck was penetrated by a bullet. Subsequently the patient became unable to shrug the left shoulder or to raise the left arm above the horizontal plane. The upper one half of the trapezius is atrophic. An attempt to abduct the arm leads to flaring of the vertebral border and to lateral displacement of the scapula. (From Haymaker, W., and Woodhall, B.: Peripheral Nerve Injuries, 2nd Ed., 1953.)

vagus are damaged by poliomyelitis, tumors, syringobulbia, vascular lesions, multiple sclerosis and amyotrophic lateral sclerosis.

The spinal accessory nerve is involved by neuritides, meningitides, extramedullary tumors and neck trauma. The nucleus is damaged by the same conditions that involve the vagus. It is important for diagnostic reasons to distinguish between trapezius palsy and palsy of the serratus anterior (Figs. 28-2 to 28-4).

The hypoglossal nerve may be affected by all the processes that involve the vagus and spinal accessory nerves. Injury to the nerve causes the tongue to deviate to the paralyzed side when it is protruded (Fig. 28-5). When the tongue lies in the mouth, however, it may deviate slightly toward the uninvolved side. Fasciculations are noted in amyotrophic lateral sclerosis and syringobulbia. In supranuclear lesions the tongue is little affected. It may deviate slightly to the paretic side on protrusion.

Guillain-Barré Syndrome

This polyradiculoneuropathy is described in another portion of the handbook. The condition is of concern to the physiatrist because it may require prolonged medical management. It has been said that it involves proximal muscles chiefly. However, Wiederholt et al.[9] point out that the distal musculature in arms and legs may be severely involved. The musculature supplied by the cranial nerves is also more often involved than is usually thought (Table 28-1).

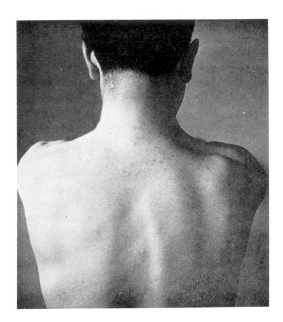

Figure 28–3 Trapezius palsy, right. Elevation of the arms in the forward plane of the body, i.e., flexion, causes lateral displacement of the scapula. Note atrophy of the superior third of the trapezius muscle and the firm approximation of the inferior angle of the scapula to the chest wall. (From Haymaker, W., and Woodhall, B.: Peripheral Nerve Injuries, 2nd Ed., 1953.)

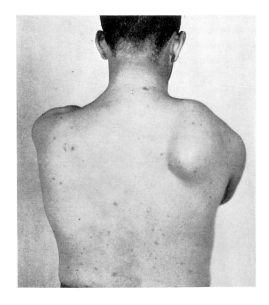

Figure 28–4 Winging of the scapula in serratus anterior palsy. When elevation of the arm is attempted the scapula becomes winged the moves upward and laterally. Abduction of the arm was not impaired. (From Haymaker, W., and Woodhall, B.: Peripheral Nerve Injuries, 2nd Ed., 1953.)

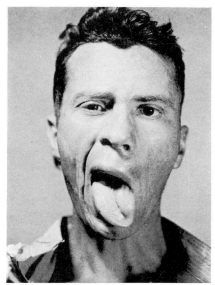

Figure 28–5 Atrophy and paralysis of the left side of the tongue due to missile wound of the left side of the neck, with missile entrance in the region of the mastoid process. The tip of the tongue deviates toward the paralyzed side. (From Haymaker, W.: Bing's Local Diagnosis in Neurological Diseases. St. Louis, The C. V. Mosby Co., 1956.)

Nerve conduction studies when done serially may accurately chart the recovery of the patient. Artificial respiration after elective tracheostomy should be considered immediately on development of bulbar signs. Steroids in the acute phase may be of help on theoretical grounds, but there is little statistical support for their use.[10] Postural hypotension is also seen.[11] It is postulated that there is involvement of the intermediolateral cell column and consequently damage to autonomic function. It is important to remember that positive pressure respiration may produce marked peripheral pooling in the absence of reflex venous constriction and thus aggravate the tendency toward hypotension.

TABLE 28–1 DISTRIBUTION OF MUSCLE WEAKNESS ON INITIAL EXAMINATION: 97 PATIENTS*

		INSTANCES
Weakness		
Both upper and lower extremity		88
Proximal and distal parts of both extremities affected	66	
Other combinations	16	
Neck		44
Facial muscles (subsequently 6 more)		28
Lower extremity (proximal and distal in 7, distal in 1)		8
Extraocular muscles		5
Upper extremity		2
Anal sphincter		2
Palate		1
Tongue		1
No weakness of upper or lower extremity		5

*From Wiederholt, W. C., Mulder, D. W., and Lambert, E. H.: The Landry-Guillain-Barré-Strohl Syndrome or Polyradiculoneurophaty: Historical Review, Report on 97 Patients, and Present Concepts. Proc. Mayo Clin., 39:427–451, 1964.

Poliomyelitis

Poliomyelitis is no longer the scourge of former years but still merits our attention as a cause of profound weakness. It has been estimated that approximately 15 per cent of the cases have involvement of the brain stem nuclei. The facial, palatal and pharyngeal muscles are most often involved but ocular and glossal muscles are also affected. Muscles of mastication are involved less often.[4]

Infantile Spinal Muscular Atrophy

This disease is one of several which affects infants and young children. It falls into the "floppy" infant category and may on occasion be confused with muscular dystrophy. Walton[12] discusses the infantile hypotonias under the headings of infantile spinal muscular atrophy, symptomatic hypotonia (which includes cerebral palsy and a host of metabolic disorders) and benign congenital hypotonia. The last category is far from clear at the present time. Such cases may on the one hand be formes frustes of Werdnig-Hoffmann disease, and on the other perhaps examples of universal muscular hypoplasia.[13]

Since some patients with infantile spinal muscular atrophy may reach adulthood,[14] it is important to be constantly vigilant against upper respiratory infection, the development of scoliosis and pulmonary insufficiency and the development of contractures. The disease is genetically determined and may afflict one in four children in any sibship.

Tetanus

The cephalic form of tetanus may cause severe involvement of cranial nerves. The cause has not been clearly elucidated, but it is thought that the toxin may act on both the neuromuscular junctions and cell bodies in the anterior horns and cranial nerve nuclei.[15] Trismus, spasm of the pharyngeal muscles and glottis and stiffness of the facial muscles are common findings. Cranial nerve palsies may develop. Aside from treatment with anti-tetanus serum, maintenance on artificial respiration is important. Muscle relaxation has been approached in various ways; curare, chlorpromazine and barbiturates are most commonly used.

Diphtheria

Diphtheritic neuropathy has some interesting characteristics. It tends to come on slowly—perhaps three weeks after infection—and involves many cranial nerves. Palatal weakness and faulty accommodation due to involvement of the ciliary muscle usually are seen first. This is followed by paralysis of the pharyngeal, facial and external ocular muscles. Palatal and ciliary involvement distinguish it from the Guillain-Barré syndrome.

Multiple Sclerosis

All sorts of combinations of brain stem involvement are possible in this disease. The clinical picture depends on the random location of the plaques. In the terminal stage bulbar palsy may be total.

Amyotrophic Lateral Sclerosis

This disease has a so-called bulbar form which may involve chiefly the bulbar nuclei. It is usually fatal in three to five years and in the terminal stages requires respiratory support and nursing care.

BRAIN STEM SYNDROMES

Basilar Artery Syndromes. The basilar artery supplies the medulla, pons, midbrain and cerebellum by way of the paramedian, short and long circumferential branches. There are various clinical pictures involving the cranial nerves and long tracts. Most common findings are hemiplegia, tetraplegia, various cranial nerve palsies, pseudobulbar palsy and respiratory disturbances. In thrombosis of the main trunk the outcome is almost invariably fatal.

Vascular Lesions of the Brain Stem. Each side of the brain stem has an independent blood supply. Syndromes may be divided into paramedian (area supplied by short vessels from the vertebral and basilar arteries) and lateral (area supplied by vessels with a long course before they enter the brain stem) (Fig. 28-6).

THE PARAMEDIAN AREA. This area contains the motor nuclei of the third, fourth, sixth and twelfth cranial nerves, the corticobulbar and corticospinal tract and the medial lemniscus. Vascular accidents produce syndromes characterized by paralysis of one or more cranial nerves on the homolateral side and paralysis or paresis on the opposite side.

Weber's syndrome is produced by damage to the third nerve and cerebral peduncle. There is ophthalmoplegia on the ipsilateral side and paralysis of the arm or leg on the opposite side.

The Millard-Gubler syndrome involves the sixth and seventh nerves on the ipsilateral side and the corticospinal tract on the opposite side (Fig. 28-7).

Foville's syndrome consists of paralysis of conjugate gaze to the side of the lesion in addition to the findings in the Millard-Gubler syndrome.

Another lesion lower in the stem produces twelfth nerve palsy with contralateral hemianesthesia and hemiplegia.

THE LATERAL BRAIN STEM AREA. Vessels supplying this area also supply the cerebellum. In addition to cerebellar dysfunction there may be involvement of the fifth, seventh and tenth motor nuclei, the fifth and eighth sensory nuclei, the spinal lemniscus and the sympathetic pathways.

Wallenberg's syndrome (posterior inferior cerebellar artery) produces dysphagia, dysarthria, impairment of pain and temperature sensation in the face, Horner's syndrome, nystagmus and cerebellar signs on the ipsilateral side. Contralaterally there is impairment of pain and temperature sensation of the body (Fig. 28-8).

Thrombosis of the anterior cerebellar artery produces homolateral deafness, facial paralysis, Horner's syndrome and loss of sensation of touch in the face. On the opposite side there is impairment of pain and temperature sensation. Homolateral cerebellar signs are also present.

Superior cerebellar artery thrombosis produces homolateral involuntary movements, loss of hearing and facial paralysis. Contralaterally there is loss of pain and temperature sensation over the entire half of the body.

Pseudobulbar Palsy. Theoretically this condition may be produced by bilateral lesions in the brain stem. The term implies, however, interruption of the

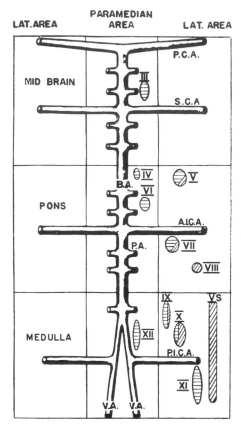

Figure 28–6   Brain stem nuclei and their blood supply. Roman numerals refer to cranial nerve nuclei. Horizontal lines in the nuclei indicate motor nuclei; diagonal lines indicate sensory nuclei. (From Holtzman, M., Panin, N., and Ebel, A.: Anatomical Localization of Common Vascular Brain Syndromes. Amer. J. Phys. Med., *38*:133–135, 1959.)

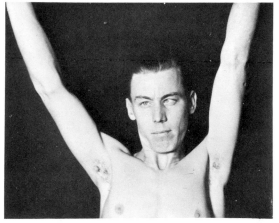

Figure 28–7   Patient with left abducens palsy and right hemiparesis. Seventh nerve palsy is not evident in this picture. (Courtesy of Dr. A. Ornsteen, Philadelphia.)

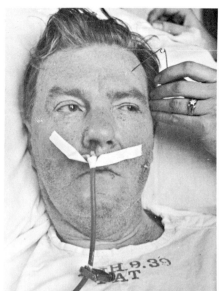

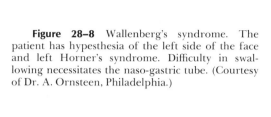

Figure 28–8 Wallenberg's syndrome. The patient has hypesthesia of the left side of the face and left Horner's syndrome. Difficulty in swallowing necessitates the naso-gastric tube. (Courtesy of Dr. A. Ornsteen, Philadelphia.)

corticobulbar pathway. The chief cause is multiple arteriosclerotic lesions in both hemispheres. There may be emotional outbursts, personality changes, aphasia, loss of memory, deterioration of intellective function and moderate difficulty in speaking, chewing and swallowing. Psychiatric evaluation and support may be necessary.

GENERAL MEDICAL MANAGEMENT

It is obvious that patients with brain stem involvement may be desperately ill and require long-term medical management. Attention must be given to nutrition and electrolyte balance, and care must be taken to prevent urinary tract and respiratory infections and thrombophlebitis.

Respiratory Management. Many of the problems discussed have in common the need for management of respiratory difficulty. Beaver[16] cites the most common causes of admission to a respiratory unit as the following: injuries to brain or brain stem, Guillain-Barré syndrome, poliomyelitis, tetraplegia, prolonged coma, virus encephalomyelitis, myasthenia gravis, myopathies and bulbar palsy. Respiratory failure has many causes. From a physiologic point of view, they can be classified as atmospheric, ventilatory, circulatory, hemotologic and cytologic.

Tracheostomy should be considered early for many reasons: (1) it enables secretions to be removed by suction, (2) it provides an obstruction-free airway, (3) it reduces the dead space by 70 cc., which may prove lifesaving, (4) it allows immediate employment of mechanical assistance, (5) it makes humidification and endobronchial medication easy, (6) in some cases, especially postoperative, it may serve as insurance against respiratory complications.

The merits of positive pressure ventilation as compared with the tank respirator have been argued. The advantages of positive pressure are definite:

the patient is less restricted psychologically and physically, nursing and physical therapy procedures are performed more easily, transport is easy and there is no difficulty with the neck seal and handling the tracheostomy. On the other hand, these machines are more delicate and there is less margin for error. There is interference with cardiovascular activity by reversal of the thoracic pump mechanism, direct tamponage of the heart and inhibition of alveolar capillary circulation when intra-alveolar tension exceeds 8 mm. Hg.

There are conditions in which the mechanical support of respiration may be contraindicated. A patient literally dying from amyotrophic lateral sclerosis can only be made uncomfortable and unhappy if life is prolonged in a senseless way. The author remembers well a young woman kept alive for a year at great cost to her family in terms of money and anxiety. This woman was far from grateful. She had not been allowed to die simply and comfortably. Tracheostomy and oxygen given through a catheter would have permitted a far more comfortable and dignified death.

REFERENCES

1. Haymaker, W.: Bing's Local Diagnosis in Neurological Diseases. Translated, revised and enlarged from the 14th German edition. St. Louis, The C. V. Mosby Co., 1956, pp. 118-224, 241-253.
2. Grinker, R. R., Bucy, P. C., and Sahs, A. L.: Neurology. 5th Ed. Springfield, Ill., Charles C Thomas, 1960, pp. 402-463.
3. Ford, F. R.: Diseases of the Nervous System in Infancy, Childhood, and Adolescence. 4th Ed. Springfield, Ill., Charles C Thomas, 1960, pp. 20-43.
4. Merritt, H. H.: A Textbook of Neurology. Philadelphia, Lea and Febiger, 1955.
5. Alter, M.: Familial Aggregation of Bell's Palsy. Arch. Neurol., 8:55, 1963.
6. Ghiora, A., and Winter, S. T.: The Conservative Treatment of Bell's Palsy. A Review of the Literature, 1939-1960. Amer. J. Phys. Med., 41:213, 1962.
7. Kettel, K.: Surgical Treatment in Atraumatic Facial Palsies. J. Laryng., 73:491, 1959.
8. Langworth, E. P., and Taverner, D.: The Prognosis in Facial Palsy. Brain, 86:465, 1963.
9. Wiederholt, W. C., Mulder, D. W., and Lambert, E. H.: The Landry-Guillain-Barré-Strohl Syndrome or Polyradiculoneuropathy: Historical Review, Report on 97 Patients, and Present Concepts. Proc. Mayo Clin. 39:427, 1964.
10. Marshall, J.: The Landry-Guillain-Barré Syndrome. Brain, 86:55, 1963.
11. Birchfield, R. I., and Shaw, C.: Postural Hypotension in the Guillain-Barré Syndrome. Arch. Neurol., 10:149, 1964.
12. Walton, J. N.: The "Floppy" Infant. Cereb. Palsy Bull., 2:10, 1960.
13. Krabbe, K. H.: Congenital Generalized Muscular Atrophies. Acta Psychiat. Scand., 33:94, 1958.
14. Brandt, S.: Werdnig-Hoffmann's Infantile Progressive Muscular Atrophy. Copenhagen, Munksgard, 1950.
15. Abel, J. J., Hampil, B., and Jonas, A. F., Jr.: Researches on Tetanus: Further Experiments to Prove that Tetanus Toxin Is Not Carried in the Peripheral Nerves to the Central Nervous System. Bull. Johns Hopkins Hosp., 56:317, 1935.
16. Beaver, R.: The Management of Respiratory Failure. In Modern Trends in Neurology—3. Ed. D. Williams. Washington, Butterworth, Inc., 1962.
17. Taverner, D., Kemble, F., and Cohen, S. B.: Prognosis and Treatment of Idiopathic Facial (Bell's) Palsy. Brit. Med. J., 4:581, 1967.
18. Alford, B. R., Weber, S. C., and Sessions, R. B.: Neurodiagnostic Studies in Facial Paralysis. Ann. Otol., 79:227, 1970.
19. Edgerton, M. T.: Surgical Correction of Facial Paralysis: A Plea for Better Reconstructions. Ann. Surg., 165:985, 1967.
20. Peiris, O. A., and Miles, D. W.: Galvanic Stimulation of the Tongue as a Prognostic Index in Bell's Palsy. Brit. Med., J., 2:1162, 1965.
21. Campbell, E. D. R., Hickey, R. P., Nixon, K. H., and Richardson, A. T.: Value of Nerve-Excitability Measurements in Prognosis of Facial Palsy. Brit. Med. J., 2:7, 1962.

Chapter 29

DEGENERATIVE DISEASES OF THE CENTRAL NERVOUS SYSTEM

by Jerome S. Tobis

A significant proportion of all diseases of the central nervous system are degenerative. These diseases are progressive and incurable. They occur most frequently in the later decades of life and include such disorders as amyotrophic lateral sclerosis, encephalomalacia associated with senility and parkinsonism. On the other hand, there are several diseases that are of hereditary origin such as Friedreich's ataxia, familial spastic paralysis, dystonia musculorum deformans and presenile dementia. Those that have a hereditary predisposition are inclined to appear at an earlier stage of life.

Many diseases are grouped under the term degenerative disease. By and large, the term signifies that the etiology is unknown. As knowledge is acquired, it is likely that specific defects of metabolic origin will be disclosed. Each of these diseases characteristically affects a specific portion of the central nervous system; however, there is no portion of the nervous system that is free of degenerative change.

For this discussion concerning physiatric management of these disorders, some of the basic principles and techniques of care will be reviewed. They will be discussed under symptomatic headings.

PROGRESSIVE CHARACTER OF THE DISEASE

The progressive degenerative pathologic changes with their accompanying progressive disabilities make these diseases tragic and difficult management

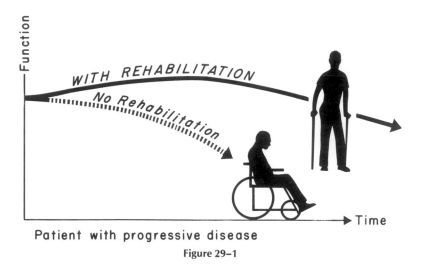

Patient with progressive disease

Figure 29–1

problems. The objectives of care of these patients are to maintain their maximal physical and psychologic function and to limit the effects of disuse. Figure 29-1 shows diagrammatically the role of a therapeutic program of physical medicine and rehabilitation in these conditions. Although physiatric measures do not affect the underlying disease process, they can prolong motor function by counteracting the consequences of disuse and deconditioning.

SENILITY

In the psychologic sphere many of these patients suffer the consequences of two underlying pathophysiologic processes, namely, the immediate effects of the neural damage and the long-term changes associated with the aging process. Many attempts have been made to differentiate the mental disturbance of arteriosclerotic dementia from intrinsic senile dementia. Elderly people may also suffer from functional psychologic disorders. One should not assume the organic nature of a psychosis even though it may appear in older age. In Table 29-1 — which is from a paper by Ehrentheil[3] — the differential diagnoses of the senile psychoses and the dementias are presented.

It should be emphasized that the organic disease processes are variable in their effects upon the personality of the patient. There is no direct relationship between the severity of the cellular change and the observable social and psychologic functioning of the patient. The effects of these organic processes may be primary, as the direct consequence of cortical disorganization, or secondary, as the result of the reaction of the individual to his disability.

Ability to Learn. An area of immediate concern to the physiatrist is the patient's capacity to learn or relearn a task. Patients who cannot be taught are incapable of deriving benefit from a rehabilitation program. However, the capacity to learn is very much dependent upon other physiologic and environmental factors. For example, psychologic and neuromuscular functions are interrelated. The presence of urinary incontinence of central origin is usually considered evidence of advanced brain damage, yet it is not uncommon to find that as the incontinent hemiplegic learns to stand and walk again, his bladder control also improves. Therapy that improves neuromuscular function is likely to have a salutary effect upon the psychologic status of the patient.

Effective Environment.   Environmental factors may significantly influence the patient's intellectual capacities. The metabolic consequences of deconditioning have been well documented. There are also psychologic counterparts. Deconditioning of brain function is likely to occur in an unsympathetic, strange and confusing environment. Those stresses with which the patient cannot cope will lead to further intellectual disorganization.

All too often the physician (especially the young house officer) interprets bizarre behavior as purely the result of an organic brain syndrome. Frequently the term encephalomalacia is assigned with a finality and irreversibility that is tragic, for it establishes an atmosphere of hopelessness and fatalism. For example, Litin[5] has defined the risk of hospitalizing an apparently normal elderly person for diagnostic evaluation. A very common reaction is delirium that is intensified at night. The delirium is associated with agitation and panic. In the more severe manifestations destructiveness and incontinence appear.

Pollack and others[6] have reported an interesting observation in their study of the results when the double simultaneous stimulation test was administered to subjects over 65 years of age in a variety of nursing homes and homes for the aged. Errors of response in this test have been interpreted as being due to brain damage. The finding of special interest in the study was that there was similarity in patterns of response in subjects within the same institution. The authors suggest that a subject-institution accommodation occurs as regards intellectual activity. In institutions where almost all the residents had a positive test response, there was an atmosphere of despair and futility.

Aring,[2] a neuropathologist, has written with great wisdom on the subject of senility. He noted that the rate of occurrence of cerebral atherosclerosis in individuals past the age of 50 would almost make it appear to be a normal finding and yet senility is not a constant in the aged. He emphasized that social factors such as isolation contribute to senile dementia.

Much has been written concerning the consequences of sensory deprivation in both the experimental and the clinical setting. Diminished sensory input from hearing, vision, position and touch loss may cause aged patients to experience the consequences of sensory isolation. An unsympathetic environment tends to compound the problem.

An optimal environment, on the other hand, is one that is well organized. Senile patients frequently have difficulty in abstract thinking. Many are unable to cope with complex problems of daily living but can function effectively in a regularized and simplified setting. Some patients may not comprehend the abstract concept of time but still may be able to carry out routine activities on a regular schedule without becoming confused.

A prerequisite for optimal psychologic activities is an environment in which the patient may function within his intellectual capacities. These patients are more likely to show evidence of deep fears in an unsympathetic or desolate environment such as may be found in the back wards of a hospital or in the home of a disinterested family. Stress with which the patient cannot cope will lead to further disorganization and confusion. The environment should be stimulating but not disruptive, sympathetic but not apathetic, well organized and scheduled.

TABLE 29–1

	AFFECTIVE, DEPRESSIVE PSYCHOSES	ARTERIOSCLEROTIC PSYCHOSIS
PATHOLOGY	No characteristic anatomic changes.	Three variants: (1) cases with evident softenings or hemorrhages; arteries at base mostly show patchy or diffuse arteriosclerotic changes. (2) cases of granular or verrucose atrophy of cortex usually associated with similar change in cortex of kidney, and with hypertension while alive. (3) cases with focal rarefaction and degeneration of the nerve cells (areas of paling) with no naked-eye changes of brain or vessels apart from slight thinning of cortex. Usually hypertension while alive.
AGE OF ONSET	At any age.	45 to 85, average 66 years.
MODE OF ONSET	Onset is often sudden, clearly defined. In reactive depression, stress situation is often obvious.	Abrupt onset very common, but may be gradual. Mental and physical stresses less commonly a precipitating factor.
HEREDITARY AND PRECIPITATING FACTORS	Menopause, involution. History of attacks of depression suggests manic depressive psychosis.	Tendency to arteriosclerotic disease in families, the relative early age of onset in many cases suggests that metabolic and toxic factors may play a role.
SEX DISTRIBUTION	In younger age group more women; in older age group more men.	Men: women = 3:1
NEUROLOGIC ABNORMALITIES	Functional disorders of the vegetative nervous system common.	Signs of local and diffuse damage to brain (see text). In pathologic variant (1) local signs; in variant (2) diffuse damage in the foreground. Isolated impairment of higher functions: agnosias, apraxias, and so on are possible. Apoplectic insults are common.
EPILEPTIFORM SEIZURES	No seizures.	Epileptiform seizures are common, also syncopal attacks, headache, dizziness.
MAIN PSYCHIATRIC SIGN	Emotional depression and mental retardation but no mental deterioration.	Lacunar type of intellectual impairment frequent with relative integrity of personality. Fluctuating course downward.
PSYCHIATRIC PICTURE	Marked depression with self-reproach, sometimes nihilistic and somatic delusions, in tune with affective disturbances. Motor activity reduced.	Memory less impaired than in senile psychosis. Confusion often varies suddenly in a day, probably depending on changes in blood circulation. Relatively good preservation of insight with depressed feelings and fears. Weakness, fatigue, emotional instability with outbreaks of weeping or laughter. Sometimes improvements lasting many years.

* From Ehrentheil, O. F.: Differential Diagnosis of Organic Dementias

DIFFERENTIAL DIAGNOSTIC POINTS*

SENILE DEMENTIA	ALZHEIMER'S DISEASE	PICK'S DISEASE
Shrinking of brain, especially gray substance in diffuse symmetric distribution. Hydrocephalus. Gliosis. Senile plaques. Often atrophy of basal ganglia. Degeneration of cells with shrinking, deposition of lipofuscin in cytoplasm and appearance of intra-cellular fibrils.	Atrophy of cerebral cortex, especially of parietal and occipital lobes. Marked hydrocephalus. Outfall of cells, particularly of three outer cortical layers. Senile plaques and intracellular fibrillar degeneration. Same microscopic changes as in senile psychosis but more marked and earlier. Changes in basal ganglia are common.	Massive circumscribed shrinkage en bloc of frontal and temporal lobes and insular region, mostly symmetric. Peculiar swelling of nerve cells (ballooning), characteristic cytoplasmic inclusions (argentophylic bodies), atrophy and reactive gliosis. Absence of senile plaques, Alzheimer, neurofibrillary changes, and absence of arteriosclerotic vascular lesions. Basal ganglia are rarely affected.
Between 60 and 90 years, average 75 years.	Age 50 to 60, average 54.	40 to 75, average 54.
Insidious, gradual failing in their work.	Not so sudden as in arteriosclerotic dementia but more sudden and less insidious than in senile dementia.	Gradual onset.
Sometimes precipitated by mental or physical stress.	"Multifactorial inheritance" (Sjoegren). Not heredofamilial (Hoff).	Dominant gene of incomplete penetrance (Sjoegren).
Men: women = 1:3	Men: women = 1:1	Men: women = 1:2
Signs mainly of diffuse damage to the brain (see text). Tremors, changeable muscular rigidity, uncertain gait may be observed.	Signs of diffuse brain damage (see text). Parietal lobe symptoms tend to appear earlier and stronger than in equivalent stage of Pick's disease. Agnosias, apraxias, amnesia, aphasia are common. Transient or progressive pareses, increase in muscle tone and unsteady gait, occasional tremor.	Signs of diffuse damage confined to one or both frontal and temporal lobe (see text).
Usually not.	Epileptiform seizures may occur.	Epileptiform attacks are rather rare and occur only in later stages but there are peculiar attacks of muscular hopotonia.
Defect of recent memory, disorientation in time and space, then increasing dementia.	Defect of recent memory, disorientation in time and space, then increasing dementia.	Affective changes, impairment of ethical and social behavior, then memory defect and increasing dementia.
Predominantly "negative" signs: failing memory, confusion, disorientation, deteriorated habits, restlessness, hallucinations. Five different types usually described but no sharp distinction: (1) simple deterioration (50% of all cases); (2) depressed and agitated type; (3) delirious and confused type; (4) presbyophrenic type (confabulations, loquacity, jovial mood, aimless restlessness); (5) paranoid type (intellectual faculties better preserved).	Predominant early memory disturbance with disorientation. Insight frequently preserved for long time, causing self-embarrassment. Mood characterized by irritability. Restless behavior, occasional delusions and hallucinations.	Insight totally lacking, often apathy and inattentiveness, no element of depression. Confabulations and hallucinations are rare. Psychiatric picture varies dependent on whether frontal or temporal lobes are predominantly affected (see text).

and Affective Disorders in Aged Patients. Geriatrics, *12:* 426–432, 1957.

(Table continues on following page.)

TABLE 29–1

	AFFECTIVE,DEPRESSIVE PSYCHOSES	ARTERIOSCLEROTIC PSYCHOSIS
COURSE	Self-limited, often responsive to shock therapy. Occasionally malignant.	Intermittent.
COMPLICATING EVENTS	Suicidal attempts.	Coronary artery disease, arteriosclerosis of aorta, urinary changes, increased NPN. Diabetes. Infections, bed sores.
DURATION OF DISEASE AND CAUSE OF DEATH	Good prognosis, high percentage of discharge, good life expectancy.	One day to sixteen years, average 3½ years; progress uneven, sometimes stormy; improvement common. Death from cerebral accident, arteriosclerotic heart disease, or infections.

ATAXIA

Ataxia may be a major factor in restricting ambulation and independence in self-care. Though there are no satisfactory techniques to limit ataxia, continued efforts to reduce its effects are warranted. Some patients, by learning substitutive techniques, maintain their motor function, including ambulation, even though the ataxia is severe. Once a patient is confined to a chair, however, his capacity to regain walking ability is quickly lost. Devices such as weighted shoes or canes may increase stability and enable the marginal patient to continue to walk. In selected cases, long leg braces may serve a similar function. In far advanced cases the ataxia may be severe enough to be disturbing to the patient even when he is in bed.

INCREASED TONE – RIGIDITY OR SPASTICITY

Spasticity or rigidity may seriously mask residual muscle power. Reduction of this increased tone may permit greater functional capacity. Pharmacologic agents such as the belladonna group for the rigidity of parkinsonism may be supplemented by an activity program to improve the motor function of the patient. The activity program includes frequent periods of walking and the performance of meaningful tasks that require the use of the upper extremities. All these measures may reduce the disability.

With the introduction of the newer pharmacologic agent L-dopa in the management of parkinsonism, many patients have had a significant reduction in symptoms related to rigidity and tremor. Many of those who respond favorably to such medication are able to maintain a functional level of motor performance that was hitherto rarely feasible.

In the presence of bradykinesia or akinesia (as when the feet feel "glued" to the ground), the patient may overcome one aspect of this problem by dorsiflexing his toes and thereby initiate walking. Occasionally the patient may facilitate movement by the use of other "trick" responses. For example, the patient who has difficulty in coming to a standing position after being seated may be taught to carry out the task in one rapid continuous synergistic movement in order to overcome the consequence of gravity.

DIFFERENTIAL DIAGNOSTIC POINTS (CONTINUED)

SENILE DEMENTIA	ALZHEIMER'S DISEASE	PICK'S DISEASE
Progressive.	Progressive.	Progressive.
Signs of old age, arteriosclerosis, infections, bed sores.	Infections, bed sores.	Infections, bed sores.
Seven months to eleven years, average 4½ years. Death may occur from infections, bed sores, cancer.	Duration a few years, about two to seven years. Death from physical decline or intercurrent disease.	Two to eleven years, average five. Death occurs from physical decline or intercurrent disease.

In the case of spasticity, local nerve blocks or injections of dilute solutions of procaine may lessen the disability so that the patient is able to use his maximal degree of voluntary motor power. Local applications of cold in the form of ice packs may reduce spasticity. In our experience no pharmacologic agent has been of value in reducing spasticity.

ADVENTITIOUS MOVEMENTS

Adventitious movements may be most disabling in conditions such as parkinsonism or dystonia. Surgical procedures such as chemothalamectomy have resulted in marked reduction in adventitious movements in a significant number of patients. The combination of rigidity, tremor and emotional depression in parkinsonism encourages disuse which leads to immobilization. Rehabilitation management focuses on the promotion and maintenance of physical activity. A conditioning exercise program is usually prescribed. Participation in social activities and meaningful work should be encouraged.

DEFORMITIES

A frequent concomitant of progressive neurologic disease is the development of contractures and deformities. Active range of motion exercises of all joints should be carried out daily if the patient's status permits. Otherwise passive range of motion exercises should be performed. These routines may be preventive as well as corrective to overcome the limitation of motion that may develop in any of the major joints of the body. Occasionally braces or splints worn at night may be employed in order to maintain satisfactory posture.

DECUBITUS ULCERS

Decubitus ulcers often develop in severely debilitated patients as a result of prolonged immobilization. This subject is discussed in Chapter 32 and will not be reviewed here. Prevention should be emphasized by turning the patient frequently, maintaining adequate nutrition and keeping the skin dry and clean. Pressure over bony prominences especially should be avoided.

DECONDITIONING

The consequences of deconditioning include metabolic factors such as muscle atrophy and osteoporosis. The effects on the cardiovascular system include reduced cardiac reserve and predisposition to phlebothrombosis. Techniques to overcome or prevent these sequelae entail maintaining or returning the patient to the maximum of activity of which he is capable. Measures that are used include: conditioning exercises, use of the tilt table for those who are bedridden, standing between parallel bars, and walking exercises for those who are able.

SUMMARY

It should be emphasized that the care of the patient with progressive degenerative disease requires sympathetic understanding on the part of those who treat him. With such care the patient may live at his maximal functional capacity and be able to retain a sense of dignity. For the patient who shows evidence of brain damage, simplification and regularity in his daily activity will permit him to function more effectively. Meaningful work or responsibilities that are stimulating yet not too stressful for him are of value.

REFERENCES

1. Allison, R. S.: The Senile Brain. Baltimore, The Williams and Wilkins Co., 1962.
2. Aring, C. D.: Senility. A.M.A. Arch. Int. Med., *100:*519-528, 1957.
3. Ehrentheil, O. F.: Differential Diagnosis of Organic Dementias and Affective Disorders in Aged Patients. Geriatrics, *12:*426-432, 1957.
4. Hoch, P., and Zubin, J.: Psychopathology of Aging. New York, Grune and Stratton, 1961.
5. Litin, E. M.: Mental Reaction to Trauma and Hospitalization in the Aged. J.A.M.A., *162:*1522-1524, 1956.
6. Pollack, M., Kahn, R. L., and Goldfarb, A. I.: Factors Related to Individual Differences in Perception in Institutionalized Aged Subjects. J. Geront., *13:*192-197, 1958.
7. Walshe, F.: Diseases of the Nervous System. Baltimore, The Williams and Wilkins Co., 1963.

Chapter 30

TREATMENT OF BACK DISORDERS AND DEFORMITIES

by Hersch L. Sachs

Back disorders and deformities arise from a variety of etiologic factors. Interpretation and analysis of the symptomatology often remains an unsolved diagnostic problem. The clinical diagnosis is made on the basis of the results of many essential and important investigations. Uncertainties in diagnosis give rise to divergent therapeutic measures. Much too often treatment procedures are empirical. We are not so presumptuous as to intend to cover the conservative treatment of all the diseases of the vertebral column in this chapter but the common problems of low back pain and scoliosis will be discussed.

LOW BACK PAIN

Although a patient with low back pain may rightly be within the realm of several specialties he is frequently referred to the physiatrist for treatment and occasionally for diagnostic procedures.

Etiologic Factors

Low back pain may be symptomatic of a general infection, of a localized lesion of the viscera or of a metastatic lesion. The pain may be arthritic, caused by a localized lesion of tuberculous arthritis, rheumatoid spondylitis or hypertrophic arthritis. Lumbar insufficiency and intervertebral lesions are common causes.

Lumbar Insufficiency. Lumbar insufficiency may be apparent or latent. Often it does not cause trouble until it is exposed by strain or injury. Congenital abnormalities, including the absence of a vertebra, an abnormal axis of a joint and spondylolysis often progressing to spondylolishthesis, and post-traumatic defects which occur at the twelfth thoracic and first lumbar vertebrae in about half of the cases are causes of lumbar insufficiency. Springback or tearing of all the posterior supportive ligaments of the lumbosacral region (particularly the supraspinous ligament) may also be a cause. It is characterized by pain on flexion. Other causes include osteoporosis of varied etiologies, such as malnutrition, vitamin deficiency, immobilization, age, Cushing's syndrome, thyroid gland disease, ovarian and testicular malformation and idiopathy; Paget's disease; and muscle atonia caused by excessive heavy work combined with chronic malnutrition or occurring slowly as a result of chronic strain such as that due to poor posture.

Intervertebral Lesions. Intervertebral lesions include prolapsed intervertebral disc, which occurs at the fourth and fifth intervertebral spaces 98 per cent of the time (only 21 per cent of the patients experience objective loss of sensation); extradural inflammatory lesions and metastatic lesions mainly from the breast and prostate; intramedullary lesions that compress the nerve roots; and extraspinal truncular pain, which is most common in arthritic patients.

Clinical Aspects of Low Back Pain

Different types of low back pain have been described. One variety of deep, dull pain is central in location and poorly localized. The pain has been assigned to ligamentous structure and is usually associated with bending and picking up objects. It is not completely disabling and goes away as soon as the activity which produced it is stopped. Another variety is the agonizing pain in the lumbar region with acute and dramatic onset. Duration of the pain is variable from a few moments to a few days, with gradual improvement. Occasionally this type of pain may be absent and the patient is comfortable as long as he is immobile. At times the pain starts in the lower back and radiates to one or both legs. In chronic cases the pain is fairly well localized but is affected by activity. Pain and stiffness appear when the patient maintains the same position for a long time. The condition improves with mild activity, but excess of activity causes a recurrence of pain.

Low back pain affects, at one time or another, a large proportion of the population. Males experience an earlier onset of symptoms than females. Obesity probably increases the frequency of pain in the lower back. Asymmetrical lumbarization or sacralization or tropism may contribute to low back pain. Differences in leg length up to 1½ inches do not affect low back pain, although back pain is relieved when leg length discrepancy has been corrected, because correction changes the statics of the spinal column.

Retroperitoneal fibrosis, occlusion of the common iliac arteries, prostatic cancer, and arachnoiditis of the cauda equina have been implicated as causes of lower back pain. Psychogenic disease must also be considered. Malingering may be encountered, especially when monetary gains are in view.

The role played by poor posture in the genesis of low back pain must be emphasized. Strain in the lumbar region occurs when the back is in constant flexion, which is common in daily life. Modern overstuffed furniture and automobile seats do not prevent the transmission of tension from the extensors of the legs upward through the extensor ligaments of the lumbar spine and tend to increase the flexion of the lumbar spine. It is common knowledge that older adults will arise from soft beds with low back pain and stiffness because of strain on iliotibial bands that is transmitted to the lumbar ligaments. Examination of such a patient will yield important information. Postural changes to protect the involved area may be found: the whole patient is bent forward with the lumbar spine flattened. Pain is usually poorly located by the patient, but radiation of the pain is commonly related to the level of the lesion. The effects of coughing, sneezing, exertion and changes in position may help in the localization or management of the condition. Examination of the spine consists of palpation of the muscle spasm, location of trigger points from the fibrositis of the muscle spasm, and observing the flattening and scoliosis of the spine. Flexion and extension of the spine are more severely affected than lateral flexion, and there is definite correlation between pain on pressure or percussion of the flexed lumbar spinous processes and back pain. Straight leg raising is a simple test to assess sciatic root involvement, but muscle wasting and sensory change will supply evidence of the level of root involvement. The possibility of overlap or of individual anatomic variation must always be borne in mind. X-ray examination may show one or several of the following findings: Intervertebral narrowing, vacuum disc phenomena and intervertebral arthritis. Anterior posterior slip-on bending may also correlate with other symptoms. Developmental abnormalities may be a contributing factor. Myelography and occasionally lumbar discography are reserved for patients in whom there is reason to suspect the presence of a tumor or when surgery is definitely being considered.

Treatment

Period of Immobilization. Assuming that acute or subacute infectious and neoplastic diseases have been excluded and that the pains are caused by injury to the soft tissue structures, immobilization can be expected to lead to the repair of the injured structure. Treatment by immobilization has not gone unchallenged. Moore, Dehne and Kiersch report 476 patients with acute back pain who have been kept ambulatory, with only two exceptions. Using ice massage and a program of exercises, they reported excellent results regarding speed of recovery and return to work.

Rest in a bed that has a firm mattress and a fracture board on the springs is prescribed. Pelvic or leg traction of 4 to 10 pounds is used. In treating patients over 60 years of age traction is usually omitted. The patient is encouraged to change his position in bed systematically. Three positions are usually comfortable: supine with a pillow behind the knees or on the right or left side, lying with a thin pillow between the knees.

Heat is applied by means of hot packs, shortwave diathermy or infrared radiation for periods of 30 minutes at a time. Only very light sedative massage is to be used in the active phase of the disease.

This conservative approach often yields satisfactory results in treating a prolapsed disk except when there are unmistakable neurologic signs. Herniated disks often recede into intervertebral spaces and protrude again on exertion or change of position. This alternating backward and forward slipping results in remissions and exacerbations of pain.

Period of Mobilization. When the patient is allowed out of bed he wears a brace for back support. All back pain is not caused by injury of the soft tissues.

Reflex spasm may sometimes be present. A program consisting of mild exercises, application of heat, stretching and manipulation is instituted. Postural training is most important. The patient usually has a tendency toward increased dorsal kyphosis and lumbar lordosis.

Exercises should be prescribed only after appraising the patient's needs. These can be determined only by muscle testing and evaluation of muscle spasm. It should be the general rule to require that exercises are performed with regularity. The therapist must regulate the number of repetitions and observe especially evidence of fatigue. Muscle pain and tiredness should not last over an hour past the time of completion of the exercise.

Caillet has summarized the aims of muscle reeducation under the following headings: (a) Improve posture with a decrease of lumbar lordosis; (b) Improve power and "tone" of abdomen and buttock muscles; (c) Improve and maintain flexibility of low back structures; (d) Proper body mechanics must be a daily way of living.

Exercises are always to be preceded by application of heat. Spasm may be relieved by ethyl chloride sprays. Sinusoidal current used alone for 15 minutes will enhance the relaxation of tense or stiff muscles, and tetanizing current has also proved very effective in painful muscle spasm. The combined use of these procedures may prove useful at times in preparation for exercise. In cases where the patient does not tolerate electrotherapy, superficial or deep heating, followed by exercise, may be equally beneficial. Massage will relax deep muscles following exercise and thus offset muscle stiffness. Painful fibrositis may be benefited by rolling massage.

EXERCISES FOR THE LOWER BACK.   Lying face down on a table, the patient contracts the gluteal muscles with a pelvic roll for a count of five and relaxes. The exercise is repeated 5 to 10 times.

The patient lies supine with his hips and knees flexed and stretches the knees down and out with his hands. He holds this position for five seconds and then relaxes. This exercise is done 5 to 10 times.

The patient lies on his back with one knee flexed and the other extended. He raises his extended leg to 90 degrees and then lowers it slowly. This is done six times with each leg. This exercise should be omitted if there is severe lumbar lordosis.

To stretch the hamstrings the patient lies on his back, flexes one hip and knee and then extends the knee and dorsiflexes the foot until he can feel a pull in the hamstring muscles. The stretching is often done forcibly by an assistant. The exercise is repeated three times for each leg.

EXERCISE FOR STRETCHING THE ILIOTIBIAL BAND.   The patient stands with his right side turned toward a table 2 feet away and leans on the right hand with the arm straight. He then stretches the right hip toward the table until he feels stretching in the right tibial fascia. The exercise is done three times on each side.

EXERCISES FOR THE ABDOMINAL MUSCLES.   Exercises to strengthen the abdominal muscles and correct lumbar lordosis must be cautiously administered and should be supervised. They should be stopped if undue pain develops.

The patient lies on his back with his knees bent and his feet flat on the floor. He inhales and draws the abdomen inward and toward the chest. As he exhales he forces the lower part of the back against the floor.

Sitting with his back against a wall, the patient pushes the lower part of the back against the wall by contracting the abdominal muscles.

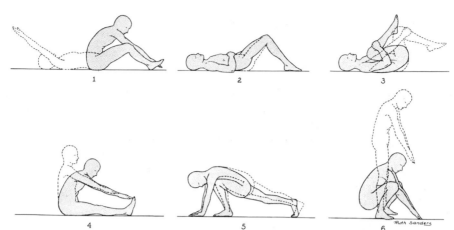

Figure 30–1   Postural exercises designed to reduce the lumbosacral angle. (From Williams, P. C.: Conservative Management of Lesions of the Lumbosacral Spine. Instruct. Lect. Amer. Acad. Orthop. Surg. *10*:90–121, 1953.)

Sit-ups performed with hips and knees flexed are helpful. The patient should start by lifting only his head and shoulders and progress cautiously to full sit-ups.

Flat-footed squats require strong flexion at the lumbosacral joint. Frequent repetition will develop the habit pattern of bending by flexing the knees rather than bending from the hips.

BACK MANIPULATION.   Back manipulation is regarded as controversial and its value has been questioned by many physicians. However the method has regained favor and controlled studies performed lately in proved cases of discogenic diseases as well as in certain other forms of low back pain, have shown improvement in 25 to 50 per cent of the cases.

The patient lies on his right side on the edge of a table. He drops the left leg forward over the edge of the table and places his left arm behind him. The manipulator places one hand on the left shoulder and the other on the iliac crest and twists the torso by pushing the shoulder backward and pulling the iliac crest forward. The procedure is repeated on the other side. Finally the patient is turned on his back and the hips and the knees are hyperflexed sufficiently to flex the lumbar spine forcibly.

This maneuver is forceful and sudden and often is accompanied by an audible and palpable crunching sound in the lower back. Dramatic improvement has sometimes been claimed following such manipulation of the back.

BACK SUPPORTS.   The value of back support has been demonstrated by experimental evidence. Morris, Lucas and Bresler showed that a corset or a regular cast increased the actual motion of the vertebrae but prevented extremes of motion. Their conclusions regarding these motions were based on strain gauge studies. Experimentally, vertebral bodies break when the spine is loaded at 1000 to 1300 pounds. In the living body the spine is part of a semi-rigid cylinder. Just by doing a Valsalva maneuver the weight on the lowest lumbar vertebra is diminished by 30 per cent, and an inflatable corset would reduce the load by about 25 per cent. Vertebral body fractures can be averted by the use of abdominal compression in fighter pilots pulling out of a dive. Intra-abdominal pressure is enhanced by wearing a corset; the corset provides something for the abdominal muscles to push against. The lessening of pressure on the disc, although not spectacular, is enough to make the difference between pain and no pain.

Although casts or braces do not increase the incidence of successful fusion in arthrodesis of the lower back, they guard against gross motion. Casts are usually of the flexion jacket type; with the disappearance of the ligamentous strain the spasm and pain will also disappear. It was long held that immobilization should extend from the dorsolumbar joint to the greater trochanter and that it had to be fairly rigid, but we now know that the spine cannot be immobilized with the rigid type of corset. Physicians today tend to avoid cumbersome rigid corsets and instead provide smaller ones, especially those with abdominal shields and straps in front for abdominal compression. This is particularly indicated for the obese patient.

SHOE LIFTS.   Asymptomatic persons with shortening of one leg of less than 1½ inches do not derive any benefit from a shoe lift, but persons with aching backs will find some improvement after correction of leg length inequality. The correction of inequality is accomplished progressively and not attempted completely at the first examination.

LIMITATION OF ACTIVITY.   During the period of rehabilitation, lifting and bending are forbidden. Short rest periods are advisable. Weight reduction is effected by diet. Even when the patient is considered fully recovered, certain athletic activities are curtailed. Bowling, handball and golf are notable instigators of low back pain. This program is often sufficient to control the symptoms for many years.

Postoperative Care

After laminectomy the patient is allowed out of bed after one or two weeks and is started on a program of muscular reeducation. Following spinal fusion the patient should be recumbent for at least six weeks and after he is out of bed he should wear a well fitting brace for at least six months. While he is in bed, all four extremities may be exercised and breathing exercises may be started.

Close cooperation between the physiatrist and surgeon is necessary for optimal results. The following postoperative exercise program, with individual adaptations, is prescribed.

Exercises.   Exercises to strengthen the weak muscles—back extensors, abdominal muscles and quadratus lumborum—are used. Disuse weakness of the hip abductors and the quadriceps must be corrected. Flexion of the trunk and sit-ups should not be prescribed during the first month. Stretching of the back extensors by pelvic roll exercises and stretching of flexion contractures of the hip and knees should be employed.

Weakness of the back extensors as a result of stretch and retraction during surgery should be remedied by postural exercises and weight reduction. An obese, protruding abdomen is a cause of lumbar lordosis.

Limitation of Activities.   The patient's activities should be limited. Initially he is allowed out of bed three or four times daily for brief periods of three to five minutes; as he progresses, the length of time is extended. The patient must be taught not to increase his activities beyond the point at which his weak muscles become fatigued.

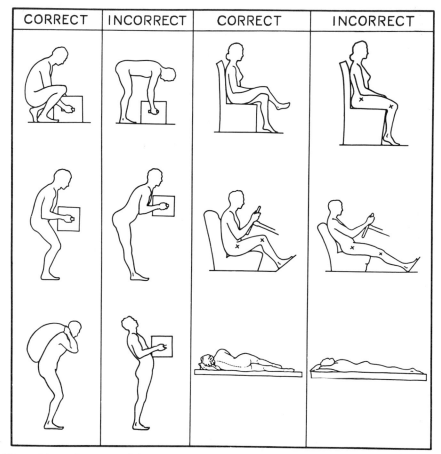

Figure 30–2 Correct and incorrect postural attitudes. (From Turek, S. L.: Orthopaedics. Philadelphia, J. B. Lippincott Co., 1959.)

If the patient has poor work habits or associated disorders they should be corrected by the use of a cane, brace, heel lift or a properly fitted orthopedic shoe.

Here are some final instructions to be given to all patients suffering from low back pain:

1. Use a firm mattress.

2. Sleep on your side with your feet drawn up.

3. To get out of bed, turn on the side, draw the knees up and then swing them over the bed.

4. Avoid soft furniture and deep sofas and do not sit with legs straight out.

5. Avoid stooping or lifting.

6. Do not lift objects in front of you above the waist line.

7. Do not bend backwards, twist to reach the phone or crouch over a low typewriter.

8. Women should avoid using very high heels.

9. Sit with the knee level higher than the hip level and the feet firmly placed on the floor.

10. Lifting, pushing and pulling should be done with hips and knees slightly flexed.

Treatment of Spinal Osteoporosis and Myofascitis

The greatest problem in treating elderly patients with spinal osteoporosis is to obtain their cooperation because they usually have been inactive for several years. Muscle reeducation and exercise to increase and maintain muscle tone are the first steps. Exercises to correct postural deformity and obtain better standing position are of utmost importance. Deep breathing exercises, exercises to strengthen the abdominal and gluteal muscles and exercises to correct other osteoarthritic deformities that involve the joints of the shoulders and upper and lower extremities and to prevent joint stiffening are also used.

When necessary, the back should be braced with a Taylor type brace, which theoretically should be the best method if the patient tolerates it, or a lighter type of orthopedic corset that gives adequate support to the lumbar spine and the abdomen.

Proper diet must be maintained and may be supplemented by a high caloric intake. Hormone therapy is usually used.

Myofascitis is treated in the same way as spinal osteoporosis. In addition, ethyl chloride sprays, local infiltration with procaine at the trigger points, kneading and crushing massage and ultrasonic therapy have been advocated occasionally.

SCOLIOSIS

Structural back disorders usually begin to develop in childhood. Scoliosis is the most common disorder of the vertebral column in children. It is a controversial and difficult entity that may be caused by congenital anomalies and deviation, developmental deformities, endocrine disturbances, metabolic defects, infections or injuries.

Definition. Scoliosis is a lateral tilt or angular deviation from the normal straight position of one or more vertebral segments of the spine. A functional curve can be completely corrected and maintained in the erect position. In structural scoliosis, however, there is intrinsic involvement of the bone, muscle or nerve elements that support the spine and complete correction is impossible.

Etiology

Functional scoliosis is compensatory to such conditions as unequal leg length, a tight iliotibial band or abduction or adduction contracture of hip.

Structural scoliosis may be osteopathic, resulting from congenital conditions, diseased conditions of the structures of the thorax or other osteopathies; neuropathic, caused by congenital disorders, residual effects of poliomyelitis or such conditions as neurofibromatosis and syringomelia; myopathic, due to congenital defects, muscular dystrophy or other myopathic conditions; or idiopathic.

Clinical Aspects of Habitual Scoliosis

Table 30-1 lists the four types of curves in paralytic and idiopathic scoliosis.

Lateral deviations of the spine must be treated as early as possible if scoliosis is to be prevented. Treatment should be preceded by a thorough clinical examination including a search for causative factors and for signs of a prominent hip, a sunken waistline, protruding ribs and scapula, a dropped shoulder, poor posture and backache. Examination is to be done in lying, sitting and standing positions. Lateral mobility of the spine in the lumbosacral region and the alignment and mobility of the rest of the spine should be studied. These studies should be followed by roentgenographic determination of the angles of the curve, either by Cobb's or Ferguson's method. Mild curves are defined radiographically as those between 0 and 69 degrees; severe curves, between 70 and 99 degrees; and very severe curves, 100 degrees or more.

Clinical Types of Scoliosis. There are two major groups, *nonprogressive* and *progressive* scoliosis. In nonprogressive scoliosis the most common forms are postural scoliosis occurring at the end of the period of growth, scoliosis secondary to obliquity of the pelvis or inequality of leg length, and reflex scoliosis associated with unilateral spasm of the erector spinae muscles. Nonprogressive scoliosis usually involves no deformity of any structural component and rarely requires lengthy treatment.

Progressive scoliosis may be congenital, but the great majority of cases are either idiopathic scoliosis or paralytic scoliosis. There are three major forms of idiopathic scoliosis: infantile, juvenile and adolescent. For the infantile form, starting between birth and the age of two years, prognosis is usually poor. Fortunately, some curves disappear without treatment within a year or two after diagnosis. The juvenile form, with an onset between 2 and 10 years, is uncommon. The earlier the onset the more severe the deformity. In adolescent idiopathic scoliosis, which comprises half of all scolioses, 40 per cent of the curves are of the lumbar pattern, with a slow pattern of deterioration and with a mean curve of 30 degrees, as opposed to curves in other forms, which reach nearly 60 degrees at maturity. In paralytic scoliosis, deterioration occurs faster

TABLE 30–1 SCOLIOTIC CURVES

Paralytic	Idiopathic
Right thoracic curve (Most common, occurs in 30% of patients)	Primary right dorsal curve (Most common)
High dorsal curve (Weakness of the shoulder girdle on the convex side)	Combined right dorsal and left lumbar curve (Apex of the curve is at the sixth to eighth thoracic vertebra)
Lumbar scoliosis (Occurs more often on the left side; the concavity is toward the stronger side unless the psoas muscle is involved)	Left total dorsolumbar curve (Apex of the curve is at the ninth or tenth thoracic vertebra)
Fixed paralytic pelvic obliquity	Primary left lumbar curve (Second most common curve; may involve the sacrum)
Prognosis	
The most obvious prognostic factor is the age at which the disease first affected the child.	The lower the location of the curve, the better the prognosis.

than in idiopathic scoliosis. The younger the patient at the onset of the curve, the more severe is the final curve.

The commonest symptoms of scoliosis are: instability of the spine, particularly in paralytic scoliosis; defects of posture evident in decompensated curves with tilting of the pelvis and flexion of one lower extremity; and pain, in later years of life. Rarely, paraplegia may occur, but without doubt the thoracic cage deformity with its resulting pulmonary disability is commonly the greatest functional impairment. Pulmonary function studies have demonstrated that exertional dyspnea is only noticeable in those with the more severe curves. Vital capacity and total lung capacity are severely diminished in those with curves of 90 degrees and above. Maximum voluntary ventilation is depressed in paralytic scoliosis with curves greater than 60 degrees. Airway resistance, previously considered uncommon, has been found to be frequent by Zorab. Pulmonary studies are important in evaluation of the operative risk in severely deformed children, especially the determination of the extent that a scoliotic patient can increase his ventilation—that is, his respiratory reserve.

Treatment of Scoliosis

The treatment of the early stages of scoliosis according to Bennett can be divided into four different parts, regional mobilization, muscle reeducation, support of the spine and limitation of activity.

Regional Mobilization.   The goal is to regain or maintain mobility in the affected region. Symmetric mobility must be obtained for successful muscle reeducation and support by bracing. Tight muscles may be stretched but there is no method of tightening the tissues on the convexity of the curve.

Manual stretching is effective and specific for the concavity of the low thoracic, thoracolumbar and high lumbar regions but not for the high thoracic region or the lumbosacral angle. To be effective it must be done very early, before the development of bony changes. The exercises should be done gently and repeated several times a day.

Stretching by plaster cast and wedging of the cast has limited value in correcting lumbosacral and high thoracic curves. Intermittent spinal traction is sometimes used. The patient holds an overhead bar and his own body weight is the stretching force.

Muscle Reeducation.   Muscle reeducation is essential in the care of scoliosis. It can be prescribed only after very accurate analysis and must be carried out only under the direct supervision of a trained therapist.

EXERCISES FOR FUNCTIONAL SCOLIOSIS.   Symmetric exercises for functional curves are done in the supine position, the prone position, or the crawling position.

In the supine position the patient is taught to realign his body symmetrically and to hold it in this position. Once he has learned to maintain his head, neck and trunk in a straight line, symmetric movements of the upper extremities are performed, alternating with movements of the lower extremities and such motions as arching the back.

In the prone position correct alignment is taught and then the patient progresses to stretching exercises, always performed symmetrically, and to

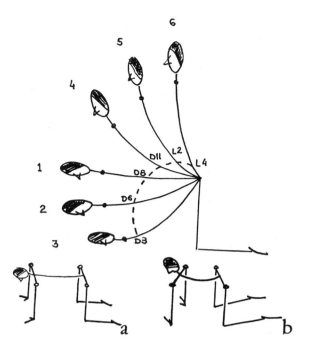

Figure 30–3 *Upper,* Diagrammatic illustration of levels of curve summits in relation to degree of lowering or straightening the plane of the back with respect to the plane of the floor. *Lower,* Horizontal quadruped: *a,* starting position; *b,* final position obtained after right lateral flexion which has created a left convex curve with summit at D8. (From Licht, S.: Therapeutic Exercise. 2nd Ed. New Haven, Conn., Elizabeth Licht, 1961.)

extension exercises of the neck, upper dorsal spine and lumbar and hip extensors. Dry swimming and cross stretching exercises are used.

In the crawling position, with his heels hooked under a stall bar, the patient assumes a kyphotic posture and, removing his arms from the floor, alternates the cross equilibrium of his body. He performs the same exercise in a lordotic posture and progresses to lateral flexion of the trunk or full extension of the spine in a kneeling position.

EXERCISES FOR STRUCTURAL SCOLIOSIS.   Knapp developed a system of exercises that have maximal effects on precise parts of the vertebral column.

If a patient supports himself on his knees and outstretched arms, motion takes place at the eighth thoracic vertebra. If elbows are semiflexed, motion takes place at the sixth thoracic vertebra. If the elbows are fully flexed the third thoracic segment is mobilized. The lower dorsal and lumbar vertebrae are mobilized when the degree of extension of the spine is lessened.

Scoliosis in the thoracic region is the most apparent, the most difficult to check and the greatest cause of embarrassment to the patient. Rotation is the only free movement possible in the thoracic portion of the spine. The purpose of derotation exercises is to shift the thorax toward the convex side and away from the concave. For the rotary exercises the patient lies over the edge of a table or on a mat where either the pelvis or the thorax can be held in a fixed position. Exercises at the stall bars and floor rolling exercises are also used.

Derotation exercises and Knapp exercises must be repeated several times a day, always under the supervision of a specially trained therapist. Frequent examinations of the patient are necessary so that progression in the exercises may be prescribed.

Support of the Spine.   Orthotic devices such as corsets, braces, adjustable frames and casts have long been used in the care of scoliosis. The aims in using

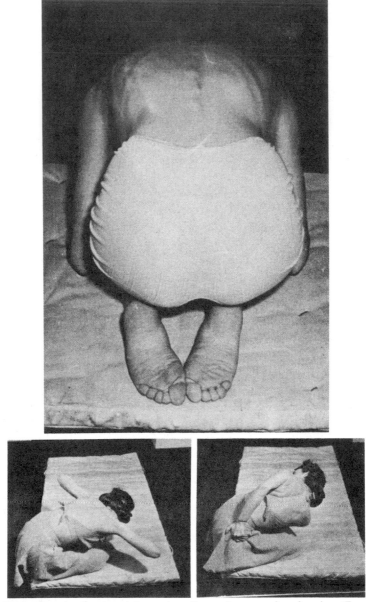

Figure 30–4   Exercise for dorsal derotation of curve in upper dorsal region. (From Woodcock, B.: Scoliosis. The Practical Approach to Treatment of Scoliosis. Stanford, Calif., Stanford University Press, 1946.)

these devices are fourfold: to support weak underlying musculature in the back and abdomen; to correct alignment by direct pressure over regions of convexity; to promote active correction by shifting the trunk and inducing the patient to maintain the correction in the sitting and upright positions; and to correct spinal alignment by distraction forces.

With the passage of time the value of the Milwaukee brace can now be better assessed: it can be used as a nonoperative treatment for scoliosis and in

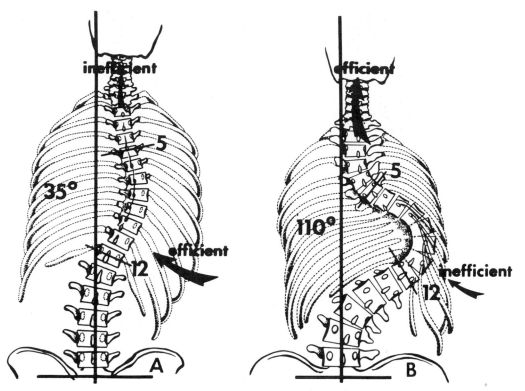

Figure 30–5   *A*, The correction of a curve of 35° is maintained principally by the holding force of the lateral pad. Distraction is an intermittent and less important force in the modern Milwaukee brace. *B*, In a curve of more than 90°, a lateral holding force compresses the ribs but is an inefficient factor in correcting the scoliosis. Distraction is more efficient and is frequently applied directly to bone by adding to the Milwaukee brace a halo and a frame for pin countertraction on the legs. (Courtesy of Dr. W. P. Blount.)

preventing spinal curves from becoming worse. The Milwaukee brace should be worn continuously and taken off only for hygienic purpose, swimming or exercises. It affords comfortable passive support by distraction and the holding force of lateral pads. A right thoracic and a left lumbar pad are usually used, with a well molded pelvic support, and a left shoulder ring is used to relieve some of the pressure at the neck. A ring flange is often used instead of a thoracic pad to counteract the tendency of the lumbar pad to increase the right thoracic curve and elevate the right shoulder. With snug fitting of the occipital support, the chin pad is placed so as to allow 3 or 4 cm. of motion to the chin. In the brace the thorax can move only in the direction of correction.

The brace is indicated for most adolescent patients who have idiopathic curves of moderate severity and for all preadolescent children, no matter what the etiology or the severity of the curve. With use of the brace, congenital curves may improve and compensatory curves may be reduced and cosmesis improved, but fusion is always possible if the curves cannot be controlled. The brace is worn until the patient is mature. If the curve is reduced to 10 degrees or less, the patient is then allowed to wear the brace at night only. Long

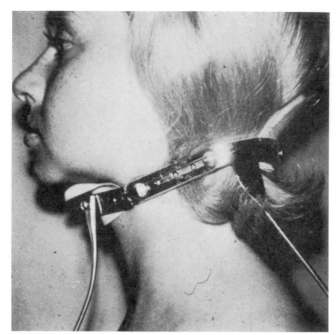

Figure 30–6 In the spring of 1969 the chin pad which had been worn low and close against the neck for several years was abandoned in favor of a more functionally designed throat mold of thermoplastic. The neck ring and occiput pad were made smaller and more closely fitting. Adequate distraction was obtained by the occiput pad as long as the head was held against it. The throat mold caused no pressure on the mandible but held against the anterior surface of the neck. The anterior projection reminded the patient to hold his chin up. The patients accepted the innovation gladly because the Milwaukee brace was now inconspicuous when a collar or scarf was worn and the hair allowed to fall over the back of the brace. (Courtesy of Dr. W. P. Blount.)

continued pressure on the mandible may cause a bite deformity. All patients should be seen by an orthodontist before initiation of the treatment, and prophylactic treatment is sometimes indicated. Exercises with the braces off are to be given daily. In the brace the child will try to shift away, actively, from the lumbar pad, arching the back. Pelvic roll exercises, energetic breathing exercises and active hyperextension exercises are indicated.

Exercises in the Milwaukee brace, as described by Blount and Bolinske:

Each exercise is held to the count of five and repeated ten times, once or twice daily.

1. Pelvic tilt, supine, with knees flexed (can be taught first with patient in quadruped position).

2. Pelvic tilt, supine, with knees straight.

3. Sit up, with pelvic tilt. Patients often need assistance to perform properly.

4. Hyperextension while lying prone. With the knees held down, tilt the pelvis and raise head and shoulder against resistance.

5. Push ups with the pelvis tilted.

6. Active correction of major curve. Ambulation with pelvis tilted and chest pulled away from the pad.

7. Tilt pelvis in standing position, inhale deeply and press backward toward the posterior bars with the chest.

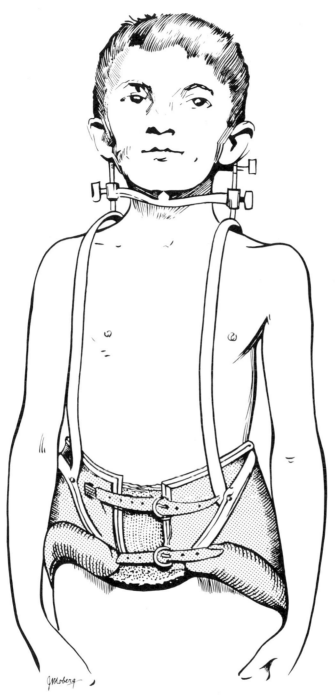

Figure 30–7   With a sharp button under the chin and another under the occiput the child had to stand up straight or else! Spitzy's brace included the head but offered no support. If the child wanted to rest from his active correction he had to lie down. The brace was not popular. (Reprinted from Orthotics, New Haven, Conn., Elizabeth Licht, Publisher, 1966.)

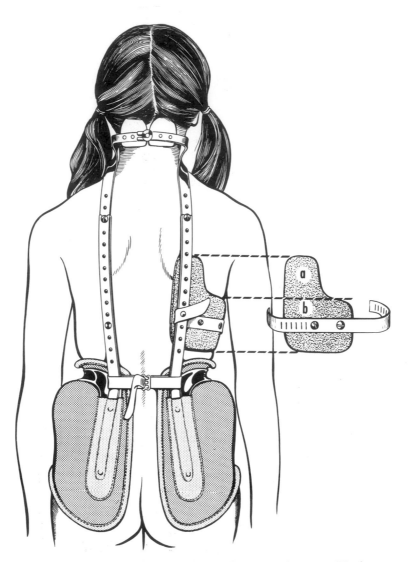

Figure 30–8   The basic thoracic pad is "L" shaped for several reasons. The lower part "B" is roughly rectangular and extends anteriorly to exert a holding force in the medial direction. It should lie snugly against the chest wall and contact the lower four ribs of the thoracic curve. If it is to maintain this position the strap must cross the middle of the rectangle.

The smaller cephalad portion "A" is backed up by the posterior upright. When the patient is recumbent, it exerts a passive corrective force on the rib hump. During ambulation its curved top edge does not traumatize the scapula as it passes under the pad and out again during arm motions. It is far enough back to be out of the way of the arm itself.

The posterior end of the strap is usually passed under and around the near bar and secured to a truss stud. The position of the strap need not often be changed and the ends can be held securely by tape. If the pad is to extend medial to the bar as it should, the posterior screw that holds the strap to the pad must be near the middle of the rectangular portion, not medial to this point. (Courtesy of Dr. W. P. Blount.)

One can foretell whether the patient will be successful after he has been wearing a brace for a certain time. Harrington described three types of brace wearers. (1) The brace rider, who refuses to exercise in the brace, develops ulcers under the chin and flaring of the teeth. (2) The second type, who lifts the chin clear out of the brace and turns his head sideways, probably to secure some relief from this peculiar position. (3) The third type of patient will constantly exercise and achieve good results. The decision to remove the brace must await the complete ossification of the vertebrae, a condition that is best determined by ossification of the iliac crest.

Demineralization and muscle atrophy must be rectified before the brace is discarded, despite completion of the ossification. This takes about three to six months and is accomplished in the following manner: the patient is initially allowed to be out of the brace for one hour three times a week, during which he is restricted to lying down, supine exercises and erect postural exercises in front of a mirror. During the following two weeks he is allowed one hour daily with the same program of exercises. In the succeeding two weeks he remains out of the brace for two hours daily; the additional hour is spent in activities of the patient's choice, except that competitive sports are forbidden. Gradually, the time spent out of the brace is extended until the patient progresses to a full day out of the brace. Maintenance of his correction should be checked by periodic x-ray examinations.

Surgical Stabilization.   Surgery is necessary in 5 to 10 per cent of the patients who have idiopathic scoliosis and in approximately 30 per cent of those with paralytic scoliosis. Surgery is indicated for a rapidly progressive curve and for the following types of curvature, according to Steindler: the long right dorsal curve; the lumbar curve that includes the sacrum; the high dorsal and cervicodorsal curve; scoliosis that causes pain in a patient who is past maturity; and the kyphoscoliotic curve that threatens to cause paraplegia.

Patients are usually placed in a Risser localizer cast. If correction is judged insufficient, the use of several additional casts or wedging the initial cast will allow further correction. Surgery is performed through a window in the cast, by fusion or by Harrington's internal fixation. This technique does not give optimal correction in severe rigid curves and in cases with severe pelvic obliquity. In those cases very favorable results have been obtained by the use of Halo femoral distraction in preparation for surgery. It must be borne in mind, however, that even surgical measures are not entirely effective in correcting structural changes. A dropped shoulder can be elevated and a hip can be made less obvious, but the deformity of prominent ribs cannot be overcome.

Pseudarthrosis is a frequent complication after spinal fusion. Significant growth in length of the fused portion of the spine is improbable and has not been convincingly demonstrated.

Limitation of Activity.   The control of activities is especially necessary in the management of paralytic scoliosis and often is completely neglected. Alignment of the patient's spine when he is at rest is important but it is more important when he is in a sitting or standing position. Specific functional training must be limited until spinal alignment has been obtained.

Rest periods should be provided while the patient is attending school with his brace on. Periods of 20 minutes every three hours are recommended. Such rest periods should take place daily four times a day in the supine position, not only on school days but seven days a week. In addition, the reclining position is to be assumed while watching television, listening to the radio and phonograph, and making telephone calls.

Conclusion

It is evident that the difficulties in the management of scoliosis are far from being solved. Persistent deviations of the spine can be dealt with successfully only if they are recognized early in the course of their development and treated competently throughout the growing years.

REFERENCES

Low Back Syndrome

Brown, T., Hansen, R. J., and Yorra, A. J.: Some Mechanical Tests on the Lumbosacral Spine with Particular Reference to Intervertebral Discs; a Preliminary Report. J. Bone Joint Surg., 39A:1135, 1957.

Caillet, R.: Rehabilitation Management of the Patient with Low Back Pain. Mod. Treatm., 5:1022-1035, 1968.

Kraus, H.: Clinical Treatment of Back and Neck Pain. New York, McGraw-Hill Book Company, 1970.

Moore, W. H., Jr., Dehne, E., and Kiersch, T. A.: Low Back Pain and its Management at the Dispensary Level. Milit. Med., May, 1960.

Morris, J. M., Lucas, D. B., and Bresler, B.: The Role of the Trunk in the Stability of the Spine. J. Bone Joint Surg., 43A:327, 1961.

Norton, P. L., and Brown, T.: The Immobilizing Efficiency of Back Braces: Their Effect on the Posture and Motion of the Lumbosacral Joint. J. Bone Joint Surg., 39A:111, 1957.

Scoliosis

American Academy of Orthopaedic Surgeons: Symposium on the Spine, Nov., 1967, pp. 188-240.

Bennett, R. L.: Classification and Treatment of Early Lateral Deviations of the Spine Following Acute Anterior Poliomyelitis. Arch. Phys. Med., 36:9-17, 1955.

Bennett, R. L.: Recognition and Care of Early Scoliosis. Arch. Phys. Med., 42:211-225, 1961.

Blount, W. P.: Scoliosis and Milwaukee Bracing. Bull. Hosp. Joint Dis., 19:152-165, 1958.

Blount, W. P.: The Principles of Treatment, According to Curve Patterns, of Scoliosis and Round Back, with the Milwaukee Brace. Post-graduate Course on the Management and Care of the Scoliosis Patient. New York Orthopaedic Hospital, 1969.

Blount, W. P., and Schmidt, A. C.: The Milwaukee Brace in the Operative Treatment of Scoliosis. J. Bone Joint Surg., 40A:511–525, 1951.

Blount, W. and Bolinske, J.: Physical Therapy in the Nonoperative Treatment of Scoliosis. Phys. Ther., 47:919-25, 1967.

Butte, F. L.: Scoliosis Treated by the Wedging Jacket. J. Bone Joint Surg., 20:1-22, 1938.

Christman, V. D., et al.: A Study of the Results Following Rotatory Manipulation in the Lumbar Intervertebral Disc Syndrome. J. Bone Joint Surg., 46A:517-526, 1964.

Cobb, J. R.: Outline for Study of Scoliosis. Instruct. Lect. Amer. Acad. Orthop. Surg., 5:261-275, 1948.

Colonna, P. C., and von Saal, F.: Study of Paralytic Scoliosis. J. Bone Joint Surg., 23:335, 1941.

Ferguson, A. B.: Roentgen Interpretation and Decision in Scoliosis. Instruct. Lect. Amer. Acad. Orthop. Surg., 7:160-167, 1950.

Gucker, T.: Experiences with Poliomyelitic Scoliosis After Fusion and Correction. J. Bone Joint Surg., 38A:1281-1300, 1956.

Harrington, P. R.: Treatment of Scoliosis-Correction and Internal Fixation by Spine Instrumentation. J. Bone Joint Surg., 44A:591-610, 1962.

Harrington, P. R.: Nonoperative Treatment of Scoliosis. Texas Med., 64:54-65, 1968.

James, J. I. P.: Idiopathic Scoliosis; Prognosis, Diagnosis, and Operative Indications Related to Curve Patterns and Age of Onset. J. Bone Joint Surg., 36B:36-49, 1954.

Kleinberg, S.: Scoliosis: Pathology, Etiology and Treatment. Baltimore, Williams and Wilkins Co., 1951.

Krusen, F. H.: Physical Medicine. Philadelphia, W. B. Saunders Co., 1941, pp. 582-587.

Mennell, J.: Back Pain. Boston, Little, Brown and Co., 1960, pp. 109-128.

Moe, J. H.: Management of Idiopathic Scoliosis. Clin. Orthop., 20:169-184, 1957.

Moe, J. H., et al.: Treatment of Scoliosis. J. Bone Joint Surg., 46A:293-312, 1964.

Moe, J. H., et al.: Harrington Instrumentation in Correction of Scoliosis. J. Bone Joint Surg., 46A:313-321, 1964.

Ponseti, I. V., and Friedman, B.: Prognosis in Idiopathic Scoliosis. J. Bone Joint Surg., *32A:*381-395, 1950.

Ponseti, I. V., and Friedman, B.: Changes in the Scoliotic Spine After Fusion. J. Bone Joint Surg., *32A:*751-766, 1950.

Risser, J. C.: Important Practical Facts in the Treatment of Scoliosis. Instruct. Lect. Amer. Acad. Orthop. Surg., *5:*248-260, 1948.

Steindler, A.: Idiopathic Scoliosis, Post Graduate Lectures on Orthopedic Diagnosis. Vol. II, pp. 101-123. Charles C Thomas, Springfield, Illinois, 1951.

Stillwell, D. L., Jr.: Structural Deformities of Vertebrae. Bone Adaptation in Experimental Scoliosis and Kyphosis. J. Bone Joint Surg., *44A:*611-634, 1962.

Willis, T. A.: Man's Back. Springfield, Ill., Charles C Thomas, 1953, pp. 129-132.

Zaoussis & James: The Iliac Apophysis and the Evolution of Curves in Scoliosis. J. Bone Joint Surg., *40B:*442-453, 1958.

Zorab, P. A.: Scoliosis. Springfield, Illinois, Charles C Thomas, 1969, pp. 30-38.

Back Disorders

Barr, J. S., and Riseborough, E. J.: Treatment of Low-Back and Sciatic Pain in Patients Over 60 Years of Age. Clin. Orthop., *26:*12-18, 1963.

Collins, D. H.: The Pathology of Articular and Spinal Diseases. Baltimore, Williams and Wilkins Co., 1950.

Freyberg, R. H., and Rogoff, B.: Diagnosis on Common Causes of Backache. Med. Clin. N. Amer., *38:*655, 1954.

Goldthwait, J. E.: The Lumbo-Sacral Articulation. An Explanation of Many Cases of "Lumbago,' Sciatica and Paraplegia. Med. & Surg. J., *152:*365-369, 1911.

Haboush, E. J.: An Anatomical Explanation of Traumatic Low Back Pain. J. Bone Joint Surg., *24:*123-134, 1942.

Haggart, G. E., and Grannis, W. R.: Management of Low Back and Sciatic Pain. Amer. J. Surg., *85:*339-346, 1953.

Hirsch, C., and Schajowicz, F.: Studies on Structural Changes in the Lumbar Annulus Fibrosus. Acta Orthop. Scand., *22:*184-231, 1953.

Keegan, J. J.: Neurosurgical Interpretation of Dermatome Hypalgesia with Herniation of the Lumbar Intervertebral Disc. J. Bone Joint Surg., *26:*238-248, 1944.

Knapp, M. D.: Low-Back Pain. Conservative Management. Arch. Indust. Hyg., *19:*577-584, 1957.

Kottke, F. J.: Evaluation and Treatment of Low Back Pain Due to Mechanical Causes. Arch. Phys. Med., *38:*395-401, 1957.

Krusen, E., and Ford, D.: Conservative Treatment of Certain Types of Back Injury. Arch. Phys. Med., *38:*395-401, 1957.

Krusen, F. H.: Physical Medicine. Philadelphia, W. B. Saunders Co., 1941, pp. 579-581.

Lewin, P.: Backache and Sciatic Neuritis. Philadelphia, Lea and Febiger, 1943.

Lindblom, K., and Hultquist, G. T.: Absorption of Protruded Disc Tissue. J. Bone Joint Surg., *32A:*557-560, 1950.

Love, J. G.: Treatment of Protruded Intervertebral Disks. Minnesota Med., *23:*692-695, 1940.

Middleton, G. S., and Teacher, J.: Injury to the Spinal Cord due to Rupture of an Intervertebral Disc During Muscular Effort. Glasgow Med. J., *76:*139-144, 1911.

Policoff, L.: Diagnostic Challenge of Back Pain. Arch. Phys. Med., *41:*441-445, 1960.

Ramsey, R. H.: Conservative Treatment of Disc Lesions. Instruct. Lect. Amer. Acad. Orthop. Surg., *11:*118-120, 1954.

Schmorl, G., and Junghanns, H.: The Human Spine in Health and Disease. New York, Grune and Stratton, 1959.

Smith, A. D., et al.: Herniation of the Nucleus Pulposus. J. Bone Joint Surg., *26:*821-828, 1944.

Steindler, A.: Lumbosacralgia, Post-Graduate Lectures on Orthopedic Diagnosis. Vol. II, pp. 81-99, Springfield, Illinois, Charles C Thomas, 1951.

Turek, S. L.: Orthopaedics. Philadelphia, J. B. Lippincott Co., 1959, pp. 746-770.

Williams, P. C.: Conservative Management of Lesions of the Lumbosacral Spine. Instruct. Lect. Amer. Acad. Orthop. Surg., *10:*90-121, 1953.

Wiig, N.: The Preoperative Clinical Diagnosis of Lumbar Disc Prolapse; Its Reliability and Practical Applicability. Acta Clin. Scand. Suppl., *295:*1-100, 1962.

Winter, E.: Lumbo-Pelvic Manipulation Technique. Vie Med., *44:*81-94, 1963.

Chapter 31

MANAGEMENT OF NEUROGENIC DYSFUNCTION OF THE BLADDER AND BOWEL

by Herbert S. Talbot

The problems arising from neurogenic dysfunction of the bladder or bowel, to be discussed in this chapter, are those encountered among patients with injury or disease of the spinal cord. Although there are neuromuscular analogies that justify their consideration together, the empiric demands of treatment make it convenient to discuss the two individually. The interrelationships will be self-evident.

THE BLADDER

The management of neurogenic bladder dysfunction is too important to be left as a matter for occasional consultation. The urologist should be an active member of the team that follows the patient day by day. By the same token, any physician charged with the over-all care of these patients, whatever his own specialty, must have an understanding of the urinary tract dysfunction and the methods available for treatment according to the needs of the individual patient. This last element cannot be overemphasized; it may provide the determining factor in many important decisions. The bladder does not exist in a vacuum and its dysfunction is not all the spinal cord injury patient has to contend with. The plan for each patient's urological care must be an integrated part of the whole plan of treatment.[8]

The basic problem is to insure urinary drainage while avoiding infection but, unfortunately, with most forms of artificial drainage infection soon appears. Yet, at least temporarily, some means of emptying the bladder must be found. Moreover, there are two corollary requirements: first, the drainage must be not only of the bladder but also of the upper tract, dysfunction of which may be insidious in onset but ultimately destructive; second, any permanent solution must insure continence, either natural or contrived, so that to the patient's well-being may be added the opportunity for socioeconomic rehabilitation. The dilemma is eased by two features. Artificial drainage may be required only temporarily, as will be described later. If this period is relatively short, infection may be avoided or, if it occurs, may clear up readily. The other encouraging observation is that infection of the bladder is not inevitably accompanied by infection of the kidneys.

The complexities of the neurophysiology of the bladder need not be considered here, nor the elaborate classifications of disturbed function which have arisen from investigation of these mechanisms. For ordinary purposes it is sufficient to consider two main categories as proposed by Bors: (1) The lower motor neuron type, with a lesion involving the region of the cord in which the spinal reflex center for micturition is located or its communicating pathways; this means lesions of the conus or cauda equina or both; (2) the upper motor neuron type, with a lesion at a level cephalad to the spinal reflex centers. In the latter case, the reflex activity of the bladder is preserved; in the former it is gone. Both groups may be further subdivided according to whether the cord transection is complete or incomplete. It is occasionally more difficult to manage the dysfunction of an incomplete than of a complete lesion. Bors suggested the word "balanced" to describe a situation in which there is a satisfactory ratio of residual urine to bladder capacity (not more than 1.5 for the upper motor neuron or 1:10 for the lower). The term, however, may be usefully applied as well in a more general context. Normal detrusor activity, both in holding and expelling the bladder content, is the resultant of a complex integration of neurogenic and myogenic activities which is easily upset by the loss or modifications of one or more; in this sense, any dysfunction represents a loss of balance. The best management is that which attempts restoration by physiologic means.[2, 3]

More refined classification, while occasionally useful for investigative purposes, may be confusing or misleading when an attempt is made to apply it clinically. Pushed too far it may lead to the intellectual Procrustean felony of stretching or trimming the case to match the category. There are remarkable variations among patients, even those with apparently similar lesions. The neurogenic dysfunction is often overlaid by secondary structural changes, the results of infection, distention, contracture or any combination of these. Treatment should be designed to prevent such changes so that there is at least a chance to deal with the neural disturbance in its pure form.

Intermittent catheterization, introduced by Guttmann, provides drainage with the lowest incidence of infection of any method yet recommended.[4] He has shown that, if a meticulous technique is employed, it is possible to catheterize patients three times a day for weeks or even months until a voiding pattern is established, the urine remaining sterile throughout in a majority of patients. Others have reported similar results.[5, 9] A disadvantage is that overdistention of the bladder may occur during the intervals between catheterizations, even though the patient be kept on a limited and regulated fluid intake. To avoid this Bors has modified the method, catheterizing as frequently as every four hours.[1]

The daily fluid intake should be held at 2000 ml., which is most easily accomplished by having the patient drink 120 ml. per hour during his waking hours. Catheterization is planned at intervals of four hours, but attempts at voiding should be encouraged just before the bladder is drained and halfway through the interval. This is done by straining or by firm pressure in the suprapubic region (sometimes, but not altogether correctly, called a Credé maneuver). The amount voided must be carefully recorded. If the total reaches 200 ml. during the four-hour period and there is no physical evidence of distention, the scheduled catheterization is omitted and the whole procedure repeated two hours later, using the same criteria to determine whether catheterization is required. It is not safe to wait longer than this because micturition, especially in the beginning, may be capricious. The patient may void well two or three times and then be unable to do so again during the rest of the day or even longer. Moreover, diuresis is often irregular. A patient who has put out 200 or 300 ml. of urine during a four-hour interval may suddenly produce 600 during half that time. For this reason, no simple rule of thumb is possible and continuing close observation is essential.

Under a consistent regimen of this type, function tends to improve and less frequent catheterization is necessary; as the amount of residual urine after voiding decreases, so also does the need for catheterization, which may be scheduled for thrice, twice and ultimately only once daily. When the residual has for several days been 60 ml. or less, catheterization may be discontinued; it is desirable to continue to check the residual, but this may be done at lengthening intervals.

The majority of patients handled in this manner will have established a good voiding function in from four to eight weeks, all other things being equal. The method is not easy; it requires trained people, meticulous techniques, accurate recording of the fluid intake and output in detail and constant exercise of judgment. All that need be said is that if it works, as it does in most cases if done well, it will have been worth the effort. In the lower motor neuron cases voiding will have to be initiated by the so-called Credé maneuver or abdominal straining or both. With an upper motor neuron lesion, the bladder empties spontaneously, being reflexly stimulated by a certain degree of distention. The frequency with which this occurs is naturally of great importance. Most patients can be trained so that micturition occurs no more frequently than is compatible with social and vocational activities. There is, however, no consensus of opinion as to how this training or reflex conditioning can best be achieved; some hold, in fact, that it is usually accomplished by the patient himself, regardless of what other efforts are made.

In general, intermittent catheterization is not the method of choice when infection of the urinary tract is present. The question then arises how to manage the patient admitted to the spinal cord injury center weeks or months after injury, which is so often the case, with an indwelling urethral catheter and infection present, at least in the bladder. If the delay has not been too great and the bladder not yet permanently contracted, tidal drainage may be of great value.[7] Although less widely used than in the past, it still has its advocates, including the author. Its hygienic effect is beneficial and it may have a conditioning influence which encourages the return of reflex micturition and the establishment of a satisfactory and consistent pattern, although this is not universally conceded. It is not used when there is marked hypertonicity or hypotonicity of the bladder. Figure 31-1 is a diagram of a simple form of

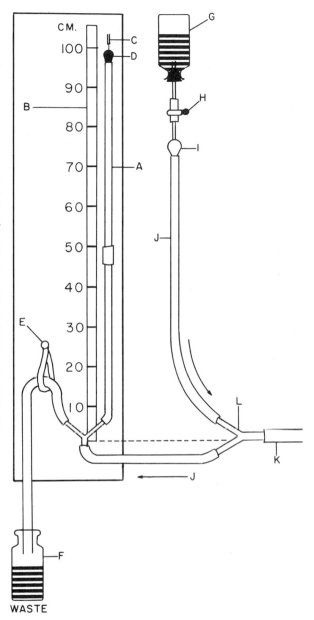

Figure 31–1 Tidal drainage. The apparatus can be mounted conveniently on a board which is fastened by clamps to a bedpost. (A) Six-mm. glass tubing. Two 50-cm. lengths jointed by a short piece of rubber tubing. (B) Centimeter scale marked on cardboard strip. (C) Hypodermic needle, about 23 gauge, inserted in rubber cap as air vent. (D) Rubber medicine cap. (E) Adjustable siphon loop suspended by a thumb tack at appropriate level. Latex tubing, 30-40 inches long; thickness of wall, 3/32″; internal diameter, 3/16″. (F) Waste bottle. The zero level on the manometer should coincide with the level of the symphysis. (G) Dispensing bottle. (H) Screw clamp to control inflow at 60-90 drops per minute. (I) Murphy bulb. (J) Latex tubing, 60-72 inches long; thickness of wall, 1/16″; internal diameter, 1/4″. (K) Catheter. (L) Glass Y-tubes.

apparatus which has proved very effective. Ordinarily the irrigant is sterile normal saline solution; when indicated, a buffered preparation such as "G" solution may be used. Various antibiotic solutions have not usually been effective in eradicating established infection, although they may be of some prophylactic value.

When tidal drainage is begun, the siphon loop should be set at 6 cm. above the level of the symphysis; when the apparatus is functioning properly, this is raised by 2 cm. every two or three days until it reaches a level of 18 cm., at which point it is maintained for a week or two. The catheter is then removed and the patient given a trial at voiding, the management being similar to that already described for intermittent catheterization. This is often a trying period and the process should be carefully explained to the patient so that his cooperation may be enlisted. He must understand that the temporary inconvenience is the price he pays for ultimate good function. If, after several days of trial, the patient is still unable to void, tidal drainage may be resumed and the whole procedure repeated. There is no way of predicting success nor of estimating how long a time may be required to achieve it. Many patients will fail on the first two or three attempts and then, for no apparent reason, succeed after the next. It is not necessary to keep the patient in bed for tidal drainage if he is otherwise able to be up. The apparatus is disconnected and the catheter clamped while he is out of bed, the bladder being drained at intervals similar to those at which it was being siphoned; making due allowance for the fact that no irrigating fluid is being added.

Regardless of what else it may or may not accomplish, tidal drainage has the important effect of keeping the bladder filling and emptying regularly, avoiding both overdistention and the risk of contracture from being continually empty. This in itself is of great importance in the physiological management of bladder dysfunction. It can, of course, be achieved by manually controlled methods of intermittent filling and emptying or even by clamping the indwelling catheter. The functional similarity of any of these procedures to early intermittent catheterization is apparent.

After reflex micturition has been established, the problem of stress incontinence must be met, for it is present, in varying degree, in a majority of patients. In a fortunate few, the bladder, although not hypotonic, is relatively tolerant to distention. These may, in fact, have difficulty in initiating micturition, but if they learn to void at regular intervals and if the residual urine is not excessive (i.e., less than 60 ml.), they get along very well. Voiding may be begun by abdominal straining, manual pressure over the lower abdomen or, more rarely, by a triggering act such as brisk tapping of the lower abdomen, squeezing the meatus, or application of any one of a number of stimuli which the patient may discover for himself. In a number of instances, particularly with high lesions, it has been found that if the patient wears a light adjustable lower abdominal girdle, he will remain continent when it is loose but be able to initiate voiding quite readily when it is tightened. There is some danger that, since he experiences no sensation, he will not remember to void frequently enough, so that in time the bladder will become overdistended and inefficient.

In another group, the bladder is more readily stimulated by distention but still accumulates a reasonable content before emptying reflexly. Among these patients, continence is possible provided the bladder is not allowed to fill to the point at which reflex micturition will occur. In such cases, some form of conditioning, however managed, is of importance, for it may thus be possible to achieve a certain consistency of capacity—a level of filling at which the reflex contraction may be anticipated. With good habit training and timed voiding, involuntary emptying may be avoided. Some individuals accomplish this readily; others, equally intelligent, cannot seem to master it. With patient effort and explanation on the part of the physician and reasonable receptiveness on the part of the patient, the discouragement and inconvenience of a poor beginning may be overcome and a satisfactory result ultimately obtained. This is difficult, trying and time-consuming, but the end is well worth the means.

There is always some risk of stress incontinence, even for the patient who has trained himself to timed voiding. Coughing, sneezing, laughter and sudden movements are most often responsible. (The bladder should always be emptied before a period of exercise.) Moreover, there are occasions when the patient may not have access to toilet facilities for a longer period than he is able to hold his urine. Against such contingencies, the best device is the so-called "C" drainage—a condom coupled by a small plastic adaptor to a latex tube which leads to a bedside urinal or one attached to the leg. The condom is best secured to the penis by a band of cement of the type used for ileostomy appliances. Since there is no pull on it, this has no other purpose than to make a water-tight fit. Straps of any kind should be avoided, for patients tend to apply them too tightly. The results include not only excoriation of the skin but periurethral abscesses and fistulas. The tubing should be of 5/16 inch external diameter and 1/4 inch internal diameter. This provides sufficient capillary action to keep the condom empty. The urinal bags should be of plastic, as strongly made as possible, and of adequate capacity. Many patients prefer rubber urinals because they are stronger, but it is difficult to keep them clean and free from odor, to which, unfortunately, the patient may become so accustomed that he does not notice it. Wearers of this apparatus must be thoroughly instructed in the hygiene of its use. A good method is to wear it for no more than 11 hours, allowing an interval of an hour during which it is removed and the skin of the penis and the meatus carefully cleansed.

"C" drainage ought to be considered a supplement to rather than a substitute for bladder training. Some require it only at certain periods—during sleep, for instance, although it is often possible for a patient to get through the night without it by being awakened to void. It is a fact, however, that the convenience of this apparatus has tempted many to use it constantly, and it is difficult to argue against this if it is properly managed. In this sense it may be considered, as one patient has put it, a portable invisible toilet.

For the female there is no similar appliance. If the incontinence is slight, the wearing of a pad with rubber or plastic panties may suffice, but if there is any considerable leakage this is disagreeable and uncomfortable. In such circumstances, an indwelling catheter may be more practicable, if not ideal. Here again, however, there is the disadvantage that the short urethra tends to dilate around the catheter and leaking occurs. Changing to a larger catheter has no more than a temporary effect, for the urethra continues to dilate. Occasionally the leakage is due to a hyperactive detrusor which may be amenable to correction. If there is active cystitis it should be managed by appropriate local or general treatment. Stones or encrustations must be removed. When no obvious pathology is noted, the activity of the bladder can sometimes be modified by hexamethonium chloride, 60 mg., three times daily at the beginning, which may be gradually increased to a dose of 240 mg. if required. Propantheline bromide, Pro-Banthine, 10 to 20 mg. three or four times a day, may be effective. Treatment by drugs should not be continued for more than two weeks. Sacral block, including the 2nd, 3rd and the 4th sacral nerves on each side, has been useful in a number of patients. Its effect is temporary but lasts longer than the expected pharmacologic effect of the agent used, and, if repeated two or three times, may last for weeks or months. All these measures, of course, may be applied to males as well when it is desired to modify excessive detrusor activity. In spite of them, the indwelling catheter in the female may continue to be unmanageable so that the patient must be offered some type of urinary diversion, such as an ileal conduit; with careful management, this should be a rare outcome.

In spite of every effort, there are patients who will be unable to void. Some of these may be helped by relatively conservative surgical procedures, such as transurethral resection or external sphincterotomy, but it is preferable to delay these for at least six months and preferably a year in order to allow full opportunity for physiologic restoration. Suprapubic cystostomy may be used, usually temporarily, in the presence of urethral complications; it is not recommended as a definitive method of permanent management. Supravesical diversion, such as a uretero-ileal conduit, should be reserved for those rare cases in which the bladder has become not only unmanageable but an actual liability.

Current experience is that about 20 to 25 per cent of patients either cannot void or cannot safely carry on with reflex micturition. The latter group comprises those who exhibit symptoms of autonomic dysreflexia (usually hypertension) when the intravesical pressure rises even moderately, or who have upper tract complications that make elevated pressures dangerous. These are usually associated with vesico-ureteral reflex, but it is incorrect to suppose that reflux in itself is an absolute contraindication to elimination of the catheter. In a mild form, and with the ureter able to empty when the bladder empties (which can be determined fluoroscopically), it is not incompatible with good reflex micturition.

When an indwelling catheter is used, a size 16 F. Foley with a 5 cc. balloon is preferred. This may be irrigated once each day, with normal saline or "G" solution, and should be changed at least once a week, or more frequently if necessary, and at once if it should become blocked. The glans, meatus and adjacent portion of the catheter should be cleansed with soap and water several times daily; dressings are unnecessary. Drainage bags or jugs should be emptied and cleansed, or replaced, at intervals of no longer than eight hours. Routine prophylactic use of antibiotics is unwise, but acidulation of the urine is desirable if it can be accomplished. The urine should be examined and cultures taken regularly, and excretory urograms done at least every six months during the first two years, then at yearly intervals. The kidney function is surveyed regularly by the usual chemical tests. During recent years, the I^{131} hippuran renogram has been found useful for following not only renal function but certain aspects of the dynamics of the urinary tract as well.

There are other problems faced by patients with spinal cord lesions which have an important bearing upon or relation to the care of the bladder; only two of which need to be mentioned here. The formation of kidney and bladder stones reflects disturbances of calcium metabolism as well as disorders of the urinary tract. So far as renal stones are concerned, their incidence can be markedly decreased by a relatively simple regimen. Musculoskeletal activity, beginning as soon as possible after injury, is of primary importance. Passive as well as active exercises may be useful, but the most effective are those which prevent rapid loss of calcium from the bones by at least simulating the stress of weight-bearing. Adequate drainage of the urinary tract has already been discussed. Except when interdicted by special circumstances, a generous fluid intake (3500 to 4000 ml. daily) will reduce the likelihood of supersaturation by providing a greater volume of solvent and is, at the same time, a useful hygienic measure. Since the usual calcium salts precipitate more readily in an alkaline medium, acidulation of the urine is desirable, although the frequent presence of urea-splitting organisms makes this difficult to accomplish. None of the commonly used acidulants is notably effective in achieving the desired pH of 5.5 to 6. Cranberry juice is as good as any and most patients find it palatable; the usual dose is 250 ml. twice a day. Ascorbic acid, in doses of 1 gm. four times a day, works well in sterile urine but has little effect when the urine is heavily infected. When effective acidulation is impossible, dilution becomes even more important.

Striated muscle spasm has variable effects upon the function of the bladder. Powerful contractions of the abdominal or thigh muscles or both may set off detrusor contraction, regardless of the level of the bladder filling, and interfere seriously with the effort to establish a consistent pattern of micturition. When the spasm involves the muscles within the urogenital diaphragm, it can prevent voiding by the resulting compression or angulation of the urethra. The treatment of spasm is not to be considered here but it must be noted that, before such treatment is undertaken, its possible further contribution to neurogenic bladder dysfunction must be carefully calculated.[6]

THE BOWEL

Although the dysfunctions are in some respects analagous, those of the lower bowel are not so immediately hazardous to health as those of the bladder. With its normally solid content and less frequent need for evacuation, the problems of reconditioning and habit training should be considerably simpler. Further, since the content is normally infected there is no such disastrous consequence of obstruction as obtains in the urinary tract. Yet, from the point of view of the patient's socioeconomic rehabilitation, to say nothing of its psychological importance, the establishment of regular evacuation without the need for regular enemas and without fear of involuntary movements is very important. Enemas should scarcely ever be necessary after the first two weeks; the fact that many patients depend upon them reflects an earlier failure to deal with bowel care.

Habit training may be begun as soon as the patient is out of shock, capable of receiving instructions, and able to take food by mouth. The diet should be such as to produce a stool of normal consistency. Diarrhea in a spinal cord injury patient is a sorry experience for himself and his attendants; any such tendency must be promptly and vigorously investigated. Scybala are prone to produce impactions which require manual extraction. A specific time of day should be established for defecation and the schedule kept closely. At first, the patient merely strains; this will naturally be facilitated by his being up, but should be started while he is bedfast. If the abdominal musculature is ineffective, a belt or binder may be worn during the effort. If this is unsuccessful, nothing more is done that day. The attempt is repeated the next day and, if there is no result, supplemented by the use of a glycerine or Dulcolax suppository. If there is still no bowel movement, nothing more is done until the third day. Then, if straining and suppository fail to work, an enema may be given. This may be with soapsuds, 250 to 500 ml., or the commercially available citrate and phosphate solutions that come ready for use in a plastic container. Whenever there is a bowel movement the patient returns next day to the first day of the schedule.

With this or a similar routine, if it is started soon enough, most patients will develop satisfactory bowel habits. Some have a daily movement but this is not essential; a regular movement every second or even every third day is quite satisfactory. Digital dilatation of the anal sphincter will often serve as well as an enema. Small doses of mild cathartics, such as milk of magnesia, as a supplement to this program may help in certain cases. Muscular activity is enormously important. The patient who is up and exercising every day is seldom constipated. In this, as in many other respects, the quadriplegic is at some disadvantage because his activity is relatively limited. A good bowel habit can still be established, but there is a tendency to chronic moderate distention, more noticeable, perhaps, on the x-ray film than on physical examination. In the investigation of a patient suspected of an intra-abdominal lesion, it is important not to interpret this as actual ileus. Once a good habit pattern has been established, involuntary defecation is unusual as long as the stool remains of normal consistency.

When an enema is required, it is best given with the patient sitting up. If he is still recumbent, the procedure is facilitated by placing him on an old Stryker frame, the slings of which have been covered with washable plastic material. Strict asepsis must be observed in the enema room. No tips or rectal stoppers should be used and all tubing and gloves should be of the disposable type and used only once. Wherever a considerable number of these patients are under treatment, there should be a team of nursing aides especially trained in this program.

REFERENCES

1. Bors, E.: Intermittent Catheterization in Paraplegic Patients. Urol. Int., 22:236–249, 1967.
2. Bors, E.: Neurogenic Bladder, Urol. Survey, 7:177–250, 1957.
3. Comarr, A. E.: The Practical Urological Management of the Patient with Spinal Cord Injury. Brit. J. Urol., 31:1–46, 1959.
4. Guttmann, L., and Frankel, H.: The Value of Intermittent Catheterization in the Early Management of Traumatic Paraplegia and Tetraplegia. Paraplegia, 4:63–84, 1966.
5. Hardy, A. G.: Experience with Intermittent Catheterization in Acute Paraplegia. Med. Serv. J. Canada, 22:538–544, 1966.
6. Talbot, H. S.: Adjunctive Care of Spinal Cord Injury. Surg. Clin. N. Amer., 48:737–757, 1968.
7. Talbot, H. S.: The Management of Neurogenic Vesical Dysfunction. Bull. N.Y. Acad. Med., 39:71–89, 1963.
8. Talbot, H. S.: The Patient and Bladder Management. Paraplegia, 8:19–26, 1970.
9. Walsh, J. J.: Intermittent Catheterization in Paraplegia. Paraplegia, 6:168–171, 1968.

Chapter 32

DECUBITUS ULCERS

by Michael Kosiak

Decubital ulcerations are localized areas of cellular necrosis of the skin and subcutaneous tissues which have been subjected to prolonged periods of supracapillary pressure. Ulcerations occur with special frequency over weight bearing bony prominences covered only by skin and small amounts of muscle and subcutaneous tissue. The areas over the sacrum, trochanters and ischial tuberosities are most frequently involved. Obviously, the distribution depends to a great extent on the patient's functional status. That is, trochanteric and sacral ulcers are more prevalent in the bedridden patient, and ischial ulcers are found almost exclusively in patients who are able to sit for long periods of time. Among the severely debilitated, ulcers over knees, heels, malleoli, scapulae and spine also occur.

Ischemic ulcers occur most frequently in the debilitated patient who is unable to change the position of his body either because he does not have the strength or because sensation is impaired with the result that he does not experience pain from pressure over the bony prominences.

The incidence of ischemic ulcers varies widely, depending primarily on the medical and nursing care provided. The occurrence in paraplegic World War II veterans has ranged from 85 per cent to 57 per cent.[7, 17, 27] Among civilians an incidence as high as 28 per cent of the total bed population has been reported.[24]

ETIOLOGY

Primary Factors

Decubital ulcers arise from prolonged tissue ischemia caused by pressure exceeding the tissue capillary pressure. Microscopic changes in muscle tissue

643

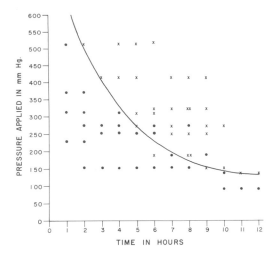

Figure 32–1 Pressure-time relationship noted in 62 separate experiments on 16 dogs: X = ulceration; • = no ulceration.

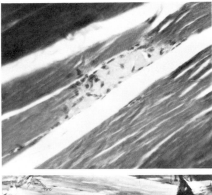

Figure 32–2 Muscle of normal rat's leg after application of 115 mm. Hg constant pressure for two hours. The section shows early involvement of an isolated fiber consisting of hyaline degeneration and phagocytosis. Stained with hematoxylin and eosin. Magnified 380 ×.

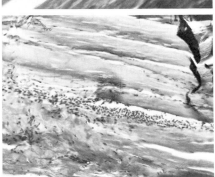

Figure 32–3 Muscle of paraplegic rat's leg subjected to 70 mm. Hg constant pressure for four hours. The section shows an isolated fiber undergoing necrosis associated with extensive phagocytosis by neutrophils and macrophages. Stained with hematoxylin and eosin. Magnified 170 ×.

have been demonstrated after the application of as little pressure as 70 mm. of mercury for only two hours. A definite inverse relationship exists between the amount and duration of pressure that normal tissue can tolerate before pathologic changes are noted (Figs. 32-1 to 32-3 and Table 32-1).

Recent studies of the changes in capillary blood flow using several experimental methods have established important facts regarding vascular hemodynamics. Remarkable instability in capillaries at low perfusion pressures with cessation or temporary reversal of flow at a low positive pressure have been demonstrated.

TABLE 32–1 MICROSCOPIC CHANGES NOTED IN MUSCLE OF ANIMALS 24 HOURS AFTER APPLICATION OF PRESSURE*

PRESSURE TRANSMITTED TO MUSCLE	TIME IN HOURS	NORMAL		PARAPLEGIC	
		Constant Pressure	Alternating Pressure (5 min. intervals)	Constant Pressure	Alternating Pressure (5 min. intervals)
35 mm. Hg	1	None	None	None	None
	2	None	None	None	None
	3	None	None	None	None
	4	None	None	None	None
70 mm. Hg	1	None	None	None	None
	2	Moderate	None	Moderate	Minimal
	3	Moderate	Minimal	Moderate	Minimal
	4	Moderate	Minimal	Marked	Minimal
115 mm. Hg	1	None		None	
	2	Minimal		Moderate	
	3	Marked		Marked	
	4	Moderate		Moderate	
155 mm. Hg	1	None	None	None	None
	2	Moderate	None	Minimal	None
	3	Marked	Minimal	Minimal	None
	4	Moderate	Moderate	Moderate	Minimal
190 mm. Hg	1	None		Minimal	
	2	Minimal		Moderate	
	3	Marked		Marked	
	4	Marked		Marked	
240 mm. Hg	1	Minimal	None	Moderate	None
	2	Moderate	Minimal	Moderate	None
	3	Moderate	None	Moderate	Minimal
	4	Moderate	Moderate	Marked	Minimal

*None = No microscopic change.
Minimal – Involvement of isolated fibers.
Moderate = Involvement of up to 10 per cent of muscle examined.
Marked = Involvement of more than 10 per cent of muscle examined.

Because the hydrostatic pressures in capillaries are relatively low (from 13 to 32 mm. of mercury) and because cessation of flow occurs even in the presence of positive arterial pressure, it would seem logical that complete tissue ischemia does occur when pressures of the order of capillary blood pressure are applied to the body.

Ulcerations occur almost exclusively over bony prominences which have been subjected to excessive pressures for varying lengths of time and the ulcerations almost inevitably will heal when the pressure is removed. Therefore it would appear that ischemia caused by supracapillary pressures is the primary factor in the production of decubitus ulcers.

Contributing Factors

Nutrition. There has been increased emphasis recently on the role of nutrition during the acute and convalescent phases of illness, especially on the negative nitrogen and calcium balance that inevitably appears after an acute insult. After almost any illness or injury, such as a fracture, tooth extraction or even a mild infection, a negative nitrogen, phosphorus, sulfur and calcium balance with evidence of osteoporosis, wasting of tissue and loss of weight generally results. The reaction is much more pronounced, of course, in a severe insult than in a mild one. This negative balance reaches its peak in about two to eight days and does not return to normal for several months. No dietary product can completely reverse the negative balance, although the degree of negativity of the nitrogen balance can be reduced.

Because of the severe alteration of body metabolism produced by almost any illness and the additional changes produced by the bed rest that usually follows injury or illness, it would seem that rather drastic changes in the dietary intake would be indicated, if only to counterbalance the metabolic losses.

Edema.   Edema of varying degrees is undoubtedly a contributing factor to the production of decubitus ulcers. An increased amount of interstitial fluid increases the distance from the capillary to the cell. Since the rate of diffusion of oxygen and food from the capillary to the cell decreases in proportion to this distance, it is clear that edema has a profound influence on the supply of nutrients to the cell.

Anemia.   Anemia is also a contributing factor of great significance in determining whether cellular hypoxia and necrosis will occur. It is obvious that the possibility for ischemic tissue to survive is greatly enhanced when the hemoglobin content and the supply of oxygen within the blood are normal even though blood flow is reduced. If in ischemia there is also a decreased oxygen content in the blood, cellular metabolism is further restricted.

The fact that ulceration may actually occur following even minimal pressures of short duration in the severely emaciated patient seems only to emphasize that well nourished tissue is more viable and can better tolerate the destructive effects of pressure and ischemia when it occurs.

PREVENTION

Because of microscopic degenerative changes which result from the application of only relatively low pressures for short periods of time, it is apparent that degenerative reaction and recovery from these changes are probably taking place simultaneously. When tissue is subjected to pressures for only short periods of time, the normal reactive hyperemic response partially compensates for the temporary ischemia with the result that the tissue does not undergo morphologic degeneration. Even when excessive pressures are applied for a sufficient period of time to result in early degenerative changes, it would appear that complete relief of pressure may often permit restoration of circulation and cellular metabolism without ulceration.

Even when adequate nursing care is available the incapacitated person is rarely turned oftener than once every two hours; thus, each trochanter, the sacrum or the iliac spine is subjected to supracapillary pressures for two hour intervals at least three times each day. Many bedridden patients develop ischemic ulcers on such a regimen, indicating that the damage produced during the time that the pressure was being exerted was not completely repaired during the intervals when the area was free of pressure. More frequent turning of the patient would result in shorter periods of compression and ischemia and more frequent periods of complete relief of pressure during which restoration of cellular function could occur.

Cushions and padding of various forms are of little value in preventing the formation of ulcers because of the relatively minute pressures which, when exerted for even short periods of time, produce ischemia and ultimate tissue necrosis. Pressures under the ischial tuberosities even when the patient is sitting on 6 inches of foam rubber cushion exceed 150 mm. of mercury.

Cutout areas intended to decrease or eliminate pressures over the bony tuberosities only tend to divert more of the weight bearing to the surrounding area.

Since it is impossible to eliminate pressure completely over all areas for any period of time, it is imperative that the pressure over part of the area be completely eliminated at frequent intervals in order to allow circulation to the ischemic tissues.

The use of an alternating pressure air mattress and more recently the use of an alternating pressure chair have proved to be very effective in the prevention of decubitus ulcers.

TREATMENT

General Measures. Since ulcerations are found exclusively over areas subjected to pressures of varying degrees, it is essential that this pressure be completely eliminated. Improvement of the nutritional status and maintenance of a positive nitrogen balance are desirable. Establishment of satisfactory hemoglobin and hematocrit levels and the elimination of edema about the involved area are necessary.

Specific Measures. Complete elimination of pressure over the ulceration must be accomplished by proper bed positioning and the use of various splints and appliances.

Scrupulous care of the involved area is important. Cleansing with bland soap and water or a mild antiseptic agent should be done at least once daily. The use of the whirlpool bath or Hubbard tank is very beneficial when available.

Ultraviolet radiation should be applied to the ulcer in bactericidal dosages to prevent growth of contaminating organisms. Ultraviolent radiation also causes local capillary vasodilatation with increased blood flow, which stimulates local healing responses.

Light stroking massage about the lesion is beneficial because it tends to promote venous return and reduce edema which might be present.

Surgical intervention is indicated only after freedom from active infection has been established and healthy granulation tissue is present. Sliding full-thickness skin flaps are usually the most successful form of surgical repair.

REFERENCES

*These articles deal especially with control and treatment of ischemic ulcers.

1. Brooks, B.: Pathological Changes in Muscle as a Result of Disturbance in Circulation. Arch. Surg., 5:188-216, 1922.
2.* Brooks, B., and Duncan, G. W.: Effects of Pressure on Tissues. Arch. Surg., 40:696-709, 1940.

3. Burton, A. C., and Yamada, S.: Relation Between Blood Pressure and Flow in the Human Forearm. J. Appl. Physiol., *4*:329-339, 1951.
4.* Cannon, B., O'Leary, J. J., O'Neil, J. W., and Steinsieck, R.: An Approach to Treatment of Pressure Sores. Ann. Surg., *132*:760-778, 1950.
5. Catell, M.: The Physiological Effects of Pressure. Biol. Rev., *11*:441-474, 1936.
6. Deitrick, J. E.: Effects of Immobilization on Metabolic and Physiological Functions of Normal Men. Bull. N.Y. Acad. Med., *24*:364-375, 1948.
7.* Dietrick, R. B., and Russi, S.: Tabulation and Review of Autopsy Findings in Fifty-five Paraplegics. J.A.M.A., *166*:41-44, 1958.
8. Goldblatt, H.: Observations Upon Reactive Hyperemia. Heart, *12*:281-294, 1925-26.
9. Griffiths, D. L.: Volkmann's Ischaemic Contracture. Brit. J. Surg., *28*:239-260, 1940.
10. Grossman, C. M., Sappington, T. S., Burrows, B. A., Lavietes, P. H., and Peters, J. P.: Nitrogen Metabolism in Acute Infections. J. Clin. Invest., *24*:523-531, 1945.
11.* Harman, J. W.: A Histological Study of Skeletal Muscle in Acute Ischemia. Amer. J. Path., *23*:551-565, 1947.
12. Harman, J. W.: Significance of Local Vascular Phenomena in Production of Ischemic Necrosis in Skeletal Muscle. Amer. J. Path., *24*:625-641, 1948.
13. Henry, J. P., Klain, I., Movitt, E., and Meehan, J. P.: The Effects of Anoxemia on the Capillary Permeability of the Human Arm. Fed. Proc., *5*:44, 1946.
14. Howard, J. E., Bigham, R. S., Eisenberg, H., Wagner, D., and Bailey, E.: Studies on Convalescence: Nitrogen and Mineral Balances During Starvation and Graduated Feeding in Healthy Young Males at Bed Rest. Bull. Hopkins Hosp., *78*:282-307, 1946.
15. Howard, J. E., Parson, W., and Bigham, R. S., Jr.: Studies on Patients Convalescent from Fracture; Urinary Excretion of Calcium and Phosphorus. Bull. Hopkins Hosp., *77*:291-313, 1945.
16.* Husain, T.: Experimental Study of Some Pressure Effects on Tissues, with Reference to the Bed Sore Problem. J. Path. Bact., *66*:347-358, 1953.
17.* Kennedy, R. H.: New Viewpoint Toward Spinal Cord Injuries. Ann. Surg., *124*:1057-1065, 1946.
18.* Kosiak, M.: Etiology and Pathology of Ischemic Ulcers. Arch. Phys. Med., *40*:62-69, 1959.
19.* Kosiak, M.: Etiology of Decubitus Ulcers. Arch. Phys. Med., *42*:19-29, 1961.
20. Kosiak, M., Kubicek, W., Olson, M., Danz, J. N., and Kottke, F. J.: Evaluation of Pressure as a Factor in the Production of Ischial Ulcers. Arch. Phys. Med., *39*:623-629, 1958.
21. Landis, E. M.: Micro-injection Studies of Capillary Permeability; Effect of Lack of Oxygen in Permeability of the Capillary Wall to Fluid and Plasma Protein. Amer. J. Physiol., *83*:538-542, 1928.
22.* Landis, E. M.: Micro-injection Studies of Capillary Blood Pressure in Human Skin. Heart, *15*:209-228, 1930.
23. Lewis, T., and Grant, R.: Observations Upon Reactive Hyperemia in Man. Heart, *12*:73-120, 1925-26.
24.* Munro, D.: Care of the Back Following Spinal-cord Injuries. New Eng. J. Med., *223*:391-398, 1940.
25. Nichol, J., Girling, F., Jerrard, W., Claxton, E. B., and Burton, A. C.: Fundamental Instability of Small Blood Vessels and Critical Closing Pressures in Vascular Beds. Amer. J. Physiol., *4*:330-344, 1951.
26. Nicoll, P. A., and Webb, R. L.: Vascular Patterns and Active Vasomotion as Determiners of Flow Through Minute Vessels. Angiology, *6*:291-310, 1955.
27.* Poer, D. H.: Newer Concepts in Treatment of Paralyzed Patients Due to Wartime Injuries of Spinal Cord. Ann. Surg., *123*:510-515, 1946.
28. Riegel, C., Koop, C. E., Drew, J., Stevens, L. W., and Rhoades, J. E.: Nutritional Requirements for Nitrogen Balance During Early Postoperative Period. J. Clin. Invest., *26*:18-23, 1947.
29.* Trumble, H. C.: The Skin Tolerance for Pressure and Pressure Sores. Med. J. Aust., *2*:724-726, 1930.
30. Zweifach, B. W., and Metz, D. B.: Selective Distribution of Blood Through the Terminal Vascular Bed of Mesenteric Structures and Skeletal Muscle. Angiology, *6*:282-290, 1955.

Chapter 33

CEREBRAL PALSY AND REHABILITATION OF CHILDREN

by Harold M. Sterling

Physicians are often surprised to learn that infants and young children may have almost any of the disorders that cause physical disabilities in older persons. Much of the material already covered in this handbook applies directly to handicapped children. The principles of physiatric assessment and management are basically similar in both groups but it is not advisable to apply to children, without modification, methods used with adults. Just as methods of treatment, dosages of medication, fluid balances and surgical techniques must be adapted for use with acutely ill infants and young children, certain modifications must be made in rehabilitation programs for young disabled persons. Perhaps the most important principles of children's rehabilitation are meticulous attention to the details of the history and physical and developmental examinations at sufficiently frequent intervals to assess the developmental level, rate of progress and potential complications (see Chapter 2).

Assessment and treatment must be pursued concurrently in three related but separable areas: (1) each element of the specific disability, (2) the specific developmental level at which the child is operating in any given activity at the moment in question and (3) any associated defects that may be present. It is useful to think of management as correction of existing problems and prevention of further complications in each of these three areas, although in practice the techniques may overlap or even may be identical.

An important principle to apply when approaching long-range plans for children with physical disorders is that one rarely can provide for complete

649

correction. Medicines and surgical procedures are rarely definitive. The physiatrist applies all his skills to lessen the effect of the disorder, to provide substitute measures, to prevent secondary complication and to allow for day-to-day function and for growth to proceed as normally as possible. Long-range management plans need to emphasize social, emotional and educational factors as the child grows, learns and adapts, because these factors are often more crucial in determining success in his ultimate rehabilitation than the specifics of physical disability and their treatment. (see Chapters 7 and 8.) The skill of the physician in helping families help their handicapped children will have great influence on the effectiveness of the management program. Because earlier chapters of this handbook have dealt with various professional roles and with specific treatment modalities in some detail, it will be possible now to outline approaches to the physical management of handicapping conditions in childhood.

The group of neuromuscular disorders in children that has been termed "cerebral palsy" can serve as a framework upon which to elaborate the basic approach to pediatric physical medicine.

Cerebral palsy is an ill-defined, diffusely characterized group of disabilities involving disorders of motor control which are congenital or which occur in early life. The basic neurological pathologic condition is, by definition, nonprogressive, but the patient's symptoms may change from hour to hour and day to day, depending on a multiplicity of physiological and emotional factors.

Usually the disability is classified according to a system which describes the symptoms of disordered motor control, such as "spasticity," "athetosis' and "ataxia," and the location, such as "hemiplegic" or "paraplegic.' Perhaps the most useful system currently used is that described by Ingram (see page 653), but there is as yet no system which has gained general acceptance or which has come into routine use. As a result, the field is plagued by a diversity of definitions and a multiplicity of descriptive terms.

The history obtained from the parents and the original physical examination should define all three of the areas mentioned. For example, what appears superficially to be nonspecific retardation may by careful history and physical examination prove to be deafness, behavior disturbance or aphasia. Similarly, children who are referred for speech problems may actually have more general neurologic problems with deficits in control of lips, tongue and breathing and in perceptual or conceptual ability. Their speech difficulties may result from relatively pure intellectual retardation or retardation on the basis of intellectual and social deprivation rather than from primary speech defects (see Chapter 5).

ASSESSMENT

History

How does one begin the assessment and treatment of a child with suspected brain damage? Starting with a careful history and physical examination is of the utmost importance. The history must include detailed prenatal and natal information as well as information about the postnatal development of the child. Eliciting familial incidence of similar or related diseases is of value.

The time at which the child began to sit, stand, walk and communicate is very useful for diagnosis and for planning the early parts of a treatment program. The child's present status—how does he stand, what does he do, how does he use his hands, what is his language level, what interests does he have—will become important as the treatment program is outlined.

Experience also indicates that questions should be directed toward such areas as fluid intake, nutritional intake, weight gain and presence of abnormal fevers. Intake and temperature control appear to present peculiar problems in children with brain damage and may lead to further damage if they are not adequately handled.

Physical Examination

One physician must be responsible for seeing that a complete physical examination is done and for assembling and interpreting all parts of the evaluation. First of all, a general and nutritional evaluation is done as with any child coming in for a well-child check-up. Second, the scalp and skull are examined for hemangioma, bony defects, premature closure of the fontanels or sutures, hydrocephalus or microcephalia. A word of warning should be inserted here: one cannot assess the intellectual capacity of a child simply by measuring the circumference of the skull.

Ears. Examination of the ears for the presence of wax plugs, for changes in the tympanic membrane and to assess hearing acuity is essential. Hearing

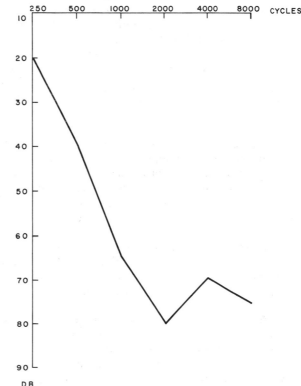

Figure 33–1 Typical RH audiogram showing severe high frequency hearing loss.

evaluation may be very difficult in children with cerebral palsy and if the physician is not fully satisfied that he can demonstrate hearing ability, a hearing test should be done by an expert. Testing by commercial hearing aid salesmen or by personnel who are not accustomed to testing these children will be more misleading than helpful. Hearing loss occurs most frequently in children with a history of jaundice and it affects high frequencies more than low, making testing difficult (Fig. 33-1).

Eyes.   Continuing the physical examination, the eyes must be examined carefully since they give many clues to the presence of neurologic damage and physical defects. The presence of nystagmus or defects in position and in conjugate movement are noted. Strabismus or lack of conjugate movement is very common in children with other evidences of brain damage. Children with spasticity are reported to show greater difficulty in balance of the rectus and oblique eye muscles. Children with athetosis, particularly of the Rh-incompatibility type, often are incapable of vertical movement of the eye. Further, examination of the lens of the eye for cataracts is indicated in cases in which the brain damage occurred as the result of infection or injury in the first trimester of pregnancy. Examination for errors of refraction as well as for retrolental fibroplasia is in order in children with a history of premature birth. Evaluation of the child's visual field is often difficult and in order to examine the fundus it may be necessary to give the child a sedative and to dilate the pupils.

Mouth.   Indications of slight motor damage can easily be obtained by examining the control of the lips, tongue and pharynx. This includes noting the ability of the child to swallow properly and the presence of drooling. In recent years much attention has been paid to enamel defects and staining which occur during the embryologic development of the teeth due to poor nutrition, general body injuries or high bilirubin levels. These defects become permanent parts of the deciduous teeth and are of some help in dating the time at which the presumed brain injury occurred. Many children with cerebral palsy have very narrow high arched palates. This should be noted and followed because of the crowding of permanent teeth that results from malformations of the jaw.

Neck.   Neck control should be evaluated. With the child lying on his back on an examining table, the physician grasps both his hands and raises him to a sitting position. If, after a very early age, the child fails to assist in or maintain head control, it is an indication of either specific weakness of the muscles in the anterior part of the neck or neurologic damage. It is also important to note the presence of asymmetric and symmetric tonic neck reflexes.

Chest.   Examination of the chest for the regularity and symmetry of respiratory motion and coordination of the upper and lower breathing muscles is important because dysrhythmia or incoordination of breathing is often present, especially in children with athetosis.

Back.   Children with neurologic damage tend to arch the back into opisthotonos. When the child is brought to a sitting position the back may form a long curve posteriorly involving the entire back from buttocks to cervical spine, with reversal of the normal lumbar lordosis. A curve of this type will cause hyperextension of the neck and of the head on the neck, producing a very uncomfortable sitting position. Children with asymmetry of neurologic signs tend to develop scoliosis and for this reason side to side symmetry of the back must be noted carefully.

Extremities. Examination of the extremities for symmetry of shape, of size, of control of motion and of position as well as for range and strength is important. Symmetry and range of motion at the shoulder and hip should be checked in children with spasticity, rigidity and dystonia. Subluxation of the hip sometimes develops in the early stages of athetosis and dislocations may occur before trouble is suspected. Shoulders are less often involved.

Neurologic Examination

Careful neurologic examination, including those procedures mentioned as part of the general physical examination, must be performed on all children with evidences of intellectual retardation, speech deficiency or slow motor development. In recording the neurologic findings it is helpful to describe them in detail since the teachers and physical, occupational and speech therapists who work with the child will need a great deal of information about his motor and neurologic disability.

Perhaps the most useful system of classification currently in use is that proposed by Ingram:

Neurologic Diagnosis	Extent
Hemiplegia	{ Right { Left
Bilateral hemiplegia	
Diplegia	

Hyptonic
       Dystonic
  Rigid or Spastic
	{ Paraplegic
	{ Triplegic
	{ Tetraplegic

Ataxic diplegia	
Hyptonic Spastic	{ Paraplegic { Triplegic { Tetraplegic
Ataxia	{ Predominantly unilateral { Bilateral
Dyskinesia	

Dystonic
    Choreoid
    Athetoid
    Tension
    Tremor
	{ Monoplegic
	{ Hemiplegic
	{ Triplegic
	{ Tetraplegic

Classification of Cerebral Palsy

Spasticity. A lower threshold to the stretch reflex, an enlarged area from which the reflex may be obtained and an exaggeration of the stretch reflex associated with a tendency to develop contractures in the antigravity muscles.

Athetosis. An abnormal amount and type of involuntary motion associated with normal deep tendon and superficial reflexes.

Dystonia. An involuntary distorted position held for periods of a few seconds to a few minutes. This is much slower than athetosis and involves the contraction of muscles on both sides of a joint usually, without reflex changes during relaxation.

Rigidity.   Resistance to slow passive movement, of a lead pipe or cogwheel type.

Ataxia.   Primary incoordination with disturbance of balance, disturbance of synergies and rebound phenomena. Again the deep tendon reflexes and superficial reflexes must not be exaggerated and may be either normal or decreased.

Hypotonia.   Weakness or lack of resting muscle tonus, often associated with exaggerated deep tendon reflexes.

Chorea.   Rapid uncontrolled movements of sudden onset producing jerky motion or bizarre postures.

Tension.   Generalized hypertonus of both flexor and extensor muscles varying in intensity over a period of time.

Tremor.   Rhythmic involuntary movement, usually distal.

Clonus is not present in athetosis, dystonia, rigidity and ataxia. The presence of more than one motor manifestation of neurologic damage, e.g., spasticity and athetosis, is not unusual in a given individual.

Textbooks and journal articles, in general, give the impression that the child's symptoms are relatively stable, and that their type and location are relatively fixed. Many so-called "systems of treatment" are predicated on these assumptions. The truth is that the nature and degree of neurologic symptoms can change with the passage of years, and that the degree of difficulty can increase or decrease significantly with a rapid change of mood or of physiologic state.

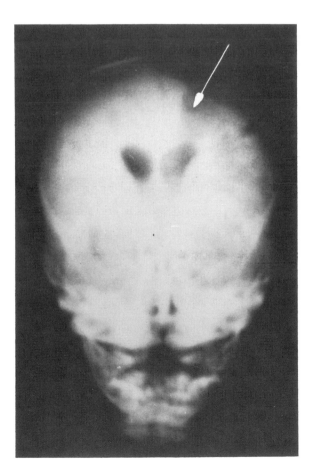

Figure 33–2   Porencephalic cyst occurring along path of ventriculography needle through cerebral cortex.

Roentgenographic Studies

Certain roentgenographic studies may be extremely helpful. Skull x-rays may or may not be useful, depending on the individual problem. A pneumoencephalogram or ventriculogram may help in evaluating the presence and extent of brain damage. Cerebral angiography may be helpful in locating suspected thromboses or vascular abnormalities. These procedures should be used sparingly, however, because experience has shown that they may be harmful (Fig. 33–2).

Since atloido-occipital subluxation, cervical fracture dislocation (Fig. 33–3), subluxation injuries of the spinal cord, congenital malformations or spinal cord tumors may masquerade as "cerebral palsy," children with evidences of long

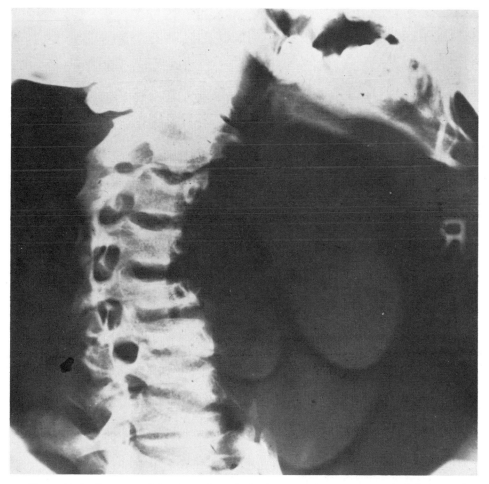

Figure 33–3   Fracture–dislocation of cervical spine secondary to traumatic delivery. Subject was managed as cerebral palsy patient for 18 years before correct diagnosis was established.

tract signs or combinations of "athetosis" and "spasticity" may require extensive examination. Certain patients with unstable fractures of the cervical spine whose progress was followed until they reached middle age have developed degenerative arthritis, instability of the cervical spine and subsequent further destruction of the cord which may progress to complete transection in the cervical region.

Speech

Since about 50 to 75 per cent of the children with known brain damage have some type of speech problem, referral for speech evaluation is usually indicated. The peripheral musculature, including the lips, tongue, pharynx, vocal cords and respiratory system, and the ability to produce sound should be evaluated and in addition central language functions and language production should be investigated. We have noted before the necessity for testing of hearing (see Chapter 5).

Psychologic Testing

Psychologic testing is an important aspect of the general evaluation. Physicians are notoriously poor at estimating intelligence, and "I.Q." scores of children with cerebral palsy are misleading (see Chapter 6). Careful testing in a number of areas—verbal, motor and perceptual—may be necessary. Since the techniques of administering tests to these children require special skill, the psychologist selected should have training and experience in the field of handicapped children. Poorly applied, the tests may do more harm than good. The experienced psychologist should also be able to help interpret behavior problems that arise from emotional difficulties.

Electroencephalography

Since by definition these children have brain damage, electroencephalography is an important part of the examination. There is a great deal of debate about the advisability of "treating the electroencephalogram" rather than treating the clinical manifestations of a seizure disorder. The types of seizures these children have may not be recognized as seizures by anyone other than professional personnel, even though they may involve a short postictal state as well as an amnesia for the immediate preictal period. Obviously these types of seizures, repeated frequently throughout the day, can hinder the child's ability to learn but if they are controlled the youngster may perform better in therapy and in the classroom.

Motor Performance

The child's motor performance, particularly in upper extremity function, eye-hand coordination and fine skills, should be evaluated and recorded since it will give many clues to the child's potential for treatment.

THERAPEUTIC PROGRAM

Having completed the detailed evaluation described, one next becomes concerned about the development of a therapeutic program. A program that deals with any specific part of the findings without including all the others at the same time is almost certainly destined to fail. An optimal program would involve treatment of the neuromotor symptoms (for example, reduction of the spasticity, athetosis or dystonia by any means available); stretching of the contractures; establishment of voluntary control; assessment of developmental level, leading the child up to the next stages of development; and treatment of visual and hearing handicaps and seizures.

Physical therapy, occupational therapy, orthopedic surgery, bracing and splinting may be needed to develop adequate range of motion in each joint. At the same time, or very shortly thereafter, development of control and sufficient strength allows purposeful function to begin. Treatment by means of the specific active exercises used routinely in older patients is very difficult, if not impossible, in children with developmental retardation. The following program is recommended as a general approach. Treatment of older children who have progressed through earlier stages can easily be taken up at their specific levels of development.

DEVELOPMENTAL CONTROL

Sitting

The first stage of developmental control in a normal infant and an essential stage of development for the child with a neuromuscular handicap is

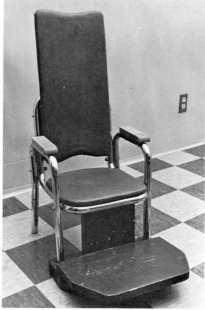

Figure 33–4 High back chair to give greater trunk support. (Courtesy of The Minneapolis Curative Workshop.)

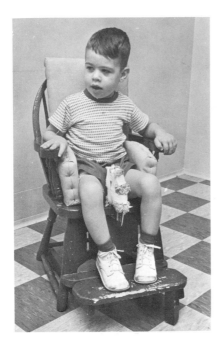

Figure 33–5   Chair with padded post to prevent adduction. (Courtesy of The Minneapolis Curative Workshop.)

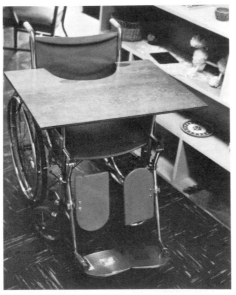

Figure 33–6   Wheelchair with removable tabletop. (Courtesy of Rehabilitation Institute of The Boston Dispensary.)

learning to sit, progressing from head control to trunk control and then to free sitting. The earliest attempt should be made with a wheelchair or wooden chair with a high back that provides head support posteriorly (Fig. 33-4). A neck pillow or side pieces may be added to the chair to give side to side head control. A chest band and knee band may be needed for control. The seat should provide comfortable support with the knees flexed.

For children who have a tendency toward adduction or adductor contractures, a large padded post on the forward edge of the chair seat will keep the hips in abduction (Fig. 33-5). The addition of a table top on the chair will allow the child to play with toys as soon as his eye control, head control, upper extremity control and mental acuity progress to a point where this is possible (Fig. 33-6). The child should be taken out of the chair when head control or trunk control begin to fail or when the child begins to be tired, uncomfortable or distraught. The amount of support that the chair provides should be decreased gradually as the child gains control of the head, neck, upper trunk, midtrunk and so forth. The child should begin to practice free sitting in a small chair that offers much less support and on the the side of the table. At all levels of training in sitting the feet should be supported.

Standing

Very shortly after head and upper trunk control begin to develop, the child can be placed in a standing chimney, which is a narrow high wooden box or table with a door on the back arranged so that the upper part of the box comes approximately at the nipple line (Fig. 33-7). A pad is placed in front of the knees and another behind the buttocks to align the child in extension at the hips and knees and the feet should be flat on the floor of the chimney. Again, the child should be removed from the chimney immediately when head and upper trunk control begins to fail, when the child begins to appear tired or when he becomes distraught. Most authorities recommend that the standing chimney not be used for periods of time longer than 30 minutes to one hour. Rather, it should be used repeatedly throughout the day.

As the child develops, the floorboard may be raised higher in the standing chimney so that less support is given to the trunk. When the thoracic spine has been brought under control the child is ready to begin either wall standing, supported in the corner so that free movement is possible only in a forward direction, or standing in a stabilizer which is arranged to give support from the

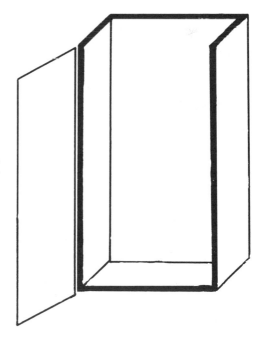

Figure 33–7 Schematic drawing of standing chimney. (Courtesy of Rehabilitation Institute of The Boston Dispensary.)

posterior thigh to allow development of the lumbar spine and hip control. Many children object to the highly constraining type of support which the stabilizer provides even though they have accepted the standing chimney. Wall standing can progress from the corner of the wall to the flat wall where the child must develop side to side as well as forward balance. When the child has developed forward balance and side to side balance, it is time to encourage him to step away from the wall to develop posterior balance.

For children who, because of ataxia, loss of position sense in the lower extremities, athetosis or spasticity, need a broader standing base, duck sole shoes (Fig. 33-8) or skis (Fig. 33-9) for the beginning stages of standing balance may be very useful.

In all of these activities of standing it is important to remember that the position of the feet must be controlled. At this point the importance of proper fitting of shoes should be pointed out. The majority of youngsters with neuro-muscular disabilities have calcaneus valgus, a few have calcaneus varus and almost none have normal heel or foot position. A high-top, steel shank, leather shoe with a fitted heel counter is the basic footwear for all of these children. When calcaneus valgus is marked, a medial heel wedge can be added. In the unusual instances when calcaneus varus is a problem, the shoe usually is corrective by itself but it may be necessary to add lateral heel wedges. For most children, $1/8$ inch wedges are sufficient.

When standing balance and strength for support have developed sufficiently the child may be placed in the parallel bars to begin progression. The parallel bars should be used rather sparingly to prevent the child from becoming habituated to them. It is extremely important to remember that the child should not pull on the bars in order to progress. If he begins to do this, it may

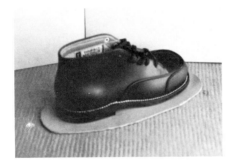

Figure 33–8   Orthopedic shoe with extended sole (duck sole) of sole leather and firm sheet metal. (Courtesy of Rehabilitation Institute of The Boston Dispensary.)

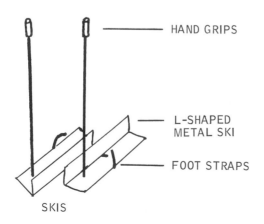

HAND GRIPS

L-SHAPED
METAL SKI

FOOT STRAPS

SKIS

Figure 33–9   Skis. (Courtesy of Rehabilitation Institute of The Boston Dispensary.)

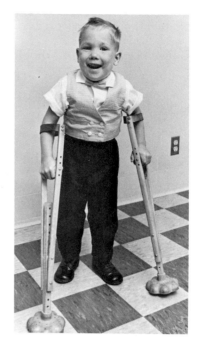

Figure 33–10 "Kenny sticks" with enlarged crutch tips. (Courtesy of Minneapolis Curative Workshop.)

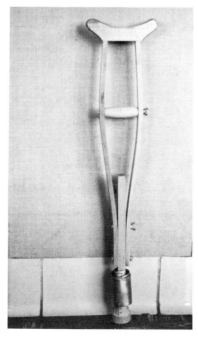

Figure 33–11 Adjustable underarm crutch with one-pound strip of lead next to base. (Courtesy of Rehabilitation Institute of The Boston Dispensary.)

be necessary to instruct him to place his hand or closed fist on the top of the bar to prevent pulling. Standing balance then can be developed in the bars, progressing to weight shifting and forward foot placement, and from there to gait training. In a short time it is possible to start training the child in standing balance either free or with crutches.

When there is a tendency for the child to lift the crutches away from the floor and lose his balance, lead weights (often amounting to several pounds) can be applied to the bottom of the sticks (Fig. 33-10). When rapid uncontrolled movement or ataxia is the problem, lead weights at the ankles to produce a lower, more posterior center of balance have been quite helpful in assisting the child to develop standing balance (Fig. 33-11).

Toeing in or toeing out usually is associated with overaction of the internal or external rotators of the hip or with contracture of these muscles. Occasionally it is related to spasticity or contracture of the adductor or gracilis muscles. "Twisters" of various sorts have generally been unsatisfactory. A more direct approach is the treatment of the contracture by stretching and by developing new positions.

Reciprocating Movement

The preceding discussions are related to the development of sitting balance and standing balance. However, very little has been said about the necessary reciprocating movement of the lower extremities. With a very young child reciprocating movements can be started passively; the therapist dorsiflexes the patient's foot and flexes the knees and hip on one side, holds the other foot in a neutral position and the knee and hip in extension and then reverses the procedure. For many years therapists have been taught to sing short nursery rhymes in association with the movements. Although it is not to be believed that the singing changes the child's ability to flex or extend, it is claimed that the child may be so conditioned from hearing the repetition of the song with the movement that singing songs may later produce reciprocating activities of the lower extremities.

As soon as there is some voluntary flexion and extension in the lower extremities with control of the head and upper extremities, the child can be placed in the creeper which supports the trunk in a canvas sling so that the hands and the knees touch the floor (Fig. 33-12). The child then is encouraged to develop creeping patterns using reciprocating movements of all four extremities.

About the same time, when head control and upper trunk control have developed and there is some active flexion and extension of the lower extrem-

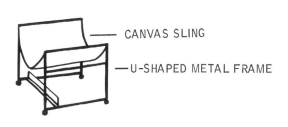

CANVAS SLING

U-SHAPED METAL FRAME

CREEPER

Figure 33-12 Creeper. (Courtesy of Rehabilitation Institute of The Boston Dispensary.)

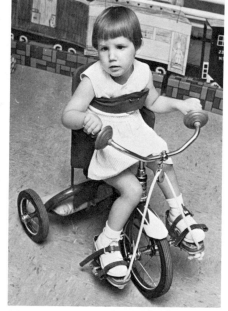

Figure 33–13 Tricycle with back, chest strap, foot plates, and pulley system to prevent plantar flexion. (Courtesy of The Minneapolis Curative Workshop.)

ities, the child can be placed in a tricycle with a built-up back and a chest strap (Fig. 33-13). The feet may be strapped to the pedals to prevent them from slipping off. It is also helpful to put a pulley over the front of the handle bars with a rope running through it to the toe of a wood plate on each pedal so that it is impossible for one foot to go into plantar flexion without stretching the gastrocnemius-soleus in the other leg. Developmental schedules indicate that children usually do not ride tricycles before they reach the age of three; however, handicapped children who are not able to move about freely in space often can ride a tricycle at two years or very shortly after that.

Having developed sitting control, standing balance, reciprocating movement of the legs, forward progression in the parallel bars and free standing, the child is ready to begin gait training either unassisted or with crutches.

Gait Training

Formal gait training is very discouraging for the therapist and for the child. Attempts at developing four-point gait may become particularly frustrating. The therapist and the parents should be encouraged not to nag the child concerning his gait but rather to devise means whereby a good erect posture and four-point or reciprocating gait of the lower extremities without crutches is developed. When dragging of the toes is a problem and there is no abnormality that prevents the child from lifting his toes, bricks or a ladder placed on the floor require the child to lift the foot up and over in order to place it for forward progression (Figs. 33-14 and 33-15). For problems of toeing in and toeing out and disparity in length of step, walking on footprints painted on the floor has been used as a game involving a number of children and works reasonably well even with fairly young children.

Often young children are reluctant to use crutches or canes until other children evince interest in them. When the crutch or cane becomes an interesting object and a matter of play with his siblings or playmates, the handicapped

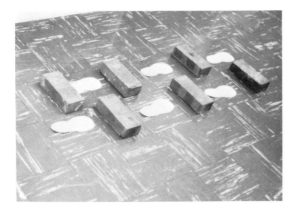

Figure 33–14 Bricks and white footprints arranged on floor to encourage hip and knee flexion, ankle dorsiflexion and proper foot placement. (Courtesy of Rehabilitation Institute of The Boston Dispensary.)

Figure 33–15 Rung ladder placed flat on floor for gait training. (Courtesy of Rehabilitation Institute of The Boston Dispensary.)

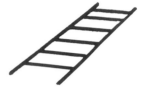

RUNG LADDER PLACED FLAT
ON FLOOR FOR GAIT TRAINING

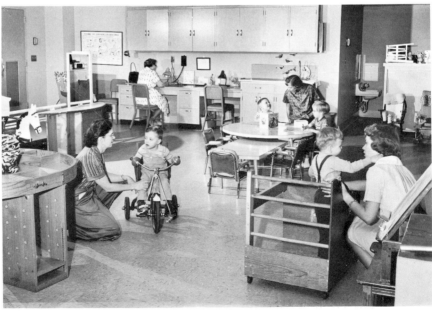

Figure 33–16 Special equipment in use in a therapeutic nursery. (Courtesy of Therapeutic Nursery of the Minneapolis Curative Workshop.)

child is much more likely to accept it. Very short adjustable "Kenny sticks" are easy to control and they stay on the arms when the child wishes to use his hands for other activities.

Figure 33-16 shows special equipment for children's rehabilitation in use.

Training for the Upper Extremities

Training for the upper extremities has been mentioned in the previous section. Specific attention should be paid to the development of range of motion, control of motion, adequate strength and active use. In the young child whose upper extremities are involved in a neuromuscular problem, grasp is usually not very well developed. Palmar grasp is often crude. When the thumb has been held flexed and adducted inside the palm with the fingers flexed over it, the web of the thumb may be shortened and it may be necessary to place a stretching splint in the web to develop abduction and extension. When flexion contractures have occurred in the finger joints, metacarpal phalangeal joints and wrist, active physical therapy and splinting may be necessary to correct the deformity. As soon as there is voluntary movement the child should engage in games that involve pushing, reaching, grasping and releasing, followed by activities that require placement and grasp, progressing from crude palmar grasp to pincer grasp. It is best to start with wooden beads, blocks and spools large enough to make prehension easy but small enough to fit in the child's hand. Progression to smaller objects, to the point where the child has relatively fine prehension, is usually rather rapid. Peg boards for the development of placement and marble games and the like are also useful.

When the child will need to use crutches for ambulation, the necessity for strengthening the shoulder depressors and the triceps should not be overlooked. Mat exercises and active games and toys that require the use of these muscles are prescribed.

Orthopedic Surgery

Supervision of the treatment program of these children involves repeated physical examinations, neurologic reevaluation and x-ray evaluation of the joints that appear not to be responding adequately to treatment. When adequate heat, massage, stretching, splinting and active exercise are not effective in overcoming weakness and contractures, orthopedic surgery often has great advantage for these children and should not be delayed. When there have been significant degrees of contracture, particularly of the hip and knee, reduction of the contracture by orthopedic surgery should be done early because as a child grows the neurovascular elements that cross the joint may not grow sufficiently in length to allow complete correction when the surgery is performed at a later date. In addition, subluxation, dislocations and outright deformities of the bones will occur.

SPASTICITY

There are various opinions, none of which is backed by much objective evidence, concerning the proper treatment of spasticity and its contractures.

Prolonged gentle manual stretching or prolonged positional stretching of short-ened structures performed by the parents or therapist have been shown to be effective in at least one study carried out over a period of many years.[9] Heat and massage make stretching easier. Only when stretching appears not to be effective after a reasonable period of trial is orthopedic surgery indicated. However, when one has spent several weeks, not years, unsuccessfully using adequate stretching procedures for the correction of the specific deformity, the orthopedic surgeon should be consulted.

Surgical release of contractures, transplantation of muscles or release of tight joint capsules may offer great advantages to children. Nerve blocks and nerve crushing properly applied have also been helpful. When adequate phys-ical therapy, positioning and soft tissue surgical procedures are performed early, bone surgery for correction of bony deformities is rarely necessary.

The use of medications for relief of spasticity has been almost uniformly disappointing. The two most effective drugs at the present time continue to be quinine and alcohol taken by mouth, and the obvious disadvantages of pro-longed use of these drugs militate against their general use. The newer "muscle relaxants" have been uniformly ineffective in spasticity in our experience, in spite of many claims to the contrary.

ATHETOSIS

Relaxation of the athetoid child before the development of voluntary control is attempted is part of almost all programs of treatment and appears to be essential. However, it does not seem reasonable to spend long periods of time, months or years, on developing relaxation in a child who will lose it as soon as he attempts voluntary movement. The child with athetosis may respond more satisfactorily to medications that cause central relaxation or that work on the muscles themselves. Meprobamate, phenobarbital and alcohol have all been useful. A word of caution: it has been said athetoid children do not develop contractures, but many children with a major diagnosis of athetosis do have limiting contractures and develop subluxation of the hip. Careful evaluation of individual patients will indicate the tendency toward contractures and the specific treatment that may be necessary.

ATAXIA

The child with ataxia generally has a better prognosis for development of physical function than children with other disabilities, assuming that his vision and intelligence are adequate. Physical therapy should be directed toward the development of control of movements and learning by visual and kinesthetic clues, insofar as possible, to develop sense of distance, sense of balance and so forth. Modifications of Frenkel's exercises are useful in this group of patients.

MIXED LESIONS

Obviously children with mixed lesions must have individualized programs for their specific neuromuscular problems and since mixed symptomatology is a common finding, systems of treatment or sets of exercises designed for universal application to all "cases" of "spasticity" or "athetosis" will serve few well and many badly. Over the years highly publicized sequences of treatment have been received with enthusiasm and applied before they have been subjected to sufficiently critical analyses to determine their effectiveness. Most of these systems have been abandoned when clinical use has shown that they do not produce the desired results.

PROGNOSIS

The child's rate of progress will be determined by his motivation and by the degree of his motor disability. The program outlined in this chapter, involving treatment of all of the associated defects—physical therapy for the specific neuromotor problems, orthopedic surgery, bracing and other methods of enhancing the child's potential functional ability—and a progressive exposure to the developmental pattern that takes place in normal children, should allow good progress and should also give evidence of the ultimate prognosis of the child. It is very difficult after only one or two examinations to assess a child's potential and to be able to give any reliable prognosis.

REFERENCES

1. Abercrombie, M. L. J.: Perceptual and Visuo-motor Disorders in Cerebral Palsy. Little Club Clinics in Developmental Medicine (11). London, William Heinemann Medical Books, Ltd., 1964.
2. American Public Health Association: Program Area Committee on Child Health Services for Children with Cerebral Palsy. New York, 1967.
3. Berenberg, W.: The Physician's Responsibility in the Education of the Cerebral Palsied Child. Pediatrics, *43:*483-485, 1969.
4. Birch, H. G.: Brain Damage in Children. The Biological and Social Aspects. Baltimore, Williams and Wilkins Co., 1964.
5. Cohen, H. J., Birch, H. G., and Taft, L. T.: Some Considerations for Evaluating the Doman-Delcato "Patterning" Method. Pediatrics, *45:*302-314, 1970.
6. Crothers, B., and Paine, R. S.: The Natural History of Cerebral Palsy. Cambridge, Massachusetts, Harvard University Press, 1959.
7. Cruickshank, W. G. (Editor): Cerebral Palsy—Its Individual and Community Problems. Syracuse University Press, 1966.
8. Egan, D., Illingworth, R. S., and MacKeith, R. C.: Developmental Screening 0–5 Years. London, William Heinemann, 1968.
9. Ellis, E.: Physical Management of Developmental Disorders. Little Club Clinics in Developmental Medicine (26). London, William Heinemann Medical Books, Ltd., 1967.
10. Foley, J.: Deterioration in the EEG in Children with Cerebral Palsy. Develop. Med. Child Neurol., *10:*287-301, 1968.
11. Frankenburg, W. R., and Dodds, J. B.: The Denver Developmental Screening Test. J. Pediat., *71:*181–191, 1967.
12. Freeman, R. D.: Psychiatric Problems in Adolescents with Cerebral Palsy. Develop. Med. Child Neurol., *12:*64–70, 1970.
13. Gesell, A., and Amatruda, C. S.: Developmental Diagnosis. 2nd Ed., New York, Hoeber, 1947.
14. Halpern, D., and MeelHuysen, F.: Phenol Motor Point Block in the Management of Hypertonia. Arch. Phys. Med., *47:*659–664, 1966.
15. Holt, K. S.: Assessment of Cerebral Palsy. London, Lloyd-Luke, Ltd., 1965.
16. Holt, K. S., and Reynell, J. K.: Assessment of Cerebral Palsy. II, Vision, Hearing, Speech, Language, Communication and Psychological Function. London, Lloyd-Luke, Ltd., 1967.
17. Ingram, T. T. S., Jameson, S., Ellis, E., and Mitchell, R. G.: Living with Cerebral Palsy. Little Club Clinics in Developmental Medicine (14). London, William Heinemann Medical Books, Ltd., 1964.
18. Ingram, T. T. S.: Paediatric Aspects of Cerebral Palsy. Edinburgh, Livingstone, 1964.
19. Klapper, Z. S., and Birch, H. G.: A Fourteen-Year Follow-up Study of Cerebral Palsy: Intellectual Change and Stability. Amer. J. Orthopsychiat., *37:*540–547.

20. Korsch, B., Cobb, K., and Ashe, B.: Pediatrician's Appraisal of His Patient's Intelligence. Amer. J. Dis. Child., *100*:478, 1960.
21. Lesny, L.: The Development of Athetosis. Develop. Med. Child Neurol., *10*:441–446, 1968.
22. Peterson, H. A., and Coventry, M. B.: Long-Term Results of Surgical Treatment of Adults with Cerebral Palsy. Develop. Med. Child Neurol., *11*:35-43, 1969.
23. Pollock, G. A., and Stark, G.: Long-Term Results in the Management of 67 Children with Cerebral Palsy. Develop Med. Child Neurol., *11*:17-34, 1969.
24. Robson, P.: The Prevalence of Scoliosis in Adolescents and Young Adults with Cerebral Palsy. Develop. Med. Child Neurol., *10*:447-452, 1968.
25. Sterling, H. M.: Pediatric Rehabilitation. Arch. Phys. Med., *48*:474-479, 1967.
26. Smith, V. H.: Visual Disorders and Cerebral Palsy. Little Club Clinics in Developmental Medicine (9). London, William Heinemann Medical Books, Ltd., 1963.
27. Wilson, B. C., and Wilson, J. J.: Sensory and Perceptual Functions in the Cerebral Palsied: I, Pressure Thresholds and Two-Point Discrimination. J. Nerv. Ment. Dis., *145*:53-60, 1967.
28. Wilson, B. C., and Wilson, J. J.: Sensory and Perceptual Functions in the Cerebral Palsied: II, Stereognosis. J. Nerv. Ment. Dis., *145*:61–68, 1967.

Chapter 34

DISORDERS OF RESPIRATION (PULMONARY FUNCTION); CHEST PHYSICAL THERAPY

by H. Frederic Helmholz, Jr., G. Keith Stillwell
and Alan D. Sessler

DISORDERS OF RESPIRATION

by H. Frederic Helmholz, Jr., and
G. Keith Stillwell

Respiration is transport. It is the process of moving oxygen from the air to the alveoli of the lungs by a mass movement of air, called ventilation, and in turn removing carbon dioxide from the alveoli by the same mass movement. Ventilation maintains a pressure (concentration) gradient between alveolar gas and venous blood so that gases exchange between blood and alveolar gas by diffusion. The circulatory system provides the transport between the lungs and the tissues.

The effort, or cost, of ventilation depends on the elastic properties of the lungs, thorax, diaphragm, abdomen complex and accessory muscles and the resistance to flow through the multiple air passages between the outside and the alveoli.

669

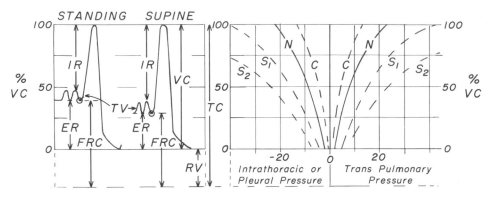

Figure 34–1 Subdivisions of total lung capacity (TC) are shown related to pressures (N) in normal respiratory maneuvers. Dotted lines indicate pressures required with different lung compliances. I R = inspiratory reserve volume; TV = tidal volume; ER = expiratory reserve volume; RV = residual volume; VC = vital capacity; FRC = functional residual capacity; C = more compliant than the normal; S_1 and S_2 = less compliant (stiffer) than the normal.

PHYSIOLOGIC BASIS OF DISORDERS OF RESPIRATION

Respiratory disorders, then, are conditions that prevent adequate transport in and out of the lungs (exchange), thereby leading to retention of carbon dioxide and to oxygen lack. These disorders may be caused by (1) muscle weakness or inefficiency or increasing stiffness of elastic components or by (2) increased resistance to air flow through the tracheobronchial tree; hence they are classified as (1) *restrictive* or (2) *obstructive*. A third category, that of conditions due to an increase in thickness of, or a decrease in area of, the alveolar diffusing membrane, is usually associated with a restrictive disorder; it leads primarily to low oxygen tension in arterial blood without carbon dioxide retention because of the much greater diffusivity of carbon dioxide in body tissues.

In Figure 34–1 the lung volume relationships and definitions are shown, and the effect of position on the end expiratory position relative to vital capacity is suggested. The end expiratory position is that at which elastic recoil of the lung is exactly balanced by the tendency of the "chest" to expand (point O, for example, in Figure 34–2). This point of equilibrium differs with position: in the supine position, the weight of abdominal contents favors expiration; in the upright position, it favors inspiration. In the weak individual, this change can be used to produce adequate resting ventilation (for example, with the rocking bed).

Restrictive Disorders

Figure 34–2 illustrates the elastic properties of the lung and "chest" (by which is meant the entire complex of thoracic cage, diaphragm, abdomen and relaxed abdominal muscles). Normally about 20 cm. of water pressure would fill the isolated lung to vital capacity size (curve L, Fig. 34–2). Thus, full inspiration requires a transpulmonary pressure of this magnitude, normally achieved

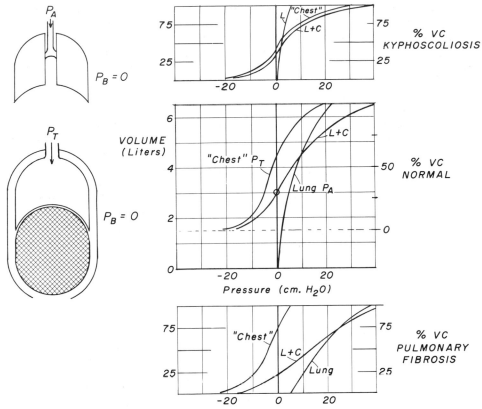

Figure 34–2 Pressure-volume diagrams of the lung alone (L; Lung; P_A), of the thoracic cavity alone ("Chest;" P_T) and of the combination (L + C) are constructed to indicate normal relationships and those found in two types of restrictive disorder. $P_B = O$ indicates that the atmospheric (barometric) pressure is the pressure to which the other pressures are referred.

by maintenance of the same pressure below atmospheric in the pleural space, i.e., the space around the lungs. (Curves N, Fig. 34–1.) The dotted curves indicate the effect of varying the lung compliance (Fig. 34–1). Curves C are for increased compliance and curves S_1 and S_1, for lungs stiffer than normal.

If the lungs were removed and pressures above and below atmospheric were applied inside the remaining cavity, the characteristic curve marked "Chest" would be obtained (Fig. 34–2).

If, in the paralyzed individual, the combination of lungs and chest were similarly treated, one would obtain the combined curve relating volume to pressure indicated by "L + C" (Fig. 34–2). Such a curve describes the elastic properties of the system and the recoil which must be overcome in breathing. For any given tidal volume, the area between the line of zero pressure and the curve to this tidal volume represents work. If the time required is specified as well, one has an expression of power, or the rate at which work is done.

In Figure 34–2 the chart above the normal indicates the effect of chest deformity in changing the elastic properties of the chest and reducing the vital capacity. Note that the chest curve is the restricting element; thus, intrathoracic (pleural) pressure is never much below atmospheric because the elastic lung is never stretched sufficiently to produce a large negative pressure.

The chart below the normal chart indicates the effect of increased stiffness of the lung (loss of compliance) in changing the elastic properties of the system and reducing the vital capacity. Note that this disorder leads to pressures well below atmospheric at all lung volumes, because of increased elastic recoil of the lung at all volumes.

Restrictive disorders are characterized by increased energy requirement to overcome elastic recoil of lung or chest structures at any given ventilation. Any disease that stiffens costovertebral or sternocostal connections or causes fibrosis of respiratory, abdominal or shoulder girdle muscles or of the lungs themselves, can lead to restrictive impairment of pulmonary function.

The same effect is produced by the loss of muscle or the loss of nerves that activate the muscles of respiration. The chart marked "normal" in Figure 34–2 shows the relationships that would occur if the vital capacity were reduced by a decrease in both the inspiratory and the expiratory reserve volumes. The restriction in such cases would be the inability to bring force to bear and do work against the recoil of the elastic system.

Obstructive Disorders

In any lung the air distribution system expands as the lung expands, and therefore there is a relationship between lung size and the resistance to gas flow (Fig. 34–3). One of the characteristics of asthma and emphysema is an increase in resistance to air flow as indicated in the curve marked "Emphysema." The dotted curve indicates the behavior in many cases of emphysema when expiration is forced. This is the phenomenon of air trapping, in which the airway develops such high resistance when transpulmonary pressure is high that air flow stops before emptying is complete. It has been shown that the obstructive phenomena in the emphysematous lung are characteristically nonuniform and are primarily brought out on expiration. Asthma tends to produce more uniform obstruction, which is evident to some extent during inspiration.

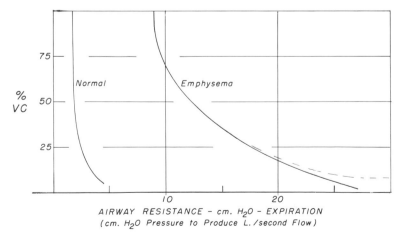

Figure 34–3   Resistance to air flow in a normal and emphysematous lung during expiration. Dotted line indicates effect of increased effort during a "forced expiration."

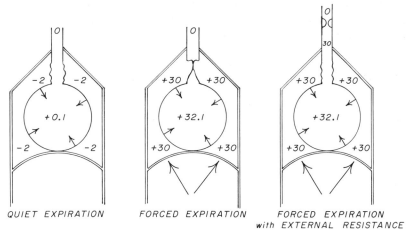

Figure 34–4 Diagram to illustrate one possible mechanism of air-trapping and effect of resistance imposed by pursed-lip or grunting expiration. (This model requires rapid onset of positive intrapleural pressure to show the phenomenon. A resistance interposed between the "alveolus" and the compliant segment of airway converts this to a better demonstration model.)

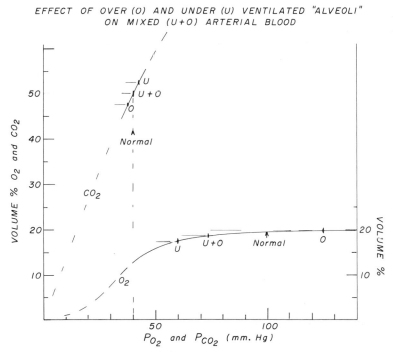

Figure 34–5 Plotting of oxygen and carbon dioxide dissociation curves together shows the effect of relative linearity of carbon dioxide solubility contrasted with alinearity of oxygen solubility on content of mixed (U + O) arterial blood content when it is made up of blood perfusing underventilated (U) and overventilated (O) areas of lung.

A simple obstructing lesion of the trachea, when intrathoracic, can simulate emphysema if the involved trachea becomes collapsible. This kind of lesion serves here as a model in understanding air trapping (Fig. 34–4). When the lung empties because of its own elastic recoil, the pressure (intrathoracic) around the nonrigid trachea remains below atmospheric and the airway remains patent. If forced expiration is attempted and intrathoracic pressure rises above atmospheric, the trachea collapses and prevents egress of the remaining air. It is theorized that multiple small air passages act the same way in emphysema. By obstruction of the airway *outside* the chest during exhalation, the pressure inside these passages is increased and the collapse is prevented. Hence, breathing out through pursed lips or grunting is often beneficial.

Obstructive disease can cause a decrease in arterial oxygen tension and retention of carbon dioxide when obstruction is relatively uniform, as in obstructing lesions of the trachea, for example.

Emphysema, however, and most cases of asthma characteristically cause a reduction in arterial oxygen tension without carbon dioxide retention because of the difference of the carbon dioxide and oxygen dissociation curves. Figure 34–5 illustrates how the retention of carbon dioxide in underventilated areas is compensated for in overventilated areas, whereas so little extra oxygen is taken up in the overventilated areas that the oxygen content and tension of arterial blood are below normal.

Diffusing Capacity Disorders

The amount of oxygen passing through the alveolar membrane of the lung depends directly on the difference between the alveolar oxygen pressure and the mean oxygen pressure of capillary blood. It depends also on the area of the membrane that separates air and blood; it is reduced by an increased distance between alveolar air and the hemoglobin of the blood (membrane thickness factor). Pulmonary fibrosis in its various forms causes thickening of the membrane and a decrease in alveolar surface, typically without obstructive disease.

Normally, increased oxygen uptake by the lung is caused by a decrease in the oxygen content of venous blood and an increase in pulmonary blood flow along with an increase in ventilation. A diffusion barrier can be compensated for to some extent by increasing ventilation, which reduces the carbon dioxide concentration in alveolar gas and thus raises the oxygen concentration (that is, pressure). In these cases the cost of maintaining a low alveolar carbon dioxide pressure is least when a rapid rate of breathing is used. Deep breathing would require excessive work because of decreased compliance.

DIAGNOSTIC CHARACTERISTICS OF DISORDERS

If the vital capacity, forced vital capacity (maximal expiratory effort following maximal inspiration) and the pattern and volume of ventilation with maximal breathing effort (so-called maximal breathing capacity) are measured with a suitable recording spirometer, the presence of obstructive disease can be detected. If no obstructive phenomena are found but dyspnea is present, the magnitude of the vital capacity may be used as an index of possible reduction in lung volume. Measurements of diffusing capacity of the lung can be made to detect abnormalities in such patients. The reader is referred to Comroe and associates[2] for details of testing procedures and, when dealing with children, to Polgar and Promadhat.[3]

Restrictive disorders are inferred when vital capacity and total capacity are reduced and no obstructive disorder is evident. Documentation of such disorders requires special tests that are beyond the scope of this presentation.

The following table gives findings in obstructive and restrictive disorders that can be obtained by a recording spirometer.

	VITAL CAPACITY	FORCED VITAL CAPACITY* (% IN 1 SECOND)	MAXIMAL BREATHING CAPACITY
Obstructive	Reduced	Less than 85%	Reduced
Restrictive	Reduced	85% or more	Normal or slightly reduced

*Many modifications of the method of estimating obstruction from a forced vital capacity are used. Any can be used when a recording is obtained.

Estimates of lung size from physical examination and chest roentgenograms will indicate that total capacity is normal or increased in obstructive disorders and reduced in restrictive disorders.

CHARACTERISTICS OF CONTROL OF VENTILATION AND CIRCULATION

Normally, the inspiratory effort causes enlargement of the thoracic cage by the contraction of the diaphragm, which decreases its doming, and by the contraction of the external intercostal muscles that raise and rotate the ribs to increase the diameter of the rib cage. The elastic lung is stretched enough to provide a rate of emptying during muscle relaxation that is adequate for alveolar ventilation at rest.

Increased oxygen demand and carbon dioxide production during muscular activity are accompanied by an increase in ventilation immediately, due to nervous impulses from active muscles and joints directly. (That due to fever is accompanied by increased ventilation as the result of increased activity of the respiratory center as the temperature rises.) Secondary mechanisms that also can increase ventilation are the effect of increased carbon dioxide tension (or fall of pH) in arterial blood on the respiratory center directly and the effect of a fall in arterial oxygen tension mediated through chemoreceptors (carotid and aortic bodies as well as specialized nerve endings on the surface of the medulla, sensitive to pH changes in the spinal fluid).

Increased activity of the respiratory center increases both the depth and the rate of breathing, and active expiration (lowering of the ribs by the internal intercostals and contraction of the abdominal muscles) begins. The stimulus to the respiratory center, if sufficiently intense, causes recruitment of accessory muscles of the neck, shoulder girdle and abdomen to aid in inspiration and expiration.

Stimulation of the respiratory center also involves the circulatory centers nearby so that increases in ventilation are accompanied by increases in cardiac output. In addition, with deeper respiration the decrease in pressure inside the thorax increases the gradient of pressure between systemic veins and the right atrium, thereby tending to increase venous return which increases the output of first the right side and then the left side of the heart.

BASIS FOR BREATHING EXERCISES

Restrictive Disorders

When the nerves are intact or remnants of the neuromuscular system are underdeveloped muscle weakness can be helped by suitable exercise. It should be emphasized that muscles of respiration cannot be put at rest and therefore they should be exercised voluntarily so that the increase in ventilation will make possible lessened activity of the muscles following therapeutic exercise. The margin between activity that will cause damage and activity that will cause hypertrophy can be narrow in patients with restrictive disorders and due caution should be observed when increased demands are put on respiratory muscles.

Chest deformities disturb the relations between the insertions and origins of respiratory muscles and may tend to flatten the diaphragm by increasing the anteroposterior dimension of the chest. Pulling in of the lower part of the rib cage with inspiration indicates inefficient use of the diaphragm. Often no increase in doming can be achieved in such patients, but the phenomenon should be noted and abdominal muscle exercises should be instituted when benefit is possible. Each case of deformity must be studied carefully before an exercise program is outlined. In many cases the only possible therapy is mechanical assistance to ventilation.

In treating any fibrosing or sclerosing disease of the chest cage and musculature the effect of loss of compliance should be kept in mind. Loosening of contractures and stiffened joints, when it is possible, decreases remarkably the work of breathing.

Loss of compliance of the lungs (fibrosis) is difficult to treat by physical means, but further development of respiratory muscles can be tried.

Obstructive Disorders

Obstructive disease is accompanied by fixation of the chest in a position larger than the normal end expiratory level, with an increase in the functional residual capacity and residual volume. This condition tends to produce a flattening of the diaphragm and thus to lessen the usefulness of this muscle in inspiration. In some cases the abdominal muscles are contracted during inspiration and work against the inspiratory effort of the intercostal, neck and shoulder muscles. In such cases help can be afforded by retraining to ensure relaxation of the abdominal muscles during inspiration. The best method is the use of exercises that contract the abdominal muscles during *expiration.*

Because the work of breathing increases rapidly when air velocity increases in obstructive disease, the following formulation is emphasized:

$$\dot{V}_A = (V_T - V_D)\, f$$

in which $\dot{V}_A$ = alveolar ventilation (liters per minute) BTPS, V_T = tidal volume (liters), V_D = dead space volume (liters) and f = frequency (breaths per minute).

Since with each breath the dead space remains constant, the amount of dead space ventilation increases as frequency increases. With each breath the volume in excess of the dead space inhaled is effective, or alveolar, ventilation; the greater the tidal volume, the less of it is dead space ventilation.

Thus, the minimal total ventilation required for a given alveolar ventilation is attained by slow, deep breathing. Air velocities are also least when a given alveolar ventilation is attained by a *maximal tidal volume* and a *minimal frequency*. Since obstruction is primarily expiratory, fast inhalation ensures the lowest frequency. In addition, the phenomenon of air trapping should be kept in mind and rapid forced expiration should be avoided except through pursed lips or the partially closed glottis or vocal cords. With these principles in mind, a rational program of breathing exercises can be worked out that will help any patient who normally uses rapid, shallow breathing through an open mouth. The patient who already breathes slowly and deeply, and who exhales through pursed lips or grunts during expiration, will be helped less but can be reassured. Training can ensure deeper expiration when exercise produces stimulation of the expiratory muscles, if emphasis is put on deeper, faster inhalation and slower exhalation through pursed lips.

Underventilation

When restrictive disorders (including loss of muscle power) and obstructive disorders are of such severity that resting ventilation is insufficient to remove metabolic carbon dioxide, alveolar concentration of this gas rises until metabolic production is removed, according to the following formula:

$$\dot{V}_{CO_2} = \dot{V}_A \times F_{ACO_2}$$

in which $\dot{V}_{CO_2}$ = liters of CO_2 exhaled per minute BTP, $\dot{V}_A$ = alveolar ventilation (liters per minute) BTPS and F_{ACO_2} = fraction of CO_2 in alveolar gas.

Underventilation produces respiratory acidosis and as carbon dioxide rises, oxygen falls to seriously low levels when air is breathed. However, cyanosis cannot be used as an index of adequacy of ventilation because of the variability in the amount of reduced hemoglobin in the superficial (visible) capillary beds. Severe oxygen deficiency in arterial blood is possible without cyanosis (for example, in peripheral vasoconstriction or anemia), and cyanosis occurs frequently in congestive failure when arterial blood is sufficiently saturated with oxygen.

Assistance to ventilation is the treatment of choice when the patient is capable of some respiratory effort. It can be accomplished by application of positive pressure to the airway during inspiration by an I.P.P.B.I. (intermittent positive pressure breathing, inspiration) machine. This device is so designed that a slight negative pressure starts a flow of gas which continues until a preset positive pressure is reached; then the flow stops and the airway is vented to the outside. The pressure setting determines the tidal volume. The patient can slow the rate or speed it up, depending on the ventilation needed. The patient's own respiratory control mechanism thus becomes effective once more in regulating alveolar ventilation to metabolic needs.

When all respiratory activity has ceased, total control of ventilation must be undertaken by applying positive pressure to the airway, or negative pressure to the body, at regular intervals. It is impossible with the equipment presently available to adjust ventilation as precisely as does the respiratory control system of the body, but estimates made periodically of arterial blood levels of pH and carbon dioxide allow one to check adequacy by the following relationship (Henderson-Hasselbalch equation for the bicarbonate-carbon dioxide system):

$$pH = 6.1 + \log \frac{[HCO_3^-]}{0.03 \ P_{CO_2}}$$

or

$$pH = 6.1 + \log \frac{[Total \ CO_2] - 0.03 \ P_{CO_2}}{0.03 \ P_{CO_2}}$$

Solution indicates that normal values approximate the following:

$$7.4 = 6.1 + \log \frac{20}{1} = 6.1 + \log \frac{24 \ mEq./L.}{0.03 \ (40) \ mM/L.} =$$

$$6.1 + \log \frac{25.2 - 1.2 \ mM/L.}{1.2 \ mM/L.}$$

$0.03 \ mM/L./mm. =$ solubility coefficient for CO_2 at body temperature.

In respiratory acidosis, P_{CO_2} goes up and pH goes down. Renal compensation will allow an increase in bicarbonate so that its ratio to P_{CO_2} increases again and pH returns toward normal.

Carbon dioxide retention can be tolerated for relatively long periods of time (though it causes narcosis when excessive), but lack of oxygen cannot; therefore, filling the lungs with high concentrations of oxygen will protect the individual from oxygen lack in emergency situations until definitive treatment can be instituted. Oxygen should always be administered first. When the lung contains only oxygen, carbon dioxide and water vapor, cyanosis will never intervene if circulation is intact; thus, once oxygen has been administered, cyanosis cannot be an indication of ventilatory insufficiency in any sense at all.

When positive pressure is applied through the airway or negative pressure around the body to expand the lungs, the intrathoracic pressure relative to systemic venous pressure is inevitably raised and venous return is decreased. The normal circulatory system can compensate for this, but when it is hampered by blood loss or other abnormalities, serious decreases in cardiac output are produced. In those forms of restrictive disorder that are due to decreased compliance of the lungs, positive pressure applied to the airway causes much less circulatory disturbance than does negative pressure around the body. In other restrictive conditions, the two methods affect the circulatory system about equally. In obstructive disease, the application of positive pressure through the airway may be expected to affect the circulatory system less than would negative pressure around the body.

In those forms of restrictive disorder in which the primary abnormality is a barrier to diffusion of oxygen from alveolar gas to blood, a simple increase in the oxygen concentration of the inhaled gas will provide adequate compensation.

By studying the charts in Figure 34–1, with the additional information that lung compliance is usually within the normal range but the "chest" curve may be moved to the left in obstructive disease, one can work out the mechanical relationships that may be expected in various forms of pulmonary disorders. The circulatory disorders that affect lung function are those that cause pulmonary venous hypertension (such as mitral stenosis or left heart failure). They produce a decrease in lung compliance and, when pulmonary edema is present, a diffusion barrier.

Chest Injuries

The special case of chest injuries merits some consideration. Loss of integrity of the lung, which causes pneumothorax, is an emergency to be handled by a thoracic surgeon, but loss of integrity of the chest cage leads to a mechanical defect that tends to prevent inspiration. For example, negative pleural pressure developed by diaphragmatic contraction causes a nonrigid rib cage to collapse, thus preventing expansion of the lungs. Fixation of the ribs has been the treatment of choice. Positive pressure applied to the airway during inspiration has many advantages in that it ensures ventilation and splints the chest without operative measures. When the ribs are intact but muscle contraction causes pain, inspiration is limited. Therefore, intermittent positive pressure breathing is the treatment of choice in chest injuries which cause underventilation. It decreases pain as it increases ventilation. Decrease in venous return is the only complication; it should be considered whenever there has been loss of blood. Fall in blood pressure or increase in pulse rate, or both, indicate the need for blood replacement.

In the use of equipment for the support of or assistance to ventilation, certain principles are often forgotten. Any pneumatic system used is effective only if forces are applied to the elastic system including the lungs. Any leaks in the system prevent this application. A leak is the most frequent cause of failure and must not be permitted. Devices designed to compensate for leaks are unrealistic and lead to slipshod therapy.

Whenever the nasal passages are by-passed (by the use of tracheal tubes, pharyngeal catheters, mouth breathing or tracheostomy), sufficient water must be added to the inhaled gas to ensure a relative humidity of 100 per cent at the body temperature of the patient. Gases below this temperature must contain particulate water. In practice, it is necessary to add heat to humidifiers in order to maintain this relative humidity.

REFERENCES

Disorders of Respiration

1. Campbell, E. J. M.: The Respiratory Muscles: And the Mechanics of Breathing. Chicago, Year Book Medical Publishers, Inc., 1958.
2. Comroe, J. H., Jr., Forster, R. E., II, Dubois, A. B., Briscoe, W. A., and Carlsen, E.: The Lung: Clinical Physiology and Pulmonary Function Tests. 2nd Ed. Chicago, Year Book Medical Publishers, Inc., 1962.
3. Polgar and Promadhat: Pulmonary Function Testing in Children. Philadelphia, W. B. Saunders Company, 1971.

CHEST PHYSICAL THERAPY

by Alan D. Sessler

Chest physical therapy is the application of physical methods to the respiratory care of patients with pulmonary disease. The range of treatment includes instruction in relaxation and breathing exercises; performance of postural drainage, percussion or clapping, and vibration; and splinting the chest or incision site to facilitate coughing. All these techniques assist in clearing pulmonary secretions. They are particularly indicated in patients with chronic obstructive lung disease manifested as asthma, bronchitis, emphysema, bronchiectasis and cystic fibrosis; after major surgery of the upper abdomen, thorax and cardiovascular system; and in all patients who are dependent on mechanical ventilation. A supportive program of chest physical therapy is necessary to assist patients with neuromuscular disease and a diminished cough reflex or effort who are unable to mobilize their pulmonary secretions. All patients immobilized in bed can benefit from instructions in coughing and breathing exercises. Surgical patients are helped if they have developed confidence in the therapist before the operation. After the operation, it is difficult to gain the cooperation of a patient who is in pain and receiving analgesics. In the acutely ill, chest physical therapy is closely allied with inhalation therapy and intensive-care nursing. A working knowledge of oxygen and humidification equipment, mechanical ventilators, intermittent positive-pressure breathing devices, and endotracheal and tracheostomy tubes is essential.

Breathing Exercises.   The therapist should instruct the patient in the techniques of breathing exercises (Fig. 34–6).

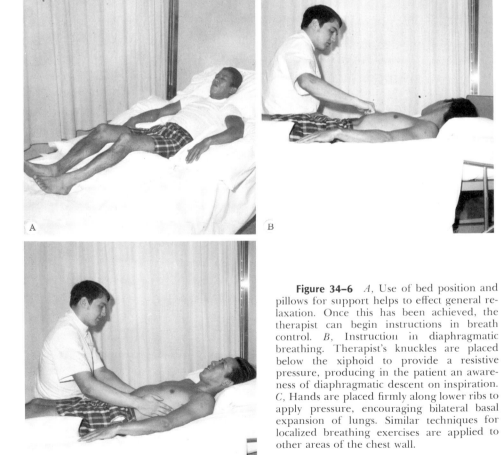

Figure 34–6 *A,* Use of bed position and pillows for support helps to effect general relaxation. Once this has been achieved, the therapist can begin instructions in breath control. *B,* Instruction in diaphragmatic breathing. Therapist's knuckles are placed below the xiphoid to provide a resistive pressure, producing in the patient an awareness of diaphragmatic descent on inspiration. *C,* Hands are placed firmly along lower ribs to apply pressure, encouraging bilateral basal expansion of lungs. Similar techniques for localized breathing exercises are applied to other areas of the chest wall.

Postural Drainage.   Optimal use of postural drainage requires a knowledge of the segmental anatomy of the lung.[4-6] Reference to more detailed manuals are listed at the end of this section. For the patient with a poor cough and widespread pulmonary secretions who is confined to bed, hourly turning from side to side may be inadequate to manage secretions. A modified program of postural drainage practical even in many critically ill patients can be developed (Fig. 34–7).

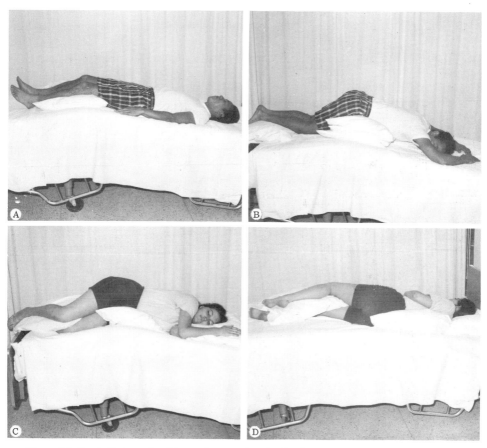

Figure 34–7   *A*, Patient should spend some time in the dependent position. Most patients will tolerate 10 to 15° of head-down tilt for a brief period, several times a day. This position facilitates drainage by gravity of the anterior basal segments. *B*, Position used for draining the posterior basal segments. *C*, Position for drainage of right lower lobe and lateral basal bronchus. *D*, Position for drainage of the left upper lobe and for lower division of the superior and inferior bronchi.

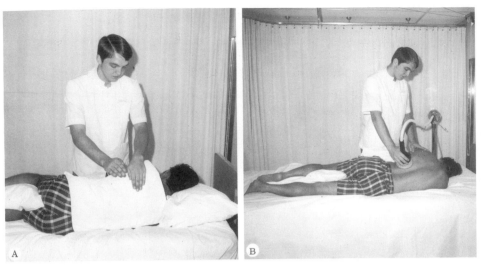

Figure 34–8 *A*, Position for chest percussion or clapping. *B*, Position for manual or mechanical vibration.

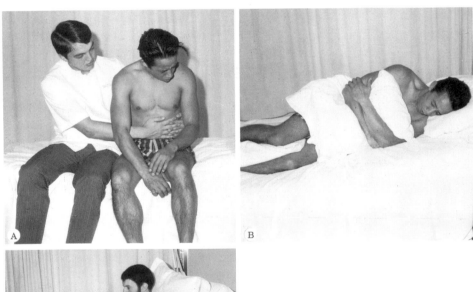

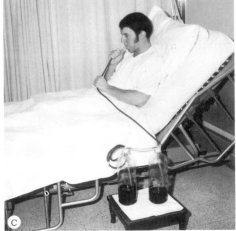

Figure 34–9 *A*, Manual splinting of chest or abdominal incision. *B*, While coughing, patient hugs pillow. *C*, Blow bottle helps lung expansion.

Other Maneuvers.   In addition to the basic postural drainage maneuvers that the patient can be taught to do for himself, chest percussion or clapping (Fig. 34–8*A*) and vibration, either manually or mechanically (Fig. 34–8*B*), are necessary and useful adjuncts in clearing secretions.

Other techniques frequently used to help postoperative patients are manual splinting of the chest or abdominal incision by the therapist (Fig. 34–9*A*), patient coughing while hugging a pillow (Fig. 34–9*B*) and use of a blow bottle (Fig. 34–9*C*) for the patient to exhale against resistance in order to aid in lung expansion. Adaptations of the techniques can be useful in small children (Fig. 34–10).

ROUTINE CHEST PHYSICAL THERAPY

In the acutely ill patient, chest physical therapy may be given as frequently as every two hours and should be closely coordinated within the overall respiratory program. For routine treatment given two to four times daily, the following sequence and procedures are ordered.

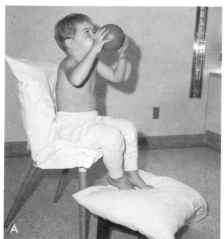
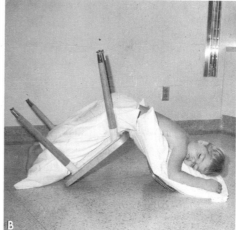
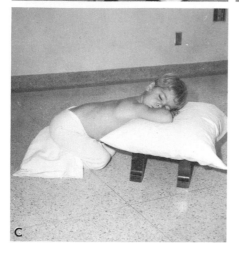

Figure 34–10 Techniques useful for small children.

1. Mist Inhalation (20 Minutes).　This will wet down the upper airways and help liquefy secretions. The mist may be cold for febrile patients but preferably is heated to deliver more water. Usually the carrier gas is oxygen-enriched air. Administration via a mask or into a tent may be by humidifier or nebulizer. Instruction for breathing exercises and cough control can be given at this time, if it is convenient for the physical therapist.

2. Intermittent Positive-Pressure Breathing (IPPB) (15 Minutes).　These treatments are given by inhalation-therapy or nursing personnel and result in a period of mild hyperventilation and an increase in lung expansion. IPPB also provides an effective means of delivering bronchodilator, decongestant and mucolytic agents to the airways and, in addition, continues to add moisture.

3. Chest Physical Therapy (20 Minutes).　After the mist and IPPB are given, postural drainage, combined with vibration and percussion, usually produces good results in clearing secretions. Supplemental maneuvers performed at this time for patients on ventilators are stimulation of cough by direct tracheal suctioning, hyperinflation with oxygen by bag and mask, and instillation of saline through endotracheal and tracheostomy tubes prior to suctioning.

Within the range of respiratory care, chest physical therapy and inhalation therapy have complementary roles. Most patients who receive chest physical therapy also will use one or more pieces of oxygen equipment and likely will receive IPPB therapy as well. The physical therapist must be familiar with the operation of this equipment, just as the inhalation therapist must have experience in the techniques of chest physical therapy.

REFERENCES

Chest Physical Therapy

4. Physiotherapy Department, Brompton Hospital, London: Physiotherapy for Medical and Surgical Thoracic Conditions. 1967.
5. Egan, D. F.: Fundamentals of Inhalation Therapy. St. Louis, Missouri, C. V. Mosby Company, 1969.
6. Department of Physical Medicine and Rehabilitation, University of Minnesota Medical School, Minneapolis: Techniques of Bronchial Drainage. 1967.

Chapter 35

COMMON CARDIOVASCULAR PROBLEMS IN REHABILITATION

by Frederic J. Kottke

CARDIAC DISEASE

The heart diseases treated in rehabilitation programs may be divided into three general types.

Mechanical Derangements. Conditions in which the valves or chambers of the heart are faulty, resulting in interference with forward flow, regurgitation or diversion of blood, fall into this category. The heart performs inefficiently like an obstructed or leaky pump. More work than normal must be performed by the myocardium to pump a given amount of blood into the arterial tree. As a consequence, there is increased myocardial strain and fatigue. If the myocardium cannot compensate by hypertrophy to meet the increased demand, cardiac failure ensues.

Increased Resistance to Blood Flow (Arterial Hypertension). In diseases of this type the heart must contract against a pressure that is greater than normal so that the myocardial work per liter of blood pumped is increased. Cardiac failure develops when the myocardium can no longer meet the increased demand for energy.

685

Decreased Energy Production. Pathologic changes in the myocardium or in coronary circulation reduce the energy output to below normal. Destruction or metabolic dysfunction of the myocardium or decreased circulation to the myocardium may limit its ability to do work. In each case the heart will be limited in its ability to respond to the demands of metabolic activities.

Work of the Heart

The function of the heart is to convert chemical energy from cellular metabolism into mechanical energy to pump the blood through the circulatory system composed of an expansible elastic-muscular network of vessels. The arteries by their elasticity and muscular tension maintain a positive pressure in the outflow system during the period between ventricular contractions and convert an intermittent, pulsatile flow into a steady flow at the capillary level. Such mechanical factors as abnormal resistance to flow through stenotic valves, regurgitation through leaky valves and abnormal flow through shunts decrease the effectiveness of the pumping action.

The work performed by the heart depends upon the quantity of blood ejected, the pressure against which it is pumped and the velocity imparted to the blood. If the valves are competent and if there are no intracardiac shunts, the work of the heart will appear as external work, represented by the formula:

$$W = QP + \frac{wV^2}{2g}$$

in which W = work of the ventricles, Q = volume of blood pumped, P = mean arterial blood pressure, w = weight of the blood pumped and V = velocity of ejected blood.

For the patient who has valvular disease with insufficiency, all of the work of the heart does not appear as external work because of the repumping of a portion of the blood. Likewise, stenotic valvular disease produces an increased resistance to flow which is not apparent in the peripheral blood pressure. Consequently, the hearts of patients with valvular disease must do more work in proportion to the external work which is accomplished and myocardial fatigue occurs more rapidly at any level of metabolic activity.

Cardiac output is determined by the volume of blood pumped per systolic contraction and the heart rate. Either or both of these may vary with the activity of the patient. For a normal healthy young adult, the maximal cardiac rate is approximately 180 to 210 beats per minute.[1] Although for each normal individual there is a linear correlation between pulse rate and metabolic work when that individual is in a constant posture, working at a nonfatiguing rate, in a steady state while working at a uniform type of work, variation of any of these factors will produce a nonlinear response.[2] Consequently, the pulse rate is not a reliable index of the demands on the heart for work during random activity. Moreover, patients with cardiac disease may differ markedly in their abilities to increase their heart rates and may be in cardiac distress at heart rates which are well within the safe working range for normal individuals.

The stroke volume of each ventricle at rest is approximately 60 to 70 cc. of the 150 to 170 cc. of blood contained in the ventricle. In trained athletes during maximal work stroke volumes of 120 to 190 cc. have been reported.[1] The resting stroke volume is greater during recumbency than it is in the erect position. The increase in stroke volume during increased muscular activity may

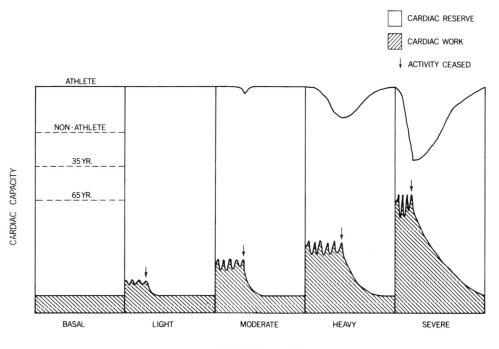

Figure 35–1   Relationship between the cardiac capacity, cardiac output and cardiac reserve of the normal heart, showing the relative decrease of cardiac capacity with age. The cardiac output of the heart of a young athlete, at maximal capacity, is approximately nine times the basal requirement for cardiac output. During heavy and severe muscular activity, the fatigue produced by the increased myocardial work causes a decrease of cardiac capacity, which recovers rapidly during the subsequent rest.

be due in part to increased diastolic volume and in part to increased systolic contraction. The cardiac patient with dilatation and hypertrophy of the heart may have a stroke volume that is considerably greater than normal.

The capacity of the normal heart to do work far exceeds the work requirement under basal conditions or during ordinary light activity. The maximal cardiac output measured in young healthy men can be increased up to nine times the resting cardiac output.[1] The myocardial work may be increased up to 15 times the resting level. In persons who are not in good physical condition because of illness or age, the maximal working capacity of the heart is greatly reduced.

The difference between the capacity of the heart to do work and the demand for cardiac work is called the cardiac reserve. With age and heart disease the cardiac reserve is reduced. During prolonged muscular work above light levels the cardiac capacity to do work is reduced by fatigue in proportion to the intensity and the duration of the work (Fig. 35-1). Therefore, the conditions of work and the intervals of rest as well as the condition of the myocardium influence the cardiac reserve. When the work required of the heart reaches the capacity of the heart to do work, a cardiac reserve no longer

RELATIONSHIP   BETWEEN   CARDIAC   CAPACITY,   CARDIAC   WORK,

AND   CARDIAC   RESERVE   IN   MYOCARDIAL   DISEASE

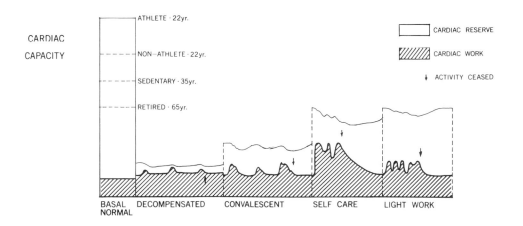

Figure 35–2 Relationship between cardiac capacity, cardiac output and cardiac reserve in myocardial disease in relation to normal. In myocardial disease cardiac capacity is severely impaired. During decompensation, cardiac output approaches cardiac capacity. Cardiac capacity gradually increases during convalescence, but activity causes cardiac fatigue with decreasing cardiac capacity, and recovery occurs more slowly during rest than it does in the normal heart.

exists and unless the work of the heart can be reduced below the capacity, the heart is decompensated and unable to continue to work at the level demanded of it.

Successful management of the patient with cardiac disease depends upon keeping the load imposed upon the heart below the cardiac capacity so that the patient maintains an adequate cardiac reserve. In myocardial disease, fatigue during muscular effort occurs more rapidly than it does in a heart in good condition. Consequently, the amount and duration of effort must be less and the period of rest during which recovery can occur must be longer (Fig. 35-2).

For the patient who has just experienced acute myocardial disease or infarction, a program must be planned that will eventually restore him to the greatest usefulness which is possible with his damaged heart. In view of the fact that 70 per cent of patients hospitalized for an acute episode of myocardial infarction survive, the initial care of the cardiac patient should include the beginning steps of the rehabilitation program anticipating the return of the patient to his home and employment. This program of restoration is long and involved. The physician must make many decisions regarding activities that the patient may perform during the acute and convalescent stages of his illness as well as the limitations he must observe when he can return to work. It becomes imperative that the clinician know the relative cardiac stresses imposed by various activities so that he can intelligently prescribe activities that fall within the patient's cardiac capacity and advise the patient against activities that cause excessive cardiac stress.

CARDIAC REQUIREMENT DURING ACTIVITY

Studies of the parameters of cardiac work indicate that changes in cardiac work are not indicated reliably by monitoring any one of these parameters. During upper extremity activity changes in cardiac work parallel changes in oxygen consumption more closely than any other single index, but there is a significant difference in these relationships during lower extremity activity[3, 4] (Fig. 35-3). The pulse rate is an insensitive index of cardiac work in normal subjects carrying out a variety of activities and is probably less reliable for patients with cardiac disease. The blood pressure does not change linearly with cardiac work. Therefore, knowledge of the cardiac work or metabolic requirements of the activities performed by cardiac patients is necessary in order to establish reasonable regulation of those activities.

Although it is customary to assume that when the patient is lying in bed he is maintained at the basal level of cardiac work, such is not the actual case. Any movement by the patient will increase oxygen consumption and cardiac output.[5] The patient who is confined to bed may move his extremities, shift his position, reach to his bedside stand, turn over or even sit erect. All of these activities require lifting of the extremities or elevation of the body and increased oxygen consumption. Even under the best of circumstances the average oxygen consumption of the patient restricted to bed is above the basal level and during certain bed activities it increases greatly. Rising from the lying position to the sitting position in bed without assistance may double the oxygen consumption above the basal level (Fig. 35-4). There is also an increase in the blood pressure because of the contraction of the abdominal muscles as the patient sits up so that the work of the heart is increased to an even greater extent.

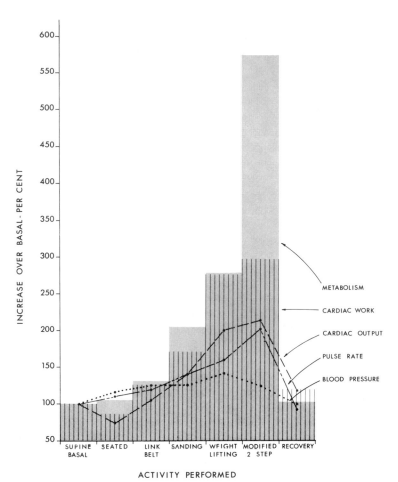

Figure 35–3 Variations of some parameters of cardiac performance during activities. Cardiac work parallels oxygen consumption more closely than any other single index of cardiac performance during upper extremity activity and then deviates widely during the lower extremity work of stair climbing. Equi-caloric activities of the upper extremities and lower extremities do not induce the same amount of work by the heart. The work of the heart is slightly less when sitting quietly than when lying supine. Light hand activities (link belt assembly) while sitting increase cardiac work to 125 per cent of the supine basal value. Bilateral arm activities (sanding) increase cardiac work to approximately 170 per cent of the supine value. Lifting a 10-pound weight through a distance of 15 inches 46 times per minute increases cardiac work to approximately 300 per cent of the supine value. The changes of the pulse rate and blood pressure do not correlate closely enough with changes of cardiac work to be good indices of cardiac work.

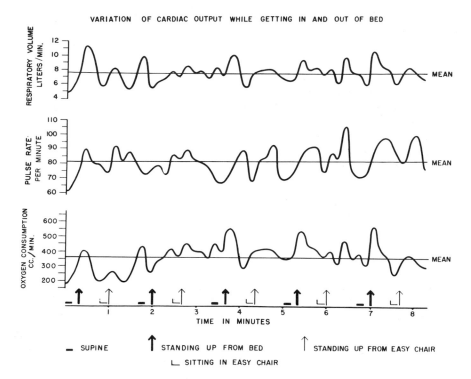

VARIATION OF CARDIAC OUTPUT WHILE GETTING IN AND OUT OF BED

Figure 35–4 Variation of demands for energy when getting out of and into bed without assistance. Sitting up from a lying position in bed requires greater energy consumption than any other phase of this activity. Standing up from sitting on the bed or on a chair also increases the oxygen consumption. The horizontal line indicates the mean value of each parameter during the eight-minute period while getting out of and into bed five times. (From Kottke, Danz and Kubicek. Arch. Phys. Med., *38:*75, 1957.)

Posture affects the work of the heart through its influence on both the cardiac output and the blood pressure. Sitting in an easy chair, fully relaxed, with support for the head, back, arms, thighs and feet is a position of minimal cardiac requirement in which the cardiac output is only approximately 85 per cent as great as when a person is lying in a supine position (Table 35-1 and Fig. 35-5). Sitting in a straight back chair or "dangling" the legs while sitting on the edge of the bed require less cardiac output than supine recumbency. Likewise, during quiet standing, cardiac output is only approximately 90 per cent of that during supine recumbency. On the other hand, when a patient is semireclining in a hospital bed (Fig. 35-6) with the backrest and the knee support elevated as is customary for patients who are bedfast in the hospital, the cardiac output is greater (110 per cent) than the value when supine, although metabolism is not increased.[5]

In estimating the cardiac work required by an activity it is necessary to take into consideration the peripheral distribution of the blood. Pooling of blood occurs when the feet and legs are dependent, decreasing the venous return and the drive on the heart. Under such conditions cardiac output is decreased. If

TABLE 35–1 THE EFFECTS OF POSTURE ON CARDIAC OUTPUT AND METABOLISM

POSTURE	METABOLISM (METS)	CARDIAC OUTPUT (COS)
Sitting in easy chair, full support	1.00 (0.90*)	0.85
Seated on straight-backed chair	1.10	0.95
Seated on edge of bed with feet supported	1.10	0.95
Standing, relaxed	1.20	0.90
Supine, basal	1.00	1.00
Lateral decubitus, up on elbow	1.10	1.00
Semireclining at 45° with knees up	1.00	1.10
Seated on high stool, forearms on table	1.25	—

COS —cardiac output, ratio to basal
METS—metabolism, ratio to basal
*Patients with old myocardial infarcts without orthopnea show a lower oxygen consumption during fully supported sitting than when lying supine.

the patient is semireclining in bed with his knees elevated, the dependent vascular bed in which pooling may occur is decreased and the splanchnic area compressed, both of which augment venous return and increase the cardiac output. The patient with heart failure who insists on "dangling" his legs over the side of the bed rather than semireclining has found that there is less cardiac effort involved even though unsupported sitting does slightly increase the demand for oxygen. The patient with myocardial insufficiency relaxes best with the least cardiac demand when he is sitting in a chair with support for his

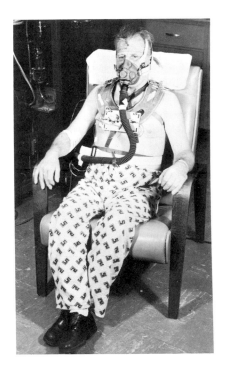

Figure 35–5 The fully supported sitting position requires less cardiac output and cardiac work than lying at supine rest in bed.

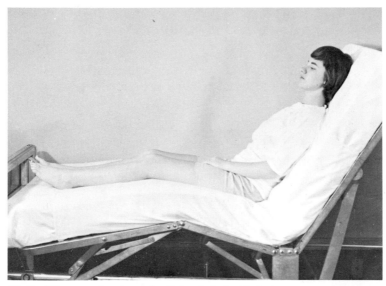

Figure 35–6   When a patient is semireclining in bed with the knee support elevated, the cardiac output is slightly greater than when the patient is lying supine.

head, back and arms but with his feet and legs dependent. If, following myocardial infarction, a 30 per cent difference in the minimal requirement for cardiac work is of significance for survival, the patient should be in the fully supported easy-chair position rather than semireclining in bed with his knees elevated.

Studies of patients with myocardial disease indicate that cardiac patients respond to positional changes as do normal individuals except that their oxygen consumption as well as their cardiac output is slightly less in a sitting position than in a recumbent position (Table 35–1).

Minimal Cardiac Activity.   Activities that require use of the hands and wrists while the patient is seated with the forearms supported increase metabo-

TABLE 35–2   MINIMAL CARDIAC ACTIVITY

ACTIVITY	POSITION	CARDIAC WORK (CUBS) OR METABOLISM (METS)	CARDIAC OUTPUT (COS)
Leather belt assembly	Sitting at table	1.25	1.10
Leather stamping	Sitting at table	1.35	1.10
Leather tooling	Sitting at table	1.30	1.20
Listening to radio	Sitting in easy chair	1.40	—
Bench assembly, light	Sitting at bench	1.40	1.10
Leather lacing	Sitting at table	1.45	—
Leather lacing	Lateral decubitus	1.55	1.20
Chip carving	Sitting at table	1.60	1.20

CUBS — cardiac work units, ratio to basal
COS   — cardiac output, ratio to basal
METS — metabolism, ratio to basal

lism and cardiac work less than 50 per cent above the supine resting level and increase the cardiac output no more than 25 per cent (Table 35-2). Since the occasional moving in bed that any patient does will produce similar changes, activities at this level have been classified as minimal. Muscular tension or an increase of blood pressure due to anxiety may increase the cardiac work far above this level. Therefore, diversional activities that cause a patient to relax will decrease his cardiac work in the early stages following a myocardial infarction.

Light Cardiac Activity.   Activity that increases cardiac work (or metabolism) from 1.5 to 2.5 times the basal value and cardiac output from 1:25 to 2.0 times the basal value has been classified as light cardiac activity. Activities that require full movement or support of the arms without a load, balancing movements of the trunk or hand work while standing fall into this category (Table 35-3).[6]

Moderate Cardiac Activities.   Moderate cardiac activities include those activities which increase cardiac work (or metabolism) 2.5 to 3.5 times and cardiac output 2.0 to 2.5 times the supine resting value. Sedentary clerical or bench-work activities requiring periodic lifting of not more than 10 pounds, dressing, showering, preparing meals, driving a car and walking at moderate speed fall into this category (Table 35-4).[7] This is the upper limit of work to which the patient with myocardial damage should be assigned. It should be noted that frequently vocational activities which have been prohibited require less cardiac work than self-care activities which the patient has been allowed to perform early in his convalescence.

TABLE 35-3   LIGHT CARDIAC ACTIVITY

ACTIVITY	POSITION	CARDIAC WORK (CUBS) OR METABOLISM (METS)	CARDIAC OUTPUT (COS)
Eating	Sitting	1.50	—
Sewing	Sitting	1.60	—
Clerical work	Sitting	1.60	—
Setting type	Standing	1.60	1.35
Getting out of and into bed	Bed to chair	1.65	1.45
Leather carving	Sitting on chair	1.70	—
Weaving, table loom	Sitting on stool	1.70	—
Clerical work	Standing	1.80	—
Writing	Sitting	2.00	—
Typing	Sitting on chair	2.00	1.35
Bimanual activity test sanding, 50 strokes/min.	Sitting on chair	2.00	1.40
Weaving, floor loom	Sitting on bench	2.10	1.75
Metal work, hammer	Standing	2.15	1.65
Printing, platen press	Standing	2.30	1.75
Bench assembly, moderate	Sitting	2.35	1.70
Hanging clothes on line	Standing — stooping	2.40	1.80

CUBS — cardiac work units, ratio to basal
COS   — cardiac output, ratio to basal
METS — metabolism, ratio to basal

TABLE 35–4   MODERATE CARDIAC ACTIVITY

Activity	Position	Cardiac Work (CUBS) or Metabolism (METS)	Cardiac Output (COS)
Playing piano		2.50	—
Dressing, undressing		2.50–3.50	—
Sawing, jeweler's saw	Sitting	1.90	2.05
Sawing, hack saw	Standing	2.55	2.00
Driving car		2.80	—
Bicycling, slowly		2.90	2.45
Preparing meals		3.00	—
Weight lifting, 10 lb. lifted 15″, 46/min.	Sitting	2.80	2.00
Walking, 2.0 m.p.h.		3.20	—
Handsawing, wood	Standing	3.50	2.35
Warm shower		3.50	—

CUBS — cardiac work units, ratio to basal
COS — cardiac output, ratio to basal
METS — metabolism, ratio to basal

Heavy, Severe and Excessively Severe Cardiac Activities. Included in the category of heavy cardiac activity are those activities which increase cardiac work 3.5 to 5.0 times or cardiac output 2.5 to 3.0 times basal values. (Table 35-5). Such activities should be avoided by the patient with myocardial disease or they should be restricted to short intervals of activity followed by prolonged periods of rest. The upper limit of this level of activity is the greatest that a normal person can maintain during daily work without evidence of metabolic deterioration and has been classified by Müller as the "endurance limit" of work.[8] Activities that require lifting, pushing, pulling and carrying may exceed this category. Activities which increase cardiac work (or metabolism) 5.0 to 7.0 times the basal value and cardiac output 3.0 to 4.0 times the basal value are

TABLE 35–5   HEAVY AND SEVERE CARDIAC ACTIVITY

Activity	Position	Metabolism (METS)	Cardiac Output (COS)
Bowel movement	Toilet	3.60	
Bowel movement	Bedpan	4.70	
Making beds	Standing	3.90	
Hot shower	Standing	4.20	
Walking fast (3.5 m.p.h.)		5.00	
Descending stairs		5.20	
Scrubbing floor	Kneeling	5.30	3.00
Master, two-step climbing test		5.70	3.00
Weight lifting, 10–20 lb. lifted 36″, 15/min.		6.50	3.50
Bicycling, fast		6.90	3.30
Running		7.40	5.10
Mowing lawn		7.70	
Climbing stairs		9.00	

METS — metabolism, ratio to basal
COS — cardiac output, ratio to basal

classified as severe, and activities which exceed these ranges are classified as excessively severe. Climbing slopes or stairs or running increase the cardiac work even further and are excessively severe cardiac work.[4, 6] Rapid work or strong emotion may transform a lighter activity to one of heavy cardiac work. Activity in a hot environment that interferes with the dissipation of the heat of the body also increases the cardiac work that must be performed. Heavy manual labor, climbing with heavy loads and many athletic activities are excessively severe and can be carried on for only short periods of time by healthy individuals (Fig. 35–7).

On the basis of studies of the physiologic parameters of cardiac function muscular activities have been classified in Table 35-6 according to the stress imposed on the myocardium. With the knowledge of the relative cardiac demands of various activities, the physician is able to protect the patient against excessive myocardial effort in the acute and subacute stages of his disease.

In the acute stage of a myocardial infarction the patient has many anxieties. Prohibition of all activity and restriction to complete bed rest increases

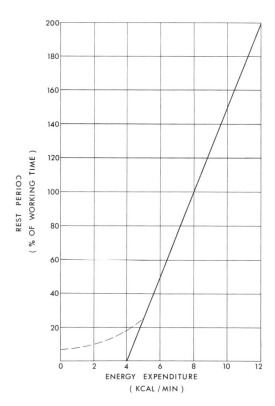

Figure 35–7   Rest allowance required in relation to the energy expended for normal work up to 2000 kilocalories per eight hour shift. Based upon a maximal work capacity of 4.0 kilocalories per minute plus basal metabolism of 1.0 kilocalorie per minute. (From E. A. Müller.[9])

TABLE 35–6 CLASSIFICATION OF NORMAL ACTIVITIES BASED ON CARDIAC OUTPUT DURING THE ACTIVITY

ACTIVITY	METABOLISM (METS)	CARDIAC OUTPUT (COS)
Minimal	<1.5	<1.25
Light	1.5–2.5	1.25–2.0
Moderate	2.5–3.5	2.0–2.5
Heavy	3.5–5.0	2.5–3.0
Severe	5.0–7.0	3.0–4.0
Excessively severe	>7.0	>4.0

COS —cardiac output, ratio to basal
METS—metabolism, ratio to basal

anxiety which in turn increases muscular tension and blood pressure so that the work of the heart is increased. Allowing the patient to sit in a chair that gives adequate support provides a psychologic reassurance at the same time that it decreases the myocardial work. If the patient is assisted to sit up in bed and stand up from the bed, the energy requirement to transfer from bed to chair is not excessive (Fig. 35-8). The performance of hand activities of the "minimal" class while the patient is sitting is diversional and will usually decrease anxieties, thereby reducing the work of the heart. During the first three weeks while an adequate scar is developing in the infarcted myocardium, the patient's exposure to cardiac work should be kept minimal.

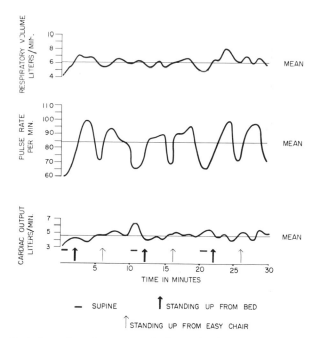

Figure 35–8 Variation of cardiac output during assisted transfer from bed to chair and back again. The patient is assisted in all activities requiring elevation of the body: rising from lying to sitting in bed, standing up from sitting on the bed, and standing up from sitting in the chair. The horizontal lines are the means of the parameters for the entire recorded period.

During convalescence the patient may be allowed to begin increasingly stressful activity. It appears that, as in skeletal muscle, the capacity of the myocardium to do work is increased by short exposures to fatiguing work followed by adequate periods of rest. Therefore, the progression from light to moderate activity for increasingly longer periods of time appears to be beneficial for redeveloping the capacity of the myocardium.

Conventional wisdom recognizes that sexual intercourse with its attendant excitement and muscular activity increases cardiac work. For many years the increased stress of sexual excitement has been listed as one of the common causes of sudden death of patients with coronary disease. However, carefully documented studies in recent years indicate that this is a relatively rare cause of sudden cardiac death. Bartlett,[44] measuring pulse rate, respiratory rate and volume, found that during coitus the heart rate and respiration were increased to near maximal levels in young men and women during orgasm and compared the response to that produced by strenuous forms of exercise. This study seemed to confirm conventional wisdom regarding the dangers of sexual activity in patients after myocardial infarction. However, Hellerstein and Friedman[45] equipped men who had had myocardial infarctions with portable electrocardiographic recorders, which they wore continuously through the working day and through the night. They found that conjugal sexual intercourse increased the pulse rate equivalent to the exertion associated with climbing two flights of stairs or walking briskly on the street. The mean maximal heart rate at orgasm was 117 beats per minute (range, 90 to 144 beats per minute). Tests of physical activity to produce a similar increase in heart rate in these patients showed that during physical activity producing an equivalent increase in pulse rate the blood pressure was 162/89 mm. Hg and the maximal oxygen consumption was less than that required for the Master two-step test. In counseling a patient regarding rehabilitation, the physician plays a key role in advising the patient regarding his sexual activity, as well as other activities. The patient's happiness and successful re-entry into the family dynamics depends upon his sexual adjustment. If the patient can exercise at the level of 6 to 8 calories per minute, such as the Master two-step test, without symptoms, abnormal pulse rate or blood pressure, or ECG changes, it is generally safe to recommend the resumption of sexual activity. Even when abnormal responses indicate caution, he may still be able to perform these activities which are comparable to the requirements for climbing two flights of stairs.

CARDIAC WORK EVALUATION

Graded exercise tests may use treadmills, bicycle ergometers or step tests, applying the principles and methods developed by work physiologists as an appraisal of the cardiac status of the patient. Maximal oxygen intake during treadmill exercise has been used as an index of maximal cardiac performance.[10, 11] The maximal oxygen intake for normal healthy young men was nearly 11 times the basal requirement (11 METS). The total oxygen intake during a multistage progressive test[11] was 450 ml./kg. body weight for trained athletes and 220 ml./kg. for normal patients. Cardiac patients had a reduced maximal oxygen intake which varied according to the functional class: Class I, 115 ml./kg.; Class II, 85 ml./kg.; and Class III, 60 ml./kg. In a multistage progressive test of cardiac capacity the individual begins the exercise with a brief period of warm-up at a level of energy expenditure which doubles that of

TABLE 35–7 AVERAGE ENERGY COSTS OF TWO MILE PER HOUR TREADMILL TEST*

METS	Kcal./min.	O$_2$ ml./kg.-min.	PULSE RATE	PER CENT GRADE
2	2.5	7.0	97	0
3	3.7	10.5	105	3.5
4	5.0	14.0	114	7.0
5	6.25	17.5	126	10.5
6	7.5	21.0	135	14.0
7	8.7	24.5	144	17.5

*The energy costs of treadmill walking at 2.0 m.p.h. at various slopes are tabulated in terms of the oxygen intake, Kcal. per minute and METS. The pulse rate figures represent average values measured in healthy, middle-aged sedentary men. (From Naughton, J., J. S. Carolina Med. Ass. 65 [Suppl.]: 96, 1969.)

the resting metabolic state. Following a short rest the individual begins exercise at a relatively low effort of energy expenditure, which is increased either intermittently or continuously until the patient approaches a predetermined end-point such as heart rate, respiration, symptoms or maximum oxygen uptake.

In the Naughton modification of the maximal aerobic work capacity the patient begins walking on a treadmill at a speed of two miles per hour at a level grade.[12] The speed is held constant while the slope of the treadmill bed is elevated 3.5 per cent every three minutes. Blood pressure and pulse rate are recorded by auscultation during the last half of each minute. A single ECG continuously monitors heart rate and regularity. Minute ventilation and metabolism are measured by collecting and analyzing expired gases. The increments of energy expenditure are in multiples of the resting metabolic states, or METS, as shown in Table 35–7. This test is adequate for most clinical appraisals, since the average man has an aerobic working capacity of 9 to 10 METS.

A bicycle ergometer may be used to evaluate working capacity either on a continuous or intermittent basis.[13] In the intermittent work capacity test, the patient begins pedaling at an energy requirement of 300 kpm.*/min. (oxygen intake approximately 500 ml. per minute) for six minutes followed by a four minute rest. Each subsequent step is increased 150 kpm. (170 ml. O$_2$ per min.), with six minutes of exercise and four minutes of rest. The patient continues the exercise until the heart rate reaches 150 beats per minute. In this test the data which should be recorded includes blood pressure, pulse rate and electrocardiogram (Table 35-8).

Another method for estimating the safe working level for the damaged heart has utilized upper extremity activities of standardized intensity and recorded the cardiovascular responses of the patient as he works through the stages from light to heavy work.[3] The demonstrated ability to carry on sustained activity at any stage without adverse effect indicates the capability of the patient to carry on the same intensity of activity at home or at work. Five levels of activity have been studied and related to the supine basal resting condition as the reference level of metabolism (METS) or cardiac output (COS). These activities in increasing order of effort are shown in Table 35-9, together with the requirements of the Master two-step test as reported by Dawson[4]. As shown

---

*Kpm. = kilopondmeter. A kilopondmeter is the work of moving one kilogram against the gravitational force of the earth through a distance of one meter.

TABLE 35–8 AVERAGE ENERGY COSTS OF UPRIGHT BICYCLE
ERGOMETER TESTS*

METS	Kcal./min.	O$_2$ml./kg.-min.	Kpm./min.	Watts
2.6	3.2	10.4	305	50
4.0	4.9	15.8	458	75
5.2	6.4	20.9	610	100
6.5	8.1	26.2	763	125
7.8	9.6	31.4	915	150
9.2	11.3	36.6	1068	175
10.5	12.9	41.9	1220	200

*The energy costs of pedaling a bicycle ergometer at various loads are compared for a 70 kg.
man in terms of METS, Kcal./min. and oxygen intake.

This table is constructed on the basis that each watt of resistance is equivalent to 6.1 Kpm. of
work and that each Kpm. requires approximately 2.4 ml. O$_2$. (From Naughton, J., J. S. Carolina Med.
Ass., 65 [Suppl]: 96, 1969.)

in Figure 35-3, none of the parameters of cardiac performance remain proportional to the cardiac work throughout these activities. Therefore it is highly desirable to measure cardiac output and blood pressure during an activity in order to have a more precise estimate of the work of the heart.

A radio-frequency impedance cardiometer has been developed, which is, in essence, a thoracic impedance plethysmograph responding to the increased column of blood in the aorta with each systole[14] (Fig. 35-9). The change of impedance provides a measure of the left ventricular systolic stroke volume. The stroke volume times heart rate gives minute cardiac output and, multiplied by blood pressure, gives potential work performed per minute by the left ventricle. During systole the impedance, ΔZ, through the chest, from neck to lower thorax, decreases (Fig. 35–10). The rate of change of impedance, dz/dt, is proportional to the stroke volume. From the record in Figure 35–10 it is clearly evident that dz/dt begins at the closure of the mitral valve and ends at the closure of the aortic valve. The magnitude of (dz/dt)$_{min}$. is directly proportional to the stroke volume. The time of maximal deviation of dz/dt is the moment of maximum energy release by the myocardium. The impedance cardiometer provides a precise noninvasive method for comparing changes of stroke volume.

TABLE 35–9 PARAMETERS OF CARDIAC PERFORMANCE OF NORMAL SUBJECTS
AT SIX LEVELS OF PROGRESSIVE ACTIVITY

LEVEL OF ACTIVITY	RESPONSE — RATIO TO BASAL				
	Cardiac Work	Cardiac Output	Metabolism	Heart Rate	Blood Pressure
I Supine, basal	1.00	1.00	1.00	1.00	1.00
II Sitting at table with forearm support	0.85	0.75	1.05	1.10	1.15
III Light hand activity with forearm support	1.25	1.05	1.30	1.20	1.25
IV Bilateral arm motion, sanding pine board	1.70	1.40	2.10	1.40	1.25
V Bimanual lifting, 10 lb. lifted 15″, 46/min.	2.80	2.00	2.80	1.60	1.40
VI Master double two-step test	3.00	2.14	5.75	2.03	1.26

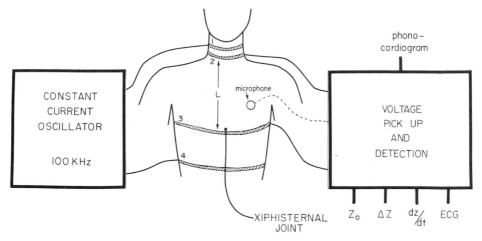

Figure 35–9   Schematic diagram of impedance cardiometer with cutaneous leads around neck and chest. Z_0, impedance through chest. ΔZ, change of impedance during systole. dz/dt, rate of change of impedance which represents rate of energy release by ventricle. (From Kubicek et al.[14])

REHABILITATION EXERCISE PROGRAM FOR CARDIAC PATIENTS

Exercise programs have been developed to restore cardiac patients to a level of physical activity compatible with the functional capacity of the myocardium. Limited programs of activity are initiated in the convalescent period and increased progressively while the patients' responses are being monitored at the prescribed levels of activity. In some cases radio monitoring has been used to allow for a greater range of activities.[15] Activities are defined by caloric value since it appears that equi-caloric activities exert essentially the same stress on the heart, with the exception that equi-caloric upper extremity activities require more cardiac work than activities performed by the lower extremities.

Patients carry on exercise programs at home as well as in hospital or gymnasium groups. The variation of exercises is almost unlimited, progressing from lower to higher energy levels as the patient improves. Calisthenics, walking, jogging, and stair climbing at increasing rates of speed for progressively longer intervals provide a means of increasing the stress on the heart.[16] Other workers have used daily self-care or working activities as the basis for prescribed activity, again increasing from low caloric to high caloric levels as the patient's condition improves.[17]

For vocational rehabilitation of the cardiac patient an occupation should be selected which is in the light or moderate activity class. The cardiac work associated with the muscular requirements of such an activity can be measured reasonably well. However, the blood pressure responses of cardiac patients may vary during occupational activities according to the amount of emotional stress associated with that activity. Repeated measurements of blood pressure should be made during work to assure that the job does not induce an increase of blood pressure which will change the cardiac work from a moderate level to a heavy or severe level.

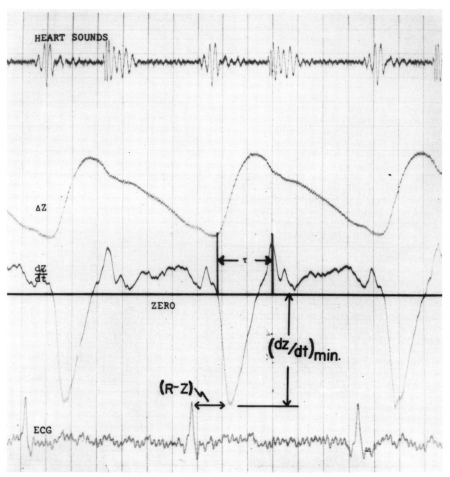

Figure 35–10   Record from impedance cardiometer. Top tracing, phonocardiogram. Second line, ΔZ, change in impedance through thorax with systole. Third line, dz/dt, rate of change of impedance with systole. Fourth line, electrocardiogram. (From Kubicek et al.[14])

PERIPHERAL VASCULAR DISORDERS

Categories of Vascular Diseases. The major arterial diseases for which physical medicine offers diagnostic or therapeutic aid are those that produce chronic organic occlusion, including arteriosclerosis obliterans with or without diabetes (this contributes 75 per cent of all cases) and thromboangiitis obliterans; those that produce acute organic occlusion, including embolic occlusion, arterial thrombosis and freezing and frostbite; and vasospastic disease.

The types of venous vascular diseases commonly treated by physical medicine are thrombophlebitis, varicose veins with venous stasis and chronic venous insufficiency.

Evaluation of the Arterial Circulation. The adequacy of the circulation through an extremity may be estimated by palpation of the peripheral pulses, color changes of the skin, trophic changes in the skin and special testing procedures.

Oscillometry provides one objective method of assessment of the patency of the larger arteries which can be correlated with functional performance.[18] When an oscillometer is calibrated and used in a standard manner, the data obtained provide a reliable index of the maximal blood flow through the arteries of an extremity. Troedsson has published standards of oscillometric readings in the lower extremity giving minimal normal values and the values relating to ability to run, walk, heal an ulcer or support the wearing of a prosthesis (Table 35-10). When reasonable attention is paid to the details necessary to provide uniformity of measurement, this method has proved to be reliable for estimation of peripheral circulation. In addition, oscillometry may be used to localize the level of arterial obstruction in an extremity.

Venous occlusion plethysmography is a method by which circulation may be measured in an extremity or a segment of an extremity.[19, 20] If the extremity is enclosed in an airtight chamber and a cuff just proximal to the chamber is inflated to prevent the return of venous blood, the inflow of arterial blood into

TABLE 35–10   RELATIONSHIP OF MINIMAL OSCILLOMETRIC INDICES AND FUNCTION IN THE LOWER EXTREMITY FOR NON-DIABETIC MEN*

| | Ambulation | | Ulcer of Foot | | | B/K Amputation | | |
| LEVEL OF MEASUREMENT | Run | Walk† | Healing | | Gangrene | Prosthesis Tolerated | Healing Only | |
			Slow	None			Yes	No
Foot, instep	0.75	0.5	tr	0.0	0.0	—	—	—
Above ankle	3.0	2.5	0.25	0.25	0.0	—	—	—
Below knee	6.5	4.0	0.5	0.5	0.125	2.0	1.5	0.5
Lower thigh		3.5						
Mid-thigh		2.5						
Upper thigh		2.5						

*From Troedsson.[18] These values have been standardized only for arteriosclerotic male patients without diabetes.

†The values to sustain walking also are the lower limits of normal. The walking index shows the circulation adequate to walk 400 yards at 120 steps per minute with only slight fatigue.

the enclosed segment of the extremity can be estimated from the change of volume or pressure in the plethysmograph chamber (Fig. 35-11). The electromagnetic impedance plethysmograph is based on the same principle but measures the change of impedance as the volume of the extremity changes.[21] Plethysmography is a valuable clinical method for estimating the response of the circulation to autonomic regulation or to the administration of pharmaceutic compounds under standardized conditions.[22]

Skin thermometry may also be used to estimate the circulation through the extremities. Skin thermistors or thermocouples with a low heat content may be used to measure the changes of skin temperatures under controlled environmental conditions (Fig. 35-12). This method is useful for evaluating vasomotor responses of the circulation.[23]

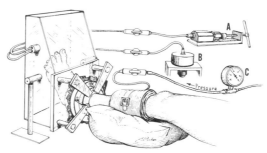

Figure 35-11 The venous occlusion plethysmograph. The foot is enclosed in an airtight plastic chamber. A cuffed latex diaphragm around the ankle seals the chamber against leaks without exerting pressure great enough to impede venous return. Pressure changes in the chamber are measured by strain gauge. B. Syringe A is used to calibrate the response of the system to known changes of volume. The pneumatic cuff is placed around the leg immediately adjacent to the plethysmograph and inflated with a pressure slightly less than diastolic pressure to prevent venous outflow.

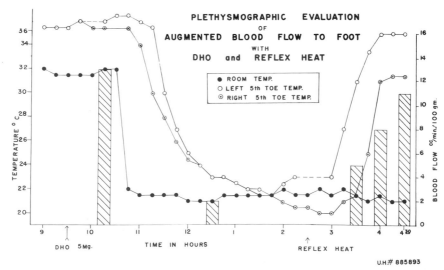

Figure 35-12 Relationship of skin temperatures of the toes and blood flow through the foot to environmental temperature and reflex heating. (From Gilbertson, Emerson and Kottke. Angiology, *11*:139-143, 1960.)

Arterial Disease

Chronic Organic Occlusion.   The management of chronic occlusive vascular diseases is similar regardless of cause of the disease. The principles of management are:

To protect the ischemic part from physical damage.

To arrest the progress of the disease if possible.

To overcome vasospasm.

To relieve local areas of arterial obstruction.

To prevent or control thrombosis.

To prevent or control infection.

To attempt to increase the collateral circulation at a rate faster than the occlusive process develops.

To amputate when adequate circulation cannot be maintained.

The extremities must be protected from environmental exposure or trauma which may cause further damage. The ischemic foot is less able than normal to tolerate stress or trauma. Excessive activity such as prolonged walking, rubbing of ill fitting shoes or other excessive wear will exceed the ability of the metabolism to effect repair. The ischemic foot is especially susceptible to extremes of hot or cold and should be kept at a neutral temperature. If the symptoms are severe, the patient should be confined to bed and a heat cradle at a temperature of 80 to 90° F. should be placed over the lower extremities. Because nicotine has a vasoconstrictive action, the use of all tobacco should be discontinued.

The head of the bed should be elevated 8 to 16 inches higher than the foot of the bed. Williams, Montgomery and Horwitz[24] have shown that for patients with ischemic feet, depressing the position of the foot 7 inches below the horizontal increased oxygen tension in the skin of the toes by 13 per cent; elevating the feet 7 inches above the horizontal decreased the oxygen tension by 22 per cent. This observation probably explains why patients who have ischemic pain in the feet when recumbent find relief when the feet are lowered below the horizontal.

There may be a variable amount of vasospasm in chronic organic obstruction. However, in approximately one-half of the cases of arteriosclerosis obliterans the amount of vasospasm is so slight that sympathetic blocking agents or sympathectomy does not improve the circulation significantly.[25, 26] If a vasodilator response cannot be demonstrated by plethysmography, neither sympathetic blocking agents nor sympathectomy are of therapeutic value. In thromboangiitis obliterans or acute organic obstruction the diminution of circulation due to vasospasm is a significant part of the problem.

PRODUCTION OF VASODILATATION BY HEAT.   A number of measures are available in physical medicine to produce vasodilatation. Heat is a powerful vasodilator and is useful in the treatment of peripheral arterial disease. It increases the circulation by direct action on the tissues locally and also by reflex action initiated from the tissues heated and from the vasodilator center.[27] In addition, heat also produces an analgesic action to relieve the pain associated with ischemic ulcers.

On the other hand, direct heat to the ischemic area raises the local tissue temperature and with it increases the metabolism and the requirement for an increased blood flow to the tissues. In severe organic vascular obstruction heat is beneficial only if it increases the circulation to a greater extent than it increases the metabolic demands for circulation. If the circulation cannot be increased as much as the metabolism, heat will be detrimental and destructive rather than beneficial.

Heat must be applied more cautiously when there is impaired circulation than when the circulation to the extremity is normal. Normally during thermotherapy heat is removed rapidly from the skin by the circulation. The rate of application of heat in standard thermotherapeutic procedures is based on the assumption that heat will be removed by the intact circulation. In an area of ischemia heat is removed less rapidly and the danger of a burn is greatly increased. In an area of hypesthesia, especially, such burns may develop before the damage is appreciated.

Heat may be applied directly to a limb with organic vascular impairment if there is some circulatory reserve or if vasoconstriction is responsible for some of the circulatory impairment. However, in severe arterial vascular disease it is dangerous to apply heat directly to the ischemic part.

Troedsson uses the oscillometric index in determining the amount of heat that can safely be applied to the extremities. A hand or foot with normal circulation will tolerate a whirlpool temperature of 43° C. (110° F.). For each 10 per cent reduction below normal in the oscillometric reading above the ankle, he decreases the temperature of the whirlpool by 1° F. When the oscillometric reading above the ankle is 0, the whirlpool temperature is not allowed to exceed 100° F. Hydrotherapy is given for 20 minutes, or less if the patient complains of the development of pain during the therapy. Heat by hydrotherapy causes vasodilatation of the collateral circulation and over a period of time may significantly increase the total circulation to the extremity.

Radiant heat, by means of a therapeutic lamp or baker, may also be applied to ischemic extremities that have some vascular reserve. The lamp at a distance of 2 to 3 feet produces diffuse heating of the skin without pressure or direct contact which might result in burns. The area being treated should be observed during the period of therapy. Conductive heating by electric pads, hot water bottles or hot packs is dangerous because pressure may increase the ischemia and produce local burns which are unobserved and unrecognized until after treatment. Shortwave and microwave diathermy or ultrasonic diathermy are highly effective methods of producing deep heating but because they cannot be adequately observed or controlled, they are dangerous in cases of severe ischemia.

Reflex heating is the safest means of stimulating the circulation in organic vascular disease. When reflex vasodilatation is produced by the application of heat to the torso or the uninvolved extremities, the increased temperature of the thermosensitive vasodilator center of the hypothalamus causes generalized vasodilatation in the skin. The only increase in temperature in the ischemic part will be that associated with flow of blood to that part. Consequently, metabolism in the ischemic tissues will not be increased more than the blood flow. Among the effective methods of applying reflex heat is the application of a diathermy coil over the abdomen with the patient well covered with blankets.[28] Reflex heating produces a mild hyperthermia which, when effective, may increase the oral temperature as much as 1 to 2° F. It should be used with caution or not at all for patients with cardiac disease since the general vasodilatation that occurs in the skin increases the work of the heart.

PRODUCTION OF VASODILATATION BY IONTOPHORESIS.   Local cutaneous vasodilatation can also be produced by iontophoresis using histamine or Mecholyl. These substances dilate the minute blood vessels and produce an active hyperemia and an increased blood flow. Iontophoresis is especially valuable for disorders with associated arterial spasm.[29, 30] To apply histamine, a thin cotton felt or filter paper pad which has been soaked in a 1:1000 solution of histamine acid phosphate is placed over the area to be treated. Over this pad is placed a sheet of metal foil, slightly smaller than the pad, to which the positive pole of the direct current generator is attached. A larger dispersive pad wet with saline is connected to the negative pole. The pads are fastened to the patient by an elastic bandage. A current of approximately 0.3 to 0.5 milliampere per square centimeter of pad surface is applied for three to five minutes. Histamine may also be applied as a 1 per cent histamine ointment rubbed onto the skin and covered with a moist saline pad electrode.

Mecholyl is applied by saturating a cotton felt or filter paper pad with a 0.2 to 0.5 per cent solution and using the technique described for histamine. The duration of treatment should be approximately 10 minutes; if the application is prolonged, systemic effects consisting of flushing, sweating, salivation, tachycardia, hyperperistalsis and hypotension may occur. The vasodilatation following Mecholyl iontophoresis may last for six to eight hours.

PRODUCTION OF VASODILATATION BY EXERCISE. Exercises have been recommended to produce reactive vasodilatation in the ischemic extremities. The Buerger-Allen exercises in which the patient alternately elevates and lowers the feet have been prescribed for many years. However, evaluation of these exercises by measuring the rate of removal of radioactive sodium injected into the belly of the gastrocnemius muscle has shown that the exercises are not effective in increasing the circulation in muscle.[31] On the other hand, contraction of the muscles against resistance such as can be obtained by plantar flexion of the feet against a footboard is an effective means of increasing blood flow during and for a short time after the exercise.

Walking also is a good exercise to increase circulation in the feet and legs of patients with chronic arterial obstruction and intermittent claudication. The walking should be continued only to the point of incipient pain. After a brief rest period either standing or sitting, the patient should resume walking until discomfort recurs. This walking exercise should be performed repeatedly each day to stimulate the development of collateral circulation until walking periods of 30 minutes twice a day have been achieved. Severe pain that produces vasospasm should be avoided. Walking exercises are contraindicated however, in the presence of rest pain, ulcers or gangrene.

The use of the suction-pressure or pavex boot or of intermittent venous occlusion has fallen into disuse with the demonstration that circulation is not increased by these methods and that any clinical effects obtained are largely due to the bed rest that is entailed.

Acute Arterial Occlusion. Acute arterial occlusion in an extremity, whether it is due to embolism or arterial thrombosis, is an emergency condition that requires immediate treatment. Usually arterial spasm is present in addition to the organic obstruction and it interferes with the establishment of collateral circulation. Management should be directed toward protection and support of the ischemic part and vasodilatation should be induced. The patients should be confined to bed with a heat cradle over the legs at a temperature of 80 to 85° F. The head of the bed should be raised 8 inches to provide the effect of dependency oxygenation.[24] Ischemia from pressure should be prevented by the use of an alternating air pressure mattress and hourly changes of the position in bed. Reflex heating should be instituted in order to stimulate collateral circulation. For the same reason, vasodilating drugs as papaverine, guanethidine or alcohol should be used. Localization of the site of the lesion followed by embolectomy or endarterectomy is the treatment of choice whenever possible.

Venous Vascular Disease

Thrombophlebitis.   The treatment for acute thrombophlebitis of a lower extremity includes rest in bed; elevation of the inflamed limb by raising the foot of the bed 6 to 8 inches; paravertebral sympathetic block with 1 per cent procaine solution to minimize vasoconstriction, pain and edema; hot packs applied to the involved extremity from foot to groin; anticoagulant therapy; and vasodilators such as guanethidine or tolazoline hydrochloride.

The patient should remain in bed on therapy until the inflammation in the veins subsides. When he becomes ambulatory an elastic bandage or stocking should be applied from the toes to the upper thigh until edema is no longer present. The major dangers of thrombophlebitis are the upward extension of the thrombus and the production of pulmonary emboli.

Chronic Venous Insufficiency.   Following thrombophlebitis chronic venous insufficiency may occur. Persisting organized venous thrombosis obstructs venous blood flow and produces stagnation of deoxygenated blood in the dependent extremity. If the thrombosed veins recanalize, the valves remain fibrosed and incompetent so that there may be a reversal of blood flow through the veins into the dependent extremity. When venous valves are incompetent the pumping action of the muscle is no longer effective to assist the return of venous blood from the dependent extremity to the heart.[32] The resulting stasis and congestion produces edema, impairment of metabolism, pain, dermatitis, pigmentation and ulceration of the skin of the lower third of the leg. Chronic edema produces interstitial and lymphatic fibrosis which decreases the rate of metabolic repair following injury. Recurrent cellulitis in the lower half of the leg frequently leads to chronic ulceration. Effective treatment to heal the ulcer requires improvement of circulation, relief of edema and protection against chronic edema.

Stasis Ulcers.   Stasis ulcers typically are indolent, superficial ulcers with a surrounding area of induration and inflammatory reaction. Like all superficial ulcers, they contain a mixed infection of the common contaminating organisms. Healing is slow because the circulation is inadequate to cope with the infection and support the epithelium. Treatment is aimed at the improvement of circulation, control of the infection, resolution of the brawny edema and support of the tissues to prevent further edema. Therapy in a whirlpool at 105° F. provides mechanical cleansing of the ulcer and stimulates arterial dilatation. This is followed by ultraviolet irradiation for its vasodilator and bactericidal actions.[33] The ulcer and surrounding 1 cm. of skin are painted with 1 per cent mercurochrome solution, masked, and irradiated with cold quartz ultraviolet radiation beginning with 1 minimal erythema dose (M.E.D.) and increasing by 1 M.E.D. each treatment to a maximum of 5 M.E.D. Friction massage is applied to the fibrotic subcutaneous tissue surrounding the ulcer and extending over the entire area of the fibrosis. Following this treatment the ulcer is covered with a sterile Telfa dressing, several layers of sterile gauze and a 1 inch foam rubber pad with beveled edges and is firmly wrapped with an Ace bandage. After the ulcer has healed, a fitted elastic stocking is prescribed to be worn at all times when the patient is up in order to prevent the recurrence of the edema. As an alternative method of controlling the edema and allowing the ulcer to heal, a gelatin-zinc oxide gauze boot may be applied and changed every week or two until the ulcer has healed.

LYMPHEDEMA

Lymphedema of the extremities may be primary or it may be secondary to the surgical removal of lymphatic vessels or obstruction by infection. In any case the water and protein balance across the capillary membrane is disturbed, resulting in the accumulation of extravascular, extracellular fluid. The endothelium of the lymph vessels is more permeable than is that of the blood capillaries. Protein molecules and particles of microscopic dimensions are able to enter the lymph capillaries and by passing through the lymph vessels are removed from the tissue spaces. The main function of the lymph vessels is to remove plasma proteins which filter through the capillaries into the tissue spaces. When the lymphatic vessels are absent or obstructed, the proteins are retained in the tissue spaces where they increase the colloid osmotic pressure, upset the water balance across the capillary endothelium and stimulate the production of fibrosis in the tissue spaces.

Movement through the lymphatics is dependent solely upon external pressures.[34] The compressive action of contracting muscles, of joints during motion or of external massage causes flow through the lymphatics. If the lymphatic valves are intact, this motion is centripetal. During normal activity lymph is moved from the feet to the thoracic duct in a few minutes.[35] During inactivity the pressure in the extravascular spaces and the lymphatics rises to a level slightly below that of the pressure in the veins.[36] The venous pressure in the inactive dependent extremity rises to equal the pressure exerted by a column of water extending from the dependent extremity to the level of the heart.[32]

Lymph contains fibrinogen and thrombin but, owing to a deficiency of thromboplastic substance, it clots more slowly than blood, usually clotting in from 10 to 20 minutes. However, if traumatized cells or bacteria are present they will provide the deficient thromboplastic substance and then thrombosis in the lymph vessels will occur readily. When a lymph vessel thromboses, the thrombi contract and shrink away from the wall of the vessel, leaving adequate space for circulation of lymph. Recurrent thrombi may completely fill the vessel, however.[37]

At a site of severe inflammation, particles of colloidal size or larger will pass through the capillary endothelium into the tissue spaces but will not be removed because fibrin thrombi in the lymphatic vessels obstruct the flow of lymph away from the inflammatory process.[38] When the protein content of lymph increases, collagen is laid down more rapidly. This fibrosis contributes to further stasis. As a result of the increased quantity of lymph and protein in the tissues, there is increased susceptibility to infection. Recurrent inflammation produces progressive thrombosis of the lymph vessels, more stasis of lymph, more fibrosis and a progressively increasing edema.

Lymphatic vessels have remarkable powers of regeneration. When a large lymphatic vessel is cut, a new channel develops across the scar of the incision and physiologic regeneration may be complete by the eighth day.[39] Collateral vessels also develop extensively. However, if the flow of lymph is so great that it markedly dilates the collateral vessels, the lymphatic valves become incompetent and the lymph flows in the direction of pressure or gravity.

Lymphedema most frequently occurs secondary to surgery in which the regional lymph nodes are extensively removed, such as in radical mastectomy with removal of the axillary lymph nodes or in surgery of the lower extremity with resection of the inguinal lymph nodes. Edema in the arm and hand causes considerable distress due to the increased weight, sensory disturbance in the skin, stiffness of the fingers and interference with the fit of clothing. In the lower extremity, lymphedema causes stiffness and discomfort and increases fatigability. In both cases resistance to infection in the edematous extremity is decreased and recurrent attacks of cellulitis occurring spontaneously or following minor trauma are common results.

Treatment of lymphedema by physiatric means involves reduction in the volume of the extremity, support of the affected area to prevent recurrence of the edema and measures to prevent recurrent infection.

The rationale for management of edema is based on knowledge of the Starling cycle of exchange of water across the capillary membrane. Movement of water across the capillary membrane into the tissue spaces is promoted by the hydrostatic pressure of the blood in the capillary and the osmotic pressure of protein in the tissue fluid. The movement of water from the tissue spaces into the capillary is promoted by the hydrostatic pressure in the tissue fluids and the osmotic pressure of proteins in the plasma. Any excess fluid and protein filtering into the tissue spaces is normally removed through the lymphatic channels. Disturbance of the normal balance by increased capillary pressure, whether it is due to venous congestion or arterial dilatation, or by increased colloidal osmotic pressure in the extravascular space must be offset by increased lymph flow or increasing edema until the increasing tissue pressure restores a balance of exchange of water across the capillary membrane. When the extremity is dependent, the flow of venous blood and lymph will be opposed by the force of gravity.

Management of lymphedema involves attempts to increase venous and lymphatic drainage and tissue hydrostatic pressure. The movement of fluid out of the limb is aided by elevation, mechanical and manual massage and increased tissue pressure by the application of elastic support.[40] In addition, it is necessary to use measures to prevent the recurrence of cellulitis and lymphangitis. The reduction of lymphedema may require several weeks of intensive therapy to be effective.

Reduction of Edema. For the treatment of lymphedema, the extremity is elevated on a bolster at an angle of 30 to 45 degrees to take advantage of gravity flow. Intermittent mechanical compression is applied by a pneumatic sleeve which is inflated to a pressure of 60 to 100 mm. of mercury for approximately 45 seconds and then deflated for 15 seconds. This mechanical pressure may be applied for periods of 30 minutes to two hours. It appears that the major effect is obtained in the first 60 minutes. Following this mechanical massage, deep stroking and kneading manual massage is applied in a centripetal direction for 10 minutes in an attempt to strip more fluid from the lymphatics. The volume of the arm may be determined by measuring the amount of water displaced from a large cylinder before and after treatment (Fig. 35-13). In addition, the circumferences along the extremity may be recorded as further indices of the effect of the treatment.

Following this therapy the extremity is snugly wrapped with an elastic

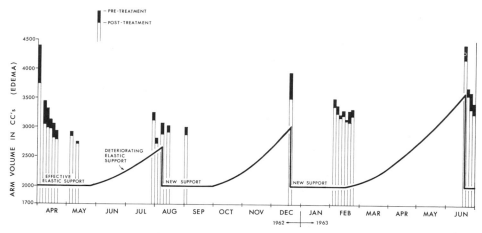

Figure 35–13   Changes in volume of an upper extremity with massive lymphedema following radical mastectomy. The volume of the contralateral normal extremity was 1700 cc. Black sections of columns indicate changes in limb volume during one to three hours of intermittent compression treatment using a pneumatic sleeve. The line graph indicates the effectiveness of elastic support of the arm from an Ace bandage or an elastic sleeve. Deterioration of the elastic support without therapy resulted in increase of the lymphedema.

bandage 4 inches wide. The patient is also instructed to hold the extremity elevated 45 degrees and perform isometric contractions of all the muscles in the extremity four times daily. These isometric contractions are held to the count of 10 and repeated four times a minute for five minutes. Following the isometric exercises the extremity should be unwrapped and wrapped again with the elastic bandage so that a firm compression is obtained. Progressive reduction in the size of the arm with decreased turgor of the tissues and decreased arm volume usually occurs over the period from about the second to the tenth day of treatment. At the end of two weeks the patient is fitted with an elastic sleeve which provides a tissue pressure of 50 mm. of mercury and is instructed to wear the sleeve throughout the day at home. She is also instructed to continue her isometric exercises four times each day at home and to sleep with the arm elevated 30 degrees on a bolster. On this regimen, patients report a continuing slow decrease in the size of the arm after they return home.

The decrease of the volume of edema during a six day period of therapy has been reported to be greater than 20 per cent in 82 per cent or more cases, greater than 30 per cent in 64 per cent of cases and 40 per cent in 41 per cent of cases.[41]

Prevention of Infection.   Frequently the patient with lymphedema has a history of recurrent cellulitis and lymphangitis. Minor trauma such as insect bites, cat scratches, needle or thorn pricks, small burns, infected hangnails and epidermophytosis are commonly associated with the history of recurrent cellulitis in the edematous extremity. Such conditions should be treated appropriately. Clinical findings of induration and increased temperature in the forearm and medial surface of the arm or in the calf, with or without pain or fever, may be taken as evidence of chronic subclinical infection. Frank cellulitis or lymphangitis obviously represents an acute infection which should be treated by penicillin or a broad spectrum antibiotic.[42] Antibiotics have also been given prophylactically to prevent recurrent lymphangitis and excellent results have been reported. Benzathine penicillin G injections of 1,200,000 units monthly; penicillin V monthly; phenethicillin potassium, 250 milligrams twice daily for five days each month; or oxytetracycline, 250 milligrams four times daily for five days each month if the patient is allergic to penicillin have been reported effective in preventing recurrent lymphangitis in cases of lymphedema.[43]

REFERENCES

1. Asmussen, E., and Nielsen, M.: Cardiac Output during Muscular Work and its Regulation. Physiol. Rev., 35:778-800, 1955.
2. Berggren, G., and Christensen, E. H.: Heart Rate and Body Temperature as Indices of Metabolic Rate during Work. Arbeitsphysiol., 14:255-260, 1950.
3. Kottke, F. J., Kubicek, W. G., Olson, M. E., Hastings, R. H., and Quast, K.: Five Stage Test of Cardiac Performance during Occupational Activity. Arch. Phys. Med., 43:228-234, 1962.
4. Dawson, W. J., Jr., Kottke, F. J., Kubicek, W. G., Olson, M. E., Harstad, K., Bearman, J. E., Canner, P. L., and Canterbury, J. B.: Evaluation of Cardiac Output, Cardiac Work and Metabolic Rate during Hydrotherapy and Exercise in Normal Subjects. Arch. Phys. Med., 46:605-614, 1965.
5. Kottke, F. J., Kubicek, W. G., Danz, J. N., and Olson, M. E.: Studies of Cardiac Output during the Early Phase of Rehabilitation. Postgrad. Med., 23:533-544, 1958.
6. Passmore, R., and Durnin, J. V. G. A.: Human Energy Expenditure. Physiol. Rev., 35:801-840, 1955.
7. Gordon, E. E.: Energy Costs of Various Physical Activities in Relation to Pulmonary Tuberculosis. Arch. Phys. Med., 33:201-209, 1952.
8. Müller, E. A.: The Physiological Basis of Rest Pauses in Heavy Work. Quart. J. Exp. Physiol., 38:205-215, 1953.
9. Müller, E. A.: Personal Communication.
10. Taylor, H. L., Buskirk, E., and Henschel, A.: Maximal Oxygen Intake as an Objective Measure of Cardio-Respiratory Performance. J. Appl. Physiol., 8:73-80, 1955.
11. Bruce, R. A., Blackmon, J. R., Jones, J. W., and Strait, G.: Exercising Testing in Adult Normal Subjects and Cardiac Patients. Pediatrics, 32:742-756, 1963.
12. Naughton, J., Sevelius, G., and Balke, B.: Physiological Responses of Normal and Pathological Subjects to a Modified Work Capacity Test. J. Sports Med., 3:201-207, 1963.
13. Hellerstein, H. K., and Hornsten, T. R.: Assessing and Preparing the Patient for Return to a Meaningful and Productive Life. J. Rehab., 32:48-52, 1966.
14. Kubicek, W. G., From, A. H. L., Patterson, R. P., Witsoe, D. A., Castaneda, A., Lillehei, R. C., and Ersek, R.: Impedance Cardiography as a Noninvasive Means to Monitor Cardiac Function. J. Ass. Advancement Med. Instrum., 4:79-84, 1970.
15. Tobis, J. S., and Zohman, L. R.: A Rehabilitation Program for Inpatients with Recent Myocardial Infarction. Arch. Phys. Med., 49:443-448, 1968.
16. Boyer, J. L.: Adult Fitness Starter Program for Individuals Considered to be at High Risk for Coronary Heart Disease. J. S. Carolina Med. Ass., 65 (Suppl. 1):99-100, 1969.
17. Kellermann, J. J., Levy, M., Feldman, S., and Kariv, I.: Rehabilitation of Coronary Patients. J. Chron. Dis. 20:815-821, 1967.
18. Troedsson, B. S.: Establishment of Oscillometric Clinical Norms for Arterial Circulation in the Legs in Arteriosclerotic Obstructive Disease. Arch. Phys. Med., 39:566-571, 1958.
19. Abramson, D. I.: Diagnosis and Treatment of Peripheral Vascular Disorders. New York, Paul B. Hoeber, Inc., 1956.
20. Goldberg, M. J., and Skowlund, H. V.: Comparison of Oscillometric Index and Blood Flow of the Foot as Measured by Plethysmography. Arch. Phys. Med., 44:308-312, 1963.
21. Nyboer, J.: Electrical Impedance Plethysmography. Springfield, Ill., Charles C Thomas, 1959.
22. Skowlund, H. V., and Kottke, F. J.: Studies of Vascular Responses of Feet of Normal Subjects to Dihydrogenated Ergot Alkaloids and Tolazoline under Controlled Conditions. Arch. Phys. Med., 44:157-166, 1963.
23. Kottke, F. J., and Stillwell, G. K.: Studies on Increased Vasomotor Tone in the Lower Extremities following Anterior Poliomyelitis. Arch. Phys. Med., 32:401-407, 1951.
24. Williams, P. G., Montgomery, H., and Horwitz, O.: Oxygen Tension of Tissues by the Polarographic Method. VI. Effect of Changes in Position on Oxygen Tension of the Skin of Toes. J. Clin. Invest., 32:1097-1100, 1953.

25. Knox, W. G.: The Value of Digital Plethysmography in Evaluating Patients with Peripheral Arteriosclerosis for Lumbar Sympathectomy. Ann. Surg., *149*:539–545, 1959.

26. Lempke, R. E., King, R. D., Kaiser, G. C., Judd, D., and Nahrwold, D.: Amputation for Arteriosclerosis Obliterans. Arch. Surg., *86*:406–413, 1963.

27. Hemingway, A., Rasmussen, T., Wikoff, H., and Rasmussen, A. T.: Effects of Heating Hypothalamus of Dogs by Diathermy. J. Neurophysiol., *3*:329–338, 1940.

28. Bennett, R. L., Hines, E. A., Jr., and Krusen, F. H.: Effect of Short Wave Diathermy on the Cutaneous Temperatures of the Feet. Amer. Heart J., *21*:490–503, 1941.

29. Abramson, D. I., Tuck, S., Jr., Zayas, A. M., Donatello, T. M., Chu, L. S. W., and Mitchell, R. E.: Vascular Responses Produced by Histamine by Ion Transfer. J. Appl. Physiol., *18*:305–310, 1963.

30. Kramer, D. W.: Peripheral Vascular Diseases. Philadelphia, F. A. Davis, 1948, p. 238.

31. Wisham, L. H., Abramson, A. S., and Ebel, A.: Value of Exercise in Peripheral Arterial Disease. J.A.M.A., *153*:10–12, 1953.

32. Pollack, A. H., and Wood, E. H.: Venous Pressure in the Saphenous Vein at the Ankle in Man during Exercise and Changes in Posture. J. Appl. Physiol., *1*:649–662, 1949.

33. Koller, L. R.: Ultraviolet Radiation. New York, John Wiley & Sons, Inc., 1952.

34. Ladd, M. P., Kottke, F. J., and Blanchard, R. S.: Studies of the Effect of Massage on the Flow of Lymph from the Foreleg of the Dog. Arch. Phys. Med., *33*:604–612, 1952.

35. Elkins, E. C., Herrick, J. F., Grindlay, J. H., Mann, F. C., and DeForest, R. E.: Effect of Various Procedures on the Flow of Lymph. Arch. Phys. Med., *34*:31–39, 1953.

36. Irisawa, A., and Rushmer, R. F.: Relationship between Lymphatic and Venous Pressure in Leg of Dog. Amer. J. Physiol., *196*:495–498, 1959.

37. Opie, E. L.: Thrombosis and Occlusion of Lymphatics. J. Med. Res., *29*:131–146, 1913.

38. Menkin, V.: Biochemical Mechanisms in Inflammation. 2nd Ed. Springfield, Ill., Charles C Thomas, 1956.

39. Middleton, D. S.: Congenital Lymphangiectatic Fibrous Hypertrophy (Elephantiasis Congenita Fibrosa Lymphangiectatica). Brit. J. Surg., *19*:356–361, 1932.

40. Stillwell, G. K., and Redford, J. W. B.: Physical Treatment of Postmastectomy Lymphedema. Proc. Mayo Clin., *33*:1–8, 1958.

41. Stillwell, G. K.: Physical Medicine in the Management of Patients with Postmastectomy Lymphedema. J.A.M.A., *171*:2285–2291, 1959.

42. Britton, R. C., and Nelson, P. A.: Causes and Treatment of Postmastectomy Lymphedema of the Arm. J.A.M.A., *180*:95–102, 1962.

43. Babb, R. R., Spittell, J. A., Jr., Martin, W. J., and Schirger, A.: Prophylaxis of Recurrent Lymphangitis Complicating Lymphedema: Preliminary Observations. Proc. Mayo Clin., *37*:485–491, 1962.

44. Bartlett, R. G., Jr.: Physiologic Responses during Coitus. J. Applied Physiol., *9*:469–472, 1956.

45. Hellerstein, H. K., and Friedman, E. H.: Sexual Activity and the Postcoronary Patient. Arch. Intern. Med., *125*:987–999, 1970.

Chapter 36

INDICATION FOR AND POSTOPERATIVE CARE IN RECONSTRUCTIVE SURGERY OF THE EXTREMITIES

by Earl C. Elkins

The following is a brief outline of the indications for and the possibilities resulting from tendon transfers and other reconstructions of the extremities performed to increase function or to prevent the development of or correct deformities. There will be no discussion of surgical techniques.

GENERAL INDICATIONS FOR TENDON TRANSFERS

Loss of function of a muscle or group of muscles is usually due to neurologic defects resulting from upper and lower motor neuron lesions, to injuries to muscles or tendons or to congenital anomalies.

Surgical procedures should be considered, in general, only for nonprogressive conditions, for the obvious reason that in progressive lesions there may be further loss of function.

The strength of the muscles that may be transferred must be carefully evaluated. In general, only tendons of normal or nearly normal muscles should

714

be used for transfers. To do otherwise may result in failure, because a transferred muscle always loses some power, and therefore if it does not have normal strength in its regular position it may not perform adequately in its new position.

RECONSTRUCTION OF THE UPPER EXTREMITY

Shoulder-Arm Complex. Paralysis of these muscles is always complicated and procedures that are likely to be beneficial are not many.

DELTOID PARALYSIS. None of the procedures designed to correct this deficiency are completely satisfactory. Most transfers for this form of paralysis have been abandoned.

ARTHRODESIS of the scapulohumeral joint is performed but this procedure is not satisfactory unless the scapular rotator muscles (particularly the trapezii and anterior serratus) are functioning normally, or nearly so. It probably should not be done in women because of the cosmetic results. It should not be done in cases in which loss of humeral rotation might interfere with the occupation of the patient, or make impossible an occupation the patient might otherwise have.

ANTERIOR SERRATUS PARALYSIS. Not many surgical procedures are available to remedy this disability. There are procedures that involve wiring the scapula to the ribs in order to stabilize scapular movement and thus allow partial abduction by the deltoid. Likewise, fascial strips may be used to tie the scapula to the ribs. These procedures may fail if the wire cuts the ribs or if the fascial transplants stretch out or break.

Transfer of the origin of the pectorals to the vertebral border of the scapula has been advocated. This transfer is difficult from the standpoint of reeducation to the desired pattern of motion, that is, rotation of the scapula forward and the outer angle upward during humeral abduction and forward flexion.

RECURRING DISLOCATION OF THE SHOULDER. Since the primary reason for the recurring dislocation is the ability of the head of the humerus to move downward and forward, the most successful operations are those that prevent these motions. The Bankart operation does this by restoring the continuity of the anterior capsule of the shoulder joint where it has been torn loose from the anterior rim of the glenoid. The Putti-Platt operation does the same thing by reinforcing and shortening the capsule and the tendon of the subscapularis muscle to prevent downward and forward displacement of the head of the humerus. Both of these operations are effective in preventing further dislocations, and both limit external rotation of the shoulder to a moderate degree.

Elbow Flexors. In cases of paralysis of the biceps brachii in which there is good or, preferably, normal function of the forearm muscles, the finger flexors, which arise from the epicondyle of the humerus, may be advanced upward (Steindler advancement), thereby enhancing the flexor component of the muscles. The transfer may increase the flexion power to several pounds antigravity. If the biceps is not completely paralyzed, some of its function may return.

It may be difficult to stretch the transferred muscles out so that there is full extension of the elbow in the absence of the triceps function.

Reeducation *after* this transfer is simple because the flexors transferred enter into the pattern of elbow flexion or any stronger flexion motions.

This transfer should not be performed unless the wrist extensors are sufficiently strong to stabilize the hand in the functional or extended position. If the hand cannot be stabilized in this position, the wrist will flex, tension will be lost and there will be little flexing action at the elbow. Occasionally, if the wrist extensors are weak, arthrodesis may be performed to stabilize the wrist.

Disorders of the Hand.   It is not possible to discuss adequately all the various indications for reconstruction of the hand. This is a highly specialized subject and requires the greatest surgical skill and judgment. Transfer of tendons, arthrodesis, arthroplasties, tenodesis and bone blocks may be indicated in traumatic conditions, upper and lower motor neuron paralysis and rheumatoid arthritis.

Wrist.   Arthrodesis of the wrist in the case of extensor paralysis has been done, but its popularity is waning. If there are flexor or other tendons that can be transferred to perform the lost function, such a procedure is preferable.

Paralysis of Wrist and Finger Extensors.   In the case of paralysis such as permanent radial palsy, the flexors of the wrist may be transferred for wrist extension and the pronator teres with a tendon graft may be transferred to the wrist or to finger extensors. Another possibility is for one wrist flexor to be transferred to the finger extensors and one to the wrist extensor.

SPINAL CORD LESIONS

Fracture or fracture dislocation of the cervical vertebrae may result in damage to the spinal cord, and the fifth or sixth cervical vertebra is possibly the most frequent area involved in such injuries of the neck. Lesions at the fifth cervical vertebra or above usually leave few muscles functioning in the forearm and hand. Lesions at the sixth to seventh cervical segments generally leave the following muscles functioning in the forearm and hand: the extensor carpi radialis and brevis, occasionally the flexor carpi radialis and palmaris, pronator teres, the brachioradialis and the supinators of the wrist. In lesions at the seventh and eighth cervical segments the finger extensors may be intact. If this is the case, more active tendons are available for transfer.

In the case of a lesion at the sixth or seventh cervical segment the following transfer, or variations thereof, may be done, the choice depending on the available active tendons.

1. Extensor carpi radialis longus to the finger extensors, with a slip to the extensor pollicis longus.

2. Pronator teres to the long flexors of the fingers.

3. Flexor carpi radialis (with tendon graft) through a pulley for thumb opposition.

4. Brachioradialis for thumb flexion. (Although this muscle is a strong one, it has a very short range of excursion; therefore, it is not satisfactory for transfer if considerable range of motion is necessary.)

5. For very supple hands it may be necessary to tie slips of the extensor tendons of the fingers into the finger extensor mechanism to prevent hyperextension of the fingers at the metacarpophalangeal joints. This tenodesis tends to replace the action of the lumbricales muscles and prevents clawing of the fingers.

These procedures may be modified. In cases in which the finger extensors have been preserved, the extensor carpi radialis may be transferred to provide opposition of the thumb and sometimes other functions of the fingers. When only the extensors of the wrist are functioning, tenodesis of the finger flexors to allow automatic flexion of the fingers on wrist extension and tenodesis of the muscles of the thumb to hold it in a position of opposition, or a bone block to hold it in position, may allow some holding or pinching when the wrist is brought into strong extension.

RECONSTRUCTION OF THE LOWER EXTREMITIES

Hip. Not many tendon transfers are applicable for the muscles of the hip. Probably the most common is transfer of the tensor fascia lata. This muscle and its fascia are freed up and attached to the trochanter of the femur and then to the large erector spinae muscles. This procedure may be indicated in cases in which the muscles of the hip and thigh are essentially flail. The muscle can be so placed as to act either as an extensor of the hip or as an abductor; generally it is used for the latter purpose. Usually the transferred fascia to the erector spinal muscles is not sufficiently strong to prevent the gluteal lurch, but it does have some "strut" effect and the patients feel that they have more stability at the hip. If some action of the gluteus medius remains, this transfer may give sufficient added strength to improve the gait considerably.

OTHER RECONSTRUCTIVE SURGERY AROUND THE HIP. Many surgical procedures are available for the improvement of hip joint function and a description of them could fill a volume by itself. Probably the most common procedure was the cup arthroplasty for degenerative disease of the hip, for osteoarthritis or, occasionally, for inactive rheumatoid arthritis. This procedure consisted of placing a Vitallium cup over the head of the femur and deepening the acetabulum if necessary. It is probably one of the oldest arthroplasty procedures used in hip reconstruction and has had varied results.

HIP PROSTHESIS. The use of a prosthesis replaced the cup arthroplasty to a degree. The head and neck of the femur are removed and a new ball and neck are inserted into the shaft of the femur. There are several different types of prostheses; the choice depends on the surgeon. The method is used in fracture of the neck of the femur, particularly in the elderly, and in degenerative changes of various types. It would appear that the results in most instances are good.

TOTAL HIP PROSTHESIS. In 1961 Charnley reported on the use of a hip prosthesis composed of an acetabular portion and a femoral head portion, which are together referred to as a "total hip." There are, in general, three different types of total hips now in use. Of these, the most recently developed is the Ring prosthesis. Ring reported in 1968 on a total hip prosthesis in which both the acetabular and femoral portions were made of chrome-cobalt alloy, which has been found to have the lowest coefficient of friction of those metals tried. The acetabular portion is held in place by a long, threaded stem seated into the pelvis along the weight-bearing line. The femoral portion is a modified Moore prosthesis.

The other two types of prosthesis are somewhat similar in their construction and use. One is the McKee-Farrar prosthesis, described in 1966. It has an acetabular portion plus a femoral portion, which is a modification of the Thompson prosthesis. Both parts are made of chrome-cobalt alloy.

The second of this type is the Charnley prosthesis, in which the cup is made of a high molecular weight polythene and the metallic femoral head is smaller than in the other two types. This combination of a smaller head on a polythene cup produces a coefficient of friction similar to that of a skate on ice and is thus referred to as a "low friction" prosthesis.

In the latter two prostheses, both the acetabular cup and the femoral portion are held in place by the use of a self-sterilizing, "cold-curing" acrylic cement placed within the cavity of the acetabulum and the upper femoral shaft. The cement cures through an exothermic reaction, but no harm is done to the bone, as most of the heat is carried off by the metal.

The procedure can be done through most of the conventional surgical approaches to the hip joint, although many find that the straight lateral approach allows the best view and working area. It has become routine procedure in some institutions to remove the greater trochanter and transplant it further distally to increase the mechanical advantage of the hip abductors. This must be kept in mind during the early stages of gait training and motion exercises, because one must await bony healing prior to active use of hip abductors.

Knee and Thigh.   There are many reconstructive surgical procedures that may be used for the knee but for purposes of this dissertation only tendon transfers will be discussed.

The most common transfer of the thigh muscle is that of one of the hamstring muscles to the quadriceps tendon in cases of quadriceps paralysis. It was used frequently when poliomyelitis was prevalent. Use of the biceps femoris, if it is powerful, is usually preferred. Some surgeons combine this procedure with transfer of one of the inner hamstrings because transfer of one hamstring alone may tend to dislocate the patella. This transfer should not be done if all of the posterior muscles of the thigh, other than the hamstrings, function poorly or are paralyzed or if the gastrocnemius-soleus muscles are not functioning. To transfer a remaining hamstring in these instances may make the knee more unstable because it cannot be held in balance without requiring hyperextension of the knee, and this may lead to genu recurvatum, especially in young patients.

Spastic Paralysis.   A common complication in spastic paraplegia or paraparesis resulting from cerebral palsy and other lesions of the central nervous system is marked spasticity of the hip adductors resulting in a "scissoring" of the lower extremities. The deformity may be severe enough to prevent walking even though there is some voluntary control. Adductor tenotomy or obturator neurectomy, either on branches of the nerve to the several adductor muscles or on the obturator nerve before it emerges from the pelvis, may be used.

Other Common Surgical Procedures of the Knee.   By far the most common operations on the knee are those done to correct the results of injury because the knee ligaments, menisci and articular surfaces are exposed and readily subject to injury. Removal of the medial or lateral menisci when they are torn is a common procedure and quickly returns the patient to the most strenuous type of physical activity. Torn major ligaments of the knee are much more serious, but they may be successfully repaired if operated on soon after the injury occurs. Late repairs often are not successful in restoring good stability to the knee.

Operations to restore reasonable function to the knee damaged by osteoarthritis, rheumatoid arthritis and lateral deformities include débridement of hypertrophic bony ridges, synovectomy and osteotomy. In each of these procedures, restoration of motion of the knee joint and of the power of the quadriceps and hamstring muscles is a major problem. Frequently the knee must be manipulated under anesthesia three to eight weeks after the operation in order to restore enough motion for good knee function and to facilitate muscle strengthening.

In spastic overaction of the gastrocnemius muscle with resulting plantar flexion of the foot so that the patient must walk on the fore part of his foot, the heel cord may be lengthened. However, the tightness is apt to recur, and therefore release of the heads of the gastrocnemius muscles, allowing the muscle to reattach below the knee, or neurectomies to the gastrocnemius and soleus muscles may be performed.

Imbalance and Paralysis of the Foot.   In hemiplegia the everters (peroneals and toe extensors) are usually not capable of function or are paretic, but the inverters, particularly, may be overactive so that the foot is in inversion and the patient tends to walk on the side of the foot or turns his ankle frequently. Occasionally, in younger patients a transfer of the anterior tibial muscle laterally will give the foot much better balance.

Imbalance of Dorsiflexors and Inverters.   In weakness or paralysis of the anterior and posterior tibial muscles with overaction of the everters and toe extensors, especially in growing children, there is frequently an eversion-pronation deformity. If the intrinsic muscles (the short toe flexors) are weak, cocking of the toes, especially the great toe, may occur. There is a shortening of all the toe extensors and the toe cannot come down in flexion to grip the floor in the toe-off phase of gait. The ball of the foot becomes prominent, and the patient bears all his weight on the metatarsal heads as he toes off. The foot with this type of deformity is prone to the development of many corns and calluses.

In the case of imbalance of the inverters alone and when the peroneus muscles are essentially normal, transfer of the peroneus longus to the insertion of the anterior tibial will frequently lead to much better balance. If there is cocking of the toes, the extensor hallucis longus may be transferred into the distal end of the first metatarsal, with arthrodesis of the interphalangeal joint of the great toe. These two procedures will frequently improve both deformities.

Gastrocnemius-Soleus Weakness or Paralysis.   In weakness or paralysis of this muscle group, gait is disturbed because the power toe-off in gait is lost and the patient walks flat-footed. The ability to climb stairs is likewise impaired. In the growing child a calcaneal deformity may occur, especially if the dorsiflexors are strong because when these muscles are unopposed the calcaneus angles downward and allows the longitudinal arc to increase and the forefoot to be higher than the heel. If this condition is allowed to progress, the foot becomes severely deformed, and the patient may walk entirely on the heel without touching the ball of the foot to the floor.

If the peroneus longus is functioning normally, or nearly so, it may be translocated. The tendon is not transferred but is moved to a groove in the posterior aspect of the calcaneus. It seems to be a better procedure than a transfer of the peroneal tendon to the Achilles tendon. In a fair percentage of cases the translocation will provide enough power to allow the patient to toe off and even if it does not, it definitely tends to prevent deformity (or further deformity) of the foot.

In cases in which the peroneus longus is not sufficiently strong to permit translocation and if there are normal or nearly normal dorsiflexors of the foot and the posterior tibial muscle is functioning, the anterior tibial muscle is transferred through the interosseus septum to the Achilles tendon. Reeducation into the patterns of gait after this transfer is extremely difficult because the normal action of the anterior tibial muscle is completely antagonistic to plantar flexion.

There are several *arthrodeses* that may be done on the foot to prevent footdrop or to prevent and correct deformities of the foot (or both). They usually should not be done until the growth centers are closed, because the growth of the foot may be disturbed. Among the most common procedures, the triple arthrodesis, so named by Ryerson, is a classic operation in which the three major joints of the posterior part of the foot, namely, the subastragalar, calcaneocuboid and talonavicular joints, are fused. It may be used for any condition in which the posterior part of the foot is unstable or is in varus or valgus position. It is frequently combined with tendon transfers. If the remaining muscle power is not sufficient for the foot to function well, some procedure is indicated to provide a mechanical block to dropping of the foot into the equinus position. An arthrodesis of the ankle (tibiotalar) joint will accomplish this, but a fused ankle causes a definite limp and requires good mobility of the joints of the foot to allow a reasonably good gait. Motion may be preserved in the ankle joint by providing a bone block from the superior surface of the os calcis against the posterior surface of the tibia to prevent plantar flexion. Other alternatives are the Lambrinudi operation, which is essentially a triple arthrodesis with tilting of the astragalus downward, and a tenodesis of the tendons, which dorsiflexes the ankle into the tibia.

Discrepancies of Leg Length.   The most common measure used to correct discrepancy in the length of the lower extremities is slowing down of the growth of the uninvolved extremity. Steel staples are placed in the epiphysis of the lower portion of the femur or upper part of the tibia. The procedure should be done before the growth centers are closed, usually between the ages of 10 and 12 years. It may be done earlier in girls than in boys because growth stops earlier in the female. This operation is generally considered if the discrepancy is as much as 1 to 1½ inches and seems to be increasing and the patient has several years in which to grow. In cases in which growth is complete, actual shortening of the femur is considered if the discrepancy is extreme. This measure is accomplished by removing a section of the femur.

POSTOPERATIVE MANAGEMENT OF RECONSTRUCTIVE PROCEDURES

Management After Tendon Transfers

There is considerable variance of opinion regarding the optimal period of immobilization following tendon transfer. Some believe the period should be six weeks or more. Some fear any motion other than active, because of the possibility of pulling off the tendon. Some do not advise use of the physical agents, for example, massage, whirlpool baths or heat, which are generally used to reduce swelling and hasten mobilization of the joints.

Possibly one of the most important factors in obtaining good results from tendon transfer is immobilization for the minimal period of time to assure healing of the newly transferred tendon and mobilization as soon as possible thereafter. Prolonged immobilization results in more scarring and in loss of range of motion of the joints involved.

In our experience, mobilization of tendon transfers can safely be started after four weeks if no bone block or arthrodesis was done at the time of the tendon transfers.

Some forms of heat, for example radiant heat or hydrotherapy (whirlpool bath with water temperatures at 102 to 104°), may be used to reduce swelling, clear the dry skin and reduce soreness. Along with this, stroking and kneading massage may be applied to reduce swelling and to attempt to loosen the adherent tissues.

Exercise should be started immediately. It should be in the form of very gentle, passive movements without force or stretching of the tendons. Of utmost importance is the beginning of reeducation of the transferred muscles to perform the new function. The patient must be carefully instructed as to which muscles were transferred, what they did before transfer and what they are expected to do in their new position. Then the patient is told to attempt to perform the function the muscle did before it was transferred. The part may have to be carefully stabilized if other muscles are present that perform movements similar to those of the transferred muscle. This movement must be done repeatedly until the patient begins to see the new movement and is performing it well.

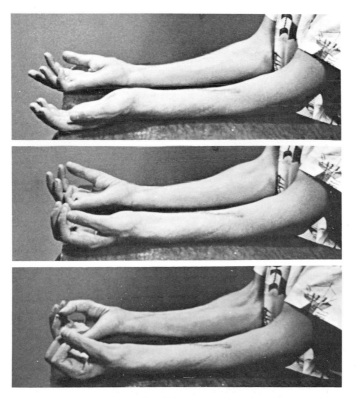

Figure 36–1   Postoperative photographs after tendon transfers showing: *top,* active extension of finger; *center,* attempted opposition of thumbs to index fingers; and *bottom,* grasping performed with fingers and opposing thumbs in a patient with tetraplegia resulting from fracture-dislocation of the sixth cervical vertebra on the seventh. (From Lipscomb, Elkins and Henderson. J. Bone Joint Surg., *40-A:*1071–1080, 1958.)

The motion of the muscle whose paralysis necessitated the tendon transfer should never be requested because then the transferred tendon will never come into action. Once the patient produces the function intended by the transferred tendon, he generally isolates the function quickly and the new pattern of motion is created.

Generally speaking, transferred muscles which were synergistic to the lost function are the most easily reeducated to the new function. However, strong antagonistic muscles that have been transferred can also be reeducated if proper care is taken to stabilize the part and to see that the transferred muscle produces visible motion of the kind intended.

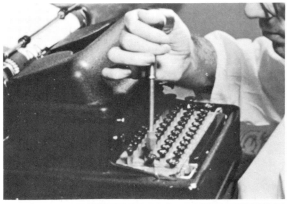

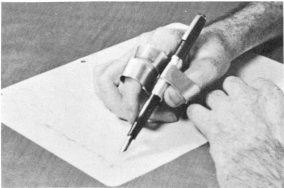

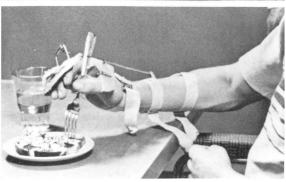

Figure 36–2 Appliances used by patients with tetraplegia prior to tendon transfers: *top*, device used for typing; *center*, device used to clamp pen or pencil; and *bottom*, appliance with movable parts controlled by springs and elastic bands to enable a tetraplegic patient to use various utensils. The assistance of an attendant for application is required. (From Lipscomb, Elkins and Henderson: J. Bone Joint Surg., *40-A*:1071–1080, 1958.)

Occasionally, because of adhesions, electrical stimulation of the transferred muscle may be beneficial if the new function cannot be established, but this is rarely necessary if careful reeducation can be started soon after surgery.

Reeducation after tendon transfers in the hands and forearms may be very effective. Figures 36-1, 36-2 and 36-3 show results that can be obtained. Transfers in the shoulder and some parts of the lower extremity are less amenable to reeducation. It may be difficult to reeducate a transferred hamstring muscle, for example, the biceps femoris for quadriceps action, not only because it is antagonistic to extension of the knee but also because its action must be isolated from its companion flexors of the knee, the inner hamstrings.

The hamstrings normally decelerate the lower leg and plant the heel on the floor during the swing-through phase of gait and when the heel is stabilized on the floor they act as extensors of the knee. The quadriceps acts as the heel strikes an instant later. Thus in walking both of these muscle groups are knee

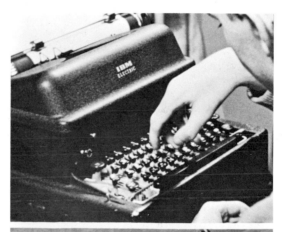

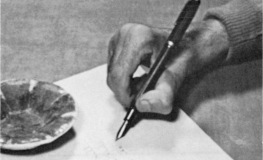

Figure 36–3 Photographs showing ability of a tetraplegic patient after tendon transfers to type, write and use eating utensils without the aid of appliances. (From Lipscomb, Elkins and Henderson: J. Bone Joint Surg., *40-A:*1071–1080, 1958.)

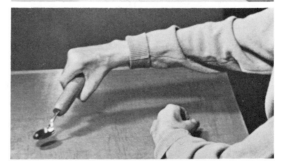

extensors. Therefore, in reeducation of the biceps femoris, patterns of motion simulating that of the patterns of gait may be used to reeducate the transferred muscle.

Postoperative management of the translocation of the peroneus longus consists mainly in stretching out the tendon and muscle. The foot must be in full plantar flexion when the tendon is placed in its new position. An attempt is made to stretch the muscle manually and by having the patient walk, in order to allow the ankle to resume its normal range of motion. Reeducation of the muscle is not difficult, because the peroneus longus is a plantar flexor and everter. When it is translocated most of the eversion component is removed.

Reeducation of the peroneus longus that has been transferred for dorsiflexion is not difficult, especially if the muscle was originally stronger. Usually, when asked to perform eversion and plantar flexion, the patient will produce fairly strong contraction of the transferred tendon. When this contraction develops, the patient is trained to cease using the other peroneus muscles and even the toe extensors. When the transferred tendon acts fairly independently, resistance exercises may be performed.

Reeducation of the transferred hallucis longus, as in the Jones procedure, is quite simple because the actual function of the muscle has not been changed.

The transfer of the anterior tibial muscle through the interosseus membrane to the Achilles tendon is one of the most difficult from the standpoint of reeducation and may take weeks of treatment. The patient must be trained to attempt dorsiflexion of the foot without using any of the toe extensors. This may be practiced first on the other foot if the anterior tibial muscle is normal. When the patient has learned to separate the action of the transferred muscle from dorsiflexion and has achieved plantar flexion action, resistance exercise is started and an attempt is made to train the patient to use the muscle during walking.

Management After Hip Arthroplasties

Opinion varies greatly regarding the postoperative care of patients with hip arthroplasties. What is done postoperatively depends on the procedure, cup arthroplasty or the use of a prosthesis, but there are differences of opinion concerning the measures to be used after each procedure. Most surgeons, however, seem to think that exercise of the hip to maintain motion and increase the power of the muscles around the hip joint is extremely important. Some carefully teach the patient how to do these exercises within a few days after operation and recommend assistive splints to help him perform the exercises in bed. The patient progresses from this assistive type of exercise to active antigravity exercise.

Other surgeons use some form of heat or hydrotherapy to lessen soreness and pain in the hip, along with active-assistive exercise started within the first 7 to 10 days. After about 10 days, progressive resistive exercise may be begun; the exercise is done with gravity eliminated and gradually advanced to include resistance against gravity. In cases of degenerative hip disease of long duration it may be necessary to reeducate the hip flexors especially. The strengthening exercise should include hip flexors, extensors, abductors and adductors. If the gluteus medius has been detached, resistive exercise possibly should be delayed two to three weeks, although opinion about this varies.

In recent years, a less conservative attitude seems to have developed toward weight bearing on the hip after arthroplasty. Some surgeons prefer partial weight bearing on the prosthesis almost immediately after operation; others advocate only minimal weight bearing for several weeks on any type of prosthesis. From a practical standpoint, early institution of strengthening exercise and some weight bearing seem to produce the best results. However, these procedures should be carefully supervised and how rapidly the patient progresses may depend upon his reaction to the treatment.

In general, then, treatment after those operations mentioned consists of the use of some form of heat or hydrotherapy after about 10 days, with sedative massage and gentle active and assistive exercise to regain normal range of motion. When a few degrees of motion have been obtained, strengthening exercise may be started. The quadriceps muscle tends to atrophy rather rapidly; therefore, it may be necessary to continue strengthening exercise for several weeks after operation.

Postoperative treatment of the "total hip" arthroplasty varies. In general, tilt table and gait training with partial weight bearing are started 5 to 8 days postoperatively. Flexion of the hip beyond 40 to 45 degrees is avoided during the first two postoperative weeks, and then during the third week, flexion up to 90 degrees and sitting in a chair are permitted but only if easily accomplished. Relief of pain and not restoration of motion is the prime goal of this surgery, and it must be stressed that motion is not to be forced during rehabilitation of the patient.

Arthrodesis of the foot generally requires no treatment other than training the patient to use crutches; later, perhaps, gait training will be necessary.

REFERENCES

1. Aufranc, O. E.: Constructive Surgery of the Hip. St. Louis, C. V. Mosby Co., 1962.
2. Campbell, W. C.: Operative Orthopaedics. 4th Ed. St Louis, C. V. Mosby Co., 1963.
3. Charnley, J.: Arthroplasty of the Hip: A New Operation. Lancet, 1:1129–1132, 1961.
4. Charnley, J.: A Biomechanical Analysis of the Use of Cement to Anchor the Femoral Head Prosthesis. J. Bone Joint Surg., 47–B:359, 1965.
5. Charnley, J.: Transplantation of the Greater Trochanter in Arthroplasty of the Hip. J. Bone Joint Surg., 46–B.191–197, 1964.
6. Elkins, E. C., Henderson, E. D., and Lipscomb, P. R.: Physical and Surgical Rehabilitation of the Quadriplegic Patient. Motion picture. (Available from Mayo Clinic, Rochester, Minnesota.)
7. Elkins, E. C., Janes, J. M., Henderson, E. D., and McLeod, J. J., Jr.: Peroneal Translocation for Paralysis of Plantar Flexor Muscles. Surg. Gynec. Obstet., 102:469–471, 1956.
8. Lipscomb, P. R., Elkins, E. C., and Henderson, E. D.: Tendon Transfers to Restore Function of Hands in Tetraplegia, Especially After Fracture-Dislocation of the Sixth Cervical Vertebra on the Seventh. J. Bone Joint Surg., 40–A:1071–1080, 1958.
9. McKee, G. K., and Watson-Farrar, J.: Replacement of Arthritic Hips by the McKee-Farrar Prosthesis. J. Bone Joint Surg., 48–B:245–259, 1966.
10. Ring, P. A.: Complete Replacement Arthroplasty of the Hip by the Ring Prosthesis. J. Bone Joint Surg., 50–B:720–731, 1968.

Chapter 37

AUDITORY DISORDERS: EVALUATION AND MANAGEMENT

by Hubert L. Gerstman, D.Ed.

Just as this text is written for the student and practitioner of Physical Medicine and Rehabilitation, so this chapter is addressed to those who desire to treat the "whole" person and his problems of "body and soul." Indeed, what patient could be more isolated, alienated, depressed and confused than one who has lost his primary sensory means of communication? Has your spouse ever attempted to engage you in conversation while you were in the shower, with the sounds of the freshly flushed toilet still noisily mingling with the spray of the shower head, the gurgle of the drain and the drone of the bathroom fan? Such noise in the communication circuitry tends to create a feeling of frustration, which usually manifests itself in extreme hostility toward the "unenlightened" and bemused individual thoughtless enough to initiate a significant human contact under such adverse conditions. So much for my family problems. We now consider the problem of the individual with permanent noise* in his communication circuitry.

This chapter attempts to place problems of hearing loss in a rehabilitation context by: (a) sketching "normal" function; (b) describing that which might destroy, weaken or otherwise modify the system; (c) drawing some behavioral correlates (test responses and effects on general "well-being"); and (d) by

---

*Noise is here used in a technical sense, as any undesirable sound that interferes with the signal or message in communication.

sampling current rehabilitative practice for various types of problems. As a practicing clinician, this author's bias is reflected in an emphasis on clinical, and thus individual, evaluation and treatment.

This approach treats each client first as an entire organism with unique needs relating to an ever-changing environment. The client's adaptation patterns lead to hypotheses formulated both for purposes of analysis of his deficiency (with emphasis on the improvement of residual function) and assistance leading to new, improved adaptation patterns. Management takes the form of frequent diagnostic efforts, with emphasis on the dynamic nature of the human organism and its propensity for change as a result of learning and practice. There is no one method stressed, but rather, current ideas, methods and systems are considered and applied when deemed relevant to the clinical hypotheses formed.

Because a major thrust in audiologic literature has been toward refined testing tools and techniques, such ongoing sampling of the auditory system has led to critical considerations of rehabilitation methods employed. Thus, no one system has been magically accepted ("eclectic" audiologists are numerous). Such developments in clinical practice closely parallel those in Physical and Rehabilitation Medicine. Audiology and Physical and Rehabilitation Medicine speak similar languages in their search for qualified and appropriate patient management. The choice of this "basic" approach was influenced by its success with resident physicians in physical medicine in recent years.

Before proceeding to the body of the text, it is probably useful to describe audiology and its contribution to the rehabilitation team and to the subgroup of professionals concerned with communication problems. Audiology is properly defined as the "science of hearing." The audiologist is usually considered as one who evaluates and recommends management and rehabilitative measures for those having difficulty "hearing." By implication, then, clinical management for problems of audition requires an understanding of the following areas: the scientific bases of the stimulus (sound); the receiver mechanism (the human ear and its neural pathway); auditory and communication behavior in general; examination and testing techniques (psycho-acoustics, signal detection theory); and instrumentation (audiometric equipment, hearing aids, calibration devices and so forth).

A chapter on the importance and clinical implications of audition similarly requires discussion of the various fundamental considerations involved in the identification, evaluation and rehabilitation of persons with reduced abilities in the reception, perception, discrimination and understanding of sound.

THE EAR

The ear is classically divided into three parts. As the sectional diagram indicates (Fig. 37–1):

1. The *outer ear* consists of the auricle, or pinna, and the external canal.

2. The *middle ear* is delineated by the tympanic membrane laterally and the oval and round windows medially. In the normal state the middle ear cavity is an air-containing space housing the ossicles (malleus, incus, stapes). The middle ear is continuous with the nasopharynx by way of the eustachian tube. Two muscles, the tensor tympani and stapedius, constitute the mechanism for the acoustic reflex. The middle ear is said to "communicate" with the air cells of the mastoid. The same mucous membrane lines the middle ear, eustachian tubes, nasopharynx and mastoid.

Sectional Diagram of
THE HUMAN EAR

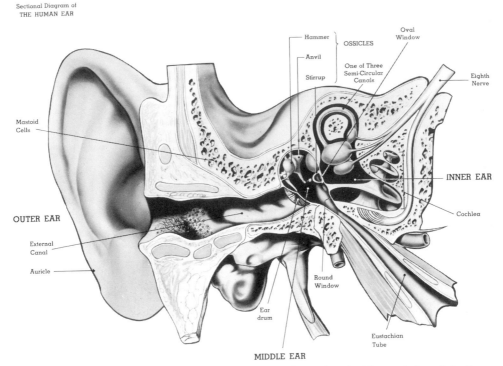

Figure 37–1   Sectional diagram of the human ear. (Reproduced with permission of the Sonotone Corp.)

3. The *inner ear* is made up of the sensory end-organ of hearing (organ of Corti), housed in the cochlea, and the sensory organ of balance, the semicircular canals. Housed within the otic capsule of the hardest bone in the body, the petrous portion of the temporal bone, these organs share the same fluid systems of perilymph in the osseus portions and endolymph in the membranous portions. The end-organ's function is dependent on the integrity of hair cells which extend into the endolymphatic fluid and which are contained and nourished by supporting cells. The hair cells generate the impulses in nerve fibers which ascend via the two branches of the eighth nerve bundle (identified as the stato-acoustic nerve).

The *cochlea* (Fig. 37-2) is housed in a bony spiral of approximately two and three-fourths turns, from base to apex; its widest portion is found at the basilar end and its narrowest at the apical. Conversely, the basilar membrane, which runs almost the entire length of the cochlea, is thickest at the narrow (apical) end of the cochlea, and thinnest at the basilar end.

The *basilar membrane* separates the scala media from the scala tympani, which ends at the round window; a thin membrane extends diagonally, separating the scala media from the scala vestibuli (which derives its name from its place of origin — the vestibule). Microscopic study of the organ of Corti, with its one row of inner and three rows of outer hair cells, has yielded information about the physiologic function of the ear and theories of hearing, which we will discuss shortly.

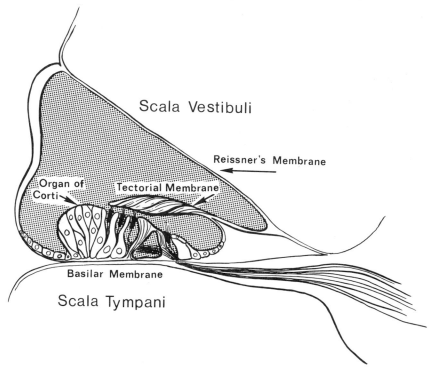

Figure 37–2   Cross section of the cochlea.

The Ear as a "Receiver"

Sound is "collected" by the pinna and proceeds medially through the external canal to the tympanic membrane. Many texts consider the pinna to be functionally useless and primarily ornamental. Recent information (Batteau;[2] Fisher and Freedman;[15] Freedman and Fisher;[16] Freedman and Gerstman[16a]) suggests that the pinna structure reflects the oncoming wave front in such a way as to create a set of delayed replications, which are fed into the auditory canal after the direct signal. Because of its three-dimensional asymmetry, the pinna can encode information relative to localization. Freedman, on the basis of his work to date and Batteau's mathematical theory, feels that localization, attention and speech intelligibility are inseparable processes.

The *tympanic membrane* (TM) reacts differentially to sounds of various frequencies and intensities. The handle of the malleus is attached to the tympanic membrane and thus moves with the tympanic membrane, setting in motion the remainder of the ossicular chain. This system, culminating in the footplate of the stapes at the oval window (of the vestibule), acts as a transforming and transducing mechanism. The lever arrangement allows transformation of the large displacements of air-borne sound into small displacements of the relatively incompressible cochlear fluid.

The *round window* allows for displacement of the perilymph, which is continuous in the scala vestibuli and scala tympani at the apical end of the cochlea. Simultaneously, this system allows transformation of small forces at the tympanic membrane into larger forces acting upon the cochlear liquid. This additional piston action provides a mechanical advantage (tympanic membrane to stapes) which is assisted by an advantage provided by the ossicles. Thus the differential responses of the tympanic membrane, the flexibility of rotational movement in the ossicles, and the ability of the footplate to rock as well as pulse at the oval window allow the fluid-borne waves to be highly complex and laden with information.

The information delivered to the inner ear is "distributed" according to its frequency and amplitude. This process has been described by von Békésy[64] (the description of which—to a great extent—won him a Nobel Prize) in terms of effects on the basilar membrane and the vibrational patterns produced. These "traveling waves" account for points of maximum amplitude (maximum impact on the hair cells) along the length of the basilar membrane; based on this process, various theories can account for some current data.

It is possible to support a *frequency theory of hearing* to a limited extent by demonstrating a point-by-point correspondence for an air-borne pure tone with responsiveness throughout the auditory mechanism and ascending pathway. Because the maximum theoretical rate of a class A neural fiber is about 1000 impulses per second, the limitations of the *frequency theory* are obvious. Nevertheless, such undifferentiated responsiveness can be demonstrated for sounds up through about 400 to 500 Hz (Hertz, or cycles per second). These low frequency stimuli have been shown by von Békésy to "travel" to the apical end of the cochlea, stimulating the hair cells in that area.

In direct contrast to frequency theory, *place theory* holds that the place of maximum stimulation determines sensation. This appears to be correct for stimuli delivered to the basilar end of the cochlea for sounds around 5000 Hz and above (the range of human hearing is usually given as 16 to 16,000 Hz or 20 to 20,000 Hz). Between these low and high tones, sensation appears dependent on the hair cells firing in volleys (at a certain area, at certain rates); thus Wever's reconciliation of theories with the *Volley Theory*.[68]

The Ascending Pathway

The auditory portion of the eighth cranial nerve is comprised of nerve fiber endings associated with the several thousand (approximately 3500 inner and 12,000 or more outer) hair cells, thus forming a well-defined collection at the spiral ganglion and emerging from the temporal bone through the internal auditory meatus in the company of the vestibular branch of the eighth cranial nerve and the seventh cranial nerve.

Much theory and speculation arises relative to the course and function of the ascending pathway because of the number of neurons involved, the number of centers involved, the crossovers of the pathway, and the number of synapses, as well as the existence of collateral routes, and the finding that there exist some descending (motor) fibers. The pathway is diagrammed in Figure 37-3.

THE NATURE OF THE STIMULUS (SOUND)

In classic psychophysics and its modern modifications, when testing sensory processes, the numerical designation of function arises from specification of the physical properties of the stimulus. We measure and assign numbers to the stimulus, which can be modified and manipulated according to knowledge

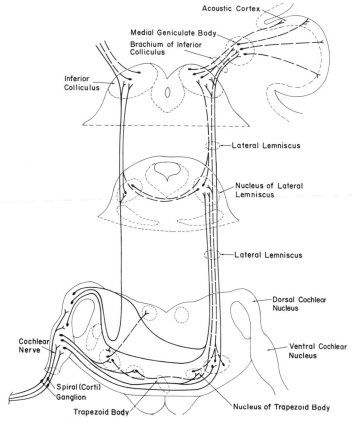

Figure 37-3   The ascending auditory pathway.

of its parameters and characteristics; then, with some agreed upon response from the subject, we are able to state that we have defined some aspect of the subject's sensation. With such behavioral methodology, it cannot be said that we measure sensation *per se*. This can become a critical point in clinical measurement. Most audiometric testing consists of a series of psychophysical experiments.

Some otologic, otoneurologic and audiologic tests are not psychophysical in nature and thus require different forms of analysis and interpretation. The discussion in this section is necessary for understanding in reading and interpreting Audiologic Reports of clients, the quantifications of which are derived from measures of the stimuli assigned, in turn, to a mutually acceptable response.

Frequency

The psychological sensation of *pitch* is related to the physical parameter identified as *frequency*, which is defined in terms of Hertz (Hz). This term (Hz) has generally replaced such previously acceptable terms as cycles per second (cps) and double vibrations (dv) and merely describes the number of times cycles of compression and rarefaction occur in a second for a given vibration. As frequency is increased, pitch is raised.

Tuning forks are calibrated to the musical "C" scale (middle C = 256 Hz) and successive octaves of 128, 256, 512, 1024, 2048 and 4096 have been used for otologic testing and experimentation. Older audiometers were similarly adjusted. Modern audiometers utilize round-numbered octaves: 125, 250, 500, 1000, 2000, 4000 and 8000 Hz, with half-octave intervals at 750, 1500, 3000 and 6000 Hz. (Most musical organizations tune to an A = 440, which is consistent with none of the above and places middle C at 261.6 Hz.) As already noted, frequency plays a critical part in auditory theory. Knowledge of frequency is also important in terms of instrumentation, analysis of speech sounds, and speech perception.

Intensity

Intensity is the physical parameter of the psychologic perception called *loudness* and is related to the amplitude of the signal. Measurement of intensity is usually reported in decibels (dB). The decibel implies a ratio and is based on a logarithmic scale to the base 10. The pressure formula for dB is: $dB = 20 \log_{10} \frac{V_1}{V_2}$ (pressure, as the square of the power, requires a "doubling" of the log scale where $dB = 10 \log_{10} \frac{W_1}{W_2}$). The fact that the "Bel" of decibel represents a logarithmic increase indicates certain relationships not readily apparent from the numbers. The range of tolerable intensity from the threshold of detectability to the threshold of pain is approximately ten million "units" or 140 dB sound pressure level (*SPL* — computed to a standard reference of 0.0002 dyne/cm^2). While the decibel does not represent a perfect mathematical model for perception of intensity, it approximates auditory function in the middle ranges and is convenient in the experimentation and calibration of the stimulus.

The Audiogram

Figure 37-4 displays the pure tone audiogram and indicates the two parameters of intensity and frequency used to sample auditory functions. Audiometric zero is represented as a flat line, equivalent at each frequency. In reality, each frequency requires a different SPL level to reach average normal threshold so that calibration of audiometers "builds in" the corrections necessary to maintain the audiometric zero relationships. A current international standard is used for this purpose (ISO), which is well explained in a number of recent publications (*e.g.*, Davis — Chapter 9 in Davis and Silverman,[10] and Goodman[23]).

Spectrum

Although we sample the receiving mechanism with pure tones, which are characterized by their regularity and periodicity, most meaningful sounds are complex and contain varying mixtures of frequency and intensity. Through a

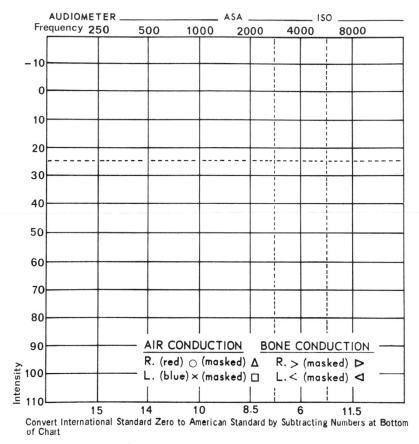

Figure 37–4 Pure-tone audiogram.

process known as harmonic analysis, we are able to describe the distribution of energy among the frequencies represented in a complex sound. This description may be called the *spectrum*. Its psychological counterpart is *quality*.

Noise is characterized by its aperiodic qualities and is usually defined as any undesirable sound. Analysis of the spectra for speech may include brief "noisy" segments. Such cues, when incorporated as part of the spectra, may offer information. If such noisy segments do not interfere with the signal, this quality is considered as part of the spectrum. Analysis of the speech spectrum contributes information to audiologic testing that aids in understanding and explaining how a specific type of hearing loss affects the behavior of the client. In discussing audiometric results, we shall refer to spectral features.

The speech scientist's study of phonetics may be further delineated as: (a) motor phonetics, in which the speech mechanism and its articulatory gestures are studied; (b) acoustic phonetics, in which the physical events are identified, described or manipulated; and (c) perceptual phonetics, in which significant features are analyzed (this area of study has also been called phonemics). In the understanding of the speech mechanism, we are able to discern the loss of control of speech experienced by the adventitiously deafened, as well as the difficulties of children with various degrees of hearing loss in their attempts at speech acquisition.

As described by Goehl, such information is utilized by the speech pathologist in devising therapeutic techniques for such persons (see Chapter 5).

The analysis of the acoustic signal allows us the luxury of manipulation of the various parameters and leads to experimentation in both evaluative and therapeutic techniques. Analysis in the perceptual areas has led us to identify certain critical facets of the spectrum, particularly in the consonant sounds. The voice generates the part of the syllable signal that is identified as the vowel, and the shaping of the speech mechanism is responsible for the vowel characteristics, while most of the information of the speech signal is carried in the releasing and arresting portion of the syllable identified as the consonant. For consonant production the on-going breathstream is interrupted. These brief moments of interruption generate certain characteristic energies, which if not fully perceived, lead to a distortion of the incoming speech material.

It has already been mentioned that the speech frequencies are usually identified as the bands of energy between 500 and 2000 Hz. Phonetic analysis further indicates that there are three major bands of energy, which scientists have called formants. The first formant (formant I) represents the lowest band of energy and is correlated with the *manner* of articulation of a given phoneme or syllable, whereas the two higher bands of energy (formants II and III) are related to the *place* of articulation.

The learning of speech requires immense amounts of imitative behavior. In an attempt at duplicating a spectrum, the child imitates all the apparent visual movement that he can and depends for the remainder of the imitation on the kinesthetic feeling in the oral area while trying to match the acoustic end-product as closely as he can. Although conscious imitation is eventually short-circuited in favor of a more sophisticated and abstract method in the learning of new words, studies have shown that the sensory processes of

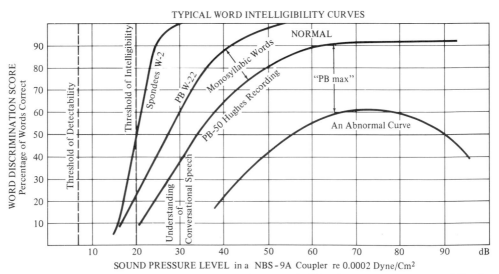

Figure 37–5 Articulation curves. (From Davis, H., and Richardson, S. R.: Hearing and Deafness, 3rd Edition, Holt, Rinehart and Winston, 1970.)

previous experience are searched, retrieved and utilized in all their dimensions when such new learning is attempted. That is, neural impulses akin to those involved in actual and conscious imitation have been reported in the learning of new words or nonsense syllables.

For purposes of analyzing the hearing mechanism, hearing scientists have borrowed from the earlier acoustic systems' scientists and engineers, who devised the concept of the articulation curve. Articulation is used in a highly technical sense and relates to the discrimination of sound syllables and the percentage correctly perceived when broadcast through an acoustic system (or the human ear) as a function of intensity. For this purpose one uses word lists that are constructed to specific criteria. The criteria dictate the steepness of such a curve and depend, for instance, on whether one wishes to investigate the discriminability or homoegeneity of certain sounds relative to a given system.

Figure 37–5 shows a series of curves for selected lists. Note the bottom curve, in which an abnormal ear reaches maximum efficiency at about 68 dB. Such a person can never understand all that is said, whatever the intensity level. This has ramifications for hearing aid fitting, which we shall discuss later.

INSTRUMENTATION

Noise has already been defined as any undesirable sound that might interfere with the informational content of the signal. Because even low energy levels of noise may interfere with threshold testing, one of the major "instruments" employed by the audiologist is the sound-treated room. The object of a specially constructed room is to minimize ambient noise levels. By controlling the sound environment in this way, the audiologist is able to understand the results of his testing with certain stimuli at given energy levels. He is thus assured that responses given to a specific stimulus are reliable (the response is not elicited by some unwanted stimulation). The repeatability of the subject's responsiveness then is an operational definition of such reliability. Face validity also is accomplished when the environment is sufficiently controlled and when the experiment is operationally defined in terms of the specific responses elicited.

One way in which the "behavior" of the subject may be analyzed is in terms of *signal detection theory*. Investigation of literature relative to the "subject's experience" indicates that, as a human organism, the subject brings to bear certain past experiences on the moment of investigation. These past experiences are essentially "uncontrolled." Rather than forcing ourselves to make assumptions about sensory thresholds, we might prefer to control for the decision-making processes of the subject. We can do this by computing the various probabilities upon which his decision may be based.

By controlling certain aspects of the signal (through our instrumentation) and by introducing and limiting specific choices available to the subject as responses, we might postulate certain distributions. Such distributions could be based on the number of "hits" and "misses" that might occur in a given series. The analysis could attempt to describe a perfect ideal observer as compared with a non-perfect non-ideal observer.

The ideal observer is one who makes use of all available information in proper proportion, as opposed to one who makes no use of any data in any reasonable proportion. Comparing the two observers, it is now possible to describe the limits of the probability that certain behavior might occur, given a specified stimulus. If we describe this as a "region of possible performance," we have criteria and measurement points to which an actual performance might be compared. Given such mathematics, we are now in a position to generate information relative to the observer's personal criteria and to describe the influence of the past experience of the observer on any current experiment. Such methodological modifications of classic psychophysics might lead us to modify instructions to an observer in an experiment (which, as we have indicated, is equivalent to the "patient" in the audiometric evaluation).

The introduction of noise into such an environment may also be controlled in that the noise would be of a known type and quantity. Thus, testing could be given in a white noise background or in a background of voices or of some other known wave form characteristic.

Pure tone audiometers vary in size, cost and complexity. The components necessary include the oscillator as a sound source; a means of selecting the frequency to be tested; an attenuation circuit for control of intensity of the signal; an amplifier and the earphones for the subject's listening by air conduction, as well as a bone conduction oscillator for placement on the skull.

Although much has been written about bone conduction testing, its rationale and practice, it will suffice for our current purposes to indicate that we are apparently able to stimulate the cochlea while by-passing the middle ear mechanism, so that it is possible to achieve an estimate of sensori-neural reserve, whether or not the external and middle ears and the conduction apparatus are properly functioning.

Most audiometers are further elaborated by the presence of a masking circuit for purposes of generating noise to the contralateral ear (the ear not being tested). This circuit may be further refined by the addition of a filtering device that allows energy to be produced on a narrow band, thus fatiguing the masked ear far less than the wide band method, and, in general, allowing for better control of effective masking for the frequency band desired. Other possible additions will be described in conjunction with the various special tests found below.

The *speech audiometer* uses either a microphone, tape recorder or phonograph as its sound source and allows for control of amplification to either loudspeakers or earphones. In actuality, any signal may be broadcast through this network (e.g., music, specialized sounds, from whistles to sirens, and other warning stimuli). Probably the critical value is the frequency response of the entire system and its ability to duplicate the live or recorded signal while maintaining the relative energies of the spectrum.

One looks for a generally "flat" response characteristic with rapid decay at the frequency cutoff points so that the system does not deliver undue emphasis to particular cues at a given frequency band, and so that points along the spectrum are not distorted.

Another machine frequently found in audiometric laboratories is the *Békésy audiometer*. This instrument is a self-recording audiometer in which a button is used to drive a motor which controls the attenuator and is, in turn, connected to a motor-driven pen, which is able to record the ups and downs of attenuation as controlled by the subject during the listening situation. We will refer to this machine later, particularly as it relates to abnormal adaptation and fatigue patterns.

The audiometer, then, is merely a calibrated network that is able either to generate a signal or to take its signal from another sound source, and is then further able to control such sound energy so that it is delivered to a subject's ear at a given intensity. An associated instrument is a device known as a *sound level meter*, or audiometer calibration unit, which is able to measure the output of an audiometric device, particularly its intensity. In this measuring instrument the frequency band is usually controllable, so that analysis of the frequency components of a given noise signal or any complex signal may be made instantaneously. The sound level measuring instrument is essentially substituted for the human ear, so that the output of an audiometric machine may be measured "at the ear." A standard coupling, duplicating the volume of the external auditory canal, is generally used when measuring the output of an earphone; thus the sound is recorded "at" the tympanic membrane of the ideal subject.

Auditory training devices consist of essentially the same types of components as the speech audiometer. These devices utilize a microphone, an amplification circuit and a set of earphones with controlled attenuation at the amplifier for specific training purposes.

The *hearing aid* is basically no different from this type of network. The hearing aid is typically a miniaturized device that is kept down to a size that is easily worn and usually is cosmetically appealing. If the hearing aid is not particularly attractive from a cosmetic standpoint, it is at least typically unobtrusive. As in the case of audiometric equipment, the primary concerns with the responsiveness of a hearing aid relate to its characteristic frequency response and the amount of amplification it is able to deliver. The amplified signal through the hearing aid circuit is referred to as "gain." Factors such as the placement of the microphone in the device and the wearing of the device itself, whether in the ear, behind the ear, or on the body, and the coupling of the instrument to the person wearing it (the end-aural insert—ear mold—or bone conduction oscillator) will be discussed as such factors relate to a particular individual and his pattern of auditory difficulty.

Another diagnostic device which has gained attention in recent years is the *acoustic impedance bridge*, which uses a test tone reflected back from the tympanic membrane. The amount reflected depends upon the acoustic impedance (mass, stiffness, resistance) of the ear. By first computing the volume of the ear and then matching (bridging) the impedance by adjusting the bridge to a null (found by listening to the reflected sound and canceling by means of the bridge adjustment), data can be gathered, without requiring a test response from the subject, that reveals information relative to the status of the middle ear.

HEARING LOSS: A PROBLEM OF DEFINITION

It has become traditional in chapters of this sort to strive somehow for common agreement concerning the terms utilized in describing hearing loss of deafness. In reviewing the literature, it is possible to conclude that finding terms that are fully acceptable to all parties approaches an exercise in futility. Nevertheless, we will attempt to integrate some generally acceptable information.

The 1967 Rehabilitation Codes stated that "hearing function implies reception and recognition of sounds within appropriate environmental limits."[12] The essence of most of the classification systems for degree of hearing loss relates to the above statement in that the dynamic qualities of human behavior are recognized. The problem arises when an attempt is made to assign numbers (dB) to such classifications. One further problem is noted when, even in the recent publications, older descriptions are used to relate the degree of hearing loss to American Standards calibration rather than to the newer International Standardization Organization (ISO) levels. Classifications using the terms normal, borderline, mild, moderate, severe, profound or terms approximating such a sequence appear acceptable. However, in ISO terms, acceptance of 25 dB as the "limits of normal" creates some confusion as to the limits of mild, moderate, and so on.

It is possible to follow the resolution of some of the confusion through the revisions from edition to edition of *Hearing and Deafness* (Davis and Silverman).[9, 10] In the second edition "deafness" was confined to hearing levels of 82 dB (or worse), and a zone of uncertainty between hearing levels of 60 and 80 dB for speech is noted. Note that if the decibel had no reference base, we could be dealing with sound pressure level (SPL), average normal hearing ASA, or average normal hearing ISO as reference.

Average normal hearing for speech — *Speech Reception Threshold* (SRT) — is around 18 to 22 dB SPL reference. The third edition[10] presents an excellent discussion of the problem by Dr. Davis (Chapters 4 and 9).

Various studies relate pure tone averages to SRT. Averaging the best two of three of the speech frequencies (500 to 2000 Hz) generally yields a good prediction of SRT using ISO pure tone reference. As indicated, the various classification schemes relate to pure-tone averages for the speech frequencies. For medico-legal purposes, American Medical Association averages (an older method) were computed for 0.5, 1, 2 and 4 KHz with a 7:1 advantage for the better ear. The American Academy of Ophthalmology and Otolaryngology (AAOO) subtracts 15 dB from American Standard (or 26 dB ISO) for average pure-tone air-conducted threshold (500, 1000, 2000 Hz), weights the better ear at 5:1, and uses 1½ per cent per dB as the multiplier. Again, the so-called "high-fence" appears at 82 dB ASA or 93 dB ISO. There exists no wholly satisfactory method of computing a percentage of hearing impairment relative to a given individual's ability to communicate and adapt. A percentage figure cannot, for example, account for variations in audiometric configurations or differences in discrimination ability.

Under the International Standard we might use the following dB-Hearing Level scheme to describe impairment:*

0–25	= Range of Normal
26–30	= Borderline
31–40	= Mild
41–60	= Moderate
61–70	= Moderately Severe
71–90	= Severe
90 to audiometric limits	= Profound

We will see possible appropriate application of such figures in following sections.

Throughout this chapter, we have used various terms for hearing problems, including "hearing loss," "impairment," "disability," "handicap" and others. *Deafness* carries a connotation of "profound" hearing loss and is usually accepted in that way, and therefore is not useful in describing partial impairment. *Hypocusis* has been suggested (Nober[44]) as a generic term for all hearing loss while *anacusis*, by nature of its prefix, denotes absence of sensation, or deafness. *Hypoacusia* has been suggested for a description of the "hard of hearing." Davis[8] prefers *dysacusis* for describing all conditions not due to simple losses of sensitivity.

---

*Similar to Silverman[59a] and Goodman[23].

TABLE 37–1 SITE OF LESION

PERIPHERAL	NON-CLASSIFIED OR MIXED	CENTRAL
Obstructive (external ear)		Ascending path
Conductive (external or middle ear)	Conductive-sensori-neural	levels
Sensory: Sense organ, cochlear hair cell	Sensori-neural-conductive-central, Sensori-neural-central etc.	Subcortical Brainstem Midbrain
Neural: Eighth cranial nerve		
Sensori-neural (or neuro-sensory)	Retrocochlear	Auditory aphasia
		Brain Auditory aphasia Wernicke's aphasia
	Overlay Psychogenic, functional, non-organic Malingering	Auditory retrieval Auditory memory

Diagnostically, one might forego such terms in favor of the "site of lesion" terminology shown in Table 37-1.

A problem arises as to the term sensori-neural or neuro-sensory. "Neural loss" should refer to the eighth nerve which is part of the peripheral nervous system, as opposed to "cochlear damage" (sensory). An audiologist will usually try to differentiate further a sensori-neural loss with such terms as "primarily cochlear," "probably eighth nerve problems" and "retrocochlear" (not cochlear and probably more central, as in the cerebello-pontine angle), or he may attempt, along with the otologist, radiologist, neurologist and others, to interpret his findings in terms of pathology or etiology as "results are not inconsistent with tumors of," "mass occupying lesion," "similar to findings in otosclerosis," "responses consistent with problems of aphasia," "the general aging process," and "presbycusis."

Mixed losses are common and do not always relate to conductive pathology. When a loss produces responses indicating a lesion that is primarily central, these responses are frequently confounded by some degree of sensori-neural impairment. The same ear may be scarred from early childhood otitis so that "mixed conductive-sensori-neural-central impairment with some degree of psychogenic overlay" is not an impossible diagnostic statement.

Conductive Hearing Loss

The external and middle ears make up a system that gathers and transmits sound to the inner ear. This system is connected and suspended in an optimal manner so that its mass and tension characteristics handle this job efficiently. Changes in mechanical impedance tend to alter such efficiency. Addition of any mass (wax, fluid, growth) restricts the system's ability to convey high frequency sounds, while alterations in tension, i.e., stiffness (caused by adhesions, scarring or early otosclerotic growth), impair its ability to respond to lower frequency sounds. Conductive hearing impairments are treatable through medical (pharmaceutical) and surgical intervention. There are numer-

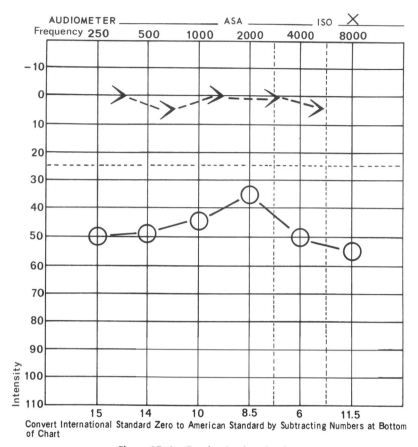

Figure 37–6   Conductive hearing loss.

ous otologic sources of information describing such treatment (e.g., DeWeese and Saunders;[11] Shambaugh[55]).

Those conductive conditions not easily treated or those for which surgical risk is too great are subject to excellent rehabilitation results using amplification (hearing aids). The operational definition of conductive impairment is the presence of the "air-bone gap." Tuning fork tests can describe (but not "measure") hearing phenomena in much the same way that audiometric testing does.

The *Rinne Test* describes air-bone differences. Tuning forks cannot be struck with sufficient intensity (without distortion) to describe severe to profound hearing losses. On the audiogram in Figure 37-6 you see the results of a pure tone examination for a right ear exhibiting a "pure" conductive impairment. That is, sensori-neural reserve is well within normal limits as shown by bone-conducted responses, while air-conducted stimuli elicit responses of 40 dB through the speech frequencies.*

Persons troubled by conductive loss suffer little or no difficulty in discrimination of words. So long as sounds are made loud enough, they are able to get all necessary cues provided in the spectrum. The major behavioral correlate of

---

*Averaging the best two of three responses at 500 to 2000 Hz; thus, 35 + 45 = 80 divided by 2 = 40.

conductive hearing loss is the loss of responsiveness to a quiet or soft sound. Such persons possess the ability to hear speech better in the presence of noise because others speak more loudly under noise conditions, while sub-threshold noise has no effect on the person with conductive impairment and super-threshold noise loses some of its "value" for him.

On occasion, bone-conduction test results will be reduced as a function of a loss of the reciprocal action afforded by the action at the oval and round windows. This occurs in advanced otosclerosis owing to total fixation of the footplate of the stapes, but is remedied by the stapedectomy procedure, which restores the reciprocal action.

Sensori-Neural Hearing Loss

When bone-conducted responses follow air-conducted responses, as in Figure 37-7, the sensori-neural loss is defined. These losses of function are typically worse in the higher frequencies. They are rarely reversible. Known exceptions are: the fluctuations associated with Menière's disease; the *temporary threshold shift* (TTS), which is not actually a hearing "loss" but is associated with exposure to intense but not traumatic noise; hearing loss caused by use of cer-

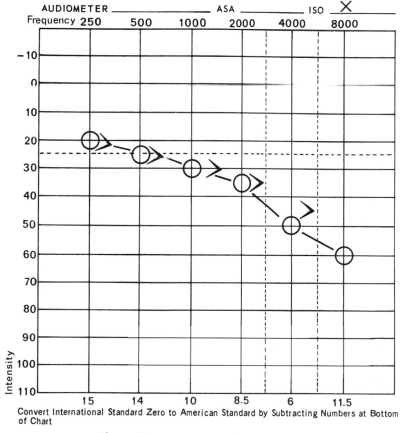

Figure 37-7 Sensori-neural hearing loss.

tain pharmaceuticals, some of which may produce a reversible loss; sensorineural loss resulting from salicylates taken orally (as in aspirins) or absorbed through the skin (as in specially-prepared, compounded ointments). Loss of discrimination for speech, to varying degrees, tends to be associated with sensorineural hearing loss, as are abnormal patterns of auditory adaptation.

With sensori-neural impairment, sounds are received at reduced intensity, and spectral cues are lost, while distortion of the signal may occur. Because audiometric configurations may vary from "flat" to "gradually sloping" to "marked high-frequency drop," and may thus reveal possible etiologic or explanatory information or help pinpoint the site of the lesion, the "pattern" of loss assumes greater relevance than absolute dB numbers. (Reliability of pure-tone audiometry is relatively "weak"—on the order of ± 5 dB—because of the many variables, referred to in an earlier section.

It is believed that cochlear losses are revealed through certain peculiarities of response. Certain tests have become standardized for this purpose:

1. Difference-Limen Testing.   *Short Increment Sensitivity Index* (SISI). This test, which is not a test of personality, has evolved from a long history of Difference-Limen (DL) testing. The difference limen investigated is that of intensity. At sufficient intensity most ears will sense small differences in intensity increment. At about 20 dB sensation level (above one's own threshold) one-dB differences are sensed typically by subjects with cochlear damage (hair cells). The physiologic correlate has apparently not been satisfactorily described.

2. Recruitment.   This phenomenon is operationally defined in terms of the *Alternate-Binaural Loudness-Balance Test* (ABLB), in which a good ear is matched for loudness against the poorer (cochlear loss) ear (Fig. 37-8).

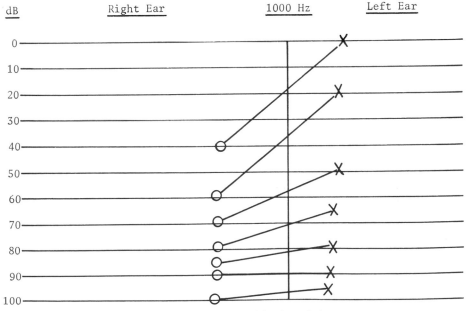

Figure 37–8   Alternate binaural loudness-balance test.

In the illustration, note how the poorer ear gains intensity value between threshold and test limit. This is called an abnormal increase in loudness. Other manifestations of recruitment relate to the reduced dynamic range and the inability of the subject to tolerate loud sounds that are handled by the normal ear with no loss of comfort. Tolerance testing *per se* is also used as a guide to the diagnosis of recruitment and thus of cochlear pathologic conditions. The presence of recruitment is critical to the rehabilitation specialist when considering the desired characteristics of an individually fitted hearing aid.

3. Characteristic Adaptation.   When the sensori-neural mechanism is functioning properly, the ear would be considered normal, or one with a conductive loss. Another measure of this function is the manner in which an ear handles sustained stimulation. The normal ear is capable of sustaining any given pure tone at or near threshold for a minute or more. If we were to allow the system to relax momentarily, that is if we were to interrupt or pulse the tone, there would be no difference in the response from continuous stimulation over a period of time. This would be equally true if we were to test at a fixed frequency or if we were to sweep across the frequency range.

Such testing may be accomplished by utilizing a clinical audiometer and manually presenting the tones at various frequencies. This test is called a *Tone Decay* Test. Earlier in the chapter we mentioned the Békésy audiometer, which is automatic and self-recording. This audiometer, made by several manufacturers, is able to present both continuous and pulsed tones to the listener's ears. The ear with cochlear involvement typically decays to a limited degree, on the order of 20 to 25 dB (Rosenberg[51a]).

Békésy audiometry yields interweaving configurations from continuous- and pulsed-tone sweep frequency testing in normal ears. With cochlear pathologic involvement, in addition to threshold loss, there is a tendency for the continuous tracing to drop at the mid-frequencies and through the higher frequencies. This occurs in a substantial number of cases; however, its absence does not obviate the possibility of cochlear damage. Upon continuous-tone tracing the peaks of amplitude tend to decrease in the same mid- and high-frequencies. This appears to relate to the DL differences described previously.

Other Considerations

Tinnitus.   Noise or ringing in the ear is a subject of a large amount of fascinating literature. However, in spite of the numbers of words written on this subject, tinnitus may be the least specific and poorest understood phenomenon that might be used as a diagnostic sign. Clinically, a ringing tinnitus is frequently associated with cochlear pathologic involvement, at least as demonstrated by other diagnostic tests. On the other hand, a sound that seems to be localized bilaterally but is the same in pitch and loudness would be difficult to explain on the basis of cochlear pathology.

Certain "rushing water" and "machinery" types of noise have been associated with vascular problems wherein the subject frequently experiences his own pulse. It is possible to have an "objective" tinnitus that is vascular or muscular in origin. Objective tinnitus can be heard by persons other than the subject. According to Goodhill[22], tinnitus may be associated with virtually every structure and function subject to lesion in the auditory system. He attempted to relate tinnitus to site of lesion. No definitive clinical protocols are broadly utilized for this purpose by otologists or audiologists; thus it does not appear that any one scheme has achieved full clinical utility. Nevertheless, questioning the subject about his head noises does occasionally yield diagnostic information.

Significance of History-Taking.   Although we have not mentioned the importance of history-taking as yet, it must be strongly emphasized that history-taking may be the most important procedure in any consideration of differential diagnosis. In the case of cochlear pathologic involvement, this becomes particularly obvious when a history reveals "spells of dizziness, intense tinnitus, periods of fluctuating hearing loss which are decreased during dizzy spells and so forth." Most physicians are familiar with such classic historical information relative to Menière's disease and, even in the absence of complete audiometric data, would predict a permanent hearing loss, cochlear in origin.

A history revealing exposure to intense noise such as cannon fire or exposure to noisy sounds over many years' duration would eliminate all the confusion that might result from audiometry displaying a "notch" at 4 KHz (see Figure 37-9). The "typicality" of noise-induced hearing loss cannot be readily diagnosed without a supporting history. Such a history, combined with a knowledge of the research literature, permits a presumptive diagnosis of cochlear hearing loss.

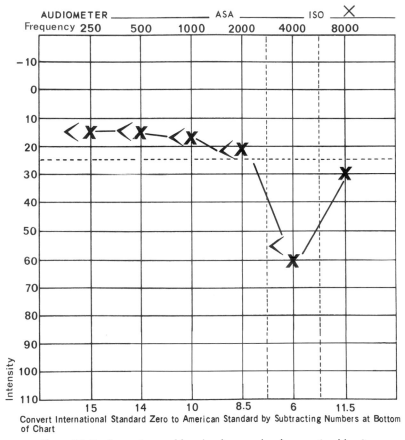

Figure 37-9   Sensori-neural hearing loss—noise damage (cochlear).

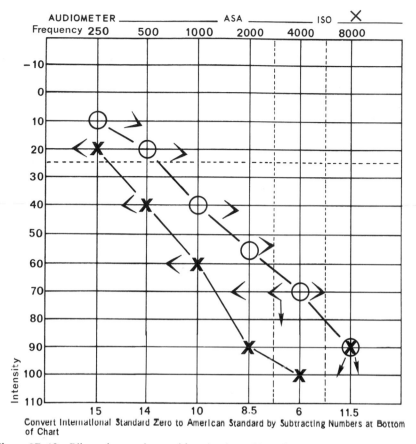

Figure 37–10 Bilateral sensori-neural hearing loss. (Note the somewhat steeper slope.)

Ototoxicity.   There are numerous substances capable of causing varying degrees of hearing loss. Effects of arsenic, lead and quinine are relatively well known and tend to be associated with neural deficit. Drugs from the mycin family tend to cause damage to hair-cells and to other structures of the cochlea (and to the eighth nerve as well). Whether sensory or neural, toxic conditions tend to cause a steeply sloping audiometric configuration (see Figure 37-10).

Viral and Bacterial Agents.   Sensori-neural loss with cochlear signs (ringing tinnitus, recruitment and so on) has been reported relative to viral infection.[43] The specific toxic mechanisms have not, apparently, been fully described, although neurotropic action and "attack" at the stria vascularis have been named as the loci of activity.[54] Sensori-neural losses in association with upper respiratory infections are frequently reported.

Careful history-taking is a common practice when attempting to associate hearing loss with specific pathologic conditions. The conductive elements of such losses are easily recognized, but sensori-neural problems associated with a disease such as influenza or meningitis are difficult to relate to specific signs associated with cochlear manifestations. These signs include hair-cell destruction or damage to other specific structures of the auditory mechanism. Such damage may result from a specific propensity of an agent for a given cell from an associated exudate; from effects on a functional system (as in endolymphatic hydrops); or possibly from a systemic pathologic condition that causes toxicity leading to either central or peripheral problems.

Cerebrovascular Accidents. According to Sataloff, "the role of blood vessel spasm, thrombosis, embolism and rupture as causes of hearing loss is still not clear."[54] Nober indicates that occlusion rather than hemorrhage is more typical.[43] Cochlear signs are also associated with such sudden hearing loss, but retrocochlear signs may be found as often; thus a differential statement relative to sensory and neural components is usually difficult to make.

Presbycusis. Apparently hearing begins diminishing at an early age. Some authors suggest that the loss in sensitivity begins at birth; others at 18 years and still others at around age 32. As with other sensori-neural loss discussed in this section, the types of degeneration may involve several sites, so that presbycusis is usually an aging of several parts of the system. In some cases the symptoms displayed are more markedly peripheral; others are more markedly retrocochlear; in others the overriding manifestations are central. The loss of discrimination has been called "phonemic regression" and implies that the difficulty in understanding found in the geriatric population cannot be explained on the basis of loss of function in the sensori-neural mechanism alone.

Neural Hearing Loss. When the eighth nerve is involved, certain audiometric patterns may help to differentiate the diagnosis. The history tends to be highly variable and such factors as vertigo may assume importance. There is typically little or no recruitment, while abnormal tone decay and a striking separation between the continuous and pulsed Békésy tracings are usually present and strikingly obvious. Ability to discriminate speech is also markedly reduced, sometimes in spite of the fact that pure-tone voluntary threshold may indicate no worse than mild to moderate involvement. Although bone-conduction thresholds always parallel air-conducted thresholds in sensori-neural loss, neural hearing loss may tend to elicit bone-conducted responses slightly below those elicited by air.

When a tumor is involved (acoustic neurinoma or neuroma, at the cerebellopontine angle) the neural symptoms are evident. Early onset is usually accompanied by tinnitus, which is reduced as the nerve is severely or totally destroyed. With growth, nystagmus, facial paralysis, ataxia, dysarthria and other cranial nerve symptoms may also appear. Similar symptoms in audiometry may be elicited in lesions of the ascending pathway.

The audiologic "state of the art" is such that current investigational effort is heavily weighted toward producing test materials that might differentiate the site of the lesion. Filtered speech tests, tests that overlap parts of words, and studies of sites of neural processing of noise will, it is hoped, allow us to quantify and qualify neural and central auditory processes for diagnostic purposes. Some questions requiring answers are: What are the processes of central summation? How is it possible to separate signals with only the subcortical system?

Psychogenic Dysacusis. There are numerous psychological problems associated with hearing loss. In the adult, depression is frequently noted following the loss, and suspicion and a feeling of alienation frequently tend to characterize behavior. Ramsdell[49] discusses three levels of hearing: the symbolic, the warning and the background. The most primitive level, the background, serves to keep us in contact with our environment, helps us perceive a dynamic world of constant activity, and at a reasonably unconscious level affords us a state of feeling "alive." Hearing loss generates an opposite feeling so that this deadened quality depresses the individual's relationship with the world at large. Loss of sounds as warnings presents fairly obvious difficulties, particularly in city traffic. At this level also we can include the aesthetic experience, particularly sounds of nature and music. At the symbolic level the utility of language and other symbol systems represents the sensory aspect of what has been described as man's greatest accomplishment.

The loss of sensitivity for audition, no matter how little, may cause serious problems for even the best adjusted person. The most frequent problem encountered in hearing testing, in general, is the functional overlay generated in reaction to hearing loss. There is perhaps a natural tendency to react in some way to the presence of such a sensory change. Many persons who may ostensibly attempt "to hide" a disability will in a test situation tend to exaggerate the impairment, possibly as a means of calling attention to it. In any case conflicting test results or test results that appear to exceed the probabilities suggested by history may frequently be considered to be a psychogenic overlay.

The rarer problem of apparent hearing loss unsupported by audiometric data also suggests a maladaptive reaction to some psychological stress (or an adaptive reaction in a situation where a reaction appears necessary and a hearing loss may seem to be the best selection of available options). Finally, there is the situation sometimes associated with compensation cases in which a conscious effort is made to simulate a hearing loss and which is frequently referred to as *malingering*. All these represent psychological problems of one sort or another whether or not they are consciously or unconsciously motivated.

There are numerous tests in the armamentarium of audiological test protocols that can detect and compute inexplicable results. Certain so-called objective test measures utilizing *galvanic skin response* (GSR), which utilizes electroshock-conditioning techniques, and *encephalographic audiometry* (EEA), which adapts EEG techniques, may further help to define the presence of psychogenic hearing loss.*

Because of the many variables involved (the relative newness of the profession of audiology and the numerous medical techniques available), medical or surgical therapy should not be determined solely on the basis of audiologic examination. As a discipline able to make significant contributions to diagnostic methods, audiology has made substantial progress over a relatively short span of time. We have not discussed the contributions of nystagmography or other procedures usually utilized by the otologist in arriving at his diagnosis. The treatment aspect of the profession of clinical audiology is in the area of rehabilitation. Such rehabilitation is invoked when it is likely that neither medical nor surgical treatment can make any further contribution, or, sometimes, as a concomitant to a medical or surgical treatment plan. The remainder of this chapter deals with management practices utilized in rehabilitation for hearing loss in terms of instrumentation, education, therapy practices and counseling.

---

*These techniques (GSR—or PGSR—and EEA) have been utilized in a wide range of cases. They are being further defined and delineated through experimental research at this time. They are not discussed more completely here because they are not considered part of the "standard minimum" instrumentation of the Rehabilitation Audiology Clinic.

HEARING AIDS

For many years it appeared that hearing aid usage would be restricted to those with normal or near normal sensori-neural reserve, whose hearing was impaired only by conductive pathologic conditions. It was common to find physicians (and even audiologists) advising their patients with "nerve" or "perceptive deafness" that "nothing can be done" or "no hearing aid will help." While this may have been true for a few, owing either to the nature of their particular hearing loss or to the lack of sophistication of hearing aids, hearing aid dealers were discovering that many persons with sensori-neural hearing loss could be helped.

As otology became more skilled and successful in alleviating the effects of middle-ear pathologic conditions, hearing aid engineers were responding to suggestions from the dealers in the field and developing more sensitive instruments. With further development of the transistor they were also able to deliver more power (gain) and better control of frequency response. This produced instruments with greater potential for refined adjustment, including better control of maximum output, so that those impaired by reduced tolerance were able to accept hearing aids more readily. Finally, the newer technology was able to enhance cosmetic appeal by virtue of miniaturization. The older, bulkier, heavier hearing aid was out and the newer, smaller, lighter instrument was "in."

One major benefit for the moderately impaired was that an aid could be made that was worn at, in or near the ear rather than on the body. Body and surface noise were vastly reduced. Because of this increased utility and the ease of wearing an aid, the industry began "talking up" the *binaural hearing aid.* Binaural amplification could now be used for *two* ears, each with its own control, as opposed to the "Y" cord (two receivers and two molds on one instrument, with one microphone, on the body) or as opposed to two bulky body instruments. The sales "pitch" was "two ears are better than one." This can sometimes be true but not invariably. Nevertheless, the binaural concept has finally gained much greater acceptance, probably owing to improved localization (spatial orientation) and the fact that monaural fitting amplifies both signal and noise to the same ear irrespective of the source or direction of these competing sounds, whereas, at the very least, the binaural arrangement may assist in such necessary "separation" of signal from noise.

With increased acceptance of the "two-ear" model, thought was directed to the individual with unilateral hearing loss. Because factors of angle and phase entered into the analysis of two ears tracking the desired signal and because these can be discerned, to some extent, on the basis of fine-time difference, the idea of receiving the sound at the location of the impaired ear and relaying it to the better ear, gained consideration and acceptance. This is an uncomplicated procedure known as CROS-fitting (Contralateral Routing of Offside Signal). Note that the acronym is spelled with one S. The ear mold is "open" (non-occluded) and the amplified sounds are delivered through a "tube." Persons with a hearing loss in both ears, but in whom one ear is "dead" or a poor candidate for fitting (because of degree of loss or very poor discrimination), may be fitted with BI-CROS (Bilateral-CROS). In this arrangement the poorer ear has a microphone on its side. The signal is routed to the contralateral side through a "closed" (occluded) mold while the signal from the better side is delivered from a microphone on its own side through its own "tube."

In addition to the many factors already discussed, we must amplify our comments on the coupler (the end-aural insert or ear mold). Because resonance patterns at the ear are largely determined by the volume of the chamber and by the length and diameter of the external auditory meatus, and are modified by the hole in the ear mold and the connective tubing to the receiver of the hearing aid, it is possible to modify the hearing aid fitting by manipulating these sizes. Thus, with an open mold it is possible to amplify the high frequency sounds without significantly affecting the low sounds. Molds or tubing can be vented for relief of pressure at the tympanic membrane (the cause of an otherwise frequent complaint), alleviating "stuffy" feelings and complaints of "echo."

Other indications for hearing aid selection for "unusual" problems include amplification for those with bothersome *tinnitus* in which the amplified signal or the increased ambient noise is used to mask the tinnitus. On occasion amplification has been recommended for aphasic children or aphasic adults to "override" the transmissive difficulties. Desk hearing aids or auditory trainers have also been used to train or retrain clients with speech difficulty but no apparent peripheral hearing loss, in order to heighten awareness of auditory feedback and improve discrimination abilities.

In *conductive hearing loss,* when the pathologic condition is inactive and surgery is not indicated, a hearing aid may be satisfactorily fitted. The limitations of such amplification are found only in the sensori-neural mechanism. When the sensori-neural reserve approaches normal limits, the hearing aid selection is based primarily on the amount of gain needed.

On occasion the external or middle ear may be troubled by an active infection so that the fitting of an end-aural insert is prohibited. In such cases a bone-conduction vibrator is fitted so that, as in pure-tone bone-conduction audiometry, the middle ear mechanism is by-passed and sound is directed to the inner ear. It is generally less desirable to utilize this fitting because of the amount of power needed to overcome the additional impedance offered by the skull and the additional power needed to drive the bone-conduction oscillator (on the order of 35 dB). For the client with sensori-neural hearing loss, hearing aids may be satisfactorily selected from a dealer's stock or, on occasion, custom manufactured.

Gain is an important consideration which, among other things, determines whether an aid may be worn at ear level or must be worn on the body, thus separating the microphone from the receiving elements so as to eliminate feedback (squeal).

Other considerations include frequency response, frequency emphasis, power limiting (control of maximum output) and the type of ear mold to be worn. Thus the subject with high frequency sensori-neural hearing loss may be fitted satisfactorily with an aid that emphasizes the highs and either passes or offers minimal amplification to the lows. The subject with unilateral loss may be "brought into balance" with an aid that improves his abilities; if the loss is severe enough, he may be offered a CROS aid. The patient with a tolerance or recruitment problem may be offered an aid that allows him satisfactory listening while controlling the amount of intensity that may reach his ear.

Though it is becoming relatively rare to find a person who cannot be helped by amplification, there are still those whose discrimination abilities are so reduced that amplification may be said to be "unwarranted." This group is most often found among those with an eighth nerve lesion, wherein discrimination is greatly reduced and "staying power" (abnormal adaptation) is very poor. Other than in such cases, the effects of amplification are well worthwhile even when the effects are limited to bringing only some background noise to the ear and nervous system. If we refer back to our brief discussion on the "psychology" of hearing loss, we will recall the rationale for such a fitting.

In cases of hereditary, congenital or early childhood profound loss, the fitting of a hearing aid assumes an important role, perhaps even a greater role. Even in the profoundest hearing loss one can generate some response to intense auditory stimulation, even if the response is a result of stimulation of the tactile sense. In fitting an aid to a preverbal child (or infant), one hopes to deliver usable portions of the sound spectrum to his ear. In the absence of this possibility we would hope to deliver some sensation that allows perception of the rhythm and stress patterns of speech and language as added cues to his learning and understanding. Any auditory or quasi-auditory experience can help in the training of the peripherally deaf child. Such fittings also contribute to the ongoing diagnostic regime in helping to rule out other disorders that resemble "deafness" (e.g., psychologic disturbance, mental deficiency, disorders of the central nervous system.)

You will note that our discussion of amplification has implied the necessity for individual approaches. The client's needs must be assessed and he must participate in the diagnostic and hearing-aid-selection process, because he is a source of information relative to factors such as those of comfort, ease of usage, perceived benefits, and maintenance of the instrument. The effectiveness of current instrumentation and procedures can be measured by the audiologist and hearing aid dealer in terms of the number of hearing aids that are "worn in the dresser drawer." To overcome reluctance to adapt to hearing aid usage, the team of specialists (discussed further on) must interact with the client to reassure him. Much that is "aural rehabilitation" is counseling rather than "teaching," "treating" or "directing."

AURAL REHABILITATION

In essence, all that we have covered thus far may be considered aural rehabilitation; however, the activities described in this section are those that more accurately describe the rehabilitation province of the audiologist. Although all rehabilitation activities for persons with hearing loss require the close cooperation of several disciplines, these are the management considerations that the audiologist is apt to recommend, to follow, and for which hc is willing to assume some ultimate responsibility. In this section we will cover hearing aid counseling, speech reading (lip reading), auditory training, speech conservation, special education, approaches to education of the deaf and hard of hearing, and counseling for adjustment.

Hearing Aid Counseling

Integrated with the process of hearing aid selection must be the dual task of eliciting a positive response to the idea of wearing a hearing aid, while educating the client to the various limitations of amplification. As in most other clinical settings, the client is typically seeking the "magic pink pill" that will cure his ailment. Indeed, the most difficult client is frequently one who has worn an aid for many years and is still seeking the instrument that will restore his hearing to "normal." We will frequently advise our clients that "the hearing aid is a very stupid instrument." While it will make sounds louder, it will not make them more easily understood.

The characteristic frequency response of a hearing aid tends to produce a sound of low fidelity, often described by the wearer as "tinny." The reason for this reaction lies not only in the hearing aid but in the user's own acoustic system as well. The coupling merely emphasizes the quality of the hearing loss on many occasions. Because the hearing aid has no curative powers as such, the individual's system does not improve. Any improvement that does take place occurs because of his own ability to adapt, sometimes in spite of his hearing aid and its fitting.

In order for learning to take place, time must pass; therefore, the hearing aid user must be convinced that he will need to become accustomed to the device and he must be forewarned not to expect immediate success in his new experience. In point of fact, the success of the aural rehabilitation program is dependent upon the development of "the experiential attitude." That is, the client must be willing to engage in trial-and-error learning and needs to be encouraged to view his "misses" not as mistakes but as learning experience. The user needs to be oriented to the factors we have previously discussed concerning separation of signal and noise, and so forth. Eventually he can learn to manipulate the volume control and generally adjust to the various environmental characteristics.

The hearing aid wearer must obviously be introduced to the mechanical elements of his instrument. He must learn to recognize when his battery has worn down and when his ear mold is dirty. He must become familiar with the various adjustments, such as the telephone induction coil, the frequency response switch and the volume control wheel. These may not be quite so simple as they sound but, with practice, the client is able to adapt to the techniques required in terms of his own particular need. If possible, the audiologist should be available to the client during the early periods of adjustment to his aid so that, if the client is placing his battery in the aid upside down, or if there is actually a malfunction, the client can be advised quickly, thereby preventing the occurrence of a "failure experience."

Speech Reading

In learning to speak, the child uses visual cues provided by the parental model. His is apt to study lip movement and facial expression and attempt to duplicate that which he sees. While such conscious imitation is eventually phased out, even the adult is apt to "hear better" when he can see the speaker. Thus each of us is prone to seek visual information from a speaker whether we are impaired by hearing loss or not. There are apparently innate differences among individuals in terms of the degree of dependence on such visual information. These differences may be found among the hearing-impaired as well.

Experience plays a role in determining the "visual awareness" of the hard-of-hearing or deaf client. This is supported by the success of oral schools for the deaf wherein many of the students are successfully trained from an early age to be able to speech-read extensively and to carry out entire conversations with a minimum of difficulty. Some of these differences among the hearing impaired may be discerned by giving "look and listen" discrimination tests. In these tests, the client is allowed to see the examiner's face while he listens to the speech under both amplified and unamplified conditions. Most test subjects will respond with a higher score when given the opportunity to look and listen but some will score significantly better than others.

O'Neill and Oyer[46] operationally define lip reading as ". . . the correct identification of thoughts transmitted via the visual components of oral discourse." They shortened this to "visual thought comprehension." Unfortunately the literature of the many disciplines concerned with "thinking" is replete with examples of problems associated with defining words like "thought,"

TABLE 37–2   VARIABLE FACTORS IN THE LIP-READING PROCESS*

SPEAKER-SENDER	LIPREADER-RECEIVER
1. Facial characteristics	1. Visual acuity and discrimination
2. Articulatory movements	2. Communication "set"
(a) Rate of speaking	3. Residual hearing
(b) Distinctness of speaking	4. Personality
3. Gesture activity	(a) Intelligence
4. Amount of voice used	(b) Behavior patterns
5. Feedback characteristics	(c) Past communicative experience
	(d) Visual feedback

ENVIRONMENT	CODE OR STIMULUS
1. Lighting conditions	1. Visibility
2. Physical arrangements	2. Familiarity
3. Number of senders	3. Structure
4. Physical distractions	4. Rate of transmission
	5. Auditory-visual aspects

*From O'Neill, J. J., and Oyer, H. J.: Visual Communication for the Hard of Hearing, Prentice-Hall, Inc., 1961.

"thinking," "meaning" and "concepts," *ad infinitum*. Until such time as it is possible to agree upon a general definition of "thought" and utilize some acceptable theory of behavior accompanied by an analysis of the physiological analogues to thinking and behavior, it will probably be impossible to generate a comprehensive theory of communication. Without such a theory, defining "visual thought comprehension" must be one of those phrases that continue to try the patience and character of the most devoted student clinician.

The deaf and hard-of-hearing need to learn to benefit from every clue available in the communication situation. In the course of training, the instructor may specify the context for his class but in unstructured situations, the speech reader will often need assistance in order to perceive the topic under consideration. This writer was once informed by a client having such contextual difficulty that "if this were real life, I'd be mad." Factors influencing the success of the speech reader in conversation are found in Table 37-2.

Methods of lip reading have been described over many years. These have attempted to account for the variables enumerated in Table 37-2. The methods have been identified as "analytic" (close observation of syllable movements and associated drill work), synthetic (stress on synthesis of ideas and training in comprehension of "whole thoughts") and combined forms (utilizing the benefits of syllable analysis while recognizing the psychology of Gestalt-type perceptions of the whole, intuitive practices and more refined learning theory).

Modern technology has made available to the teacher of speech reading a vast array of tools and techniques applicable to the learning and improving of speech reading skills. However, these modern methods should not obscure that very important relationship necessary to the motivational environment—the human-to-human contact shared by the client and his clinician and all that this relationship implies.

Auditory Training

Auditory training, like speech reading, has a long history; but unlike it there have been few formal systems developed either to restrict or to further

TABLE 37–3   MAN'S RESPONSE TO THE WORLD OF SOUND*

WORLD OF SOUNDS	MAN

I. Inanimate sounds of environment
  a. Horns   d. Motors
  b. Bells   e. Wind
  c. Music   f. Rain, etc.
	Awareness level
	  (Sound Reception)
	
	Crude filtering
	First identifications

II. Nonhuman animate sounds
  a. Dogs barking   c. Birds chirping
  b. Cows mooing   d. Chickens cackling, etc.
	(Gross discriminations—separating out in
	  large categories)
	Fine filtering

III. Human sounds
  a. Mother calling   f. People laughing
  b. Whistling   g. Humming
  c. Singing   h. Group chattering
  d. Radio and TV   at social events
     announcing   i. Crowds cheering and
  e. Teacher talking   booing, etc.
	Fine discrimination of speech sounds, voice
	  qualities, inflections, etc.
	
	Final judgments concerning acoustical
	  events

*From Oyer, H. J.: Auditory Communication for the Hard of Hearing, Prentice-Hall, Inc., 1966.

progress. Table 37-3 suggests some of the ways in which people need discrimination awareness for audition.

As with speech reading, the amount of training and the selection of what might be called "teachniques" are at least partially dependent on the degree of hearing loss, the pattern of loss and the particular individual affected. Some children and adults have difficulty discriminating sounds (or rhythm or stress patterns). Such persons, even when hearing loss is slight may also benefit from training in sound discrimination. Indeed, one physician of the author's acquaintance chose dermatology as a specialty because of its need for greater visual orientation rather than attempt to deal with problems of cardiology, which required a rather refined listening skill.

Sound recognition in noise and utilization of various amplification equipment (including hearing aids) and materials are considerations in planning the course of study for the client. Work and practice usually proceed from gross and unrefined sound stimuli to refined and sensitive speech material, depending on the degree of hearing loss. Most hearing-impaired persons will benefit from such training. In point of fact, far too few clinics offer sufficient auditory training. Because such training is particularly needed for hearing aid users, it should be made part of the clinical activity associated with hearing aid counseling. An emphasis on the improvement of *residual* auditory abilities tends to have an assuring effect, thereby creating a more positive attitude toward the hearing aid fitting and the rehabilitative process in general.

With the availability of good recording devices, it is possible to program auditory training with relative ease. Materials may be purchased as a package from a large commercial source or may be tailored to fit the amount of time the clinician has left open for such purposes. Recordings may be multi-track and may be fed through a variety of circuits in order to simulate a multiplicity of circumstances. As a concomitant to discrimination training, habits of improved listening, attention and communication may also be taught. As with efforts in the other rehabilitation areas, auditory training should be more concrete, experiential and meaningful instead of consisting of merely the "telling about," abstract type of instruction found in a chapter such as this.

Speech Conservation

Elsewhere in this text Goehl discusses general problems of speech and language. Here, we need only point out that, as one of the mechanisms of speech monitoring, hearing is necessary to the maintenance of meaningful vocal characteristics and to the precision necessary to intelligible consonant production. Lacking such feedback, those with impaired hearing require assistance in the use of compensatory techniques. For example, the deaf need to be shown how kinesthesis may be utilized for oral shaping and positioning. Early training should help demonstrate the need for conservation of speech skills, and periodic evaluation and counseling will usually enable the client to continue to function with a modicum of success in a world in which communication is so necessary.

Educational Concerns

In this section, no attempt is made to trace the lengthy and extremely interesting history of education in auditory problems—a history that antedates the Christian era. The relationship between deafness and muteness, and the consequent stigma relating lack of speech to lack of intelligence or to lack of emotional stability, is associated with some of educational history's least savory moments. On the other hand, many heroic and inspiring relationships have accrued to those who have dedicated themselves to the process of discovery in finding ways of helping the deaf and hard-of-hearing to a life of reasonable productivity and meaning.

It is generally conceded that education starts at birth, or possibly before. It necessarily follows that early identification of hearing problems or identification of those whose history marks them as "high risks" for such problems is crucial to programs seeking to provide assistance to such individuals. Whenever someone is faced with a hearing loss or deafness, no matter what the cause or age, the earlier it is discovered—identified—(i.e., the earlier a positive diagnosis can be made), the more it is possible to effect adequate counseling (to the client or the parent) and the easier it is to institute an educational management plan.

Programs of audiometry designed to identify those with hearing problems have been demonstrated to be effective in work settings where noise appears to be a hazard, in public schools as a regular screening procedure, in mobile clinics using a cruising van or bus, and even in maternity hospitals where each newborn is screened. This type of activity appears to be the major preventive effort in the range of professional services offered by the "aural rehabilitation team." We feel that the audiologic examination should be routinely given to all patients undergoing evaluation in the specialty of Physical and Rehabilitation Medicine.

If early evaluation and diagnosis are basic to the management of the hearing-impaired client, then continuing diagnostic activity is critical to the process as well. The client, whether child or adult, continually changes as he learns new ways of adapting to his environment. This dynamic quality forces the therapist or teacher to revise and update his approaches for each individual. We have already discussed modification of amplification, conservation or speech, learning experiences for language, speech reading and auditory training as processes that need to be presented as part of the education, habilitation or rehabilitation of the client. With these processes in mind we may more effectively attend to approaches and issues relevant to the deaf and hard-of-hearing.

Of necessity, because of the small numbers of trained teachers and deaf clients, many residential schools for the deaf were established over the years. The issue of institutions offering surrogate parentage for resident children versus day school education has continued; parents have primarily been opposed to their essential loss of the child in a resident program. With early diagnosis, amplification, home programs and day school and preschool nursery education, the parent has been able to develop a close bond with the deaf child that was not possible just a few years ago. The consensus among those involved in the problem appears to be that a form of continuing day school education would be preferable—if possible. Although the resident school can offer "education" during all of the child's waking hours, it is difficult to assess the impact of the parental deprivation on parents and child.

We may find that eventually clinicians will be forced to make a judgment about children who are saddled with guilt-ridden parents or parents who are otherwise inadequate and would therefore *benefit* from residential placement, as opposed to "adequate" parents who should retain the child and move closer to available day school programs. Such a choice is not always possible at this time because there are not enough facilities of either type capable of handling the entire load, particularly when one considers the almost total lack of services for the child who is multi-handicapped.

Schools have been divided into three basic approaches (although the categorizations are arbitrary and often include more than one type): manual, oral and mixed. Ideally, the peripherally deaf child, given essentially normal intelligence and opportunity, might be forced into dependence on auditory reception via his hearing aid, accompanied eventually by speech reading. This mandatory acceptance of verbal expression has yielded fine results and has become official government policy in some countries. Unfortunately, the system does not work with a good many children. In our own practice we have seen many oral school graduates dispense with their hearing aids the day after graduation. These same young adults often then gravitate to groups utilizing some form of manual expression.

While it has been often argued that manual education (signing, finger spelling, mime) tends to isolate the deaf, thus causing the formation of a subculture that propagates genetically determined deaf offspring, it is also argued with equal validity that this group is happier and much more secure than the deaf in an unsegregated society. It does appear that once "manualism" is permitted, oral efforts tend to deteriorate. Nevertheless, it has been observed that even in oral school the deaf tend to generate much non-verbal communicative behavior that is not predicted or accepted by the confirmed oralist. Under such circumstances, the advice of one past professor is recalled: "If it works, use it."

Silverman and Lane[60] differentiate between those who would try to produce a happy deaf child and those whose educational efforts would result in a poor, unhappy imitation of a better educated child with normal hearing. In such a comparison there are indeed implications that might be noted throughout the rehabilitative professions.

Looking back to our previous discussions, we noted some difficulty in defining language, conceptualization and so forth. A critical factor in viewing the education of the deaf supersedes the considerations of speech and hearing in themselves. Language, whatever its meaning, is the supreme tool. Language facilitates the ability to move from the concrete—the here and now—to the abstract. Can the creative mind soar to lofty heights without adequate symbols to shortcut and assist in the process of "thinking?" If the deaf adult communicates poorly through the oral mode, can he still use his pen for self-expression? Experience is the basis for thought and language. The educational process must provide a graded set of profitable experiences that eventuate in conceptualization, language and then, it is hoped, speech. The loss in efficiency of this process is operationally defined by the typical two to three years' educational retardation commonly predicted for the progression of the deaf child.

Modality training may proceed on a "one-at-a-time" basis, which is sometimes, probably mistakenly, referred to as a unisensory approach, or on a "several-at-a-time" basis, described as a multisensory approach. As these approaches are reviewed they frequently appear alike in their stress of visual and kinesthetic cues. The objective is to strengthen residual abilities for compensatory purposes. More recently a unisensory approach utilizing audition has acquired a number of advocates. In its various forms the approach has been identified as "acoupedics" (Pollack and Downs[48]), "verbo-tonal" (Guberina[26]) and "auditory-emphasis" (Luterman and Karp[36]). Concern with the problem of attention—the ways in which deaf children pay attention—contributes to the rationale for proceeding with such training. This is further supported by Ling[35] who has been attempting to fit the deaf with milder-gain hearing aids (about 40 dB) in binaural units at ear level. It appears not to be so much a question of how much (gain) but how it is used.

For the hard-of-hearing youngster, educational concerns have also tended to center about the "how much" question. While degree of hearing loss is a critical matter, a child with impaired hearing may adapt to the classroom with some extra help (tutoring, speech training and so on), so long as he has received training as described throughout this chapter, and counseling relative to his difficulty (as described in the next section).

Counseling

In our discussion of this rehabilitation area there is no intent to usurp the function of "other disciplines" of the rehabilitation team. As already indicated, it is part of the author's bias that counseling is the natural adjunct of any clinical attempt. The client (patient) has questions. The family has questions. The expert is presumed to have information, if not answers. Any information supplied by the expert will tend to carry with it an attitudinal aura. The client's future course of action will be affected by his response to information provided by the expert as well as by the "advice" generated. The language used by the expert affects the perception of the client, and the client's response, in turn, structures the language, and thus the performance, of the client. The "give and take" of this procedure is "counseling," whether or not it is formalized or so designated.

The object of counseling is to assist the client to adapt to all the variations of life style that ensue when a problem is discovered or becomes evident. In order for counseling to be meaningful the counselor must know something of the so-called "disability," the residual functions, the client's strengths and potentials, and so forth. Once the diagnostic information has been reviewed and general management approaches chosen (as discussed in the previous portions of this chapter), the counseling task is reduced to a question of trust or positive regard. Both counselor and client must have a relationship that is honest so that a problem can be confronted and a satisfactory solution concluded. For the deaf and hard-of-hearing this means their needs require a listener who is able to communicate readily, whatever the mode or skill in speaking, signing or hearing.

Although data indicate that intelligence and manual skills are normally distributed among the hearing-impaired populations, according to many anecdotal reports the deaf face barriers to their acceptance for vocational training and employment that are similar to the barriers against racial, religious and social minorities, as well as other more subtle forms of discrimination. While public education is needed to dissipate stereotypical thinking concerning those with impaired hearing, counseling, in the interim, must help the client to function effectively in his activities of daily living.

Counseling, then, is a continuing, dynamic process that takes into account the degree and type of hearing loss, the associated compensatory practices (hearing aids, other aural rehabilitation), personality, intelligence, family constellation, vocation and community; and counseling also focuses on the client's motivation. Both before and after counseling begins, such motivation helps in defining goals and in shaping a rehabilitative program. With technology progressing so rapidly and new training required for each new adaptation form—vocational or social—the attitude best held and utilized must be one of "willingness to try." Both client and counselor must be willing to experiment and to continue to trust, relate and interact until each considers the term of rehabilitation *completed*.

SUMMARY

The mechanisms of human hearing must be understood in order to establish a criterion against which hearing "loss" may be measured, and which may be used as an aid to understanding the individual with such loss—one who, after all, must compete and relate in the "hearing" world. Residual function is measurable in various ways. Various means of restoration, modification and adaptation are utilized. Primary influencing factors include:

1. The nature of the hearing mechanism
2. The nature of the stimuli with particular emphasis on:
   a. Speech parameters (frequency, intensity and spectrum) and complexity
   b. Noise
3. The nature of instrumentation:
   a. Test devices
   b. Amplification devices
   c. Measurement devices relative to physical stimuli
4. Aural pathology—means of evaluation
5. Modality training and general principles of learning as applied to so-called "aural rehabilitation"

The passage of time and the acquisition of experience are requisites to satisfactory adaptation to changes in physical and emotional status. Various methods of approach to rehabilitation for auditory disorders—including individual (clinical) approaches—should be employed. Stressing the client's role as part of the "team" enables the audiologist to assist the client satisfactorily in utilization of maximum residual auditory function. The discussion offered in this chapter is by no means a complete review of all factors contributing to the auditory process nor does it reveal the complete range of medical or audiologic evaluation. It is obvious that all audiologic rehabilitation practices cannot be outlined in a chapter of this length. We have attempted to describe enough to give a "flavor" of audiologic practice and to entice the reader to pursue his specific interests. Finally, it must be stressed that consideration of auditory status is a critical and integral part of the *total* evaluation of the Physical and Rehabilitative Medicine patient. It is hoped that future editions of this publication may find improved evaluation and rehabilitation techniques for the hearing impaired, and thus improved interactional and interpersonal human adaptations.

REFERENCES

The author is indebted to many on the following list who have not been sufficiently credited by reference in the text. No attempt was made in this chapter to credit all the opinions and approaches discussed as the various issues were surveyed. Although certain paraphrases or charts were specifically acknowledged, it was impossible to identify the sources of each datum or idea because, most frequently, these were shared by many authors and investigators. My apologies, therefore, to those requiring them.

H.L.G.

1. Alpiner, J. G.: Aural Rehabilitation and the Aged Client. In Maico Audiological Library Series, Vol. IV. Maico Hearing Instruments, Inc., 1967, pp. 9–12.
2. Batteau, D. W.: Listening with the naked ear. In Freedman, S. J. (Ed.): The Neuropsychology of Spatially Oriented Behavior. Homewood, Ill., Dorsey Press, 1968.
3. Brubaker, R. S.: Experimental Phonetics. In Rieber, R. W., and Brubaker, R. S.: Speech Pathology. Amsterdam, North-Holland Publishing Co., 1966, pp. 77–99.
4. Clarke, F. R., and Bilger, R. C.: The Theory of Signal Detectability and the Measurement of Hearing. In Jerger, J. (Ed.): Modern Developments in Audiology. New York, Academic Press, 1963, pp. 371–408.
5. Collins, R. D.: Illustrated Manual of Neurologic Diagnosis. Philadelphia, J. B. Lippincott Co., 1962.
5a. Corso, J. F.: Age and Sex Differences in Pure Tone Thresholds. J. Acous. Soc. Amer., *31:*498–507, 1959.
6. Davis, H.: Psychophysiology of Hearing and Deafness. In Stevens, S. S. (Ed.): Handbook of Experimental Psychology. New York, John Wiley & Sons, Inc., 1951, pp. 1116–1142.
7. Davis, H.: Abnormal Hearing and Deafness. In Davis, H., and Silverman, S. R. (Ed.): Hearing and Deafness (3rd Ed.). New York, Holt, Rinehart and Winston, 1970, pp. 83–139.
8. Davis, H.: Hearing Handicap, Standards for Hearing and Medico-legal Rules. In Davis, H., and Silverman, S. R. (Ed.): Hearing and Deafness (3rd Ed.). New York, Holt, Rinehart and Winston, 1970, pp. 253–279.
9. Davis, H., and Silverman, S. R. (Ed.): Hearing and Deafness (Rev. Ed.). New York, Holt, Rinehart and Winston, 1966.
10. Davis, H., and Silverman, S. R. (Ed.): Hearing and Deafness (3rd Ed.). New York, Holt, Rinehart and Winston, 1970.
11. DeWeese, D., and Saunders, W. H.: Textbook of Otolaryngology (3rd Ed.). St. Louis, Missouri, The C. V. Mosby Co., 1968.
12. Eagles, E., and Hardy, W. G.: Human Communication: The Public Health Aspects of Hearing, Language and Speech Disorders. Public Health Service Publication No. 1754, 1968.
13. Feldmann, H.: Experiments on Binaural Hearing in Noise: The Central Nervous Processing of Acoustic Information. Translations of the Beltone Institute for Hearing Research, No. 18, 1965.
14. Fisher, H. G., and Freedman, S. J.: Localization of sound during simulated unilateral conductive hearing. Acta Otolaryng.: *66:*213–220, 1968.
15. Fisher, H. G., and Freedman, S. J.: The Role of the Pinna in Auditory Localization. J. Aud. Res., 1968, 15–26.
16. Freedman, S. J., and Fisher, H. G.: The Role of the Pinna in Auditory Localization. In Freedman, S. J. (Ed.): The Neuropsychology of Spatially Oriented Behavior. Homewood, Ill.: Dorsey Press, 1968.

16a. Freedman, S. J., and Gerstman, H. L.: The Role of the Pinna in Speech Intelligibility. In press, 1971.

17. Frisina, D. R.: Measurement of Hearing in Children. In Jerger, J. (Ed.): Modern Developments in Audiology. New York, Academic Press, 1963, pp. 126-167.

18. Gardner, E.: Fundamentals of Neurology (5th Ed.). Philadelphia, W. B. Saunders Co., 1968.

19. Glorig, A.: Audiometry: Principles and Practices. Baltimore, The Williams & Wilkins Co., 1965.

20. Goehl, H.: Speech and Language Disorders. In Krusen, F. H. (Ed.): Handbook of Physical Medicine and Rehabilitation. Philadelphia, W. B. Saunders Co., 1966, pp. 111-136.

21. Goldstein, R.: Electrophysiologic Audiometry. In Jerger, J. (Ed.): Modern Developments in Audiology. New York, Academic Press, 1963, pp. 168-193.

22. Goodhill, V.: Pathology, Diagnosis and Therapy of Deafness. In Travis, L. E. (Ed.): Handbook of Speech Pathology. New York, Appleton-Century-Crofts, Inc., 1957, pp. 313-388.

23. Goodman, A. C.: Reference Zero Levels for Pure-tone Audiometers. In Maico Audiological Library Series, Vol. IV. Maico Hearing Instruments, Inc., 1967, pp. 20-22.

24. Graham, A. B. (Ed.): Sensori-Neural Hearing Processes and Disorders. Henry Ford Hospital, International Symposium. Boston, Little, Brown and Co., 1967.

25. Green, D.: Threshold Tone Decay. In Katz, J. (Ed.): Handbook of Audiology. Baltimore, Williams & Wilkins Co., 1970.

26. Guberina, P.: Verbotonal Method and Its Application to the Rehabilitation of the Deaf. In Report of the Proceedings of the International Congress on Education of the Deaf, June 22-28, 1963. Washington, D.C., U.S. Gov't. Printing Office, 1964, pp. 279-293.

27. Harford, E.: Recent Developments in the Use of Ear-level Hearing Aids. In Maico Audiological Library Series, Vol. V. Maico Hearing Instruments, Inc., 1968, pp. 10-13.

28. Hearing Loss, Hearing Aids, and the Elderly. Hearings Before the Subcommittee on Consumer Interest of the Elderly of the Special Committee on Aging, U.S. Senate, 90th Congress (2nd Session), Washington, D.C., July 18-19, 1968.

29. Hirsh, I. J.: The Measurement of Hearing. New York, McGraw-Hill Book Co., Inc., 1952.

30. Kendall, D. C.: Auditory Problems in Children. In Rieber, R. W., and Brubaker, R. S. (Ed.): Speech Pathology. Amsterdam, North-Holland Publishing Co., 1966, pp. 210-258.

31. Kodman, F.: The Team Approach to Hearing Problems. Maico Audiological Library Series, Vol. II. Maico Hearing Instruments, Inc., 1967.

32. Krusen, F. H. (Ed.): Handbook of Physical Medicine and Rehabilitation. Philadelphia, W. B. Saunders Co., 1966.

33. Licklider, J. C. R.: Basic Correlates of the Auditory Stimulus. In Stevens, S. S. (Ed.): Handbook of Experimental Psychology. New York, John Wiley and Sons, Inc., 1951, pp. 985-1039.

34. Licklider, J. C. R.: The Perception of Speech. In Stevens, S. S. (Ed.): Handbook of Experimental Psychology. New York, John Wiley and Sons, Inc., 1951, pp. 1040-1074.

35. Ling, D.: Research on Speech Discrimination by Profoundly Deaf Children. Unpublished presentation at Emerson College, Boston, May 7, 1970.

36. Luterman, D., and Karp, E.: An Auditory Emphasis Program for Training Children with Impaired Hearing. 1970 (unpublished).

37. Matzker, J.: Attempt at Explanation of Directional Hearing on the Basis of Very Fine Time-Difference Registration. Translations of the Beltone Institute for Hearing Research, No. 12, Nov., 1959.

38. McDonald, E. T.: Articulation Testing and Treatment: A Sensory-Motor Approach. Pittsburgh, Stanwix House, Inc., 1964.

39. Miller, M. H.: Clinical Hearing Aid Evaluation (Parts 1 and 2). Maico Audiological Library Series, Vol. III. Maico Hearing Instruments, Inc., 1967, pp. 24-26.

40. Myklebust, H. R.: Your Deaf Child: A Guide for Parents (2nd Ed.). No. 94, American Lecture Series. Springfield, Ill., Charles C Thomas, 1954.

41. Naunton, R. F.: The Measurement of Hearing by Bone Conduction. In Jerger, J. (Ed.): Modern Developments in Audiology. New York, Academic Press, 1963, pp. 1-29.

42. Newby, H. A.: Audiology (2nd Ed.). New York, Appleton-Century-Crofts, 1964.

43. Nober, E. H.: Physiogenic Auditory Problems in Adults. In Rieber, R. W., and Brubaker, R. S. (Ed.): Speech Pathology. Amsterdam, North-Holland Publishing Co., 1966, pp. 149-151; 182-209.

44. Nober, E. H.: Psychogenic Auditory Problems in Adults. In Rieber, R. W., and Brubaker, R. S. (Ed.): Speech Pathology. Amsterdam, North-Holland Publishing Co., 1966, pp. 337-353.

45. O'Neill, J. J., and Oyer, H. J.: Applied Audiometry. New York, Dodd, Mead and Co., Inc., 1966.

46. O'Neill, J. J., and Oyer, H. J.: Visual Communication for the Hard of Hearing. Englewood Cliffs, N.J., Prentice-Hall, Inc., 1961.

47. Oyer, H. J.: Auditory Communication for the Hard of Hearing. Englewood Cliffs, N.J., Prentice-Hall, Inc., 1966.

48. Pollack, D. C., and Downs, M. P.: A Parent's Guide to Hearing Aids for Young Children. Volta Review, *66:*745-749, 1964.

49. Ramsdell, D. A.: The Psychology of the Hard of Hearing and the Deafened Adult. In Davis, H., and Silverman, S. R. (Ed.): Hearing and Deafness (3rd Ed.). New York, Holt, Rinehart and Winston, 1970, pp. 435 to 448.

50. Rieber, R. W., and Brubaker, R. S. (Ed.): Speech Pathology. Amsterdam, North-Holland Publishing Co., 1966.

51. Rosenberg, P. E.: Auditory Rehabilitation. Maico Audiological Library Series, Vol. I. Maico Hearing Instruments, Inc., 1967, pp. 26-29.

51a. Rosenberg, P. E.: Tone Decay. Maico Audiological Library Series, Vol. VII. Maico Hearing Instruments, Inc., 1969, pp. 17-20.

52. Ross, M.: Changing Concepts in Hearing Aid Candidacy. Maico Audiological Library Series, Vol. VII. Maico Hearing Instruments, Inc., 1969, pp. 36-40.

53. Rudmose, W.: Automatic Audiometry. In Jerger, J. (Ed.): Modern Developments in Audiology. New York, Academic Press, 1963, pp. 30-75.

54. Sataloff, J.: Hearing Loss. Philadelphia, J. B. Lippincott Co., 1966.

55. Shambaugh, G. E.: Surgery of the Ear (2nd Ed.). Philadelphia, W. B. Saunders Co., 1967.

56. Siegenthaler, B. M., Pearson, J., and Lezak, R. L.: A Speech Reception Threshold Test for Children. J. Speech Hearing Dis., *29:*360-366, 1954.

57. Siegenthaler, B. M., and Strand, R.: Audiogram-average Methods and SRT Scores. J. Acoust. Soc. Amer., *36:*589-593, 1964.

58. Silverman, S. R.: Clinical and Educational Procedures for the Deaf. In Travis, L. E. (Ed.): Handbook of Speech Pathology. New York, Appleton-Century-Crofts, Inc., 1957, pp. 389-425.

59. Silverman, S. R.: Clinical and Educational Procedures for the Hard of Hearing. In Travis, L. E. (Ed.): Handbook of Speech Pathology. New York, Appleton-Century-Crofts, Inc., 1957, pp. 426-435.

59a. Silverman, S. R.: Hard of Hearing Children. In Davis, H. (Ed.): Hearing and Deafness. New York, Holt, Rinehart & Winston, 1960.

60. Silverman, S. R., and Lane, H. S.: Deaf Children. In Davis, H., and Silverman, S. R. (Ed.): Hearing and Deafness (3rd Ed.). New York, Holt, Rinehart and Winston, 1970, pp. 384-425.

61. Stetson, R. H.: Motor Phonetics: A Study of Speech Movements in Action. Amsterdam, North-Holland Publishing Co., 1951.

62. Stevens, S. S.: Mathematics, Measurement and Psychophysics. In Stevens, S. S. (Ed.): Handbook of Experimental Psychology. New York, John Wiley and Sons, Inc., 1951, pp. 1-49.

63. von Békésy, G.: Experiments in Hearing. New York, McGraw-Hill Book Co., Inc., 1960.

64. von Békésy, G., and Rosenblith, W. A.: The Mechanical Properties of the Ear. In Stevens, S. S. (Ed.): Handbook of Experimental Psychology. New York, John Wiley and Sons, Inc., 1951, pp. 1075-1115.

65. Vosteen, K. H.: New Aspects in the Biology and Pathology of the Inner Ear. Translations of the Beltone Institute for Hearing Research, No. 16, July, 1963.

66. Ward, W. D.: Auditory Fatigue and Masking. In Jerger, J. (Ed.): Modern Developments in Audiology. New York, Academic Press, 1963, pp. 241-286.

67. Wever, E. G., and Lawrence, M.: Physiological Acoustics. Princeton, N.J., Princeton University Press, 1954.

68. Wever, E. G.: Theory of Hearing. New York, John Wiley and Sons, Inc., 1949.

Chapter 38

PSYCHIATRIC REHABILITATION OF THE PHYSICALLY DISABLED, THE MENTALLY RETARDED AND THE PSYCHIATRICALLY IMPAIRED

by Carl D. Herman, Richard A. Manning and Edward Teitelman

INTRODUCTION

In this chapter, three relatively discrete areas of functioning will be discussed — psychiatric rehabilitation of (1) the physically disabled, of (2) the mentally retarded, and of (3) the psychiatrically impaired. These three areas are linked by a common bond in that the psychiatric and related personnel are involved in a blending of their traditional functions of diagnosis and treatment with the relatively new challenge of rehabilitation. It is not enough to be satisfied with relief of symptoms and with emotional balance or insight into one's mental mechanisms. Rather, the ultimate goal of effective assimilation into the family and community becomes equally important.

761

PSYCHIATRIC REHABILITATION OF THE PHYSICALLY DISABLED

by Carl D. Herman

Each illness or trauma resulting in physical disability possesses its unique constellation of threats to the personality. Hemiplegia is an outstanding example, as, probably more than any other disability (except massive brain damage or trauma), it can potentially effect the largest number of body symptoms.

1. Defects of the Motor System.   By definition, hemiplegia involves paralysis of muscle groups innervated by the pyramidal tract. Thus the means for control and manipulation of the environment is jeopardized. Included are defects in hand grasp, locomotion and activities of daily living (feeding, dressing, washing and so forth). Dependency on others—and, implicitly, regression to a more childlike relationship with others—is inevitable, at least temporarily.

2. Loss of Sensation, Perception and Awareness.   At a time when alertness and reception of stimuli from the external world, as well as from the remaining integral parts of the body, must be optimal, these very capacities may be compromised by confusion, hemianopsia or position-sense loss. Critical channels of contact are hence lost, resulting in the frequently seen blank, masked facies and constricted affect. Although statistical studies have been inconclusive, it appears from clinical observation that perception of the environment and integrated visual motor performance are more frequently impaired in left hemiplegics (right parietal lobe damage) than in right hemiplegics. Whereas motor strength may return or be compensated for by bracing, the individual with perceptual losses may be unable to function effectively as a result solely of these losses.

3. Aphasia.   There is an ancient mystical belief that one can master that which he can name; the achievement of the faculty of speech itself is experienced as the acquisition of a great power. Among the infant's earliest approval-experiences is the reaction of his parents to his first babblings and especially his first meaningful verbal productions. Speech is soon perceived as a means for extracting gratification from the significant beings in the environment and for manipulating them. With the loss of speech, one of our most potent instruments for relating to people is removed, followed by the consequent reversion to more primitive techniques of controlling the environment: thus the frustrated stuttering of the aphasic who, without the use of language, regresses to childish insistence and infantile temper tantrums.

Others retreat to a depressed dependency and call on us to care for them as infants. Still others react with gross anxiety. Unable to comprehend the nature of their impairment they fear that they have lost their mind and wonder if we recognize their plight and will respond to their needs. Yet others are so afflicted that they will withdraw into a state of encapsulated apathy, a defensive maneuver aimed at avoiding all stress.

4. Incontinence. Another of the earliest milestones of childhood development centers around sphincter control. The child, as he develops control over bowel and bladder, will frequently learn to use this capacity to extract approval from or mete punishment to his parents. His attitudes regarding cleanliness, maturity and shame are all intimately involved in the process of developing continence. Should this vital function be impaired in adult life, there is likely to be a return to former well-entrenched attitudes. Thus, shame, feelings of uncleanliness and not being adult, or fear of displeasing others result. The reactions of those assigned to the bodily care of the impaired person are critical in proving or disproving his self-doubts.

5. Intellectual Resources. The chronic brain syndrome seen in many hemiplegics is manifested by one or more of the following: disorientation to the external environment; inability to attend and concentrate and remember newly learned material; poor judgment; inability to plan for the future; and defect in abstract conceptualization. Various compensatory mechanisms may come into play in reaction to the patient's conscious or unconscious awareness of his deficiencies, such as denial, withdrawal, and confabulation.

6. Loss of Esteem. Values are established through such functions as speech, physical strength, vocational skill and independence. With these impaired, the sense of value is lessened and there is a consequent fall in self-esteem. Not only self-esteem but the esteem looked for from others is put to task by the stigmatizing effects of disability. The patient sees himself, and is viewed by others, as incompetent, inadequate, infantile and, at times, insane.

7. Decrease of Relatedness. Any diminution of our channel of contact with people, as by confusion or aphasia, leads to the breaking off of previously meaningful and supportive ties with family, friends and coworkers.

8. Change in Body Image. The psychic conceptualization one has developed of his body since infancy is disturbed by any change in function or structure, and a vast readjustment and adaptation is required. One's body image is particularly threatened by the facial paresis, limp arm and awkward gait of hemiplegia, or by the loss of a body part through amputation.

9. Separation and Role Change. Often the disabled person is separated from home, family and work—and the social roles he has played in these areas—because of admission to a hospital or rehabilitation center. Thus he loses, at least temporarily, these valuable sources of gratification, esteem, security and identity.

MODES OF REACTION

How an individual reacts to disability is dependent on a complex of factors. What does the disability mean to him? Is it a threat to his control over the environment, a threat to his concept of himself as masculine (or, in the case of a woman, feminine) and competent, or is it a punishment for sins, real or imagined? Is it perhaps a socially acceptable means of escaping from a conflictive life-struggle? Techniques for dealing with stress that the individual has developed since childhood and which he has learned from those important in his development will most likely be mobilized.

1. Regression. The patient, facing major physical and intellectual disaster and unable to use his usual physical and personality resources, regresses or reverts to techniques he found successful in the past, at times returning to the most primitive methods. Thus he may become jealous of the care of other patients and subtly or overtly become seductive to doctor or nurse, recalling the sibling rivalry of an earlier time. Or he may attempt to control or manipulate or angrily punish staff members by his obstinacy as he did at an even earlier epoch.

A more extreme regression is manifested by gross dependency and depression, desire to be taken care of, pleading for love in the guise of requests for special permission to use supportive devices or bed rest beyond his need. Excessive dependency is frequently seen in two superficially dissimilar personality types: (a) the individual who has always been dependent, in whom disability is merely a concrete, demonstrable reason for continued dependency; and (b) the compulsively independent person who has never allowed expression of his dependency needs, in which case disability opens the door to a reservoir of previously repressed needs.

2. Denial. The disabled person may deny his impairment—a rather gross departure from reality, usually seen in conjunction with some degree of organic brain dysfunction—or, more commonly, he may deny the affect associated with the illness. Thus, his behavior expresses the idea, "I am disabled, but I am not upset or concerned." Here again is a defensive device for controlling anxiety, useful if it does not hinder participation in therapy or if it does not permanently mask reality.

3. Anxiety. There is no greater source of anxiety than the awareness of the fact that one's continuance is threatened. The knowledge that one has been so close to death and the fear of a recurrence may prey on the mind of the hemiplegic.

4. Hostility. Hostility may be expressed in two ways: (a) inwardly—"What did I do to deserve this? What a failure I am. My life is not worth living."; or (b) outwardly "It is not my body that has failed me; it's their fault, family, doctors and nurses; they are responsible and inadequate, not me."

5. Depression. Depression is a reaction to loss. With all the losses experienced by the disabled, it is no surprise that he manifests gross depression. In fact, if this does not become apparent at some point, it is cause for concern; the patient may be undergoing denial or the satisfaction of deep psychologic needs (dependency, self-punishment, punishment of others).

6. Withdrawal. The disabled person, rather than cope actively with the challenge of reality, may consciously or unconsciously choose to retreat totally into profound passivity or apathy, preferring an almost fetus-like existence.

7. Psychosis. Many factors can contribute to the development of a major break from reality: cerebral hypoxia, as in cerebral arteriosclerosis; loss of brain tissue, as in brain trauma; pressure effects, as in brain tumor; sudden loss of body parts from amputation; drug effects (steroids, anti-Parkinsonism agents); lack of familiar surroundings; and fear-evoking diagnostic and surgical procedures.

The type of reaction will likewise vary with the differing personality constellations, but it may include acute confusional or delirious states (fearfulness, agitation, disorientation, visual and tactile hallucinations), psychotic depression (mutism, refusal to eat, psychomotor retardation, suicidal behavior), or schizophrenic reactions (delusions, hallucinations, catatonic withdrawal or excitement).

8. Healthy Adaptation.   Here the individual accepts reality and works in constructive, goal-directed activities toward recovery of functions. Minor upsets and regressions may occur, but they are brief and are followed by renewed acceptance of the challenge.

PHASES OF ADAPTATION

The person faced with the loss of major bodily functions or parts proceeds through a succession of adjustment reactions, all designed to handle the flood of feelings at each particular stage. While there is variation from person to person—some remaining longer in certain phases than others, some skipping an entire phase—most patients manifest a rather similar progression.

1. Shock.   This is a time when the patient is unsure not only of his body and its functions but of the continuity of life itself. This first reaction may be displayed by complete emotional withdrawal even to the point of mutism or by agitation or by marked dependency on staff personnel. All three reactions represent regressive measures by which intolerable feelings are either blocked from consciousness or diverted.

2. Denial.   Shortly thereafter, restitution via denial occurs, giving the personality resources a period of time to recoup and mend. As mentioned previously, the patient may deny the illness itself or the feelings associated with it. In either case, too early challenge can be detrimental by destroying the tenuous emotional balance established by this defense. Support and gentle, gradual reality-confrontation is much more effective, especially as return of bodily functions proves the possibility of at least partial recovery.

3. Turbulent Awareness.   Especially, but not exclusively, in younger patients who have not yet learned to control or sublimate their aggressiveness, a period of marked internal turmoil (depression) or external turmoil (anger, manipulativeness) ensues. Patient, consistent efforts by all staff members are more frequently mandatory than in any other phase. Intra-staff conflicts are quickly perceived and used by the patient to project his hostilities away from himself.

4. Working Through.   This is the longest phase in duration. Faith and trust in the staff's empathy and understanding develop if the previous phases have been well-handled, and the patient enters into a therapeutic alliance with the staff against his disability and dependence. He explores reality, retreating again in areas of frustration but probing further into avenues of hope.

5. Separation Anxiety.   Prior to discharge, there is likely to be a brief recurrence of emotional turbulence recalling phase 3 as the patient realizes that he must face the outside world and that he may not have been restored to his pre-illness status. Increased support and environmental manipulation (vocational planning, family counseling, physical modification of home environment) help ease the separation from the protective, accepting hospital milieu.

6. Adaptation.   Gradually the patient tests out his home environment and the community's reaction to him. His reaction depends to a large degree on the confidence and self-esteem he has developed during his rehabilitation program and to an equal degree on the receptivity and acceptance of his family, employer and society.

MANAGEMENT

1. Time.   An incubation period is necessary (varying in length for each individual) during which time the patient must come to a confrontation with the meaning of his disability to him. This is primarily an internal struggle but requires secondary support from family and staff. This period of time commences with the first perception of what losses have occurred through trauma or illness and terminates when the patient enters the working-through phase.

2. Patience, Tolerance and Understanding.   These are most necessary in the earliest stages of adaptation when the patient is at the lowest ebb of self-confidence and is feeling most helpless. During the turbulent-awareness phase, these three qualities should be stressed to the maximum. They are of greatest significance in forging a therapeutic liaison between patient and staff.

3. Education and Orientation.   Demonstrating to the patient that there is a predictable and structured course to his recovery inspires trust and confidence in the staff's ability to enhance this recovery. Whether through doctor-patient bedside chats, team conferences to which the patient is invited or didactic lecture-discussions to large groups of patients, the imparting of knowledge about his disability helps the disabled to confront reality in gradual doses and to recognize those areas in which recovery of function can or cannot be expected.

4. Allowing Control.   As the patient improves, he needs to reverse the course of regression and to progress from dependence to control of self and, in some ways, of others. His feelings and ideas must be respected and considered in any decisions affecting his program.

5. Therapy Modalities.   Here the patient is reoriented to activity instead of passivity. Restoration of function is stressed rather than preoccupation with loss, success rather than failure, release of pent-up aggressive impulses rather than suppression through bed rest and inactivity.

6. Atmosphere of Hope, Optimism and Respect.   Even when adequate recovery of function is not attained in the program, the return home should be proposed as an opportunity to allow natural restorative processes to operate, with the hope that future active rehabilitation efforts may then be possible.

7. Milieu.   Resocialization and stimulation must be fostered, but there must also be respect for the patient's need for times of solitude. An activity program emphasizing the patient's assets should be provided, and long periods of unscheduled time avoided. Especially for the elderly, a well-structured constant environment is helpful in avoiding confusion from frequent changes of room or personnel or procedures.

8. Keeping the Patient Informed.   The passivity that disability forces upon an individual should not be compounded by the staff's treating him as the completely passive recipient of a program which vitally concerns him. Although his permission need not be solicited for every detail of the program, the rationale should be presented explicitly so as to add meaning to his participation.

9. Psychotherapy and Psychoactive Drugs.   Initially, supportive measures are frequently needed to help the patient accept disability and dependency as a temporary way station on the road to recovery and to allow some regression while the weakened ego mends its decompensated defenses and prepares for the rigorous phases ahead. Techniques at this time include reassurance, opportunity for ventilation and suggestion, persuasion and environmental manipulation (change of room, change of roommate, presentation of limited goals). In later phases of rehabilitation, and with the more verbal, psychologically facile individual, insight-directed psychotherapy may be indicated to help the patient understand the meaning of his disability and his reactions and to provide the psychologic environment for self-appraisal and revision of coping techniques.

STAFF REACTIONS TO DISABILITY

How the physician interprets and reacts to the disabled is the principal subject discussed here, but these remarks can also be generalized to apply to all personnel working with this group of patients—nurses, therapists, orderlies and so forth.

The physician may perceive the disabled person primarily as dependent. Dependency may be ill-tolerated by some physicians: for example, the young resident who is struggling with his own feelings about dependency on his wife and parents. To others, disability may stimulate fearful fantasies of mutilation (recall the psychoanalytic concept of castration anxiety).

Many physicians can cope with any situation except chronic incurable disease, as this may jeopardize their "rescue fantasies." Disability may conjure up the specter of old age to some; conflicts involving the physician's parents may be transferred to the disabled patient. Finally, disability, if it can be interpreted as partial death, brings the physician face to face with the ultimate victor in the struggle against disease.

The physician may be challenged or threatened by the preceding factors and the feelings they stimulate. Just as the patient has a repertoire of techniques available to him from his past life-experiences and habit-formations, so too does the physician consciously, and to a larger degree unconsciously, retreat to anxiety-control mechanisms. Often seen are reactions of omnipotence and omniscience in which an aura of power and intellectual pseudomastery substitute for empathy and involvement with the patient. An opposite retreat into feelings of inadequacy and impotence may occur in some. Hostility, rejection and ultimate withdrawal from the threatening patient may be seen in others. However, with proper awareness of their feelings, most physicians, as they develop experience and comfort in dealing with the disabled, will be able to utilize the same techniques of healthy adaptation and reality-confrontation that they expect their patients to use.

ROLE OF THE PSYCHIATRIST IN A REHABILITATION SETTING

The psychiatrist, either on a staff basis or as a part-time consultant, can provide a multitude of valuable services. An early psychiatric evaluation of the patient's emotional and personality resources and deficits can provide important clues to the most effective rehabilitation approach. For example, recognizing in a patient long-term dependent trends which existed prior to the disability will serve to caution staff members against emphasizing total self-care too early in the rehabilitation course—gradual weaning to independence will be more effective. On the other hand, for the individual who evidences a basic need to control and manipulate his environment, participation in staff decisions regarding his course will enable him to cooperate more fully than if he were to see himself merely as a passive recipient.

Direct patient services by the psychiatrist may be required, such as psychotherapy or use of psychoactive medications for depression, anxiety and other adjustment reactions. Of greater and broader relevance is the orientation of the rehabilitation team members toward recognizing the patient as unique, an individual who presents not only a physical disability and assorted medical-surgical entities, but also a reservoir of psychologic needs and drives. The team members must recognize also that there are identifiable techniques for handling such needs and drives. Thus a psychologic prescription follows from evaluation and observations designed to individualize the rehabilitation program for each patient.

REFERENCES

Psychiatric Rehabilitation of the Physically Disabled

1. Adams, G. F., and Hurwitz, L. J.: Mental Barriers to Recovery from Strokes. Lancet, 2:533, 1963.
2. Golden, J., and Wahl, C.: Psychosis in the Hospitalized Patient. Hospital Medicine, April 1, 1967, pp. 120-129.
3. Herman, C.: Behavior in Hemiplegia—A Study in Regression. Albert Einstein Med. Center, 13:248, 1965.
4. Meerloo, J. A.: Modes of Psychotherapy in the Aged. J. Amer. Geriat. Soc., 9:225, 1961.

MANAGEMENT OF PSYCHIATRIC COMPLICATIONS OF MENTAL RETARDATION

by Richard A. Manning

HISTORY OF DIAGNOSIS AND MANAGEMENT OF THE RETARDED

The history of the diagnosis and care of the mentally defective is, indeed, an interesting one, marked with uncertainty, inconsistency and emotionalism. Before the nineteenth century little mention is made of mental deficiency in the medical literature—even in papers and books dealing with psychiatric differential diagnosis. Throughout other literature, obvious references are made to mentally defective individuals, although little that could be interpreted as special care for them is described.

Even before the time of Christ, mental defectives were apparently utilized as personal and court jesters, buffoons and fools for the entertainment of their masters, and some attained widespread reputations for their antics. Other defective individuals were often felt to be especially gifted and blessed by God and able to give prophecies and speak with divine revelation. There are passages in the Bible which support this notion.

However, these were probably the few more fortunate victims of this age-old malady, and no one really wrote about the fate of the less fortunate, although it is likely that they were often left unmolested and regarded superstitiously as "infants of God." The only indication of special attention given the retarded in much earlier times is that Saint Nicholas Thaumaturgos, Bishop of Myra, in the fourth century was described as the protector of the feebleminded. However, he has also always been regarded as the patron saint of all children and served in some way, presumably through his deeds, as the prototype for the modern-day Santa Claus.

However, during the Reformation the lot of the feebleminded was not nearly so good and they, along with many others suffering from psychiatric disorders, became victims of demonism. Even such notable reformers as Martin Luther and John Calvin considered the defectives as having no soul and as being possessed by the devil in the very site within them where their souls should reside.

Although the reformers had an easy and ready-made explanation for mental deficiency, medicine seemed completely unconcerned until the first half of the nineteenth century. This was a time in history when men all over the world were raising their voices against all forms of oppression and maltreatment of fellow human beings. Numerous cries and vehement accusations were made against the treatment of slaves, prisoners, the insane, the blind, the deaf and the intellectually impaired. The sudden spurt of interest in the mentally defective seemed to follow on the coattails of special interest given to the care and education of deaf-mutes and, indeed, the first schools for the training of idiots were housed in institutions for the deaf and blind.

Jacob Pereire, who pioneered the teaching of deaf-mutes to read and write during the eighteenth century, was the main inspirational force behind those who became interested in working with the retarded. Most notable among these physicians was Jean Itard. Itard rapidly became prominent in the medical field as a result of his painstaking efforts with Victor, the Wild Boy of Aveyron.[6] Victor was brought to Itard in 1800 at the age of 11 or 12. He had been known for several years as a naked boy who roamed the woods around Aveyron, France, exposed to extreme cold and living off roots and acorns. Victor spoke no language, walked on all fours, drank water while lying flat on his face, and bit and scratched anyone who dared to interfere with him. Although he was discouraged from accepting the task by his teacher, Philippe Pinel, Itard undertook the task of civilizing Victor. He worked for five years with the boy, and although his accomplishments were far below the original goals he had set for himself, he nevertheless received special commendation from the French Academy of Science for the very positive contributions he had made to educational science. He proved that even the severely defective can be taught and gave many insights into useful techniques.

In 1840, Johann Guggenbühl founded an institution in Abendberg, Switzerland, for cretins. This was the first attempt at institutional treatment and rehabilitation of the mentally defective. At the time, most medical authorities considered all forms of idiocy as due to the same cause, cretinism, and attempted to differentiate only the degree of the impairment. Guggenbühl made an all-out effort to help his patients in a most humane fashion. He believed that pure mountain air, a good diet, plenty of exercise and special educational techniques, as well as kindness and interested female attention, were all necessary ingredients of the treatment plan.

He also tried a variety of medications, including many mineral preparations, especially calcium, zinc and copper. He attempted to develop better sensory perception in his patients by devising techniques for obtaining responses to progressively more complex stimuli. Guggenbühl's fame rapidly spread far and wide, and his techniques began to be utilized with all the mentally defective. His institution at Abendberg became the site of many pilgrimages by physicians, educators and writers from all parts of the world. Many returned to their own countries and pressured their governments to establish institutions patterned after Abendberg.

Guggenbühl himself rapidly became in great demand as a consultant and lecturer and spent an increasing amount of time away from Abendberg because of his travels. This fact, along with the rapidity of his acquired fame, was probably primarily responsible for the short life of the Abendberg institution. By 1860, the institution was closed, and both it and Guggenbühl were then subjected to much criticism because of the deterioration of the quality of the personnel employed and the patient treatment, poorly kept or nonexistent patient records, a loosening of admission requirements, and the general dismay at the fact that no cretin had ever actually been "cured." Still, the institutions founded in other lands were flourishing, and Guggenbühl must be recognized as the founder of institutional treatment for the mentally defective.

At about the same time that Guggenbühl was active in Switzerland, Edouard Séguin, a pupil of Itard's, had undertaken the treatment and education of many feebleminded children at the Hospital of the Incurables in France. He had met with much success and had had the foresight to invite examination of his pupils both before and after he had worked with them. He wrote a classical textbook on the instruction of idiots and he, too, won widespread fame and his techniques were observed by many interested professional people from other parts of the world. He emigrated to the United States during the mid-nineteenth century revolution in France. For a short time he was head of the Pennsylvania Training School for Idiots, but then settled in New York City, where he continued to play a major role as a consultant to those interested in establishing institutions for the treatment of the retarded.

In the United States, however, the main force behind the early institutional care of the feebleminded was Samuel Gridley Howe, a physician who was intensely interested in and dedicated to the care of all handicapped individuals. He was instrumental in the founding of the first institutional care for the retarded in this country, that is, a wing of the Perkins Institute for the blind in Boston, Massachusetts, which opened in 1848. He served as the institution's director and when dealing with the retarded he adhered to the principles set forth by Guggenbühl and Séguin, both of whom he had visited and with whom he had consulted. Pennsylvania founded the third institution for the mentally defective in the United States. It was initially called the Pennsylvania Training School for Idiots and was located in the Germantown section of Philadelphia. Several years later the institution was moved to Media, Pennsylvania, and renamed the Elwyn Training School. It is presently called the Elwyn Institute; Dr. Gerald Clark is its president.

Probably because the "cures" and hopes for "normalcy" originally sought by Itard, Guggenbühl, Séguin and others were never realized, attitudes toward the feebleminded began to change by the end of the nineteenth century. Almost insidiously, the focus changed from the needs of the patients to what came to be conceived as the needs of society. A feeling began to prevail that society, through its tolerance of the feebleminded, was actually fostering the problem, and that society was in danger of being overrun by the mentally defective. As Dr. Kanner[9] writes, "The mental defectives were viewed as a menace to civilization, incorrigible at home, burdens to the schools, sexually promiscuous, breeders of feebleminded offspring, victims and spreaders of poverty, degeneracy, crime and disease." It was, therefore, felt necessary to isolate the feebleminded from the rest of society with a life-long commitment to an institution.

Several other events in the early 1900's fostered greatly the general feeling of ill-will against the retarded. Alfred Binet's newly developed tests for measuring intelligence, although giving much needed standardization to intelligence estimates and introducing academic and medical personnel to the area of minimal, mild and borderline mental deficiency, also seemed to substantiate the idea that criminal behavior and feeblemindedness go hand in hand. In addition to this, many articles began to appear in the literature relating crime, moral degeneration and mental deficiency to heredity. The classic family studies of the Jukes,[3] the Kallikaks,[5] the Zeros,[7] the Nams[4] and the Hill Folk[1] caused further alarm and now, in addition to segregation, methods of preventing reproduction seemed imperative. Laws permitting sterilization of mental defectives began to appear in many states, and in some states this procedure is still carried out.

It was not until the early 1930's that the tide again began to change in favor of the feebleminded. When Binet's intelligence tests were restandardized during World War I and again administered to inmates of penal institutions, it was found that their intelligence scores did not vary significantly from that of the general population. In addition to this, when studies were carried out on retarded people who had escaped from institutions, it was found that the majority had made adequate community adjustments. Perhaps the greatest event in this era that aided the treatment of the retarded, however, was Dr. Fölling's discovery in Norway, in 1934, that phenylketonuria, a metabolic disturbance associated with mental retardation, was treatable with proper dietary regulation. This discovery again made mental deficiency a respectable area for medical and biological research.

During World War II, many retarded individuals proved that they were capable of being trained and gave excellent performances to meet an urgent labor shortage, and this helped also to temper past ill feelings. Major forces in the present impetus for improved care of the mentally retarded include the formation of the National Association for Retarded Children, in 1950, and, later, the Joseph P. Kennedy, Jr., Foundation, as well as relatively recent government legislation at all levels.

DIAGNOSTIC CLASSIFICATIONS OF MENTAL DEFICIENCY

As stated earlier, even as late as the mid-1800's, all feeblemindedness was attributed to cretinism and diagnoses given were in these terms—"cretin" or a descriptive modification of this, such as "cretin, mongoloid type." Also some classification of the degree of mental retardation present would be made, largely on the basis of speech development. For example, if little or no speech was present, the term "idiocy" was applied, while "imbecility" would denote somewhat better speech development and imply a higher intelligence.

It was not until 1866 that John Down described, as a syndrome separate from cretinism, the Mongolian type of idiocy that appeared in about 10 per cent of his patients.[2] In addition, he further subdivided the classification of idiocy into three major groups, i.e., congenital idiocy when present from birth, developmental idiocy when deterioration occurred after a satisfactory start, and accidental idiocy when it is related to injury or illness. By the end of the 1800's, numerous pathological reports of autopsies done on mental defectives showed some to have lesions of the central nervous system and the diagnoses of neurofibromatosis, tuberous sclerosis and so forth emerged. Autopsy findings and family studies by Tay[16] and Sachs[15] led to the piecing together of the syndrome named after them and much enlightenment as to the etiology of the mental deficiency seen in these patients.

Still, because of the general lack of enthusiasm on the part of physicians for the field of mental deficiency and with the emergence of Binet's testing and ultimate formation of classification on the basis of psychological testing, the medical classification of mental deficiency remained inadequate. Psychological classifications gained favor and were, and still are, widely used for descriptive, administrative and educational purposes. Such terms as mild, moderate, severe, educable, trainable and dependent are widely used and have replaced the older terminology of moron, imbecile and idiot to a large extent.

The following chart gives rough estimates of intelligence quotient scores obtained through psychological testing and the descriptive names generally applied to each group:

Intelligence Quotient Score	Descriptive Terms Applied		
Greater than 120	Superior Intelligence		
80 to 120	Normal Intelligence		
75 to 80	Borderline Intelligence		
50 to 75	Mild Mental Retardation	Educable	Moron
25 to 50	Moderate Mental Retardation	Trainable	Imbecile
0 to 25	Severe Mental Retardation	Dependent	Idiot

As a physician, I believe that we cannot be satisfied with such descriptive diagnoses. It has been inherent in my medical education to seek out cause and to strive for etiological classification of illnesses. One of the leading figures in the United States at present in the differential diagnosis of mental deficiency is Dr. George A. Jervis. In a chapter in the American Handbook of Psychiatry, Volume II,[8] he classifies mental deficiency into Physiological and Pathological categories. He defines Physiological Mental Deficiency as "a large group of defective individuals who show no pathological conditions which might interfere with normal functioning of the brain and no clinical manifestation aside from the intellectual impairment." This group usually tests in the I.Q. range of 50 to 75, and at the present time is thought to comprise about 75 per cent of all people deemed mentally defective. As to etiology, it is felt that the deficiency in this group is the end result of all the genetic factors that go into the making up of the individual's intelligence. Thus the causes of such variations in intelligence are in the same categories as the factors that bring about superior intelligence.

Pathological Mental Deficiency may result either from Endogenous or Exogenous causes. Endogenous Pathological Mental Deficiency relates to genetic problems and is further subdivided into three groups: (1) illnesses due to single dominant genes, such as the group of neuroepidermal syndromes including neurofibromatosis, Sturge-Weber's disease and tuberous sclerosis, and a group of lesions involving bony structures such as acrocephaly, Marfan's syndrome and achondroplasia; (2) single recessive genes, commonly seen as metabolic abnormalities, such as galactosemia, phenylketonuria, Wilson's hepatolenticular degeneration, "maple sugar disease," Tay-Sach's disease, Gaucher's disease, primary microcephaly, macrocephaly and some cerebellar atrophies; most of these diseases are thought to be associated with enzymatic defects brought about by genetic errors; (3) mental defects caused by undetermined genetic mechanisms. In this group, Dr. Jervis includes mental retardation associated with idiopathic epilepsy, and mental retardation due to congenital brain malformations for which a dominant gene pattern has not been indicated. Such conditions as anencephaly, agyria, agenesia of the corpus callosum and congenital hydrocephalus are in this group and the latter malady, of course, is the most common brain malformation.

To these three groups delineated by Jervis, I would add a fourth group which might be titled "Other Chromosomal Aberrations"—this group offers an especially interesting and stimulating challenge at the present time. In 1956, when it was first discovered how to burst a cell nucleus while leaving the chromatin material intact,[18] a great impetus was given to the study of diseases associated with mental retardation, as well as to many other areas of medicine.

Chromosomal karyotyping has led to the discovery of many hitherto unknown and often unthought of facts. For example, a new dimension was added to the already long history of mongolism in medicine when it was discovered that mongoloids possess 47 chromosomes in their cell nuclei instead of 46—there is an extra chromosome number 21. Hence, the syndrome previously called mongolism or Down's syndrome, has assumed yet another name, trisomy 21.

In relatively recent epidemiological studies investigating the relationship of the incidence of mongolism to viral epidemics, a high incidence of mongoloid births was reported in mothers who were afflicted with viral hepatitis in the early months of pregnancy. It has been hypothesized that viral infections may interfere in some manner in the metaphase of gamete cell division, making the separation of the chromosome pairs more difficult. Perhaps the chromosome pair designated as number 21 is more susceptible than other chromosome pairs to the effects of the presence of the virus, although the trisomy phenomenon is known to exist also with other chromosome pairs, such as trisomy 15 and trisomy 18.

A striking and intimate similarity is reported to exist in the chemical compositions of viruses and of chromosome material—a similarity which leads us to wonder what role, if any, this might play in the development of chromosomal aberrations.

Other chromosomal aberrations which are often, although certainly not always, associated with mental retardation, are those involving the sex chromosomes. The exciting discovery by Dr. Murray Barr[14] of the dark-staining sex chromatin material (the so-called Barr bodies) that is present in the periphery of the nucleus of each female's cell may aid in the diagnosis of this type of retardation. The buccal smear with its staining procedure is an extremely simple and inexpensive test and in many cases eliminates the need for the more costly and time-consuming chromosomal karyotyping.

Deletion of or reduplication of either or both sex chromosomes is now known to occur. The previously known Klinefelter's syndrome of men was found to be associated with the presence of one or, rarely, two extra X (female) chromosomes. In Turner's syndrome, the absence of one X chromosome gives a karyotyping in these females of XO instead of XX as in normal females. In addition, new syndromes have been discovered, such as that of the so-called "super female" who possesses one or even two extra X chromosomes. The so-called "super male" possesses an extra Y chromosome in his cells. The latter syndrome is certainly one that every psychiatrist and psychologist should be familiar with, since it has been associated with delinquent acts, often of a sexual nature. These males, as the Klinefelter males, tend to be quite tall and gangling and have often been first detected in penal institutions. However, although all of the other chromosomal aberrations referred to are often associated with mental retardation, I know of no studies to date that link the XYY (super male) syndrome with mental deficiency.[17]

The Exogenous Pathological Mental Deficiency group is further subdivided by Jervis into six categories according to the environmentally induced etiology. These six categories are: (1) infection, either intrauterine, such as with German measles, or postnatal, such as with the various encephalitides; (2) toxic agents, such as radiation, lead, and others; (3) trauma—prenatal, perinatal or postnatal; (4) endocrine disorders, such as hypothyroidism, hypopituitarism and so forth; (5) psychosis in infancy or childhood; and (6) sociocultural deprivation, or so-called pseudofeeblemindedness.

A CHILD PSYCHIATRIST LOOKS AT MENTAL RETARDATION

Since working in the field of mental retardation, I have been continually struck by the confusion which exists even in the mere defining of the terms mental retardation or mental deficiency. If one reads the literature, one can't help but be impressed with the large number of behaviors, reactions, personality characteristics, learning problems and so forth, which are at times mentioned as occurring, together or separately, in persons diagnosed as mentally retarded, mentally defective or mentally deficient. In some countries, the diagnosis of persons as mentally defective suffices even when the symptoms are more related to faulty social interaction—including a lack of awareness of social graces, immaturity in social responses, or delinquent behavior—than they are to less than average intelligence.

It is both confusing and alarming when such terms are used so loosely, and it leaves one with the feeling that he can't be certain he understands what the author intends to relate, and more importantly, with little certainty that he understands the true nature of the malady being discussed. Classically and traditionally, the terms mental deficiency, mental defective and mental retardation were meant to pertain to one's intelligence and lack thereof. To avoid further confusion, at least within professional groups, these terms should be reserved for this meaning and this meaning alone. Without such clear definition of the words "mental deficiency," we tend to do what children do when they refer to others as "retard" or "reject" in describing behavior which is very often not related to a lack of intelligence.

In suggesting that we restrict the meaning of such terms as mental retardation, mental deficiency and mental defective to a measure of intelligence, I am now confronted with a question that has often been posed to me by others working in this field, especially other physicians. That question is: "Does the diagnosis of mental deficiency belong in the field of medicine and psychiatry at all?" And they ask, "Is mental retardation any more of a medical diagnosis than mental superiority, or the definition of a genius?" Mental retardation can be either a diagnosis itself or only a symptom or part of a symptom complex that occurs with certain maladies.

One must remember that presently in only 20 to 25 per cent of those found to be mentally retarded is an etiological factor known. Probably in not a single case, except perhaps for those individuals with brain damage in which actual tissue destruction is known to have occurred, can we actually pinpoint how the interference with intellectual performance takes place. In this brain-damaged group, mental retardation accompanies other signs and symptoms resulting from trauma, toxicity, infection involving the central nervous system or from genetic errors. This is the group Jervis refers to as having Pathological Mental Deficiency. Thus, in the case of the mongoloid, mental retardation is part of the total picture along with the short stature, the peculiar facies, the simian crease and, of course, the finding of an extra chromosome number 21 upon chromosomal karyotyping.

Although further etiological factors pertaining to mental retardation will doubtless be discovered, it is likely, purely on a statistical basis, that the other group of mental retardates, i.e., the other 75 per cent, will not be significantly reduced in number. With this group, which Jervis designated as having Physiological Mental Deficiency, it is believed that the deficiency is a result of the sum total of all the genetic factors that determine one's intelligence, and thus the cause is of the same order as that which brings about intellectual superiority. This group naturally falls on the lower side of the bell-shaped curve of intelligence.

Even in this area there is a ray of hope: recent medical advances in virology suggest the possibility of controlling the amino acids and proteins that go into the synthesis of genetic material and substituting superior genetic material for that which may be less beneficial. However, as matters now stand, this group of 75 per cent of all mental retardates falls primarily into the area designated as mildly defective. It is probably true that the great majority of these individuals never seek medical or psychiatric help because of their retardation per se. By and large, those retarded individuals whom I have seen for psychiatric consultation or who have been committed to an institution have severe social, emotional and behavioral problems, and upon careful evaluation are found to have major concomitant problems, usually related to the cause of the mental retardation.

For the most part, I believe this group of 75 per cent of all retardates struggles along, perhaps passing through school in remedial classes or other classes for slow learners, eventually receiving vocational training either on a formal or informal basis, sometimes marrying and forming families of their own, or perhaps remaining at home with their parents even in adulthood. Does this then mean that, since it is likely that the majority of all retardates do not seek psychiatric help for unconscious conflicts related to their retardation, that mental retardation is not a psychiatric problem and, therefore, should not be part of the differential diagnoses of psychiatric problems? Is mental retardation a medical problem only when it is part of a symptom complex resulting from involvement of several body systems? I believe that the answer is "no" to both questions. All mental retardation is part of every physician's business, and when mental retardation is unaccompanied by any other clinical manifestation, it is especially the concern of the psychiatrist, psychologist, social worker and others who are intensely concerned with normal psychological growth and development.

If a child is slow to learn from birth, one may expect that his entire growth and development will be affected. Although mild degrees of mental retardation are often first detected when the child begins school and is unable to perform adequately, the slowness to learn doesn't begin then. In most instances, it is present since birth and probably is first revealed by the infant's slowness to learn that it is mother who has been bringing him the bottle which is so satisfying and pleasurable to him and that she is a separate individual from himself; that the object which passes in front of his eyes is his hand and that it is connected to an arm that is connected to his shoulder and that he is able to learn control over the entire mechanism; that when mother leaves, she'll be back and that he'll continue to exist in the meantime.

It probably means a slowness to learn what words mean, and especially a slowness to give up the usage of global words in favor of a larger vocabulary in which each word possesses a more definitive meaning; a slowness to put words together in a sentence; a slowness to know what mother means when she points to the toilet and shows much disgust with his soiled diaper time and again; and a slowness to realize that the bad dreams he experiences at night and the frightening thoughts he has during the day aren't real and that no harm will come to him.

I purposely have used the words "probably means" because much of what I have proposed here seems logical but has not really been substantiated. A careful perusal of histories of mentally retarded individuals, in my experience, suggests that all these things occur. However, these histories are usually recollected many years later, when the diagnosis is first made, and there is seldom an opportunity for direct observations of the early years of a child who is mildly mentally retarded. In addition, it seems likely that the mother-child relationship is affected in an adverse way, i.e., in much the same manner that we find with brain-damaged children. These mothers, too, are often cheated of an expected, age-appropriate response from their child, and are burdened not only by having to give much extra care, patience and guidance to their youngster but also by tremendous feelings of guilt and responsibility that so often accompany maladies of this nature.

Although I have not examined large numbers of individuals who have only lower intelligence as a finding and my impressions have largely been formed through examination of individuals with multiple handicaps, usually brain damage of one degree or another, I believe that mental retardation has been a very significant contributing factor to the impairments found.

THE MAJOR EFFECTS OF MENTAL RETARDATION ON CHILD GROWTH AND DEVELOPMENT

The major aberrations of normal child growth and development which are related to mental retardation are pre-latency personality fixations and disturbances in ego development. The term "pre-latency personality fixation" is not as yet commonly used in the literature.[10, 11] The psychological meaning of "fixation" as defined by Freud and as typically used in psychological writings refers to developmental barriers in the forward progressive movement of libido. Thus, Freud likened libido and its forward progression to an army of invading soldiers and pointed out how important it is for some soldiers to remain behind at highly strategic and tactically important areas of the invaded land in order to maintain and fortify these areas while the remainder of the army continued to advance.

He further described how these fortified areas serve as logical places to which the army could return, should it meet insurmountable opposition at the front line and if retreat were required. Thus, the army could again dig in at this previously acquired and fortified position in an attempt to withstand the onslaught of the opposition there and, indeed, to turn the tide and enable progression to take place again. In this sense, then, fixation refers to opposition that confronts the normal progressive movement of libido, to the extent that part of the libido must remain at the point of opposition and continue to wage the battle for growth and development at that level or stage, in order that the major part of libido can move on.

Further, these minute levels of libido fixation also serve as logical areas for retreat when the major, advancing portion of libido is confronted with intra-psychic stresses that it cannot manage. In this manner, then, "fixation" is inti-mately bound to the psychological concept of regression, implying a *return* to a previously acquired position from a position of higher or more advanced libido development. It should also be noted that individuals experiencing this phenom-enon usually have the potential to advance again to a higher level of attain-ment if the regression is brought on by psychic trauma (and not by irreparable trauma, such as some forms of central nervous system damage) and especially if given the benefit of therapeutic intervention where required.

The term "pre-latency personality fixation" and the alternate term "devel-opmental personality arrest" refer to those conditions in which the reciprocal of what Freud described in defining "fixation" takes place, i.e., most of the army of soldiers remains behind to wage battle while relatively few are able to advance. "Fixation" is also an adequate term to describe this phenomenon, but as used in this context, it implies a much broader and more severe develop-mental problem in libido progression than was defined by Freud. Indeed, as applied here, "fixation" refers not only to libido progression but to every facet of human growth and development related to one's psychic development, including libido, ego, superego, personality and so forth.

In persons exhibiting this phenomenon, chronological age and usually physical growth continue but broad-scale emotional stagnation exists. Regres-sion is not implied, but rather a lack of progression. This condition can be caused, wholly or in part, by any of the innumerable factors that tend to impede normal growth and development, but especially brain damage, mental retardation, irreversible constitutional and hereditary maladies, cultural depri-vation, an excess or lack of early stimulation, and inadequate or insensitive maternal care. Because of the broader implications of the word "fixation" as utilized here, and to avoid confusion with "fixation" as originally implied by Freud, "developmental personality arrest" is used here to describe these condi-tions.

Far too often this finding of a personality arrest, as well as the disturbances in ego development, is taken for granted as being just part of what one expects to find in a mentally retarded individual — even to the extent that we're often willing to consider these findings as a relatively unimportant part of the total diagnostic picture. However, lower than normal intelligence is not in itself sufficient to explain why such a person's personality remains infantile, or why his ego development is faulty. Although one is born with a certain potential for the development of intelligence and this potential is inherently dependent on one's genetic make-up as well as the integrity of his central nervous system, the same cannot be said, at least not to the same extent, about one's personality development.

Aside from various constitutional factors that are discussed in the literature and have to do with individual differences in strength of impulses, by and large, a person is not born with a specific personality potential. Rather, the personality develops throughout the formative years and it is much more dependent on environmental guidelines than is an intelligence quotient. A far more satisfactory explanation is that the slowness to learn and the lowered maximum potential for learning that exist make the early growth and development of these children fraught with age-inappropriateness, confusion, disorientation and high levels of anxiety, so that personality development often never goes beyond the pregenital years to a significant degree. Also, the ego development of these children, upon close inspection, almost invariably shows significant aberrations from normal.

In view of the intense interest, in recent years, in the rather fuzzy areas of the ego disturbances and developmental personality problems in child psychiatry, the following explanation for these dual findings in the retarded is offered. It is in no way a coincidence that these dual findings exist together, but rather, they are intimately related—even in a cause and effect relationship. The personality arrest itself, often, along with the mental retardation, the most striking manifestation to the untrained observer, is a result of and actually a symptom of the faulty ego structure. In all personality arrests, regardless of cause, it is the ego that should be incriminated, since it is surely one's ego, utilizing whatever skills have been developed throughout its many important functions, that allows personality formation and progression to take place.

Ego development is related to personality development in at least three ways: *first,* what constitutes the personality is at least in part a reflection of the level at which the ego is functioning. Or, stated another way, what we call personality is in part (and probably in large part) the outward manifestations of the internal stresses a person is struggling with and of the manner in which the ego is attempting to cope with these stresses.

Secondly, it is basically the ego's job to maintain a person sufficiently anxiety-free so that personality formation and progression ensue, and this includes a vigilant, intense interest in the progressive libidinal dictates. The development of higher-level defenses to manage the changing intrapsychic stresses is imperative, and these higher-level defenses then not only allow for further growth of the personality but are themselves reflected as part of the personality. Thus, early reaction formations not only defend against anal impulses and allow one to begin to approach sexual impulses more comfortably but are themselves incorporated in the very structure of the developing personality. A extreme example of this, of course, is seen most vividly in the obsessive-compulsive personality.

Thirdly, one's ego has the further task of self-inspection and is expected to view the personality with a critical eye and make whatever adjustments might seem necessary for what would be considered a "normal" personality, on the basis of its own criteria as well as those of the social environment.

Very often in individuals "suffering" with developmental arrests, the early ego development appears to be so hampered that there is a marked persistence of oral and anal drives which may never be adequately mastered—and the mastering of these drives is itself inherent in further ego development. In its attempts at mastery, the ego consistently utilizes the more primitive defense mechanisms, such as regression, withdrawal, imitation and identification, and this reliance on such primitive defense mechanisms, along with the persistence of the early libidinal drives and anxieties, is reflected in the personality as immaturity, dependency, impulsivity and similar traits. Little development of higher-level defense mechanisms may take place, since the intrapsychic, libidinal dictates may never advance beyond the pregenital stages to a significant degree. Also, in these individuals, especially if mental deficiency is of etiological significance, there seems to be little awareness of and little concern for the state of the personality and the level of its development.

These three ways in which ego development and personality development are related are all factors primarily referable to qualitative aspects of the ego. Developmental arrests can also occur with a quantitative lack of ego development. This might occur, for instance, in the mentally retarded, in whom deficient intelligence may severely impede or make impossible the development of certain ego functions such as reality testing, the ability to integrate and to synthesize environmental stimuli, and the ability to learn. It may also occur in the brain-damaged child in whom central nervous system excitation can lead to an inability to develop proper control of motility, or faulty neuronal pathways may lead to misperceptions of reality and a disruptive body image.

Proper personality formation and progression constitute one of the more important ego functions. The diagnosis of personality arrest is a descriptive diagnosis that implies a core problem in the ego, much as a diagnosis of a psychoneurosis not only provides some understanding of the manifest symptomatology but also implies a core problem of an oedipal conflict.

CHARACTERISTICS OF PERSONALITY ARRESTS IN THE MENTALLY DEFECTIVE

Although personality arrests can occur at any stage of growth and development, and in the retarded the degree of arrest depends to a large extent upon the degree of mental retardation, quite often the personality is found arrested in the pregenital years. Thus, one often finds many derivatives, as well as direct expressions, of the oral and anal periods of life when examining a retarded individual. Higher levels of development are not uncommon, but when present one usually finds a particularly supportive and stimulating environment present since birth, as well as an I.Q. in the upper limits of what is classified as mild mental retardation. Some of the descriptive findings from each of the early stages of growth and development—oral, anal and phallic-oedipal—are discussed in the following paragraphs.

Oral Stage. The individual remains whiny, dependent and clingy, often becoming overly anxious when separated from anyone he has formed an attachment to, and such attachments are often formed indiscriminately. This latter finding is especially pronounced if the individual is separated from the primary love object for an extended period of time, as through death or institutionalization. He will often maintain a pronounced interest in food and in all objects that suggest food, as well as retaining a fondness for putting a variety of objects in his mouth to gum on, suck on, lick or taste. Insatiable appetites for both food and affection are common. If angered, physical biting, or biting remarks with oral-aggressive content are often employed as weapons.

There is a general lack of spontaneity and motivation present, especially to learn, where positive action is required. The major fear of the individual seems to be the loss of the love object, and coping with this fear appears to embrace all of the person's energies as well as his goals. Transitional objects are often retained from childhood, and the relationship of the individual to the object commonly appears to involve separation anxiety.

Anal Stage.   Various personality traits which are derivatives of this stage of growth and development may be found. The individual may be overly sensitive, easily slighted, irritable, anxious or withdrawn. He might be argumentative, rebellious, stubborn, and passive-aggressive. Fits of temper are common, and temper tantrums are not uncommon. Speech disturbances may be present, such as stuttering, inadequate vocabulary, and many mispronunciations, as well as numerous slips of the tongue which betray a greater than usual retention of primary process thinking. Increased speech is often used to ingratiate, while decreased speech (and silence) is used to express anger. There is often a complete lack of concern and awareness about a disheveled appearance.

Difficulties with toileting may take the form of either constipation or soiling or enuresis, as well as inadequate toilet habits. There is great interest in bowel movements and in all substances that suggest feces. Often useless articles or articles of little practical value are collected and stored. Many articles are automatically smelled as part of a routine inspection, and great exhilaration as well as open pleasure is experienced in response to flatus.

As with the oral derivatives, a lack of spontaneity and motivation may be present. The major fears appear to be the loss of the love object and the loss of the love object's love. The individual's whole being appears to be directed toward means of coping with the anxiety associated with these fears. One of the most common and striking derivative manifestations of this process is seen in an individual's almost total investment in the discovery, handling and storage of a collection of articles that exhibit little or no value, aside from an obvious emotional significance to the collector.

Phallic-Oedipal Stage.   Those manifesting personality arrest at this level often retain intense interest in childish combative games, such as "cops and robbers" and "cowboys and Indians," and in toys which retain a marked phallic significance for them. A great deal of daydreaming, restlessness and other overt signs of anxiety are often present. These individuals tend to be "loners" in play (setting up combative situations in a variety of different but often repetitive ways), or are able to play comfortably only with younger, oedipal children or those in early latency. Excessive masturbation often occurs, as well as the continuance of childish nightmares and fears, although the latter tend to be more numerous and general in nature and not well delineated as is more typical of the psychoneurotic phobic child.

Fear of bodily injury (castration anxiety) persists as the major fear these individuals struggle with, and they continue to be plagued with disproportionately intense anxiety feelings when injured or threatened with injury, even of a slight degree. Conscience formation appears to remain at a primitive, precursor stage, harsh in nature, and more related to fantasized introjects than to reality-oriented demands. Thus, these individuals can become quite depressed at times and burdened with feelings of low self-esteem and worthlessness, while at the next moment, they may feel put upon or treated unfairly by the environment and may feel few qualms about taking things that don't belong to them or giving distorting information to meet their personal needs.

The feelings of depression, low self-esteem and worthlessness appear to be related not only to the stagnated conscience formation but also to the fact that these individuals have reached a somewhat higher level of development than the pre-oedipal stages. Therefore, they have increased awareness of their surroundings and their own personal comparative shortcomings, as well as higher-level object relationships, especially with the mother.

I have met many institutionalized persons with personality arrestments, some at pre-oedipal levels and some at the phallic-oedipal level, and often wonder which person is worse off. The individual with pre-oedipal personality arrest is usually dull, often apathetic, and concerned only with the immediate task at hand. He seems to get upset only when his food or lodging or a relationship with an individual he is especially attached to is threatened in some way. The individual with phallic-oedipal personality arrest, on the other hand, seems never to be able to overcome the feelings of being rejected by his parents by their act of institutionalization. He constantly suffers with intense feelings of being bad, defective and worthless, as well as intense feelings of being deprived and not loved. He remains exquisitely sensitive to the least slight or critical comment, and is especially jealous of siblings and sibling surrogates.

These latter individuals often come from good homes, where they've been given a great deal of extra care and love in their early years by parents exceptionally sensitive to the increased demands of their child. This somewhat disturbing, paradoxical situation, should not suggest that extra love and attention should not be given to the child because it sometimes leads to greater depression and anxiety on the child's part. That would be a decided step backward. However, it does demand that professionally trained people develop further techniques to help these children cope with and master these intense feelings that cause such suffering, and thereby help lift (or push) them into a higher level of growth and development—a latency period.

In the school situation, the child with phallic-oedipal arrest rarely forms good peer relationships, nor does he make a good school adjustment. He is usually restless, playful, unmotivated to learn, and is generally described by his teacher as "immature." Regardless of his age then, the history and interviews reveal that he has never experienced a true latency period, with the necessary repression of the oedipal conflicts, sublimation of drives, and displacement of affects that are typical of that period.

Differential Diagnosis of Personality Arrests and Psychoneuroses

The differential diagnosis of the developmental arrests and the psycho-neuroses primarily concerns the phallic-oedipal stage of development. However, the element of regression must be constantly kept in mind. It is entirely possible for an acute psychoneurotic reaction to be manifest primarily by regressive symptomatology, and the individual overtly can resemble a person with personality arrest at any of the three levels previously described. On the other hand, it is also possible for a child with a primary personality arrest, later, under stress, to show additional regressive symptomatology, typical of a still earlier stage of development.

Although the person with a personality arrest at the phallic-oedipal level and the person with a psychoneurosis have the same core to their problem— that is, an unresolved and inadequately repressed oedipal conflict with the associated oedipal fantasies—and both show derivatives of the conflict in their symptoms, including regression, the ego of the neurotic individual appears stronger and more intact. His ego at least partially channels the anxiety aroused into one or more of the well-established neurotic symptom formations; i.e., a phobia, conversion-hysteria, depressive reaction, obsessive-compulsive reaction, and so forth. Thus, although the individual is suffering, handicapped, and unable to perform up to his potential, he is usually able to maintain a fairly adequate school or work situation and peer relationships, and personality development usually proceeds or is maintained, at least temporarily. This is not, however, always the case, and anyone who has worked much with neurotic individuals has seen many examples of a neurosis which can massively impede a person in all areas of growth and productivity.

When presented with the overall picture of the two diagnostic categories, one cannot help but be impressed with the fact that the person with phallic-oedipal arrest, in contrast to the psychoneurotic, never really leaves the oedipal period emotionally. The struggles and characteristics of this period of growth and development become part of his total character and personality, and thus invade his total self. A careful, detailed history of the present illness, as well as the individual's overall past development can be most helpful in establishing all the important circumstances and thus a proper diagnosis.

One might ask why the preceding discussion on differential diagnosis is important to this presentation on mental retardation. Although it is possible for some mentally retarded persons to develop psychoneurotic reactions, no evidence suggests that mental retardation predisposes the person to form a psychoneurotic reaction. Quite the reciprocal is true, however, in the case of developmental arrests. Here, mental retardation may be of prime etiological significance by its constant undercutting effects on normal growth and development. If the mental retardation is mild, a higher-level personality arrest may develop. But if the degree of retardation is more than mild, or if it is associated with or results from disturbances of the central nervous system or genetic abnormalities, then the likelihood of personality arrest at the pre-oedipal levels is greatly increased.

Pain.   The concept of developmental arrest can make an interesting contribution to our understanding of the constituents of pain. It had long been observed by members of the medical staff at the Elwyn Institute that the general population of students enrolled there (a resident setting with many students having mental retardation associated with central nervous system abnormalities or genetic abnormalities, and pre-oedipal developmental arrests) had markedly elevated pain thresholds. Many of these students would undergo dental extractions, the lancing of abscesses and other minor surgery, as well as other painful medical and dental procedures, with little or no anesthesia.

Members of the staff often speculated on the reasons for this readily observable phenomenon and wondered if, somewhere between the epidermis and the cerebrum in this population, there is a difference in the pain recognition processes. They wondered if the findings suggested by Margaret Mahler[12, 13] as being important in explaining a seemingly similar phenomenon observed in autistic children, played a role here also. Doctor Mahler feels that the dramatic insensitivity to pain often found in autistic children is attributable to a lack of early peripheral body cathexis, a severe ego defect. I suggest that the phenomenon observed in the group of patients I'm discussing has to do with the arrestment of libido and personality development present.

Since the arrestment so often occurs at the pre-oedipal stage of development, these individuals never experience intense oedipal conflicts with overwhelming castration anxiety and the need to resolve the conflict or eventually submit it to repression. As a result, they are spared the apprehension, inner turmoil and anxiety that are normally aroused at an unconscious level by such medical and dental procedures. What is amazing to me is the extent of the contributions of these unconscious sources to pain—contributions which appear to outweigh by far the real, conscious components of physical pain.

DISTURBANCES IN EGO DEVELOPMENT

Mental retardation typically leads to some disturbances in ego development. However, it is generally agreed that both the ego-disturbed child and the developmentally arrested child show significant disturbances in ego development. If the degree of mental retardation is greater than mild, or if the retardation is associated with other abnormalities—especially impairments of the central nervous system, however subtle—a frankly ego-disturbed child may result. When a child is diagnosed as ego-disturbed, it is generally because he shows greater disturbance over a broader range of ego functions; i.e., control of motility is tenuous, object relationships poor, and there is often a marked involvement in fantasy life, which is not well differentiated from reality. The ego deficits combine to give the child a bizarre, confused and disoriented appearance, whereas the developmentally arrested child often comes across as immature, dull, bland and apathetic.

Ego-disturbed children often appear to be struggling with impulses and conflicts from every level of psychosexual development at once, whereas the developmentally arrested child reflects primarily the struggles of one psychosexual level. Whether the presenting picture in a child and the degree of disturbances in ego development found are most compatible with the diagnosis of developmental personality arrest or of ego disturbance or whether another diagnostic entity is present is for the clinician to decide after his evaluation.

The disturbances in ego functions found associated with mental retardation can be described without considering the degree of impairment. The degree of impairment is naturally quite dependent on the severity of mental retardation, and other maladies that may be associated with it. The following list of the various ego functions indicates how the disturbance of each tends to manifest itself.

1. Control of Motility. One often finds a lack of control over one or another of the bodily functions, such as soiling or enuresis, and even daytime wetting. Impulsive behavior is evident, in that normal automatic restraints are easily overcome by a minor stimulus such as food. Control of total body musculature is often not completely developed, and a general awkwardness, clumsiness, poor fine coordination and a lack of physical finesse are not uncommon findings. Control of the musculature involved in speech often appears incompletely developed, and poor articulation and pronunciation with slurring of words is rather commonly found. Contrary to findings with brain-damaged children, the mentally retarded child who does not have brain damage will often appear slow motorially also. His gait is usually slow, and he is generally docile, being able to sit for hours, perhaps just rocking in a chair. However, when he is aroused and anxious, environmental controls, either by actual physical restraint or verbally by repetitive reminding, are often needed.

2. Object Relationships. An inability to form meaningful, mature attachments to others is striking. Attachments are most often of the dependent type, even among themselves, and good peer relationships are uncommon. Not only is the ability to empathize with the feelings of others usually lacking, but these children often appear unaware of or unconcerned with the physical needs of others. They demand to receive a great deal, but are unable to give comfortably in return.

3. Reality Testing.   In these children the ability to distinguish reality from their fantasies is often tenuous. However, depending on the level of psychosexual development, their fantasies are often more infantile and deal with fears of and feelings about being abandoned or rejected. They tend to retain and keep alive all their childhood fears. They easily misinterpret situations and tend to make distortions that reflect an immediate struggle, involving, as often as not, separation anxiety.

4. Defense Mechanisms.   Signal anxiety often appears to be over-active or of little use. When the mentally retarded are confronted with relatively little stress, defense mechanisms falter easily and impulsive behavior ensues. They often cannot tolerate the unexpected. Defense mechanisms tend to be primitive, including a major use of imitation and projection. Even identification, although appearing to be constantly sought, is often a difficult defense mechanism for the retarded to incorporate successfully. Avoidance and denial are commonly seen. When the child is more ego-disturbed and fears of disintegration are paramount, compulsive-type defenses are often prominent, such as sameness, orderliness, rigidity and perserveration; increased structuring of the environment, either self-devised or externally produced, often provides much relief. However, reaction formation, isolation of affect, and intellectualization are less often seen.

5. Body Image.   An unawareness or uncertainty of body boundaries, with a general confusion in body orientation, is often found. These children tend to retain very immature and unsophisticated ideas of the total body structure, as well as of the individual body parts, and often develop little correct understanding of various bodily functions, especially those involving the internal structures. Many of these findings are easily demonstrated in conversations with the retarded about their bodies, and in the numerous distortions and deletions so often present in their drawings of persons.

6. Synthesis.   The main emphasis in these children is often on the synthesizing of a structured environment which is bland and undisturbing. Thus, they are often unable to see various, related events as being related, whereas on other occasions they will relate happenings in a primary process manner, i.e., according to infantile, concrete associations. Because they tend to become overwhelmed by changes in their environment and tend to misinterpret situations readily, in these children various simultaneous environmental stimuli are often not synthesized (as parts of a whole) at all. Even when the stimuli are related, it is often not done in an economical, meaningful or appropriate manner, and confusion persists.

PSYCHIATRIC CONTRIBUTIONS TO THE MEDICAL MANAGEMENT OF THE RETARDED

The functions of a child psychiatrist should include treatment of mentally retarded children, both as outpatients and as inpatients in an institutional setting. By and large, psychiatric outpatient clinics have been negligent in the care they have offered these children. Because the great majority of mentally retarded children are not candidates for insight psychotherapy, they have often been dismissed from clinic contact after the initial evaluation has been completed. Some are referred to other agencies for help, but further ongoing service rendered by the referring clinic itself is unfortunately rare.

Psychiatric Evaluation

Our psychiatric outpatient clinics have a great deal to offer these children and their families in addition to a careful, complete psychiatric evaluation. A careful, complete psychiatric evaluation is emphasized because the child psychiatrist's service begins here, not just from a diagnostic standpoint, but also from the standpoint of detecting the specific neurological, academic and ego deficits of the child. One must evaluate carefully all areas of growth and development of a mentally retarded child and make individual estimates of levels of functioning in relation to mental age, physical development, libidinal progression, ego and superego development, and the level of motor functioning. Comparisons can then be made with normal levels for the child's chronological age, and where discrepancies are found, one can comb the developmental history to evaluate possible factors causing or contributing to the arrest, fixation, or delay in the development of each, or in any one area of growth and development. Logically, this would be the first step in instituting corrective measures that might be utilized to overcome or improve the deficits or discrepancies found.

To carry out such an evaluation, one must have access to psychological testing, neurological examinations, electroencephalography, audiometric studies, ophthalmological examination, chromosomal karyotyping, buccal smears, speech and reading evaluations, dermatoglyphics, biochemistry studies (especially for amino acid surveys), and endocrinological consultations. Certainly, the evaluation of one child does not usually call for all these studies to be completed. However, it is not at all unusual that a good number of them will be necessary, in addition to routine physical and psychiatric examinations, in order to complete the diagnostic studies.

Of course, milder or minimal signs of brain damage, when present—and they are not uncommonly seen in association with varying degrees of mental retardation—are not only often difficult to detect but also may be the defects that require the most ingenuity when planning a corrective program. The importance of these defects cannot be overemphasized and one must attempt to institute corrective measures for them and not be influenced into minimizing their effects merely because present-day terminology uses such terms as "mild" and "minimal" in making a descriptive diagnosis, whether of minimal brain damage or of mild mental retardation.

In many cases, these terms in no way reflect the degree of the actual overall impairment but merely the number of physical signs we delineate with present-day techniques. Although the outward manifestations of such impairments may be minimal and seem minor, and even the physical brain damage itself appear to be minimal, these impairments may have a major detrimental influence on the development of the child. Without a careful evaluation, it is difficult to know, or even estimate, the effect that even a mild disturbance in perception or visual-motor coordination or an intelligence quotient in the mildly defective range may have on any or all areas of the child's development.

Coordination of Therapeutic Program

After the initial evaluation, the child psychiatrist should assume the role of a medical coordinator for the program he initiates for the child. Too many of these children get lost in the shuffle between various agencies and even when many of their needs are met, it is done in a less organized and less beneficial manner than is possible. As a member of a team doing diagnostic evaluations on children for the Pennsylvania Eastern Diagnostic and Evaluation Center, I was constantly impressed with the need for professionally trained people who could coordinate a broad program for the benefit of these children. Too often, the child must be referred to a special school, while medications are prescribed by the family physician, and parental counseling is provided through a family service agency. A child psychiatrist could oversee the entire therapeutic program. He would need to regulate medications, counsel parents, refer the child to special educational and vocational programs, and meet with the child intermittently for a periodic evaluation of the effectiveness of the program.

Medications.   The use and choice of medications depend largely on the level of anxiety, behavior characteristics and degree of ego disturbance that the child presents. If the child shows high levels of anxiety, difficult or bizarre behavior patterns, or severe pressure from his fantasy life, and his reality testing is tenuous, trifluoperazine hydrochloride (Stelazine) in low doses, even 1 to 2 milligrams per day, is often quite helpful. If reality testing is relatively good and anxiety is usually held in check, but the main problem is hyperkinetic behavior in a brain-damaged child, the amphetamines are quite useful. Some recent studies carried on at Johns Hopkins on the use of amphetamines with brain-damaged children seem to indicate that these drugs may aid the learning of brain-damaged children, whether hyperkinetic behavior is present or not. If there is a problem with high levels of anxiety, but no major defects in control of motility or reality testing, low doses of thioridazine (Mellaril) may prove to be helpful.

Counseling.   The counseling of parents of mentally retarded children is an essential but difficult part of the program. Supportive therapeutic measures must be used to relieve huge amounts of guilt and anxiety that are so typically present in parents of mentally retarded and brain-damaged children and to release quantities of this psychic energy for more beneficial purposes. Although the therapist's relationship with the parents is certainly being established from their very first meeting and throughout the evaluation, the parental conference when the evaluation is discussed and recommendations are made is often crucial in solidifying this relationship. These parents are often so anxious about what they imagine you'll be telling them, and how it may establish their long feared notion that they are responsible for their child's problems, that it is usually best to allow them to ventilate first by bringing you up to date on developments since they last met with you.

If this is not done, and sometimes even if it is, the parents' anxiety often remains at such a high pitch that they are unable to be attentive to your discussion of their child's problems, and they will continually interrupt — often asking seemingly irrelevant questions which really reflect their immediate concern, i.e., are they responsible? A discussion of the dynamics and evaluation of the child's problems in words that are palatable and understandable to the parents is then often helpful.

The results of the other tests performed as part of the evaluation, both negative and positive, should be reviewed within the limits of the parents' understanding, tolerance and good supportive technique. The extent to which one can elaborate on the etiology of the disturbance varies greatly, but the parents should be given an honest evaluation of the child's situation, whether it involves minimal impairment of the central nervous system or some degree of mental retardation or both. In almost all cases, however, it is usually best to leave the parents with the distinct impression that their child's problem was not caused by factors that they had control over. If it seems appropriate at this time, the therapist may even want to indicate to the parents that he had the feeling that they had felt responsible for a long time for causing the child's problem and that he's very happy to be able to relieve them of this burden.

The therapist can then focus on how this malady, usually present since birth, has affected the growth and development of the child, and it is often helpful to cite examples from the history in the parent's own words to verify these effects. In addition to pointing out how it has made growing up so much more difficult for the child, the therapist should also point out how this has naturally affected the child's relationship with the parents, and how it has immensely increased the demands made upon them as parents. One can empathize with the parents because of the constant drain the child's problems has put on the parents' time, energy and resources, often while the parents received little in the way of positive feedback via the child's emotional responses and progressive maturation. The therapist is usually then in a position to impress upon the parents that, even though their child has problems and they are serious ones, this does not mean that the child can't be helped.

The therapist must emphasize that the child needs a great deal of extra help and every reasonable effort must be made to afford him this help at this time. This aspect of the discussion is equally as important as the therapist's attempts to relieve the parents' intense guilt and anxiety, because it undercuts the parents' conscious and unconscious attempts to attribute all of the child's problems to the mental retardation. When this happens, the negative side of the parents' ambivalence toward the child tends to take over and they may feel that the die is cast and that there is little they can do to remedy the situation. Therefore, it is extremely important to focus on the child's immediate problems and stress to the parents their responsibilities in attempting to help their child master his handicaps now.

After solid relationships are formed with the parents, they can be further educated about the nature of their child's malady and advised about how they can better and more reasonably deal with the child's impulsiveness and disruptive behavior. Moreover, specific suggestions can be made to the parents as to how they can actively support the child's special school program and help their child better utilize his free time in constructively mastering his deficits. At these counseling sessions, discussion can include such things as encouraging the child to work with scissors or squeeze a hard rubber ball to improve fine motor coordination of his hands; having the child examine pictures of himself in various positions and encouraging him to investigate his body in the mirror may help to improve body image; teaching the parents how to utilize the child's various senses at the same time, such as visual, auditory and tactile, in teaching him letters and numbers and the meaning of words.

This type of activity does not have to be an impingement on the child's free time or play time at all, since there are numerous ingenious ways of combining this work with play. The game "Simon says" and the dance called the "Hokey Pokey" are really very enjoyable ways for a child to learn his right from his left, up from down, and in from out. The use of cards in the game "Concentration" can be a most enjoyable manner of improving a child's attentiveness and ability to concentrate. Moreover, this type of interaction can offer the added benefits of improving the child's interpersonal relationship with parents and peers and can also help him to develop a competitive spirit, which is so often lacking in these children. If the toys and games utilized are carefully chosen and in tune with the child's functioning psychosexual level of development, they may stimulate further personality growth and aid the child in mastering his emotional and conflictual problems.

Special Training and Education.   The medical coordinator should have a thorough knowledge of what special educational and vocational facilities are available in his area. Actual visits to these resources are highly desirable whenever possible, for they give a much clearer picture of what each facility is equipped to do, as well as provide an opportunity for the medical coordinator to begin to establish a relationship with the authorities there. He will doubtlessly have need for future contact with these people, both in the continuing evaluation of the child's overall treatment program, and for consultation with the school authorities regarding the establishment and maintenance of an academic program which will best meet with all the child's needs.

In most parts of the country the demand for service is much greater than the supply of special academic facilities, especially if one is dealing with a family of low to moderate income. With these children, the greatest part of the load falls upon the shoulders of the public school authorities, and although special classes are maintained for the retarded educable, retarded trainable, and brain-damaged children, in most cases the number of available seats cannot approach the number of children needing special attention. More often than not, child psychiatric coverage or services are not utilized with these classes. This is probably as much a result of the lack of availability of talented child psychiatrists as it is of conditions within the school system.

This is another important service that the child psychiatrist can offer to retarded children, i.e., to serve as a consultant to the public and private school systems. Through his guidance and influence, more appropriate class placement for these children could be accomplished with subsequent better utilization of an individual teacher's talents; in the long run, more effective utilization of school funds could result. Again, the need to meet each impaired child's individual needs by introducing workable variations of standard teaching techniques should be emphasized.

In addition to having a thorough knowledge of the special academic facilities available for the mentally retarded in his area, it is very important that the medical coordinator also be familiar with other community resources which might be of service to him in planning the child's therapeutic program. Such programs as those of the Big Brothers of America, the Boy Scouts and Girl Scouts, and summer camps can be immensely helpful in stimulating and supporting further growth and development. Tutoring services can offer an exceptionally good growth experience for the child, especially if the tutor is advised of some of the child's special academic needs by the medical coordinator. A tutor can offer the child a warm, friendly, understanding interpersonal relationship as well as specific help with his academic problems.

The medical coordinator should see the child intermittently, perhaps every six to eight weeks, to maintain a personal, continuing familiarity with the child's progress. This would enable him to institute whatever modifications in the program become necessary either because of the child's progression to a higher level of functioning or because of the child's failure to respond to the techniques presently being used.

In addition to the medical coordinator's own estimate of the effectiveness of the program set up for a child, periodic neurological examinations and psychological testing would be helpful in delineating which parts of the program may need reinforcement or modification.

A child psychiatrist may also be involved in the management of mentally retarded children as a consultant to residential institutions. Again, a careful appraisal of the past history as well as the present situation is the best approach, whether in attempting to evaluate an application for admission or an acute upset in a resident student, or in placing a long-standing institutional policy under scrutiny. The services the child psychiatrist or psychologist can best render are similar to those he offers a child and his family on an outpatient basis. The main difference is that he is dealing with the institution's staff instead of the child's parents.

Educating the staff—especially those who are directly in charge of the students, such as child care workers, counselors, houseparents and teachers—regarding the normal growth and development of children, as well as pathological aberrations, is essential. This information must be put in understandable as well as acceptable form for them. Such information is of immense value not only in educating these core, front-line institutional personnel, but in helping them to be more empathic with the children through learning about how the child's present predicament evolved.

Staff education, to a large degree, reduces tendencies to look upon the child's present behavior, or indeed, the child himself, as being "bad," "evil," "naughty," "spoiled" or "impossible." Many of these children already feel that they are "bad" or "evil," and that it was their "badness" that brought about their present maladies. These feelings constantly eat away at their self-esteem and the therapist must use all techniques possible to counteract them. All institutional workers, as well as parents, should strike the word "bad" from their vocabularies when dealing with mentally retarded and brain-damaged children. Instead, such words as "not helpful," "not desirable," or "upset" should be used.

Coordinated Staff Evaluation and Therapy.   When the child psychiatrist or psychologist working in an institution for the retarded is asked to evaluate a child and the problems he is presenting, the psychiatrist must realize that, in most instances, he is not dealing with an acute situation. Although certain, immediate shifts he might make in the child's routine may relieve the pressures which led to the request for consultation, he usually can offer more. The best approach is a careful evaluation of the child, including perusal of past history, houseparents' reports, and medical records; current discussions with houseparents, child-care workers and counselors regarding their present concerns for the child; discussions with the child's teachers; and, of course, interviews with the child.

To gather all this necessary information to allow him to arrive at a dynamic formulation of the child's problems, it is often very helpful to request a "staffing" on the child. All professional and nonprofessional personnel who come in contact with the child, or who should be involved in the evaluation, should be invited to contribute freely to the discussion. Such a "staffing" needs structure for best results, and the best format for order of presentation includes: a summary of the past history as gathered by the child psychiatrist or social worker; the current history presented by the child care workers and in an academic report; a medical report; a social service report; psychological testing; and psychiatric interviews. The latter two reports should be withheld until the end, for if these presentations are made early in the "staffing," they tend to intimidate others' views, and one may not get a true impression of the way key personnel feel about the child and how they visualize his behavior.

Out of such a "staffing" should come a "prescription," individualized to meet the child's needs while remaining within the framework of what the institution is able to provide. Besides recommending shifts in the use of medications, environmental changes (such as encouraging more contact from the child's home, or a change in work assignment) and further studies that should be carried out, the prescription must include specific, *workable,* therapeutic suggestions to the teachers and child care workers regarding the management of the child. These suggestions should stem naturally from the explanation of the dynamics involved and most often, as is the case with parents, it is most helpful to utilize recent incidents, as related by the child care worker himself, in describing how a child might best be managed and why. Such a "staffing" can be completed in approximately one and a half hours. Although it is often costly in both money and time, if properly run, such a staffing will pay great dividends not only for the child involved but for the institution—by giving education, training and support to its staff.

In addition to these "staffings," it is most helpful, productive and enlightening to meet with groups of child care workers for "troubleshooting" sessions regarding the overall functioning of children under their care. Such meetings, especially if held at least weekly, allow opportunities to give continuous education and support to the staff, and permit the psychiatrist or psychologist to follow through with and make modifications in the "prescriptions," arranged for in the "staffings" held on children.

Although most mentally retarded children are not candidates for intensive psychotherapy, it should not be implied that these children are not often in need of a one-to-one relationship. Quite to the contrary, many mentally retarded children, especially those who are institutionalized, are in need of a supportive, therapeutic relationship. However, because of his intellectual and ego deficits, the retarded child is often severely handicapped in developing insight into his emotional problems, or even the therapeutic relationship necessary to bring about such insight. Therefore, at the Elwyn Institute, we recognized that the need for supportive counseling was great, but we did not feel that this counseling required the direct participation of a psychiatrist. Indeed, since such an effort would be poor utilization of the time of a person trained to do intensive, insightful psychotherapy, we began a "counseling pool."

This "pool" consisted of staff members from various departments of the institution who had the time, desire and necessary maturity and emotional adjustment to meet with a child, usually on a weekly basis. These persons would be asked to write a summary after each of their counseling sessions with the child, and the counselor would then meet with a psychiatrist from our staff once a month to discuss the meetings and receive suggestions on how to proceed. Through such a program, we were able to provide, under direct psychiatric supervision, high-level counseling to many children with a great variety of emotional problems, with little increase in cost to the institution.

I am not sure how such a program might be instituted for children seen on an outpatient basis, although a similar program has worked quite admirably with tutors and school counselors. However, some organizations, including the Bureau of Vocational Rehabilitation (which, by and large, provides outstanding services for the handicapped), presently provide psychiatric services to many retarded individuals and pay average psychiatric fees. It is certainly apparent that if psychiatric consultation and supervision of counseling services which provide supportive, therapeutic relationships were utilized instead, these organizations could provide equally adequate service on a broader basis and for less money.

REFERENCES

Management of Psychiatric Complications of Mental Retardation

1. Danielson, F. A., and Davenport, C. B.: The Hill Folk; Report on a Rural Community of Hereditary Defectives. Eugenic Record Office Memoir, No. 1. Cold Spring Harbor, R.I., 1912.
2. Down, J. L. H.: Observations on an Ethnic Classification of Idiots. London Hospital Reports, 1866, 3, 25. J. Ment. Sci., *12*:121-123, 1867.
3. Dugdale, R. L.: The Jukes. New York, Putnam, 1877.
4. Estabrook, A. H., and Davenport, C. B.: The Nam Family; A Study in Cacogenics, Eugenics Record Office Memoir, No. 2. Cold Spring Harbor, R.I., 1912.
5. Goddard, H. H.: The Kallikak Family; A Study in the Heredity of Feeblemindedness. New York, Macmillan, 1912.
6. Itard, J.: The Wild Boy of Aveyron, translated by G. and M. Humphrey; New York, Appleton-Century-Crofts, 1962.
7. Järger, J.: Die Familie Zero. Arch. f. Rassen-u Gesellschaftsbiofogie, *2*:494-559, 1905.
8. Jervis, G. A.: The Mental Deficiencies. American Handbook of Psychiatry, Vol II, 1959, pp. 1289-1314.
9. Kanner, L.: A History of the Care and Study of the Mentally Retarded. Springfield, Illinois, Charles C Thomas, 1964.
10. Kolansky, H.: An Overview of Child Psychiatry. Journal of the Albert Einstein Medical Center, Volume 16, Autumn, 1968.
11. Kolansky, H., and Stennis, W.: Focus of Training in Child Psychiatry, Journal of the Albert Einstein Medical Center, Volume 16, Spring, 1968.
12. Mahler, M. S. Discussion remarks to papers by Anna Freud and Ernst Kris. Symposium on Problems of Child Development, Stockbridge, Mass. Psychoanal. Stud. Child, Vol. 6, 1951.
13. Mahler, M. S.: On Child Psychosis and Schizophrenia, Autistic and Symbiotic Infantile Psychoses. Psychoanal. Stud. Child, *7*:286-305, 1952.
14. Moore, K. L., and Barr, M. L.: Smears from the Oral Mucosa in the Detection of Chromosomal Sex. Lancet, *2*:57, 1955.
15. Sachs, B. A.: Family Form of Idiocy, Generally Fatal, Associated with Early Blindness. J. Nerv. Ment. Dis., *23*:475-479, 1896.
16. Tay, W.: Symmetrical Changes in the Region of the Yellow Spot in Each Eye of an Infant. Transact. of the Ophthalmol. Society of London. 1881, pp. 1, 55.
17. Telfer, M. A., Clark, G. R., Baker, D., Richardson, C. E., and Schmauder, E.: Diagnosis of Gross Chromosomal Errors in Institutional Populations. Penna. Psych. Quarterly, No. 4, Vol. 7, 1968.
18. Tjio, J. H., and Levon, A.: The Chromosome Number of Man. Hereditas, *42*:1, 1956.

REHABILITATION OF THE PSYCHIATRICALLY IMPAIRED

by Edward Teitelman

Although the physiatrist, general practitioner or allied health worker in physical medicine will not usually be involved *directly* with the rehabilitation of psychiatric patients, his understanding and support can often be of great importance. An increased awareness of this aspect of rehabilitation may also allow referral of patients at an earlier stage of disability, when change can be effected more easily and with less residual of social and psychological damage.

Consideration of the topic might best be approached by first reviewing three cases which represent the range of problems as well as some of the techniques currently available.

Case 1. *Mr. B.* was referred for psychiatric evaluation by the State Rehabilitation Service. Because of severe anxiety, he was having increasing difficulty working at a relatively simple job. This had become almost paralyzing when his wife left him about a month earlier. Interview revealed that he had remained in his current job for seven years because he was so preoccupied with mistrust and jealousy of his wife that he needed isolation and low pressure at work to allow time to phone her frequently and "worry." His demands upon her had eventually led to the separation. Other relationships, especially with his father, were seen also to reinforce his longstanding insecurity. However, Mr. B. not only seemed to have resources that, when mobilized, would get him through his current difficulties, but also gave promise of a more productive future if some of his neuroses were resolved. After evaluation, the Rehabilitation Service agreed to sponsor treatment.

A limited course of psychotherapy (25 sessions) and the initial use of an anti-anxiety medication, fluphenazine hydrochloride (Prolixin, 2 mg. a day), comprised the treatment. During the course of therapy his symptoms gradually disappeared, and he became reconciled with his wife. At the end of the treatment he had attained some clarification of feelings and conflicts and some understanding of his neurotic defensive patterns.

No further psychiatric treatment was considered necessary. However, he had expressed a lifelong desire to work as a bricklayer, and it was felt such employment would not only strengthen his sense of self-esteem, but would more nearly match his capacities. The Rehabilitation Service subsequently sponsored his training. He has now been two years in his new work, enjoys it and has had no need for further medication or psychiatric contact.

Case 2.   *Mrs. S.*, mother of two school-aged children, is a young housewife, who experienced her second schizophrenic psychosis. After a six-week hospitalization, she was improved enough for discharge but remained unable to concentrate and was frightened by the responsibility of caring for her house and children. She also was beset with strong impulses to get deeply involved again with what had been a frustrating experience attempting to sell mutual funds; these impulses in turn resulted in feelings of guilt about "not wanting to stay at home."

As there was no real reason why she had to be at home all of the time, and work did provide her with real satisfaction and a sense of importance, treatment was directed toward getting her comfortable enough for a realistic part-time job. With continued medication and weekly supportive psychotherapy, she gradually became well enough to begin working as a Red Cross Volunteer. She found satisfaction with the work and was better able to deal with her home responsibilities, but still did not want to risk the more intensive pressures of a paid position.

However, she stopped taking her medications because she "felt so good," and after a month suffered a mild relapse. Return to medication and prompt placement in a Day Care Program resulted in return to her prior level of adjustment after several more months. She subsequently took a part-time retail sales position which, although "not as exciting as mutual funds," seemed more realistic and stabilizing, and was in fact quite satisfying to her. With continued administration of trifluoperazine hydrochloride (Stelazine, 15 mg. per day) and monthly supportive psychotherapy, she has remained in remission, functioning at a fairly high level at home, at work and in the community.

Case 3.   *Mr. Q.* has had ten psychiatric hospitalizations since age 17 when he first showed a paranoid psychosis. Now 30 years of age, he has never been in the community for longer than five months between hospitalizations, which have lasted up to two years in length. After his most recent hospitalization he was sent to the day program of a Psychiatric Rehabilitation Center. He was severely regressed socially, with no vocational skills and extremely unsure of himself.

He gradually got involved with the program of the Center. This included workshop experience, group counseling, and education in such areas of individual living as shopping, food preparation and budgeting. Because his parents, with whom he had lived, tended to infantilize him, he was encouraged to move into the Center's residence, and later into an apartment which he obtained with another client. He continued on chlorpromazine (400 mg. of Thorazine per day) and was seen for brief interviews at a Community Mental Health Center monthly.

After about ten months in the program, he found a job in a stockroom of a factory, and continues working there after 18 months. He has remained in contact with the Center through its evening social program and still receives maintenance medication through the Mental Health Center. He recently obtained his high school diploma following attendance at night school. He is quiet, does not venture much, and is still uncertain in interpersonal relationships, but is considered to be in stable remission — in a useful and relatively independent situation in the community.

As these cases suggest, psychiatric illness often involves a chronic pattern of maladaptation in addition to the acute condition which may require immediate attention or bring the patient for treatment. Even in seemingly healthier persons there is often a hidden disability: the patient usually has limited his life in various ways to avoid anxiety or conflict. Sometimes dependence on alcohol or drugs has developed as an effort at self treatment, or vocational or interpersonal expectations have been lowered. In persons who have suffered more severe disruptions, as in psychosis, this avoidance of psychic pain often results in marked withdrawal from meaningful interpersonal relationships. A cycle may come into operation in which withdrawal leads to social or vocational failure, lowering self-esteem further, and leading to still more chronic withdrawal.

The pessimistic attitude toward mental illness which persisted from 1850 until the past several decades often reinforced disability by adding a social breakdown syndrome to the preexisting illness. A mutually dependent interaction between patient and staff intensified the protective withdrawal of the sick person and allowed no chance to restore social resources. This syndrome led to the apathetic, untidy, dilapidated, unresponsive creature we traditionally associate with the back wards of custodial care institutions.

Recently, especially with the introduction of effective antipsychotic medications in the 1950's, there has been a rediscovery of the importance of social expectation and manner of approach in the minimizing of disability from mental illness. Essentially this marks a return to the effective philosophy of the early nineteenth century mental hospitals, often called Moral Treatment, which involved a high level of expectation of normal behavior in a supportive humane social setting. The importance of work and social interaction was realized and value was placed upon healthy behavior rather than fulfillment of a role as "mentally sick." The difficulty of transition from the shelter of the hospital to the demands of the "normal" world was appreciated and the return to the community facilitated with halfway houses and frequent visits home prior to discharge. A return to the real therapeutic involvement, if not the specific institutions, of this earlier period, has probably been the major phenomenon in psychiatry in recent years. Unfortunately, this movement has not yet fully penetrated many chronically understaffed and underfunded state facilities and, for this reason, secondary iatrogenic disability must still be dealt with all too often.

The return to therapeutic enthusiasm has led to development of a number of rehabilitation services, some of which were illustrated in the cases presented. Although medication and psychotherapy still remain central to psychiatric treatment, it is now realized that they are not sufficient by themselves to deal with the moderately or severely disabled. Thus the psychiatrist evaluating such a disabled patient must not only determine that patient's positive and negative psychological resources, but must also determine the treatment resources available in the community. Thus he will attempt to bring into play all appropriate programs to achieve the quickest and most complete rehabilitation or to keep disability to a minimum in the more acute processes. Most programs are not directly medical in orientation and problems with communication must be anticipated.

Application of high expectation programs in many inpatient facilities, use of new techniques such as operant conditioning with severely regressed patients, and fiscal pressure to keep public hospital populations down have led to release into the community of large numbers of severely disabled persons who are able to survive outside the hospital but unable to do so with any great success or ease.

Also contributing to the shift out of hospitals has been the sometimes unrealistically arbitrary goal of treating patients "at home in the community" — tragic, when, as is often the case, there is a severe lack of community treatment resources. Thus, especially stimulated by the growing population of disabled outside of hospitals, much recent effort has been directed toward establishment of a variety of options for treatment, ranging from simple outpatient psychotherapy to full-time inpatient hospitalization.

For those requiring some of the advantages of a hospital setting, day hospitals have been most beneficial. These provide formal medical and psychiatric attention, although they are less institutional than conventional hospitals, and allow the patient to spend a large part of his time at home and on his own.

Night hospital, or weekend care programs, are variations of the partial hospitalization concept, especially useful when patients are fully employed but can benefit from the additional support of periods of residential care.

Halfway houses, with or without therapy programs, as well as boardinghouses or foster homes catering to former mental patients, have also grown increasingly in variety and numbers.

Probably the most unique of these institutions is the psychiatric rehabilitation center. By 1970 there were some 40 such agencies in the United States; Fountain House in New York City, established in 1948, is probably the earliest and most widely known. Like most of these organizations, Fountain House grew out of the initiative of former hospital patients who initially simply wanted a place to socialize and relax. Gradually more formal programs developed for what was clearly a clientele with multiple problems, so that today the agency offers such services as counseling, education and vocational training and placement.

Fountain House pioneered with an interesting Transitional Employment program, in which employers such as restaurants and banks designate one or more of their regular jobs for Fountain House. Instead of working in a sheltered workshop, clients begin on these jobs on a less than full-time basis, with several clients filling a given position during the day. They are supervised by a Fountain House counselor and receive support and guidance from him, but gain their confidence and work skills in a reality setting.

Horizon House, established in Philadelphia in 1953, has a somewhat more conventional workshop program, but has combined it with a high expectation multidisciplinary approach in which advancement is stressed with a time-limited, phased program. Closely integrated with direct client service is a research and evaluation unit, which is attempting to gather information that is so generally lacking in this field. A small experimental program for those too disabled to make progress in the regular program has also recently been added. In all cases, these agencies stress a non-institutional setting with an orientation that attempts to combine the warmth and understanding of a home with the colder, more formal, expectation of the industrial or commercial world.

Special rehabilitation programs for such disabilities as drug or alcohol dependence have also multiplied in recent years. These frequently are oriented around multidisciplined therapeutic teams. As in the general field of psychiatric rehabilitation, the number of treatment facilities is woefully inadequate for the need, and our level of expertise is far short of what is required for really effective care.

Although statistics in the psychiatric rehabilitation field are neither extensive nor especially sophisticated, there is reasonable evidence of the value of the programs of the psychiatric rehabilitation centers. Twelve month follow-ups on unselected patients discharged from state mental hospitals indicate that about 40 per cent are rehospitalized within a year with conventional follow-up techniques. Figures from Horizon House, Fountain House and Hill House (Cleveland, Ohio) show a hospital readmission rate of about 30 per cent for their clients during the same post-hospital period. In a recent (1970) six month follow-up at Horizon House, 55 per cent of patients graduating from the program were employed and none were rehospitalized, while only 13 per cent of persons who had dropped out of the program were working and 24 per cent were rehospitalized. These figures show how poorly even the best of our current rehabilitation efforts cope with the multiple needs and limitations of the psychiatrically disabled. They do suggest that we are moving in the right direction, but it is likely that dramatic gains in the field must await vastly better provision of psychiatric care than currently it seems realistic to expect. Ultimately, real advances in the field will come only with increased understanding of the mechanisms—social, psychological and chemical—of psychiatric illness itself.

REFERENCES

Rehabilitation of the Psychiatrically Impaired

1. Fountain House Foundation, Inc.: Two Year Report, 1967 and 1968, New York, 1969.
2. Hyde, R. W., Bockoven, J. S., Pfautz, H. W., and York, R. H.: Milieu Rehabilitation. Butler Health Center, Providence, R.I., 1962.
3. Rothwell, N. D., and Doniger, J. M.: The Halfway House. In Masserman, J. H. (ed.): Current Psychiatric Therapies—1965. New York, Grune & Stratton, Inc. 1965, pp. 240–246.
4. Rutman, I., and Loeb, A.: Comprehensive, Community-Based Rehabilitation Services for the Psychiatrically Disabled—Final Report, July, 1970. Horizon House, Philadelphia, 1970.
5. Silverstein, M.: Psychiatric Aftercare. Philadelphia, University of Pennsylvania Press, 1968.
6. Sinnett, E., and Sachson, A. (ed.): Transitional Facilities in the Rehabilitation of the Emotionally Disturbed. Lawrence, Kansas, University of Kansas Press, 1970.
7. Zusman, J.: Some Explanations of the Changing Appearance of Psychotic Patients. Int. J. Psychiat., 3:216–247, 1967.

CONCLUSION

Specialists working with the psychiatric rehabilitation of the physically disabled are most frequently centered in a physical medicine and rehabilitation hospital or hospital wing or private health agency. Those working with the psychiatrically impaired are usually associated with progressive public and private psychiatric hospitals, private health agencies and halfway houses.

Rehabilitation services for the mentally retarded can be found in institutions for the mentally retarded, private health agencies and newly formed special clinics within many pediatric departments. The United States Social and Rehabilitation Service with its associated state offices has been instrumental in stimulating services in all three areas. Also, with the development of community mental health centers, more and more impetus can be anticipated at the local community level. Finally, a small number of private practitioners are pioneering in rehabilitation psychiatry as an unofficial psychiatric subspecialty, but one which is destined to become integrated into the full range of services offered to all persons in need.

Part IV

BASIC CONSIDERATIONS
OF IMPORTANCE IN
TOTAL REHABILITATION

Chapter 39

REHABILITATION OF THE BLIND

WHAT PHYSICIANS AND OTHER REHABILITATION SCIENTISTS SHOULD KNOW, IN GENERAL, REGARDING PERSONS WHO ARE BLIND OR VISUALLY HANDICAPPED

by Robert C. Goodpasture

It is somewhat ironic that so little is known by the general practicing physician, as well as by the layman, about blindness and the rehabilitation of blind persons. Few physical ailments have been more widely studied in the history of mankind than has blindness. Starting in the earliest days of civilization, society has evidenced a special sympathy and concern for those who are blind. From biblical days to the present, blind people have been a source of concern for all and an object of charity for most.

In spite of these facts, there continues to be much misunderstanding regarding the rehabilitation potential of blind persons, even on the part of medically trained specialists. However, a cadre of specialists has developed throughout the world with rehabilitation of the blind as its special concern. In many ways, the United States has been a forerunner of this new professionalism in service to blind persons. As a result, in the United States extensive facilities and talent are now available to the physician as he contemplates the problems of a blind patient. In this chapter, an effort will be made to catalogue the wide range of services that can be utilized in the evaluation of problems of the blind, and in their resolution. The most reliable sources of information that can be called upon will be listed. It is not the intention here to explain the complexities of blindness or how the blind person should be approached by the physician. There are abundant local resources available for consultation on these matters.

CHARACTER AND EXTENT OF BLINDNESS

To most people, the word "blind" seems to connote complete inability to see. "Blind" and "sightless" are frequently interpreted as synonymous. In reality, however, the legal definition of blindness does not necessarily preclude some ability to see. A number of federal laws relating to subsidized services to blind persons are predicated upon compliance with this legal definition in order to establish client eligibility. Most states have patterned their definition of blindness upon that used by the federal government.

The most widely accepted definition of "blind" is "a person having visual acuity not to exceed 20/200 in the better eye with correcting lenses, or visual acuity greater than 20/200 but with a limitation in the fields of vision such that the widest diameter of the visual field subtends an angle no greater than 20 degrees."* Under this definition, a blind person can have sufficient vision with corrective lenses to make it possible to distinguish size, shape and color, and even to read large print.

Professionals in the field generally agree that there are also some persons who do not meet the legal definition of blindness but who are effectively "visually handicapped" from a social and vocational standpoint. As a consequence, many agencies and programs which serve blind persons also cater to the visually handicapped and, in some instances, the names of these agencies and programs incorporate the term "visually handicapped."†

The National Society for the Prevention of Blindness, New York, estimates that 400,000 American citizens are within the legal definition of blindness. This figure must be considered a rough approximation, as many persons are embarrassed or otherwise hesitant to acknowledge their blindness or the blindness of someone in their immediate family. Even though such factors are taken into consideration in the preparation of estimates, it is still important to emphasize that precise figures on blindness are not available.

The extent of visual impairment is even more difficult to assess fully. Leading national agencies, such as the Department of Health, Education and Welfare, and the American Foundation for the Blind, endeavor to estimate the number of persons with visual impairment in order that various service programs can be adequately financed and staffed. The consensus of these and other agencies, as well as experienced professionals in the field, tends to confirm that another 600,000 Americans suffer some degree of handicap as a result of deficient sight.

It is startling to discover that many well-educated, experienced and enlightened persons carry gross misapprehensions regarding blindness. These misconceptions vary from the extreme of believing that it is a contagious disease to social rejection of the blind as physically unattractive. The fact is that blind

---

*Paragraph 51–1. 1(a), Code of Federal Regulations, Title 41 — Public Contracts and Property Management.

†As an example, the Virginia Commission for the Visually Handicapped, Richmond, Virginia. This state-owned agency is the principal vehicle through which blind persons in Virginia receive a broad range of evaluation, training and rehabilitation services.

persons are no different from nonblind persons—except that they happen to be blind. Some are brilliant, some are dull. Some pleasant, some not. By virtue of blindness a person does not develop other physical or mental impairments. The blind person's principal problem, in addition to his visual impairment, is often the reaction of his fellow man toward him and his problem.

According to the National Society for the Prevention of Blindness, the incidence of blindness averages 2.14 per 1000 of population. This figure varies from one section of the nation to another: the State of Hawaii has an estimated rate of 3.98 and the comparable figure for Utah is 1.39. The absolute number of blind persons in the United States is steadily increasing due, in large part, to the fact that blindness is predominantly a problem of age. As medicine and science extend man's life, they create more elderly persons vulnerable to certain causes of blindness.

Although approximately 40 per cent of the United States population is under 21 years of age, only 10 per cent of the blind population is in this age category. Conversely, about half of the blind persons in the United States are at least 65 years of age.

CAUSES OF BLINDNESS

According to the National Society for the Prevention of Blindness, the three most prevalent causes of blindness are cataract, glaucoma and diabetes. Almost 40 per cent of all blindness is the result of one of these. The balance of known causes includes (but is not limited to) injuries, poisoning and infectious diseases such as syphilis.

Cataracts are the largest single cause of blindness. Although they can develop in young persons, they are directly connected with the aging process and, in varying degree, are the most common form of blindness among "senior citizens." Fortunately, this problem can be remedied through surgery, and the success rate for such operations is very high.

Whereas cataracts cause blindness by making the lens more opaque, it is through damage to the retina and the optic nerve that glaucoma blinds. The damage is caused by increased pressure in the fluid within the eye. The damage is not reparable, and since it is a slowly developing and generally painless process, it often catches its victim unawares. Therefore, regular eye examinations are highly recommended for persons over 40. Once detected, the glaucoma can usually be contained.

Cataracts and glaucoma account for about 30 per cent of all blindness. Approximately 12 per cent is attributable to diabetes; in these cases there is usually damage of one form or another to the retina. The exact causes of this deterioration are not known.

SPECIAL SERVICES AVAILABLE

Federal and State Governments

The Department of Health, Education and Welfare (HEW) has, within the Rehabilitation Services Administration, a Division of Services to the Blind. This office is the focal point at the federal level for both the development of information relating to blindness and also the establishment and implementation of most subsidy programs through which the federal government assists in the resolution of problems of the blind and the extension of services to blind persons throughout the nation.

The Division of Services to the Blind is by no means the only federal office concerned with and active in the rehabilitation of blind persons. HEW's Office of Research, Demonstration and Training frequently finances grants relating to blindness. Other departments of the government are participants in the national effort to resolve problems of blindness. The Library of Congress has a Division for the Blind which compiles and distributes a variety of reading matter through disc records, tapes, braille and large type print. Special record players are furnished by the government at no cost. This office also is a focal point for generalized information relating to blindness and other physical handicaps, and can be very helpful in directing inquiries to other proper sources of information.

Every state in the nation provides specialized services to blind persons, the cost of which is shared by the state and federal governments. Federal allotments per state are determined by population and per capita income. In about three quarters of the states, responsibility for this program is vested with a special Division of Services to the Blind. Elsewhere, it generally rests with the state Division of Vocational Rehabilitation. In either case, there is clear responsibility at the state level for various forms of services to blind persons. Both the quality and extent of these services vary widely throughout the country. A list of some of the types of services offered at the state level is shown below:

Types of State Agency Services
Child education
Evaluation
Parent counseling
Personal adjustment
Placement services
Physical restoration
Reader services
Transportation
Vocational counseling

National Agencies

Functioning on a national basis are several important private non-profit agencies, whose goals are to help improve services to blind persons and to expand the technology and literature devoted to this important field. Since blindness has for so many centuries been a special cause of concern for mankind, it has spawned many kinds of private agencies. The variety and range of character of the national private agencies is extensive. There has evolved also a degree of independence among these agencies and, in certain instances, a lack of clear definition of areas of responsibility and adequate coordination of programs. Notwithstanding these facts, there remain some generally recognized areas of function and influence.

American Association of Workers for the Blind (AAWB).   This is the principal national association of professionals and lay persons who serve the blind people of this nation. The AAWB was established in 1895 and through its 75-year history has been the sponsor of many important new programs for the blind. Its level of influence has varied considerably. At the present time it is in a period of resurgence, partly because of a move to decentralization, which includes the sponsorship of state chapters and regional meetings. The AAWB maintains a headquarters office at 1511 K Street, N. W., Washington, D. C. 20005. Inquiries may be directed there regarding any and all matters relating to blindness and the correspondent can rest assured that he will be referred to a reliable source if the information is not immediately available at AAWB.

American Foundation for the Blind (AFB). The American Foundation for the Blind was established in 1921 and has its headquarters at 15 West 16th Street, New York, N. Y. 10011. This organization enjoyed and prospered from intimate association with Helen Keller and it became, in time, a respected advocate of the blind person and a successful sponsor of his needs. AFB has a sizable staff, including field representatives located throughout the nation. Consultation is provided to state and local agencies on virtually all facets of service programs to the blind. AFB is also an important research resource and it has pioneered in the development of numerous types of aids and appliances for blind persons. AFB maintains an extensive library on blindness and can be an indispensable source of information, guidance and help.

American Printing House for the Blind. The American Printing House, at 1839 Frankfort Avenue, Louisville, Kentucky 40206, is the world's largest publisher of books for the blind. It is subsidized, in part, by the federal government and in its 112-year history has become a giant among the organizations which most effectively serve the nation's blind.

Association of Educators of the Visually Handicapped (AEVH). This association brings together persons who serve as instructors and teachers of the blind. Its primary focus is on educational programs and techniques designed to serve the particular needs of blind students. The AEVH has its national office at 1604 Spruce Street, Philadelphia, Pennsylvania 19103. It sponsors national meetings on an annual basis and it is periodically involved in the promotion of local and regional gatherings of its members.

National Accreditation Council (NAC). Considering the lengthy history of service programs for blind persons, it is surprising that a program of standards and accreditation was not forthcoming until the decade of the 1960's. However, that is the fact. At a very recent date, primarily through the joint efforts of the American Foundation for the Blind and the Department of Health, Education and Welfare, a Commission on Standards and Accreditation was established. The Commission (generally referred to as COMSTAC) produced an excellent set of standards to use in evaluating service programs for blind persons. Subsequently, the National Accreditation Council of Agencies Serving the Blind and Visually Handicapped (NAC) was incorporated as COMSTAC's successor, and for more than three years it has been actively involved in the accreditation of agencies throughout the country. It is generally believed that, in due time, NAC accreditation will be a necessary prerequisite to the development of community support, the implementation of fund-raising programs and the receipt of subsidies from state and federal governments. Inquiries regarding accreditation and accredited agencies can be directed to the National Accreditation Council, 79 Madison Avenue, New York, N. Y. 10016.

National Industries for the Blind (NIB). National Industries for the Blind is primarily concerned with evaluation of the vocational potential of blind persons and their subsequent training and employment. NIB serves as an association headquarters for a group of 80 special facilities, which are frequently referred to as "sheltered workshops." These facilities are operated either by states or by local non-profit corporations and they provide, among other services, remunerative employment opportunities for the blind. NIB has a staff of over 100 persons which provides technical help and consultation in connection with problems of finance, marketing, vocational rehabilitation, engineering, product development, quality control and other matters normally connected with an industrial business operation. NIB has its headquarters at 50 West 44th Street, New York, N. Y. 10036, and maintains branch offices in four other cities, including Washington, D.C.

National Society for the Prevention of Blindness (NSPB).   With headquarters at 79 Madison Avenue, New York, N.Y. 10016, the NSPB is primarily concerned with studies and dissemination of information relating to the character, extent and cause of blindness. On subjects of this kind, the NSPB is widely accepted as the most reliable authority and source of data.

Local Agencies

In most of the principal cities of the nation, there is a local agency for the blind operating under a name generally indicative of the character of the organization. Perhaps the most prevalent name is Lighthouse but, in many cities, the term Association for the Blind has been adopted. If necessary, the agency can usually be traced through the classified telephone directory. An excellent source of information regarding the names, addresses and services of local agencies is a publication of the American Foundation for the Blind entitled Directory of Agencies Serving Blind Persons.

Local agencies vary greatly in the scope and quality of their services. The most comprehensive offer to the public many of the following:

Types of Agency Services

Aids and appliances	Personal management
Braille and large type books	Placement and follow-up
Communication skills	Prevocational and vocational
Consultation services to children	training
and parents	Psychological testing
Eye health	Reader services
Group work	Recreational services
Home economics	Residence for trainees
Homemakers	Talking books
Nursery school	Vending stands
Orientation and mobility	Workshop

One finds virtually any and all combinations of the above-listed services, depending upon the size of the community, the caliber and number of other related social agencies and the level of special community support engendered for blind persons.

In most instances, the local agencies are independent non-profit corporations, the trusts of which are carried by community leaders who serve as board members on a voluntary basis. The management of these agencies is the responsibility of a professional director and the subordinate staff can number anywhere from zero to 200. Fundamental to the local agency is the fact that its sole mission is service to the community and, more particularly, to the blind members of the community. As a consequence, it can be assumed that local agencies will respond to any inquiry for help.

Children's Services

In earlier times, there was a lag in the functional development of blind children owing to deprivation of experience which was then common among them. Pioneering agencies recognized this deficiency and endeavored to minimize or even overcome it. The first organized efforts toward this goal were made by special teachers who worked with the children and their parents. Principal problems faced initially by those working with blind children were the children's lack of confidence, lack of skills of daily living and lack of experience in day-to-day activity. This led to the conclusion that programs with emphasis on adjustment and training were needed in order to meet the minimum needs of the blind child.

As these problems have become better understood, a variety of special services have been developed by agencies for the blind. The resultant programs evolved through a combination of know-how and a certain amount of experimentation. They generally include the following:

Mobility

Physical usefulness and improvement of posture

Mental usefulness or the development of concrete thinking

Communication skills

Skills of personal care

Domestic science

Environmental orientation

One of the most important factors in the planning of children's services is the realization that they cannot be provided in isolation from other services to blind persons. Although the children have special problems and needs, their programs must be woven into the total fabric of the agency.

Experimentation in this area has been most successful when conducted with the knowledge and cooperation of the parents of the children and with safeguards in the form of frequent evaluation. Programs for blind children are now beginning to serve as a basis for instruction of public school teachers, school health personnel and special education teachers as well as the parents and blind children themselves. Conscientious efforts are made to present each new experience as a thoroughly enjoyable activity and not as another kind of instruction imposed upon the blind child. Such programs do not lend themselves well to large groups. Hence, there is considerable expense involved because of the high ratio of instructors to children. The agencies realize, however, that to offer children's services with insufficient school personnel or less intensity of personal contact would substantially destroy their value.

LEGISLATIVE SUPPORT

A number of federal laws have been enacted which are designed exclusively around the needs of blind persons. No other handicapped group has enjoyed the level of legislative favors extended to blind persons. Perhaps one of the most widely known of these legislative benefits is the special exemption given to blind persons in the filing of federal income tax returns. However, this is by no means the most important of these benefits. Among those which do warrant special note are the following:

Barden-LaFollette Act. The Barden-LaFollette Act of 1943 was responsible for a tremendous expansion of vocational rehabilitation programs for the handicapped. Earlier laws provided for distribution of federal funds among the states to help subsidize the rehabilitation of the disabled. However, it was not until the tragic influx of wounded veterans from World War II that rehabilitation received its most important boost.

The Barden-LaFollette provisions covered programs for blind persons and authorized administration of state plans by established "Commissions" or agencies serving blind persons. This gave new life and established new dimensions of goals for these local agencies. And through the local agencies, the contribution of the federal government has been immeasurable.

As the American Association of Workers for the Blind reported in its publication "Blindness 1966," rehabilitation services were broadened to include hospitalization, surgery and mental treatment to reduce or remove a handicapping condition. The law also provides economic maintenance to assist an individual to take advantage of other vocational services in addition to those which had been authorized by previous Acts.

The net result was an unprecedented increase in the range of rehabilitation services for blind persons and in the development of programs to place blind persons in competitive employment. Subsequent amendments only served to further extend and strengthen this important legislation.

Randolph-Sheppard Act. A 1936 statute, popularly known as the Randolph-Sheppard Act, provides to blind persons the special privilege of operating vending stands in federal buildings. There have been subsequent amendments to the basic Act, all designed to strengthen and improve its value to blind persons. The law is administered at the state level, and under this statute approximately 3341 blind persons now enjoy the status of independent proprietors through the operation of small businesses selling food, tobacco, soft goods, newspapers and magazines in public buildings. This has been an extremely popular and successful program and is reported to provide approximately $18 million of net income to blind persons each year.

Social Security Disability. The Social Security Act acknowledges the severity of the handicap of blindness by making blind persons eligible under certain conditions for disability benefits. The Social Security Administration of the Department of Health, Education and Welfare reports that approximately 30,000 blind persons and 15,000 of their dependents receive disability payments totaling $40 million per year.

Blindness alone does not qualify a person for benefits. A variety of conditions and combinations of conditions make a blind person eligible. The primary goal of this program is to provide financial assistance to a blind person who, because of his blindness, is unable to perform substantial gainful work in keeping with his age, education and work experience.

The law has special provisions for persons who become blind before the age of 31 and other provisions for blind persons who are over 55 years old. Some of the special provisions of the Act affecting blind persons are complex and each individual case is best discussed with someone intimately familiar with the program.

State-Use Laws. A number of states have passed laws patterned after the federal Wagner-O'Day Act. Under these statutes, certain requirements of the state governments are supplied by blind-made products produced by agencies within the state. These laws have been extremely popular and quite effective in providing material support to the employment of blind and handicapped persons through the broadening of markets for their products.

Wage and Hour Law. In recognition of the limited earning potential of certain severely handicapped persons, the federal government has passed a law which authorizes the payment of special statutory minimum wages. The administration of this law is the responsibility of the United States Department of Labor, which operates an Office of Handicapped Worker Problems within its Wage and Hour and Public Contracts Division. Employers of blind and other handicapped persons, whether they be private industrial firms or publicly operated "sheltered workshops," may apply to the Department of Labor for exemption certificates. If the applicant can verify that a blind person is incapable of earning the statutory minimum of $1.60 per hour, the Department of Labor will issue a certificate authorizing hourly rates of pay down to as little as 50 per cent of the statutory minimum.

In certain cases, agencies can establish "Work Activity Centers" in which blind and other handicapped persons can work under certificate rates of less than 50 per cent of the statutory minimum. These Centers are generally reserved for multi-handicapped persons, such as deaf-blind and mentally retarded blind. However, even in these settings, it has been found that many handicapped persons can benefit substantially from the experience of a work environment where other persons with similar handicaps are also trained to become as productive as they are able.

Wagner-O'Day Act. In 1938, the Congress passed a law which obligated the government to buy certain blind-made products from non-profit agencies for the blind. A presidentially appointed committee is responsible for the selection of suitable products to be included under relevant provisions of the Wagner-O'Day Act, and this committee also establishes the fair market price of these products. The government's Committee on Purchases of Blind-Made Products has, since 1938, utilized the services of National Industries for the Blind in connection with the implementation of this law. NIB is responsible for allocation of all government orders and provides a variety of other services to the Committee on a non-compensatory basis.

The Wagner-O'Day Act has helped generate employment of approximately 4500 blue-collar blind workers in 80 shops throughout the country. The value of their annual production approximates $50 million.

SCIENTIFIC ADVANCES

A marked degree of sophistication has emerged in work for the blind in the post-World War II period. This is evident in many ways, perhaps none more important than the extensive teaching of "scientific" means of travel. All major agencies now offer courses in travel training. They may vary widely in the extent to which they can be called "scientific," but, nonetheless, there is always considerable science involved. Personal independence and mobility are so fundamental to social and vocational success that this type of training is scheduled early in the rehabilitation program.

There are several techniques of cane travel and, when any of them is properly utilized, a totally blind person can move about public buildings and through city streets with complete confidence. These programs depend not only upon the effective use of the physical aid but, more importantly, upon the thoughtful use of senses other than sight. Invaluable knowledge can thereby be imparted to blind persons regarding special relationships between mobile as well as fixed objects. In addition to sound, a trained person can derive important information from vibrations of vehicular traffic, odors of plant life, predominating winds and numerous other communicators.

Although originating in pre-World War II days, the training and use of guide dogs has proliferated since the war. There are now several guide dog organizations in different parts of the nation. It is recognized that the use of guide dogs is not the best solution for all blind persons, but they serve successfully and effectively for many. They seem to be especially valuable to blind persons who are traveling by foot over constantly changing and unfamiliar routes.

Through the mid-1940's, scientific research into problems of blindness was undertaken primarily by persons and agencies directly involved in this field. The scope and the success of these efforts were somewhat modest in those days. The rising national concern for disabled World War II veterans changed this situation. Suddenly a number of federal agencies initiated new approaches and new sources of funding. Research organizations not primarily devoted to problems of blindness commenced applying their knowledge and expertise to the field.

An important new element in this Research and Development endeavor has been the involvement of universities as well as large private laboratories. In time, this produced a growing "pool" of technical talent, a portion of which became diffused throughout the professional agencies for the blind. Thus, some interesting developments resulted, such as the following:

Automated braille production as a by-product of computer technology;

Commercial adaptations of radar and sonar used in guide devices;

Compressed speech utilizing modern techniques of speech transmittal and computerized analysis.

Much of the more sophisticated work remains in the developmental stage and has had little direct impact on the average blind person. However, earlier research has produced a variety of relatively simple items which are in everyday use. They include braille calendars, labels, tags, thermometers, watches, timers, embossed paper, script-writing utensils and recreational materials such as brailled games.

Several less commonly known items are:

Braille Communicator.   This device has a keyboard similar to a typewriter. Pins are operated mechanically in a recessed spot where the person who is both deaf and blind may gently rest his finger and read the constantly changing brailled message.

Electronic Cane.   The cane has been modified with an electronic sensing device which detects steps and holes. The device measures the capacitance to the ground and transmits the information auditorily or tactilely through the handle.

Magnascope Projection Reader.   Blind persons with limited vision can use a machine which magnifies printed material to 24 times its original size. Light from a 200-watt bulb projects the text through two mirrors to a ground glass screen. The reader can manually manipulate the printed material in all directions.

Visotoner. This is a portable reading machine which scans ordinary print and transforms the letter images into tones which can be recognized and interpreted.

The present range of scientific aids is considerable, but the potential for technological advances in the field of blindness seems limitless. Local agencies and the American Foundation for the Blind are excellent sources of information regarding the status of these technological programs.

REFERENCES

Note: The following list of references is intended as recommended supplementary reading and not as a list of sources for the information in this chapter.

1. *Aids and Appliances for the Blind.* American Foundation for the Blind, New York, 1968.
2. *Blindness—Ability Not Disability.* Maxine Wood, Public Affairs Pamphlet #295A, American Foundation for the Blind, New York, 1968.
3. *Caring for the Visually Impaired Older Person.* The Minneapolis Society for the Blind, Minneapolis, Minnesota, 1970.
4. *Diabetes and Blindness, Contemporary Papers, Vol. V.* American Association of Workers for the Blind, Washington, D.C., 1969.
5. *Disability Benefits for Blind People.* U.S. Department of Health, Education and Welfare, Social Security Administration (SS1-2), April, 1969.
6. *Estimated Statistics on Blindness and Vision Problems.* The National Society for the Prevention of Blindness, New York City, 1966.
7. *Facts About Blindness.* American Foundation for the Blind, New York, 1967.
8. *If You Become Disabled.* U.S. Department of Health, Education and Welfare, Social Security Administration (SS1-29), January, 1969.
9. *The IHB Way, An Approach to the Rehabilitation of Blind Persons.* The Industrial Home for the Blind, Brooklyn, New York, 1961.
10. *Opportunity for the Blind and Visually Impaired.* U.S. Department of Health, Education and Welfare, Social and Rehabilitation Service, Rehabilitation Services Administration, Washington, D.C., 1969.
11. *State Vocational Rehabilitation Agency, Fact Sheet Booklet.* U.S. Department of Health, Education and Welfare, Social and Rehabilitation Service, Rehabilitation Services Administration, Washington, D.C., 1969.
12. *When Your Patient Is Blind.* The Industrial Home for the Blind, Brooklyn, New York, 1970.

Chapter 40

ENGINEERING PRINCIPLES IN REHABILITATION MEDICINE

by Roy W. Wirta and Donald R. Taylor, Jr.

The increasing collaboration between the medical and engineering professions during the past two decades is a natural outgrowth of the combined application of the life and physical sciences to improve the sustenance and quality of life for the patient. It has been demonstrated that the engineer brings to the clinical situation certain problem-solving capabilities which add new dimensions to rehabilitation medicine.

Although engineering has been defined in a variety of ways, the following definition seems to encompass the essence in a meaningful manner:

Engineering is the profession in which a knowledge of mathematical and physical sciences gained by study, experience, and practice is applied with judgment to develop ways to utilize, economically, the materials and forces of nature for the benefit of mankind.*

The term bioengineer, used frequently, simply denotes the engineer who applies his skills in an environment dealing with living things.

It has been said that a driving force within all engineers is to try to create order out of what might seem like a mass of confused ideas. This is generally so because engineers insist on reducing variables to numbers in order to solve problems. It can be presumed that this is the reason that engineers have begun to be invited into problem-solving circles in the medical professions. The engineer's insistence on accurate measurements consequently leads to the devel-

*_Mechanical Engineer_, Vol. 91, No. 6, p. 81, June, 1969.

opment of instrumentation that is vital in improving diagnostic and therapeutic practices.

What, one might ask, does the engineer bring to the clinical situation in which there exists a recognized problem? The answer may be summarized in the following seven salient attributes which an engineer brings to the situation:

1. Problem-solving approach.
2. Basic skill in the application of laws of physical sciences.
3. Skill in mathematics to apply to problem solving.
4. Consideration of economics.
5. Knowledge of hardware implementation.
6. Experience and judgment.
7. Ability to organize and manage an undertaking.

If the increasing utilization of engineering skills in rehabilitation medicine that has occurred over the past two decades is to continue, it is imperative that both the medical and engineering professions establish means of communication among one another in order to be able to reach meetings of the mind in the definition and solution of problems. This is one of the objectives for which this chapter has been prepared; another objective of this chapter is to serve as a reference to the non-engineering person. Certain principles and concepts of the physical sciences are interpreted with the hope that each person can do his job more effectively to provide better care for the patient.

The scope of the chapter has been purposely limited to only three general aspects of physics: *mechanics, materials* and *electronics.* These topics were chosen because they seem to encompass those physical sciences which are in most critical need of interpretation at this point in time. It is anticipated that some time in the future the subject matter may be elaborated to include additional topics.

MECHANICS

The branch of physical science called mechanics is so commonplace and accepted that it often goes completely unnoticed. Our bodies are constantly affected by various forces in the conduct of everyday activities. The normal person is usually unaware of the intricacies of bodily position and movements. However, some impairment of health, such as cerebral palsy or a cerebrovascular accident, can render movement patterns ineffective. Thorough understanding of the laws of mechanics is indeed relevant to improving the care offered these patients.

Mechanics is defined as that branch of physical science that deals with energies and forces and their effect on bodies. The term *biomechanics* may be defined as the science that deals with the effect of energies and both internal and external forces on human and animal bodies in movement and at rest.

The fundamentals of theoretical mechanics, anatomy, kinesiology and physiology (of the musculoskeletal system) are used to relate the forces in muscles, bones and joints with externally applied loads; such externally applied loads may result from the pull of gravity on the body parts or from some resistance which may be applied to a segment. Applied biomechanics is concerned with the more practical problems of improving movements and posture in rehabilitation medicine and in everyday living activities.

The whole subject of mechanics covers three basic areas:

1. *Statics,* which deals with bodies at rest or in equilibrium as a result of the forces acting upon them.

2. *Kinematics*, which deals with displacements, velocities and accelerations without considering the attendant forces involved.

3. *Dynamics*, which deals with moving bodies and the forces that act to produce the motion.

A person standing upright, and relatively motionless, illustrates a *static condition*, in which the forces caused by gravitational pull of the earth are borne by the musculoskeletal system and transferred downward onto the floor. All the downward forces are just exactly countered by the upward forces and the body is said to be in static equilibrium. A body moving at constant velocity is said also to be in equilibrium, if there are no unbalanced forces present to create a change in velocity.

A person walking illustrates both *kinematics* and *dynamics*. The body and limb displacements, changes in joint angles, and the movement of the body center of gravity are classified as kinematics, while the forces generated by the muscles, ground reaction forces, the exchanges of energies causing accelerations and decelerations of limb segments, work done and the power used all come under the consideration of dynamics.

Laws of Motion

Concepts of motion are not difficult to visualize, since they involve considerations of speed, velocity and acceleration. All these consist of a displacement in space with respect to time. Although speed and velocity are sometimes used interchangeably, there is a clear distinction. Speed is a scalar quantity and velocity is a vector quantity; hence, speed is a measure of magnitude only, whereas velocity includes both magnitude and direction. Acceleration is simply the rate of change of speed or velocity per unit of time.

The study of motions in themselves is in the category of kinematics, but the study of the causes of the motions of a body is in the category of dynamics. The motion of a body is the result of work having been done on it by an expenditure of energy. Before terms such as work, energy and power are discussed, it would be appropriate to introduce first two very important constituents, namely, *mass* and *force*.

Mass is a quantitative measure of inertia. Inertia is a property of matter which causes an object to resist change in velocity; if the body is at rest, it tends to stay at rest, and if moving, it tends to resist being speeded up or slowed down. In order to effect a change in the state of condition of the body, work must be done on it to overcome the effect of the inertia. Sir Isaac Newton is credited with formulating the basic ideas governing all motion, and, accordingly, three laws of motion in mechanics are named for him.

Newton's first law states that a body remains at rest or in uniform motion until acted upon by an unbalanced set of forces.

Newton's second law states that the acceleration of a particle is proportional to the unbalanced force acting upon it and inversely proportional to the mass of the particle. This law may be expressed mathematically:

$$a = \frac{F}{m}$$

whence

$$F = ma \tag{1}$$

or,   force = mass × acceleration,

where F is the force acting on a body of mass, m, which undergoes a change in velocity by acceleration, a.

Newton's third law states that to every action force there is an equal and opposite reaction force.

To illustrate Newton's laws of motion, consider a wheelchair with a patient in it. To move the patient to some new location, a person would have to exert force to get the wheelchair into motion, in accordance with Newton's first law. The magnitude of the force is proportional to the mass of the wheelchair plus the patient (plus the force needed to overcome friction) and proportional to the acceleration imparted to the mass, in accordance with Newton's second law. Since the inertia of the wheelchair and patient resist a change in velocity, there is an opposing *reaction* force developed against the action force supplied by the person pushing the wheelchair, in accordance with Newton's third law. To render the terms of equation (1) into a less abstract form, consider an example in which the mass of the wheelchair and patient is 80 kg., and the average acceleration is 0.3 meter/second²; then the force needed (neglecting friction) is:

$$F = 80 \times 0.3 = 24 \text{ newtons}$$

The newton is a unit of measure of force, and will be defined in the succeeding section devoted to the nature of forces.

Application of Newton's second law also distinguishes between weight and mass. Mass is the quantitative measure of the inertia of a body, and weight is the force developed by the gravitational pull of the earth on the body. The relationship between weight and mass is derived from equation (1) and is expressed as:

$$W = mg$$

where, W = weight of the object (a force term), m = mass of the object (measure of inertia), and g = acceleration effect of gravity.

Note that a patient in a Hubbard tank may be weightless, yet he possesses and retains his mass or inertia. Accordingly, in the strictest sense, a patient does not *weigh* 60 kg., for example, but his *mass* is 60 kg. By Newton's second law, the weight of the patient is equal to the force developed by the acceleration of the earth's gravitational field acting on the body, which is 9.8 meters/second², or:

$$F = 60 \times 9.8 = 588 \text{ newtons}$$

Hence, the reported weight of a patient whose mass is 60 kg. should be 588 newtons.

Force

Force is one of the basic concepts in the subject of mechanics. The notion of force is easy to recognize, but it is difficult to define; it is the agent or influence which changes or tends to change the state of rest or of motion of a body. Force comes about by virtue of stored energy, such as potential energy due to a gravitational field, a coil spring, an electrical charge, a magnetic field or the conversion of stored chemical energy into tension in a muscle.

The units of measure of force magnitude may be expressed in dynes, newtons or pounds, and they are defined as follows:

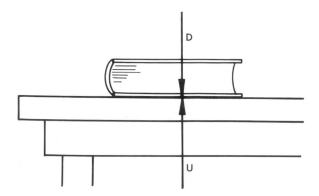

Figure 40–1   An object resting on a table illustrates the linear force system, where the downward force, D, is in equilibrium with the upward force, U. U = D.

Dyne is an amount of force that, acting on a 1 gram mass, will give it an acceleration of 1 centimeter per second per second.

Newton is an amount of force that, acting on a 1 kilogram mass, will give it an acceleration of 1 meter per second per second.

Pound is an amount of force, that acting on a 1 slug mass, will give it an acceleration of 1 foot per second per second.

Force has four characteristics that must be given to define it completely:

1. *Magnitude,* expressed in units, such as dynes, newtons or pounds.
2. *Action line,* which may be vertical or horizontal.
3. *Direction,* which may be upward along the vertical or downward along the vertical.
4. *Point of application* — for example, at the heel of the foot.

Force, in addition to having four characteristics necessary to define it, may act on bodies or systems in the following four different ways:

1. *Linear,* in which all the forces occur along the same action line, as shown in Figure 40-1.
2. *Parallel,* with all the forces parallel and occurring in the same plane but not along the same action line, as shown in Figure 40-2.
3. *Concurrent,* in which all the forces meet at a point, as shown in Figure 40-3.
4. *General,* with all the forces in a plane but not arranged as in any of the other three, as shown in Figure 40-4.

Resolution and Composition of Forces.   Force systems representable by linear and parallel configurations are readily solved by simple consideration of tensile or compressive actions (linear) or by concepts of levers (parallel) and

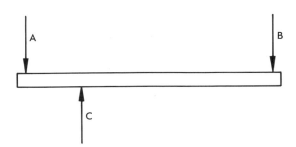

Figure 40–2   A lever application illustrates the parallel force system, where A + B = C.

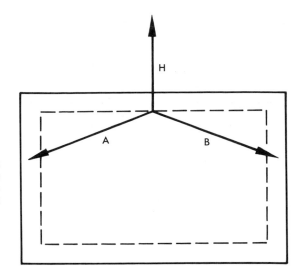

Figure 40–3 A picture hung by a wire and supported by a hook on the wall illustrates the concurrent force system, where $A \rightarrow B = H$ ($\rightarrow$ denotes vector addition).

moment arms. However, in many situations, these are not representative of the actual conditions. In the body, for example, muscles are arranged so that their action lines are applied at many different angles to the bone. Furthermore, as a segment moves through its range of motion, the action line of a given muscle attached to the part constantly changes. External forces are applied from many directions. Therefore, methods are needed to deal with forces which are not arranged in linear or parallel fashion.

In solving problems in biomechanics, the primary task is to recognize the factors involved and to set up the problem properly for solution. The setup of the problem as a *free body diagram* permits conversion into mathematical expressions that can be solved. This is accomplished by processes called resolution and composition of forces. *Resolution* is the operation of replacing a single force by a system of components. The single force is the *resultant* of its components. *Composition* is the operation of replacing a system of forces by its resultant. Stated differently:

1. Replacing a single vector by two or more equivalent vectors, whose combined effect is equal to that of the original force, is termed *resolution* of a force.

2. Adding two or more vectors together so that their combined effect is shown by a single vector is termed *composition* of forces.

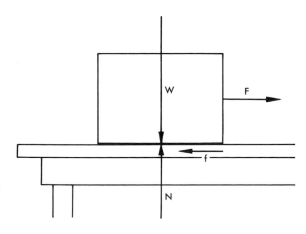

Figure 40–4 An object being slid on a surface at uniform velocity illustrates the general force system, where $W = N$ and $F = f$.

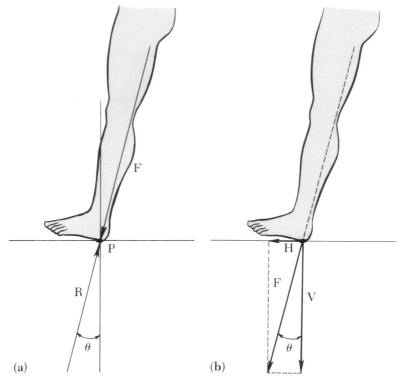

Figure 40–5, *a* and *b*.   Resolution of forces. Force F can be resolved into two component forces: vertical, V, and horizontal, H.

To illustrate the resolution and composition of forces, consider the point in the gait cycle when heel strike occurs, as shown in Figure 40-5, *a*. At that instant there is a force, F, transmitted down the leg and onto the ground. Equal and opposite to the transmitted force, F, is a ground reaction force, R. The force F may be thought of as consisting of two component forces, namely, a vertical force, V, and a horizontal force, H, as shown in Figure 40-5, *b*. This consideration of the single force as a product of the two component forces is the process of resolution of forces. Consider, on the other hand, that the same subject is walking in a laboratory equipped with a force plate to measure the vertical (V) and horizontal (H) forces; then the two forces can be combined vectorially to determine F. This process is known as composition of forces.

To resolve the force F in Figure 40-5, *a*, into its components requires more information than just its magnitude. One must also know its direction (otherwise it would not be a vector). If by some means the angle which the force makes with the ground is known, as illustrated by angle θ, then the calculation may be made as follows:

$$V = F \cos \theta \qquad\qquad (2)$$

$$H = F \sin \theta \qquad\qquad (3)$$

To determine the magnitude of force F by having available measured values of H and V, the Pythagorean Theorem may be applied:

$$F = \sqrt{V^2 + H^2}$$

Alternately, one might also solve for F by use of trigonometry by first calculating the value of angle θ, and then using versions of equations (2) and (3) as follows:

$$\tan \theta = \frac{H}{V}$$

Having found the value of θ, then the following apply:

$$F = \frac{V}{\cos \theta}$$

or

$$F = \frac{H}{\sin \theta}$$

Note that for solving these problems, in each case, a free body diagram is drawn to represent the forces and their directions on an arbitrary set of reference axes. In Figure 40-5, the arbitrary axes chosen were the horizontal and vertical lines drawn through the point of intersection of the force vector F and the ground at P. One could just as easily call these reference axes X and Y. Such notation is entirely up to the individual, although if the calculations are to be submitted for study by some other persons, then certain conventions become useful in helping convey information. In keeping with mathematical practice, the vertical axis (ordinate) is noted as Y, and the horizontal axis (abscissa) is noted as X.

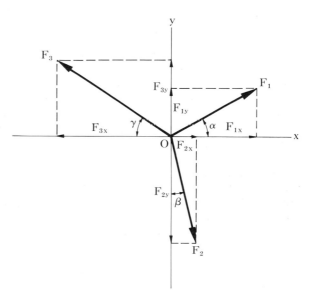

Figure 40–6 Composition of forces. Three concurrent forces, F_1, F_2 and F_3, as shown, can be treated by addition of vectors (composition) into a single vector.

Sometimes a concurrent force system does not lend itself readily to assigning one or more of the component forces into one of the reference axes. Such might be the case in analyzing the nature of the forces at the hip joint. Then a free body diagram may be drawn in a form resembling the general diagram shown in Figure 40-6. Here three concurrent forces are depicted going through point O, and labeled as F_1, F_2 and F_3. If the directions of the three forces are known, then a set of reference axes may be assigned, as illustrated, with the forces F_1, F_2 and F_3 making angles α, β and γ with the reference axes as shown. Now the X and Y components of each force may be calculated and added to find the resultant. The resultant may be calculated in the same manner as shown in equation (4), using the Pythagorean Theorem by inserting the squares of the X and the Y summations of the three force vectors:

$$R = \sqrt{(\Sigma\, F_x)^2 + (\Sigma\, F_y)^2}$$

where the symbol Σ represents the algebraic summation. By algebraic summation is meant taking into account the sign of the component—that is, whether to treat it as a plus or a minus value. For example, F_{2y} would be treated as a minus value while F_{1y} and F_{3y} would be treated as plus values.

The angle which the resultant vector R makes with the reference axis may be calculated in the manner given in equation (5), using the tangent function:

$$\tan \theta = \frac{\Sigma\, F_y}{\Sigma\, F_x}$$

To illustrate the solution of the concurrent force problem given above, assume the following values for the terms:

Let $F_1 = 20$ newtons and $\alpha = 45°$
Let $F_2 = 30$ newtons and $\beta = 30°$
Let $F_3 = 40$ newtons and $\gamma = 30°$

Then
$$\begin{aligned}
\Sigma\, F_x &= F_1 \cos 45° + F_2 \sin 30° - F_3 \cos 30° \\
&= (20)(0.707) + (30)(0.50) - (40)(0.866) \\
&= 14.14 + 15.00 - 34.64 \\
&= -5.50 \text{ newtons}
\end{aligned}$$

and
$$\begin{aligned}
\Sigma\, F_y &= F_1 \sin 45° - F_2 \cos 30° + F_3 \sin 30° \\
&= (20)(0.707) - (30)(0.866) + (40)(0.50) \\
&= 14.14 - 25.98 + 20.00 \\
&= +8.16 \text{ newtons}
\end{aligned}$$

Composition
$$\begin{aligned}
R &= \sqrt{(-5.50)^2 + (8.16)^2} \\
&= \sqrt{30.2 + 66.6} \\
&= 9.84 \text{ newtons}
\end{aligned}$$

Angle
$$\tan \theta = \frac{8.16}{5.50} = 1.483$$

$$\theta = 56.5° \text{ from the horizontal}$$

(See Figure 40–7.)

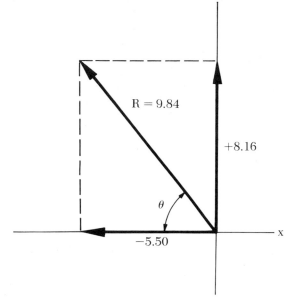

Figure 40–7 Resultant vector produced by composition of forces.

Friction

Friction is generally necessary in the conduct of our daily activities. Walking, for example, requires adequate friction between the sole of the shoe and the floor so that the foot will not slip forward or backward. Friction is necessary in the use of canes and crutches. It is also necessary in the operation of vehicles like wheelchairs and automobiles, even though in each of these vehicles there are devices used to reduce friction at locations where it is considered undesirable, such as in the bearings for the wheels.

When two surfaces are pressed together, as shown in Figure 40-8, a force directed parallel to the surface is required to make one surface slide over the other. The force of the sliding friction, f, is proportional to the total normal (perpendicular to surface) force, N, and is independent of the area of contact. The relationship may be expressed by the following.

$$f = \mu N \tag{6}$$

where the Greek letter μ is introduced as the proportionality constant called *coefficient of friction*. By knowing the value of μ for any given pair of surfaces, one may calculate the force of friction in terms of the normal force, N. For

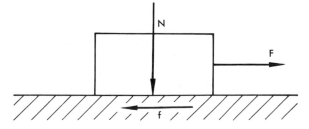

Figure 40–8 The force of sliding friction, f, is proportional to the normal force, N.

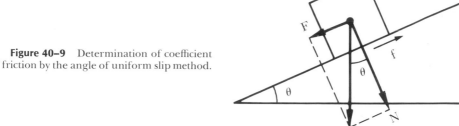

Figure 40–9   Determination of coefficient of friction by the angle of uniform slip method.

example, if the coefficient of friction between a box and the floor is 0.20 and the box weighs 100 pounds, then the force needed to slide the box along the floor is

$$F = \mu \, N = (0.20) \, (100) = 20 \text{ pounds}$$

Sometimes the coefficient of friction is reported to have been determined by the angle of uniform slip method. This is a simple and often convenient way to determine the coefficient of friction by using gravity to provide the force, F, needed to develop uniform motion. This is illustrated in Figure 40-9. If a test object is placed on a plane and the plane is slowly tilted, an angle will ultimately be reached at which the test object starts to slide down the slope with constant velocity. Under the constant velocity condition, the gravity component, F, of weight, W, is just equal in magnitude to the opposing friction force, f. By equation (6), $\mu = \dfrac{f}{N}$, and under the condition of force equilibrium, where F = f, then $\mu = \dfrac{F}{N}$. From the right triangle in Figure 40–9, the relationship of F to N is:

$$\frac{F}{N} = \tan \theta$$

Therefore, the expression for the coefficient of friction is:

$$\mu = \tan \theta \tag{7}$$

where the angle θ is the so-called angle of uniform slip. For example, if the angle of uniform slip was found to be 14°, then the coefficient of friction is:

$$\mu = \tan 14° = 0.25$$

As another example, if the coefficient of friction, μ, between a rubber heel and a floor tile is about 0.50, then during heel strike, a longitudinal shear force of about 80 pounds could be sustained when the body weight of a 160 pound person is borne at the beginning of the stance phase. Although such a large force may in reality not occur, the high coefficient of friction provides adequate reserve to assure safety. Water spilled on the floor, for example, will reduce the coefficient of friction between the heel and the tile, thereby reducing the magnitude of the friction force, f, the available force to oppose relative motion, and slippage may occur. Another example in which the coefficient of friction is deliberately increased may be noted in occupational therapy when sandpaper is used between a sliding block and the work surface just to increase the load. On the other hand, in machines, wheel bearings and orthotic pivot joints, an effort is made to reduce friction in order to gain higher efficiency by reducing wasted energy. Lubricants and rolling types of bearings are in common use to reduce friction in these applications. For example, dry steel rubbing on dry steel may have a $\mu = 0.20$, whereas, when lubricated, the same surfaces may have a $\mu = 0.05$; by contrast, a ball bearing rolling on a steel surface may have a $\mu = 0.002$.

Friction in a gas or a liquid manifests itself when the fluid is made to flow around a stationary object. It makes no difference whether the fluid is considered flowing and the object standing still or vice versa. It is only necessary to specify that there is relative motion between the two. At relatively low velocities, the flow of a fluid is smooth and regular and is said to be laminar; under such conditions, the fluid friction is proportional to the velocity:

$$f = Kv \qquad (8)$$

where K is a proportionality constant. As the velocity increases, turbulence sets in and the force of friction changes drastically and becomes proportional to the square of the velocity:

$$f = Tv^2 \qquad (9)$$

where T is a proportionality constant. The friction force represents a loss of energy, and it is quite apparent that the losses are small when the flow is laminar and increase greatly at high velocities when the flow is turbulent.

Moment

The concept of a moment or torque is one of the more commonly found manifestations of applied force in the musculoskeletal system. The principal motion about all bodily joints is rotary in nature. The tendency to produce a rotation is called a moment. The moment may be defined as that which produces or tends to produce rotation or torsion and whose effectiveness is measured by the product of the force and the perpendicular distance from the line of action of the force to the axis of rotation:

$$M = F \times r \qquad (10)$$

$$\text{or, moment} = \text{force} \times \text{lever arm}$$

This principle is illustrated in Figure 40-10, which depicts a wheel of radius r acted upon by a tangential force F at its rim. The moment tending to rotate the wheel clockwise is

$$M_{\underset{\smile}{)}} = F \times r$$

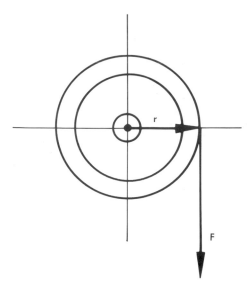

Figure 40–10 Concepts of moment illustrated by a wheel and axle with a force F acting tangentially at the rim at a distance r from the axle.

The units of measure of moment (or torque) are the dyne-centimeter and newton-meter in the metric system and the pound-inch or pound-foot in the engineering system.

A biomechanical application of the concept of a moment may be seen in the illustration of walking, as depicted in Figure 40-5 *b*, and redrawn for clarity in Figure 40-11. To calculate the moment about the knee joint, consider that the vertical and horizontal ground reaction forces, V and F, act about the knee joint at distances a and b, respectively. The moment tending to extend the knee at this point consists of two components, one clockwise (↘) and the other counterclockwise (↖) as follows:

$$M_\downarrow = M_\downarrow \longmapsto M_\uparrow$$
$$M_\downarrow = V \times a - H \times b$$

Note that a direction for positive moment for this illustration is chosen to be clockwise; therefore, the clockwise component $V \times a$ is considered positive, and the counterclockwise component $H \times b$ is considered negative.

The concept of torque is evident in the consideration of rotational dynamics, in which a rigid body is acted upon by an unbalanced rotational force. The torque necessary to accelerate angularly or decelerate a mass is proportional to the mass distribution and proportional to the angular acceleration. Analogous to equation (1) for Newton's second law, $F = ma$, the expression for torque is:

$$T = I\alpha$$

where T is the torque, I is the mass moment of inertia and α is the angular acceleration in radians per second per second. During the swing phase of the gait cycle, the shank and foot undergo angular accelerations and decelerations, while pivoting about the knee joint. The torques necessary to develop these changes in angular velocity come from the flexor and extensor muscles at the hip and knee. Consider, for example, the effect that a walking cast can have

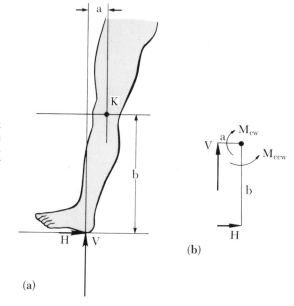

Figure 40–11, *a* and *b*   Moment at the knee joint, K, is the algebraic sum of the moments developed by ground reaction forces H and V at heel strike during walking.

upon gait. Because of the size and location of the added mass, the total mass moment of inertia of the lower extremity is increased substantially. The direct effect is to cause the following tendencies: greater torques, T, are required and the angular accelerations, α, about the joints are decreased. Although a walking cast represents an extreme instance in altering the mass moment of inertia of the lower extremity, the design of orthotic and prosthetic appliances also commands careful attention so as not to affect deleteriously the gait, metabolic cost and safety.

The mass moment of inertia, I, is a description of the body in terms of how the mass is distributed about the axis of rotation. It is calculated as the integral of the mass of each elemental particle of the body multiplied by the square of its distance from the axis of rotation, and may be expressed by:

$$I = mr^2 \tag{12}$$

This means that the inertial property of the body to resist change in angular velocity is dependent upon both the amount of mass that the body possesses and upon the distribution of that mass. Imagine a long rod and a cube both having the same mass. Almost intuitively one would recognize that it would be much easier to spin the cube than to spin the rod, end over end. To illustrate the effect of mass distribution, Figure 40-12 shows a number of common shapes and the mass moment of inertia, I, associated with each shape.

Levers

The musculoskeletal arrangement in the human body consists of a system of levers ingeniously connected together to give the human organism a high degree of mobility and strength. The arms, legs and spine all include bony structural members which are joined by flexible tissues to form articulate joints; these members are moved by forces developed in the attached muscle tissues.

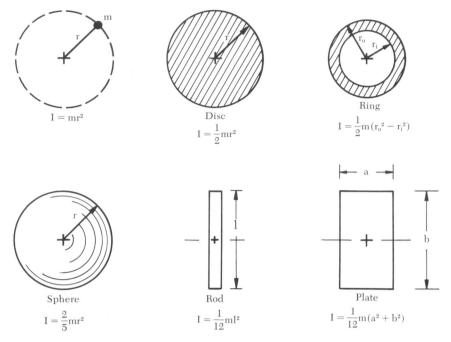

Figure 40–12   Formulas for the mass moment of inertia for six common regularly shaped bodies.

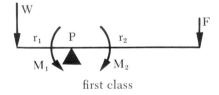

first class

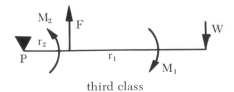

second class

Figure 40–13   Three classes of levers commonly used.

third class

The lever is one of the simplest of all mechanical devices and employs the concept of moments in its principle of operation. Depending upon the arrangement of the load, the applied force and the fulcrum, levers can be classified into three categories, as shown in Figure 40-13. In each illustration, P is the *fulcrum,* or the axis about which the lever is made to pivot; W is the *weight,* or load to be moved; and F is the *applied force,* or effort. The distance r_1 is called the lever arm of the load, and the distance r_2 is the lever arm of the applied force. The moment developed by the product of the force times the lever arm is M_1 for the load, and M_2 for the applied force. Note that in each case the two moments are in opposite directions, and that under conditions of equilibrium the moment tending to produce a clockwise rotation must just equal the moment tending to produce a counterclockwise rotation. For each of the lever arrangements shown in Figure 40-13, the moments may be expressed by:

$$M_1 = M_2$$
$$W \times r_1 = F \times r_2$$

As an example in biomechanics, consider the forearm in the function of supporting an object in the hand, as shown in Figure 40-14, *a.* Imagine that the object weighs 10 pounds, and that the elbow is flexed 30°. Assume that the biceps is attached 2 inches from the nominal center of rotation of the elbow joint, and that the load is applied 14 inches from the center of rotation. A free body diagram of this problem is shown in Figure 40-14, *b.* To determine the magnitude of the force T, it is necessary to find first the perpendicular

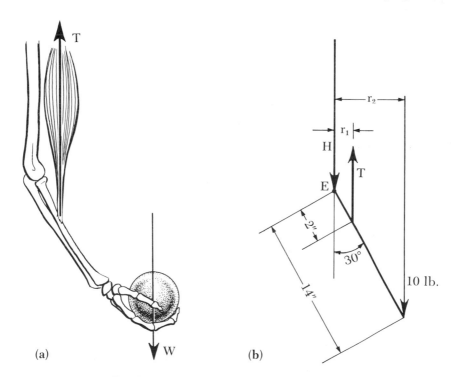

(a)   W   (b)

Figure 40–14 Diagram illustrating the forearm acting as a lever to support a weight, W, by biceps tension, T. The freebody diagram gives pertinent information to solve for biceps tension and the force of the humerus on the ulna, H.

distances of the two force action lines from the center of rotation, depicted as r_1 and r_2.

$$r_1 = 2 \times \sin 30° = (2)\ (0.5) = 1 \text{ inch}$$
$$r_2 = 14 \times \sin 30° = (14)\ (0.5) = 7 \text{ inches}$$

By equation (10),

$$T \times r_1 = W \times r_1$$

$$T = \frac{r_2}{r_1}$$

$$T = (10)\left(\frac{7}{1}\right) = 70 \text{ pounds}$$

By summation of vertical forces, the upward forces must equal the downward forces:

$$T = H \times W$$

Hence,

$$H = T - W = 70 - 10 = 60 \text{ pounds}$$

The resolution of forces can be illustrated using the example of the previous problem, as shown in Figure 40-15. The tension force developed by the biceps can be thought of as two components, namely, a rotary component, R, acting perpendicular to the forearm, and a stabilizing component, S, acting longitudinally along the ulna. These component forces may be calculated, using the values in the previous solution.

$$R = T \sin 30° = (70)\ (0.500) = 35.0 \text{ pounds}$$
$$S = T \cos 30° = (70)\ (0.866) = 60.6 \text{ pounds}$$

Contemplation of the two forces reveals that the magnitudes of R and S vary as a function of the angle of flexion. When the elbow is extended and the angle is small, then the biceps tension is manifest almost entirely as a stabilizing force with almost no rotary component. When the elbow is flexed to 90°, the biceps tension is totally rotary and the stabilizing force is zero. When the elbow is flexed beyond 90°, the rotary component begins to diminish and the stabilizing component becomes negative.

Work and Energy

There is little doubt that one of the most important concepts in all nature is energy. It represents a fundamental entity common to all forms of matter in

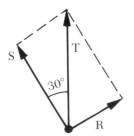

Figure 40–15   Resolution of the force T, shown in Figure 40–14, into a rotary component, R, and a stabilizing component, S.

all parts of the physical world, and it is important because all human life depends upon energy.

Energy is the capacity for doing work. Work is a term used to describe the expenditure of energy which has been stored in one form or another in a body.

Mechanical energy is divided into two categories: *potential energy* and *kinetic energy*. A body is said to have potential energy if, by virtue of its position or state, it is able to do work. A body is said to have kinetic energy if, by virtue of its motion, it is able to do work. Work is defined as the product of force times the distance through which the force acts.

Because of the reciprocal nature of work and energy, both have the same units of measure. In the metric and engineering systems, work and energy units are:

Centimer-gram-second (cgs) system: dyne-centimeter, also called the erg;
Meter-kilogram-second (mks) system:newton-meter, also called the joule;
Engineering system: foot-pound

Examples of potential energy can be seen in work done to lift a weight some distance from the floor, or to compress a spring. This work input is stored as potential energy in the weight or in the spring, and can be returned as work output by releasing the weight or by releasing the spring.

A moving body, because of its mass and motion, has kinetic energy. For instance, to bring a moving body to rest, a force must be exerted in a direction opposing the motion, and this force must act through some distance in order to stop the body. Obviously, the reverse is also true: in order to set the body in motion, work had to be done *on* the body to give it the kinetic energy in the first place.

Disregarding any losses due to other reasons, such as friction, the input work used to develop the potential energy or the kinetic energy can all be realized as output work by returning the stationary body to its lower potential or by slowing down the moving body.

The relationships of the factors in both work and energy are shown in the following equations:

$$\text{work} = F \times d \tag{13}$$

$$\text{potential energy (P.E.)} = w \times h \tag{14}$$

$$\text{kinetic energy, translational (K.E.)} = \tfrac{1}{2}mv^2 \tag{15}$$

$$\text{kinetic energy, rotational (K.E.)} = \tfrac{1}{2}I\omega^2 \tag{16}$$

where   F= force   I = mass moment of inertia
        d = distance ω = angular velocity
        m = mass   w = weight of object
        v = velocity   h = height to which weight, w, is lifted

Note that the energy in the kinetic energy equations expresses the velocity to the second power. This means that if the velocity is doubled, then the energy is quadrupled. This is a very important consideration in the study of human motion.

Conservation of Energy.   One of the most important laws of nature is the law of conservation of energy, which states that the amount of energy in the universe is always the same. It can neither be increased nor decreased but only transformed. Here are some examples: the decrease in potential energy of a falling object transforms into kinetic energy; burning fuel transforms chemical energy into heat energy; and an electric motor transforms electrical energy into mechanical energy.

In the study of human locomotion, there is a subtle but very real process of transformation of energies. This transformation occurs not only in the metabolic cost needed to develop forces and movement but also in the interchanges between potential and kinetic energies of the moving parts of the body segments as they change velocities and heights from the ground.

Power.   The mechanical concept of power is loosely analogous to the metabolism rate in the human body. It relates the amount of energy expended in a period of time; hence, power is the time rate of doing work. The unit of measure in the metric system is either ergs per second or joules per second. In the engineering system power is expressed in foot-pounds per second, and in some cases, horsepower. In the physical sciences, power is often discussed in terms of three forms of energy, namely, mechanical, thermal and electrical. Some of the commonly used conversion factors relating these forms of energy and power are the following:

$$1 \text{ kg.-cal.} = 4186 \text{ joules}$$
$$1 \text{ joule/sec.} = 1 \text{ watt}$$
$$69.77 \text{ kg.-cal./min.} = 1 \text{ watt}$$

$$1 \text{ British thermal unit (Btu)} = 778.3 \text{ ft.-lb.}$$
$$1 \text{ horsepower} = 550 \text{ ft.-lb./sec.}$$
$$1 \text{ horsepower} = 746 \text{ watts}$$

Glossary of Terms Used in Mechanics

Dynamics is that branch of mechanics which deals with the effect of unbalanced external forces in modifying the motion of bodies.

Energy of a body (or a system of bodies) is the amount of work it can do, by virtue of its motion or position, against forces applied to it, while changing to a standard state.

Fluid friction is that resistance developed by a stationary object tending to oppose flow of an adjacent fluid.

Force is that which changes or tends to change the state of rest or of motion of a body.

Impulse is the product of the average value of force and the time during which it acts (being equal to the change in momentum produced by the force).

Inertia is that property of a body by virtue of which it tends to continue in the state of rest or motion until acted upon by some force.

Kinematics is that branch of mechanics which deals with the motion of bodies without consideration of the mass and force. It considers only concepts of geometry and time.

Kinetic energy of a body is its capacity to do work by virtue of its velocity.

Kinetic friction is that friction which opposes motion when one body is slipping off the surface of another.

Mass is a quantitative measure of inertia.

Mechanics is that branch of physical science that deals with energy and forces and their effect on bodies.

Moment, or *torque,* is that which produces or tends to produce rotation or torsion and

whose effectiveness is measured by the product of the force and the perpendicular distance from the line of action of the force to the axis of rotation.

Momentum is the product of the mass of a body and its velocity. The momentum of a
moving body determines the length of time required to bring it to rest when
under the action of a constant force or moment. (See also *Impulse.*)

Potential energy of a body is its capacity to do work by virtue of its position or state.

Power is the time rate of doing work.

Rolling friction is that friction developed when one body rolls over the surface of
another.

Static friction is that friction which opposes motion when there is no slipping.

Statics is that branch of mechanics dealing with the relations of forces that produce
equilibrium among material bodies.

Weight is the force by which a body is attracted toward the earth by gravitation. Weight is
equal to the product of the mass and the local gravitational acceleration.

Work is the product of force and the distance through which the force acts.

MATERIALS

Those serving in the rehabilitation practices deal constantly with various
materials and substances. Characteristic qualities of these substances are of
importance to the practitioner, whether solid mechanics are involved in orthotic or prosthetic devices, properties of liquids in hydrotherapy, or gas dynamics
in pulmonary care. It is important to have a good working knowledge of the
reaction of these materials to conditions in use, so that the practitioner's skills
may be more effectively applied to patient care.

The properties of solid materials will be discussed in this section to acquaint the reader with some of the physical characteristics which need to be
considered when applying such materials. In order to gain insights into the
subject of materials and to become familiar with concepts of properties and
their relationship to each other, certain terms will be defined and then
examples will be given to illustrate their utilization. Terms such as elasticity,
strength and stiffness may seem so familiar that they hardly require definition;
however, these terms together with others make up a vocabulary that is needed
to convey the meanings germane to a thorough understanding. Such an understanding is necessary if one is to advance the state of the art in practice.

Terms and Properties of Solids

Elasticity.   A material is said to be elastic when it is able to deform under
load and to return to its original shape upon removal of the load. Regardless of
the amount of the deformation, the ability to recover its original form is the
criterion of elasticity.

Hooke's law states that stress is proportional to strain. This is understood
to hold only within the elastic limit of the material. By stress is meant the
intensity of force distributed over a cross-sectional area, and by strain is meant
the amount of physical distortion distributed over a unit dimension. The stress
set up within an elastic body is directly proportional to the strain caused by the
applied load (see Figure 40-16) and may be expressed as

$$K = \frac{\text{stress}}{\text{strain}} \tag{17}$$

This proportionality of stress to strain is called the *modulus* of elasticity. In a sense, the modulus of elasticity denotes the relative stiffness of the material.

By definition, stress is the force, F, per unit area, A.

$$stress = \frac{F}{A}$$

and strain is the elongation, e, per unit length, L.

$$strain = \frac{e}{L}$$

When these defining equations are substituted into the expression for Hooke's law, the modulus of elasticity, K, is called Young's modulus, written as E, and expressed by:

$$E = \frac{F/A}{e/L} = \frac{FL}{Ae} \tag{18}$$

Young's modulus E is a very practical constant, for, if its value is known for any given material, the amount of stretch, bending or compression produced in that material by an applied load can be calculated.

Elastic Limit.   The elastic limit is the maximum unit stress to which a material may be subjected and still be able to return to its original form upon removal of the stress. In Figure 40-16 the elastic limit is denoted by the part of the curve designated between points a and b.

Yield Strength.   The yield strength of a material is defined as the unit stress at which the material exhibits a specified limiting permanent set and is a measure of the useful limit of the material. In Figure 40-16 the yield strength is denoted by point c, where, upon removal of the applied stress, the body returns only partially toward its original form and thereby acquires a permanent deformation, designated by point a'.

Yield Point.   The yield point of a material is the unit stress at which the deformation first increases markedly without a proportional increase in the applied load. The yield point is always beyond the proportional limit and the true elastic limit, as designated by point d in Figure 40-16.

Ultimate Strength.   The ultimate strength, tensile or compressive, of a material is the highest unit stress it can sustain before rupture. This point is designated by point e in Figure 40-16.

Ductility and Malleability.   Ductility and malleability, often considered to be almost synonymous, indicate the ability of a material to undergo large permanent deformations without rupture. Ductility of a material is commonly thought of as the property which enables a material to be drawn into a wire, whereas malleability is the property which permits it to be beaten or rolled into thin sheets. Hence, ductility is frequently more specifically defined as the ability to undergo large permanent deformations in tension, and malleability the ability to undergo large permanent deformations in compression.

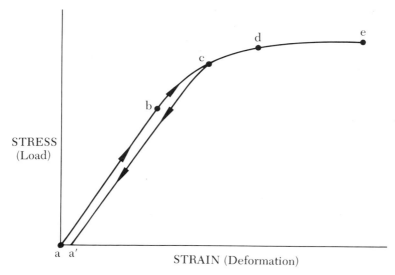

Figure 40–16 Stress-strain curve for a ductile material. The elastic range of the curve is between points a and b. Point b represents the elastic limit of the material. At point c some plastic deformation has taken place and, upon removal of the load, a permanent set of magnitude a' may be noted. Continued loading beyond point c will further deform the material until it ruptures at point e.

Brittleness. A material which can be only slightly deformed without rupture is termed brittle. Brittleness is relative and no material is perfectly brittle — that is, capable of no deformation before rupture. Many materials are brittle to a greater or lesser degree; glass is one of the more brittle materials.

Plasticity. A material is plastic if the smallest load produces a deformation which persists even after the load is removed. A completely plastic material is nonelastic and has no ultimate strength (like chewing gum) in the ordinary meaning of the term. Plasticity, like brittleness, is relative, and no material is completely plastic. However, the degree of plasticity varies from material to material and under differing conditions of externally applied energies, such as at elevated temperatures or at certain rates of deformation beyond the elastic limit. Plasticity and brittleness are opposite terms.

Toughness. Toughness is the ability to withstand a high unit stress together with a great unit deformation without complete rupture. The distinction between ductility and toughness is that ductility pertains only to the ability to deform, whereas toughness considers both the ability to deform and the stress developed during the deformation.

Stiffness. Stiffness is the ability to resist elastic deformation under stress. The modulus of elasticity is the criterion of stiffness.

Hardness. Hardness is the ability to resist very small indentations, abrasion and plastic deformation. There is no single measure of hardness, for it is not a single property but a combination of several properties.

Creep.   Creep is a form of plastic or inelastic action by means of which some solids flow appreciably under small stresses. Creep is a temperature-dependent quality, higher temperatures being conducive to higher creep rates.

Atomic Theory.   The understanding of concepts such as elasticity, elastic limit, yield strength and ultimate strength requires an appreciation of the constitution of matter. For this reason, it is appropriate to begin consideration of this topic with the smallest divisions of matter, that is, on the atomic and the molecular scale.

The atomic theory of matter holds that all matter consists of very small particles called atoms, and that these particles are at all times in a rapid state of motion. The nature of this motion depends upon the temperature of the substance and upon its state of matter, that is, whether it is in the solid, liquid or gaseous form. The atom is the smallest division of matter that has distinct chemical characteristics. Atoms of elements may combine chemically to form molecules. A compound is a substance that consists of molecules of two or more atoms. Molecules may range in their number of atoms from two (diatomic) to the many hundreds of atoms that make up the very complex molecules found in living organisms.

Most atoms, whether in their elemental state or as chemically combined molecules, tend to cling together or cohere, depending on temperature and, to an extent, upon the surrounding pressure. They cling together at some equilibrium distance which is in the order of 3×10^{-8} cm. To push them closer together or to try to pull them apart requires work. The characteristic force needed to displace atoms from their equilibrium position is illustrated in Figure 40-17. Note that to try to push them closer together requires a greater and greater force because of the repulsive force developed between the atoms. On the other hand, pulling them apart requires a force that first increases but which on further separation diminishes and eventually goes to zero. This occurs when the cohesive force is overcome and the substance physically ruptures.

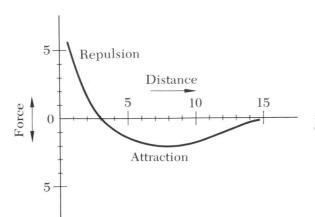

Figure 40-17   Typical relationship of the force between two atoms of a diatomic molecule.

Divisions of Materials

Matter that can be recognized as being of a certain type or kind, such as an alloy, plastic or wood, is said to be a material. To understand some of the useful properties of materials, it is helpful to classify them into categories. One way of classifying materials is depicted in Figure 40–18, which shows them divided first into two categories: metals and nonmetals. Each of the two divisions may be further subdivided into two additional categories. Under the classification of metals, one may consider two divisions: ferrous and nonferrous. Under the classification of nonmetals, one may consider two divisions: organic and inorganic.

Metals are chemical elements which are usually solid, crystalline bodies. Most metals have a silvery color, are shiny and are usually denser than water. Most of them conduct heat and electricity well. Many of the more important metals can be rolled into thin sheets and they are described as malleable. They can also be drawn out into wires and are called ductile.

Nonmetallic materials, as contrasted to metallic, are not shiny, are poor conductors of heat and electricity, and are not in the same sense considered malleable or ductile. Common nonmetallic materials considered here include plastics, adhesives, lubricants, surface protective and cosmetic materials, thermal and electrical insulators and refractories.

Metals. Desirable physical properties and cost are two of the most important factors to be considered in the choice of materials for construction. From the technical standpoint, the two properties of metals and alloys which most influence their selection as the preferred material for construction are, first, strength combined with ductility, and second, the ready ability to be shaped, that is, to be changed in size or shape. Shaping includes machining as well as welding and soldering, which are techniques for joining metals. Other techniques used in shaping include casting, extrusion, rolling, wire drawing and spinning. Some other important properties of metals are hardenability, electrical and thermal conductivity, magnetic permeability, magnetic retentivity, and resistance to corrosion, staining or rusting.

Metals comprise a large part of materials expected to provide properties of strength, toughness, abrasion resistance and other qualities not usually asso-

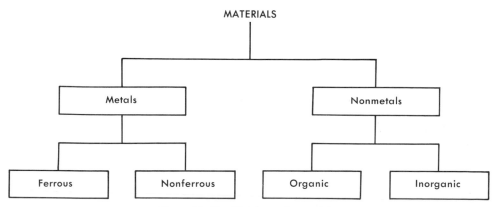

Figure 40–18 Divisions of materials.

ciated with nonmetallic materials (See Table 40-1.). Among metallic materials two divisions are identified: *ferrous* and *nonferrous*. Ferrous metals are those which contain iron, whereas nonferrous, such as aluminum, copper or nickel, are those which do not contain iron. Besides the differences in physical and chemical properties of ferrous and nonferrous metals, there are wide economic differences.

Almost all metals find use not so much in their pure state but rather as some intimate combination of two or more metallic elements called alloys. Alloys have been devised to provide certain unique physical and chemical properties, such as high strength, corrosion resistance and good machineability, not possessed by any one of the elements by itself.

FERROUS METALS.   Ferrous metals are often classified into two categories: carbon steels and alloy steels. The carbon steels contain small amounts of carbon (up to about 1.7 per cent carbon) and trace amounts of other elements. They are widely used for structural shapes, tools, springs, fasteners, containers and machinery. By varying the amount of carbon, the heat treatment and the cold working of carbon steel, one can obtain a large variety of physical properties. The strength of the steel varies with the amount of carbon contained in it; however, if the percentage exceeds about 2 per cent (the minimum percentage for cast iron), the material becomes hard and brittle and cannot be worked at any temperature.

Alloy steels have been developed for a large variety of special properties, each of which has its own peculiar advantage. Certain materials are added to the steel to enhance its magnetic quality, other materials are added to increase its corrosion resistance, and still other materials are added to make the steel

TABLE 40-1   PHYSICAL PROPERTIES OF SOME COMMON MATERIALS

SUBSTANCE	DENSITY (lb./in.³)	SPECIFIC HEAT (Btu/lb./°F.)	THERMAL CONDUCTIVITY*	YIELD STRENGTH (1000 psi)	MODULUS OF ELASTICITY (Millions psi)
Aluminum					
1060-H15	0.098	0.098	1580	15	10
2024-T3	0.098	0.100	830	50	10
6061-T4	0.098	0.098	1060	40	10
Brass	0.30	0.09	350 to 1700	22–125	15
Copper	0.32	0.095	2650	30	16
Iron	0.284	0.123	460	40	29.7
Lead	0.41	0.032	241	1.7–3.0	2.1–2.5
Magnesium	0.063	0.250	1090	27	37
Steel, mild	0.28	0.117	310	30	29
Steel, tool	0.28	0.117	300	80–120	29
Steel, 18-8 SS	0.29	0.12	113	80	28
Titanium	0.163	0.113	105	40–75	16
Acetal	0.051	0.35	1.58	9	0.4
Methyl Methacrylate	0.043	0.35	1.44	7–11	0.45
Nylon	0.04	0.40	1.68	9–12	0.2–0.4
Polycarbonate	0.044	0.28	1.32	8–9.5	0.32
Polyethylene	0.034	0.55	3.45	3–5.5	0.06–0.15
Polypropylene	0.032	0.46	0.83	4–5.5	0.16–0.2
Polystyrene	0.038	0.32	0.30	3.5–6.5	0.3–0.45
Polyvinyl chloride	0.05	0.25	0.14	5–9	0.35–0.6
Polytetrafluoroethylene	0.08	0.25	0.17	2–3	0.06

*Thermal conductivity in Btu/hr./ft.²/in./°F.

almost as hard as diamond. One of the common corrosion-resistant steels is called "18-8" stainless steel and it consists of about 18 per cent chromium, 8 per cent nickel and 74 per cent iron. This type of stainless steel is commonly used for applications in which rusting and tarnishing are not desired. The material may be procured in a large variety of shapes and forms of raw stock as well as finished products such as hardware, screws, nuts and washers. Its corrosion-resistant properties often override its disadvantages of additional cost and increased difficulty of machineability, as compared to carbon steels.

Often easily machined, inexpensive materials such as brass and steel are plated to give protection from corrosion and to enhance their appearance. Such plating, usually applied electrolytically, consists of nickel, chromium or cadmium.

NONFERROUS METALS.   The subject of nonferrous metals is of large scope, far greater than can be fully discussed in the context of this publication. Aluminum is used for its low density, copper for its high electrical conductivity, bronze for its good bearing qualities, and brass for its excellent machineability. Suffice it to say that a large variety of physical properties differing from those of the ferrous metals (see Table 40-1) are available to the designer who may want to select those properties which most nearly meet the requirements of the intended application.

Nonmetallic Materials.   The nonmetallic materials include a host of substances such as wood, glass, plaster, rubber, fabrics, paper, oils and gases. While all these substances are utilized in rehabilitation, many of the more useful materials are included in the general classification of plastics. The word plastic comes from the Greek *plastikos*, "fit for molding." Today, plastic products include not only molded things but useful articles made in many other ways. Fabrics may be woven from plastic fibers—the synthetic rubber for automobile tires is a plastic—and a multitude of shapes and forms are cast from resins.

The plastics industry uses seven principal processes for making articles of plastic. They are compression and injection molding, laminating, extrusion, blow molding, casting, fabrication and calendering. Available for use in the field of rehabilitation are stock materials and finished items made by these processes. Such stock materials as sheets and rods, as well as finished products such as containers, bearings, gears and insulators, may be obtained from distributors.

The choice of type and physical form of plastic depends upon the use for which it is to serve. Consideration of color, strength, rigidity, ease of fabrication, frictional characteristics and cost are among the criteria for making the choice. Some of the physical properties of several common plastics are shown in Table 40-1.

Some plastics harden when they are heated, while others harden only when they are cooled below their melting points. By this distinction, the plastics are frequently referred to as the *thermosetting* and *thermoplastic* types, each having certain useful characteristics to serve specific needs. Among the so-called thermosetting plastics—those which cannot be softened by heating—are the phenolics, ureas, melamines and epoxies. Almost all the remaining widely used plastics are in the thermoplastic family—those which soften on heating and reharden when cooled. Among the thermoplastic materials are cellulose, cellulose acetate, acrylic resins, vinyls, polyethylene, polystyrene, polyamide, silicones, trifluoroethylene and polytetrafluoroethylene.

The physical properties of plastics are varied by the manufacturer by the degree of polymerization, compounding, addition of fillers and plasticizers,

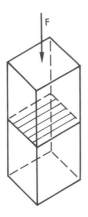

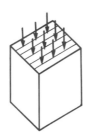

Figure 40–19 Normal stress. A distributed force acting in a direction perpendicular to a given area.

and other treatments. To use any of these materials properly, one should consult specifications provided by the manufacturer regarding the specific material to be used.

Mechanics of Materials

Materials for construction are arranged by fabrication into some suitable physical geometric shapes in order to serve a specific desired purpose. These geometric shapes consist of a variety of generally familiar forms, such as tubes, beams and columns. To meet design requirements, one must consider appropriate physical properties of matter such as yield strength, modulus of elasticity, density, hardness, thermal or electrical conductivity, ease of fabrication, and hygienic and cosmetic qualities.

External forces acting upon an object can cause stresses within the object. These stresses may result from any one or a combination of four types of loading; compressive, tensile, shear and torsional. While the loading may be distinguishable by four possible modes, the resulting stresses consist of only two types: *normal* stress and *shear* stress. Normal stress (see Figure 40-19) results from a force acting perpendicular to the area being considered, while shear stress (see Figure 40-20) results from a force acting parallel to it.

Stress, like pressure, is measured in units of force per unit area. Stresses, in simple tension or compression, may be related to the force, F, acting on the cross-sectional area, A, as shown in the following equation:

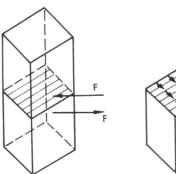

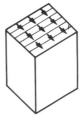

Figure 40–20 Shear stress. A distributed force acting in a direction parallel to a given area.

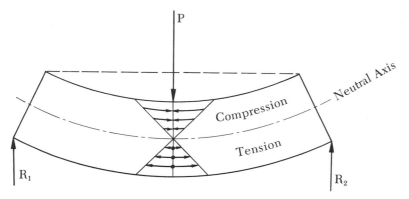

Figure 40–21   Stress distribution in a beam under a single, concentrated lateral load.

$$S = \frac{F}{A} \tag{19}$$

which simply states that the stress is equal to the force per unit area. If the force is increased, the stress is increased; if the area is increased, the stress is decreased.

Stresses in bending and in torsion are somewhat more complicated than in simple compression or tension. Figure 40-21 depicts a beam supported at its ends and an applied load at the center of the span. To help visualize the stresses within the beam, one might think of the beam as consisting of a bundle of fibers; the fibers near the concave surface are in compression, those near the convex side are in tension, and those at the center, the neutral axis, are unstressed.

The stress in a beam is related to the dimensional characteristics of the beam and to the magnitude of the applied load, and may be expressed by:

$$S = \frac{Mc}{I} \tag{20}$$

where M is the bending moment at the section through the point under consideration, c is the distance of the point from the neutral axis, and I is the area moment of inertia. Equation (20) is the basis of the design and investigation of beams and is one of the most important relationships in use. The bending moment is the product of the applied load and the distance of the point under consideration from the nearest support. The area moment of inertia is an expression of the distribution of material in the cross-sectional area under consideration. The area moment of inertia is that property of the cross-sectional area that takes into account not only the amount of area but also the disposition of the area with respect to the neutral axis. For instance, a flat slat like a paint stirrer is much more readily bent in its flat dimension than in its wide direction. Area moments of inertia of four common shapes are given in Figure 40-22. This concept becomes very important in the consideration of shaping materials in the construction of splints and braces. To obtain maximum rigidity, it is necessary to locate the material as far from the neutral axis as possible. Although the simple shapes shown in Figure 40-22 are not always

Rectangle, axis through center

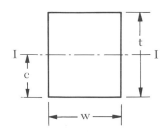

$$A = wt$$

$$c = t/2$$

$$I = \frac{wt^3}{12}$$

$$r = \frac{t}{\sqrt{12}} = 0.289\, t$$

Hollow rectangle, axis through center

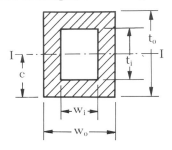

$$A = w_o t_o - w_i t_i$$

$$c = t_o/2$$

$$I = \frac{w_o t_o^3 - w_i t_i^3}{12}$$

$$r = \sqrt{\frac{w_o t_o^3 - w_i t_i^3}{12(w_o t_o - w_i t_i)}}$$

Circle, axis through center

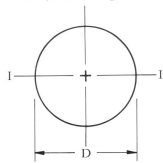

$$A = \frac{\pi D^2}{4} = 0.785\ D^2$$

$$c = D/2$$

$$I = \frac{\pi D^4}{64} = 0.0491\ D^4$$

$$r = \frac{D}{4}$$

Hollow circle, axis through center

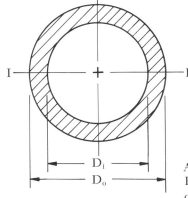

$$A = \frac{\pi}{4}\,(D_o^2 - D_i^2)$$

$$c = D_o/2$$

$$I = \frac{\pi}{64}\,(D_o^4 - D_i^4)$$

$$r = \sqrt{\frac{(D_o^2 + D_i^2)}{4}}$$

A = Area of section
I = Area moment of inertia about axis I-I
c = Distance from axis I-I to remotest point of section
r = Radius of gyration

Figure 40–22   Area moments of inertia of four common shapes.

directly applicable to a given problem, nevertheless, understanding the principles involved should be very helpful in dealing with many applications.

Bending. The beam is one of the more common shapes used in structural members; one such use in rehabilitation medicine is an upright bar for a leg brace. A beam by definition is a bar or structural member subjected to transverse loads that tend to bend it. Two of the most common types of beams encountered are the simple beam and the cantilever beam. Figures 40-23 and 40-24 illustrate these two beam configurations, which differ in their means of support and manner of loading. Equations relating the factors to be considered in beam design are the following:

(Simple beam)
$$d = \frac{P\,L^3}{48\,E\,I} \tag{21}$$

and by direct substitution for the area moment of inertia, I, from Figure 40–22:

$$d = \frac{PL^3}{4\,Ewt^3}$$

where d is the deflection, P is the applied load, L is the length, E is the modulus of clasticity, w is the width of the beam, and t is its thickness.

(Cantilever beam)
$$d = \frac{PL^3}{3\,E\,I} \tag{22}$$

and by direct substitution for I as previously:

$$d = \frac{4\,PL^3}{Ewt^3}$$

For each type of beam, certain conclusions regarding the characteristics of the beam may be drawn. The following may be said of the deflection, d:

1. The deflection is directly proportional to the applied load, P. Doubling the load doubles the deflection.

2. The deflection is directly proportional to the cube of the length. By doubling the length of the beam, the deflection is increased eight-fold ($2^3 = 8$) for the same load.

3. The deflection is inversely proportional to the modulus of elasticity. By doubling E, through choice of a different material of construction, the deflection is halved under the same load.

Figure 40–23 Simple beam is one which is supported at each end; the load is applied between the supports.

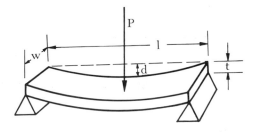

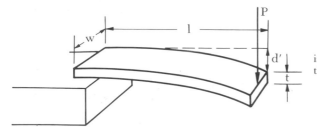

Figure 40–24   Cantilever beam is one which is supported at one end; the load is applied to the other end.

4. The deflection is inversely proportional to the width of the beam. By doubling the width of the beam, the deflection is halved under the same load.

5. The deflection is inversely proportional to the cube of the thickness. By doubling the thickness of the beam, the deflection is reduced to $\frac{1}{8}$ under the same load.

These statements simply say that the relative stiffness of a beam—that is, the relationship of the deflection, d, to the applied load, P—can be altered by changing any one or more of the terms identified in equations (21) and (22). The deflection-to-load relationship is very sensitive to varying the thickness or the length as compared to varying the width, for example. Note also that if both length and thickness are changed proportionately, the relationship of the deflection to the load remains constant, because the term for length, L, is in the numerator and the term for thickness, t, is in the denominator.

Equations (21) and (22) deal with beams of rectangular cross-section. If one should consider a circular cross-section, then the equations for deflection become, by direct substitution of the area moment of inertia for a circular cross-section from Figure 40-22:

(Simple beam) $$d = \frac{4\ PL^3}{3\ E\pi D^4} \tag{23}$$

(Cantilever beam) $$d = \frac{64\ PL^3}{3\ E\pi D^4} \tag{24}$$

where D is the diameter of the round beam or rod. Note that the diameter is related by its fourth power to the deflection. Because the diameter is related by its fourth power, it becomes apparent that the material in the center of a solid rod does not contribute substantially to the stiffness of a rod or beam. For this reason, economies in weight and cost can be effected by making the section hollow. By considering tubing for the application for which the outside diameter is D_o and the inside diameter is D_i, then equations (23) and (24) become:

(Simple beam) $$d = \frac{4\ PL^3}{3\ E\pi(D_o^4 - D_i^4)} \tag{25}$$

(Cantilever beam) $$d = \frac{64\ PL^3}{3\ E\pi(D_o^4 - D_i^4)} \tag{26}$$

For example, if the inside diameter of the tube is one half of the outside diameter, that is, $D_i = 0.5D_o$, then the weight is reduced to 75 per cent of that of the solid rod, and the deflection for the same applied load is only 7 per cent greater. Further, if the inside diameter were to be $0.8\ D_o$, then the weight would be reduced to 36 per cent of that of the solid rod, and the deflection for the same applied load would be 69 per cent greater. Since the fourth power of the diameter is used, the loss in stiffness by hollowing out the rod can readily be compensated by a very small increase in outside diameter. For example, considering the above sample, by increasing D_o by 14 per cent, while retaining the $D_i = 0.8\ D_o$ ratio, the weight is 44 per cent of the solid rod of the original D_o and the deflection is no more than a solid rod of the original D_o. In other words, a tube of 1.14 inches outside diameter and 0.91 inch inside diameter is as stiff as a solid rod of 1.00 inch outside diameter and weighs only 44 per cent as much.

Torsion.   Another form of flexural deflection is axial twisting of a structural member. Such twisting is called torsion. Within the elastic limit, the angular displacement is expressed by the following:

$$\theta = \frac{32\ \mathrm{TL}}{\mathrm{E_s}\,\pi \mathrm{D}^4} \tag{27}$$

for a solid rod, and for a hollow rod or tube:

$$\theta = \frac{32\ \mathrm{TL}}{\mathrm{E_s}\,\pi(\mathrm{D_o^4} - \mathrm{D_i^4})} \tag{28}$$

where

$\theta =$ angular displacement in radians
$\mathrm{T} =$ torque applied
$\mathrm{E_s} =$ shear modulus of elasticity, which is usually different from the tensile or compressional value
$\mathrm{L} =$ length of the rod or tube

Stress in Bending and Torsion.   Elastic deformation of a body, whether in bending or in torsion, causes stresses within the body. Bending and torsion illustrate the two types of stress identified earlier. Bending produces normal stresses within the body, whereas torsion produces shear stresses.
    The stress occurring in any part of the cross-sectional area of a beam can be calculated by use of the general formula for flexure. Refer to equation (20):

$$S = \frac{Mc}{I}$$

It holds true, of course, only if the longitudinal fiber stress, S, does not exceed the proportional limit of the material. By direct substitution of other terms for M, c and I in the equation, the following expressions for the bending stress in a rectangular beam may be derived:

Simple beam

Letting $\qquad\qquad\qquad\qquad M = \dfrac{PL}{4}$

assuming the load, P, to be applied to the center of the span of length, L, and

$$c = \frac{t}{2}$$

and

$$I = \frac{wt^3}{12} \quad \text{(from Figure 40-22)}$$

$$S = \frac{Mc}{I} = \frac{\frac{PL}{4} \times \frac{t}{2}}{\frac{wt^3}{12}} = \frac{6\ PL}{wt^2}$$

Cantilever beam

Letting

$$M = PL$$

and the other terms as above

$$S = \frac{3\ PL}{2\ wt^2}$$

By similar direct substitution, the stress equations for beams of round cross-section may also be derived to yield the following:

(Simple beam)

$$S = \frac{8\ PL}{\pi D_o^3}$$

(Cantilever beam)

$$S = \frac{32\ PL}{\pi D_o^3}$$

The shear stress induced into a shaft by a twisting action may also be calculated. The expressions for this shear stress for a solid and a hollow rod are the following:

(Solid)

$$S_s = \frac{16\ T}{\pi D_o^3} \tag{29}$$

(Hollow)

$$S_s = \frac{16\ T\ D}{\pi (D_o^4 - D_i^4)} \tag{30}$$

The expressions for the calculation of stresses within beams and shafts are valid just so long as the elastic limit of the material is not exceeded. If the elastic limit of the body is exceeded, then a permanent set will take place, or if the ultimate strength of the material is reached, then the object will rupture. The stress formulas are used in design to calculate physical dimensions of components. A safety factor is normally applied to the yield strength value of the material selected so as to arrive at dimensions adequate to assure mechanical integrity of the component in its expected use.

As in the discussion on bending, the reader may draw certain conclusions about the various terms in the expressions as to the sensitivity of their contribution to the relative strength of a beam or shaft. If, for example, a beam type of structural member fails by taking a permanent set, then one might select a material of higher elastic limit or alter the physical dimensions in a manner which will preserve the integrity of the beam in its application by reducing the stress developed by a given load.

This discussion on mechanics of materials is quite elementary and obviously does not cover the flexural properties of the varied shapes that are to be found in the "real" world. To attempt to cover the multitude of shapes, and to include consideration for combined stresses due to both bending and torsional loading of structural members such as splints and braces, would extend beyond the scope of this publication. However, the basic technology offered in this section should acquaint the reader with physical concepts and terminology that should enable him to apply his skills to patient care more effectively.

ELECTRONICS

Webster's Collegiate Dictionary defines electronics as a branch of physics that deals with the emission, behavior and effects of electrons. The principal technological developments have taken place in only the last fifty years. In spite of this fact, electronics has drastically altered the life of civilized man by providing widespread communication facilities, easy access to entertainment, news, education and art forms, and by providing improved means of lower-cost manufacturing of goods and methods of carrying on commerce.

The application of the technology of electronics in medicine has been slower to develop, although the trend to exploit the tools of this branch of science is growing and will continue to do so at an accelerated rate. Even now, in physical medicine, electronic devices are found in almost every aspect of the diagnosis, treatment, care and rehabilitation of the patient. In electrodiagnosis the electrocardiogram, electroencephalogram and electromyogram provide the clinician with information and measured parameters on phenomena too minute to be observed in any other way. In treatment, the use of diathermy, ultrasound and electrical stimulation of denervated muscle provides modalities not otherwise available. In hospital care of the disabled, monitoring of the patient by closed circuit television and by attached instruments for cardiac, renal and pulmonary function indicators permits a quality of care not previously available. Control methods for externally powered assistive devices in prosthetics and in orthotics give rehabilitation potential not formerly achievable. The ability to measure and evaluate objectively a patient's function, his needs and the results of treatment provides powerful tools for advancing the treatment of physical dysfunction caused by neuromuscular damage.

The following sections can hardly serve as either a course in electronics or a complete exposition on its application to medicine. A number of selected topics are presented with the hope that they may be useful in teaching something of the principles and the jargon of the technology, and a few of the basic considerations involved in using electronic equipment are given.

Basic Electronic Concepts

Electrons and Electron Flow. The electron is a fundamental particle of matter possessing a negative charge and a very small mass. In the Bohr model of the atom, the central nucleus consists of protons and neutrons, particles having large mass and electrical charges of positive and zero respectively, while the electrons are pictured as satellite particles orbiting the central nucleus at a distance of some ten thousand times the nuclear diameter. In some solid materials, those known as good electrical conductors, the outermost planetary electrons are loosely bound to their orbits. In the Bohr atomic model such electrons may characteristically transfer their orbits to paths around adjacent atomic nuclei if influenced by an external force which may be thermal, mechanical, chemical or electrical in nature. Thermal agitation ordinarily produces a random orbital exchange, whereas an electrical force, if oriented in a uniform direction, produces a net movement of electrons through the material in the direction of the applied force.

The net movement of electrons through a material may be likened to what occurs in a row of billiard balls in a trough; if a new ball is added at the end, another is ejected at the far end to make room for the added ball. Viewed externally, it appears as though the electron has made an almost instantaneous transit through the material. However, viewed internally, the emerging electron is not the original one at all but rather the end electron in a series of progressive transferences of orbital electrons from atom to atom.

A net movement of electrons through a material is called an electric current and its unit of measurement is the ampere. The ampere is defined as the flow of 6.24×10^{18} electrons per second. The electromotive force which must be applied to produce such a flow of electrons is called a volt.

The number of amperes flowing in a substance is dependent upon the applied voltage and upon the geometry and the conduction characteristics of the substance, just as the flow of water in a pipe is dependent on the applied pressure, the pipe's diameter and length and the smoothness of the internal walls. The ease or, more properly, the difficulty with which electron flow takes place in a circuit is called *resistance* and is measured in units called ohms. Accordingly, an electrical circuit which possesses high resistance will show a smaller flow of electrical current than one with low resistance with the same applied voltage. The relationship among voltage, current and resistance is stated very simply in *Ohm's Law*:

$$I = \frac{E}{R} \qquad (31)$$

where

$$
\begin{aligned}
I &= \text{current in amperes} \\
E &= \text{number of applied volts} \\
R &= \text{resistance in ohms}
\end{aligned}
$$

A mechanical analogy of this relationship may be found in considering a water supply to a community, as illustrated in Figure 40-25. The height of water in a city's water supply tower determines the pressure that forces water to flow through the system of pipes and corresponds to the electromotive force called voltage. The frictional characteristics of the pipe, its length and diameter determine the resistance (R) to water flow and therefore, the rate of discharge (I) obtained by the available pressure (E).

Electrical Circuits. Electronic circuits are not ordinarily composed of single elements. Often there are several branches with different resistances. The current in any branch can be calculated if the individual resistances are

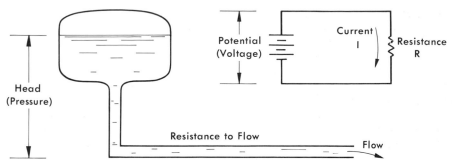

Figure 40–25 Hydraulic analogy of electrical flow.

known and if the applied circuit voltage is also known. The branching of current takes place in the same way that water flow does in passing through series and parallel portions of a piping system or in the branching of a stream. The total flow in must equal the total flow out, and the rules for division of the total current follow from the relative resistances of each branch. High resistance branches, like small diameter pipes, carry little current; low resistance branches, like large diameter pipes, carry more of the total flow. The rules for combining resistances in series and in parallel are:

Add resistances in series directly,

Add resistances in parallel according to the reciprocal rule:

$$\frac{1}{R_p} = \frac{1}{R_1} + \frac{1}{R_2} + \frac{1}{R_3} \cdot \cdot \cdot \cdot + \frac{1}{R_n} \text{ or, } R_{parallel} \frac{1}{\dfrac{1}{R_1} + \dfrac{1}{R_2} + \dfrac{1}{R_3} \cdot \cdot \cdot + \dfrac{1}{R_n}}$$

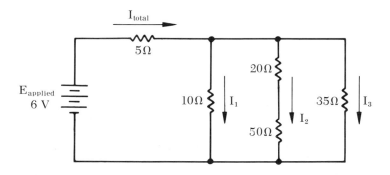

$$I_{total} = \frac{6 \text{ V}}{R_{total}} = I_1 + I_2 + I_3$$

$$= \frac{6}{5 + \dfrac{1}{\dfrac{1}{10} + \dfrac{1}{20 + 50} + \dfrac{1}{35}}} = \frac{6}{5 + 7} = \frac{6}{12} = \frac{1}{2} \text{ Amp}$$

Figure 40–26 Example of series-parallel resistive circuit.

Using these combining rules, Ohm's Law and simple arithmetic allows the series-parallel circuit in Figure 40–26 to be solved for the total current flowing as a result of the applied voltage.

Power. Electrical energy may be converted into other forms of energy. An electric current flowing through the fine high resistance wire of an electric light bulb is converted into both heat and light; an electric current flowing through an electric motor is converted into mechanical energy. The rate of energy conversion is called *power* and is measured in joules per second. A joule per second is equal to a watt and may be calculated from the voltage and the current flow by the simple formula:

$$\text{Power, watts} = \text{Volts} \times \text{Amps} \qquad (32)$$
$$\text{or, } P = E \times I$$

Other expressions for electrical power may be derived by using Ohm's Law (31) to obtain

$$P = \frac{E^2}{R} \quad \text{and} \quad P = I^2 R$$

Note in the latter expressions that doubling the current or doubling the voltage in a circuit results in quadrupling the power.

Almost all the basic quantities of measure in electronics, thermodynamics and hydraulics can be related to one another and converted to equivalent units by proportionality factors. An air conditioner, for example, may be variously rated in terms of its volts and amps (and therefore its wattage), its horsepower (746 watts equals one horsepower), its cooling capacity in BTU's (British thermal units) or in terms of the tonnage of ice it can freeze in a day. In each case, the power, or rate of doing work, is being expressed. For further equivalents, consult the section on mechanics and one of the engineering handbooks listed in the References at the end of the chapter.

Electric Current and Magnetic Field. A magnetic field is a phenomenon of nature which is associated with an electron in motion. A wire carrying an electric current (flow of electrons) is surrounded by a magnetic field, the strength of which depends upon the magnitude of the current.

The magnetic field developed by a current in a wire can be intensified if the wire is wound into a coil, and further concentrated if a piece of iron or steel is placed in the coil. The electromagnet so formed, besides behaving like any other magnet as long as the current continues to flow, exhibits some other interesting properties. For example, an ammeter connected in series with the coil will show that the current does not start to flow instantly when the battery is connected; the current builds up from zero to its final value over a measureable period of time. In addition, if after establishing this current flow, the battery connection is suddenly removed and replaced with a short circuit, the ammeter will show that the current requires a comparable period of time to subside. This interaction of the magnetic field and the current in an electromagnet, or inductor, is called *self-induction*, and behaves very much the same as its mechanical equivalent of inertia. The electrical equivalent of mass is *inductance*, which is measured in henries, millihenries (10^{-3} henry), and microhenries (10^{-6} henry). The symbol for inductance is L.

The flow of electrons in a coil stores energy in the magnetic field it produces. The energy stored by a current in an inductance is expressed in the following equation:

$$W = \frac{1}{2} L I^2 \tag{33}$$

where

W = stored energy in joules
L = inductance in henries
I = current in amperes

The mechanical concept of kinetic energy, K.E. = $\frac{1}{2} mV^2$ from equation (15), is a direct analog, where m and L represent the inertia and V and I represent the rate of displacement with respect to time.

Another property of magnetic fields and electron flow in a wire is that force or motion can be produced. If a wire is placed between the poles of a strong permanent magnet and then connected to a battery, the wire will tend to move. The magnetic field caused by the electric current interacts with the field of the permanent magnet to produce a force. An electric motor uses this phenomenon to turn electrical energy into mechanical force and motion. This interaction of motion, current and magnetic field is also manifested in the corollary generator effect. If a closed loop of wire is moved rapidly through the jaws of a large permanent magnet, an electron flow is produced by the interaction of motion and magnetic field. Generators employ this phenomenon to produce electrical voltage from mechanical motion. In this case, the generated voltage is directly proportional to the magnetic flux and to the velocity of motion. A small generator can therefore be used to measure velocity and can be calibrated in terms of volts per feet per second or volts per revolution per minute.

Voltage and Electrostatic Field.   The phenomenon of current flow is described in terms of the movement of the loosely bound planetary electrons in conductive materials. The result of an impressed voltage—that is, one applied from an outside source—is to cause transference of electrons from atom to atom. In a non-conducting or insulating material, on the other hand, the outermost electrons are tightly bound to the orbits around the nucleus to which they belong, and an applied electromotive force is usually not sufficient to overcome the binding forces and produce atom hopping of the planetary electrons. In this case, an applied potential to the material causes an internal stress but no continuous flow of electrons between atoms or molecules of the material.

Two plates separated by an insulator form a capacitor. A voltage applied across these plates results in an initial momentary electron displacement in the direction of the applied voltage. The effect in the conducting plates is to move electrons from the positive plate through the source of voltage to the negative plate, until the internal electrostatic forces in the insulator are in equilibrium with the applied voltage. If the source of voltage is then removed, the electrostatic tension remains and is evidenced by a sustained voltage difference across the plates. The capacitor is said to be charged. Applying an external conductive circuit from one plate to the other will then result in a momentary return current flow as the interatomic forces resume their original undisturbed conditions.

Capacitance is the analog of mechanical elasticity or compliance and is measured in farads, microfarads (10^{-6} farad), and picofarads (10^{-12} farad). It can be defined in terms of the net number of electrons transferred from one plate of the capacitor to the other through the external circuit as a result of the applied voltage:

$$C(\text{farads}) = \frac{\text{Number electrons transferred}}{6.24 \times 10^{18} \times \text{applied voltage}}$$

$$\text{or} \quad \frac{\text{Current (amps)} \times \text{Time (sec.)}}{\text{Voltage}}$$

The energy stored in the dielectric, or insulator, of a capacitor is the analog of potential energy and can be calculated from the formula:

$$W = \frac{1}{2} CV^2 \qquad (34)$$

where

W = stored energy in joules
C = capacitance in farads
V = volts

Electrical Resonance.   If a spring is hung from a hook in the ceiling and a weight is hung from the spring, the elastic properties of the spring and the inertial properties of the mass will allow the weight to bob up and down at some fixed rate of oscillation, if it is mechanically disturbed. At the lowest point of the oscillation, the potential energy of the system is stored in the elongation of the spring. As the mass moves upward, this potential energy decreases because a portion of it is being transformed into the kinetic energy of the moving mass. This kinetic energy is then transferred to potential energy again as the weight rises to its highest point in the cycle. The rate at which this energy is transferred back and forth between the stretching of the spring and the velocity of the moving weight can be calculated from the spring constant and the mass.

In view of the analogs drawn between elasticity and capacitance and mass and inductance it is not surprising that a similar situation occurs electrically when these two elements are connected in a circuit. If a charged capacitor containing stored potential energy by virtue of its charge is connected across an inductance, an oscillatory flow of current results. The potential energy stored in the capacitor is transformed into kinetic energy of current flow through an inductor. The frequency of this electrical resonance can be calculated from the values of L and C by means of the formula:

$$\text{Resonant frequency, } f = \frac{1}{2\pi \sqrt{L \times C}} \qquad (35)$$

where

f = frequency in hertz (cycles per second)
L = inductance in henries
C = capacitance in farads

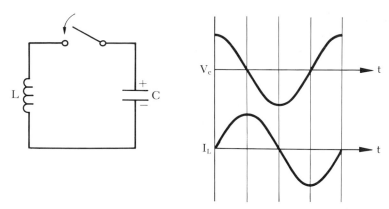

Figure 40–27 Electrical resonance of a coil and capacitor.

Both the voltage across the capacitor and the current flowing in the circuit vary sinusoidally with time. If you remember that the maximum electric current, I, is due to the maximum energy stored in the inductance while maximum voltage, E, is due to the maximum energy stored in the capacitor, the fact that these two events alternate in time and that the voltage and current waveforms go through their maxima at instances displaced in time is not surprising. The appearance of these two waveforms is the same as if one were a sine wave and the other a cosine wave, since they are displaced by 90 degrees, or one-quarter cycle. (See Figure 40-27.)

AC and DC. The oscillatory waveform of voltage and current observed in electrical resonance is an example of alternating or wave motion. This example of a current which alternately flows in one direction and then in the other differs from a direct, or unidirectional, current in the same way that the motion of the surf at the seashore differs from the motion of a waterfall, and in the same way that a sound vibration differs from a steady barometric pressure. Pressure and flow are manifest in both types of phenomenon and can be described similarly.

Alternating sinusoidal voltages can be described by stating their frequency and amplitude. The frequency is usually stated in hertz (cycles per second), kilohertz (10^3 hertz), megahertz (10^6 hertz), or gigahertz (10^9 hertz). The amplitude of the voltage is changing at every instant in time and may be stated in several ways: the peak or maximum voltage may be given; the peak to peak or total excursion may be used as a measure of amplitude; or you can determine the magnitude of an equivalent DC voltage which produces the same heating effect in a resistance as does the alternating voltage. This equivalent voltage, called the RMS or root-mean-square voltage, can be found by integrating the product of the alternating voltage with the alternating current flow through the resistor over one complete cycle of the waveform. The resulting RMS voltage for a sinusoidal shape is equal to 70.7 per cent of the peak voltage (see Figure 40-28) and is the measure of alternating voltage waveform amplitude ordinarily given. The 60 hertz AC power line voltage of 115 volts RMS is a sinusoidal voltage waveform with a peak value of 163 volts. Its heating effect is the same as the heating effect of 115 volts DC.

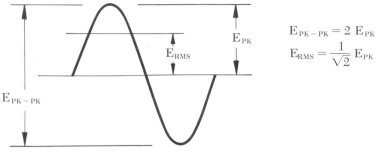

$$E_{PK-PK} = 2\, E_{PK}$$

$$E_{RMS} = \frac{1}{\sqrt{2}}\, E_{PK}$$

Figure 40–28   AC voltage measurement.

Alternating current is often the preferred form of electrical energy in use because the wave motion phenomenon gives it additional properties that direct current does not have. For example, a device called a transformer may be used with alternating current; the constantly changing amplitude of current flowing in the primary winding of the transformer produces the equivalent of a relative motion between the magnetic field and the wires of the secondary winding. This relative motion of magnetic field and conductor results in a voltage being generated in the secondary winding. The relationship of the voltage generated in the secondary winding to that applied to the primary winding is determined by the efficiency of the magnetic circuit and the ratio of the number of turns wound on each coil. It is therefore possible to "step up" or "step down" alternating voltage with a simple device called a transformer, which consists of two coils wound on a magnetic core material.

By the same mechanism, it is possible to generate a small voltage in a coil by virtue of the alternating magnetic field produced by a radio transmitter some distance away and thus to transmit and detect high frequency signals for use in communications. The home radio uses just such a coil to "pick up" the transmitter's magnetic field, then amplifies it and turns it into an audible signal.

Reactance and Impedance.   Resistors, inductors and capacitors behave differently in alternating current circuits. The resistor dissipates energy in the form of heat whereas both the capacitor and the inductor temporarily store energy in their respective electrostatic and magnetic fields and then must return this energy to the circuit. Furthermore, an AC voltage applied to a resistor results in a current which is in phase, or in step, with that voltage, but the same voltage applied to an inductor results in a current which lags behind the voltage by 90 degrees, or one quarter cycle. The same AC voltage, if applied to a capacitor, results in a current which appears to lead the voltage by 90 degrees. These leading and lagging currents are commonly called reactive currents.

In a circuit containing a resistor, or inductor and a capacitor in parallel, the net current from the source of voltage will contain components in phase and 90 degrees out of phase with the applied voltage. These circuits are combined vectorially in a manner similar to that used for combining forces acting at different angles. In this situation, however, resistive current is always assumed to act at zero degrees (that is, in phase), inductive current is assumed to add as a vector placed at $+90$ degrees, and capacitive current is always added

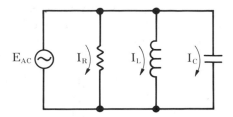

Figure 40–29   Vector addition of resistive and reactive currents.

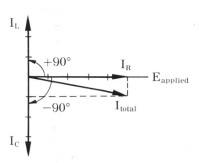

as a vector at −90 degrees. The total current must be determined by vector addition, as shown in Figure 40-29.

The reactive currents result from the property of inductors and capacitors that is referred to as reactance. Just as resistance indicates the difficulty encountered by a current flow through this device, reactance indicates the difficulty of AC current flow through either an inductor or a capacitor. Reactance and resistance in a circuit must be combined vectorially to obtain the net *impedance*. The impedance, then, may be stated as a magnitude, in ohms, at an angle whose tangent is equal to the ratio of the reactance to the resistance. It is frequently represented by stating the two components separately, however. The two equivalent notations are shown as follows:

$$\text{Impedance} = Z = \text{ohms } \underline{/\theta}, \text{ degrees or } Z = R + jX_L$$
$$\text{or } R - jX_c$$
$$\text{where } j = \sqrt{-1}$$

If the frequency of the applied sinusoidal voltage waveform is known, then inductive reactance and capacitive reactance may be calculated by the simple formulae:

$$X_L = 2\pi fL \tag{37}$$

where
$$f = \text{frequency in hertz}$$
$$L = \text{inductance in henries}$$
$$\text{and } X_L = \text{inductive reactance in ohms}$$

$$X_c = \frac{1}{2\pi fC} \tag{38}$$

where
$$f = \text{frequency in hertz}$$
$$C = \text{capacitance in farads}$$
$$\text{and } X_c = \text{capacitive reactance in ohms}$$

Vacuum Tubes and Transistors. Most electronic circuits, whether they are amplifiers, oscillators or some other functional element, employ either vacuum tubes or transistors to provide the vital function of gain. In the British Isles the vacuum tube has traditionally been called a valve; the term is very descriptive of the function. Both vacuum tubes and transistors function by controlling a current flowing through them by means of a much smaller current or voltage applied to the input terminal.

The vacuum tube may contain several internal elements but the basic function of amplification is best demonstrated by the three element or triode tube (Fig. 40-30). It consists of a heated cathode, a control grid and an anode structure. The cathode's function is to supply a source of free electrons by "boiling" them off from a special coating on the metal cathode structure. A positive DC potential is applied to the anode; the electrons are thus drawn across the intervening space, and they impinge on the anode and then flow through the external circuit. A control grid is interposed between the cathode and anode structures. This grid consists of an open wire structure through which the electrons may pass. The application of a negative potential to the control grid causes a decrease in the anode current by repelling some of the electrons back to the cathode before they manage to pass through the grid structure. The net result is that a varying voltage applied to the control grid causes a similarly varying current to flow in the anode circuit. The most significant characteristic of the vacuum tube is the ratio of the change in anode current to the causative change in voltage applied to the control grid. The parameter is called transconductance and is given in units of mhos, millimhos or micromhos.

The transistor performs a similar function but by a different mechanism. It generally has three elements: the emitter, base and collector (Fig. 40–31). Functionally, these perform similarly to the cathode, grid and anode of the vacuum tube. The important differences between the vacuum tube and transistor are that no heated source of electrons is required in the transistor (they are supplied by the properties of the semiconductor material), the device is much

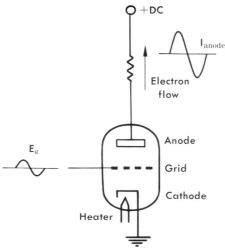

Figure 40–30 The triode vacuum tube.

$$\text{Transconductance, } g_m, \text{ in Mhos} = \frac{\Delta I_A}{\Delta E_g}$$

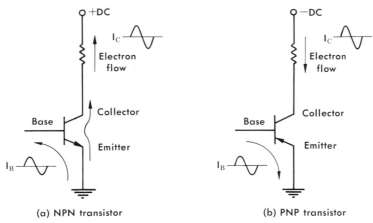

(a) NPN transistor   (b) PNP transistor

Figure 40-31   The transistor.

smaller physically and it functions basically as a current amplifier. A DC potential applied between the emitter and the collector results in no current flow until a current flow is also provided between the base and the emitter. The collector current flow is approximately proportional to the base current flow but many times larger. The most important transistor characteristic is its current gain, which is defined as the ratio of the resulting collector current to the base current. The most common name for this current gain is the beta of the transistor. It is a unitless number since it is a ratio of two currents. Typical betas range from ten to several hundred.

Most transistors are of two basic types: NPN or PNP, the letters indicate the relative polarities of the semiconductor materials comprising them. The NPN transistor is operated with positive collector voltage supplies and requires a positive input voltage to cause base current flow. The PNP is exactly the reverse, that is, negative voltages with respect to the emitter must be applied to obtain current gain. The symbol for the device indicates the type by the direction of the emitter arrow (Fig. 40-31).

The transistor is rapidly replacing the vacuum tube for most circuit functions (but not all) because of its reliability, low power requirements (it needs no heating power), small size, and economy in mass production.

Functional Electronic Systems.   The world of electronic circuits is an invisible, motionless, silent world. An operating circuit makes no sound, just sits there and appears to do nothing, unless, of course, you should touch it and receive a shock or unless it should decide to burn itself up! To make its operation perform a useful function for us and also to make it sensitive to the external world, an electronic circuit must usually be equipped with a transducer at its input and another at its output. Transducers are devices which communicate into and out of electrical circuits by turning some form of energy like sound, light or motion into an electronic current flow input and by converting the modified electrical output signal back into a form detectable by the senses. A functional system, then, consists usually of an input transducer, an electronic circuit, an output transducer and a source of electrical power (Fig. 40-32).

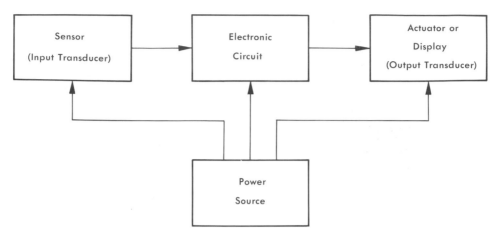

Figure 40–32 Block diagram of an electronic circuit.

Many electrical transducers are bidirectional devices. A loudspeaker, for example, is used to produce audible sound from an electrical signal from an amplifier. It may also be used to perform the reverse operation, that of turning an audible sound into an electrical signal. Most office intercom systems do exactly this; the loudspeaker is switched either to the amplifier input terminals when sending or to the output terminals when receiving a communication over the interconnecting wires. More frequently, however, a transducer is specially designed to function better in one mode than the other. The loudspeaker and the microphone are both electroacoustic devices, for example, but each has been specially designed to be better at one function than the other. Input transducers are frequently called sensors and are specially designed to turn a physical parameter into an electrical signal so that it can be amplified, modulated, rectified, gated or otherwise operated upon by electronic circuitry. Output transducers perform the reverse function and are often described as display devices, actuators, output indicators, monitors or recorders.

Sensors and Input Transducers. Input transducers can be broadly categorized as either electromechanical, electrochemical, electroacoustic, photoelectric, thermoelectric or bioelectric. The microphone and phonograph pickup are of the electroacoustic type. The photocell (or electric eye), the solar cell and the TV camera are examples of photoelectric transducers. The electrogoniometer, the tachometer, the switch and the strain gauge are electromechanical transducers. The thermistor and thermocouple are thermoelectric devices. The electrocardiograph and myoelectric sensors are not transducers like the others; they are simply specially designed contacting devices for observing bioelectric phenomena.

The *electrogoniometer* is a device that converts an angular position into an electrical signal. It is an electrical protractor which delivers an electrical signal proportional to the angular position of its two mechanical arms (Fig. 40–33). Although not the only type available, the most common form of electrogoniometer is the potentiometer. A potentiometer is a device with fixed linear resistance arranged in a circular form and equipped with a slider that is free to move its point of contact from one end of the resistance to the other. If a voltage is applied across the total resistance of the potentiometer, then the

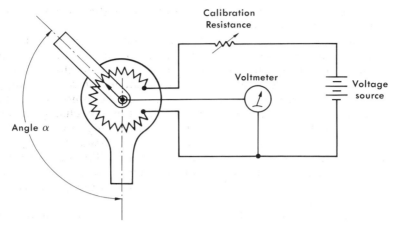

Figure 40–33   Typical electrogoniometer schematic.

portion of the total applied voltage picked off by the slider will be a direct measure of its position. The device is almost identical to the volume control used on radios and TV sets.

The important thing to know about the selection of the electrogoniometer is its linearity, its accuracy and its calibration or sensitivity in volts per degree of angle. Potentiometers used for electrogoniometers should be precision devices to provide true readings of angular position over their entire range. Look for linearity and repeatability specifications from the manufacturer of fractions of a percentage point and mechanical operating torques low enough to guarantee easy movement. The sensitivity of the device can be regulated by adjusting the voltage applied to the unit (Fig. 40-34). It is a very simple device and has the

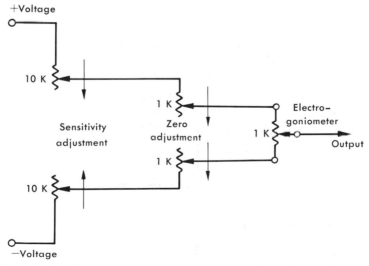

Figure 40–34   Electrogoniometer circuit with zero and sensitivity adjustments

advantage of providing a high level output signal that often can be used directly without further amplification.

The *strain gauge* is usually a very fine wire laid down in a back and forth pattern; the wire can be cemented to a structural member to measure the small deflection or strain produced when a force is applied to that member (Fig. 40–35). The stretching of the fine wire causes a small resistance change that is proportional to the total deformation within the elastic limits of both the wire and the member upon which it is mounted. Since the total change in resistance for an applied load is small, strain gauges are usually operated in bridge circuits, which serve to cancel the reading of fixed resistance and provide an output proportional only to the change in resistance. To enhance the output reading further, gauges are usually operated in pairs—one on each side of the structural member undergoing deformation, so that as one gauge is stretched the other is compressed.

Since the resistance of the fine wire used in strain gauges is temperature

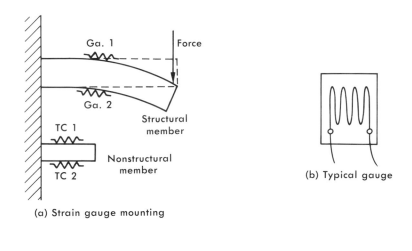

(a) Strain gauge mounting

(b) Typical gauge

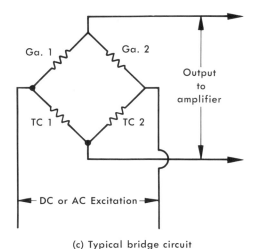

(c) Typical bridge circuit

Figure 40–35 Schematics of typical strain gauge application.

sensitive, it is usual to employ temperature compensating (TC) elements for the inactive elements of the bridge circuit. A good way to do this is to mount two additional gauges on an identical nonstructural member near the member being measured.

Since the output level of a strain gauge circuit will generally be in the order of millivolts, additional amplification is usually required before the output reading is displayed. In addition, a sensitivity adjustment control and a bridge balance control are usually provided to adjust the circuit prior to making a measurement. The calibration of the circuits for force measurements should be carried out with known weights applied to the beam.

Microphones convert sound or vibration energy into a minute electrical signal for use in electronic circuits. Although carbon granule types are still used in some telephone equipment, most high quality microphones are either of the piezoelectric, magnetic or capacitive type. The piezoelectric microphone has good sensitivity and is economical to manufacture. It is used in most commercial sound equipment for general applications and is the type usually supplied with home tape recorders. The active element is a small piece of Rochelle salt or barium titanate material, which possesses the property of responding to mechanical strain by generating a small electrical voltage. This is called the piezoelectric effect. A magnetic, or dynamic, microphone produces electrical output by coupling the acoustical energy to a magnetic circuit element which changes the magnetic flux sensed by a small coil. It is, therefore, a miniature alternating current generator. A capacitive microphone, on the other hand, uses the incident acoustical energy to vibrate one plate of a capacitor, changing the separation of the two plates and thus the total capacitance of the structure. This parameter change is then sensed by electronic circuits designed to convert capacitance change into an electrical output signal.

Important characteristics of microphones are their sensitivity, uniformity of response with frequency, and their directionality. In choosing an electro acoustical transducer for instrumentation systems, the specifications of the device must be compared with the characteristics of the phenomenon to be observed. Almost any microphone with adequate sensitivity and response in the audible range can be used to provide input for spoken voice annotation of a magnetic tape recording, since intelligibility is the only factor of importance. For recording of instrumental and vocal music, however, the fidelity of the recording depends on the choice of a transducer with uniform frequency response, and on directional characteristics suitable to the geometry of the performing area. For instrumentation systems which monitor or record the phonocardiogram, a microphone with exceptionally good low frequency response is required in order to transduce accurately the low frequency valvular and contractile sounds of the heart in the chest cavity. An ordinary tape recorder microphone in this case would not respond to the essential information being sought. For audiometric work a subaudible range of frequencies is not as important as uniformity and calibration accuracy in the microphone used for measurement. Here the transducer must be one specified by the audiometer manufacturer if the measurements are to be accurate.

Thermistors are temperature-sensitive resistors with known characteristics. Their sensitivity is relatively high and they are ordinarily used to measure moderate temperature ranges like those of the human body and of the environment. These transducers can be made quite small and are admirably suited to measuring local temperatures in implanted or ingested devices. A temperature probe using two thermistors can be made directional to detect the flow of heat by subtracting the output of the unit on one side of a probe from the output of the unit mounted on the other side. Ambient temperature effects are thus largely ignored and only local temperature gradients are sensed.

Photocells convert incident radiant energy into an electrical output. Their peak response to incoming energy can be controlled by the materials used to make them, so that their measuring capabilities can extend both below and above the narrow range of radiant energy frequencies to which the human eye is sensitive. They are generally of either the *photoconductive* or *photovoltaic* type.

The photoconductive, sometimes called photoresistive, transducer varies its resistance with the amount of incident light. Common materials used are lead sulfide, cadmium sulfide and cadmium selenide. These transducers are characterized by high sensitivity but suffer from an inability to respond quickly to changes in light intensity. Their most frequent application is in "electric eye" devices, which are used to turn lights on and off at dusk and sunrise, and to detect the presence of objects within a light path. Many elevators use these devices to prevent the closing of the elevator door if a light beam across the entrance is interrupted by an object or person.

The photovoltaic cell generates an electrical voltage in response to incident radiation and is therefore a direct converter of energy from one form into another. Solar cells, which may be used in sufficient numbers to power electrical equipment, are photovoltaic devices. They are also frequently used to measure the presence or absence of light in devices like punched card readers, which must respond quickly to the presence or absence of radiant energy. Their sensitivity is much lower than the photoresistive cell.

Photodiodes and *phototransistors* comprise a third classification of photocells frequently used in electronic equipment. They respond much faster than the photoresistive type and have intermediate sensitivity to light. In each of these two devices, a normally backbiased semiconductor junction responds to incident radiant energy by allowing a current to flow from an applied source of voltage.

Surface electrodes are used for detecting electrical activity on the skin surface; these should utilize the simplest input sensor since transduction is not required. Poor and unreliable recordings are often obtained, however, because the nature of the contact and the effect of the amplifier used are not considered, Since body tissue can be considered as aqueous salt solution, the nature of the contact to be made is that of a metal to an electrolyte or ionized solution. This interface can contribute unwanted noise if it is not mechanically and chemically stable. The quality of the contact with the tissues below the surface can be enhanced by cleaning the skin adequately to remove surface oils and also by means of a slight abrasion or by the use of a small amount of salt gel or electrode paste. The electrode material should be chosen for its ionic and chemical stability in contact with the chloride ion, and relative motion at the interface should be avoided. Silver electrodes or specially chloridized silver electrodes are frequently used for their desirable characteristics and are held in place in ways designed to minimize motion at the metal-to-salt interface. Remember, too, that the connecting leads to the subsequent amplifier, although they should be as short as possible to minimize stray electrical pickup, must be arranged so that they do not pull on the electrode. In addition, cable "microphonism" and spurious signal pickup may be introduced if the amplifier is not close to the site of observation.

By far the most important consideration is the input impedance or input resistance of the amplifier which receives the minute signal from the electrodes. An equivalent circuit for the situation (omitting the capacitive elements) is shown in Figure 40-36.

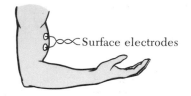

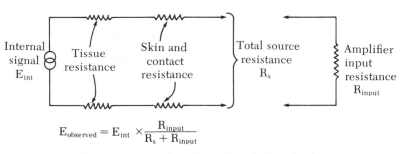

$$E_{observed} = E_{int} \times \frac{R_{input}}{R_s + R_{input}}$$

Figure 40–36   Surface electrode equivalent circuit.

It can be seen that the tissue resistance and the skin and contact resistance are in series with the internal source of signal and form a voltage divider with the input resistance of the amplifier. The voltage actually observed by the amplifier input terminals will be that given by the equation in Figure 40-35. Since the portion of the actual source signal observed is determined by the ratio of input resistance of the amplifier to the total resistance, it is desirable that it be substantially higher than the source resistance elements. If the equivalent source resistance of the signal is between 1000 and 100,000 ohms (it is usually not accurately determined and can easily vary this widely, depending on skin preparation and the subject), then an input resistance of at least a megohm is required to make the observed signal 90 per cent of the actual source signal. In practice it is desirable that it be higher than this, say ten megohms, to ensure that the observed signal is substantially that which is available for any reasonable contact resistance.

Amplifiers.   Electronic circuits are available to perform a large variety of functions. Oscillator and timing circuits, modulators and demodulators, pulse generators, counters, multipliers, squarers, integrators, differentiators, sweep generators, quantizers and scalers are but a sampling of applications attainable with the use of a relatively small category of components such as resistors, coils, capacitors, transistors, diodes, vacuum tubes and ordinary wire. Many of these are electrical analogs of mechanical and hydraulic devices as familiar as the abacus, the clock and the hydraulic ram. Although not unique to electronics, the most useful and versatile functional element is the amplifier. It appears many times over again in slightly different forms in radio and television receivers, public address and hi-fi systems, servo controls, remote controls and in almost every electronic apparatus put together. Certainly it is the most frequently encountered functional component in instrumentation and assistive electronic systems used in medicine and in rehabilitation.

The basic function of an amplifier circuit is to magnify a small electrical signal into a larger one so that it can be observed or so that it can be used to control power sufficient to operate a motor, loudspeaker or other output device.

Amplifiers can be most easily classified by the portion of the frequency band of the electromagnetic spectrum that they are designed to amplify and by their total gain or magnification. A DC amplifier can amplify a small DC voltage into a larger one and may also be designed to function not only at DC but also well up into the audio range of frequencies. Audio amplifiers are specifically designed for the audible range, which does not include DC but covers approximately the range from 10 hertz to 20 kilohertz. Video amplifiers, in addition to the audio range, function well up into the megahertz region. Selective amplifiers using resonant circuits are designed to respond only to a discrete frequency or a very narrow band of frequencies surrounding a center frequency in order to "select" this specific signal from among all others. Selective amplifiers are most often used in radio, telephone and television communications systems, whereas the DC amplifier and the bandpass amplifier are most commonly encountered in biomedical instrumentation systems and in audiovisual equipment.

Whether a particular amplifier is appropriate for a given application may be determined by examining its gain or amplification, by comparing its frequency response characteristics to those of the phenomenon to be amplified, and by comparing its other characteristics with the particular circumstances of its intended usage. As a guide to choosing appropriate instrumentation amplifiers, Table 40-2 lists the approximate frequency ranges of commonly encountered signals for which an amplifier might be desired. The listed ranges are only approximate and may not match perfectly those listed by others investigating certain details of the phenomena.

Having chosen an amplifier with appropriate gain and frequency response characteristics, several other factors need to be considered. These are: input impedance, linearity, dynamic range, maximum input and output levels, noise figure, output impedance, and overload and recovery characteristics. In addition, if the equipment is to be battery operated, the power consumption of the device should be examined and chosen to be consistent with the battery capacity and replacement period or allowable recharging intervals.

TABLE 40–2 FREQUENCY RANGES OF PHYSICAL PHENOMENA

PHENOMENON	APPROXIMATE FREQUENCY BAND
Electroencephalogram	0.01 to 100 hertz
Electrocardiogram	0.01 to 200 hertz
Electromyogram	10 hz to 10 khz
Galvanic Skin Response	DC to 10 hertz
Phonocardiogram	0.1 hz to 1 khz
Speech and Hearing	10 hz to 20 khz
Radio and television transmission	100 khz to 300 mhz
Ultrasonic	20 khz to 5 megahertz
Video (TV picture content)	DC to 10 megahertz
Radar	300 mhz to 30,000 mhz (30 Gigahertz)
Infrared (heat)	30 Ghz to 30,000 Ghz
Visible light	30,000 Ghz to 3×10^6 Ghz
Ultraviolet	3×10^6 Ghz to 3×10^8 Ghz
X-rays	3×10^8 Ghz to 3×10^{10} Ghz
Gamma radiation	3×10^{10} Ghz to 10^{12} Ghz
Cosmic rays	10^{12} Ghz to 10^{14} Ghz

In general, it is desirable that a voltage amplifier have an input impedance at least one to two orders of magnitude higher than the signal source impedance from which it receives the signal to be amplified. Otherwise, the input signal may be reduced by the voltage divider relationship between driving source impedance and amplifier input impedance. Although there are exceptions to this statement in audiovisual signal distribution systems and in some low noise amplifier applications in communications, it is well to adhere to this requirement unless the supplier of an input sensing device specifies otherwise.

The linearity of an amplifier determines how much distortion of the input signal waveform occurs in passing through the device. Since it is sometimes difficult to design for very wide dynamic ranges, it is usual to specify this parameter over a range of output levels. If the range of input voltage to be presented to the amplifier is known, then the gain of the amplifier can be used to calculate the expected range of output level and this can be compared to the specifications for the device. Linearity is usually specified in terms of percentage of deviation from true linearity, but may often be stated by quoting the amount of distortion of the input signal incurred in passing through the amplifier (this is usually the way sound equipment is specified).

Output impedance of an amplifier is important when considering the connection of the amplifier to a succeeding amplifier or to an output transducer. Generally it is desirable that the output impedance of a voltage amplifier be low so that the gain and output voltage swing are not affected by the output device being driven. Power amplifiers, on the other hand, are usually designed to operate into a specified load impedance prescribed by the designer and stated in place of a specification on the amplifier output impedance. For example, in audio equipment it is usual to specify the speaker impedance that the power amplifier is designed to drive in order to obtain stated power output levels and distortion figures.

Two amplifier characteristics that are often neglected are the overload and recovery characteristics. Although these are not important as long as the amplifier is being continuously operated at signal output levels below the maximum specified by the manufacturer, in some applications, artifact signals occur in the input to the amplifier and may drive it up to or beyond its full output level. The result is to produce a grossly distorted replica of such signals. In addition, it is possible that internal DC operating levels may be shifted and may not return to normal conditions for some time after the transient phenomenon has disappeared. During this recovery period the amplifier is not operating normally and may be completely unresponsive to information present at its input terminals. An instance in which this would happen might be in the testing of neuromuscular function by means of a stimulating pulse applied to a motor nerve and an amplifier used to observe the resulting myoelectric signal from electrodes placed into or over a muscle site. The stimulating signal may be in the tens of volts while the electromyographic response may be in the microvolt range. The overload or upset of the amplifier that occurs as a result of the stimulating signal may completely mask the resulting electromyographic response if the recovery time of the amplifer is too long. It is obviously important in such an instrumentation application to choose an amplifier with good recovery characteristics if the information to be obtained is to be accurate.

Output Transducers and Display Devices.   Electromechanical devices form the most important category of output transducers among direct applications of electrical and electronic controls to patient-applied assistive devices, while recorders and display devices are the most prominent transducers in instrumentation systems. The solenoid, the relay and the electric motor are prime examples of electromechanical devices. They are all based in principle on the production of a magnetic field by the flow of current through a wound coil and the interaction of the field so created with either magnetic materials or another magnetic field. The *relay* is an electromagnet with a movable piece of iron or steel which is attracted by the magnetic field set up by the current flowing in a coil. A set of contacts mounted on the movable elements, called the armature, can be opened or closed by the movement of the armature in response to coil current. The useful thing about a relay is that the controlling coil and its circuit are completely independent of the electrical circuits to which the contacts are connected. The result is good isolation of the controlling electronic elements (to which a patient may be attached) and the final use of the relay switch contacts. It is also apparent that large quantities of current in the contact circuits can be controlled by much smaller amounts of power applied to the relay coil.

The *solenoid,* again, is basically an electromagnet. The central iron core over which the coil is wound is arranged to be loose so that it is free to move into and out of the coil assembly. A current introduced into the coil sets up a magnetic field which tends to draw the metal core (again called an armature) into the coil assembly. The armature, of course, can be attached to a mechanical device, such as the knee-locking mechanism of a brace, so that energizing the coil of the solenoid produces a pull on the mechanical linkage. The force obtained is directly proportional to the current in the coil and varies with the relative position of the armature within the coil.

The *electric motor* is an electromagnetic device in which the field set up by the passage of current through a coil interacts with a stationary magnetic field to produce attraction and repulsion of the two mechanical members on which they are mounted. The form of the motor is familiar: a freely rotating central shaft carries the coil windings to which current is applied, and the surrounding metallic structure, the stator, carries the fixed magnetic field with which the armature's field reacts. In addition, a set of rotary contacts called a commutator is arranged so that, as the armature rotates relative to the stator, the direction of current flow in the coil of the armature is reversed as the north pole of the armature comes into line with the south pole of the stator. In this way, the attractive force exerted on the armature pole as it approaches the stator pole is changed to a repulsive force as it leaves the stator pole, and the exerted force is always maintained in the direction of desired rotation.

In instrumentation systems for measurement of physiological parameters the most important types of output transducer are the meter, the oscilloscope, the chart recorder and the magnetic tape recorder. *Meter* displays and *pen recorders* are electromagnetic devices very similar in operating principle to the electric motor. The shaft, to which either a pointer and scale or a writing pen is attached, is really the output shaft of a small electric motor; the shaft is free to rotate over only a limited range. The net deflection obtained is directly proportional to the input current so that a meter may be directly calibrated in terms of the applied input and a direct reading scale may be placed behind the pointer. The pen recorder calibration, on the other hand, must be stated in terms of millimeters per milliamp or millimeters per volt so that the tracing can be interpreted. Because of the relatively high inertia of the moving parts, meters and pen recorders are limited in response to a maximum of about 100 hz. The pen recorder is used most frequently for recording the electrocardiogram, electroencephalogram, galvanic skin phenomena and respiration waveforms.

The *photo-optical recorder* is a similar but lower inertia device which produces a line tracing on photosensitive paper by deflecting a light beam from a small mirror and thereby avoids the high inertia added by a mechanical pen assembly. Its upper frequency limit may be as high as 10 kilohertz and thus it is a useful output recorder for phenomena that require a wider frequency range, such as in electromyography.

A more complicated output device is the *cathode ray oscilloscope*. The cathode ray tube, which performs the transducer function, is the same device as the picture tube in a television set. The viewing end of the tube consists of a glass screen coated on the inside with a material called a phosphor. At the other end of the tube is a heated filament which emits free electrons that are focused and accelerated in an electrostatic device called an electron gun. The electron gun sends a slender stream of high velocity electrons toward the phosphor screen. The impact of these electrons on the phosphor surface causes the phosphor to emit light, or glow, at the point of impact. The emission of light, which occurs when the electron beam strikes the phosphor, continues as long as the beam is present and fades out gradually when the beam is removed. This afterglow is called persistence.

Cathode ray tubes used for monitoring physiological parameters are usually equipped with longer persistence phosphor screens than those used for television sets, since the repetition of a trace on the screen is much less frequent in time. In addition, the intensity is only manually adjustable and the information is usually displayed as a vertical deflection of the trace so that a graphlike presentation is produced. Instrumentation oscilloscopes provide amplifiers that are accurately calibrated to indicate the vertical deflection sensitivity to an input signal in volts or millivolts per centimeter.

Multichannel monitoring scopes present traces of the same kind that pen recorders do but have the advantage of not requiring large supplies of paper. They can also display rapidly occurring phenomena much better than the electromechanical device, since the inertia of the electron beam is minute. If the cathode ray oscilloscope is used for cases in which a permanent record is required, of course, photographs of the screen presentation must be made.

Tape Recorders. Acoustical, mechanical and visual display classifications include most output devices used in electronics. The principal exception is the *magnetic tape recorder*. It is not truly a display device but rather a memory device which allows the information fed into it to be subsequently re-created. It operates by altering the magnetization pattern of metal oxide particles on plastic tape. As the moving tape passes over the recording head, the permanent magnetization induced in the oxide material follows the direction and intensity of the electrical current flowing in the coil of the recording head. If the recorded tape is then allowed to pass a replay magnetic head, the minute changes in magnetization of the metal oxide particles as they pass the reading station induce a small electrical signal in the reading coil; this signal can then be amplified to re-create the original recorded signal. Important things to consider in using a tape recorder in scientific instrumentation are adequate frequency response for the phenomena to be recorded, the amount of distortion added to the recovered signal, and the amount of frequency variation or flutter due to unsteadiness in the mechanism transporting the tape through the magnetic heads. A good tape recorder suitable for instrumentation incorporates flutter compensation circuits to minimize this source of error. In addition, if DC or very low frequency information is to be handled adequately, then the recorder must be of the frequency modulation (FM) rather than the direct type. Recordings of the electrocardiogram, for example, cannot be adequately

TABLE 40–3 FREQUENCY RANGES OF DISPLAY DEVICES

Display Device	Approximate Frequency Range
Meter displays	DC to 100 hertz
Pen recorders	DC to 100 hertz
Photo-optical recorder	DC to 10 kilohertz
Oscilloscope and camera	DC to beyond 10 megahertz (depending on type)
Magnetic tape recorder	
Direct recording	50 hertz to 500 khz
FM recording	DC to 50 khz (depending on type and tape speed)

made on a home entertainment type of tape recorder without special circuitry to convert it to an FM recording. Table 40-3 gives a brief summary of the approximate useful frequency ranges of different recording and display devices.

Power Sources. Most electronic equipment requires a source of DC power in order to operate its transducers, amplifiers and output devices. For laboratory and other fixed location equipment the source of the DC power is ordinarily obtained by means of a transformer, rectifier and filter circuit operated from the AC power line. The transformer makes it possible to obtain a wide range of voltages by proper choice of the ratio of primary to secondary turns and can also provide excellent isolation from the power line for minimizing or eliminating safety hazards normally associated with power line operation. The rectified direct current may be filtered and regulated to any degree desired to provide ripple-free voltage for equipment operation.

For portable equipment with applications in instrumentation and for assistive or replacement devices worn by patients, a battery is ordinarily the source of DC power. These electrochemical devices convert the energy released in chemical reactions directly into electrical energy. There are many types of batteries in general usage. The most common types are listed in Table 40-4, together with their approximate energy-to-weight ratios and typical applica-

TABLE 40–4 BATTERY TYPES, THEIR APPLICATIONS AND SPECIFIC ENERGIES

Type	Applications	Approx. Watt-hrs./lb.	Approx. Cycles of Charge/ Recharge Life
Leclanché dry cell	Flashlights, toys, transistor radios	5 to 20	0
Alkaline-manganese	Portable electronic equipment, photo-flash, portable radios	10 to 30	0
Mercury	Hearing aids, portable electronic equipment, automatic cameras	40 to 50	0
Lead-acid	Automobiles, electric wheelchairs, portable power packs	5 to 10	100 to 200
Nickel-cadmium	Electric toothbrushes, pacemakers, portable stimulators, prostheses	15	1000
Silver-zinc	Portable transmitters, aerospace applications, prostheses, military equipment	50	20 to 80
Zinc-air (in development)	Applications similar to silver-zinc	70 to 90	0

tions. Although the specific energy of a battery is one of its most important characteristics, there are other factors which should be considered in choosing a particular type. Cost, general availability of replacements, rechargeability, shelf life, current drain, and schedule of usage are all important factors influencing the selection.

The Leclanché cell, more commonly referred to as the dry cell, is the most universally used and most familiar of all the batteries listed. It comes in sizes ranging from the penlight variety to the larger types used in camping lanterns. It performs best with intermittent usage, has reasonable shelf life and is relatively inexpensive. It is not efficiently rechargeable (although a portion of the energy can be restored for a very few rechargings) but has the useful characteristic of recovering between periods of heavy drain. The terminal voltage varies with current drawn and with battery lifetime so that this must be taken into account in circuit design. The total watt-hour capacity is also affected by the current drain and the usage schedule. It is therefore best to consult a manufacturer's manual in choosing the particular battery to be used. A readily available manual of this type is listed in the references at the end of this chapter.

The alkaline-manganese battery offers higher energy per pound and also differs from the Leclanché cell in being able to withstand higher current drains. The total energy available from the alkaline-manganese system is also less dependent on the schedule of discharge and on current level. Although it will outperform the conventional Leclanché cell in almost any type of service, the alkaline-manganese battery is more expensive for relatively light current drains and for intermittent service. It is not rechargeable and must be replaced at the end of its life.

The mercury battery sustains a very constant terminal voltage over its lifetime, has a relatively constant watt-hour rating independent of discharge schedule, and will sustain its terminal voltage under heavy discharge rates. Its specific energy in watt-hours per pound is higher than either the Leclanché or alkaline-manganese types and the volumetric efficiency is also higher. This last characteristic makes it a logical choice for use in hearing aids where space is severely limited. It is not rechargeable and is more expensive than the Leclanché and alkaline-manganese types.

Next to the dry cell, the most familiar battery is the lead-acid battery, used in almost all automobiles. Its distinguishing features are its rechargeability, high current capacity, easy availability and modest cost in terms of capacity and total lifetime. It is more difficult to seal against leakage of the sulphuric acid electrolyte, as any car owner knows from the tendency of the battery terminal connectors to corrode, and is relatively low in watt-hour rating per pound, since the lead used in its construction is one of the heaviest elements. It is not a good choice for low current drain devices, for which the Leclanché excels, but is the most economical battery for high current drain and large ampere-hour applications.

The nickel-cadmium battery is initially more expensive than the lead-acid type but has a much longer lifetime in cycles of charging and discharging. It is available in a sealed unit which prevents electrolyte (in this case, potassium hydroxide) spillage problems. It can be applied either to low current or high current demands, although its total capacity and lifetime are influenced by discharge rates and recharging techniques. Outside of automotive applications, in which the lead-acid type reigns, the nickel-cadmium cell is the most economical for rechargeable portable power.

If initial cost is not of paramount importance but rather high energy-to-weight ratio and rechargeability, then the silver-zinc battery is an excellent choice. Voltage versus current drain is relatively stable and the battery is available in a wide range of ampere-hour ratings. It is not as long-lived as either the lead-acid or nickel-cadmium types but has a distinct advantage in terms of its energy-to-weight ratio and size.

The zinc-air battery is just appearing on the market and is still under development in the laboratory. It promises eventually to provide the most compact and lightest source of portable power for applications requiring relatively high energy storage. In its present form it is not rechargeable although rechargeable units are under development. It is hoped that eventually it will be competitive economically for applications in which lead-acid, nickel-cadmium, and silver-zinc batteries now dominate because of their low cost per watt-hour.

To summarize roughly the batteries listed, the lead-acid, silver-zinc and zinc-air batteries are generally used for high current and high capacity purposes like automobiles and electric wheelchairs. The dry cell, alkaline-manganese and mercury batteries are usually used for much lighter loads and for operating electronic circuits. Nickel-cadmium batteries are found in both types of application; their size and weight determine their appropriateness.

Electrical Safety Hazards. Treatment modalities used by physicians and therapists often involve the use of electrical equipment. Whirlpool baths, diathermy machines, ultrasound equipment and muscle stimulators are examples. Care should be taken to see that such apparatus is equipped with a three-wire type of grounded power plug used with a properly installed receptacle; also, a check should be made to ensure that the cord, plug and receptacle are in good condition and that the equipment is functioning normally before it is ever applied to the patient. The three-wire grounding plug is now used by almost all manufacturers of metal-cased electrical equipment. The third, grounding wire protects the user by providing a current return path to earth for leakage or faulty currents which may be present in the device or which might develop during use. To bypass or avoid using this protective feature is to invite trouble. If treatment equipment is brought into the home, make sure that the household electrical outlet is of the three-wire grounding type. Unfortunately, older houses are not usually so equipped. If a treatment device is to be used in this situation, insist that a proper outlet be installed by a licensed electrician before using the apparatus. Don't be tempted to use one of the three- to two-wire adapters with a small green wire to be connected to the screw on the outlet cover plate. The cover and the box may not be connected to earth through the house wiring and a potential hazard will exist in the use of the equipment.

Safety hazards in electrical or electronic equipment assume an even greater importance when equipment of any kind is used by the rehabilitation patient himself. The greater the disability, the greater the potential danger, since the patient is less able to deal with unexpected situations. Fortunately, most prosthetic, orthotic and assistive devices used or worn by rehabilitation patients are battery operated, since such devices must be portable, and thus they entail very little electrical hazard.

The greatest potential dangers for the patient exist with the more common, everyday devices he may use in the home. By far the most dangerous of these are the television set and the home radio. Most of these sets are designed with the internal metal chassis connected directly to one side of the power line. The two-wire line cord may usually be plugged into the wall outlet in one of two directions so that there is no way of knowing whether the chassis is connected to the low or the high side of the line. The plastic case and plastic knobs on the operating controls protect the user from accidentally contacting the internal chassis structure. If one of these knobs is missing, however, or has been replaced with a metal knob from some other appliance, it is possible that the metal shaft of the control, usually attached to the internal chassis, may be touched. If this occurs while the user is leaning on a radiator, refrigerator, kitchen stove or plumbing fixture, or if he has his feet or hands in the washbowl or tub, then a bad shock or even an electrocution can result. Another potential hazard with these sets exists if they are placed on radiators. If the plastic case softens or melts, the internal metal chassis may contact the radiator and a fire may result. If radio or television sets are to be used at home by a disabled person, the sets should be located sensibly away from plumbing and heating fixtures and should be kept in good repair.

Two methods of avoiding potential risks with home entertainment devices are to choose a television set that is equipped with a wireless remote control unit which the patient can operate from his bed, and to supply radio entertainment by means of a battery operated portable. The occasional battery replacement for the portable is a small price to pay for the safety of the device and for its additional usefulness in providing outside world contact in case of a local emergency and power failure.

REFERENCES

1. Eshbach, O. W.: Handbook of Engineering Fundamentals. 2nd Ed. New York, John Wiley and Sons, 1952.
2. "Eveready" Battery Applications and Engineering Data. Union Carbide Consumer Products Company, Division of Union Carbide Corporation, New York, N.Y.
3. Frankel, V. H., and Burnstein, A. H.: Orthopaedic Biomechanics. Philadelphia, Lea and Febiger, 1969.
4. Kent, R. T.: Mechanical Engineers' Handbook. Design and Production. New York, John Wiley and Sons, 1950.
5. Wells, K. F.: Kinesiology. 5th Ed. Philadelphia, W. B. Saunders Co., 1971.
6. Westman, H. P. (Ed.): Reference Data for Radio Engineers. 5th Ed. Indianapolis, Ind., Howard W. Sams & Co., 1968.
7. White, H. E. et al.: Physics: An Experimental Science. New York, Van Nostrand-Reinhold Books, 1968.
8. Williams, M., and Lissner, H. R.: Biomechanics of Human Motion. Philadelphia, W. B. Saunders Co., 1962.
9. World Book Encyclopedia. Chicago, Field Enterprises Educational Corporation.

Chapter 41

THE EDUCATION OF PHYSICIANS AND HEALTH-RELATED PROFESSIONALS IN PHYSICAL MEDICINE AND REHABILITATION

by Leonard D. Policoff

THE DEVELOPMENT OF THE SPECIALTY

The adequate education of all physicians and health-related professionals in the principles of physical medicine and rehabilitation would be a significant contribution to the improvement in the quality and scope of health care services which our society is so urgently seeking at this time. "The physician in practice today, the academician teaching in the medical school, and the medicial student who is his product, represent the ultimate development of the concept of medical training and care which began with the Oslerian clinical clerk and terminated in the complete discrediting of the family physician in favor of the white-coated, laboratory-based, applied physiologist who is well versed in all of the technical minutiae required for diagnosis of his patients' problems but has little or no interest in the patient himself."[1]

In opposition to this approach, educators in the field of physical medicine and rehabilitation have constantly sought to achieve a holistic, person-oriented concept of medicine which concerns itself with the patient's total ecological accommodation or adaptability. It is, however, most difficult for a physician or allied health professional trained in the traditional manner, without exposure to an educational experience in rehabilitation medicine, to make the transition from a biomolecular to a humanistic approach, particularly in the care of the chronically ill and disabled.

A few who have through their own experiences become aware of the values of such a transition have been able to make major contributions to the development of the specialty of physical medicine and rehabilitation and to its incorporation into the curricula of medical schools. But the process has been painfully slow and much more remains to be done, primarily because of a failure of many medical educators to understand what it is that needs to be taught to the undergraduate. In part this results from the fact that, as a specialty, physical medicine and rehabilitation is still relatively new, and that it presents unique conceptual pathways that are not shared with most other medical disciplines. But it results equally from the broad scope of the spectrum of physical medicine and rehabilitation today and the fact that its practitioners may differ widely in individual areas of interest and expertise.

The specialty of physical medicine and rehabilitation was conceived originally as a narrow form of applied biophysics, utilizing a variety of physical forces for the diagnosis and treatment of disease. For the past two decades the character of the specialty has been insidiously evolving from the primary study of the biological effects of physical forces to an increasing concern, first, with the psychosocial and vocational aspects of disability and, more recently, with the ecological problems of the socially, culturally and economically deprived and disadvantaged. Despite this shift in the character of the spectrum of the specialty, the basic structure remains.

The developments in the "state of the art" which moved the physiatrist upward from the status of electrotherapist and heliotherapist[2] gave him the tools to provide better methods of management for the disabled. The applied physical measures were able to improve function and restore or prolong varying degrees of independence in the disabled within the protected institutional milieu, but this only made the problems of returning the involved human being to his former family, socio-cultural and community status more pressing and, perforce, the biophysical applicators became problem managers and medical sociologists.

The physiatrist today is trained in the management of both acute and chronic long-term disability, regardless of disease etiology. He should be the medical management consultant to all other physicians faced with long-term patient care in disability-prone disorders where his expertise may be able to forestall or avoid incipient disability as well as to ameliorate the already established disability. Despite heroic efforts by many dedicated physiatrist-educators, it appears unlikely that physiatrists can be educated in sufficient numbers to meet the total needs of the disabled in the burgeoning population of the last quarter of the twentieth century. Many of these needs will have to be satisfied by the work of the "new" family physician specialist, by members of the other existing health-related professions and perhaps even by professionals of a new genre not yet developed.

It is clear that all physicians and many of the allied health professionals will require basic training and competence in physical medicine and rehabilitation and that the emphasis of educational efforts in this field must turn in this direction, recognizing potential role shifts of all health-related professions rather than emphasizing purely specialty education. The specialty of Physical Medicine and Rehabilitation has now come of age. The American Board of Physical Medicine and Rehabilitation was founded in 1947 and has passed its majority. The expressed requirement by the late Bernard Baruch to Dr. Frank H. Krusen, when the Baruch Committee on Physical Medicine was established in 1943, that this new specialty could not survive or grow unless arrangements were made "to teach teachers who can teach others"[3, 4] has been satisfactorily met, although much remains to be done before physiatrists can rest on their laurels.

The recommended structure and content of specialty residency training have been well defined by the American Board of Physical Medicine and Rehabilitation and by the American Academy of Physical Medicine and Rehabilitation[5] and need not be discussed further here. Early in 1964, through the joint efforts of the American Board of Physical Medicine and Rehabilitation, the American Academy of Physical Medicine and Rehabilitation and the American Congress of Rehabilitation Medicine, the Commission on Education in Physical Medicine and Rehabilitation was created. Each of these professional organizations is represented on the Commission by three delegates.

THE COMMISSION ON EDUCATION IN PHYSICAL MEDICINE AND REHABILITATION

The Commission was initially charged with carrying out a study of the undergraduate teaching programs in Physical Medicine and Rehabilitation in the nation's medical schools. However, the interests and activities of the Commission have now been broadened to encompass the full range of undergraduate and graduate education in this specialty. The present work of the Commission also includes a study of the definition and nature of Physical Medicine and Rehabilitation.[6]

The Commission employs a research staff which is presently housed with the American Rehabilitation Foundation in Minneapolis and has successfully carried out a variety of studies resulting in published bulletins.[7] Other studies in pedagogic principles and resources relating to physical medicine and rehabilitation are in current progress. Bulletin No. 2 of the Commission on Education in Physical Medicine and Rehabilitation provides some cogent definitions of the field and its content which can serve as a focus for discussion.[7]

This discipline consists of elements derived from several disciplines including general medicine, physiology, physics, psychology, sociology, and so forth. The structure of this field inheres in the theory which guides the selection of "mix" of elements required to achieve predetermined clinical goals. Thus, unlike chemistry or mathematics, which "carry their structure along with them," physical medicine and rehabilitation combines elements of various disciplines to achieve its goals.

Physical medicine and rehabilitation is essentially an applied clinical discipline. It utilizes a continuing process of assessment, management and reevaluation in achieving its patient treatment goals. Its treatment goals derive from the nature of the limitations associated with severe and continuing disease processes or physical disability. Although less frequently concerned with acute and episodic conditions, some of its diagnostic and therapeutic tools and methods find application at these levels of illness, as well.

The treatment goals seek adaptation of the human organism to customary or attainable life patterns within the limits imposed by the disabling conditions. Conventional and curative medical resources, while essential to physical medicine and rehabilitation, are not sufficient for the management of those disease processes which result in loss or defect in normal human functions such as mobility, self-care and communications skills; such defects limit personal, social, recreational and economic activities. His patients' needs may be so broad that, in addition to applying his specialized clinical medical skills, the physiatrist must be able to incorporate the contributions of many medical, medically related and behavioral sciences in the restorative process. In this context, the physiatrist is the coordinator of a complex group process. This medical discipline, like others, is supported by a body of scientific knowledge. Scientific study and applications in the following areas are essential to the clinical practice of the physiatrist:

A. The structural and functional characteristics of the human organism in relation to mobility, self-care and other normal human activities.

B. The physiological and biochemical responses of tissues, organs and body systems to external physical sources of energy and to internal energy production in exercise, which enhance and aid the healing process and the restoration of useful function.

C. Pathology of neuromusculoskeletal systems and the physiologic disturbances produced thereby.

D. Electrophysiology as applied to the diagnosis of neuromuscular disease and measurement of impaired function (electrodiagnosis).

E. The compensatory mechanisms.

1. The prescribed use of drugs and exercise to increase, enhance and substitute for useful function.

2. The substitution of mechanical devices, such as braces, splints, artificial limbs, assistive devices, wheelchairs, etc., for lost or impaired functions or strength.

3. Behavorial sciences—psychopathology, motivation and learning—in relation to adjustment to and compensation for lost or impaired mental, social or vocational abilities associated with physical disability.

Like all clinical medicine, physical medicine and rehabilitation is concerned with prevention, diagnosis and treatment. However, for the physiatrist prevention takes on special meaning. It includes methods of avoiding preventable secondary conditions which result in increased disability. Diagnosis adds to the pathological label the assessment of deficits or limitations, as well as of residual potential, of mobility, self-care, communications skills and similar normal human functions. Treatment is centered around the amelioration of the consequences of disease in the context of previously mentioned normal human functions. . . .

Physical medicine and rehabilitation is a unique pattern of elements drawn largely from several scientific and medical disciplines and modified to its special purpose. In the practice of medicine, some overlapping of content between specialties is inevitable. Thus, the physiatrist shares in common with other physicians the general skills and knowledge required of all medical practitioners. He also has certain skills in common with several medical specialists. Such overlapping in medicine is not unusual, and is desirable, since it tends to reinforce the treatment and management procedures required in complex cases in which collaborative and interdisciplinary efforts are required for their solution.

EDUCATIONAL REQUIREMENTS

If the validity of these statements is accepted, certain educational requirements are also necessary. Firstly, physical medicine and rehabilitation must be taught as a clinical discipline. Secondly, its structure and content are so broadly based that it draws skills and technologies in varying degrees from most basic sciences and clinical specialties, and in turn makes a significant contribution to them. To ensure that the educational effort is effective and productive, physical medicine and rehabilitation must be taught in two distinct but concurrent patterns—as an isolated medical specialty for its own unique body of knowledge and as general principles of a ubiquitous holistic and humanistic orientation which can serve as the catalyst to effect cohesion and coherence in a variety of multidisciplinary educational efforts.

Skills Required of the Competent Physician

Dr. Paul Sanazaro, then Director of the Division of Education of the Association of American Medical Colleges, emphasized that the major purpose of medical education is to supply physicians who are competent in providing care to patients.[8] He stressed that in addition to being able to take a reliable and adequate history, to perform an accurate physical examination, to obtain information by special tests and to make a diagnosis and administer therapy, the competent physician must be skilled in the following:

Treating more than immediate health problem
  1. Modifying patient's physical or social environment
  2. Dealing with problems of patient and family
  3. Instituting preventive measures

Working with health care team
  1. Making appropriate use of health care team
  2. Integrating efforts of team members

Providing follow-up care
  1. Providing for rehabilitative care
  2. Planning home care or self-care
  3. Instructing patient and family in home care

A detailed review of these basic requirements for competence in the practice of comprehensive medicine, in the light of previous definitions, supports the view that, based on a matrix of teaching in physical medicine and rehabilitation, such principles can be imparted superbly well. Without such a basis, results in many medical schools will continue to be poor and additional generations of physicians will develop inappropriate patterns of behavior with regard to the already disabled and to those with chronic or acute illness whose potential disabilities may be preventable.

Reports on the Teaching of Physical Medicine and Rehabilitation

From 1955 through 1960 the National Foundation sponsored a series of annual "Conferences on Teaching of Rehabilitation," each of which resulted in the publication of a loose-leaf proceedings report. These reports did little to modify the patterns of medical school curriculum planning because they failed to focalize the teaching of rehabilitation medicine in the hands of the physiatrist but left it as a free-floating concept which was the concern of all medical academicians and hence the responsibility of none.

Over a period of several years the New York Academy of Sciences, through its Interdisciplinary Communication Program, also sponsored a series of five conferences on rehabilitation. Of these the most pertinent, held in Princeton, New Jersey, in 1965 and 1966, resulted in widely circulated mimeographed reports which attempted to define objectives for teaching programs in rehabilitation medicine.[9, 10, 11]

Dr. Frederic Kottke has also written cogently on rehabilitation teaching concepts, many of which have been widely adopted. He states:

Physical Medicine and Rehabilitation is not merely a philosophical system separate and apart from the orthodox concept of medicine but is, instead, an integral component of the total medical care needed to restore the patient with a disability to an optimal level of function. The goal of medicine is the prevention or cure of disease—therefore, the maintenance or restoration of health. It has often been tacitly assumed that when pathology has been removed health will be restored; for acute diseases this is frequently true. On the other hand, in a chronic disease or disability in which there is no longer a specific pathology of organs which can be removed or corrected, major physiological and psychological adaptations of the entire individual must take place before he can function at his optimal level. The unique emphasis of rehabilitation is upon the compensatory adaptations of the body to the pathophysiology of disease. In this role physical medicine and rehabilitation deals with the problems of evaluation, restoration, and management of patients who have chronic impairment of neuromusculoskeletal and vascular function. The evaluation of such patients includes assessment of residual abilities and capacity for compensation, in addition to diagnosis and assessment of pathological loss. Rehabilitation management of chronic disability attempts to enhance the compensatory adaptation by every possible means—pharmacological, physical, psychological, substitution of mechanical devices, and alteration of environmental conditions.[12]

Integrated and Correlated Teaching Plus a Core Curriculum

If one can accept this concept of the ubiquity of physical medicine and rehabilitation in comprehensive medical care, it becomes clear that effective teaching in this field can be done only by providing the same universality in teaching. Thus physical medicine and rehabilitation cannot be taught as an isolated lecture series inserted near the end of the clinical curriculum of a medical school program but must be integrated and correlated with all other aspects of medical care with which it is contiguous. However, a subject material which is taught only in relation to other subject materials loses its identity. To establish in the mind of the medical student that there exists a body of knowledge unique for the specialty of physical medicine and rehabilitation, it is necessary that a clearly defined core curriculum in physical medicine and rehabilitation be identifiable in the medical school curriculum. In the present era of experimental curricula, which differ so widely between institutions, it becomes difficult to recommend allocation of curriculum time on a chronological basis during the four years of undergraduate medical education. It appears more rational to deal with the problem of curriculum relationship on a topical basis.

Correlation with Anatomy. A sound teaching program will, therefore, begin in complete correlation with the basic sciences. In the classic curriculum anatomy is the usual starting point for a medical education and it is at this time in the curriculum that the principles of functional anatomy and kinesiology in both the physiological and pathological state should be taught. This type of instruction becomes even more meaningful to the patient-hungry young medical student if clinical correlations with the basic science program can be established by providing exposure to actual patient material which demonstrates the functional anatomical principles involved.

Correlation with Physiology. The educational program in physiology must include study of the physiology of exercise in health and disease and the physiological effects on living tissue of heat, cold and the energies of the electromagnetic spectrum.

Correlation with Pharmacology. Similarly, when pharmacology and therapeutics are taught, the use of physical modalities as therapeutic agents must be discussed and demonstrated. This has been widely done in European medical curricula and the failure to do so on a widespread basis in American medical colleges has often relegated the use of physical modalities to irregular practitioners.

Correlation with Physical Diagnosis. Included in the teaching program for physical diagnosis must be the principles of evaluation of normal and pathological gait, stance, posture, range of motion and stability of joints and the use of the manual muscle test and of functional testing in the evaluation of disability.

Correlation with Community Medicine. With community medicine, the specialty of physical medicine and rehabilitation shares a strong interest in the unique problems of the physically disabled in an urban industrialized society and the even more devastating problems of those disabled not by physical disease but by the diseases of our society. Teaching in physical medicine and rehabilitation, properly utilized, can enhance teaching in community medicine while demonstrating to the student the vast resources available in most communities for the management of these types of disorders.

Correlation with Psychiatry and Behavioral Sciences. Coordinated with teaching in psychiatry and behavioral science, a review of the psychological problems of the disabled, and of the disturbed interpersonal family relationships that may be present secondarily, can have dramatic impact on the awareness of the medical student of these problems in his future relationships with patients.

Correlation with Other Medical Specialties. It seems gratuitous to point out that the physiatrist should be permitted to make his significant contribution to the teaching programs in rheumatology, pulmonary and cardiovascular disease, orthopedics, neurology and neurosurgery as well as pediatrics.

MANAGEMENT OF DISABILITY

Physical medicine and rehabilitation, as a medical discipline, has acquired the most expertise in the management of the long-term problems of the disabled. Management as used in this context is a concept quite apart from the usual problem-solving approach to acute medical care. Instead of providing a solution for the conundrum of a specific disease process, it proposes to assist the patient—who may be considered an *organism* altered as a result of a disease process which may no longer be active—to adjust totally to all aspects of his environment, both now and in the future. This orientation to person rather than to disease is shared by physical medicine and rehabilitation with psychiatry. On this orientation has been built a system of management that can be demonstrated and transmitted in principle to the medical student. The failure of some medical schools to do so in the past has left many practicing physicians incapable of coping with chronic disease and disability, to the detriment of patient care and the aggrandizement of the cultists and quacks. To make such teaching really effective, however, the physician teaching the medical student must be qualified as a sound clinician who commands faculty respect and with whom the medical student can identify and thus emulate.

The Multidisciplinary Approach to Management

This discussion has centered on the basic education in rehabilitation medicine which is required to enable every physician to cope effectively with the problems of disability management. Such management, as currently practiced in the most enlightened centers of excellence in this field, utilizes a closely-knit team of health-related professionals, working, each from his own vantage point of expertise, toward a common goal: maximum achievement for the disabled patient. While the component professions represented on such a health care team are a variable which is dependent upon the needs of the institution and the needs of the particular patient, a typical team may include not only the physiatrist but the physical therapist, the occupational therapist, the clinical psychologist, the medical social worker, the rehabilitation nurse and the speech therapist. A health care team of this kind, working from the vantage point of a true understanding of mutual interdependence and provided with appropriate leadership, can deliver health care to the disabled at the most effective level.

The educational experiences which qualify the diverse members of the health care team for their professional roles are so variable that the members often approach their professional problems sharing only a desire to help the disabled individual. Cohesiveness and esprit-de-corps are often achieved only through a long and painful process. There is a popular aphorism to the effect that "Those who pray together stay together." I should like to paraphrase this concept a bit with relation to the education of the health care team dealing with the disabled individual. It is clear that if they were educated together, their ability to work effectively together would be enhanced and their productivity often markedly increased. This then is a plea for educators to revise some common preconceptions and to recognize that, even though some participants in such a health care team are trained in graduate programs and others in undergraduate programs, the similarity in their objectives and interests warrants a greater effort to provide shared educational experiences.

Shortage of Personnel

The physiatrist and the members of the health-related professions who work in the field of rehabilitation share all the limitations and problems that exist throughout the field of health care delivery in our complex society. Foremost among these problems has been what appear to be inadequate numbers of health professionals to satisfy the demands for health care delivery engendered by a rising level of expectation in our populace. The resulting outcries from many sources demand that medical schools and schools of the allied health professions dramatically increase their enrollment in order to satisfy the needs. While enrollment increases where feasible would indeed provide some relief, the basic truth is that it is not the deficits in the numbers of health professionals which create the problem but a failure to utilize personnel effectively and with optimum efficiency.

In certain quarters the demands are not for increased numbers of health professionals but for the creation of new kinds of health professionals, and we have seen a multiplication of training programs for the so-called "physician's assistant." At this juncture no one has been able to establish satisfactory criteria, either for the qualifications of such personnel or for their educational programs. The first obstacle that must be overcome before a rational solution to the shortage problem can be visualized is the limitation of vertical mobility and, to a lesser extent, of horizontal mobility which exists in all the health-related professions and which serves to prevent a numerical increase in the higher echelons of the health care professions.

Need for Educational Program Permitting Progression

If the educational and legal barriers could be broken so that it might be possible to enlist able young people into programs of health care training at the lowest educational level and then enable them to acquire additional educational experiences while employed, thus permitting them to rise to higher levels of professional responsibility and authority, a good deal of the health care problem could be ameliorated. It seems to me much more logical to visualize a continuum of educational experiences in our particular sphere of interest relating to the disabled patient; such training would make it feasible for persons to achieve varying degrees of expertise in rehabilitation methodology and technology.

Each of the existing health care professions that relate to the care of the disabled and the activities of rehabilitation teaching need to be given opportunities for developing increased educational resources to improve their capacities in the areas of education, administration, patient care and research. At the same time each profession should develop within it professional assistants of sufficient educational achievement so that to them can be delegated those portions of the workload of the health care team requiring lesser skills and responsibilities.

Need for Loosening Barriers Among Involved Disciplines

I spoke earlier of shared educational experiences which would ensure a wholesome interrelationship between the members of the health care team, but I would like to see this carried even further. The present artificial divisions which separate the members of the various health care teams into tight compartments need to be loosened somewhat. There is no reason why the physical therapist should not be capable of carrying on some of the functions of the occupational therapist and vice versa. There is no reason why the function of the clinical psychologist and the medical social worker need to be entirely separate operations. Each of these individuals — and this really applies to all such professional compartmentalization — should acquire sufficient expertise in the most closely related of the other professions to be able to supplement the activities of the other health professions in a supportive way so that a more equitable workload division can occur with varying demands and circumstances.

Expansion of the Roles of Allied Health Professionals

Earlier in this chapter I noted that a shift in the roles of all health-related professionals who work in the field of rehabilitation medicine might become necessary. I strongly believe this to be true. I am not advocating that the work which is appropriate for a physician should be delegated to a nonphysician but rather that a very careful analysis be made of those activities in the field of rehabilitation medicine which really require the intensive efforts of the physician and of those activities which can be selectively transferred and become responsibilities of other allied health professions. In order for this achievement to become possible, it is necessary that each of the existing health-related professions should continuously work to upgrade the quality of professional instruction that it affords its aspirants. At the same time each health-related profession should maintain and increase the professional standards which it demands of its practitioners.

Interdependence of the Members of the Rehabilitation Team

From time to time there have appeared in the literature reports which editorialize with regard to purported areas of competition between the physiatrist and members of other health-related professions working in the field of rehabilitation. Such concepts are inimical to the best development of all such professions and to the fulfillment of their responsibility to the health care needs of the disabled individual. Each of the health-related professions which participate in the activities of the rehabilitation team has a significant professional contribution to make. No one contribution can be considered consistently of greater value than any other. It is clear that, with varying professional demands based upon the needs of the patient, one or other of the health-related professions may at times make a more important contribution. However, when the next problem is presented, it may then fall to the lot of one of the other health professions to make this type of major contribution. The health care team under these circumstances can function well only if they recognize their total interdependence and offer each other appropriate support and respect. This does not preclude a continuing reappraisal of existing professional roles and goals and of possible alternate relationships and responsibilities which might enhance the achievement of team objectives.

SUMMARY

I can best sum up my philosophy with regard to education in physical medicine and rehabilitation by reiterating that I consider this a core concept which must eventually permeate the entire spectrum of education for undergraduate medical students, as well as for the health-related professions. In order for this to occur there must exist an individual whose professional objective it is; that individual does exist, in the form of the physiatrist. However, the physiatrist, while educating sufficient numbers of competent academicians to ensure the survival and growth of the specialty, must not lose track of the fact that his primary mission is to provide a unifying patient-oriented, humanistic thread of continuity which will properly orient future physicians toward the provision of the highest quality of self-care for the chronically ill and the disabled. At the same time the physiatrist must recognize as a corollary mission the development of a supportive role for those educators working in the field of the health-related professions, to assist them in continuously upgrading the quality standards of educational experiences provided in those professions. The roles of the participating members of the rehabilitation health care team should be redefined to provide each member with increased professional responsibilities and stature, to the ultimate benefit of the health care consumer.

REFERENCES

1. Policoff, L. D.: Future Perspectives in Physical Medicine and Rehabilitation. J.A.M.A., *198:*1017–1018, 1966.
2. Krusen, F. H.: Physical Medicine. Philadelphia, W. B. Saunders Co., 1941.
3. Krusen, F. H.: Personal communication.

4. Report of the Baruch Committee on Physical Medicine and Rehabilitation. Privately printed. January 1, 1948-June 30, 1949.
5. Residents' Manual of the American Academy of Physical Medicine and Rehabilitation.
6. Commission on Education in Physical Medicine and Rehabilitation. Privately printed. Bulletin 6, 1967. Physical Medicine and Rehabilitation. Career Information for Medical Students and Physicians.
7. Commision on Education in Physical Medicine and Rehabilitation. Privately printed.
  Bulletin 1, 1966. A Study of Undergraduate Teaching Programs in Rehabilitation Medicine in American Medical Colleges.
  Bulletin 2, 1966. The Structure of the Discipline of Physical Medicine and Rehabilitation.
  Bulletin 3, 1966. Standards for Academic Career Training in Physical Medicine and Rehabilitation.
  Bulletin 4, 1966. Estimates of Need for Physiatrists in the United States.
  Bulletin 5, 1966. The Vocational Interests, Values and Career Development of Specialists in Physical Medicine and Rehabilitation: A Preliminary Report.
  Bulletin 7, 1969. Fellowship Programs in Rehabilitation Medicine.
  Bulletin 8, 1968. Rehabilitation Medicine in American Medical Colleges: Recommendations for Teaching Programs.
8. Sanazaro, P. J.: Education for Patient Care. Federation Bulletin, *53:*No. 11, 1966, pp. 350-358.
9. Report of the Third Conference in Basic Principles of Rehabilitation as These Relate to the Teaching of Undergraduate Medical Students. The New York Academy of Sciences, 1965.
10. Report of the Fourth Conference on Basic Principles of Rehabilitation as These Relate to the Teaching of Undergraduate Medical Students, to Patient Care and To Research. The New York Academy of Sciences, 1966.
11. Report of the First Conference on Implications of Stroke: Diagnosis — Management — Rehabilitation. The New York Academy of Sciences, 1966.
12. Kottke, F. J.: Contemporary Concepts in the Teaching of Physical Medicine and Rehabilitation. J. Med. Educ., *39:*935-945, 1964.

Chapter 42

THE EPIDEMIOLOGY OF DISABILITY AS RELATED TO REHABILITATION MEDICINE

by Masayoshi Itoh
and
Mathew H. M. Lee

The word epidemiology is derived from the Greek *epidēmios*, meaning "among the people." Thus, it is no coincidence that in the early twentieth century C. O. Stallybrass defined epidemiology as "the science which considers infectious diseases—their course, propagation, and prevention."[66] This rather narrow and restricted definition, though obsolete, has a historic value since it characterized epidemiology as a science.

Hippocrates stressed meteorological variations and seasonal characteristics as the fundamental elements that determine cyclic variations in epidemic diseases.[59] Until the seventeenth century this theory was widely accepted as the dominant concept for explaining the causes of transmissible disease. Few supported Fracastoro[18] in the sixteenth century when he theorized that infection was a course and epidemics were a consequence. He further recognized three modes of contagion: (1) by direct contact from person to person; (2) by an intermediate agent; and (3) through the air. Sydenham in the seventeenth century suggested that there were intercurrent diseases which were dependent on the susceptibility of the human body.[59]

Beginning with ancient civilizations, the practitioners of medicine, the church and governments struggled against epidemics by using theory, superstition, authority and religion to compensate for lack of scientific knowledge. Throughout the medieval period, it was generally assumed that sorrow and suffering create a particularly favorable environment for the rise and spread of disease. The panic which erupted during epidemics was regarded as furthering the spread of the disease. Thus, municipal authorities in many European cities felt it advisable to forbid tolling the customary death knell, as it would be ringing continuously night and day. Since epidemics were attributed to the sins of man, elders of the church went from house to house hounding those suspected of religious irregularities and immoral conduct. Numerous men and women were expelled from the community in disgrace for minor offenses since it was believed that eradication of sin and the sinful would halt an epidemic.[22]

As outrageous and primitive as it may sound, these and similar preventive measures were guided by contemporary medical beliefs and prevailed until the twentieth century. Yet, we are not too far away from the day when tuberculosis and epilepsy were considered shameful afflictions. Even today, many still view venereal diseases as a sign of immorality; and superstition and fear doom patients with leprosy to life as social outcasts in many communities of the world. Because of such stigmatization, early discovery in these diseases remains extremely difficult. This is not meant to belittle or negate the tremendous amount of epidemiologic knowledge that has been accumulated in this century. It does, however, suggest that in centuries to come, our present-day knowledge on causation and prevention of diseases and morbid conditions may be considered as primitive as the witch hunt or voodoo rite.

W. H. Welch defined epidemiology as a study of the natural history of disease.[76] Lilienfeld described it as the study of the distribution of a disease or condition in a population, and of the factors that influence this distribution.[42] In these definitions, epidemiology is not restricted solely to the study of transmissible diseases but can embrace all types of diseases as well as disabilities, whether physical or mental.

This chapter on epidemiology discusses conceptual aspects, the classic theory of the natural history of disease, and practical application of an epidemiologic approach to the daily practice of rehabilitation medicine in the office, hospital, extended care facility, or home.

SPECTRUM OF HEALTH

The noted English biographer Izaak Walton stated in his famed *Compleat Angler*, "Look to your health; and if you have it, praise God, and value it next to a good conscience; for health is the second blessing that we mortals are capable of; a blessing that money cannot buy." Benjamin Disraeli, the great English statesman, said in 1877, "The health of people is really the foundation upon which all their happiness and all their powers as a state depend." "Health is an essential preliminary to the best success in the best work, and to the highest attainment in the widest usefulness. Without it there is sadness at the hearthstone, silence and sorrow, instead of cheerful words and happy heart."[17] Whether considered as personal treasure or national strength, health has long been regarded as the prime factor of human welfare. Therefore, prior to a discussion of disease and disabilities, some thought should be given to the concept of health.

One of the most frequently quoted and dynamic definitions of health was issued by the World Health Organization: "a state of complete physical, mental and social well-being and not merely the absence of disease or infirmity."[78]

This rather simply phrased definition contains two distinct thoughts. The words "complete physical, mental and social well-being" imply an infinite number of variables relative to the present and to the ever changing future. Rogers, in his Health Status Scale,[58] terms this state "Optimum Health" and notes that it is seldom maintained for a prolonged period. The second important aspect of the W.H.O. definition is the phrase "absence of disease or infirmity." This recognizes the existence of a state of health that is neither Optimum Health nor actual illness, and which may be called Suboptimum Health. Suboptimum Health can best be illustrated by the patient undergoing the incubation period of bacterial or viral disease or the person with latent diabetes mellitus.

Usually it is not too difficult to recognize the state of Overt Illness or Disability. However, in those diseases with insidious onset, such as multiple sclerosis or arteriosclerosis, it is often difficult to detect this state. When the process of disease threatens life, man reaches the state of Approaching Death. Today, however, this state does not necessarily mean that a man is going to die. A cardiac pacemaker, organ transplantation or exchange transfusion may bring a man back to Suboptimum Health.

In spite of advancements in scientific knowledge and technology, man reaches a state of Death, which is absolute and irreversible, when all vital organs cease to function. The fundamental goal of medical science is not to produce an immortal man but to maintain man in Optimum Health as long as possible, ideally until death.

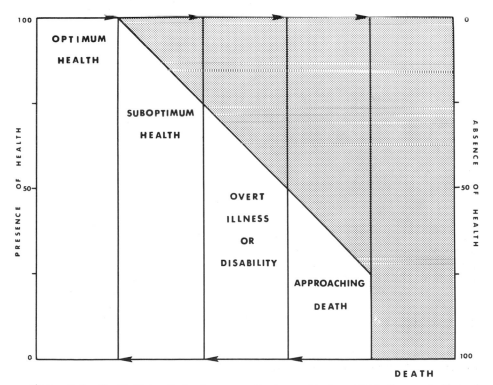

Figure 42–1   Health Status Scale. Arrows on the top and bottom of this diagram indicate declining and improving health respectively. (Modified from Rogers, E. S.: Human Ecology and Health. New York, The Macmillan Company, 1960.)

The most important aspect of Rogers' Health Status Scale (Fig. 42–1) is that no man can stay in one particular spot on this scale for an indefinite period. If we assume that the sum of the word health is constant as is the word "weather," then ill health is discord, while health is concord. Thus, as a man's health status declines, a portion of health decreases and that of ill health increases. As a train on a funicular railway, a man's health status constantly goes up and down from the peak of health to the edge of the valley of death.

This concept of health can easily be applied to the diseases or conditions that are observed in a rehabilitation service. Let us take as an example the case of a 60-year-old female who fell and sustained a subcapital fracture of the femur. Prior to the accident, this woman most likely had postmenopausal osteoporosis and possibly impairment of reflexes, of body balance and of musculoskeletal coordination. Although the patient might have thought she was in perfect health, the presence of these conditions indicates that her health status classification at the time of the fall was, at best, Suboptimum.

Now she is obviously in a state of Overt Disability. If this case is mismanaged, i.e., with prolonged bed rest subsequent to traction, then hypostatic pneumonia and possibly decubiti may develop. Thus, this woman's health enters the Approaching Death stage and may decline until it reaches Death. Not too long ago, this was the most commonly expected course after this type of accident.

The prognosis for subcapital fracture is poor if the fracture is treated with the Smith-Petersen nail, because the head of the femur will inevitably develop aseptic necrosis within a few months. In order to avoid this disaster and to bring the patient back to Suboptimum Health as rapidly as possible, replacement of the femoral head is the logical treatment.

Such surgical treatment, with proper restorative care, will return the patient to her normal state, Suboptimum Health, in a period of a few weeks. This model of the health status scale is applicable to every disabling condition, including loss of limbs or body organs.[28]

In the case just discussed, even the loss of the femoral head can be analyzed by use of the health status scale. The femoral head initially was in Suboptimum Health. Trauma from the fall resulted in Approaching Death of the femoral head. Its removal by surgery, since it could no longer function, is tantamount to Death of the femoral head. Insertion of the prosthesis, though it does not restore any portion of health to the femoral head, does restore a portion of health to the patient. In fact, it restores the patient to the level of health she enjoyed prior to the accident. Thus, Death of the femoral head prevented the patient from sliding to a lower level on the Health Status Scale.

NATURAL HISTORY OF DISEASE

In this concept of health it is obvious that there is a specific mechanism by which health changes from one direction to the other. The history of medicine clearly indicates that our predecessors made a great effort to identify the causation of illness. In early times, strange reasons were advanced as the causes of disease. Virtually anything that was beyond human control was, at one time or another, considered as the cause of some disease or affliction. Astrology and religions held that evil spirits and sins were responsible for the rise and fall of plagues. Evil spirits rising with the stench from sewage or stagnant water were thought to be the cause of epidemics. The initial use of smelling salts by European ladies may well have been an early but vague recognition of environment as a causative factor of disease.

It was not until the seventeenth century that the idea of human susceptibility emerged. During the onslaught of epidemics in the medieval period, the "sinful" people who fell victim to epidemics were obviously highly susceptible to the disease. Those who survived were naturally less susceptible but not necessarily any less sinful.

As early as the mid-seventeenth century, existence of the microorganism as a causative agent of illness was suspected. It was not until the nineteenth century, however, that this obscure theory was proved. Identification and isolation of a specific microorganism as a responsible agent of a particular disease enforced the concept of a single cause of disease, and less attention was focused on causes related to the host and environment.[39]

In the early twentieth century, various epidemiologic investigations on outbreaks of transmissible diseases were conducted. These studies revealed that mere exposure of the human host to a specific agent did not inevitably produce the state of Overt Illness. Thus, the modern epidemiologic concept that illness is caused by simultaneous interaction of host, agent and environment was established.

In order to comprehend this triad theory, which is highly relevant to later discussions in this chapter, it is essential to analyze each causative factor. The host, being human, has various characteristics: age, sex, race, chromosomal variety, body constitution, immunity, marital status, education, occupation, habit and custom, psychological state and so forth. The significance of host characteristics may be illustrated by the fact that certain diseases or conditions are more prevalent in persons with similar characteristics than in others lacking those characteristics.

Biological, chemical, mechanical, genetic, nutrient and physical elements are often cited as qualitative agent factors that may vary in their virulence. It is also important to note the value of the quantitative aspect of agent factors. Quantity may be understood in two categories: *dosage* and *frequency*. Frequent exposure to a low dosage of the agent could develop either of two opposing results: increased resistance or a cumulative effect. Increased resistance is exemplified by tuberculosis in the New World. White settlers had been exposed to *M. tuberculosis* for centuries in Europe and thus had developed resistance. Despite many hardships in America, there was no marked increase of tuberculosis among the white settlers. At the same time, American Indians and the imported black slaves in Argentina suffered greatly and some tribes and groups were virtually wiped out.

Similarly some childhood diseases may afflict adults, who have had little exposure to them and thus offer low resistance. On the other hand, chronic pulmonary silicosis, which is produced only after years of silica duct inhalation, is common among mining workers[47] but one visit to a coal mine cannot result in silicosis.

Environment may be viewed in terms of physical, biological, socioeconomic, political and other aspects. Physical environment may refer to the physical characteristics of the immediate surroundings or to atmospheric conditions such as climate, atmospheric pressure, gaseous composition and quality of air. Such characteristics of socioeconomic environment as education, customs and nutritional habits may greatly influence host susceptibility.

Paul[52] recognized two types of epidemiologic climate: micro-climate, described as the social climate and representing intimate living conditions within the home or place of work; and macro-climate, which represents climate in the ordinary meteorological sense of temperature, humidity and rainfall. The concept of micro-climate is more individualized in its interpretation of environment and includes some host characteristics which are related to socioeconomic conditions. For example, certain political climates could make one group of hosts more or less deprived in a socioeconomic sense.

When a disease or condition is analyzed, the factors of host, agent and environment must be carefully considered. An acceptable and perhaps innocent clinical statement such as "Fracture of the neck of femur is commonly seen in elderly people, mostly women"[29] is far short of satisfactory in an epidemiologic sense. Mere age and sex cannot accurately represent the host characteristics. Such characteristics in an aging female may involve body constitution—for example, postmenopausal osteoporosis, diminished vision, and a propensity for falling—in other words, an impaired sense of body balance. This could be caused by cerebral arteriosclerosis or by medications being administered for hypertension. But this is still a limited analysis. Custom and habit can also contribute to this injury and disability. Many women at home customarily wear house slippers, which cause a shuffling gait and make the wearer more susceptible to falling accidents. Some investigators[3, 74] claimed hip fracture is common among whites but another[57] disputed this by citing a large number of cases among Negroes. Thus even the racial factor must be considered when discussing the prevalence of this condition.

Since most hip fractures occur inside the home, the peculiarities of the environment must be studied. Highly waxed or wet floors, slippery throw rugs or a dangling telephone cord may become menacing obstacles. Cluttered floors, poor lighting, sagging floors or steps, defective hand rails on staircases or crowded housing indicating a hazardous physical environment may be host characteristics related to the socioeconomic and educational factors.

The agent in the accident discussed as an example is mechanical force, which exerted extreme stress to body structure.[10] Unsuccessful attempts to regain body balance resulted in the fall, and stress produced the fracture.

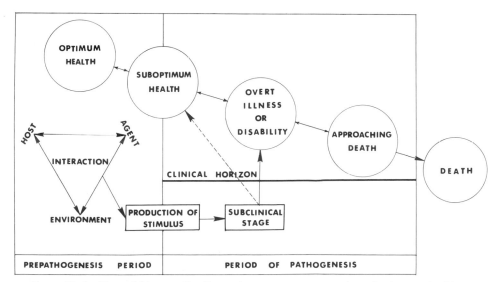

Figure 42–2 Natural history of a disease in man, as constructed on the Rogers' health status scale shown in Figure 42–1. Not every disease appears above the clinical horizon. Man may recover from the subclinical stages directly to suboptimum health.

However, one can easily ascertain that various host characteristics and environmental factors had existed for some time prior to this accident. Most likely, there had been episodes of loss of balance or near accidents before this incident. The fact that injury did occur at this particular time indicates that the three causative factors — host, agent and environment — sufficiently and simultaneously interacted and resulted in fracture.

The period when these three causative factors exist independently and have not completed interaction is called the Prepathogenesis Period (Fig. 42-2). Upon completion of simultaneous interaction, a disease stimulus is produced. At this stage, Early Pathogenesis, a man's health status changes from Optimum to Suboptimum Health. However, until the disease process reaches above the Clinical Horizon, the presence of illness is not recognizable. Once reaching the state of Overt Illness, man may recover to Suboptimum and, hopefully, Optimum Health, at which time he returns to the Prepathogenesis Period and commences another cycle for other disease. This model of the natural history of disease is applicable to virtually all diseases and conditions and is the basis for the epidemiology of disability.

LEVELS OF PREVENTION

Health care includes preventive and clinical medicine. Any health care that attempts to halt man's slide down the slope of the health status scale is termed preventive and any attempt to push it up toward the peak, Optimum Health, is called therapeutic. This definition is essential to conceptualization of the Levels of Prevention. While activities in preventive medicine have no direct therapeutic value, every measure administered in therapeutic or clinical medicine has its preventive aspects. Vaccination or fluoridation of drinking water protects populations from disease but does not cure any disease. On the other hand, antibiotics are therapeutic agents that can also prevent septicemia and death. Similarly, internal fixation of hip fracture is a therapeutic surgical treatment but also prevents pulmonary and peripheral vascular complications.

Within this frame of reference, the total spectrum of health care is classified into three levels of prevention: Primary, Secondary and Tertiary. Primary prevention is applicable during the prepathogenesis or Optimum Health periods. The other two levels cover the period of pathogenesis or, let us say, all gradations of the health scale from Suboptimum Health to Approaching Death.

Each level of prevention consists of various representative activities. Table 42-1 shows a comparison of the activities at each level, as interpreted by the authors at this chapter and by others. All the listed authors agree wholly on activities basic to Primary prevention and agree in part with our interpretation of Secondary prevention. Our interpretation of rehabilitation and limitation of disability activities differs from that of the other authors, and they also differ from each other in interpretation of these measures.

Rehabilitation is defined as "the ultimate restoration of a disabled person to his maximum capacity — physical, emotional and vocational."[61] It is widely believed that rehabilitation must be started at the earliest possible time in order to ensure the best results. Thus, the diagnosis must be established in the earliest possible phase of disease and all necessary treatment, including rehabilitation, must be initiated at that time. The belief that rehabilitation should commence after termination of specific treatment of a disease or condition which results in disability is the basis for classifying rehabilitation at the Tertiary prevention level. And the writers admit that this idea is regrettably widespread, and such procedure is common practice. But this is obviously a misconception. Inasmuch as rehabilitation should be administered in conjunction with specific medical or surgical treatment of diseases or conditions which can result in disablement, rehabilitation should be considered an integral part of Secondary prevention.

Disability limitation (Table 42-1) refers to preventing an increase in the intensity or scope of an existing disability. This measure, therefore, becomes necessary after termination of active medical or surgical treatment and rehabilitation. Disability limitation is generally known as maintenance treatment. It is particularly indispensable for those who are chronically ill or disabled and absolutely mandatory for geriatric patients. Another example of disability limitation is recreation therapy. Eventually, lack of stimuli, regimented daily life and hopelessness can mold the population of a chronic disease institution into a depressed, docile, apathetic mass. Recreation therapy, through programs designed to stimulate both groups and individuals, can prevent this kind of psychological crippling.

We have included custodial care in our table of health care. The purpose of custodial care is to make man as comfortable as possible for the last few years or days of his life. When custodial care is indicated there is usually no hope for reversal or cure. This does not mean disability limitation is not indicated. It is warranted because it prolongs activity and comfort and it should be listed as an independent entity in Tertiary prevention.

The model of Levels of Prevention that is described here can be applied to each individual disease or condition. Thus, in reality, a man may be subjected to various levels of prevention simultaneously. For example, a 65-year-old man has had a cerebrovascular accident secondary to arteriosclerotic heart disease. He complains of fatigue and shortness of breath after exercise and experiences pitting edema. He was recently discharged to his home from a rehabilitation service and is able to ambulate with a short leg brace but his upper extremity is spastic and non-functional. The time is late November and the city health department predicts influenza epidemics during the coming winter.

The cardiac condition receives priority attention; early diagnosis and prompt treatment for cardiac decompensation is in order. This is Secondary prevention. The patient is advised to wear the short leg brace daily and is given a static splint for his upper extremity. Further, ambulation commensurate with his tolerance is encouraged and a visiting physical therapist gives passive exercise to his upper extremity to prevent contracture of fingers. These are disabil-

TABLE 42–1 LEVELS OF PREVENTION

AUTHORS	PRIMARY	SECONDARY	TERTIARY
Leavell and Clark[10]	Health promotion Specific protection	Early diagnosis Proper treatment Disability limitation	Rehabilitation
Columbia University[15]	Health promotion Specific protection	Early diagnosis Proper treatment	Disability limitation Rehabilitation
Itoh and Lee	Health promotion Specific protection	Early diagnosis Proper treatment Rehabilitation	Disability limitation Custodial care

ity limitation measures. The attending physician would probably give influenza vaccine to prevent any danger to the patient from the threatened epidemic. This is Primary prevention.

Another example is cardiac surveillance of elderly disabled who are undergoing a rehabilitation program. Solomon and associates[69] found that over 25 per cent of geriatric lower extremity amputees who had no previous history of ischemic heart disease showed changes indicative of myocardial ischemia on telemetric dynamic electrocardiograms taken during ambulation exercise. This finding provides information necessary for regulating the patients' physical activity within the limits of cardiac tolerance so that ischemic heart disease might be prevented. While these patients are obviously receiving rehabilitation, the Secondary preventive care, the surveillance program promotes the "specific protection" of Primary prevention.

The purpose of this epidemiologic approach to patient care is to provide the tools that seek and analyze all factors contributing to disease and disability. It demonstrates a rational and individualized approach that assures that no factor is overlooked and no question remains unanswered.

FUNCTIONAL DIAGNOSIS

Prevention consists of two interrelated processes: the anticipation of future events and the action to thwart occurrence. Anticipation is possible only if there is some recall from past experience. When experience is documented in detail and carefully analyzed, prognostication can be reasonable and accurate. Epidemiology systematically studies the process of a disease or condition and demonstrates a chain of events which is known as the natural history. Once the natural history of a disease is established, the weakest link in the chain of events is the point where the attack to prevent the disease should start.

In the early part of this century epidemics of an unknown malady became prevalent in the southern part of the United States. An epidemiologic investigation was launched and certain characteristics regarding the prevalence of the disease were uncovered. Thus, the disease caused by a deficiency of niacin and now known as pellagra was identified.[19, 23] The methods used to discover the identity of pellagra were identical to the approach that previously had been applied only to transmissible diseases. The most important aspect of the pellagra investigation is that the whole epidemiologic study was based solely upon accurate clinical documentation of the condition of each patient so afflicted.

Rehabilitation, one of the secondary levels of prevention, focuses its attention on disability. Other specialties in therapeutic medicine require early and precise diagnosis in order to institute the most effective treatment. The same logic applies to rehabilitation, and the disabled should be given early evaluation and intensive treatment to prevent permanent disability.[37] Dynamic rehabilitation care can be administered only when an explicit early diagnosis of the disability has been established.[70] The longer explicit diagnosis is delayed, the less effective the consequent restorative care becomes.

For example, right hemiplegia due to cerebral artery thrombosis is not sufficiently accurate as a diagnosis to be utilized in making an effective rehabilitation care plan. Because the ultimate goal of rehabilitation is total restoration, the total person, physically, emotionally, vocationally and socially, must be considered in the diagnosis. Most medical records and case histories do not indicate the physical, mental or socioeconomic ability of a man.[72] There are no two identical hemiplegics. The aforementioned diagnosis, although medicolegally acceptable, does not indicate the extent of brain damage or note cultural background, which will directly influence the patient's ability to comprehend, retain instruction or respond to the rehabilitation process. Thus, the conventional non-illuminating diagnostic nomenclature for statistical purposes[79] is insufficient for dynamic rehabilitation care.

Diagnosis of disability may be expressed either in terms of the amount of disability or in terms of the amount of remaining function. The former category is commonly called the disability evaluation or rating. In the latter category, functional diagnosis is the preferred terminology. Regardless of choice, the sum of the results from either system remains constant. It is universally agreed that disability evaluation is, in reality, a quantitative diagnosis as contrasted with the more familiar qualitative diagnosis.[13, 35, 36, 80] Evaluation of disability has long been important in the legal field.[1, 35, 45, 75] Since no single standard wholly fulfills the specific needs of all programs concerned with disability,[55] various rating systems according to diagnostic groups have been reported.[2, 24, 53, 80] One of the most widely used is the cardiac classification ratings of the American Heart Association. A variety of disability scales to evaluate the injured in liability or workmen's compensation cases were developed in the first half of this century.[7, 8, 20, 46, 83]

Countless methods to assess the extent of disability pursuant to a treatment plan and to evaluate the progress of a patient in a rehabilitation program are in the literature. Some are more ingenious or sophisticated than others. Moskowitz and McCann[48] developed a physical profile called PULSES which utilizes a set of ordinal scales. PULSES expresses general physical condition, the function of upper and lower extremities, sensory status, continency and emotional status by six representative digits. The Sokolow method[67] rates physical, social, emotional and vocational capacity, but a national field trial[68] revealed this method contributes little of significant value to vocational counseling. For the past two decades numerous Activities of Daily Living (ADL) scales have been reported.[4, 6, 9, 12, 25, 26, 34, 38, 41, 44, 63, 81] While ADL scales are mainly in the domain of the occupational therapist, Pool and Brown[54] selected certain activities which a physical therapist could evaluate.

A large volume of data must be collected in order to produce one comprehensive functional diagnosis. The accumulation of voluminous information inadvertently necessitates involvement with the problem of effective format and storage which will permit easy retrieval of all the data. In this regard, electronic data processing techniques have been found to be most advantageous.[67, 70]

The expression of disability evaluation or functional diagnosis varies according to the method. The most common method is a numerical presentation in either percentage or digit based upon a specific scale. The other common method is a graphic presentation. Unlike Lawton's method[38] for ADL, Huddleston and colleagues[27] produced a graph called the Patient Profile Chart, on which the value of muscle power and comparative functional capacities were arranged. In reviewing all these methods, there are more numerical presentations than descriptive ones. This tendency is perhaps owing to the fact that the use of digits gives simplicity and provides mathematical advantages such as weighting.

The ordinal scale is becoming more popular than the nominal scale. However, one must recognize that a well-conceived nominal scale is superior to a haphazard ordinal scale despite the use of digits. One pitfall in the nominal scale is that innovators sometimes become trapped in their own jargon. There is a need to eliminate or replace vague stereotyped expression with more realistic and accurate terminology.[5] A good example of this type of ambiguous phraseology is "partial independent" or "minimum assistance." The ideal functional diagnosis should be:

1. Simple enough so that rapid evaluation is possible;
2. Reproducible so that constancy may be maintained;
3. Objective and using measurable factors so that the results are statistically more reliable;
4. Descriptive so that the actual situation is accurately reflected;
5. Comprehensive so that the diagnosis is completely and specifically utilizable in the direct care of patients and is practicable for epidemiologic investigation.

To date there is no single standard which measures disability with precision nor is there any set of precise biological units, free of subjective influences, which uniformly convey universally acceptable measuring criteria.[35]

In relation to functional diagnosis, Wylie and White[82] stated:

In each field of knowledge, such as medicine or public health, a new measuring instrument commonly results in new studies and observation: from these we evolve new hypotheses, and further instruments are invented to test these ideas. . . . When the field knowledge is still in a rudimentary stage, often a scarcity of measuring instruments delays this cycle.

Thus, the use of epidemiology in rehabilitation can aid in defining the natural history of physical disabilities in mankind and it is well recognized that there is a hiatus in our knowledge of human incapacitation. Better "instrument" or better functional diagnosis means that new studies, new observation and new hypotheses will emerge.

SECONDARY DISABILITY

In the daily practice of rehabilitation medicine in a hospital-based service or private office, there is a tendency to view disability in a simplistic or superficial way. Excluding iatrogenic disability and physical disability due to psychiatric illness,[40] two types of disabilities exist. Disabilities which are direct consequences of a disease or condition are called primary disability. Paraplegia, quadriplegia following spinal cord injury, hemiplegia, hemianopsia, aphasia due to cerebral vascular accident, or traumatic fracture are examples of primary disability. On the other hand, disabilities which did not exist at the onset of the primary disability but subsequently developed are called secondary disabilities.[62] The secondary disability is indirectly related to the disease or condition which is responsible for the primary disability. Examples are joint contracture, subluxation of shoulder joint in hemiplegia, disuse muscle atrophy and decubiti.

The epidemiology of primary disability, a subject outside the province of conventional rehabilitation medicine, will be discussed later in this chapter, under Preventive Rehabilitation. Since the secondary disability develops while the patient is under the physiatrist's care, it is important to discuss it in depth. However, literature related to the epidemiology of secondary disability is minimal. Abramson et al.[1] claimed that among injured workers there is a correlation between the degree of disability, the circumstances of injury, and the sex, age, employment status, economic status and place of residence of the injured. This finding should not be interpreted as proof of the existence of malingering among workers covered by workmen's compensation but rather as proof that many complex factors are responsible for disablement. The group of secondary disabilities commonly found in cases of Hansen's disease has received intensive epidemiologic study,[49, 71] perhaps because the nature of the illness requires that a large number of epidemiologists be engaged in control of the disease.

An epidemiologic analysis of secondary disability reveals certain characteristics in the causative factors. Elderly people and those who have had a primary disability for an extended period are more susceptible to a secondary disability. Further, when the disease or condition causing the primary disability is accompanied by pain or spasticity, the prevalence of secondary disability increases. The frequency of flexion contracture in the hip joint of above-knee amputees or the multiple contractures in rheumatoid arthritis or multiple sclerosis are examples of these. On the other hand, if the original disease diminishes skin sensation, particularly pain or temperature, the patient is also predisposed to the secondary disability. Decubiti in paraplegics, plantar ulcers in patients with Hansen's disease and in diabetics or absorption of fingers among leprous patients are representative. When nutrition is poor, certain disabilities such as decubiti are more easily developed. Socioeconomic and vocational factors may have indirect relationship to the causation of secondary disability. The level of intelligence, often related to cultural and educational background, and individual motivation are other indirect causative factors.

The environmental factor involved in the development of secondary disability is simply the position of the body itself. The idea of considering body position as an environmental factor may be unorthodox. However, positioning of either hemiplegic extremities or the stump after an amputation is external to the host and thus constitutes a contrived man-made environment. Negligence or ignorance on the part of paramedical personnel or family members results in placing the disabled in positions which foster secondary disability. Certain body positions that involve maintaining a particular position for a prolonged period may well prevent one disability but inadvertently cause another. Placing on wheelchairs elderly patients with above-knee amputations or fractured hips is an effective measure to prevent pneumonia but tends to result in flexion contracture of the hip joint.

Another important factor affecting the "environmental body is the condition of the objects with which it has direct contact. Materials that are rough surfaced, rigid and minimally ventilated also predispose the host to secondary disability.

The most intriguing part in epidemiologic observation of secondary disability is identification of the agent. The agent is sometimes mechanical force, which may be either excessive or totally absent. Excessive and concentrated force to the skin area may result in decubitus, and the absence of force may cause demineralization of bone or disuse atrophy of muscle. At times this force may simply be the natural presence of gravity. Equinus deformity in flaccid foot drop and subluxation of the shoulder joint in hemiplegics are some examples of secondary disability related to gravity. The concept of the natural history of secondary disability specifies that the three causative factors (agent, host and environment) must interact frequently or for a prolonged period. The time element is perhaps the key to the occurrence of disability stimuli.

The characteristics of secondary disability in the period of pathogenesis are always insidious and the symptoms are non-specific, regardless of the primary disability and its causative disease or condition. The process is always progressive and if not checked can at some point become irreversible. The secondary disability is usually painless but may sometimes be fatal if allowed to developed to the ultimate. The most usual result is a severe curtailment of function. There seems to be little seasonal variation and there is no known immunity to this condition.

IMMOBILIZATION

One universally recognized condition that severely damages the disabled is immobilization. According to the United States Public Health Service, disability due to immobilization was one of ten leading preventable health problems in 1960. Merely by utilization of present knowledge such disability in the United States could be reduced by 50 to 75 per cent.[56] Correlation between the amount of damage from immobilization and the duration of the immobilization is a controversial subject.[51, 65] In general, the greater the size of the body segment and the longer the period of immobilization, the greater the intensity of the pathologic condition and the number of organ systems that become involved.

The discussion of the agent factor provides the basis for understanding the mechanism of immobilization as one of the causes of secondary disability. Undoubtedly, immobilization is associated with the absence of mechanical force, the one stimulus so essential to maintenance of proper body function. Osteoporosis, the loss of bone density, is the most commonly known pathological change due to immobilization. This change is often detected in patients after a long-term plaster cast immobilization and is also found in the lower extremities of paraplegics. If the absence of force as a stimulus is the agent factor for osteoporosis, then it should be possible to produce this pathologic condition in normal individuals in a simulated environment. This hypothesis was proved correct by the distinct decrease in bone density and increase in calcium excretion in the astronauts during the 14-day Gemini VII voyage.[43, 77]

Many experimental immobilizations have revealed similar results. Mechanical stress, such as is produced by weight-bearing and muscle tension, is necessary for maintenance of the normal skeletal mass. During prolonged bed rest or extended conditions of zero gravity, the static stress distribution and its metabolic requirements are altered. The absence of normal mechanical stress on the skeletal system removes some of the stimuli necessary to bone formation.[33] Moreover, previously discussed causative factors of secondary disablement are also applicable to immobilization. The deleterious effect of immobilization cannot be considered as a primary disability.

Every pathophysiological change starts its development at the onset of immobilization, just as the aging processes begin at birth. It is interesting to review the literature which seeks to establish the exact point wherein these changes become recognizable. The cardiac rate at rest increases approximately 0.5 beat per minute per each day of immobilization and the loss of muscle tone resulting from complete disuse is estimated to be 10 to 15 per cent of strength per week.[73] After a few days of immobilization, an increase in bone blood flow was detected by means of radioactive strontium uptake and it was suggested that this may favor bone atrophy.[64] Similarly, within six to ten days following immobilization, the nitrogen balance of healthy male subjects reverses to a negative balance.[11] Significantly, the tendon capillary bed decreases after a six week period of immobilization but nothing of significance was observed in the muscle capillary bed. Because of this finding it is advisable to mobilize the recently repaired or reconstructed tendon as soon as possible, consistent with the limits of healing tensile strength.[60]

Events resulting in immobilization may be classified in various ways. Inadvertent and therapeutic immobilizations[31] are probably the most inclusive classifications. Bed rest and confinement to chair or wheelchair belong to the former category. Post-traumatic or post-surgical states, acute infection or inflammation, the convalescent period from non-surgical ailments and so forth constitute the latter category. In either group, immobilization is artificially forced upon the patients. On the other hand, there may also occur unavoidable immobilization, such as is caused by severe pain, neuromuscular impairment or psychiatric illness. Irrespective of the reason, the pathophysiological changes and clinical symptoms of immobilization are non-specific.

These changes and symptoms continue progressively throughout the immobilization, and reversal is not always spontaneous upon termination of the restriction. Even if the changes are reversible, the period of recovery from these effects is much longer than the period of immobilization. An experiment determined that young healthy men confined in bed for three weeks need five weeks after resumption of normal activity to regain normal cardiovascular response to the upright position.[73] It is conceivable that those who have deteriorated physically, particularly the elderly, need a longer recovery period. Besides the time element, the manpower and money required for restoration is enormous. Pathological changes of immobilization superimposed upon the primary disability often create totally dependent persons out of patients who initially would have been self-sufficient. This can be devastating to the families and the socioeconomic well-being of a community. Since total immunization against the ill effects of immobilization has not been developed, simulation of mechanical stimuli to the human body during immobilization is the most effective preventive measure.

PREVENTIVE REHABILITATION

All clinical specialties focus their interest and effort toward restoration of man's health from the state of Overt Illness to Optimum Health. In this sense, if the definition of rehabilitation is accepted, all clinicians practice "the act of rehabilitation."[28] Care provided through rehabilitation medicine consists of restoration of function and prevention of disability. Diverse therapeutic exercises are instrumental in anatomic and physiological restoration of function. Though this type of physical rehabilitation is ideal, the outcome depends heavily upon natural recovery from the lesion responsible for the disability and this goal is not always attainable. When anatomic and physiological restoration has failed, a compensatory body mechanism or an orthotic or prosthetic device substitutes for the lost function. Although the goals of nursing and physical and occupational therapy are primarily directed toward complete restoration or functional substitution, in actuality this may mean that they predominantly engage in prevention of secondary disability. As the greater portion of the time and energy of rehabilitation professionals is devoted, intentionally or unintentionally, to prevention of secondary disability, rehabilitation medicine should certainly become more emphatically involved in the epidemiologic approach and its application to preventive measures.

The term "Preventive Rehabilitation" has been introduced in response to this need.[28, 30, 32] Until the mid-twentieth century, the stigmatizing deformities commonly seen in patients with Hansen's disease were believed to be primary disabilities. Careful and painstaking clinical investigation and epidemiologic analysis revealed the natural history of these disabilities: they are secondary disabilities caused by trauma and infection. They result from the neglect and ignorance of both patients and medical professionals. Modifications in activities of daily living, simple self-administered daily exercise, early case finding, and regular, adequate specific chemotherapy can prevent these disabilities. Heretofore, the only alternative was reconstruction by skilled plastic surgery after these disabilities had become irreversible. "Preventive Rehabilitation" became a component of conventional rehabilitation in leprosy control programs.[50]

In recent years epidemiologists have become progressively involved in the clinical epidemiology of diseases which result in physical disabilities, and clinicians have become increasingly aware of the epidemiologic approach to clinical problems. Feinstein[16] characterized clinical epidemiology as being not restricted by type of disease, age, locale or any particular form of data collection. Clinical epidemiology may be viewed as ecologic medicine, social medicine or community medicine. The concept of health and the model for the natural history of disease were derived from experience in transmissible disease and they are essential to any analysis of non-infectious diseases or conditions such as disability. The fundamental purpose of epidemiology is the prevention and eradication of diseases and conditions through a better understanding of causation. If complete prevention or total eradication is not possible, containment is the second choice.

In this new concept of Preventive Rehabilitation, the scope of expertise and the role of the physiatrist must be enlarged. Prevention of disability does not start at birth or after a primary disability occurs. Disability due to genetic defects or genetic incompatibility can be prevented by means of genetic counseling. During the early gestation period, expectant mothers must be protected from rubella and from certain pharmaceutical products. Amniotic fluid analysis may provide vital information pertinent to the discovery of potentially disabling diseases in the newborn. These are measures to prevent primary disability. However, artificial termination of pregnancy to eliminate the fetus with suspected deformities should not be considered as prevention of primary disability. The justification for advocating artificial abortion in these cases is preponderantly psychosocial and economic and not medical. Cerebral palsy due to intracranial damage in a high forceps delivery should concern the physiatrist as much as it involves the obstetrician. Although modern health care provides many deterrents to primary disability (Fig. 42-3), prevention has mainly involved public health specialists and allied health professionals but not the physiatrist.

Current population growth, particularly a rapid increase of the aged, predicts a sharp rise in our disabled population in the near future. It is well documented that there is a great shortage of medical and paramedical professionals to care for the disabled and we cannot even meet present demands. Unless more effective methods of specific prevention are developed to protect the population from primary disability in the future, the newly disabled will face a critical situation. The cumulative shortage of health manpower will cause them to be without benefit of rehabilitation services, and superimposed secondary disabilities will render them totally dependent. This will not only result in insurmountable personal tragedy, but will create infinite economic problems for families, communities and nations.

Exploration into the epidemiology of disability, the causative factors, the natural history of secondary disability, the epidemiology of immobilization and the importance of functional diagnosis exposes the urgency for a reassessment

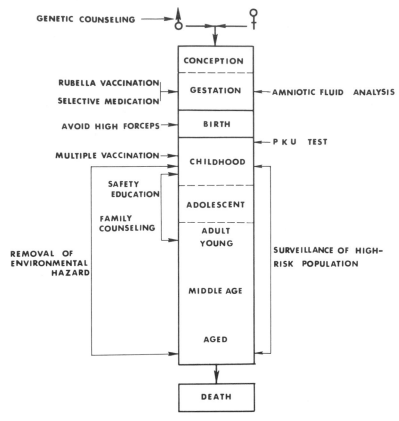

Figure 42–3 Prevention of primary disability in the life of man. Items on the left side of the column indicate specific protection against primary disability. Measures on the right side are for early detection and probable prevention of potential primary disability.

of rehabilitation medicine. Our professionals, medical and paramedical, have played rather passive roles in clinical medicine and comprehensive health care.* Though rehabilitation medicine has pioneered in vocational and legislative areas and contributed immeasurably to the welfare of the handicapped, it has not played the same spectacular role in the delivery of health care. Laymen, through the efforts of rehabilitation medicine, are now sensitive to and aware of the social and vocational needs of the disabled, and many laymen are now capable of furthering the principles that we initiated. It is now time for the science-oriented medical rehabilitation community to develop and promote its more scientific aspects, to explore every phase of disability and disability prevention, and to contribute epidemiologic investigation that will make it possible for those engaged in rehabilitation to prevent epidemics of disability in much the same manner that we are now able to prevent communicable disease.

---

*Comprehensive health care is defined as care that is provided to the patient according to his needs in appropriate, continuous and dynamic pattern.[14]

REFERENCES

1. Abramson, J. H., Mann, K. J., Nizan, A., and Goldberg, R.: Epidemiology of Disability after Work Injuries. Arch. Environ. Health, 9:572-580, 1964.
2. Alba, A., Trainor, F. S., Ritter, W., and Dacso, M. M.: A Clinical Disability Rating for Parkinson Patients. J. Chronic Dis., 21:507-522, 1968.
3. Boyd, H. B., and George, I. L.: Fracture of the Hip. Result Following Treatment. J.A.M.A., 137:1196-1199, 1948.
4. Brown, M. E.: Daily Activity Inventory and Progress Record for Those with Atypical Movement, I. Amer. J. Occup. Ther., 4:195-204, 1950.
5. Bruett, T. L., and Overs, R. P.: A Critical Review of 12 ADL Scales. Phys. Ther., 49:857-862, 1969.
6. Buchwald, E.: Physical Rehabilitation for Daily Living. New York, McGraw-Hill Book Co., 1952.
7. Burns, R. M.: Rating of Industrial Disabilities. J. Lancet, 58:17-20, 1939.
8. Carter, R. M.: Estimation of Disability. Industr. Med., 8:52-54, 1939.
9. Carroll, D.: The Disability in Hemiplegia Caused by Cerebrovascular Disease. J. Chron. Dis., 15:179-188, 1962.
10. Clark, E. G.: The Epidemiological Approach and Contribution to Preventive Medicine. In Leavell, H. R., and Clark, E. G., eds.: Preventive Medicine for the Doctor in His Community. New York, McGraw-Hill Book Co., 1965, Chapter 3.
11. Deitrick, J. E., Whedon, G. D., and Shorr, E.: Effects of Immobilization upon Various Metabolic and Physiologic Functions of Normal Men. Amer. J. Med., 4:3-32, 1948.
12. Dennerstein, A. S., Lowenthal, M., and Dexter, M.: Evaluation of a Rating Scale of Ability in Activities of Daily Living. Arch. Phys. Med., 46:579-584, 1965.
13. Dristine, M. J.: Disability Evaluation. Principles of Quantitative Diagnosis. Northwest Med., 61:1041-1042, 1962.
14. Division of Chronic Disease, Public Health Service: The Concept of Comprehensive Care. In Lilienfeld, A. M., and Gifford, A. J., eds.: Chronic Disease and Public Health. Baltimore, Johns Hopkins Press, 1966.
15. Division of Epidemiology, Columbia University, School of Public Health and Administrative Medicine: Principles, Methods and Uses of Epidemiology. New York, 1965.
16. Feinstein, A. R.: Clinical Epidemiology, I. The Populational Experiments of Nature and of Man in Human Illness. Ann. Intern. Med., 69:807-820, 1968.
17. Fowler, C. H., and DePuy, W. H.: Home and Health and Home Economics. New York, Phillips and Hunt, 1880.
18. Fracastoro, G.: *De contagione et contagiosis morbis et eorum cruratine, Libri III.* Translated and notes by Wilmer Cave Wright. New York, G. P. Putnam's Sons, 1930.
19. Goldberger, J., Wheeler, G. A., and Sydenstricker, W.: A Study of the Relation of Diet to Pellagra Incidence in Seven Textile-Mill Communities of South Carolina in 1916. Pub. Health Rep., 35:648-713, 1920.
20. Goodwin, W. M.: Meaning of Functional Disabilities. Int. J. Surg., 37:540-548, 1924.
21. Gorden, E. E., and Kohn, K. H.: Evaluation of Rehabilitation Methods in the Hemiplegic Patient. J. Chron. Dis., 19:3-16, 1966.
22. Gordon, B. L.: Medieval and Renaissance Medicine. New York, Philosophical Library, Inc., 1959, Chapter XXII.
23. Gordon, J. E., and LeRiche, H.: The Epidemiologic Method Applied to Nutrition. Amer. J. Med. Sci., 219:312-345, 1950.
24. Greenseid, D. Z., and McCormack, R. M.: Functional Hand Testing. A Profile Evaluation. Plast. Reconstr. Surg., 42:567-571, 1968.
25. Hoberman, M., Cicenia, E. F., and Stephenson, G. R.: Daily Activity Testing in Physical Therapy and Rehabilitation. Arch. Phys. Med., 33:99-108, 1952.
26. Hoff, W. I., and Mead, S.: Evaluation of Rehabilitation Outcome. An Objective Assessment of the Physically Disabled. Amer. J. Phys. Med., 44:113-121, 1965.
27. Huddleston, O. L., Moore, R. W., Rubin, D., Humphrey, T. L., Campbell, J. W., and Balanchetter, R.: Evaluation of Physical Disabilities by Means of Patient Profile Chart. Arch. Phys. Med., 42:250-257, 1961.
28. Itoh, M., and Lee, M. H.: The Future Role of Rehabilitation Medicine in Community Health. Med. Clin. N. Amer., 53:719-733, 1969.
29. Itoh, M., and Dacso, M. M.: Rehabilitation of Patients with Hip Fracture. A Clinical Study of 126 Cases. Postgrad. Med., 28:134-139, 1960.
30. Itoh, M.: Preventive Rehabilitation for Leprosy—A New Approach to an Old Problem. Rehab. Rev., 19:13-14, 1968.

31. Jebsen, R. H.: Therapeutic Exercise in Motion Problems, I. Northwest Med., *65:*742-747, 1966.
32. Karat, S.: Preventive Rehabilitation in Leprosy. Leprosy Rev., *39:*39-44, 1968.
33. Kazasian, L. E., and Von Gierker, H. E.: Bone Loss as a Result of Immobilization and Chelation. Preliminary Results in *Macaca Mulatta*. Clin. Orthop., *65:*67-75, 1969.
34. Kelman, H. R., and Muller, J. N.: Rehabilitation of Nursing Home Residents. Geriatrics, *17:*402-411, 1962.
35. Knapp, M. E.: Disability Evaluation, 1. Postgrad. Med., *46:*184-186, 1969.
36. Knapp, M. E.: Disability Evaluation, 2. Postgrad. Med., *46:*201-203, 1969.
37. Krusen, E. M.: Rehabilitation of the Elderly. Southern Med. J., *51:*225-228, 1958.
38. Lawton, E. B.: Activities of Daily Living: Testing, Training and Equipment. New York, Institute of Physical Medicine and Rehabilitation, New York University Bellevue Medical Center, Monograph No. 10, 1956.
39. Leavell, H. R., and Clark, E. G.: Levels of Application of Preventive Medicine. In Leavell, H. R., and Clark, E. G., eds.: Preventive Medicine for the Doctor in His Community. New York, McGraw-Hill Book Co., 1965, Chapter 2.
40. Lerner, J.: Disability Evaluation in Psychiatric Illness and the Concept of Hysteria. Canad. Psychiat. Ass. J., *11:*350-355, 1966.
41. Linn, M. W.: A Rapid Disability Scale. J. Amer. Geriat. Soc., *15:*211-214, 1967.
42. Lilienfeld, B. E.: Epidemiologic Methods and Inferences. In Hilleboe, H. E., and Larimore, G. W., eds.: Preventive Medicine. Philadelphia, W. B. Saunders Co., 1965, Chapter 43.
43. Lutwak, L.: Chemical Analysis of Diet. Urine, Feces and Sweat Parameters Relating to the Calcium and Nitrogen Balance Studies During Gemini VII Flight (Exp. M7). NASA Contractor Report, NAS 9-5375, 1966.
44. Mahoney, F. I., Wood, O. H., and Barthel, D. W.: Rehabilitation of Chronically Ill Patients. Influence of Complication of Chronically Ill Patients. Southern Med. J., *51:*605-609, 1958.
45. Mann, K. J., Abramson, J. H., Nizan, A., and Goldberg, R.: Epidemiology of Disabling Work Injuries in Israel. Arch. Environ. Health (Chicago), *9:*505-513, 1964.
46. McBride, E. D.: Disability Evaluation—Principles of Treatment of Compensable Injuries. 4th Ed. Philadelphia, J. B. Lippincott Co., 1942.
47. Milby, T. H.: Pneumoconioses. In Occupational Diseases, A Guide to Their Recognition. Washington, D.C., U.S. Dept. of Health, Education and Welfare, Public Health Service. Public Health Service Publication No. 1097, 1964, Section V.
48. Moskowitz, E., and McCann, C. B.: Classification of Disability in Chronically Ill and Aging. J. Chron. Dis., *5:*342-346, 1957.
49. Noordeen, S. K., and Srinivasan, H.: Epidemiology of Disability in Leprosy, I. A General Study of Disability Among Male Patients Above Fifteen Years of Age. Int. J. Leprosy, *34:*159-169, 1966.
50. Pan American Health Organization: Consolidated Report on Item III, Determination of Objectives and Preparation of Timetables, 1968.
51. Patel, A. N.: Disuse Atrophy of Human Skeletal Muscles. Arch. Neurol. *20:*413-421, 1969.
52. Paul, J. R.: Clinical Epidemiology. Chicago, The University of Chicago Press, 1966.
53. Pederson, E.: A Rating System for Neurological Impairment in Multiple Sclerosis. Acta Neurol. Scand., *41:*Suppl. 13:557-558, 1965.
54. Pool, D. A., and Brown, R. A.: A Functional Rating Scale for Research in Physical Therapy. Texas Rep. Biol. Med., *26:*133-136, 1968.
55. Price, L.: Medical Disability Standards. J. Occup. Med., *8:*542-547, 1966.
56. Public Health Service: Public Health Service Hearing before the House Subcommittee on Appropriations, Eighty-sixth Congress, Second Session, 1960, pp. 1205-1212.
57. Robey, L. R.: Intertrochanteric and Subtrochanteric Fracture of the Femur in the Negro. J. Bone Joint Surg., *38A:*1301-1312, 1956.
58. Rogers, E. S.: Human Ecology and Health. Introduction for Administrators. New York, Macmillan Co., 1960.
59. Rosen, G.: A History of Public Health. New York, MD Publications, 1958.
60. Rothman, R. H., and Slogoff, S.: The Effect of Immobilization on the Vascular Bed of Tendon. Surg. Gynec. Obstet., *124:*1064-1066, 1967.
61. Rusk, H. A., and Hilleboe, H. E.: Rehabilitation. In Hilleboe, H. E., and Larimore, G. W., eds.: Preventive Medicine, Philadelphia, W. B. Saunders Co., 1965, Chapter 33.
62. Ryder, C. F., and Daitz, B.: Prevention of Disability. In Selle, W. A., ed.: Restorative Medicine in Geriatrics. Springfield, Ill., Charles C Thomas, 1963, Chapter 14.
63. Schoening, H. A., and Iverson, I. A.: The Kenny Selfcare Evaluation: A Numerical Measure of Independence in Activity of Daily Living. Minneapolis, Kenny Rehabilitation Institute, 1965.
64. Semb, H.: Effect of Immobilization on Bone Blood Flow Estimated by Initial Uptake of Radioactive Strontium. Surg. Gynec. Obstet., *127:*275-281, 1968.

65. Sevitt, S., and Gallagher, N.: Venous Thrombosis and Pulmonary Embolism. Brit. J. Surg., *48:*475–489, 1961.
66. Smillie, W. G.: Preventive Medicine and Public Health. New York, Macmillan Co., 1952, Chapter 18.
67. Sokolow, J., Silson, J., Taylor, E. J., Anderson, E. T., and Rusk, H. A.: A Method for the Functional Evaluation of Disability. Arch. Phys. Med. Rehab., *40:*421–428, 1959.
68. Sokolow, J., and Taylor, E. J.: Report of a National Field Trial of a Method for Functional Disability Evaluation. J. Chron. Dis., *20:*896–909, 1967.
69. Solomon, M., Itoh, M., Clarke, C. P., and Goldstein, J. M.: Telemetric Electrocardiogram as a Tool for Dynamic Cardiac Evaluation in Physical Therapy. Arch. Phys. Med. Rehab., *15:* 730, 1970.
70. Spencer, W. A., and Vallbona, C.: A Preliminary Report on the Use of Electronic Data Processing Technics in the Description and Evaluation of Disability. Arch. Phys. Med., *43:*22–35, 1962.
71. Srinivasan, H., and Noordeen, S. K.: Epidemiology of Disability in Leprosy. Int. J. Leprosy, *34:*170–174, 1966.
72. Stinson, M.: Medical Care and Rehabilitation of the Aged. Geriatrics, *8:*266–299, 1953.
73. Taylor, H. L., Henschel, A., Brozek, J., and Key, A.: Effects of Bedrest on Cardiovascular Function and Work Performance. J. Appl. Physiol., *2:*223–239, 1949.
74. Van Demark, E. G., and Van Demark, R. E.: Hip Nailing in Patients of Eighty Years or Older. Amer. J. Surg., *85:*664–668, 1953.
75. Vorwald, A. J., Robin, E. D., Gordon, B. L., Moteley, L., and Noonan, T. B.: Evaluation of Disability. Arch. Environ. Health, *8:*889–897, 1964.
76. Welch, W. H.: Institute of Hygiene. In Rockefeller Foundation Annual Report, New York, 1916, pp. 415–427.
77. Whedon, C. D., Lutwak, L., and Neuman, W.: Calcium and Nitrogen Balance. In a review of medical results of Gemini VII and related flights. J. F. Kennedy Space Center, Florida, NASA SP-121, 1967.
78. World Health Organization: Constitution of the World Health Organization. Geneva, World Health Organization, 1964.
79. World Health Organization: Manual of the International Statistical Classification of Diseases, Injuries and Causes of Death. 1965 Revision, Vol. 1. Geneva, World Health Organization, 1967.
80. World Health Organization: Classification of Disabilities Resulting from Leprosy, for Use in Control Program. Bull. W.H.O., *10:*609–612, 1969.
81. Wylie, C. M.: Administrative Research in the Rehabilitation of Stroke Patient. Rehab. Lit., *25:*2–7, 1964.
82. Wylie, C. M., and White, B. K.: A Measure of Disability. Arch. Environ. Health, *8:*834–839, 1964.
83. Yamshon, L. T.: Industrial Injury. Practical Need for Evaluation of Capacity, J.A.M.A., *165:*934–938, 1957.

INDEX